A

COMPREHENSIVE

MEDICAL DICTIONARY:

CONTAINING THE

PRONUNCIATION, ETYMOLOGY, AND SIGNIFICATION

OF

THE TERMS MADE USE OF IN MEDICINE AND THE KINDRED SCIENCES

With an Appendix,

COMPRISING A COMPLETE LIST OF ALL THE MORE IMPORTANT ARTICLES OF THE MATERIA MEDICA, ARRANGED ACCORDING TO THEIR MEDICINAL PROPERTIES.

ALSO

AN EXPLANATION OF THE LATIN TERMS AND PHRASES OCCURRING IN ANATOMY, PHARMACY, ETC.; TOGETHER WITH THE NECESSARY DIRECTIONS FOR WRITING LATIN PRESCRIPTIONS, ETC. ETC.

BY

J. THOMAS, M.D.

AUTHOR OF THE SYSTEM OF PRONUNCIATION IN LIPPINCOTT'S PRONOUNCING GAZETTEER OF THE WORLD.

PHILADELPHIA:

J. B. LIPPINCOTT & CO.

1876.

PREFACE.

THE present work is designed to supply a want which has long been felt by those commencing the study of medicine and the collateral sciences.

An acquaintance with the dead languages, or at least with Latin, was formerly, and in some parts of Europe is still, considered absolutely necessary for a graduate in medicine as well as in the other learned professions. Although in the United States a classical education is not made an indispensable condition for conferring a medical degree, yet, so long as the great majority of professional terms are in Latin, some knowledge of this language may be said to be absolutely requisite for the medical student. The fact that multitudes of our young men commence the study of medicine without any previous acquaintance with Latin or Greek, renders it important that the elementary works intended for the use of students should be adapted to meet this exigency.

To supply the want above indicated has been one of the chief objects of the present work. In fulfilling this object, the editor has aimed,—

First: to give a full explanation of the etymology of the various words defined in the Dictionary. The importance of etymology in furnishing, as it generally does, a sure clue to the true signification of scientific terms; in limiting and fixing their meaning, thus guarding against looseness or vagueness of application; and lastly, and not least, in assisting the memory of the learner, since, by acquiring a knowledge of a comparatively few elements or roots, he is thus enabled to determine the signification of a multitude of compound words,—can scarcely be overestimated. It is admitted, indeed, that terms not unfrequently occur of which it is difficult or impossible to give an entirely satisfactory etymology. In a few of the most doubtful cases of this kind, it has been deemed best to make no attempt to explain the derivation, since an etymology which is purely fanciful or speculative, seems far more likely to mislead or perplex than to instruct the student. It may be proper to add that, in fulfilling this important part of his task, the editor has not been content with merely following the generally received authorities in etymology, but has made it a rule, in every case of doubt or uncertainty, to examine the subject anew, and particularly to consult the best classical and modern (foreign) dictionaries upon the point in question.

Secondly: to give, whenever practicable, a literal translation of the various Latin phrases, sentences, etc. occurring in the work: such, for example, as *Extensor Digitorum Communis*, *Motores Oculorum*, *Hydrargyrum cum Cretâ*, etc. etc. The importance of such explanations in giving clear and definite ideas to those who may be unacquainted with the Latin tongue, is too obvious to require to be enlarged upon.

For an explanation of some of the most important elements and principles of the Latin language, designed chiefly for those who have not had the advantage of a classical education, the reader is referred to the Appendix, page 660. Connected with, and immediately following, this portion of the work, will be found rules and directions for the writing of Latin prescriptions.

Another feature in the work, and one which it is hoped will prove of great practical importance, is the pronunciation of the various terms given in the Dictionary. What correct spelling is to the writer, correct pronunciation is to the speaker. If either should be wholly neglected, the most perfect language would soon become a babel, and fall into utter corruption. Every one who takes the trouble to reflect on the subject must be aware that if it were not for the constant effort or aim to conform our speech to a common standard, the language which we call English would in the course of a few years be spoken so differently in different parts of the world, as to be with difficulty understood, and in two or three centuries it would, in all probability, become wholly unintelligible, except to those few who might happen to be familiar with the local dialect. He, therefore, who is willing to take the pains to speak correctly, not only acquires an accomplishment which will raise him in the estimation of all educated men, but he contributes his portion towards exalting and extending the incalculable blessings which language, the great vehicle of thought and knowledge, is capable of conferring on mankind.

The various terms employed in medicine may be divided into two principal classes. The first class consists of those which are properly English or have an Anglicized termination, whether derived from the Saxon, as, *Blood*, *Forearm*, *Nightmare*, *Rickets*, etc.; from the French, as, *Bandage*, *Viable*, etc.; from the Latin, as, *Abdominal* (from *abdominalis*), *Abortion* (from *abortio*), *Astringent* (from *astringens*), *Ferruginous* (from *ferruginosus*), etc.; or from the Greek, as, *Apoplexy* (from ἀποπληξία), *Artery* (from ἀρτηρία), *Asthmatic* (from ἀσθματικός), etc.

The second class comprises all such terms as are Latin or Latinized Greek, as, *Abdomen*, *Amaurosis*, *Ammonia*, *Asthma*, *Cerebrum*, *Laryngitis*, *Œsophagus*, *Sternum*, *Vertebra*, etc. etc.

The pronunciation of the former class of words is attended with no particular difficulty. Those of the second class, however, though usually very easy with respect to the accentuation, and perfectly uniform as to the sounds of the consonants, present a very serious difficulty in regard to the pronunciation of the vowels. At the University of Oxford in England, and at Harvard in the United States, it is the usage to pronounce all Latin words with the English sounds of the vowels: for example, *a* when long (as the second *a* in *ama're*, *ama'bam*, *ama'tum*) has the same sound as our *a* in *fate* (never like *a* in *far*); long *i* is pronounced as in *pine*; and so on. But many of the institutions of learning in this country have adopted what is termed the "continental" pronunciation, according to which, the vowels are pronounced, not after the English sound, but according to that of the languages of Continental Europe. As, however, there is some diversity respecting the vowel sounds of the different European tongues, the

Italian, which of all the modern languages is perhaps most nearly related to the Latin, has generally been adopted as the standard. According to this system, *a* should be sounded nearly like *a* in *far*, *e* as in *there*, or like *a* in *fate*, *i* as in *marine*, or like *e* in *mete*, *u* like *oo*, and *y* like *i*, that is, like our *e*. In some portions of our country, particularly in the Middle States, there unfortunately prevails a third system, consisting of a sort of mixture of the other two already described. According to this system,—if such it may be called,—the vowel *a* is sounded as in *fast* or *fat* (never as in *fate*); *i*, when long, is usually pronounced as in *pine*, though sometimes as in *marine;* all the other vowels being uniformly sounded as in English. The improper diphthong *æ*, which in every other modern language corresponds in sound either exactly or very nearly to *e*,* is on this system sounded like our *a* in *fate*.

As may readily be imagined, these three different systems existing together in the same country, have had the effect to introduce almost unlimited confusion into the pronunciation of Latin words. Those who aim at correctness or propriety in speaking should, we think, adopt either the Oxford pronunciation or the continental; and whichever they adopt should be carried out consistently. It is greatly to be desired, however, that some common standard of Latin pronunciation might be fixed upon for the whole United States: it would be of immense advantage even were its application limited to scientific terms and phrases.

Under the existing state of things, the editor has not felt justified in attempting to lay down any positive rules for the pronunciation of the vowels occurring in Latin terms. He has, accordingly, for the most part confined his labors in regard to this class of words, to marking the accent and syllabication, and to indicating such vowel sounds (*e.g.* short *i* and short *y*) as are essentially the same whether they are pronounced according to the continental or

---

* That is, to the sound of *e* in the respective languages; *æ* in French being equivalent to the French *é*, *æ* in Spanish to the Spanish *e*, and so with the rest. To sound *æ* differently from *e* tends to great confusion, inasmuch as a multitude of words are now written almost indifferently with the diphthong or the vowel: as, *Ædile* or *Edile*, *Ætiology* or *Etiology*, etc. However such words may be written, the pronunciation ought, unquestionably, to remain the same.

the English mode. The most important point of all is the accent, which can, for the most part, be readily ascertained, and, depending as it does upon the *quantity** (not on the *quality*) of the vowels, remains the same under all the different systems and in all the various tongues of the world. The principal rules for Latin accentuation are the following:—

RULE 1.—In trisyllables or polysyllables, if the penultima be long, the accent must fall upon it: as, *Abdo'men*, *Coni'um*, *Duode'num*, *Porri'go*, *Scapula'ris*, etc.

RULE 2.—If the penultima be short, the accent must fall on the antepenultima: as, *Aç'idum*, *Abdom'inis*, *An'ima*, *Assafœt'ida*, *Chimaph'ila*, *Cimicif'uga*, *Hydroceph'alus*, *Polyg'ala*, etc.

RULE 3.—Dissyllables always take the accent on the penultima; as, *A'cor*, *Co'ma*, *Li'quor*, &c.

It may be observed that whenever the accent of a Latin word falls on the antepenultimate vowel followed immediately by a single consonant, the accent is usually placed after the consonant, and the vowel is made what in English we term "short." (See examples under Rule Second.) Accordingly, we pronounce *Abdominis—abdom'inis*, *Assafœtida—assafet'ida*, etc., although in both of these instances the penultimate syllable is long in Latin.† The only important exception to this rule occurs in words having *u* for the antepenultimate vowel; as, *Alu'mina*, *Sulphu'ricus*, etc., in which case the accent should always be placed before the consonant, the vowel retaining its full or long sound.‡

It has until recently been the almost universal usage among

---

* The quantity is determined chiefly by the usage of the Latin poets, and certain recognized rules of derivation.

† It is very important to bear in mind the essential difference between a long vowel in English and a long vowel in Latin or Greek. In the former case the word "long" refers to the *quality* of the vowel, in the latter always to the *quantity*. The pronunciation of a long vowel in Latin or Greek is estimated to occupy just twice as much time as is spent in uttering a short vowel. In the present work, however, when the term "long" is employed in reference to the pronunciation of a word, it is to be understood in the English sense, if the contrary be not distinctly stated.

‡ The plural of Greek nouns in *-oma* are, by common usage, excepted: as, *aro'mata* (from *aro'ma*), not *arom'ata*. If the penultima be a vowel followed immediately by another vowel, the antepenultimate syllable is usually made long: as, am-mo'ni-a, ci-ne're-us.

classical scholars to pronounce the ancient Greek (like the Latin) according to the quantity of the vowels; but within a few years some institutions of learning of the highest character, both in Europe and in this country, have adopted the modern Greek accentuation; that is, they pronounce according to the Greek accent, without the slightest reference to quantity. For example, *σοφία* ("wisdom"), and *ὠλέκρᾶνον* (the "elbow"), formerly called so'fe-a and o-le-kra'non, would, according to the new mode, be pronounced so-fee'a and o-lek'ra-non. How far this new system should affect our pronunciation of Latinized terms derived from the Greek may be considered an open question.*

As already intimated, the accent is the chief, if not the sole, point in Latin pronunciation about which there is no dispute among the learned. It has accordingly come to be regarded as one of the essential tests by which a finished scholar may be known. Our readers need scarcely be reminded that many Latin phrases and sentences have become, so to speak, parts of our own

---

* While it must be admitted that all, or nearly all, the best English authorities on classical pronunciation recognize no other principle than quantity for the accentuation of this class of words, it may be observed that in Italian and Spanish,—languages much more nearly related to the Latin than ours,—words and names derived from the Greek almost invariably follow the accentuation of the original, while those of Latin derivation are as uniformly accentuated according to the quantity of their Latin primitives. Not only is the name *Sofia* (from the Greek *σοφία*, whence our *Sophi'a*) pronounced *so-fee'a* (though in Greek the penultima is short), and its derivative *filosofia* ("philosophy") *fe-lo-so-fee'a*, but the numerous class of Italian and Spanish words ending in *-grafia* (Greek *-γραφία*), and *-logia* (Greek *-λογία*) always have, like the Greek, the accent on the penultima, although this is invariably short in the Greek; as *cosmografi'a* (cosmography), *geografi'a* (geography), *ortografi'a* (orthography), &c.; and *analogi'a* (analogy), *filologi'a* (philology), etc. etc. *Insania* takes the antepenultimate accent, because the penultima of the Latin (*insa'nia*) is short; while *mania*, with the same termination, has the penultimate accent (ma-nee'a), simply because the Greek (*μανία*) is so accented ☞ The remark made above, that words in Italian and Spanish derived from the Latin follow the Latin quantity, while those from the Greek conform to the Greek accentuation, should of course be limited to such as have not become materially changed or corrupted. It will be seen that in the examples above cited no change has taken place, except substituting *f* for *φ*, which does not in the slightest degree affect the pronunciation.

language. He, therefore, who aspires to the character of a correct and polished speaker, cannot, without serious danger to his reputation, neglect this important branch of orthoepy. It is true that a very few words of Latin origin (as *Au'ditor*, *Or'ator*, *Sen'ator*,* etc.) have, on becoming Anglicized, without any change in the spelling, lost the original penultimate accent. But the large majority of Anglicized words retain the classical accentuation, as *Acu'men*, *Albu'men*, *Aro'ma*, *Cogno'men*, *Deco'rum*, *Dicta'tor*, *Fari'na*, *Farra'go*, *Hori'zon*, *Sali'va*, *Specta'tor*, etc., all of which have resisted the general tendency of our language, which is to throw the accent on the antepenultima in such words: indeed, we not unfrequently hear uneducated people say, *Ar'oma*, *Cog'nomen*, *Sal'iva*, etc. If, then, Anglicized Latin words, which are in everybody's mouth, are generally pronounced according to the original accentuation, scientific terms ought unquestionably to be always so pronounced. This principle is, indeed, fully recognized in the accentuations given in the last edition of our Pharmacopœia, in which, we believe, not a single instance occurs of a Latin name that does not conform to the classical pronunciation; although, if English analogy were allowed to have any influence, we should scarcely pronounce *Coni'um*, *Mati'co*, etc., with the accent on the penultima.

Of such Latin words as were used by the ancients, there is generally no difficulty in determining the accentuation. But the case is different with respect to Latin terms (consisting chiefly of botanical and other scientific names) of modern origin. Among these there are a number of which the etymology is obscure or uncertain, and the accentuation is, in consequence, more or less doubtful. In such cases, the editor has not only sought to avail himself of the light which general analogy might shed upon the point in question, but he has carefully consulted all the best works accessible to him, relating to such subjects. Among these he would express his particular obligations to GRAY'S "Manual of Botany," MAYNE'S "Expository Lexicon," WITTSTEIN'S "Etymologisch-Botanisches Wörterbuch," and, above all, to DUNGLISON'S "Medical Dictionary," which in relation to these difficult questions

**Anemo'ne*, when used as an English word, is always pronounced *anem'one*.

exhibits a degree of accuracy, as well as judgment, unsurpassed, if not unequalled, among scientific works of reference.

Those who take a particular interest in such subjects are referred to the "Table of Disputed Pronunciations" (see Appendix, pp. 698–9), containing a list of the most important terms occurring in medical works, respecting the accentuation of which there is a difference among the best orthoepical authorities.*

Respecting the plan of the Dictionary, it may be observed that immediately after the term itself, if this be English, is inserted the Latin synonym, then the etymology, both being enclosed in brackets. If the term be Latin, it is immediately followed by the etymology, enclosed in brackets. (Compare *Ablactation*, *Apoplexy*, *Artery;* also, *Abdomen*, *Ablepsia*, etc.) The French synonyms of important medical terms are also given, excepting such as are essentially the same as the English or Latin: for example, *Ablactation* ("ablactation"), *Bandage* (a "bandage"), *Utérus* (the "uterus"), etc.; or such as differ only very slightly, as *Apoplexie* ("apoplexy"), *Artère* ("artery"), *Hépatite* ("hepatitis"), *Œsophage* ("œsophagus"), etc. As these would, for the most part, be readily understood without a dictionary, they have generally been omitted. By adopting this plan, the attention of the student is particularly directed to those French terms which it is most important for him to acquire; that is, to such as are essentially different from the Latin or English, and therefore not likely to be understood unless explained. Of this class of words the following examples may be given:—*Cœur* ("heart"), *Clou* ("clove"), *Cou* ("neck"), *Main* ("hand"), *Œil* ("eye"), *Poumons* ("lungs"), *Toux* ("cough"), etc.

A considerable portion of the Appendix is occupied with the

---

* In speaking of "authorities" in regard to questions of this kind, we do not, of course, allude to those persons, however illustrious, who are merely distinguished for their scientific attainments or for their general learning, but to *such only as have paid particular attention to the subject of orthoepy.* It is not to be denied that some, who are justly regarded as ornaments of science, either from never having given any attention to such subjects, or from mere carelessness, are most untrustworthy guides in all that relates to correctness of language, whether written or spoken. They seem to forget that thoughts are like jewels: the greater their value, the more important it is that they should be well set, that their beauty may be exhibited to the best advantage.

"Table of Materia Medica," containing the names of all, or nearly all, the medicinal articles of any importance, arranged according to their medical properties. Such a classification, it is believed, will be found extremely useful, at least to those who have not had time or opportunity to make themselves thoroughly acquainted with the vast resources of our Materia Medica.

Besides the articles already mentioned, included in the Appendix, it contains a tolerably complete Table of Doses, prepared with great care. It also contains a synopsis of the respective Nosologies of Cullen and Good. Although at the present time neither of these systems is generally followed, both have exerted great influence upon medical nomenclature, and may, therefore, justly claim some notice at our hands. It was believed that in no other way could an idea be given of them so clearly and so briefly as by means of synoptical tables.

Among the multitude of works which the editor has had occasion to consult in the preparation of this Dictionary, justice requires that he should express his great obligations to a few to which he is especially indebted. His acknowledgments are pre-eminently due to MAYNE'S "Expository Lexicon" (London, 1860); a Dictionary of Medicine, original in its plan, and evincing in its execution much diligence, learning, and research. He would also express his important obligations to GRAY'S "Structural and Systematic Botany," and "Manual of Botany," to which he has generally had recourse as his chief authorities on all questions relating to botanical science. To HOBLYN'S "Medical Dictionary" he is indebted for the matter of a number of articles, particularly those relating to chemistry. The notices of the natural orders of plants and animals have mostly been taken from that justly popular work, BRANDE'S "Encyclopædia of Science, Literature, and Art."

Nor can he omit to mention his great and important obligations to WOOD and BACHE'S "United States Dispensatory," a work which justly ranks among the first of its kind that have ever been published in this or any other country.

EXPLANATION OF THE SIGNS, ABBREVIATIONS, ETC. USED IN THE PRESENT WORK.

ā, ē, ī, ō, ū, ȳ, are long, as in *fate, mete, pine, note, tube, fly.*

ă, ĕ, ĭ, ŏ, ŭ, y̆, are short, as in *fat, met, pin, not, tub, mystic.*

ȧ, ė, and ȯ, are like ā, ē, and ō, except that the sound is less prolonged.

ạ, ẹ, are obscure, as in the final syllables of *America, writer,* etc.

ḡ = *g* hard.

ç is to be sounded like *s* or *ss;* Ģ and ġ like *j;* ṡ has the sound of *z.*

ch̶ is to be sounded like *k;* but *ch* without any mark should be pronounced as in *chill* or *child.*

N, M, and Nᵍ are used to represent the French nasal sound, somewhat resembling that of *ng* in *long.* R (small capital) implies that the *r* should be trilled: ü denotes the sound of the French *u;* U, that of the French *eu,* similar to the sound of *u* in the English word *fur.*

An asterisk (*) affixed to a word or phrase denotes that it is either Latin or Latinized Greek, etc.

= signifies "equivalent to." Thus, *Cath.* = *Catharticus* implies that *Cath.* is equivalent to, or stands for, *Catharticus* ("Cathartic").

‖ placed after the phrase "Pharmacopœial name" denotes that the name belongs alike to the British and United States Pharmacopœias.

An acute accent denotes a primary, a grave a secondary, accent.

☞ As a general rule, no marks have been placed on the vowels in cases where these would naturally be pronounced correctly without any mark.

☞ When a reference is made to some other part of the Dictionary, the word referred to is put in small capitals: hence, if small capitals are used, a reference is always implied. See *Hæmatiasis, Hæmatopoiesis,* etc. in the Dictionary.

ABBREVIATIONS.

Abl.	ablative.	Fr.	French.	N. or neut.	neuter.
Acc.	accusative.	Gen.	genitive.	Nom.	nominative.
Br. or Brit.	British.	Ger.	German.	Ph. or Pharm.	Pharmacopœia.
Dat.	dative.	Gr.	Greek.	Pl.	plural.
Dub.	Dublin.	i.e. (*id est*)	that is.	Pron.	pronunciation.
Ed.	Edinburgh.	Lat.	Latin.	Sp.	Spanish.
e.g. (*exem'pli gra'tiâ*)	for example.	Lond.	London.	U.S.	United States.
F. or fem.	feminine.	M. or masc.	masculine.	Voc.	Vocative.

To render these explanations complete, a table of the Greek alphabet is subjoined.

Letter.	Name.	Power.	Letter.	Name.	Power.	Letter.	Name.	Power.
Α α	Alpha	a	Ι ι	Iōta	i	Ρ ρ	Rho	r
Β β ϐ	Beta	b	Κ κ	Kappa	k	Σ σ ς	Sigma	s
Γ γ	Gamma	g *hard*	Λ λ	Lambda	l	Τ τ	Tau	t
Δ δ	Delta	d	Μ μ	Mu	m	Υ υ	Upsīlon	u or y
Ε ε	Epsīlon	ĕ *short*	Ν ν	Nu	n	Φ φ	Phi	ph
Ζ ζ	Zeta	z	Ξ ξ	Xi	x	Χ χ	Chi	ch *hard*
Η η	Eta	ē *long*	Ο ο	Omĭcron	ŏ *short*	Ψ ψ	Psi	ps
Θ ϑ θ	Theta	th	Π π	Pi	p	Ω ω	Omĕga	ō *long*

REMARKS.—Γ followed immediately by another *γ,* by *κ,* or by *χ,* sounds like *n:* hence, *αγγεῖον,* a "vessel," should be rendered by *angeion* or *angīon,* if Roman letters are used; *ἀγκύλος* ("bent"), by *ankylos* or *ancylos; ἄγχω* (to "choke"), by *ancho,* etc. Υ, though usually considered to be equivalent to *u,* is almost invariably rendered by *y,* in Latin. See *ἀγκύλος,* above given. K is usually replaced in Latin by *c,* as *κυνάρα* or *κινάρα, cynara* or *cinara* (a kind of "artichoke"). As in Latin words of Greek derivation *y* is sounded like *i,* and not like *u,* ☞ so *c* should in such words be pronounced with its proper Latin sound,—always like *s* before *e, i,* and *y.*

☞ Αι (in Greek) when changed into Latin, becomes *æ;* and *οι, œ;* as *αἰθίοψ, æthiops, οἴδημα, œdema,* etc.

☞ *H* is represented in Greek by ʽ, called the "rough breathing" (*spir'itus as'per*), as in *ὑπό,* "under," *αἷμα,* "blood," etc. All Greek words beginning with a vowel have either the rough or smooth breathing (*spir'itus le'nis*). Compare *αἰθίοψ,* "black," *αἰτία,* "cause," etc. The smooth breathing indicates simply the natural sound of the vowel.

PRONOUNCING

MEDICAL DICTIONARY.

A, or *an* before a word beginning with a vowel or with *h*. [*α* or *αν*.] A prefix in compound words of Greek derivation, having a negative or privative force: as, *tonic*, "possessing or imparting tone;" *a-tonic*, "without tone;" *a-cephalous*, "without a head;" *an-æsthetic*, "without perception;" *an-hydrous*, "without water."

A is also a French preposition, signifying "to" or "at," and forming a part of certain surgical and medical phrases, as *à deux temps*, å duh tōnᵍ. "At two times." Applied to the operation of lithotomy, in which the calculus, from certain causes, cannot be immediately extracted, and is therefore let alone till during the suppurating stage, when extraction may be more easily effected.

AA. A contraction of the Greek word *ana* (ἀνά), signifying, literally, "up through" or "throughout;" sometimes equivalent to "OF EACH." Written in prescriptions after the names of several different medicines, to denote an equal quantity of each.

AAA. Abbreviation for AMALGAM.

Ab. A Latin particle signifying "from," "off," "away."

Ab-ac'tus Ven'ter,* or **Ven'ter Abac'tus.*** [From *ab*, "from," and *a'go*, *ac'tum*, to "drive," to "force."] Literally, a "belly expelled" or emptied by forcible means. A term in Medical Jurisprudence for abortion induced by art.

Ab'a-cus.* [From ἄβαξ, ἄβακος, a mathematical table on which lines and figures were drawn.] An old name for a table used for medicinal preparations.

Abalienation, ab-āl-yen-ā'shun. [**Abaliena'tio, o'nis**; from *ab*, "from," and *alie'no*, *aliena'tum*, to "estrange."] Formerly used for decay of the whole or part of the body; also, loss or failing of the senses or of the mental faculties.

Abanga, ăb-ăng'ga. The name of the fruit of a palm-tree growing in the island of St. Thomas (West Indies). The seeds are considered very useful in diseases of the chest.

Ab-ar-tic-u-lā'tion. [**Abarticula'tio, o'nis**; from *ab*, "from," and *articula'tio*, "articulation."] A kind of articulation admitting of free motion. See DIARTHROSIS.

Ab-bre'vi-āt-ed. [**Abbrevia'tus**; from *abbre'vio*, *abbrevia'tum*, to "shorten."] Shortened, as when the cup is shorter than the tube of the flower.

Ab-bre-vi-ā'tion. [**Abbrevia'tio, o'nis**; from the same.] A part of a word shortened by cutting off one or more of its latter syllables. Applied to many initial and medial letters, and contractions, of medical terms, which will be found in their alphabetical order.

Abcès. See ABSCESS.

Abdom. Abbreviation for ABDO'MEN.

Ab-do'men,* gen. **Ab-dom'i-nis.** [From *ab'do*, *ab'dere*, to "hide."] The largest cavity of the body; the belly. The same region in the lower animals. See ALVUS, IMUS VENTER, VENTER.

Ab-dom'i-nal. [**Abdomina'lis**; from *abdo'men*.] Belonging to the abdomen; ventral.

Abdom'inal Aor'ta. That portion of the aorta situated below the diaphragm.

Abdom'inal Ap-on-eū-ro'sis. The conjoined tendons of the oblique and transverse muscles on the anterior portion of the abdomen. See APONEUROSIS.

Abdom'inal Gang'lia (găng'gle-ạ). The semilunar ganglia, so named from their situation.

Abdom'inal Ring. [**An'nulus Abdom'inis.**] The fancied ring-like opening on each side of the abdomen, external and superior to the *pubes*. Through it, in males, passes the spermatic cord. It is also called the IN'GUINAL RING.

Ab-dom-ĭ-na'lis.* [From *abdo'men.*] Pertaining to the abdomen; abdom'inal; ventral. In the plural (*Abdomina'lēs*) it forms the name of an order of fishes having the ventral fins under the abdomen and behind the pectorals.

Ab-dom-i-nos'co-pȳ. [**Abdominosco'pia;** from *abdo'men*, and σκοπέω, to "observe."] The examination of the abdomen by percussion, inspection, measurement, or manual examination.

Ab-du'cent. [**Abdu'cens;** from *ab*, "from," and *du'co, duc'tum*, to "lead," to "draw."] Applied to muscles by which the members or limbs are drawn from the mesial line (or axis of the body); also to the sixth pair of nerves.

Ab-duc'tion. [**Abduc'tio, o'***nis;* from the same.] That movement by which one part is moved from another, or from the axis of the body.

Ab-duc'tor, o'r*is.** [From the same.] Applied to a muscle which performs, or assists in performing, abduction.

Abelmoschus,* ā-bel-mos'kŭs. [From the Arab. *ab-el-mushk;* literally, the "father of musk."] Musk-seed; the specific name of the *Hibiscus abelmoschus.* The seeds of this plant, called *grana moschata* ("musk-seeds"), are employed in the East in forming the *Poudre de Chypre*, or *Cyprus powder*, used for flavoring coffee.

Ab-ĕp-ĭ-thȳm'ĭ-ạ.*[From *ab*,"from," "off," and ἐπιθυμία, "desire."] A faulty term (partly Latin and partly Greek) for paralysis of the solar plexus, cutting off communication between the nervous system and abdominal viscera, the supposed seat of the appetites and desires.

Ab-er-rā'tion. [**Aberra'tio, o'***nis;* from *ab*, "from," and *er'ro, erra'tum*, to "wander."] Applied to a disordered state of the intellect. Applied also to the rays of light when refracted by a lens, or reflected by a mirror, so that they do not converge into a focus.

Ab-e-vac-u-ā'tion. [**Abevacua'tio, o'***nis;* from *ab*, "from," and *evac'uo, evacua'tum*, to "empty out," to "empty."] A medical term usually applied to a partial or incomplete evacuation, but by some writers employed to denote an immoderate evacuation.

A'bĭ-ēs,* gen. **A-bi'e-tis.** [Supposed to be from *ab*, "from," and *e'o*, to "go," on account of the great height which it goes or extends from the earth.] The specific name of the *Pinus Abies*, or fir-tree. See PINUS.

A'bies Excel'sa.* One of the plants from which the *Thus*, or frankincense, is obtained.

A'bies La'rix.* The tree which affords Venice turpentine.

Ab-ĭ-et'ic. [**Abiet'icus;** from *a'bies.*] Belonging to the fir-tree.

Abietin, or **Abietine,** a-bī'ẹ-tin [**Abieti'na;** from *a'bies.*] A resinous substance, also called the resin *Gamma*, or third in order, obtained from Strasbourg turpentine.

Abi'ĕtis Rĕs-ĭ'nạ.* The resin of the fir-tree; the *Thus*, or common frankincense; spontaneously exuded by the *Pinus Abies.* See FRANKINCENSE.

Abietite, ạ-bī'ẹ-tīt. [**Abieti'tes;** from *abies*, and λίθος, a "stone."] A genus of fossil coniferous plants in the Wealden and Greensand formations.

Ab-ĭr-ri-tā'tion. [**Abirrita'tio, o'***nis;* from *ab*, "from" or "away," and *irri'to, irrita'tum*, to "irritate;" denoting the passing "away" or absence of irritation or of vital irritability.] Diminished irritability in the various tissues, and so slightly distinct from ASTHENIA.

Ab-lac-tā'tion. [**Ablacta'tio, o'***nis;* from *ab*, "from," "away," and *lac, lac'tis*, "milk." See LACTATION.] The weaning of a child. Some writers make a distinction between *ablactation* and *weaning.* By the former they mean the termination of the period of suckling as regards the mother; by the latter, the same period with reference to the child.

Ab-lā'tion. [**Abla'tio, o'***nis;* from *au'fero, abla'tum* (from *ab*, "from," "away," and *fe'ro, la'tum*, to "carry," or "take"), to "take away."] The removing of any part by excision, extirpation, or amputation.

A-blep'sĭ-ạ.* [From *a.* priv., and βλέπω, to "see."] Want of sight; blindness: ablep'sy.

Ab'lu-ent. [**Ab'luens;** from *ab*,

"from" or "away," and *lu'o, lu'tum,* to "wash."] That which washes away or carries off impurities. See ABSTERGENT.

Ab-lu'tion. [**Ablu'tio, o'**nis; from the same.] The separation of extraneous matters by washing. Anciently an internal washing by administering profuse libations of milk-whey.

Ab-nor'mal. [**Abnor'mis;** from *ab,* "from," and *nor'ma,* a "rule;" denoting a departure from the "*rule,*" course, or custom of nature.] Contrary to the natural condition; unnatural.

Ab-o-ma'sum,* or **Ab-o-ma'sus.*** [From *ab,* "from," and *oma'sum,* the "paunch."] The fourth stomach of the *Ruminantia.* From this part of calves, lambs, etc., *rennet* is prepared.

Aborigenis,* ab-o-rij'e-nĭs. [More frequently used in the plural (*Aborigines,* ab-o-rij'e-nēz); from *ab,* "from," and *ori'go,* the "beginning."] Native or original of a country: abori̲g'inal.

Ab-or'sus.* [From *abo'rior, abor'tus,* to "miscarry."] A miscarriage in the first or early months. More properly ABORTUS, or ABORTION, which see.

Ab-or'ti-cīde. [**Aborticid'ium;** from *abor'tus,* and *cæ'do,* to "kill."] The destroying of the *fœtus in utero.* See FŒTICIDE.

Ab-or'tient. [**Abor'tiens;** from *abo'rior.*] Miscarrying. Applied synonymously with STERILIS. See STERILE.

Ab-or'tion. [**Abor'tio, o'**nis; from *abo'rior, abor'tus,* to "miscarry."] The morbid expulsion of an immature *fœtus;* a miscarriage. In Botany, imperfect development.

Abor'tion, CRIMINAL. Fœticide.

Ab-or'tive. [**Aborti'vus;** from the same.] Causing abortion. Sometimes applied to treatment adopted for preventing further or complete development of disease.

Abortus.* [From the same.] See ABORTION.

Abrachia,* ab-ra̲-kī'a̲. [From *a,* priv., and βραχίων, the "arm."] A sort of monstrosity, consisting in the absence of arms.

Abranchia,* a-brank'e-a̲. [From *a,* priv., and βράγχια, the "gills" or "respiratory organs."] Literally, having no organs of respiration. A name given by Cuvier to an order of *Anellidæ* having no external organs of respiration.

Abranchiata. See ABRANCHIA.

A-bra'sion. [**Abra'sio, o'**nis; from *ab,* "from" or "off," and *ra'do, ra'sum,* to "scrape."] A term for the partial tearing off or fretting of the skin.

Abrotanum. See ABROTONUM.

Abrotonum. See ARTEMISIA.

Ab-rot'o-num Mas.* Another name for ARTEMISIA ABROTONUM, which see.

Ab-rupt'. [**Abrup'tus;** from *ab,* "from," "off," and *rum'po, rup'tum,* to "break."] Applied to leaves and roots that seem broken off at their extremity.

A'brus Pre-ca-to'ri-us.* [From ἁβρός, "delicate," "elegant," and *preca'tor,* "one who prays," alluding to its use for rosaries.] Called also Wild Liquorice, Liquorice Bush, Red Bean, and other names. A small shrub growing in the West Indies, Central America, and also in Egypt, having beautiful scarlet seeds, which are employed for rosaries, necklaces, etc. The roots and leaves contain mucilage, and are sometimes used as demulcents.

Abs. A Latin particle, having the same force as AB, which see.

Ab'scess. [**Absces'sus;** from *abs,* "from," and *ce'do, ces'sum,* to "go;" because the matter "goes from" or separates itself from the rest of the body.] (Fr. *Abcès,* åb'sȧ'.) A tumor or swelling (usually large and deep) containing pus.

Abscissa, Vox. See VOX ABSCISSA.

Ab-scis'sion. [**Abscis'sio, o'**nis; from *ab,* "from," "away," and *scin'do, scis'sum,* to "cut."] Applied to a fractured bone when a part of it is cut off and removed, or to the cutting off of any soft part, as of a nerve, or the prepuce, etc.

Absconsio* (ab-skon'she-o), **o'**nis. [From *abs,* "away," and *con'do,* to "hide."] A term formerly denoting the same as *Sinus:* an abscon'sion.

Abs. febr. = *Absen'te fe'bre.** "Fever being absent," or, in the absence of fever.

Ab-sin'thāte. [**Absin'thas, a'**tis.] A combination of absinthic acid with a base.

Ab-sin'thic. [**Absin'thicus;** from *absin'thium.*] Belonging to *Absinthium;* applied to an acid obtained from it.

Ab-sin'thin. [**Absinthi'na.**] The bitter principle discovered in *Absinthium.*

Ab-sin'thi-um.* [Gr. ἀψίνθιον.] The Pharmacopœial name (Lond. and Ed. Ph.) for Wormwood, the *Artemisia absinthium,* and (U.S. Ph.) for its tops and leaves. See ARTEMISIA.

Absin'thium Com-mu'ne.* Another name for the *Artemisia absinthium,* or Wormwood.

Absin'thium Ma-rit'i-mum.* Another name for *Artemisia maritima.*

Absin'thium Pon'tĭ-cum,* **Absin'thium Ro-ma'num.*** Other names for ARTEMISIA PONTICA, which see.

Absin'thium San-ton'ĭ-cum.* Another name for *Artemisia santonica.*

Absin'thium Vul-ga're.* Another name for *Artemisia absinthium.*

Ab'so-lute Al'co-hol. Alcohol as free from water as it can be obtained. See ALCOHOL.

Ab-sor'bent. [**Absor'bens;** from *ab,* "from," and *sor'beo, sorp'tum,* to "sip or suck."] Sucking up or absorbing. Applied to the lacteal and lymphatic vessels, and to the origins of vessels on the roots of plants. Applied to medicines which neutralize acidity in the stomach and bowels, as magnesia, chalk, etc.

Absor'bent Sys'tem. A term used to denote *collectively* the vessels and glands which perform the function of absorption.

Ab-sorp'tion. [**Absorp'tio, o'***nis;* from the same.] The sucking up of substances applied to the mouths of absorbent vessels. In Chemistry, the sucking up or imbibition of a gas or vapor by a liquid or solid.

Absorption, Cutaneous. See CUTANEOUS ABSORPTION.

Absorption, Interstitial. See INTERSTITIAL ABSORPTION.

Ab-ste'mĭ-ous. [**Abste'mius;** from *abs,* "from," and *teme'tum,* an old Latin word for "wine:" others derive it from *abs,* "from," and *ten'eo,* to "hold" or "keep," *n* being changed to *m.*] Strictly, abstaining from wine; but generally applied also to moderation in diet.

Ab-ster'gent. [**Abster'gens, en'***tis;* from *abster'geo, abster'sum,* to "cleanse."] Cleansing; abluent; abstersive. Applied to medicines which cleanse from foulness or sordes.

Ab'stĭ-nence. [**Abstinen'tia;** from *abs,* "from," and *ten'eo,* to "hold" or "keep;" to "abstain."] The refraining from, or sparing use of, food, liquors, etc.

Abs-trac'tion. [**Abstrac'tio, o'***nis;* from *abs,* "from," "away," and *tra'ho, trac'tum,* to "draw."] The separating of a fluid from a salt, etc. That mental power by which one particular idea may be dwelt upon to the exclusion of others; also, that by which general ideas may be formed from those of particular objects. Applied also to the drawing of blood from a blood-vessel.

Ab'sus.* A species of Cassia, the seeds of which, being powdered and mixed with sugar, are used in Egypt as an application to the eyes in ophthalmia.

A-bu'ta.* Another name for the PAREIRA BRAVA, which see.

A-bu'til-on.* Called also the Indian or yellow mallow. It is mucilaginous, and sometimes used for diarrhœa in cattle.

Abvacuation. See ABEVACUATION.

Acacia,* a-ka'she-a; gen. **Acaciæ,** a-ka'she-ē. [From ἀκή, a "sharp point;" the name having been given on account of the prickles or thorns with which the tree abounds.] A genus of the Linnæan class *Polygamia,* natural order *Leguminosæ.* Also, the Pharmacopœial name ‖ for gum-arabic.

Aca'cia Al'tera Trifolia'ta. See SPARTIUM SPINOSUM.

Acacia Arabica. See ACACIA VERA.

Aca'ciæ A-rab'ĭ-cæ Gum'mi.* The Pharmacopœial name (Dub. Ph.) of gum-arabic, obtained from *Acacia vera,* and other species of *Acacia.*

Aca'cia Cat'e-chu.* The systematic name of the plant which affords catechu.

Aca'cia In'dica.* See TAMARINDUS INDICA.

Aca'cia Ve'ra.* [From *ve'rus,* "true."] The "true acacia." The Egyptian thorn, or gum-arabic tree; called also *Acacia Arabica.* Also, the expressed juice of the unripe pods of the *Acacia verarel.*

Aca'cia Ver'a-vel.* A species affording the juice called *Acacia vera.*

Aca'cia Zey-lon'ĭ-ca.* A name for *Hæmatoxylon Campechianum.*

Acajou, ǎ'kǎ'zhoo'. The ANACARDIUM OCCIDENTALE, which see.

Ac-a-le'phe.* [Gr. ἀκαλήφη.] The nettle. See URTICA.

Ac-a-le'phus.* [From the same.] Belonging to a nettle. In the neuter plural (*Acale'pha*) applied to a class of the *Radiata,* from the stinging pain felt on touching them.

A-cal'ȳ-cine. [**Acalyci'nus, A-cal'ycis;** from *a,* priv., and *ca'lyx.*] Having no calyx.

A-camp'sĭ-a.* [From *a,* priv., and κάμπτω, to "bend."] An inflexible state of a joint. See ANKYLOSIS.

A-can'tha.* [Gr. ἄκανθα; from ἀκή, a "sharp point."] Applied formerly to the spine of the back, or rather of a *vertebra,* by the regular arrangement of the series of which the former is constituted. A thorn, spine, or prickle.

Acanthaceæ,* ak-an-tha'she-ē. The name of a natural order of plants resembling the *Acanthus.*

A-can'thi,* the plural of ACAN'THUS, forming the Jussieuan name of a natural order, now ACANTHACEÆ, which see.

A-can'thine. [**Acan'thinus;** from ἄκανθα, a "thorn."] Belonging to a thorn; thorny, prickly.

A-can'thi-um.* [From the same.] The specific or trivial name for the *Onopor'dium Acan'thium.*

A-can-tho-çeph'a-lous. [**Acanthoceph'alus;** from ἄκανθα, and κεφαλή, the "head."] Having a spiny head. The Latin term in the neuter plural (*Acanthoceph'ala*) is applied to a family of the *Entozo'a parenchym'ata.*

Acantho'des. See ACANTHOID.

A-can'thoid. [**Acanthoi'des;** from ἄκανθα, a "thorn," and εἶδος, a "form."] Having the form of a thorn or spine; resembling a spine.

Acanthophorous, ak-an-thof'o-rŭs. [**Acanthoph'orus;** from ἄκανθα, a "thorn," and φέρω, to "bear."] Beset with spines or coarse hairs.

A-can-tho-po'di-ous. [**Acanthopo'dius;** from ἄκανθα, and πούς, a "foot."] Having spinous petioles.

A-can-thop-te-ry̆ġ'i-i.* [From ἄκανθα, a "thorn," and πτερύγιον, a "little wing," a "fin."] The name of an order of fishes having spiny fins.

A-can'thu-lus.* [From ἄκανθα, a "thorn."] An instrument for extracting thorns, or *spiculæ* of wood, bone, etc., from wounds.

A-can'thus.* [From ἄκανθα, a "thorn."] Bear's breech. A genus of the Linnæan class *Didynamia,* natural order *Acanthaceæ.*

Acan'thus Mol'lis.* The systematic name of Bear's breech.

A-car'di-a.* [From *a*, priv., and καρδία, the "heart."] The condition of a monster-fœtus, born without a heart, or, rather, deficient as to the whole thorax.

Acardiohæmia,* a-kar-de-o-he'me-a. [From *a*, priv., καρδία, the "heart," and αἷμα, "blood."] A deficiency of blood in the heart.

A-car-di-o-ner'vi-a.* [From *a*, priv., καρδία, the "heart," and *ner'vus,* a "nerve."] A deficiency of nervous action in the heart, evinced by the sounds being inaudible.

A-car-di-o-tro'phi-a.* [From *a*, priv., καρδία, and τροφή, "nourishment."] Atrophy of the heart.

Ac-a-ro-i'dēs.* [From *ac'arus,* and εἶδος, a "form."] Resembling the *Acarus:* ac'aroid.

A-car'pous. [**Acar'pus;** from *a*, priv., and καρπός, "fruit."] Having no fruit.

Ac'a-rus.* [From ακαρής, that which cannot be cut on account of its smallness; from *a*, priv., and κείρω, to "cut."] A genus of minute insects infesting the skin.

Ac'arus Au-tum-na'lis.* The harvest-bug; the wheal-worm.

Ac'arus Do-mes'ti-cus.* The domestic tick, found on the human body.

Ac'arus Riç'i-nus.* The dog-tick.

Ac'arus Sac'cha-ri.* ("Acarus of Sugar.") An animalcule found in sugar, causing "grocer's itch."

Ac'arus Sca-bi-e'i.* ("Acarus of Itch.") The itch animalcule.

A-cat'a-lep-sy̆. [**Acatalep'sia;** from *a*, priv., and καταλαμβάνω, to "apprehend."] Uncertainty in diagnosis, etc.

A-cat-ap'o-sis.* [From *a*, priv., and καταπίνω, to "swallow."] Difficulty in swallowing. See DYSPHAGIA.

A-cau'lis.* [From *a*, priv., and *cau'lis,* a "stem."] Having no stem: acau'line.

Ac-çel-e-ra'tion. Increased rapidity of the pulse, respiration, etc.

Ac-çel-e-ra'tor, o'ris.* [From *accel'ero, accelera'tum,* to "hasten."] Applied to a muscle of the penis (*Accelera'tor uri'næ*) whose action propels the urine; also named *Ejacula'tor sem'inis,* from a similar office as to the semen.

Ac-çes'sion. [**Acces'sio, o'nis;** from *acce'do, acces'sum,* to "go to," to "approach," to "be added to."] The approach, or onset, of diseases, or of fits, paroxysms or exacerbations in fevers, etc.

Accessorii Willisii,* ak-ses-so're-i wil-lis'e-i. The "accessory nerves of Willis," so named from the discoverer. The superior respiratory nerves, a pair arising from the spinal cord and joining the *par vagum.*

Ac-çes'so-ry̆. [**Accesso'rius;** from the same.] Usually applied to muscular appendages that assist the action of larger muscles.

Ac'çi-dent. [**Ac'cidens;** from *ac'cido,* to "happen."] A familiar word used by the French as synonymous with *symptom.* See ACCIDENTIA.

Ac-çi-den'tal. [**Accidenta'lis;** from the same.] Adventitious; happening unexpectedly. Applied by French and some English writers to textures resulting from morbid action.

Acciden'tal Col'ors. A series of optical phenomena, so named by Buffon, and now known by the name of Ocular

Spectra. If the eye be steadily directed for some time to a white wafer upon a dark ground, and be then turned aside, a well-defined image of the wafer will be perceived, with the colors reversed: the wafer will appear dark, the ground white. This new appearance is termed the accidental color, or ocular spectrum. By using differently colored wafers we obtain the following results:—

Color of wafer.	Color of spectra.
Black	White.
Red	Bluish-green.
Orange	Blue.
Yellow	Indigo.
Green	Violet with a little red.
Blue	Orange-red.
Indigo	Orange-yellow.
Violet	Bluish-green.

Darwin classes the Spectra under the two heads of *direct* and *reverse;* the former depending on the permanence of the impression, the latter upon exhaustion.

Accidentia,* ak-se-den′she-ạ. [From *ac′cido,* to "happen," *ac′cidens,* "happening," "that which happens."] A chance or occurrence happening to one unexpectedly: an ac′cident.

Ac-çip′ĭ-ter.* [From *accip′io,* to "take."] A bird of prey. In the plural (*Accipitres,* ak-sip′e-trēz) applied to an order of birds, including the hawk, eagle, etc., called also *Rapa′ces,* and *Rapto′res,* from their rapacious or predatory character.

Ac-clī′mat-ed. [**Acclima′tus.** Fr. *acclimaté,* ak‵kle‵må‵tȧ′.] Thoroughly accustomed to a climate.

Ac-clī-mạ-tĭ-zā′tion. [**Acclimatiza′tio, o′***nis.*] The process or state of being acclimated.

Ac-clī′vis.* [From *ad,* "to," and *cli′vus,* the "side of a hill."] "Sloping upwards." Applied to a muscle of the abdomen, from the oblique ascent of its fibres, the *Obli′quus inter′nus.*

Accouchement (Fr.), ak‵koosh‵mŏɴᵍ′. [From *accoucher,* ak‵koo‵shȧ′, to "put to bed," to "deliver."] The act of being delivered; delivery.

Accoucheur, ak‵koo‵shᴜʀ′. [From the same.] A man-midwife; an obstetrician.

Ac-cre′tion. [**Accre′tio, o′***nis;* from *ad,* "to," and *cres′co, cre′tum,* to "grow."] The process by which nutrient particles are added to the various tissues. The adhering together of parts naturally separate, as the fingers, etc.

Acephala. See Acephalus.

Acephalia,* as-e-fa′le-ạ. [From *a,* priv., and κεφαλή, the "head."] A form of fœtal monstrosity, consisting in the want of the head.

Acephalobrachia,* a-sef‵ạ-lo-brạ-ki′ạ. [From *a,* priv., κεφαλή, the "head," and βραχίων, the "arm."] A form of fœtal monstrosity, consisting in the absence of head and arms.

A-çeph‵ạ-lo-brạ-chi′ŭs.* [From the same.] A monster-fœtus, having neither head nor arms.

A-çeph‵ạ-lo-car′dĭ-ạ.* [From *a,* priv., κεφαλή, the "head," and καρδία, the "heart."] A form of monstrosity, consisting in the absence of head and heart.

A-çeph‵ạ-lo-car′dĭ-us.* [From the same.] A monster-fœtus, without head and heart.

Acephalochirus,* or **Acephalocheirus,*** a-sef‵ạ-lo-kī′rŭs. [From *a,* priv., κεφαλή, the "head," and χείρ, the "hand."] A monster-fœtus, without head and hands.

Acephalocyst,* a-sef′ạ-lo-sĭst. [**Aceph‵alocys′tis;** from *a,* priv., κεφαλή, the "head," and κύστις, a "bladder."] The headless hydatid, formed like a bladder.

A-çeph‵ạ-lo-gas′ter.* [From *a,* priv., κεφαλή, the "head," and γαστήρ, the "stomach" or "belly."] A monster-fœtus, without head, chest, and upper part of the belly.

A-çeph‵ạ-lo-gas′trĭ-ạ.* [From the same.] A form of monstrosity, consisting in the want of head, chest, and belly.

A-çeph‵ạ-lo-po′dĭ-ạ.* [From *a,* priv., κεφαλή, the "head," and πούς, ποδός, the "foot."] A form of monstrosity, consisting in the absence of head and feet.

A-çeph‵ạ-lop′o-dus.* [From the same.] A monster-fœtus, without head and feet.

Acephalorachia,* a-sef‵ạ-lo-ra′-ke-ạ. [From *a,* priv., κεφαλή, the "head," and ῥάχις, the "spine."] A form of monstrosity, consisting in the want of head and spinal column.

A-çeph‵ạ-lo-ra′chĭ-us.* [From the same.] A monster-fœtus, without head and spinal column.

Acephalostoma. See Acephalostomus.

A-çeph‵ạ-lo-sto′mĭ-ạ.* [From *a,* priv., κεφαλή, the "head," and στόμα, a "mouth."] A form of monstrosity, consisting in the want of a head, but with an aperture like a mouth.

A-çeph'a-los'to-mus,* or **A-çeph'a-los'to-ma.*** [From the same.] A monster-fœtus, without a head, but having an aperture like a mouth.

A-çeph'a-lo-tho-ra'cĭ-a.* [From *a*, priv., κεφαλή, the "head," and θώραξ, the "chest."] A form of monstrosity, consisting in the want of head and chest.

A-çeph'a-lo-tho'rus.* [From the same.] A monster-fœtus, without head and chest.

A-ceph'a-lus.* [From *a*, priv, and κεφαλή, the "head."] Without a head: aceph'alous. In the neuter plural (*Aceph'ala*) applied to a class of *Mollusca* having no appearance of a head.

A'çer.* The maple.

Aç'era,* the plural of A'CER, a "maple-tree,"—forming the Jussieuan name of a natural order of plants. See ACERACEÆ.

A'çer Sac-cha-ri'num.* The sugar-maple-tree.

Aceraceæ,* as-e-ra'she-ē, or **A-çer-in'e-æ.*** [From *a'cer*, the "maple-tree."] A natural order of plants including the maple.

Aç'e-rāte. [**Ace'ras, a'***tis.*] A combination of aceric acid with a salifiable base.

A-cer'bi-tȳ. [**Acer'bitas, a'***tis;* from *acer'bus*, "crude," "harsh."] Sourness, with harshness.

A-cĕr'ic. [**Acer'icus;** from *a'cer*, the "maple-tree."] Pertaining to the *Acer*. Applied to an acid obtained from the juices of *A'cer campes'tre*, and *A'cer pseu'do-plat'anus.*

Acerineæ. [From the same.] See ACERACEÆ.

Aç'er-ōse. [**Acero'sus;** from *a'cus, aç'eris*, "chaff."] Chaffy; like chaff.

A-cer'vu-lus.* [Diminutive of *acer'vus*, a "heap."] The collection of sand-like particles found in the pineal gland: an acer'vule.

A-cĕs'çent. [**Aces'cens;** from *aces'co*, to "grow sour."] Becoming sour.

A-ce'ta,* the plural of ACE'TUM, "vinegar," applied in Pharmacy to preparations of vinegar.

Aç-e-tab'u-lum.* [From *ace'tum*, "vinegar."] A little cup used by the ancients for holding vinegar. Applied, in Anatomy, to the round cavity in the *Os innominatum* which receives the head of the *Os femoris.*

Aç'e-tal. A compound of aldehyde with ether; formed by the action of platinum black on the vapor of alcohol with the presence of oxygen. It is a colorless, very fluid liquid, having a peculiar odor, suggesting that of Hungary wines.

Aç-e-ta'rĭ-um,* plural **Aç-e-ta'rĭ-a.** [From *ace'tum*, "vinegar."] A salad made of roots or herbs mixed with oil, salt, and vinegar.

Aceta'rium Scor-bu'tĭ-cum.* A kind of pickle for scorbutic patients.

Aç'e-tāte. [**Ace'tas, a'***tis.*] A combination of acetic acid with a base.

A-cet'ic. [**Acet'icus;** from *ace'tum*, "vinegar."] Belonging to vinegar. Applied to an acid the product of acetous fermentation.

A-cet'ĭ-ca.* [From the same.] Pharmaceutical preparations of vinegar.

Acet'ic Aç'id. [**Aç'idum Acet'icum.**] The sour principle which exists in vinegar. It occurs ready-formed in several products of the vegetable kingdom; it is also generated during the spontaneous fermentation of many vegetable and animal juices. Two kinds are known in Pharmacy,—viz.: *Aç'idum acet'icum dilu'tum*, "dilute acetic acid," or common distilled vinegar, with very minute portions of uncombined mucilage and extractive. *Aç'idum acet'icum for'tius*, "strong acetic acid." This variety is obtained by distillation from wood, generally that of oak coppice deprived of its bark, and is then termed pyroligneous acid; also by decomposing the acetates by sulphuric acid; it is then termed radical vinegar; and when mixed with camphor and essential oils, it is called "Henry's Aromatic Essence of Vinegar," and Marseilles or Thieves' Vinegar, or *Vinaigre des Quatre Voleurs* (vȧ'nēgʀ' dȧ katʀ vo'lʊʀ'). See GLACIAL ACID.

A-cet'ĭ-fĭ-cā'tion. [**Acetifica'tio, o'***nis;* from *ace'tum*, and *fa'cio*, to "make."] The act or process of making vinegar.

Aç'e-tīte. [**Ace'tis, i'***tis;* from *ace'tum.*] An erroneous name for the salt of *acetous acid*, in distinction from that of *acetic acid*, given when these acids were supposed to be different. The proper term is ACETATE, which see.

Aç-e-tom'e-ter. [**Acetom'etrum;** from *ace'tum*, and μέτρον, a "measure."] An instrument for ascertaining the strength of vinegar.

Aç'e-tōne. A substance found, as an impurity, associated with pyro-acetic spirit, or naphtha.

Aç-e-to'sa.* [From *a'ceo*, to "be

sour."] The specific name of *Rumex acetosa*.

A-ce-to-sel'la.* [From *aceto'sa*.] The former Pharmacopœial name (Lond. Ph. 1836) for the *Oxalis acetosella*.

A-ce'tous. [**Aceto'sus;** from *ace'tum*.] Pertaining to vinegar; acetic.

A-ce'tum.* [From *a'ceo*, to "be sour."] Acetic or acetous acid in a very diluted state; common vinegar. The varieties of vinegar known in commerce are three:—Wine vinegar, Malt vinegar, and Sugar vinegar. The strongest malt vinegar is termed *proof* vinegar, and is called by the manufacturer No. 24; it is estimated to contain 4.73 per cent. of real acetic acid. See ACETIC ACID.

Aç'e-tȳl. A hypothetical radical, produced by the abstraction of two atoms of oxygen from ethyl, by oxidating processes. It pervades a series of compounds, including acetic acid, from which it derives its name.

Achænium,* a-kē'ne-ŭm; written also **Ache'nium.** [From *α*, priv., and χαίνω, to "open."] An *indehiscent* fruit: it is one-celled and one-seeded, dry, and having the integuments of the seed distinct from it.

Acheir, a-kīr', or **Acheirus.** See ACHIRUS.

Achillea,* ak-il-le'a. A genus of syngenesious plants. The *A. ager'atum* has properties similar to those of tansy. The *A. millefo'lium*, common yarrow or milfoil, is sometimes used in dyspepsia, flatulence, etc.; also in hæmorrhage.

A-chil'lis Ten'do.* (The "Tendon of Achil'lēs.") The strong tendon of the *gastrocne'mii*, or *gastrocne'mius* and *solæ'us* muscles. Also called CHORDA MAGNA, or the "great sinew."

Achirous, a-kī'rŭs, or **Acheirous.** [**Achi'rus,** or **Achei'rus;** from *α*, priv., and χείρ, the "hand."] Having no hands.

Achlamydeous, ak-la-mĭd'e-ŭs. [**Achlamyd'eus;** from *α*, priv., and χλαμύς, a "short cloak."] Without calyx or corolla.

Achne,* ak'ne. [Gr. ἄχνη.] A shred of lint. A flake of mucous-like substance on the cornea.

Acholous, ak'o-lŭs. [**Ach'olus;** from *α*, priv., and χολή, "bile."] Without bile; deficient in bile.

A'chor,* plural **A-cho'rēs.** [Gr. ἀχώρ, "scurf" or "dandruff."] A small pustule containing a straw-colored fluid, and forming scaly eruptions about the head of young children; a species of scald-head.

Achoristus,* ak-o-ris'tŭs. [From *α*, priv., and χωρίζω, to "separate."] A sign or symptom which is inseparable from (or which invariably accompanies) a particular state of health or disease.

Ach'ro-a.* [From *α*, priv., and χρόα, "color."] A colorless state of the skin, caused by the absence of the usual coloring matter of the *rete mucosum*. Compare DYSCHROA.

Ach'ro-mat'ic. [**Achromat'icus;** from *α*, priv., and χρῶμα, "color."] That which does not admit the colors of the solar spectrum. Lenses in which the prismatic aberration of light (caused by refraction) is corrected, are termed achromatic.

A-chro'ma-tĭsm. [**Achromatis'mus;** from the same.] The correction of the aberration of light arising from refraction.

Ach-ro'ma-top'sĭ-a.* [From *α*, priv., χρῶμα, "color," and ὄψις, "vision."] Inability to distinguish colors: achro'matopsy.

Achylosis,* ak-e-lo'sis. [From *α*, priv., and χυλός, "juice," and hence "chyle."] Deficient chylification.

Achymosis,* ak-e-mo'sis. [From *α*, priv., and χυμός, "chyme."] Deficient chymification.

Acia,* a'she-a. [From *a'cus*, a "needle."] A word used by Celsus, supposed to mean the thread in a needle with which a suture is made to join the lips of a wound; also, the suture itself.

A-cic'u-la,* plural, **A-cic'u-læ.** [Diminutive of *a'cus*, a "needle."] A little needle: an aç'icule. See SPICULA.

A-cic'u-lar. [**Acicula'ris;** from *acic'ula*.] Like a small needle; spicular.

A-cic'u-lā-ted. [**Acicula'tus.**] Having *aciculæ*.

Aç'id. [**Aç'idus, Aç'idum;** from *a'ceo*, to "be sour."] Sour; sharp to the taste, like vinegar. As a noun it signifies a compound substance which unites in definite proportions with alkaline bases, and has the property of turning vegetable blues to red.

Aç'ida,* the plural of ACIDUM, an acid.

Aç'ĭ-dif'er-ous. [**Acidif'erus;** from *aç'idum*, an "acid," and *fe'ro*, to "bear."] Bearing or containing acid.

A-cid'ĭ-fī'a-ble. [**Acidifiab'ilis:** from *aç'idus*, "sour," and *fi'o*, to "become."] Capable of becoming acid.

A-cid'ĭ-fĭ-cā'tion. [**Acidifica'tio, o'nis.**] The act or process of forming, or impregnating with, acid. See next article.

A-cid'ĭ-fȳ. [From *aç'idus,* "sour," and *fa'cio,* to "make."] To make sour or acid; to convert into an acid.

A-cid'ĭ-fȳ-ing. [**Acidif'icus;** from *aç'idus,* and *fa'cio,* to "make."] Making acid; converting into an acid.

Acid'ifying Prin'ci-ple. That which forms an acid.

Aç-id-im'e-ter. [**Acidim'etrum;** from *aç'idum,* an "acid," and μέτρον, a "measure."] An instrument for measuring the strength of acids or the amount of free acid. See next article.

Aç-id-im'e-trȳ. [**Acidime'tria;** from *aç'idum,* "acid," and μετρέω, to "measure."] The process by which the strength of acids is measured, or by which the amount of uncombined or free acid is determined.

A-cid'ĭ-tȳ. [**Acid'itas, a'tis;** from *aç'idus,* "sour."] The quality of sourness. See Acor.

Acidometer. See Acidimeter.

A-cid'u-lā-ted. [**Acidula'tus;** from *acid'ulus,* "slightly acid."] Slightly blended with acid.

A-cid'u-lous. [**Acid'ulus;** from the same.] Slightly acid; subacid.

Aç'ĭ-dum,* plural **Aç'ĭ-da.** [The neuter form of *aç'idus,* "sour."] An Acid, which see.

Acies,* a'she-ēz or a'se-ēz. [From ἀκή, a "sharp point."] A name for iron or steel.

Aç-ĭ-naç'ĭ-form. [**Acinacifor'mis;** from *acin'aces,* a "scimitar."] In the form of a scimitar.

Aç-ĭ-ne'sĭ-a,* or **Ak-ĭ-ne'sĭ-a.*** [From α, priv., and κίνησις, "motion."] Loss of motion in the whole or part of the body.

Aç'ĭ-ni.* The plural of Acinus, which see.

A-cin'ĭ-form. [**Acinifor'mis;** from *aç'inus,* a "grape" or "grape-stone."] Having the appearance of a grape or grape-stone. See Acinus.

Aç'ĭ-nōse, or **Aç'i-nous.** [**Acino'sus;** from the same.] Having *acini,* or full of *acini.*

Aç'ĭ-nus,* or **Aç'ĭ-nos.*** [Gr. ἄκινος, the "stone of grapes;" a "grape."] Applied in the plural (*aç'ini*) to the small granulations composing the substance of the liver and other glandular bodies. Also a term used in Botany to denote the small berries which form the fruit of the bramble, rasp, etc. Also a species of thyme.

Aç-ĭ-pen'ser.* The sturgeon, a genus of fishes from which isinglass is prepared. See Ichthyocolla.

Ac'me.* [Gr. ἀκμή, the "point," "top," "period of greatest vigor."] The highest degree, or height, of a disease; the crisis.

Ac'ne.* [Supposed to be derived from *ac'me,* because it is apt to affect those who are in the bloom of life.] A papular eruption, mostly occurring on the face, but sometimes extending to the neck, shoulders, or breast.

Ac'ne Rosa'cea*(ro-za'she-a). Pimples on the face; the conspicuous eruption, of a bright rosy hue, on the nose and contiguous parts of the face, in drunkards. Called also *Gut'ta Ro'sea,* or Rosy-drop.

Accelius,* a-se'le-ŭs, or **Acœ'lios.*** [From α, priv., and κοιλία, the "belly."] Having no belly; wasted to such a degree as to have this appearance.

A-col'o-ġȳ. [**Acolo'gia;** from ἄκος, a "remedy," and λόγος, a "discourse."] The doctrine or science of remedies. By some the term is limited to the consideration of surgical and mechanical remedies.

A-con'dȳ-lous. [From α, priv., and κόνδυλος, a "joint."] Without joints.

Ac'o-nīte. The common name for Aconitum Napellus.

Aconitia,* ak-o-nish'e-a, or **A-con'ĭ-tin.** [**Aconiti'na;** from *aconi'tum.*] An alkaloid constituting the active principle of aconite. It is a powerful poison.

Ac-o-nit'ic Aç'id. An acid obtained from aconite.

Ac-o-ni'ti Fo'lĭ-um.* ("Leaf of Aconite.") The Pharmacopœial name (U.S. Ph.) for the leaves of *Aconi'tum napel'lus.*

Aconi'ti Ra'dix.* ("Root of Aconite.") The Pharmacopœial name ‖ for the root of *Aconitum napellus.*

Ac-o-ni'tum.* [From *Ac'onæ,* a place in Bithynia where it was common.] The Pharmacopœial name (Br. Ph.) for the leaves and tops of *Aconitum napellus.*

Aconi'tum Na-pel'lus.* The systematic name of aconite.

A'cor, o'ris.* [From *a'ceo,* to "be sour."] Acidity, as in the stomach from indigestion.

A-co'rĭ-a.* [From α, priv., and κορέω, to "satisfy."] Insatiable hunger.

A-cor'mous. [**Acor'mus;** from α, priv., and κόρμος, the "trunk of a tree."] Having no stem.

Ac'o-rus,* Ac'o-rum.* [Gr. ἄκορον.] The Pharmacopœial name (Lond. Ph. 1836) for *Acorus calamus.* A Linnæan genus of the class *Hexandria*, order *Monogynia*, Jussieuan system *Aroideæ*.

Ac'orus A-sĭ-at'i-cus, Ac'orus Ve'-rus.* Other names for *Acorus calamus*.

Ac'orus Cal'a-mus.* The systematic name of the common sweet flag. See preceding article.

Acotyledon,* a-kot-ĭ-lē'don. [From *α*, priv., and κοτυληδών, όνος, a "seed-lobe."] A plant having no seed-lobe: without a cotyledon. In the plural, applied to a division of the Jussieuan system. See next article.

Acotyledones,* a-kot-ĭ-lē'do-nēz. [From the same.] Acotyledonous plants; plants whose seeds have no distinct cotyledons. The term is usually applied to what are more commonly named cryptogamic plants, such as ferns, mosses, lichens, etc., in which there are no seeds, properly so called, but which are propagated by undivided spherical bodies called spores.

A-cot-ȳ-led'o-nous. [Acotyledo'-neus, Acotyle'donus; from the same.] Having no cotyledon or seed-lobe. See Cotyledon.

Acoumeter, a-koo'mę-ter or a-kow'-mę-ter. [**Acou'metrum;** from ἀκούω, to "hear," and μέτρον, a "measure."] An instrument for estimating the extent of hearing.

Acouophonia,* a-koo-o-fo'ne-ạ. [From ἀκούω, to "hear," and φωνή, a "voice" or "sound."] A mode of auscultation in which the observer places his ear on the chest and analyzes the sound produced by percussion.

A-cous'ma, a*tis*.* [From ἀκούω, to "hear."] A species of depraved hearing, in which sounds are imagined as if really heard.

Acoustic, a-koos'tik or a-kow'stik. [**Acous'ticus;** from ἀκουστής, a "hearer."] Pertaining to sound, or the sense of hearing. Anciently applied to remedies (called *acoustica medicamenta*) for deafness.

Acoustic Duct. See Meatus Auditorius.

Acous'tic Nerve. The auditory nerve, or *Portio mollis* of the seventh pair.

A-cous'tics. [Acous'tica; from ἀκούω, to "hear."] The doctrine of the theory and principles of sound: the science of sound.

Ac-quis'ĭ-tĭve-ness. According to Phrenology, that faculty or propensity which impels to the acquisition of property.

Acræpalus,* a-krĕp'ạ-lŭs, or **A-cræp'a-los.*** [From *α*, priv., and κραι-πάλη, "drunken or gluttonous excess."] Correcting the effects of excess in eating or drinking.

A-cra'nĭ-ạ.* [From *α*, priv., and κρανίον, the "cranium."] A species of defective development consisting in partial or total absence of the cranium.

Acratia,* a-kra'te-ạ. [From *α*, priv., and κράτος, "strength."] Weakness, impotency.

Ac'rid. [From *a'cer*, or *a'cris*, "sharp."] A term applied to substances producing a disagreeable sense of irritation or burning on the tongue or in the fauces.

Ac'rĭ-mo-nȳ. [Acrimo'nia; from *a'cris*, "sharp," "acrid."] A sharp, acrid, corrosive quality, biting to the tongue.

Ac'rimony of the Hu'mors. A change supposed to take place in the fluids of the body, causing disease.

A-crin'ĭ-ạ.* [From *α*, priv., and κρίνω, to "discern," to "secrete."] A diminution or total suppression of the secretions.

A-cri'sĭ-ạ.* [From *α*, priv., and κρίσις, a "judgment."] A state of disease in which there is either no crisis, or in which no judgment or opinion can be formed.

Ac'rĭ-tạ.* [From *α*, priv., and κρίνω, to "discern," to "perceive," to "judge."] A subdivision of the *Radiata* of Cuvier, including animals which have no trace of any organs of perception or of any nervous system. It comprehends Polypi, Infusoria, and other animals of the very lowest type.

A-crit'ĭ-cal. [Ac'ritus; from *α*, priv., and κριτός, "judged," from κρίνω, to "judge."] Having no regular crisis.

Ac-ro-bȳs'tĭ-ạ.* [From ἄκρον, "extremity," and βύω, to "cover."] The prepuce.

Ac'ro-dont. [Ac'rodon; from ἄκρον, "extremity" or "summit," and ὀδούς, ὀδόντ-ος, a "tooth."] Applied by Owen to scaly *Saurii* having teeth ankylosed to the summit of the alveolar ridge.

Ac-ro-dȳn'ĭ-ạ.* [From ἄκρον, "extremity," and ὀδύνη, "pain."] Acute rheumatism of the extremities, head, hands, or feet.

Ac'ro-ġen. An acrogenous plant. See next article.

A-croġ'e-nous. [Acroġ'enus; from ἄκρον, "summit," and γένω, to "be born."] Growing from their tops. The Latin term in the plural feminine (*Acrogenæ*, a-krŏj'e-nē) is applied to plants which grow from their external points, and whose increase is in length mainly.

Ac-ro-ma'nĭ-ạ.* [From ἄκρος, "extreme," and μανία, "madness."] Confirmed or incurable madness.

A-cro'mĭ-al. [**Acromia'lis.**] Pertaining to the acromion.

A-cro'mĭ-on.* [From ἄκρον, "extremity" or "summit," and ὦμος, the "shoulder."] The projecting process of the *Scapula*.

Ac-rom-pha'lĭ-on,* Acrom'phalon.* Ac-rom-pha'lĭ-um,* Acrom'phalum.* [From ἄκρον, "summit" or "point," and ὀμφαλός, the "navel."] The centre of the navel, to which the cord is attached in the fœtus.

Acron'yeal. See ACRONYCTOUS.

Ac-ron-ȳc'tous. [**Acronyc'tus;** from ἄκρον, "extremity," and νύξ, νυκτός, "night."] Applied to stars appearing at sunset and disappearing at sunrise (sunset and sunrise being the two "extremities of the night"); in other words, to stars or planets when opposite the sun.

Ac'ro-spīre. [**Acrospi'ra;** from ἄκρον, "extremity," "end," and σπεῖρα, any thing wound round another.] A sprout or *plumule* from the end of seeds when germinating.

A-crot'ic. [**Acrot'icus;** from ἄκρος, "extreme," "outermost part."] Belonging to the external surface. Applied in the plural neuter (*Acrot'ica*) to an order of the class *Eccritica*, in Good's classification.

Ac'ro-tĭsm. [**Acrotis'mus;** from α, priv., and κρότος, the "pulse."] A defect of the pulse.

Ac-tin-ĭ-for'mis.* [From ἀκτίν, or ἀκτίς, a "ray."] Exhibiting the form or appearance of rays. The same as ACTINOIDES.

Ac'tin-ĭsm. [**Actinis'mus;** from ἀκτίν.] That branch of Natural Philosophy which treats of the radiation of heat or light (Mayne); but more usually the *chemical* power of the sun's rays as distinguished from light or heat.

Ac-tin-o-car'pous. [**Actinocar'pus;** from ἀκτίν, a "ray," and καρπός, "fruit."] Having trophosperms radiated like the rays of fruit.

Ac-tin-oç'er-āte, Ac-tin-oç'er-ous. [**Actinocera'tus, Actinoç'erus;** from ἀκτίν, and κέρας, a "horn."] Having parts like radiated horns.

Ac-tin-o'dēs. The same as ACTINOID.

Ac'tin-oid. [**Actinoi'des;** from ἀκτίν, a "ray," and εἶδος, a "form."] Resembling rays, or a ray.

Ac-tin'o-lite. [**Actinol'ithus;** from ἀκτίν, a "ray," and λίθος, a "stone."] A species of mineral composed of radiated crystals.

Ac-tin-om'e-ter. [**Actinom'etrum;** from ἀκτίν, a "ray," and μέτρον, a "measure."] An instrument for indicating the strength of the sun's rays.

Ac-tin-o-zo'um,* or **Ac-tin-o-zo'on*** (plural **Actinozo'a**). [From ἀκτίν, and ζῶον, an "animal."] The name of certain *Acephala Gastrica* having appendages, and often the *areæ* of the surface, radiated.

Ac'tion. [**Ac'tio, o'***nis;* from *a'go, ac'tum*, to "do," to "act."] The exercise of an active power; a faculty or function of the body.

Ac'tĭve. [**Acti'vus;** from the same.] Acting with energy. Applied to treatment of the sick, to certain medicines, and to surgical remedies.

Ac'tu-al Cau'te-rȳ. [From καίω, to "burn;" or καυτήριον, a "red-hot iron," a "branding-iron."] A red-hot iron, or fire, used by surgeons as a cautery, because it really *burns* away the part or surface to which it is applied, in contradistinction to caustic substances, termed potential cauteries, which produce a similar result without actual burning. Also called *Ignis actualis*, "actual fire." See CAUTERY.

A-cu'le-āte. [**Aculea'tus;** from *acu'leus*, a "prickle."] Having prickles.

A-cu'le-us.* [From *a'cus*, a "needle."] A prickle arising from the bark or epidermis of any part of a plant, and which may be peeled off with the bark.

A-cu'mĭ-nāte. [**Acumina'tus;** from *acu'men, acu'minis*, a "point," "sharpness."] Pointed; tapering to a point.

Ac-u-pres'sion. [**Acupres'sio;** from *a'cus*, a "needle," and *pre'mo, pres'sum*, to "press."] Dr. J. Y. Simpson's plan of securing against hæmorrhage in wounds or operations, by inserting a needle through the skin below the divided vessel, and returning its point to the cutaneous surface again, the ends being left *out* to a sufficient extent.

Ac-u-punc'ture. [**Acupunctu'ra;** from *a'cus*, a "needle," and *pun'go, punc'tum*, to "prick."] A small puncture made with a needle.

A'cus Can-nu-la'tạ.* A trochar: a cannulated needle used in surgery.

A'cus In-ter-punc-to'rĭ-ạ.* A couching-needle, used in operating on the eye.

A'cus Oph-thăl'mĭ-cạ.* A couching or ophthalmic needle.

A'cus Tri-que'tra.* A trochar: a three-cornered needle.

Ac-ŭt-an'gu-lar, or **Ac-ŭt-an'gu-lāte.** [**Acutangula'ris, Acutangula'tus;** from *acu'tus,* "sharp," and *an'gulus,* a "corner."] Having sharp angles.

A-cūte'. [**Acu'tus;** from *ac'uo, acu'tum,* to "sharpen," to "point."] Ending in a point. Applied also to diseases having violent symptoms attended with danger, and terminating within a few days.

Ac-u-te-nac'u-lum.* [From *a'cus,* a "needle," and *tenac'ulum,* a "handle."] A handle for a needle. Also called *Porte-aiguille.*

A-çy'ạ-no-blep'sĭ-ạ.* [From *a,* priv., κύανος, "blue," and βλέπω, to "look," to "see."] Defect of vision by which blue color cannot be distinguished.

Acyesis,* as-i-e'sis. [From *a,* priv., and κύησις, "pregnancy."] Sterility in women.

Ad. A Latin preposition signifying "to," "at," "by," "towards," "near," "with," etc. In compound words the *d* is usually changed to correspond with the following letter. Thus, *ad* becomes *ac* before *c, al* before *l, ap* before *p,* etc.

Ad. or **Add.** = *Ad'de, adda'tur,** etc. "Add," or "let there be added."

Ad Def. Animi = *Ad defectionem animi** (ad de-fek-she-o'nem an'e-mi). "To fainting."

Ad Deliquium* (de-lik'we-ŭm), or **Ad Deliq'uium An'ĭmi.*** "To fainting." Used in directions for venesection.

Ad 2 Vic. = *Ad du'as vi'ces.** "At two times," or "at twice taking."

Ad Lib. = *Ad libi'tum.** "At pleasure."

A-dac'rȳ-ạ.* [From *a,* priv., and δάκρυον, a "tear."] A deficiency of the lachrymal secretion.

Adæmonia,* a-de-mo'ne-ạ. [From *a,* priv., and δαίμων, "fortune."] Restless or unhappy thoughts; anxiety.

Ad'ạ-mant. [**Ad'amas, Adaman'tis;** from *a,* neg., and δαμάω, to "subdue."] Literally, "that which [on account of its hardness] cannot be subdued." Diamond, the hardest of all substances.

Ad-ạ-man'tĭne. [**Adaman'tinus;** from the preceding.] Having the hardness or lustre of adamant.

Adam's Apple. See POMUM ADAMI.

Ad-ap'ter. A tube used in Chemistry for increasing the length of the neck of a retort, or for connecting the retort with the receiver, where the orifice of the latter is not large enough to admit the beak of the retort.

Ad-de-pha'ġĭ-ạ.* [From ἄδην, or ἄδδην, "abundantly," and φαγεῖν, to "eat."] Voracious appetite, or *Bulimia.*

Ad'di-son's Dis-ease'. The *Melasma supra-renale,* first described by him.

Ad-dĭ-tạ-men'tum.* [From *ad'do, ad'ditum,* to "add" or "adjoin."] A small suture sometimes found added to the lambdoid and squamous sutures.

Ad-du'cens.* [From *ad,* "to," and *du'co,* to "lead," to "draw."] Drawing together: addu'cent.

Ad-duc'tion. [**Adduc'tio, o'nis;** from the same.] That movement by which one part, as a limb or finger, is drawn to another, or to the mesial line.

Ad-duc'tor, o'ris.* [From the same.] Applied to muscles that perform adduction. See ANTITHENAR.

A'den,* gen. **Ad'enis.** [Gr. ἀδήν, a "gland."] A gland. A bubo.

Ad-en-ăl'ġĭ-ạ.* [From ἀδήν, a "gland," and ἄλγος, "pain."] Pain in a gland: adenal'gy.

Ad'en-em-phrax'is.* [From ἀδήν, a "gland," and ἔμφραξις, "obstruction."] Glandular obstruction.

Ad-en'ĭ-form. [**Adeniform'is;** from *a'den,* a "gland."] Formed like a gland; glandiform. See ADENOID.

Ad-en-i'tis, idis.* [From ἀδήν, a "gland."] Inflammation of a gland; bubo.

Ad'en-o-dȳn'ĭ-ạ.* [From ἀδήν, ἀδένος, a "gland," and ὀδύνη, "pain."] Pain in a gland. See ADENALGIA.

Ad-en-og'rạ-phȳ. [**Adenograph'ia;** from ἀδήν, a "gland," and γράφω, to "write."] A treatise or dissertation on the glandular system.

Ad'en-oid. [**Adenoi'des;** from ἀδήν, a "gland," and εἶδος, a "form."] Resembling a gland.

Ad-en-ol'o-ġȳ. [**Adenolo'gia;** from ἀδήν, a "gland," and λόγος, a "discourse."] The doctrine of the glandular system. The science which treats of glands or of the glandular system.

Ad'en-o-me-nin'ġe-us.* [From ἀδήν, a "gland," and μῆνιγξ, a "membrane."] Applied to mucous or pituitous fever (*Febris adenomeningea*), because the membranes and follicular glands of the intestines were held to be the chief seat of the complaint.

Ad'en-on-co'sis,* or **Ad'en-on-ko'sis.*** [From ἀδήν, a "gland," and ὀγκόω, to "puff up" or "swell."] Swelling of a gland.

Ad'en-o-ner'vous. The same as ADENONEUROSUS, which see.

Ad'en-o-neū-ro'sus.* [From ἀδήν, a "gland," and νεῦρον, a "nerve."] Applied to the plague (*Febris adenoneurosa*), because situated in the nerves and lymphatic glands of the axilla and groin: adenonerv'ous.

Ad'en-o-phăr-ȳn-ġi'tis, *idis.** [From ἀδήν, a "gland," and φάρυγξ, the "pharynx."] Inflammation of the tonsils and pharynx.

Ad'en-oph-thăl'mĭ-ạ.* [From ἀδήν, a "gland," and ὀφθαλμός, the "eye."] Inflammation of the Meibomian glands: adenophthal'my.

Ad'en-o-phy'mạ.* [From ἀδήν, a "gland," and φῦμα, a "tumor."] The swelling of a gland. When it occurs in the liver it is called *hepatophyma.*

Ad'en-o-scle-ro'sis.* [From ἀδήν, a "gland," and σκληρόω, to "harden."] A hard, indolent swelling of a gland, not of a scirrhous character.

Ad'en-ōse. [**Adeno'sus;** from *a'den,* a "gland."] Having many glands; glandulous.

Ad-en-ot'o-mȳ. [**Adenoto'mia;** from ἀδήν, ἀδένος, a "gland," and τέμνω, to "cut."] Dissection of the glands.

Adephagia. See ADDEPHAGIA.

A'deps, gen. **Ad'ĭ-pis.*** A Latin term, signifying fat, animal oil.

A'deps An-ser-i'nus.* Goose-grease.

A'deps O-vil'lus.* Fat of the sheep; mutton-suet.

A'deps Præ-pa-ra'tus.* Prepared lard.

A'deps Su-il'lus.* Hog's lard; *Axungia porcina.* The same as LARDUM.

Ad-he'sion. [**Adhæ'sio, o'**nis; from *ad,* "to," and *hæ'reo, hæ'sum,* to "stick."] That property by which certain bodies attract others, or their particles adhere to each other. One of the terminations of inflammation.

Ad-he'śĭve. [**Adhæsi'vus;** from the same.] Having the property of adhesion. See GLUTINOUS, VISCOUS.

Adhe'sive In-flam-mā'tion. [**Inflamma'tio adhæsi'va.**] The process by which the sides of incised wounds, being brought into exact contact, unite without suppuration, constituting *union by the first intention.*

Ad-he'sive Plas'ter. [**Emplas'trum Adhæsi'vum.**] Common name for the EMPLASTRUM RESINÆ, which see.

Ad-ĭ-an'tum.* [Gr. ἀδίαντον; from α, priv., and διαίνω, to "moisten;" so named because less juicy than many other ferns, or because the leaves are not easily moistened.] A genus of ferns called maiden-hair, from which a syrup termed *capillaire* is prepared. See CAPILLAIRE.

A-dĭ'ạ-pho-re'sis.* [From α, priv., and διαφορέω, to "perspire."] Deficient cutaneous perspiration. See ADIAPNEUSTIA.

A-dĭ-aph'o-rus.* [From α, priv., and διαφέρω, to "differ."] Formerly applied to medicines which did neither good nor harm; also to neutral salts: adiaph'orous.

A-di'ap-neus'tĭ-ạ.* [From α, priv., and διαπνέω, to "breathe through," to "evaporate."] The absence, obstruction, or diminution of perspiration.

Adipocere, or **Adipocire,** ad'e-po-sēr'. [**Adipoce'ra;** from *a'deps, ad'ipis,* "fat," and *ce'ra,* "wax."] A peculiar substance like fat, or spermaceti, formed by the spontaneous conversion of the flesh of man or other animals when placed for a considerable period in moist situations or under water; also called Grave-wax.

Ad'ĭ-pōse. [**Adipo'sus;** from *a'deps, ad'ipis,* "fat."] Of the nature of fat; fatty.

Ad'ipose Ar'te-ries. The branches of the diaphragmatic, capsular, and renal arteries, because they supply the fat round the kidneys.

Ad'ipose Mem'brane, Ad'ipose Tis'sue. Cellular membrane with fat collected in its cells.

Ad-ĭ-po'sis.* [From *a'deps.*] The growth of fatness or obesity.

A-dip'sĭ-ạ.* [From α, priv., and δίψα, "thirst."] Absence of thirst; a genus of the order *Dysorexiæ,* class *Locales,* of Cullen's nosology.

A-dip'sous. [**Adip'sus,** or **Adip'sos;** from the same.] Allaying thirst. Applied to medicines and fruits which so act.

Ad'jec-tĭve. [**Adjecti'vus;** from *adjic'io, adjec'tum,* to "add to."] Applied to coloring matters which require to be fixed through the addition of another substance termed a *mordant.*

Ad'ju-vant. [**Ad'juvans;** from *ad'juvo,* to "assist."] Assisting other remedies.

Ad-mix'ture. [**Admistu'ra;** from *ad,* "to" or "with," and *mis'ceo, mis'tum* or *mix'tum,* to "mix."] A mixing or blending one substance with another.

Admov. = *Admo've,** "apply," or *Admovea'tur,** "let there be applied."

Adnata. See TUNICA ADNATA.

Ad'nāte. [**Adna'tus;** from *ad*, "to," and *nas'cor, na'tus*, to "be born," to "grow."] Connected or grown together.

Ad-o-lĕs'cence. [**Adolescentia,** ad-o-les-sen'she-ạ; from *adoles'co*, to "grow," to "grow up to maturity."] Youth; the period between puberty and full development: from fourteen or fifteen to about twenty-five in males, and from twelve or thirteen to twenty-one in females.

Ad-op'ter. The same as ADAPTER.

Ad-os-cu-lā'tion. [**Adoscula'tio, o'**nis; from *ad*, "to" or "towards," and *os'culor, oscula'tus*, to "kiss."] The impregnation of plants by the pollen coming in contact with the pistils; the joining or inserting one part of the plant into another. Also the external contact of the genital organs of the opposite sexes in birds and fishes during impregnation, instead of the insertion of that of the male.

Ad Pon'dus Om'nĭ-um.* "To the weight of the whole." Used in prescriptions to indicate the proportion of some particular ingredient.

Adragantlin. See TRAGACANTHIN.

Adst. Fe'bre = *Adstan'te fe'bre.** "Fever being present," or when the fever is on.

Ad'ult. [**Adul'tus;** from *ado'leo, adul'tum*, to "grow up."] Applied to animals arrived at maturity; also sometimes applied to plants. See ÆTAS.

Ad-ul-te-rā'tion. [**Adultera'tio, o'**nis; from *adul'tero, adultera'tum*, to "adulterate," to "counterfeit."] The corrupting of pure ingredients with others resembling them, but of inferior value.

A-dus'tion. [**Adus'tio, o'**nis; from *adu'ro, adus'tum*, to "burn," to "scorch."] A synonym of cauterization; the application of the actual cautery to any part of the body. See AMBUSTIO.

Adventitious, ad-ven-tish'ŭs. [**Adventi'tius;** from *adve'nio, adven'tum*, to "come to," to "come to accidentally."] That which is accidental or acquired, in opposition to what is natural or hereditary.

Ad-ver-sĭ-fo'lĭ-ate. [**Adversifo'lius;** from *adver'sus*, "against," and *fo'lium*, a "leat."] Having leaves against or opposite to each other.

Ad-y̆-na'mĭ-ạ.* [From *a*, priv., and δύναμις, "power."] Loss or deficiency of vital power; adyn'amy.

Ad-y̆-nam'ic. [**Adynam'icus.**] Pertaining to *Adynamia.*

Ædœitis (e-de-i'tis), **i**dis.* [From *αἰδοῖα*, the "parts of generation," the "pudenda."] Inflammation of the pudenda.

Ædœodynia,* e-de-o-din'e-ạ. [From *αἰδοῖα*, the "pudenda," and ὀδύνη, "pain."] Pain in the genital organs, from whatever cause.

Æ-dœ-o-gra'phĭ-ạ.* [From *αἰδοῖα*, the "pudenda," and γράφω, to "write."] Description of the parts of generation.

Æ-dœ-o-lo'ġĭ-ạ.* [From *αἰδοῖα*, the "pudenda," and λόγος, a "discourse."] A treatise on the parts of generation, their structure and functions; also that branch of Anatomy or Physiology treating of the same.

Æ-dœ-op-so'phĭ-ạ,* or **Æ-dop-so'phĭ-ạ.*** [From *αἰδοῖα*, the "pudenda," and ψοφέω, to "make a noise."] The sound caused by the escape of wind from the womb *per vaginam*, or from the bladder *per urethram*, in females.

Æ-dœ-os'co-py̆. [**Ædœosco'pia,** or **Ædœop'sia;** from *αἰδοῖα*, the "pudenda," σκοπέω, to "see;" ὄψις, "vision."] Examination or inspection of the pudenda.

Æ-dœ-ot'o-my̆. [**Ædœoto'mia;** from *αἰδοῖα*, the "pudenda," and τέμνω, to "cut."] The anatomy or dissection of the parts of generation.

Æ-gag-ro-pi'lus.* [From αἴγαγρος, the "wild goat," and πῖλος, "hair wrought into felt."] A concretion found in the stomach of goats, deer, cows, etc., composed of hair collected on the tongue of the animal in licking itself, and swallowed.

Ægilops (ej'il-ops), **o'p**is.* [From αἴξ, αἰγός, a "goat," and ὤψ, the "eye."] A sinuous ulcer under the inner angle of the eye, so called from its resemblance to the *larmier* or infra-orbital glandular sac of goats: now considered to be only a stage of the *fistula lachrymalis.*

Ægobronchophony, e-go-bron-kof'o-ne. [**Ægobronchopho'nia;** from αἴξ, a "goat," and *bronchopho'nia.*] The bleating and bronchial voice; the principal symptom in pleuro-pneumonia. See BRONCHOPHONY.

Æ-go'nĭ-ạ.* (Contraction of *Ægopho'nia.*) A minor degree of ægophony, or a resonance of voice intermediate between well-marked bronchophony and ægophony.

Ægophony, e-gof'o-ne. [**Ægopho'nia;** from αἴξ, αἰγός, a "goat," and φωνή, the "voice."] In auscultation, a strong resonance of the voice, jerking and tremulous, like that of the goat or kid.

Æolipile, e-ol′e-pīl. [From *Æ′olus*, the "god of the winds," and *pi′la*, a "ball."] Literally, "Æolus's ball." A hollow ball of metal with two orifices on opposite sides. If water be placed in such a ball and converted to steam, the escape of the latter reacting on the atmosphere may be made to communicate a rotary motion to the ball.

Æora,* e-o′ra. [From *αἰωρέω*, to "raise into the air."] A species of gestation; swinging.

Æquilibrium,* e-kwĭ-lib′bre-ŭm. [From *æ′quus*, "equal," and *li′bro*, to "balance," to "weigh."] Literally, a "balancing of forces." That rest which occurs when many forces applied to the same body are equally opposed. In Medicine it signifies the harmonious action of the organs of the body.

Æ′qui-valved. [**Æquival′vis;** from *æ′quus*, "equal," and *val′væ*, "folding doors."] Having equal valves. Applied to a dehiscent pericarp so formed.

A′er.* [From *ἀήρ, ἀέρος*, "air," the "atmosphere."] The natural air we breathe: atmospheric air.

Aerate, ā′er-āt. [From the preceding.] To impregnate with carbonic acid gas.

A′e-rāt-ed. [**A′eratus.**] Applied to liquids impregnated with carbonic acid gas.

A′er Fix′us.* Fixed air, or carbonic acid gas.

A-e′rĭ-al Aç′id. Carbonic acid gas.

Ae′rial Plants. Certain plants which can live by absorption from the atmosphere, without requiring their roots to be fixed to any place; as the *Flos a′eris*. See AEROPHYTUM.

Aeriferous, ā-er-if′er-ous. [**Aer′ifer;** from *a′er*, "air," and *fe′ro*, to "bear," to "carry."] Air-bearing. Applied to the air-passages, the windpipe, bronchi, etc.

A′er-ĭ-fĭ-cā′tion. [**Aerifica′tio, o′nis;** from *a′er*, "air" or "gas," and *fa′cio*, to "make."] The converting of a body into gas.

A′er-ĭ-form. [**Aerifor′mis;** from *a′er*, "air" or "gas."] Having the form of air or gas: gaseous.

A-er-o-dȳn-am′ic. [**Aerodynam′i-cus;** from *ἀήρ*, and *δύναμις*, "power."] Pertaining to the force of the air.

A-er-o-dȳn-am′ics. [**Aerodyn-am′ica;** from the same.] The doctrine of the air and its properties while in motion.

A-er-og′ra-phȳ. [**Aerograph′ia;** from *a′er*, "air," and *γράφω*, to "write."] A description of the air.

Aerolite, ā′er-o-līt; written also **A′e-ro-lith.** [From *ἀήρ*, the "atmosphere," and *λίθος*, a "stone."] A certain meteoric stone which falls from the heavens: an aërolite or aërolith. Also termed a *Meteorolite*. See BRONTOLITH.

A-er-ol′o-ġȳ. [**Aerolo′gia;** from *ἀήρ*, "air," and *λόγος*, a "discourse."] A treatise or consideration of the properties of air.

A-er-om′e-ter. [**Aerom′etrum;** from *ἀήρ*, "air," and *μέτρον*, a "measure."] An instrument for ascertaining the mean bulk of gases.

A-er-om′e-trȳ. [**Aerome′tria;** from the same.] The ascertaining of the physical properties of atmospheric air, their nature and history.

A-er-o-pho′bĭ-a.* [From *ἀήρ*, "air," and *φόβος*, "fear."] A dread of any current of air; because in hydrophobia and some other diseases it induces a paroxysm: aëroph′oby.

Aerophyte, ā′er-o-phīt. [**Aeroph′-ytum;** from *ἀήρ*, "air," and *φυτόν*, a "plant."] A plant that lives in the air without being rooted in the earth. See AERIAL PLANTS.

A-e-ros′co-pȳ. [From *ἀήρ*, "air," and *σκοπέω*, to "survey," to "examine."] The investigation of the air.

Ærose, ē′rōs. [**Æro′sus;** from *æs*, *æ′ris*, "copper" or "brass."] Of the nature of copper; coppery.

A-er-o-stat′ic. [**Aerostat′icus;** from *ἀήρ*, "air," and *σтατική*, the "science of weights."] Pertaining to the science of the weight of air, or *Aërostatics*.

A-er-o-stat′ics. [**Aerostat′ica;** from the same.] The doctrine of air, its specific gravity, and properties in a state of rest.

A-er-os-tā′tion. [**Aerosta′tio, o′nis;** from *a′er*, and *sto*, *sta′tum*, to "stand."] Literally, "standing (or being suspended) in the air." The raising and supporting of heavy bodies by the buoyancy of heated air or light gases received into a spherical bag called a balloon.

Æ-ro′sus La′pis.* ("Coppery Stone.") A name for *lapis calaminaris*, from the notion of its being a copper ore.

Æ-ru′ġin-ous, or **Æ-ru-ġin′e-ous.** [**Æruginо′sus;** from *æru′go*, *æru′ginis*.] Pertaining to copper-rust, or verdigris. Applied to a bluish-green color like verdigris, or like the leaves of some pine-trees.

Æ-ru′go,* gen. **Æ-ru′ġin-is.** [Contraction of *æ′ris rubi′go*, the "rust of copper." See Æs.] The rust of a metal, especially copper. The Pharmacopœial name (Lond. and Ed. Ph.) of the impure subacetate of copper. See VERDIGRIS.

Æs,* gen. **Æ'ris.** The Latin term for "copper" or "brass."

Æs Co-rin'thĭ-um.* [*Æs*, "brass," and *Corin'thius*, belonging to "Corinth."] A kind of brass produced, as it is said, by an accidental mixture of metals at the burning of Corinth. It appears, however, from Pliny, to have been in use in Corinth long before the burning of that city.

Æs Us'tum.* [*Æs*, "copper," and *us'tus*, "burnt;" from *u'ro*, *us'tum*, to "burn."] Burnt copper; a preparation consisting of equal parts of copper and rough brimstone, laid in strata, with a small quantity of common salt sprinkled on each layer, and exposed to the fire till the brimstone is burned out. It has been called *Æs Ven'eris* (*Venus* being one of the ancient names for copper), *Æs crema'tum, Ci'nis æ'ris, Cro'cus Ven'eris*, etc.

Æsculin, or **Æsculine,** ĕs'ku-lin. An alkaloid lately discovered in the bark of the *Æsculus Hippocastanum*, or horse-chestnut; supposed to be a febrifuge.

Æstates,* ĕs-ta'tēz. [The nominative plural of *æs'tas*, "summer."] Heat-spots; freckles; sunburnings. See EPHELIS.

Æsthesia,* ĕs-the'se-ạ. [From αἰσθάνομαι, to "perceive," to "feel."] Perception; feeling; sensibility.

Æsthesis,* ĕs-the'sis. [From the same.] Feeling or sensibility; also, sense or sensation.

Æs-thet'ic. [**Æsthet'icus;** from the same.] Pertaining to the understanding, or mental perception. The Latin term, in the plural neuter (*Æsthet'ica*), forms the name of an order of the class *Neurotica* in Dr. Good's arrangement.

Æs-thet'ics. [**Æsthet'ica;** from the same.] Literally, the science of the sensations or perceptions. The science which explains the cause of the pleasure or displeasure derived from the contemplation of the works of nature or art.

Æs-tĭ-vā'tion, or **Es-tĭ-vā'tion.** [**Æstiva'tio, o'nis;** from *æsti'vo, æstiva'tum*, to "spend the summer," to "retire for the summer season."] The state in which the different parts of the flower are folded in the bud: prefloration.

Æs-tu-a'rĭ-um.* [From *æs'tus*, "heat," "boiling water," the "tide."] Literally, a place where there is boiling or raging water: hence, an estuary (*i.e.* an arm of the sea, or part of a river in which the tide rises). A stove for applying dry heat to all parts of the body at once; also a vapor-bath.

Æstus,* ĕs'tŭs. (See preceding article.) Heat, as well natural heat in intense degree, as that which is the effect of inflammatory disease.

Æs'tus Vo-lat'ĭ-cus.* The sudden flushing of the face; also *Strophulus volaticus*, or wild-fire rash of children.

Æ'tas,* gen. **Æ-ta'tis.** "Age." Different writers have designated different stages in the life of man; but perhaps the most usual division is into five periods, as follow:—

1. INFANCY (*infan'tia*), generally considered to extend to about the seventh year, or to the second dentition. 2. CHILDHOOD (*pueri'tia*), extending from the seventh to the fourteenth or fifteenth year, the period of puberty. 3. ADOLESCENCE (*adolescen'tia*), or YOUTH, reaching in males from the age of about fifteen to twenty-five; in females, from thirteen to twenty-one. 4. ADULT AGE, or MANHOOD (*viril'itas* or *æ'tas viri'lis*, the "manly age"), extending from the close of adolescence to about the fiftieth year. 5. OLD AGE (*senec'tus*), which comprehends the declining portion of life.

The Roman writers again subdivided Manhood into different stages, as Æ'TAS FIRMA'TA, the prime or full strength of man,—the age from thirty to thirty-five; Æ'TAS MATU'RA, the age of maturity or prudence,—the age of fifty.

Old age was variously subdivided, as Æ'TAS PROVEC'TA, advanced age; Æ'TAS INGRAVES'CENS, the age when the weight of years begins to be sensibly felt; Æ'TAS DECREP'ITA or CREP'ITA, decrepit age: reckoned from the sixtieth year, and ending in death.

Æ-the're-ạ.* [Neuter plural of *æthe'reus*, "ethereal."] The Pharmacopœial name (U.S. Ph.) for preparations of ether. See ETHER.

Æ'thĭ-ops,* or **E'thĭ-ops.*** [From αἴθοψ, "black."] A name anciently given to several black powders.

Æ'thiops An-tĭ-mo-nĭ-a'lis.* A term applied to a compound of Æthiops mineral with the sulphuret of antimony.

Æ'thiops Mar'tial. An old name for the deutoxide of iron.

Æ'thiops Min'e-ral. The black sulphuret of mercury (*Hydrar'gyri Sulphure'tum Ni'grum*). As an anthelmintic, it has been called *Poudre Vermifuge Mercurielle* (poodʀ vĕʀ'me'füzh' mĕʀ'kü're-ĕll').

Æ'thiops per se* (pẹr sē). The name given by Boerhaave to the gray oxide formed by long agitation of mercury in a bottle half full of air.

Æ'thiops Veg-e-tab'i-lis.* A name given to a species of charcoal, prepared by burning the *Fucus vesiculosus* in the open air and reducing it to a black powder.

Æth'o-gen. [From αἶθος, "fire," or "light," and γεννάω, to "produce."] A compound of boron and nitrogen, which gives a brilliant phosphorescent light when heated before the blow-pipe.

Æ'thri-scope. [From αἴρθα, the "clear sky," and σκοπέω, to "observe."] An instrument invented by Sir John Leslie for indicating the power of the clouds in preventing radiation. It consists of the differential thermometer, having one of the balls excluded from the light and the other placed in a polished metallic cup. Exposed to a clear part of the sky, the heat radiated from it escapes rapidly, and the temperature falls; exposed to a cloud, the radiated heat is restored and there is no reduction of temperature.

Æ-thu'sa Cy-na'pi-um.* Lesser Hemlock, or Fool's Parsley; a plant of the order *Umbelliferæ*, possessing poisonous properties. It yields an alkaloid called *cynapia*.

Æ-ti-ol'o-gy. [**Ætiolo'gia;** from αἰτία, "cause," and λόγος, a "discourse."] The science of the causes of disease.

Aetites,* a-e-ti'tēz. [From ἀετός, an "eagle," λίθος, a "stone," being understood.] Eagle-stone. A clay-ironstone, hollow, and containing another substance within it of variable composition.

Af-fec'tion. [**Affec'tio, o'nis**; from *affi'cio, affec'tum*, to "affect," to "disturb."] Nearly synonymous with "disease," as inflammatory, nervous, or rheumatic affection, etc.

Af'fer-ens.* [From *ad*, "to," and *fe'ro*, to "bring."] Applied to the lymphatic vessels, or *Vasa afferentia*: afferent.

Afferentia,* af-fer-en'she-ạ, the plural neuter of AFFERENS, which see.

Af-fin'i-ty. [**Affin'itas, a'tis**; from *ad*, "to," "on," and *fi'nis*, "boundary:" *affi'nis*, "on the boundary," "near," "connected with," "neighboring."] Literally, "connection by marriage." That kind of attraction by which different classes of substances combine to form *new* substances, as in the case of an alkali with an acid, forming a salt. As marriage unites persons of different or opposite sexes, so affinity unites substances of different and often opposite qualities: *e.g.* a supporter of combustion with a combustible, an alkali with an acid, etc. Affinity is sometimes used, but less appropriately, to denote attraction in a more general sense. See AFFINITY OF AGGREGATION.

SINGLE OR SIMPLE AFFINITY is the power by which two elementary bodies combine.

ELEC'TIVE AFFINITY denotes the preference which one body manifests in combining with another rather than with a third or fourth, etc.

DOUBLE ELECTIVE AFFINITY occurs when two compounds decompose each other and two new compounds are formed by an exchange of elements. Thus, when sulphate of zinc and carbonate of potassa are mixed, the sulphuric acid leaves the zinc and unites with the potassa, forming sulphate of potassa, while the carbonic acid combines with the zinc, producing carbonate of zinc.

QUIES'CENT AFFINITY is that which tends to maintain the elements of a compound in their present state, preventing decomposition.

DIVEL'LENT AFFINITY (from *divel'lo*, to "pull apart," to "separate") is that which tends to arrange the particles of a compound in a new form, producing decomposition. In mixing different compounds, if the sum total of the *divellent* be more powerful than that of the quiescent affinities, decomposition takes place.

DISPOSING AFFINITY is that which promotes the tendency of bodies to combine in a particular way, by presenting to them a third substance which exerts a strong attraction to the compound they form: when the combination has been effected, the third substance may be withdrawn. Some writers call this tendency to unite the *affinity of intermedium*, or intermediate affinity. Berthollet styles it "reciprocal affinity."

Affin'ity of Ag-gre-gā'tion. A force by which two substances tend to combine and form an aggregate, without their properties being changed. Another term for the attraction of cohesion.

Affin'ity, Chem'i-cal, or **Affin'ity** proper. That property or attraction by which different elements unite with each other, forming new substances. See AFFINITY.

Affinity, Intermediate. See AFFINITY (DISPOSING).

Affin'ity, Vi'tal. That power which forms the solids and fluids from the common circulating fluids.

Af-fla'tus.* [From *ad,* "to," "upon," and *flo, fla'tum,* to "blow."] Applied to a species of erysipelas, as if blown upon by an unwholesome blast.

Af-flux'us.* [From *ad,* "to" or "towards," and *flu'o, flux'um* or *fluc'tum,* to "flow."] Af'flux; a name given in former times to a supposed reciprocal influence of terrestrial bodies: it was compared to the effect of a magnet on iron, and of amber on chaff. *Affluxus* or afflux is also used to denote the flow or determination of blood or other fluid of the body to a particular part.

Af-fu'sion. [**Affu'sio, o'**nis; from *ad,* "to," "upon," and *fun'do, fu'sum,* to "pour."] The pouring of water on a substance to cleanse it. Applied to the pouring on a patient, in certain fevers, of a liberal quantity of cold water: the cold affusion. To this head some writers refer LOTIONS, ASPERSIONS, SHOWER-BATHS, which will be noticed in their alphabetical places.

Af'ter-Birth. The common English term for the placenta, cord, and membranes, or *secundines.*

Af'ter-Pains. Those pains, more or less severe, after expulsion of the after-birth, from the contractile efforts of the uterus to return to its normal condition.

Agalacta'tio. See AGALACTIA.

Ag-a-lac'ti-a.* [From *a,* priv., and γάλα, γάλακτος, "milk."] Deficiency of milk after child-birth.

A-gam'i-cus.* [From *a,* priv., and γάμος, "marriage."] Sometimes applied, in Botany, to plants the sexual organs of which cannot be detected: cryptogamic.

Ag'am-ous. [From the same.] Sexless. A term applied to the cryptogamous plants, from the notion that they possess no sexual characters.

A-găr'i-cum.* [Said to be derived from *Aga'ria,* or *Ag'arum,* a region of Sarmatia, where it was first discovered.] The agaric, a species of mushroom.

A-găr'i-cus.* [See preceding article.] The generic name of the mushroom family, order *Fungi,* class *Cryptogamia.*

Agar'icus Cam-pes'tris.* The Linnæan name of the common eatable mushroom of Europe.

Agar'icus Chi-rur-go'rum.* ("Surgeon's Agaric.") See AGARICUS QUERCUS.

Agar'icus Min-e-ra'lis.* ("Mineral Agaric.") The *mountain milk* or *meal* of the Germans; one of the purest of the native carbonates of lime, found in clefts of rocks, etc. It is named from its resemblance to an agaric in texture and color.

Agar'icus Quer'cus.* ("Agaric of the Oak.") *Bole'tus Ignia'rius,* or Touchwood: a fungus formerly used for arresting external hæmorrhages.

Ag'ate. [From *Acha'tes,* a river of Sicily where agates, it is said, were first discovered.] A hard siliceous stone, used by lapidaries for engraving seals, cameos, and other objects of ornament. It is composed of chalcedony blended with jasper, quartz, and other minerals.

A-ga've A-mer-i-ca'na.* The American Aloe.

Aga've Cu-ben'sis.* A species of American aloe, the roots of which resemble the red sarsaparilla of the shops.

Age. See ÆTAS.

Agedoite. See ASPARAGIN.

Agenesia. See AGENNESIA.

A-gen'e-sis.* [From *a,* priv., and γεννάω, to "beget," or γένω, to "be born."] Applied to anomalies of organization, consisting in the absence or imperfect development of parts.

Agennesia,* aj-ĕn-ne'se-a, or **A-gen'ne-sis.*** [From the same.] Impotence, sterility.

A'gent. [**A'gens;** from *a'go,* to "act" or "do."] Any power or influence which produces an effect on the human body. Thus, we speak of a "morbific agent," that is, something which causes disease. In Chemistry, a substance capable of producing chemical action or a change in the composition of bodies.

Agerasia,* aj-e-ra'se-a. [From *a,* priv., and γῆρας, "old age."] The non-appearance of the effects or infirmities of old age: a green old age.

A-ger'a-tum.* [Gr. ἀγήρατον.] See ACHILLEA AGERATUM.

Ageusia. See AGEUSTIA.

Ageustia,* a-gūs'te-a. [From *a,* priv., and γεῦσις, "tasting."] Loss of taste. A genus of the order *Dysæsthesiæ,* class *Locales,* of Cullen's Nosology.

Ag-glom'er-ate, or **Ag-glom'er-āt-ed.** [**Agglomera'tus;** from *ag-glom'ero, agglomera'tum* (from *ad,* "to," "on," and *glo'mus,* a "ball"), to "wind upon a ball," to "gather into a ball."] Applied to glands. Applied also to the stamens of plants when collected in a globular form; and to *amenta,* or catkins, similarly disposed.

Ag-glu'ti-nant. [**Agglu'tinans;** from *ad,* "to," and *glu'tino, glutina'tum,* to "glue."] Applied to external applications of a gluey nature, which favor the healing of parts by keeping them together.

Ag-glu-ti-nā'tion. [**Agglutina'tio, o'**nis; from the same.] A gluing or joining together: also the action of an agglutinant substance. See COLLESIS.

Agglutina'tion, Im-me'di-ate. Union by the first intention.

Agglutina'tion, Me'di-ate. The interposing of some substance between the lips of a wound, or the flaps after amputation; as agaric, charpie, or lint, on which cerate is first spread.

Ag'gre-gāte. [**Aggrega'tus;** from *ag'grego, aggrega'tum* (from *ad,* "to" or "together," and *grex, gre'gis,* a "herd," "flock," or "crowd"), to "crowd together," to "gather together."] Applied to flowers which have a number of smaller flowers collected into clusters. Applied also, in Chemistry, to several substances of the same kind producing one, its chemical properties not differing from theirs. In the plural neuter (*Aggrega'ta*) it forms the name of a family of the *Mollusca, Acephala nuda,* which are united in a common mass. See AGGLOMERATE.

Ag'gregate. A body or mass made up of smaller bodies or masses. The smallest parts into which an aggregate can be divided without destroying its chemical properties are called *integrant parts.*

Ag-gre-gā'tion. [From the same.] A collection of many individual particles, etc., into a cluster or mass. Also, a form of attraction, commonly called that of *cohesion,* by which the particles of bodies are *aggregated,* or retained in the state of a solid.

Ag-i-tā'tion. [**Agita'tio, o'**nis; from *ag'ito, agita'tum,* to "shake," to "agitate."] The act of putting into active or violent motion. Mental emotion, from the violence of some prevailing passion.

Ag'li-a.* [Gr. ἀγλίη.] A whitish speck on the cornea of the eye.

Ag-lo-bu'li-a.* [From *a,* priv., and *glob'ulus,* a "globule."] Decrease or diminution in the quantity of blood-globules.

Ag-lu-ti'tion. [**Agluti'tio, o'**nis; from *a,* priv., and *glu'tio, gluti'tum,* to "swallow."] Inability to swallow. See DYSPHAGIA.

Ag-ni'na Mem-bra'na.* [From *ag'nus,* a "lamb," and *membra'na,* a "membrane."] The name given to one of the membranes of the fœtus, on account of its tenderness. The same as the *amnion.*

Agni'na Tŭ'nĭ-ca.* [From *ag'nus,* a "lamb," and *tu'nica,* a "coat."] The lamb's coat; the *amnion.*

Agnoea,* ag-nē'a. [From ἀγνοέω, to "be ignorant."] The state of a patient who does not recognize persons or things.

Ag'nus Cas'tus.* The chaste tree, a species of *Vitex,* formerly celebrated as an antaphrodisiac. This name has also been given to *Castor Oil,* or the oil of *Ricinus communis,* from its effects upon the body and mind.

A-gom-phi'a-sis.* [From *a,* priv., and *gompho'sis,* the "insertion of the teeth in their sockets."] Looseness of the teeth.

A-go'ni-a.* [From *a,* priv., and γόνος, "seed," "offspring."] Sterility, or barrenness.

Ag'o-nȳ. [From ἀγών, a "contest," a "struggle."] The last struggle of life, closing in death.

A-gres'tis.* [From *a'ger, a'gri,* a "field."] Pertaining to a field; the specific name of many plants.

A'gri-a.* [Gr. ἀγρία, the "holly." Another name for the *Aquifolium,* or holly.

A'gria.* [From ἄγριος, "wild," "untamable."] A pustular eruption, with redness and erosion; named from its intractability.

Ag-ri-am'pe-los.* [From ἄγριος, "wild," and ἄμπελος, the "vine."] Another name for the *Bryonia alba,* or wild vine.

Ag'ri-mo-nȳ. [**Agrimo'nia Eupato'ria.**] A plant of the order *Rosaceæ,* used as an astringent and stomachic.

Ag-ri-o-rig'a-num.* [From ἄγριος, "wild," and ὀρίγανον, "marjoram."] The *Orig'anum vulga're,* or wild marjoram.

Ag-ri-o-thym'i-a.* [From ἄγριος, "wild," and θυμός, "passion," "rage."] Furious insanity.

A-grip'pa.* [As if *Ægrippa,* from *ægrè partus,* "born with difficulty."] A term applied to children born with the feet foremost. Hence the name of some celebrated Romans.

Ag-ros-tog'ra-phȳ. [**Agrostogra'phia;** from ἄγρωστις, a kind of "grass," and γράφω, to "write."] A treatise on grasses.

A-grўp'nĭ-a.* [From *a*, priv., and ὕπνος, "sleep."] Sleeplessness; watchfulness, or wakefulness.

A-grўp-no-co'ma, *atis*.* [From ἄγρυπνος, "sleepless," and κῶμα, "lethargy."] A lethargic state of wakefulness, with low muttering delirium, aptly expressed otherwise by the term *Coma-vigil*.

A'gūe. [Supposed to be derived from the Gothic *agis*, "trembling."] The common name for intermittent fever.

A'gue-Cake. [**Placen'ta Febri'lis.**] Enlargement of the spleen, the effect of protracted ague.

A'gue-Drop. A solution of arseniate of potash; Fowler's tasteless ague-drop, for which the *Liquor arsenicalis* is substituted. It is used as a remedy in intermittent fevers.

A'gue-Tree. Another name for sassafras, given on account of its virtues as a febrifuge.

A-gyr'ta.* Formerly, a mountebank; a person who collected a crowd about him; a quack.

Ah-rī'zous. [**Ahri'zus;** from *a*, priv., and ῥίζα, a "root."] Applied to certain *acotyledonous* plants, because reproduced by *sporulæ*, without radicles, striking root from any part of their surface.

Air. [Lat. **A'er, A'eris:** Gr. ἀήρ; from ἄω, to "breathe."] The natural air, or atmosphere: atmospheric air. When pure, it consists of about 20 parts (in the hundred) of oxygen and 80 of nitrogen; it contains also a small quantity of carbonic acid, the proportion of which varies greatly according to circumstances, being far more abundant in the air of a densely peopled city than in the country.

Air Bag, or **Air Bladder.** See VESICA NATATORIA.

Air, Fixed. [**A'er Fix'us.**] Carbonic acid gas.

Air, In-flam'ma-ble. Hydrogen gas.

Air Pump. A machine by which the air in a vessel may be withdrawn.

Air, Vi'tal (formerly called dephlogisticated air, empyrial air, etc.) is a term applied to oxygen gas, from its being indispensable to life.

Akinesia. See ACINESIA.

Al. The Arabic article signifying "the," prefixed to many terms formerly in use; as *al-chemy, al-kahest, al-cohol*, etc.

A'la,* plural **A'læ.** [Supposed to be a contraction of *axil'la*, the "armpit."] A wing. Applied, in Anatomy, to parts, from their resemblance to a wing, as *alæ nasi*, "wings of the nose," etc.; also, to the armpit. In Botany it is applied to the side petals of papilionaceous flowers, and angles formed by leaves or stalks with their branches, etc.

Al-a-bas'ter. [Lat. **Alabastri'tes,** and **Alabas'ter;** Gr. ἀλάβαστρος, and ἀλάβαστρον.] A species of white gypsum (sulphate of lime), used for ornamental purposes. The name is also sometimes applied to a form of carbonate of lime.

Al-a-bas'trum.* [From the same.] A term applied to the five green leaves forming the calyx of some flowers before the expansion of the bud, from a supposed resemblance to an alabaster box.

A'læ Ma-jo'rēs.* ("Larger Wings.") Another term for the *labia externa* of the pudenda. See LABIA PUDENDI.

A'læ Mi-no'rēs.* ("Lesser Wings.") A term applied to the two small folds formed by the nymphæ.

A'læ Na'si.* ("Wings of the Nose.") The lateral or movable cartilaginous parts of the nose.

A'læ Ves-per-til-ĭ-o'nis.* ("Bat's Wings.") The broad ligaments situated between the uterus and the Fallopian tubes.

Alæformis. See ALIFORM.

A-la'lĭ-a.* [From *a*, priv., and λαλέω, to "speak."] A defect of articulation.

A-lan'tĭne. A starch-like powder, obtained from the *Angelica Archangelica*.

A-la'res Ve'næ.* [See ALARIS.] The superficial veins at the bend of the arm.

A-la'rĭ-a Os'sa.* The lateral processes of the sphenoid bone.

A-la'ris,* plural **A-la'rēs** and **A-la'rĭ-a.** [From *a'la*, a "wing."] Wing-like: applied to the pterygoid processes of the sphenoid bone, to a ligament within the knee-joint, and to the inner veins of the bend of the arm.

A'late. [**Ala'tus;** from *a'la*, a "wing."] Winged, as certain stems and leaf-stalks having side membranes.

Al'bĭ-cans,* neuter plural **Albican-tia,** al-be-kan'she-a. [From *al'bico*, to "grow white."] Applied (in the plural) to two small bodies on the base of the brain, the *Corpora albicantia*.

Al-bĭ-cau'lis.* [From *al'bus*, "white," and *cau'lis*, a "stem."] Having a white stem: albicau'line.

Al-bĭ-dac'tў-lus,* or **Al-bo-dac'tў-lus.*** [From *al'bus*, "white," and δάκτυλος, a "finger."] Having white, digitated wings.

Al-bĭ-flo′rus.* [From *al′bus*, "white," and *flos, flo′ris*, a "flower."] Having white flowers.

Al-bĭ-ner′vus.* [From *al′bus*, "white," and *ner′vus*, a "nerve."] Having white nervures.

Al′bĭ-nism. [From *al′bus*, "white."] A diseased state, in which the skin is of a uniform dull, milky white color; the hair resembles bleached flax or silk; the iris is pink, and the retina and choroid, seen through the pupil, present another shade of the same color; the sight is weak, and strongest in the dark.

Al-bī′no. A term applied to an individual marked by the above characteristics. There is the *Ethiopian* variety, found among negroes, and the *European*, found among Europeans and other white nations. See LEUCOPATHIA.

Albino-Skin. See ALBINISM.

Al′bīte. [Probably a contraction of *al′bus*, "white," and *li′thos*, a "stone.] *Soda Felspar*, a silicate of alumina, resembling felspar in its properties, with the substitution of soda for potash.

Al-bĭ-ven′ter,* **Al-bĭ-ven′tris.*** [From *al′bus*, "white," and *ven′ter*, the "belly."] Having a white belly.

Al-bu-ġin′e-ous. [**Albugin′eus;** from *albu′go, albu′ginis*, the "white of the eye."] White like the sclerotic coat of the eye; also, pertaining to albumen, or white of egg. Applied to a membrane of the eye, also to a covering of the testicles, each named *Tu′nica albugin′ea.*

Al-bu′go,* gen. **Al-bu′gi-nis.** [From *al′bus*, "white."] The white of the eye; sometimes the white of egg, or albumen. A white opacity of the cornea, not superficial, but affecting its very substance; also called the "pin and web." See ARGEMA and LEUCOMA.

Al′bum Græcum* (grē′kum). *Ster′cus ca′nis.* The white and solid excrement of dogs which subsist chiefly on bones. It consists, for the most part, of the earth of bones or lime, in combination with phosphoric acid. It was formerly used in medicine; it is now sometimes used to soften leather in the process of dressing it after the depilatory action of lime.

Al′bum Ni′grum.* The excrement of mice and rats; formerly used both externally and internally as a remedy, but now very properly abandoned.

Al-bu′men,* gen. **Al-bu′min-is.** [From *al′bus*, "white."] The white of an egg. A peculiar constituent principle, of essentially the same character as the albumen of an egg, found in the animal and vegetable kingdoms. It is distinguished by its property of coagulability on the application of heat.

Animal albumen is the chief solid ingredient in the white of eggs: it also enters largely into the composition of blood, muscles, etc. It may be obtained pure by coagulating the white of an egg with alcohol, washing thoroughly with that fluid, and then drying it at the temperature of 120° Fahrenheit.

Albumen, Vegetable. See VEGETABLE ALBUMEN.

Al-bu′mĭ-noid. [**Albuminoi′des;** from *albu′men*, and εἶδος, a "form."] Resembling albumen. Often used in the sense of *Proteinaceous.* See PROTEIN.

Al-bu′mĭ-nose. [From *albu′men.*] A product of digestion found in the chyle and blood. It differs from albumen in not being coagulable by heat.

Al-bu′min-ous. [**Albumino′sus.**] Containing or resembling albumen.

Al-bu-min-u′ri-a.* [From *albu′men*, and *uri′na*, "urine."] An albuminous state of the urine. See NEPHRITIS ALBUMINOSA.

Al-bur′num.* [From *al′bus*, "white."] The soft white substance between the inner bark and the wood of trees. See SAP-WOOD.

Alcana. See ALKANA.

Al-car′ġen. Another name for CACODYLIC ACID, which see.

Alchemy, al′kẹm-e. [**Alche′mia,** or **Alchym′ia.** Supposed to be derived from the Arabic definite article *al*, and χύμα, a "melting" or "pouring."] A chimerical art which proposed to find out the means of effecting the transmutation of metals and preparing a remedy for all diseases.

Alchornea Latifolia. See ALCORNOQUE.

Alchymy. See ALCHEMY.

Al-cĭ-cor′nis.* [From *al′ce*, an "elk," and *cor′nu*, a "horn."] Having horns, or similar objects, like those of the elk.

Alcoate. See ALCOHOLATES.

Al′co-hol, or **Al′ko-hol.** [From the Arabic definite article *al*, and *kohol*, an "impalpable powder," "something very subtle."] The Pharmacopœial name (U. S. and Br. Ph.) for rectified spirits. A term applied to the pure spirit obtained by distillation from all liquids which have undergone vinous fermentation. When diluted with an equal weight of water, it is termed *Proof spirit*, or *Spiritus tenuior* of the Pharmacopœia.

The first product of distillation is technically called *low wine,* and is again subjected to distillation. The latter portions of what comes over are called *feints,* and are reserved for a further process in the wash-still. The second product is termed *raw spirit,* and when again distilled is called *rectified spirit.* The strongest alcohol which can be procured is termed *Absolute Alcohol,* or *Anhydrous Alcohol,* to denote its entire freedom from water.

Alcohol, Absolute. See ALCOHOL.

Al'cohol Am-mo-nĭ-a'tum.* The *Spir'itus ammo'niæ aromat'icus.* A combination of alcohol and ammonia, prepared by passing ammoniacal gas into alcohol, which must be kept cool.

Alcohol Amylicum. See FUSEL OIL.

Al'co-hol-ātes. [From *al'cohol.*] Applied to officinal medicines, differing from alcoholic tinctures first, in the menstruum containing the volatile principles of medicinal substances, and, secondly, in their mode of separation, which consists in impregnating the alcohol with medicinal principles, first by maceration and then by distillation.

Al-co-hol'ic. [**Alcohol'icus;** from *al'cohol.*] Pertaining to alcohol.

Al'co-hol-ĭsm. A diseased condition of the system resulting from the use of alcoholic drinks.

Al-co-hol-ĭ-zā'tion. The development of alcohol in a liquid.

Al-co-ho-lom'e-ter. [**Alcoholom'etrum;** from *al'cohol,* and μέτρον, a "measure."] An instrument for ascertaining the quantity of alcohol in any fluid.

Alcohometer. See ALCOHOLOMETER.

Alcornoque, al'kor'nok'. (Fr.) The bark of the *Alchornea latifolia,* growing in the West Indies and South America. It is bitter and tonic, and has by some been regarded as a specific in phthisis.

Al'çy-on,* gen. **Al-çy'o-nis.** [Gr. ἀλκυών; from ἅλς, the "sea," and κύω, to "conceive," because said to hatch its eggs in the sea.] A bird of the swallow kind, found in Cochin China and the Philippine Islands, whose nest, composed chiefly of a gelatinous matter, possesses nutritious properties, is esteemed as an article of diet in China, and used as an analeptic and aphrodisiac.

Al'de-hȳde. [From *al,* first syllable of *al'cohol,* and *de-hyd,* first two of *dehydrogena'tus,* "deprived of hydrogen."] A colorless liquid of a suffocating odor, and readily absorbing oxygen from the atmosphere.

Al-de-hyd'ic. [**Aldehyd'icus;** from *al'dehyde.*] Pertaining to aldehyde.

Alder. See ALNUS.

Ale. The fermented infusion of pale malted barley, usually combined with infusion of hops.

Al-ec-tru'rous. [**Alectru'rus;** from ἀλέκτωρ, a "cock," and οὐρά, a "tail."] Having a tail like the cock's.

A-lem'bic. [**Alem'bicus;** from the Arabic *al,* and ἄμβιξ, a "cup" or "pot."] A glass, metal, or earthenware utensil, fitted to receive volatile products from retorts.

A-lem'broth. [Said to signify, in Chaldaic, the "key to art or knowledge."] The Salt of Wisdom of the Alchemists. A muriate of mercury and ammonia, corresponding to the *Hydrar'gyrum præcipita'tum al'bum* of the London Pharmacopœia. It is a compound of bichloride of mercury and sal ammoniac.

Al'e-tris Far-ĭ-no'sa.* Star-grass. A plant of the natural order *Asphodeliæ.* It is intensely bitter, and is used as a tonic.

Al-ex-an'drĭ-a.* [Named from the place of its growth.] The name for the *Pru'nus laurocer'asus;* the Alexandrian laurel.

Alexipharmacon. See ALEXIPHARMIC.

A-lex-ĭ-phar'mic. [**Alexiphar'micus;** from ἀλέξω, to "ward off," to "protect," and φάρμακον, a "poison."] Antipharmic; neutralizing the effects of poison.

A-lex-ĭ-py-ret'ic. [**Alexipyret'icus;** from ἀλέξω, and πυρετός, a "fever."] Driving off fevers: febrifuge.

Alèze, or **Alèse,** å'låz'. [From ἀλέξω, to "protect."] A cloth folded several times in order to protect the bed from discharges of blood, etc.

Al'ga.* An herb or weed growing on the sea-shore: sea-weed.

Algaceæ,* al-ga'she-ē. An order of plants including the *Algæ* or sea-weeds. They consist of leafless, flowerless plants, without any distinct axis of vegetation, growing in water.

Algæ,*al'jē, the plural of AL'GA, a "sea-weed," forming the Jussieuan name of a natural order of plants. See FUCACEÆ.

Al'ga-roth. [From *Victor Algarotti,* a physician of Verona.] The oxide of antimony in the form of a white powder.

Al-ge'do, d'inis.*[From ἄλγος, "pain."] Violent pain about the urethra, testes, bladder, perinæum, and anus, caused by sudden stoppage of severe gonorrhœa.

Al'ġid. [**Al'gidus;** from *al'geo*, to "be cold," to "suffer from cold."] Chilled with cold.

Al'ġid Chol'e-ra. [**Chol'era Al'gida.**] Applied to Asiatic cholera, on account of the diminution of temperature, this being one of its chief characteristic symptoms.

Al'ġi-da Fe'bris.* A term for a malignant remittent fever, the *Fièvre algide* (fe-âvR' âl'zhèd') of the continent, characterized by icy coldness on the surface.

Al-go-i'dēs.* [From *al'ga*, a "seaweed," and εἶδος, a "form."] Resembling the *al'gæ:* al'goid.

Al'gor, o'ris.* [From *al'geo*, to "be cold."] The sense of coldness in the onset of fever: chillness. See Rigor.

Al'ĭ-ble. [**Alib'ilis;** from *a'lo*, to "nourish."] Nutritious.

Al'ĭ-ca.* [From the same.] A kind of grain like wheat, supposed to be spelt, from which the ancients made their *tisanes;* also a kind of pottage made of this.

Alices,* al'e-sēz. [From ἀλίζω, to "sprinkle."] Spots on the skin preceding the eruption of small-pox.

A'lien-ate, or **A'lien-āt-ed.** [**Aliena'tus;** from *alie'no, aliena'tum*, to "estrange," to "withdraw," to "put away."] Applied in Botany to first leaves, which give way to others different.

Alienation, āl'yen-ā'shŭn. [**Aliena'tio, o'nis;** from the same.] Any species of derangement or wandering of the mind.

Aliena'tion of Mind. Applied more especially to *insanity*, as distinct from derangements symptomatic of some other disease, as delirium, etc.

Al'ĭ-form. [**Alifor'mis;** from *a'la*, a "wing."] Having the form of a wing: pterygoid.

Al'ĭ-ment. [**Alimen'tum;** from *a'lo*, to "nourish."] That which affords nourishment. See Alitura, Pabulum.

Al-ĭ-men'ta-rў. [**Alimenta'rius;** from *a'lo*, to "nourish."] Pertaining to aliment; nourishing.

Alimen'tary Ca-nal'. The entire passage (from the mouth to the anus) through which the aliment or food passes.

Alimen'tary Duct. [**Duc'tus Alimenta'rius.**] A name sometimes applied to the thoracic duct.

Al-ĭ-men-tā'tion. [**Alimenta'tio, o'nis;** from *alimen'tum.*] The act of taking or receiving nourishment.

Al-ĭ-pæ'nos,* Al-ĭ-pæ'nus.* [From *a*, priv., and λιπαίνω, to "make fat."] Applied to very lean persons; also to dry external remedies, as powders, etc.

Alipede, al'e-pēd. [**Al'ipes;** from *a'la*, a "wing," and *pes, pe'dis*, a "foot."] Having winged feet. See Cheiropterus.

A-lis'ma Plan-ta'go,* or **Plan-ta'go A-quăt'i-ca.*** The water-plantain, a medicinal plant formerly regarded as efficacious in cases of hydrophobia.

Al-is-mā'ceous. [**Alisma'ceus;** from *alis'ma*, the "water-plantain."] Having an arrangement similar to that in the *alis'ma*. In the plural feminine (*Alismaceæ*, al-is-ma'she-ē) applied to a natural order of plants.

A-lis'moid. [**Alismoi'des;** from *alis'ma*, and εἶδος, a "form."] Resembling the *alisma*.

Al-ĭ-sphe'noid. [**Alisphenoi'des;** from *a'la*, a "wing," and os *sphenoi'des*, the "sphenoid bone."] Applied by Owen to the middle or great wing of the sphenoid bone.

Al-ĭ-tu'ra.* [From *a'lo, al'itum*, to "nourish."] The process of assimilation or nutrition; food or nourishment; aliment.

Alizarin, or **Alizarine,** â-liz'a-rin. [**Alizari'na.**] A coloring matter extracted from madder (*Ru'bia tincto'rum*), called in France *alizari* (â'le'zâ're').

Al'ka-hest. The pretended universal solvent or menstruum of the ancient chemists. But, if it dissolves all substances, in what vessels can it be contained?

Al-ka-lĕs'çent. [**Alkales'cens;** from *al'kali*, and *-es'co*, a Latin termination signifying to "grow," to "become."] Having slightly alkaline qualities: becoming alkaline.

Alkali, al'ka-le. [From the Arabic *al*, definite article, and *ka'li*, the plant from which soda was first obtained.] A substance of peculiar properties, uniting with acids in definite proportions, thus forming salts, and having the power to change vegetable blues to green. It may be said to be the reverse of an acid, the properties of which, by combination, it neutralizes.

Al'kali, Caus'tic. [**Al'kali Caus'ticum.**] An alkali in a pure state; in which it possesses strong caustic powers. Usually, caustic potash.

Al'kali, Fixed. Applied to potash

and soda, because they are permanently in a solid state.

Al'kali, Fos'sil; Al'kali, Min'e-ral. Other names for *soda.*

Al'kali, Phlo-gis'ti-căt-ed; Al'-kali, Prus'sian. Applied to a fixed alkali when mixed with an animal substance, and lixiviated, because it is then found to be saturated with Prussic acid; and from a former theory of this combination it received the first name.

Al'kali, Veg'e-tą-ble. Another term for *potash.*

Al'kali, Vol'ą-tĭle. Another name for *ammonia,* given on account of its volatile nature.

Al-ką-lig'en-ous. [**Alkalig'enus;** from *al'kali,* and γεννάω, to "generate."] Producing alkaline qualities.

Al-ką-lim'e-ter. [**Alkalim'e-trum;** from *al'kali,* and μέτρον, a "measure."] An instrument for ascertaining the quantity of alkali in impure potash or soda.

Al-ką-lim'e-trȳ. [**Alkalime'tria;** from *al'kali,* and μετρέω, to "measure."] The process by which the amount of free alkali in various substances is determined.

Al'ką-līne. [**Alkali'nus;** from *al'kali.*] Having the properties of an alkali.

Al-ką-lin'ĭ-tȳ. [**Alkalin'itas, a'tis.**] The peculiar properties of an alkali.

Al-kal-ĭ-zā'tion. [**Alkaliza'tio.**] The act of imparting alkaline qualities.

Al'ką-loid. [**Alkaloi'des;** from *al'kali,* and εἶδος, a "form."] Resembling an alkali. Applied as a noun to the alkaline principles found in vegetables.

Al'ką-ną, or **Al'cą-ną.** The name of the root and leaves of the *Lauso'nia Iner'mis,* a plant employed in the East for dyeing the nails, teeth, hair, garments, etc. See HENNE.

Al'ką-net Root. [From the Arabic *al'kanah,* a "reed."] The root of the ANCHUSA TINCTORIA, which see.

Alkekenge, al'ke-kenj. Winter-cherry; the fruit of the *Phys'alis Alke-ken'gi,* used in nephritis, dysuria, ascites, etc.

Alkohol. See ALCOHOL.

Al'lą-nite. The name of a mineral containing *cerium,* found in Greenland, and named in honor of Mr. Allan, who first distinguished it as a species.

Al-lan-to'ic. [**Allanto'icus;** from *allan'toïs.*] Belonging to the allantoïs.

Allanto'ic Aç'id. The substance ALLANTOIN.

Al-lan'toid. [**Allantoi'des;** from ἀλλᾶς, ἀλλᾶντος, and εἶδος, a "form."] Resembling a sausage.

Allan'toid Mem'brane. A membrane communicating with the bladder by the *urachus,* and containing the fœtal urine: it exists in almost all the *Mammalia.* Also termed *Allantoïs.*

Al-lan'to-in. [**Allantoi'na;** from *allan'toïs.*] The nitrogenous constituent of the urine of the fœtus of the cow. Also termed *Allantoic Acid.*

Al-lan'to-is, ĭ'dis.* [From ἀλλᾶς, ἀλλᾶντος, a "sausage," and εἶδος, a "form."] The human allantois is a small, very vascular vesicle, sprouting from the end of the embryo. Also synonymous with *Allantoid membrane.*

Al-lan-to-tox'ĭ-cum.* [From ἀλλᾶς, and τοξικόν, a "poison."] A poison developed in putrid sausages made of blood and liver, often proving speedily fatal.

Alliaceous, al-le-ā'shus. [**Allia'-ceus;** from *al'lium.*] Of the nature of garlic.

Al'lĭ-um.* [From ἀλέομαι, to "avoid;" because of its offensive smell.] The Pharmacopœial name (Ed. and U. S. Ph.) of *Allium sativum.* A Linnæan genus of the class *Hexandria,* natural order *Liliaceæ.*

Al'lium Ce'pą.* The common onion.

Al'lium Por'rum.* The leek.

Al'lium Są-ti'vum.* Garlic.

Al-lœ-o'sis.* [From ἀλλοιόω, to "alter."] A constitutional change.

Al-lo-path'ic. [**Allopath'icus.**] Belonging to allopathy.

Al-lop'ą-thȳ [**Allopathi'a;** from ἄλλος, "other," and πάθος, "affection"]; written also **Al-lœ-op'ą-thȳ.** The curing of a diseased action by inducing a different kind of action, yet not necessarily diseased. See HOMŒOPATHY.

Al-lo-trĭ-oph'ą-ġȳ. [**Allotrio-pha'gia;** from ἀλλότριος, "another's," "foreign," "not proper," and φάγω, to "eat."] Depraved appetite, or a desire for improper food.

Al-lo-trop'ic. Pertaining to ALLOTROPISM.

Al-lot'ro-pism. [**Allotropis'mus;** from ἄλλος, "other," and τροπή, "conversion."] The existing of the same compound in two or more conditions, with different physical and chemical properties; as sulphur melted at a high temperature, which, before bright yellow and brittle, becomes dark, tenacious, and may be drawn out into threads like caoutchouc.

Al-lox'an. A new product obtained in the oxidation of uric acid by nitric acid.

Al-lox'a-nate. [**Allox'anas, a'**_tis._] A combination of alloxanic acid with a base.

Al-lox-an'ic. [**Alloxan'icus;** from _allox'an._] Of or belonging to the product alloxan. Applied to an acid into which alloxan is converted when brought into contact with soluble alkalies.

Al-lox-an'tin. [**Alloxanti'na.**] A substance obtained by boiling and evaporating a concentrated solution of alloxan.

Al-loy'. [Fr. _aloyer,_ to "mix metals."] A combination of any two metals, excepting mercury, etc., the least valuable being called the alloy. See AMALGAM.

All'spice. The fruit of the _Myrtus pimenta._

Al-lu'vi-al. [**Alluvia'lis;** from _allu'vium._] Applied to rocks or beds of recent formation, which still acquire the matter deposited by the waters.

Al-lu'vi-um.* [From _al'luo,_ to "wash."] The formation of new earths or islets by the action of water accumulating mud and debris in particular situations.

Almond, å'mand. [**Amyg'dala.** Fr. _amande,_ å'mônd'.] The fruit, both bitter and sweet, of the _Amygdalus communis._

Al'mond-Oil. A bland, fixed oil, obtained usually from bitter almonds by the action of a hydraulic press, either cold, or by means of hot iron plates.

Al'mond-Tree. The _Amygdalus communis._

Al'monds of the Ears. The small external glands near the ears. See AMYGDALÆ.

Al'monds of the Throat. The tonsils.

Al'nus.* The Alder; a tree of the order _Betulaceæ._

Al'nus Glu-ti-no'sa.* A tree growing in many parts of Europe. The leaves and bark are bitter and astringent, and as a tonic are used in intermittent fevers.

Al'nus Ser-rat'u-la.* The American alder, possessing properties like the preceding.

Al'o-e,* gen. **Al'o-ës,** in English **Aloes,** ăl'ōz. A genus of plants of the order _Asphodeliæ,_ characterized by an intensely bitter taste, belonging to the Linnæan class _Hexandria,_ natural order _Liliaceæ_ (or _Asphodeleæ_ of some writers).

Al'oë Bar-ba-den'sis.* The Pharmacopœial name (Lond. Ph.) of Barbadoes aloes, or inspissated juice of the cut leaf of the _Aloë vulgaris._

Al'oë Ca-pen'sis.* The Pharmacopœial name (U.S. Ph.) for the inspissated juice of the leaves of _Aloë spicata,_ and of other species of _Aloe._

Al'oë He-pat'i-ca.* The name of a kind of aloes the source of which is uncertain.

Al'oë Per-fo-li-ā'ta.* The tree formerly believed to yield Socotrine aloes.

Al'oë Soc-o-tri'na.* ("Socotrine Aloes.") The Pharmacopœial name ‖ of Socotrine aloes, obtained from the _Al'oe Socotri'na_ (U.S. Ph.); but according to the British Pharmacopœia, from one or more undetermined species.

Al'oë Spi-ca'ta.* The tree which yields a kind of aloes used in place of the Socotrine.

Al'oë Vul-ga'ris.* The tree believed to afford common hepatic aloes, but said (Lond. Ph., 1851) to be from an uncertain species.

Aloes, al'ōz. The English name for the juice of the several species of _Aloë,_ reduced to an extract.

Aloes, Socotrine. See ALOE SOCOTRINA.

Al'oes Wood. A fragrant resinous substance, consisting of the interior of the trunk of the _Aquilaria ovata_ and _A. agallochum._

Al-o-et'ic. [**Aloet'icus;** from _Al'oë,_ "aloes."] Applied to any medicine containing a large proportion of aloes.

Al-o-got'ro-phy. [**Alogotro'phia;** from ἄλογος, "without proportion," and τρέφω, to "nourish."] Applied to the morbid or excessive nutrition of any part.

Al'o-in. [**Aloi'na.**] The cathartic principle of aloes.

Al-o-pe'ci-a.* [From ἀλώπηξ, a "fox," because subject to loss of hair.] The falling off of hair from the beard and eyebrows, as well as the scalp; baldness the effect of disease, and so distinct from _Calvities:_ alop'ecy.

Alouchi, al-loo'che. The name of a gum obtained from the tree of the _Canella alba._

Al'phi-ta* [the plural of ἄλφιτο, "meal"]. Another name for barley-meal; barley-meal fried.

Al'phoid. [**Alphoi'des;** from _al'-_

phos, a "skin-disease," and εἶδος, a "form."] Like *Alphos*, as *Lepra alphoides*.

Al-phon'sin. [From *Alphon'so* Fer'ri, of Naples, its inventor.] An instrument for extracting balls from wounds.

Al'phos,* **Al'phus.*** [From ἀλφός, "white."] A species of leprosy; the *Lepra alphos*.

Al-pho'sis.* [From the same.] Albino-skin.

Al-pi'ni, Bal'sa-mum.* [After Prosper *Alpinus*.] The "balsam of Alpinus." The balsam produced by the *Amyris Gileadensis*.

Al-pin'i-a.* [Named in honor of *Alpinus*.] A Linnæan genus of the class *Monandria*, natural order *Scitamineæ*.

Alpin'ia Car-da-mo'mum.* The plant said (Lond. Ph. 1836) to produce the lesser Cardamom seeds, formerly referred to the *Amomum cardamomum*, and now to the *Elettaria cardamomum*.

Alterantia,* ăl-ter-an'she-a. See ALTERATIVE.

Alteran'tia Ner-vi'na.* ("Nervous Alteratives.") A class of substances, as spirituous liquors and narcotics, which produce gradual changes in the brain, attended by disturbance of the intellectual functions.

Al'ter-a-tive. [**Al'terans;** from *al'tero, altera'tum*, to "vary."] Applied to medicines (Lat. *Alteran'tia*) which re-establish the healthy functions of the system without any sensible evacuation.

Altern. Horis = *Alter'nis ho'ris.** "At alternate hours,"—that is, every other hour.

Al-ter'nate. [**Alterna'tus;** from *alter'no*, to "interchange."] Applied to leaves or branches recurring by turns with those of the opposite side.

Al-thæ'a.* [Gr. ἀλθαῖα, from ἄλθω, to "heal."] A Linnæan genus of the class *Monadelphia*, natural order *Malvaceæ*. Marsh-mallow.

Althæ'a Of-fiç-i-na'lis.* The marsh-mallow, the root of which is ordered for use in the Pharmacopœia (Lond. Ph.); the leaves and root (Ed. and Dub. Ph.); and the flowers and root (U S. Ph.).

Al-the'in. [**Althæi'na;** from *althæ'a*.] An alkaline substance discovered in the marsh-mallow, similar to *Asparagin*.

Al-tim'e-try. [**Altime'tria;** from *al'tus*, "high," and μετρέω, to "measure."] The art of measuring heights or altitudes.

Aludel, al'oo-dĕl. A pear-shaped vessel used by the earlier chemists, resembling the head of an alembic, with the exception of the beak, etc. A series of these vessels, joined together, is used for distilling mercury in Spain.

Al'u-la.* [Diminutive of *a'la*, a "wing."] A little wing. Applied in the plural (*al'ulæ*) to the membranous scales above the *halteres* in certain *Diptera*, and under the *elytra* of some aquatic *Coleoptera*.

Al'um. [From *alu'men*.] The *Persulphas aluminæ et potassæ*. See ALUMEN.

Al'um, Am-mo-ni'a-cal, is a double salt, consisting of the sulphates of ammonia and of alumina, in which ammonia takes the place of the potassa of common alum.

Al'um Curd of Ri-ve'ri-us. [**Albu'men Alumino'sum.**] A coagulum formed by briskly agitating a drachm of alum with the white of an egg.

Al'um Oint'ment. A preparation consisting of common turpentine, lard, and powdered alum.

Al'um Wa'ter. A solution of alum in water, used by painters in water-colors.

Al'um Whey. [**Se'rum Alumino'sum.**] A whey made by boiling two drachms of alum with a pint of milk, and then straining.

Al-u'men,* gen. **Al-u'min-is.** Alum. The *Sulphas aluminæ et potassæ*, a double or sometimes a triple salt, consisting of sulphuric acid and alumina, with either potassa or ammonia, or frequently both. The alumen of the Pharmacopœias is prepared from schistose clays. In Italy this salt is procured from *alum stone*, a mineral substance occurring in most volcanic districts.

Alu'men Ex-sic-ca'tum vel Us'tum.* Dried alum (or burnt alum); the Pharmacopœial name of alum when it has undergone watery fusion and parted with all its water of crystallization by the action of heat. Its chief use is as an escharotic for destroying fungous flesh.

Alu'men Ro-ma'num.* Roman alum; the purest variety of alum, containing no ammonia in its composition.

Alu'men Ru'pe-um.* [From *ru'pes*, a "rock."] Roche or rock alum. A variety of alum brought from Roccha, formerly called Edessa, in Syria That which is sold under this name is common English alum, artificially colored.

A-lu'mĭ-na.* [From *alu'men,*"alum."] The base of *alumen:* al'umine.

A-lu-mĭ-na'tus.* Containing *alumen:* alu'minated.

A-lu-mĭn-if'er-ous. [**Aluminif'erus;** from *alu'men,* and *fe'ro,* to "bear."] Bearing or having alum.

Aluminium. See ALUMINUM.

Al-u'min-ous. [**Alumino'sus;** from *alu'men.*] Pertaining to alum.

A-lu'mĭ-num.* The metallic base of *Alumina,* sometimes spelled *Aluminium.*

Al'ums. [**Alu'mina,** the plural of **Alu'men.**] A group of salts having a constitution similar to that of common alum.

Alun, å'lŭNᵍ'. The French term for *Alum.* See ALUMEN.

A-lu'sĭ-a.* [From ἀλύω, to "become insane."] Hallucination; illusion; mental deception, error, or misconception.

Alu'sia Elatio* (e-la'she-o). Sentimentalism, or mental extravagance. See ELATION.

Alu'sia Hyp-o-chon-dri'a-sis.* Low spirits, or hypochondriacism.

Alutaceous, al-u-tā'shŭs. [**Aluta'ceus;** from *alu'ta,* "dressed leather."] Applied to the leaves of plants resembling a soft, tanned skin.

Alv. Adst. = *Al'vo Adstric'tâ.** "The bowels being bound."

Al-ve-a'rĭ-um.* [From *alvea're,* a "beehive."] That part of the external meatus of the ear where the *cerumen* is secreted.

Al-ve'o-lar. [**Alveola'ris.**] Belonging to the *alveoli,* or sockets of the teeth.

Al-ve'o-lar Struc'ture. A term applied by Hewson to minute superficial cavities found in the mucous membrane of the stomach, œsophagus, and small intestine, and which he compared to the cells of honeycomb. They are distinct from the follicles.

Al-ve'o-late. [**Alveola'tus;** from *alve'olus.*] Having little troughs or cavities.

Al-ve'o-li.* [See ALVEOLUS.] The alveolar processes, or the sockets of the teeth. Hence the term *alveolar* as applied to the arteries and veins of the sockets of the teeth.

Al-ve'o-lĭ-form. [**Alveolifor'mis;** from *alve'olus.*] Formed like *alveoli.*

Al-ve'o-lus,* plural **Al-ve'o-li.** [Diminutive of *al'veus.*] A little hollow. The socket of a tooth, or other cavity.

Al've-us.* [From *al'vus,* the "belly."] A trough or channel; any large hollow, such as the hold of a ship. Applied to tubes, canals, especially their enlarged portions, through which some fluid flows.

Al'veus Am-pul-lĕs'çens.* [See AMPULLA.] The dilated portion of the thoracic duct at its commencement from the *receptaculum chyli.*

Al'veus Com-mu'nis.* The communication of the *ampullæ* of the semicircular canals of the ear.

Al'vĭ-du'ca.* [From *al'vus,* the "belly," and *du'co,* to "lead," to "move."] Medicines which promote evacuation of the contents of the intestines.

Al-vĭ-flux'us.* [From *al'vus,* the "belly," and *flu'o, flux'um,* to "flow."] Diarrhœa; a flux or discharge of the contents of the intestines.

Al'vine. [**Alvi'nus;** from *al'vus.*] Belonging to the belly, stomach, or intestines.

Al'vine Con-cre'tion. [**Enterol'ithus.**] A calculus in the stomach or bowels. See BEZOAR.

Al'vus.* The belly, stomach, paunch, or intestines. See ABDOMEN, VENTER.

Al'vus As-tric'ta.* [From *astrin'go, astric'tum,* to "bind."] A costive state of the bowels.

Al'vus Co-ac'ta.* Literally, hardbound belly. The state of costiveness.—(CELSUS.)

Al'vus Flu'ĭ-da.* A loose state of the bowels.

Amadou (Fr.), å'må-doo'. Literally, "touch-wood," a kind of fungus. A substance used in graduated compresses; also to support varicose veins, and protect abraded surfaces, etc.

A-măl'gam. [**Amal'gama;** from ἅμα, "together," and γαμέω, to "espouse."] A combination of mercury with any other metal.

A-mal-ga-mā'tion. [**Amalgama'tio, o'nis.**] The process of combining mercury with a metal, or forming an amalgam.

A-man'ĭ-tin. [**Amaniti'na;** from ἀμανῖται, "fungi," or "mushrooms."] The poisonous principle of *fungi.*

A-ma'ra.* [Neuter plural of *ama'rus,* "bitter."] Bitters; medicines with a bitter flavor and tonic property, as chamomile, gentian, etc.

Amaranthaceæ,* am-a-ran-tha'-she-ē, or **Am-a-ran-ta'ce-æ.*** [From *amaran'thus,* or *amaran'tus.*] A natural order of plants, mostly tropical. It comprises the *Amaranthus* and other flowers which are always dry and not liable to fade.

Am-a-ran'thi,* the plural of **Amaran'thus.** A natural order of plants. See AMARANTHACEÆ.

Am-a-ran'thus.* [From *a*, priv., and *μαραίνω*, to "wither," or "fade."] A genus of plants with unfading flowers. Written also AMARAN'TUS.

Am'a-rin. [**Amari'na;** from *ama'rus*, "bitter."] The bitter principle of vegetables.

Am-a-ryl-li-da'ceæ* (-da'she-ē). A natural order of plants, including the *Amaryl'lis*.

Amatoria Febris. See CHLOROSIS.

Am-a-to'ri-us.* [From *a'mo, ama'tum*, to "love."] Belonging to love: am'atory. Applied to the oblique muscle of the eye, used in ogling.

Am-au-ro'sis.* [From *ἀμαυρόω*, to "darken."] Partial or total loss of vision, from paralysis of the retina, usually attended with paralysis and dilatation of the iris, though occasionally it is rigidly contracted. It is also termed *Gut'ta sere'na*. The term Amaurosis was originally used in the sense of obscurity or dimness of vision; but now it is employed to denote a particular disease.

Am-au-rot'ic. [**Amaurot'icus.**] Belonging to *amaurosis*.

Am'bē.* [Gr. *ἄμβη*, a "rising," "something elevated."] An old machine for reducing dislocations of the shoulder.

Am'ber. [**Suc'çinum.**] A transparent bituminous substance, of a yellow or orange color, having electric properties; anciently called *ἤλεκτρον*, whence the word *electricity*.

Am'ber, Aç'id of, or **Suc-çin'ic Acid,** is obtained from amber by dry distillation. It is a delicate reagent for separating red oxide of iron from compound metallic solutions.

Am'ber Cam'phor. A yellow, light sublimate, obtained by the destructive distillation of amber in a retort or alembic. It has been termed *volatile resin of amber*.

Ambergris, or **Ambergrease,** am'ber-grēs. [**Ambragri'sea;** from the French *ambregris* (ŏM'br-grè'), or "gray amber."] A concrete bituminous substance, of a grayish or ash color, inflammable, and when heated emitting a fragrant odor. It is found about the sea-coast of warm countries, or floating on the surface of the ocean, also in the intestines of the *Physeter macrocephalus*, and is supposed to be a morbid secretion of that and perhaps other species of the *Physeter*. Chiefly valuable as a perfume.

Am-bi-dex'ter.* [From *am'bo*, "both," and *dex'ter*, "right-handed," "skilful."] One who uses his left hand as well as his right.

Am-blo'sis.* [From *ἀμβλόω*, to "have an abortion."] Miscarriage. Hence the term *amblot'ic* (*amblot'icus*, plural *amblot'ica*), as applied to medicines supposed to cause abortion.

Am-bly-a'phi-a.* [From *ἀμβλύς*, "blunt," and *ἁφή*, "sense of touch."] Blunted or dulled sense of touch.

Am-bly-o'pi-a.* [From *ἀμβλύς*, "blunted," and *ὤψ*, the "eye."] Impaired vision from defective sensation of the retina; incomplete amaurosis, or the weakness of sight attending certain stages and forms of this disorder.

Am'bon.* [Probably from *ἀναβαίνω*, to "rise," to "ascend."] Literally, an "elevation." The margin of the sockets in which the heads of the large bones are lodged.

Am'bre-āte. [**Am'breas, a'tis.**] A combination of ambreic acid with a base.

Am-bre'ic Aç'id. A peculiar acid obtained by digesting ambrein in nitric acid.

Am'bre-in. [**Ambrei'na;** from the Fr. *ambre*, "amber."] A fatty substance forming the base of ambergris, and differing slightly from cholesterin.

Ambrosia,* am-bro'zhe-a. [From *ἄμβροτος*, "immortal."] Literally, the "food of the gods," that which confers immortality or life. Applied to several plants, on account of their good qualities, as tansy, wormwood, etc. Applied also to several alexipharmic medicines.

Am-bu-la'crum.* [From *am'bulo*, to "walk."] The space between two *strigæ*, or each *striga*, formed by the small holes on the shell of the *Echinus*, as of a walk or path.

Am'bu-lance. [From the French *ambulant*, "ambulatory."] The kind of movable hospital accompanying an army. In popular language, a wagon or carriage for conveying wounded soldiers.

Am-bus'tion. [**Ambus'tio, o'nis;** from *ambu'ro, ambus'tum*, to "burn."] A burn or scald on any part of the body.

Am'e-lin. [**Ameli'na.**] A new base precipitated in the alkaline solution from which melamin has been deposited, on being supersaturated with acetic acid.

A-men-o-ma'ni-a.* [From *amœ'nus*, "pleasant," and *ma'nia*.] A hybrid term (half Latin and half Greek) denoting a gay or cheerful form of mania.

Amenorrhœa,* a-men'o-rē'a. [From

a, priv., μήν, a "month," and ῥέω, to "flow."] Absence or stoppage of the menstrual discharge, including *Emansio mensium* and *Suppressio mensium*.

A-men'ta,* the plural of AMENTUM, which see.

Amentaceæ,* am-en-ta'she-ē. [From *amenta'ceus*. See next article.] The Jussieuan name of an order of plants now distributed among different orders.

A-men-tā'ceous. [**Amenta'ceus;** from *amen'tum*.] Having an *amentum*.

Amentia,* a-men'she-a. [From *a*, priv., and *mens*, the "mind."] Idiocy; fatuity; imbecility of mind. A genus of the order *Vesaniæ*, class *Neuroses*, of Cullen's Nosology. See DEMENTIA.

A-men'tum,* plural **A-men'ta.** [From ἅμμα, a "thong."] A catkin, or imperfect flower, somewhat like a rope or cat's tail. Also termed *Nucamentum*.

Amer (Fr.), å'maiR'. ("Bitter.") The bitter principle produced by digesting silk in nitric acid.

American Balsam. See BALSAM OF PERU.

American Gamboge. See GAMBOGE.

A-mer'i-can Sen'na. The common name for *Cassia Marilandica*.

Am'e-thyst. [**Amethys'tus;** from *a*, priv., and μεθύσκω, to "make drunk."] A violet-colored gem, a species of rock crystal. Its name is derived from its reputed virtue of preventing intoxication: topers were formerly in the habit of wearing it about their necks. It consists almost entirely of silica.

Am-i-an'thoid, or **Am-i-an'toid.** [**Amianthoi'des,** or **Amiantoi'des;** from *amian'thus* or *amian'tus*, a fossil, fibrous stone.] Resembling *amianthus*.

Am-i-an'thus.* [From *a*, priv., and μιαίνω, to "defile."] Literally, "that which cannot be defiled;" because cloth made of it could always be purified by burning. Mountain flax; an incombustible mineral, consisting of very delicate and regular silky fibres. See ASBESTOS.

Amide, å'mēd'. A saline compound, in which a compound of nitrogen and hydrogen occurs, containing an atom less of hydrogen than ammonia.

Am'i-din. [**Amidi'na;** from the French, *amidon*, "starch."] A substance intermediate between gum and starch, obtained by the solution of the latter in hot water.

Amilen or **Amilene,** am'e-lĕn. A liquid hydro-carbon, obtained by distilling hydrate of oxide of amyl repeatedly with anhydrous phosphoric acid.

Ammi. See SISON AMMI.

Am-mo'ni-a.* The volatile alkali; ammoniacal gas. A transparent, colorless, pungent gas, formed by the union of nitrogen and hydrogen. By Priestley it was called *alkaline air*; it is called "the volatile alkali" to distinguish it from the fixed alkalies,—soda and potash. Its present name is derived from sal ammoniac, of which it constitutes a basis, and which received its appellation from being first prepared in the district of Ammonia, in Libya.

Am-mo-nī'a-cal. [**Ammoniaca'lis.**] Belonging to *ammonia*.

Ammoni'acal Al'um. A double salt, consisting of the sulphate of ammonia and alumina, the potassa of common alum being replaced by ammonia.

Ammoni'acal Gas. *Ammonia*, the volatile alkali.

Am-mo-ni'a-cum.* [From Ἄμμων, a name of Jupiter, who had his temple in a part of Libya, where the tree chiefly grew.] The Pharmacopœial name ‖ of a gum resin, from the *Dore'ma ammoni'acum*: ammo'niac, or gum-ammo'niac.

Am-mo'ni-æ Li'quor.* ("Liquor of Ammonia.") The name of the concentrated solution of ammonia. One volume of water takes up about 750 times its bulk of the gas, forming a liquid possessed of similar properties, and termed *spirits of hartshorn* from its being produced by distillation from that substance.

Ammoniaque, am'mo'ne-åk'. The French term for AMMONIA, which see.

Am'mo-nite. [**Ammoni'tes;** from Jupiter *Am'mon*; worshipped as a ram.] A kind of petrified shell, like a horn or snake. From its resemblance to the horns of the statues of Jupiter Ammon, it is called *Cor'nu Ammo'nis*, "horn of Ammon." From its coiled form it is popularly known as snake-stone.

Am-mo'ni-um.* The supposed metallic base of ammonia.

Ammoniuret, am-mōn'yu-rĕt. [**Ammoniure'tum.**] A combination of ammonia with a metallic oxide.

Am-ne'si-a,* **Am-nes'ti-a.*** [From *a*, priv., and μνῆσις, "remembrance."] Want of memory; forgetfulness.

Am'ni-i, Li'quor.* The fluid contained in the amnion.

Am'ni-on.* [From ἀμνός, a "lamb."] The soft, most internal membrane, containing the waters which surround the *fœtus in utero*. Also called *Agnina tunica*.

Am'ni-o-tāte. [**Amni'otas, a'tis.**] Amniotic acid combined with a base.

Am-nĭ-ot′ic. [**Amniot′icus.**] Pertaining to the amnion.

Amniot′ic Aç′id. Same as allantoic acid.

A-mo′me-us.* Having an arrangement as in the *Amomum:* amo′meous.

A-mo′mum.* [From ἄμωμος, "blameless."] A Linnæan genus of the class *Monandria,* natural order *Scitamineæ.*

Amo′mum Car-da-mo′mum.* The former name of the lesser Cardamom seed plant; now ascertained to be the *Alpinia cardamomum.*

Amo′mum Gra′na Par-a-di′si.* Grains of Paradise Amomum: a plant of the order *Scitamineæ,* the fruit of which is well known under the name of *Grains of Paradise* or Mellegetta Pepper.

Amo′mum Re′pens.* The plant producing the Cardamom seed; but this is chiefly obtained from the *Alpinia cardamomum.*

Amo′mum Zin′gĭ-ber.* The ginger-plant, or *Zingiber officinale.*

A-mor′phism. [**Amorphis′mus;** from α, priv., and μορφή, "form."] The state of being amorphous.

A-mor′phous. [**Amor′phus;** from α, priv., and μορφή, "form."] Wanting form; shapeless.

A-mor′phous Quĭ-nine′. The substance *Quinoidine;* so named because its salts cannot be crystallized. See Quinia.

Am-pel′ic Aç′id. An acid obtained by Laurent from the oils of bituminous schist. The term *ampelin* has been also applied to an oily matter prepared from the same substance.

Am′pe-los-a′grĭ-a.* [From ἄμπελος, a "vine," and ἄγριος, "wild."] The *Bryonia alba,* or wild vine.

Am-phem-e-ri′na,* or **Am-phim-e-ri′na.*** [From ἀμφί, "on" or "by," and ἡμέρα, a "day."] Applied to a fever, such as a quotidian ague, or hectic, occurring "day by day,"—that is, every day.

Am′phi (ἀμφί). A Greek preposition, signifying "on both sides," "about;" sometimes "on," "at," or "by." It is nearly allied to ἄμφω, "both," and to ἀμφίς, "on both sides," "in both directions," "around."

Am-phĭ-ar-thro′sis.* [From ἄμφω, "both," and ἄρθρον, a "joint," an "articulation."] A movement partaking both of *Diarthrosis* and *Synarthrosis,* as in the tarsal and carpal bones, and the *vertebræ.*

Am-phib′ĭ-o-lite, or **Am-phib′ĭ-o-lith.** [**Amphibiol′ithus;** from *amphib′ius,* and λίθος, a "stone."] A fossil relic of an amphibious animal.

Am-phib-ĭ-ol′o-ġy̆. [**Amphibiolo′gia;** from *amphib′ius,* and λόγος, a "speech."] A treatise on amphibious animals; the science of amphibious animals.

Am-phib′ĭ-us.* [From ἄμφω, "both," or ἀμφί, "on both sides," and βιόω, to "live."] Amphibious. Applied to plants and animals that live in both elements,—on land or in the water. In the neuter plural (*Amphib′ia*) it forms the name of the second class of the *Encephalata,* or vertebrated animals. The animals of this class commence their larva state as fishes, and undergo various degrees of metamorphosis in advancing to the condition of reptiles.

Am-phĭ-dĭ-ar-thro′sis.* [From ἀμφί, "on both sides," and διάρθρωσις, an "articulation."] Applied to the articulation of the lower jaw with the temporal bone, because partaking both of the nature of *ginglymus* and *arthrodia.*

Am-phĭ-ga′mĭ-us.* [From ἀμφί, "on both sides" (and hence "doubtful"), and γάμος, a "marriage."] In the neuter plural (*Amphiga′mia*) applied to plants (the *Cryptogamia*) whose fructification is unascertained and may be of both sexes.

Am-phip′o-dous. [**Amphip′odus;** from ἀμφί, "about," and πούς, ποδός, a "foot."] Having feet round about. Applied to certain *Crustacea.*

Amphiscius,* am-fish′e-ŭs. In the plural, **Amphiscii,** am-fish′e-i. [From ἀμφί, "on both sides," and σκία, a "shade" or "shadow."] Having their shadow to the north one season, to the south another. Applied to the people within the Torrid Zone. Amphis′cians.

Am-phis′to-mous. [**Amphis′tomus;** from ἀμφί, "on both sides" or "both ends," and στόμα, the "mouth."] Applied to certain *Entozoa,* having a cup at each extremity, by which they adhere to the intestines.

Am-phit′ro-pal, or **Am-phit′ro-pous.** [**Amphit′ropus;** from ἀμφί, "about," and τροπέω, to "turn."] Applied to the embryo of any seed when it extends round the albumen.

Am′pho-ra.* [From ἀμφί, "on both sides," and φέρω, to "carry;" because carried by two handles.] An ancient wine-vessel with two auricles, containing about nine English gallons.

Am-phŏr′ic. [**Amphor′icus.**] Belonging to the *amphora;* resembling that of an *amphora*. Applied to a sound (the amphoric resonance) in auscultation, resembling that heard on blowing into a decanter.

Am-plex-i-cau'lis.* [From *amplec'tor, amplex'us*, to "surround," and *cau'lis*, a "stem."] Surrounding the stem: amplex'icaul, or amplexicau'line.

Am-pul'la,* plural **Am-pul'læ.** A big-bellied jug or bottle used by the Romans for containing wine. In Anatomy, applied to the trumpet-mouthed portions of the semicircular canals of the ear. See ALVEUS COMMUNIS. Also a small membranous bag attached to the roots and immersed leaves of certain aquatic plants.

Ampullaceous, am-pul-lā'shus. [**Ampulla'ceus.**] Appearing like an *ampulla*.

Am-pul'lu-la.* [The diminutive of *ampul'la*.] Applied to a canal or bag slightly enlarged in the centre.

Am-pu-tā'tion. [**Amputa'tio, o'nis**; from *am'puto, amputa'tum*, to "cut off."] The operation of cutting off a limb, or projecting part of the body, as the breast, etc.

Am'u-let. A supposed charm against infection or disease: such are anodyne necklaces, used in teething of infants.

A-my-e'li-a.* [From *a*, priv., and μυελός, "marrow," "spinal marrow."] The condition of a monster fœtus, born without the spinal marrow. Such a fœtus is said to be *amy'elous*. When the encephalon also is absent, the fœtus is termed *amyenceph'alous*. There may be absence of the encephalon,—of the cerebrum and cerebellum only; in this case the fœtus is called *anenceph'alous*. Or the cerebrum merely may be in a state of defective development, or *atrophy*, more or less partial or extensive.

Amyelous. See preceding article.

A-mÿg'da-la.* [Gr. ἀμυγδάλη.] The fruit of *Amyg'dalus commu'nis*, the sweet and bitter almond.

A-mÿg'da-læ* (the plural of the preceding). A popular name for the exterior glands of the neck and for the tonsils.

Amÿg'dalæ A-ma'ræ,* and **Amÿg'dalæ Dul'cēs.*** Bitter and sweet almonds; the fruit of two varieties of the *Amyg'dalus commu'nis*. The bitter almond contains prussic acid, and enters into the liquor or composition called *noyau*.

Amÿg'dalæ Pla-çen'ta.* "Almond-cake;" the substance left after the expression of the oil, which when ground forms *almond-powder*, so generally used for washing the hands.

Am-ÿg-da'le-us.* Having an arrangement as in the *Amygdalus*. Amygda'leous.

Am-ÿg-dal'ic. [**Amygdal'icus**, from *amyg'dala*, an "almond."] Belonging to the almond. Applied to an acid obtained from amygdalin.

A-mÿg-da-lif'e-rous. [**Amygdalif'erus**; from *amyg'dala*, an "almond," and *fe'ro*, to "bear."] Bearing almonds. Applied to a *geode* with a movable kernel.

A-mÿg'da-lin. [**Amygdali'na**; from *amyg'dala*, an "almond."] A white crystalline substance obtained from the bitter almond.

A-mÿg'da-line. [**Amygdali'nus**; from the same.] Belonging to the almond.

A-mÿg-da-li'tis.* [From *amyg'dalæ*, the "tonsils," and *i'tis*, denoting inflammation.] Same as TONSILLITIS.

A-mÿg'da-loid. [**Amygdaloi'des**; from *amyg'dala*, an "almond," and εἶδος, a "form."] Having the form of an almond.

A-mÿg-da-loi'dal. The same as the preceding.

A-mÿg'da-lus.* [Gr. ἀμύγδαλος, the "almond-tree."] A Linnæan genus of the class *Icosandria*, natural order *Rosaceæ*.

Amÿg'dalus Com-mu'nis.* The tree which yields the almond, both bitter and sweet.

Amÿg'dalus Per'si-ca.* The peach-tree.

Am'ÿl. The hypothetical radicle of a series of compounds, of which the hydrate of the oxide has long been known as *fusel oil*, or as the *oil of grain-spirit* or *potatoes*, as it is produced in the fermentation of unmalted grain and potatoes.

Amylacea Corpora. See NEUROGLIA.

Amylaceous, am-e-lā'shus. [**Amyla'ceus**; from *am'ylum*.] Starch-like.

Am'ÿ-len. A substance obtained by distilling fusel oil with chloride of zinc. It is a narcotic poison.

A-mÿl'ic. [**Amyl'icus**; from *am'ylum*, "starch."] Applied to an acid obtained from starch.

Amylin. The same as AMIDIN.

Am'ÿ-loid. [**Amyloi'des**; from *am'ylum*.] Resembling *amylum*, or starch.

Amyloid Degeneration. See LARDACEOUS DEGENERATION.

Am'ÿ-lum.* [Gr. ἄμυλον, "fine meal."] The Pharmacopœial name ‖ for starch, being the fecula of the seeds of *Triticum vulgare;* (Dub. Ph.) the *Seminis feculæ.*

Am'ylum Ma-ran'tæ.* Arrowroot,—a nutritive starch prepared from the *Maranta arundinaceæ.*

Am'ў-ous. [**Am'ўus;** from *a*, priv., and μῦς, μυός, a "mouse;" also a "muscle."] Without muscle; fleshless.

Amyridaceæ,* am-ĭr-e-da'she-ē. An order of dicotyledonous plants, abounding in fragrant resin.

Am'ў-ris.* [From *a*, intensive, and μύρον, a "sweet-scented juice."] A Linnæan genus of the class *Octandria*, natural order *Amyridaceæ* (formerly a division of *Terebinthaceæ*).

Am'yris El-e-mif'e-ra.* The systematic name of the tree which yields gum-elemi.

Am'yris Gil-e-a-den'sis.* The systematic name of the tree which affords balm or balsam of Gilead. See ALPINI BALSAMUM.

An (αν). A Greek particle having a privative force. See **A.**

Ana (ἀνά). A Greek particle, signifying "through," "up through," "upwards," "again;" sometimes "according to."

For the use of *ana* in medical formularies, see **AA.**

An-ab'a-sis.* [From ἀνά, "up," and βαίνω, to "go."] Literally, an "ascending." The increase of a disease or of a paroxysm. See ACME.

An-a-bat'ic. [**Anabat'icus.**] Pertaining to anabasis.

Anacardiaceus,* an-a-kar-de-a'she-ŭs. Having an arrangement as in the *Anacardium* (cashew-tree:) anacardia'ceous. Applied in the feminine plural (*Anacardiaceæ*, an-a-kar-de-a'she-ē) to an order of dicotyledonous plants, including the cashew-tree, the sumach, etc.

An-a-car'di-um.* *Anacardium Occidentale.* Cashew-nut, or marking-nut. The nut contains, between its rind and shell, a red, inflammable, and very caustic liquor, or oil. See CASHEW-TREE.

An'a-ca-thar'sis.* [From ἀνά, "up," and καθαίρω, to "purge."] Literally, a "purgation upwards." A term used to denote cough with expectoration, or expectoration simply.

An-a-ca-thar'tic. [**Anacathar'ticus;** from the same.] Promoting expectoration or vomiting.

An-a-cўc'lus Pўr'e-thrum.* The Pharmacopœial (Lond. and Ed. Ph.) name for *Anthemis Pyrethrum.*

An-ad'ro-mous. [**Anad'romus;** from ἀνά, "up," and δρόμος, a "course."] Swimming up into rivers from the sea.

An-æ'mĭ-a.* [From αν, priv., and αἷμα, "blood."] Deficiency of blood: more correctly written ANHÆMIA.

An-æm'ic (or **Anem'ic**), or **An-æ'-mĭ-al.** [**Anæm'icus,** or **Anæmia'lis;** from the same.] In a state of *anæmia.*

An-æ-mot'ro-phў. [From *anæ'mia*, and τροφή, "nourishment."] By this term and *hæmotrophy* are implied simply a deficiency and an excess of sanguineous nourishment. *Atrophy* and *hypertrophy*, as commonly understood, include the idea of diminished and increased magnitude; while *anæmia* and *hyperæmia* have reference only to the quantity of blood present, without regard to its nutritive properties.—(PROUT.) See ANÆMIA.

Anaëroid. See ANEROID.

Anæsthesia,* an-es-the'se-a. [From αν, priv., and αἰσθάνομαι, to "perceive," to "feel."] Loss of feeling or perception: an'æsthesy. A genus of the order *Dysæsthesiæ*, class *Locales*, of Cullen's Nosology.

Anæsthetic, an-es-thet'ik. [**Anæsthet'icus;** from *anæsthe'sia.*] Having no perception nor sense of touch.

Anæsthet'ics. [From the same.] A term applied to certain medicines, such as chloroform, ether, &c., having the power of rendering the recipient insensible to pain.

A'nal. [**Ana'lis.**] Pertaining to the *anus.*

An-a-lep'sis.* [From ἀναλαμβάνω, to "take again," to "recover."] Recovering of strength after sickness.

An-a-lep'tic. [**Analep'ticus;** from the same.] Belonging to *analepsis.*

Analep'tics. [From the same.] Restorative medicines.

A-nal'o-gous. [**Anal'ogus;** from ἀνά, "according to," and λόγος, "ratio" or "proportion."] Literally, "proportionate:" hence, corresponding to in a general way.

Analogue, an'a-lŏg. [From the same.] Applied in Comparative Anatomy, by Owen, to a part or organ in one animal having the same function as another part or organ in a different animal.

A-nal'o-ġў. [**Analo'gia;** from the same.] The relation of things or parts of a different nature, but similar in their function, and so contradistinguished from the term *Homology.*

A-nal'ў-sis.* [From ἀναλύω, to "undo."] The process of separating any compound substance into its constituents.

An-a-mir'ta Coc'cu-lus.* The

plant which affords the *Cocculus Indicus* fruit (Ed. Ph.).

An-am-nes'tic, An-am-nes'tĭ-cal. [**Anamnes'ticus;** from ἀναμνήσκω, to "recall to mind."] Recalling to memory.

An-an'drous, or **An-an'drĭ-ous.** [**Anan'der,** or **Anan'drius;** from αν, priv., and ἀνήρ, ἀνδρός, a "man," a "male."] Applied to plants which have no male organs.

Anaphrodisia,* an-af-ro-diz'e-ą. [From αν, priv., and ἀφροδίσια, "things pertaining to Venus."] Impotence; incapability of sexual intercourse, from whatever cause.

An-ą-plas'tic. [**Anaplas'ticus.**] Of or belonging to anaplasty.

An'ą-plas-tȳ. [**Anaplas'tia;** from ἀνά, "again," and πλάσσω, to "form" or "fashion."] Literally, forming anew. Surgical operations for the restoration of lost parts, or for the reparation of certain deformities or natural defects in the structure of the body.

An-ą-ple-ro'sis.* [From ἀναπληρόω, to "fill again," to "supply."] The supplement of parts destroyed, as in wounds, cicatrices, etc.

An-ą-ple-rot'ic. [**Anaplerot'icus.**] Belonging to anaplerosis; supplementary.

An-ą-sar'cą.* [From ἀνά, "through," and σάρξ, the "flesh."] Dropsy in the integuments of the body. General dropsy, as distinguished from dropsy of some particular organ or part.

An-ą-stal'tic. [**Anastal'ticus;** from ἀνά, "upwards," and στέλλω, to "set," "send," "contract."] Formerly applied to medicines that were styptic.

An-as'to-mo'sis.* [From ανα, "by," "through," and στόμα, a "mouth."] The communication of branches of vessels with each other.

An-as-to-mot'ic. [**Anastomot'icus.**] Of the nature of *anastomosis.*

An-ą-tom'ĭ-cal. [**Anatom'icus.**] Belonging to anatomy.

A-nat'o-mist. [From ἀνά, "through," "up," and τέμνω, to "cut."] A dissector of organized bodies, whether human, brute-animal (then called Zoötomist), or vegetable (then Phytotomist).

A-nat'o-mȳ. [**Anato'mia;** from the same.] Generally, the dissection of organized bodies, whether human, brute-animal, or vegetable.

Anat'omy, Ar-ti-fiç'ial. [**Anato'mia Artificia'lis.**] Imitated dissections in wax, etc.

Anat'omy, Com-păr'a-tive. [**Anato'mia Comparati'va.**] The dissection of the lower animals, plants, etc., to illustrate those general principles of organization which are common to an order, class, grand division, etc.

Anat'omy, De-scrip'tive. [**Anato'mia Descripti'va.**] Details of the situation, form, and relative attachments of the various parts.

Anat'omy, Gen'e-ral. [**Anato'mia Genera'lis.**] Description of the structure and nature of the various tissues, apart from any consideration of the organs they compose.

Anat'omy, Hu'man. [**Anato'mia Huma'na.**] Dissection of man.

Anat'omy, Med'i-cal. [**Anato'mia Med'ica.**] Embracing *Descriptive, Physiological,* and *Pathological Anatomy.*

Anat'omy, Path-o-log'i-cal. [**Anato'mia Patholog'ica.**] The investigation of changes in the structure of organs by disease, or from congenital malformation.

Anat'omy, Phȳs-ĭ-o-log'i-cal. [**Anato'mia Physiolog'ica.**] The examination of the organs of animals to understand their respective functions in the healthy state.

Anat'omy, Speç'ial. [**Anato'mia Specia'lis.**] Properly, the anatomy of a single species, as the anatomy of man, of the horse, etc.—Cruveilhier. In this sense it is contradistinguished from Comparative Anatomy; but, according to most writers, it is that branch of Anatomy which treats of the particular organs or parts (in a state of health) as contradistinguished from General Anatomy, which treats of the tissues, etc., common to the various organs.

Anat'omy, Surg'ĭ-cal. [**Anato'mia Chirur'gica.**] The examination of the various organs, muscles, nerves, and blood-vessels, their precise situation and relations to each other, with a special reference to surgery.

Anat'omy, Tran-scen-den'tal. [**Anato'mia Transcendenta'lis.**] That branch of Anatomy which treats of the development of parts, their analogies, their primary model or type, approximation to, or deviation from, that model; also termed Philosophical Anatomy.

An-at'ro-pous. [**Anat'ropus;** from ἀνατρέπω, to "subvert."] Applied in Botany to the ovule, in which the *hilum* and internal *umbilicus* are opposed to each other.

An-au'dĭ-ą.* [From αν, priv., and

ἀνωδή, "speech."] Dumbness; privation of voice; catalepsy.

An-a-zo-tu'rĭ-a.* [From αν, priv., *azo'tum*, "azote," and οὖρον, "urine."] A variety of chronic *diuresis*, in which there is a deficiency of urea. See UREA.

An'ceps.* [From *am*, contraction of ἀμφί, "on both sides," and *ca'pio*, to "take," to "compass."] Ancip'ital. Having the sides sharp like a two-edged sword. A term used in Botany.

An'chĭ-lops.* [From ἄγχι, "near to," and ὤψ, the "eye."] Supposed to be a stage of *fistula lachrymalis* before the inflamed swelling bursts; afterwards called *ægilops*.

An'cho-ne.* [From ἄγχω, to "strangle."] The sensation of strangling, in *hysteria*.

An-cho-ra'lis.* [From *an'chora*, an "anchor."] Applied to the coracoid process of the scapula. See ANCYROIDES.

An-chu'sa.* [From ἄγχω, to "choke," to "constringe the fauces."] A Linnæan genus of the class *Pentandria*, natural order *Boragineæ*.

Anchu'sa Tinc-to'rĭ-a.* [From *tin'go, tinc'tum*, to "dye."] Dyers' alkanet; a plant of the order *Boraginaceæ*, the root of which abounds in the red coloring-matter called *alkanet*, used by dyers; also for imparting a deep red to oils, ointments, and plasters.

Anchusin, an'ku-sin. [**Anchusi'na.**] A red-colored principle obtained from *Anchusa tinctoria*, termed by some Anchusic acid.

Anchylosis. See ANKYLOSIS.

Ancipitius,* an-se-pish'e-ŭs. The same as ANCEPS.

An'con.* [From ἀγκών, the "elbow."] The elbow; the olecranon process of the ulna.

An-co'nad. Applied the same as anconal used adverbially.

An-co'nal. [**Ancona'lis.**] Belonging to the *ancon*. Applied by Dr. Barclay, of Edinburgh, in his proposed nomenclature, as meaning towards the *ancon*.

Anconeus,* ang-ko-ne'ŭs, or an-ko'-ne-ŭs. [From *an'con*.] Pertaining to the elbow. Formerly applied to various muscles attached to the olecranon; now limited to one.

An'co-noid. [**Anconoi'des**; from *an'con*, and εἶδος, "a form."] Resembling the *ancon*.

Ancyloglossia. See ANKYLOGLOSSIA.

Ancylosis. See ANKYLOSIS.

An-çȳ-ro-i'dēs.* [From ἄγκυρα, an "anchor," and εἶδος, a "form."] Resembling an anchor. See ANCHORALIS.

An-dra-nat'o-mȳ. [**Andranato'mia**; from ἀνήρ, ἀνδρός, a "man," and ἀνατέμνω, to "cut up."] Dissection of the human body, particularly the male.

Androgynous, an-droj'e-nŭs. [**Androg'ynus**, or **Androgyn'ius**; from ἀνήρ, ἀνδρός, a "man," and γυνή, a "woman."] Partaking of both sexes; hermaphrodite.

An'droid. [**Androi'des**; from ἀνήρ, a "man," and εἶδος, a "form."] Resembling a man.

An-dro-ma'nĭ-a.* [From ἀνήρ, a "man" or "male," and μανία, "madness."] Same as *Nymphomania* or *Furor uterinus*.

An-droph'o-rus.* [From ἀνήρ, a "man" or "male," and φέρω, to "bear."] The slender pillar which supports the united anthers in monadelphous and diadelphous plants.

An-drot'o-mȳ. [From ἀνήρ, a "man" or "male," and τέμνω, to "cut."] The same as ANDRANATOMY, which see.

An'drum.* [Probably derived from *and*, a Hindoo word signifying "testicle."] A species of hydrocele, peculiar to the south of Asia, and described by Kæmpfer.

An-eī-lop'ter-us.* [From ἀνειλέω, to "unroll," and πτέρον, a "wing."] Applied to insects with four wings, the two superior of which are flexible: aneilop'terous.

A-nel-la'ta,* or **A-nel'lĭ-dēs.*** [From *anel'lus*, a "little ring."] The fifth class of the *Diploneura* or *Helminthoida*, consisting of long, cylindrical, mostly aquatic worms, with red blood, covered with a soft and more or less segmented and annulated skin. The earth-worm belongs to this class. Also called ANNULATA, ANNULIDA, and ANNELIDANS.

Anemia. See ANÆMIA.

Anemic, Anemial. See ANÆMIC, etc.

An-e-mog'ra-phȳ. [**Anemogra'phia**; from ἄνεμος, "wind," and γράφω, to "write."] A description of the winds.

An-e-mol'o-ġȳ. [**Anemolo'gia**; from ἄνεμος, the "wind," and λόγος, a "discourse."] The doctrine or science of the winds.

An-e-mom'e-ter. [**Anemom'etrum**; from ἄνεμος, the "wind," and μετρέω, to "measure."] An instrument for measuring the strength or velocity of the wind.

An-e-mom'e-trȳ. [**Anemome'tria**; from the same.] The art of ascertaining the rapidity and direction of the winds.

A-nem'o-scope. [**Anemosco'pi-um;** from ἄνεμος, the "wind," and σκοπέω, to "examine."] An instrument which shows the direction of the wind; a weather-vane.

An-en-çe-pha'li-a.* [From αν, priv., and ἐγκέφαλος, the "brain."] A kind of fœtal monstrosity characterized by absence of the brain.

An-en-çe-phal'ic. [**Anencephal'-icus;** from the same.] Pertaining to a monster-fœtus born without a brain.

An-en-çeph'a-lous. [**Anenceph'-alus.**] The same as ANENCEPHALIC.

An-en-çeph'a-lus.* A monster-fœtus without brains.

An-en'ter-ous. [**Anen'terus;** from αν, priv., and ἔντερον, an "intestine."] Without intestines.

An-ep-i-thy̆m'ĭ-a.* [From αν, priv., and ἐπιθυμία, "desire."] Loss of any of the natural appetites, as hunger, thirst, etc.

An'e-roid, written also **An'aeroid.** [From αν, priv., and ἀήρ, "air."] A defective term, meaning "without air." See next article.

An'eroid or **An'aeroid Ba-rom'e-ter.** An apparatus consisting of a flat, circular box of some white metal, having the upper and under surfaces corrugated in concentric circles. This box, being exhausted of air, is affected by every variation of pressure in the atmosphere, the corrugations on its surface giving it greater elasticity.

An'e-sis.* [From ἀνίημι, to "relax."] A remission or relaxation of a disease or symptom.

A-ne'thum.* [Gr. ἄνηθον.] The Pharmacopœial name (Br. Ph.) of *Ane'-thum grav'eolens,* or dill.

Ane'thum Fœ-nic'u-lum.* Sweet fennel; also called *Fœniculum dulce, F. Germanicum, F. Vulgare* or *Officinale, Marathrum.*

Ane'thum Grav'e-o-lens,* **Ane'-thum Vul-ga're.*** The common dill plant.

An-et'ic. [**Anet'icus;** from ἄνεσις, a "remission."] Applied to soothing medicines.

A-net'ĭ-ca.* Soothing medicines. See ANETIC.

An'e-tus.* [From ἄνεσις, a "remission."] Applied by Dr. Good as a generic name for intermittent fever.

An-eū-ral'ğī-con.* [From α, priv., νεῦρον, a "nerve," and ἄλγος, "pain."] An apparatus used by Dr. Downing for applying warmth and sedative vapor for relief of neuralgia.

An'eū-rism. [**Aneuris'ma, a**tis; from ἀνευρύνω, to "enlarge."] Fr. *Anévrisme,* a'nå'vrèzm'. A tumor filled with blood, from the rupture, wound, ulceration, or simple dilatation of an artery; also applied to dilatation of the heart.

The old distinction was between *true* and *false aneurism:* the former comprehends dilatation without rupture of any of the arterial coats; the latter, dilatation with rupture of some of the coats.

FALSE ANEURISM admits of some distinctions. When the extravasation is diffused, the disease has been termed a *diffused false* aneurism; when circumscribed, a *circumscribed false* aneurism. The French writers term the former *anévrisme faux primitif,* the latter *anévrisme faux consécutif.*

An'eurism by An-as'to-mo'sis. A mulberry-colored mark, in children, caused by an anastomosis of the minute arteries. It sometimes increases in size, and is at length attended with pulsation.

An'eurism of the Heart. Enlargement or dilatation of the heart.

An'eū-ris'mal Nee'dle. A slender instrument for passing a ligature under an artery in order to tie it. Used in operations for aneurism.

Aneuris'mal Va'rix. [**Va'rix Aneurisma'lis.**] The dilatation and pulsation of a vein from the passing of blood into it from an artery; both, with the fascia, having been wounded in the act of blood-letting, all the openings having become united into one by adhesive inflammation.

Aneurysm. See ANEURISM.

Anévrisme. See ANEURISM.

An-frac-tu-os'ĭ-ty̆. [**Anfractuos'-itas;** from *anfrac'tus,* a "winding, bending, or turning of a way."] A term applied to the furrows or *sulci* between the convolutions of the brain.

An-frac'tus,* plural **An-frac'tus.** The same as the preceding.

Angeiospermia,* an-jī-o-sper'me-a. See ANGIOSPERMIA.

An-ğel'ĭ-ca.* [From *an'gelus,* an "angel;" named from its virtues.] Garden Angelica. A Linnæan genus of the class *Pentandria,* natural order *Umbelliferæ.* Also, the Pharmacopœial name (U.S. and Ed. Ph.) for the root of *Angelica archangelica.*

Angel'ica Arch-an-ğel'ĭ-ca.* The plant called garden angelica.

Angel'ica A-tro-pur-pu're-a.* A species possessing the same properties as the garden angelica.

An-gĭ-ec'ta-sis.* [From ἀγγεῖον, a "vessel," and ἔκτασις, "extension."] Dilatation of a vessel, as aneurism, varix, etc.

An-gĭ-i'tis.* [From ἀγγεῖον, a "vessel."] Piorry's term for inflammation of vessels, particularly of the capillaries.

An-gĭ'na.* [From ἄγχω, to "strangle."] Applied to diseases attended by a sense of suffocation, or by sore-throat.

Angina Maligna. See CYNANCHE MALIGNA.

Angina Parotidæa. See PAROTITIS.

Angina Pectoris,* an-jī'na pek'to-ris. Spasm of the chest. A disease attended by acute pain, sense of suffocation, and syncope. It has been called also *Asth'ma dolorif'icum, Sternal'gia, Sternodyn'ia syncopa'lis, Sternocar'dia*, etc.

Angina Tonsillaris. See TONSILLITIS.

An-gĭ-no'sus.* [From *angi'na*.] Having *Angina*, or accompanied by *Angina*.

An-gĭ-o-car'pi.* [From ἀγγεῖον, a "vessel," and καρπός, "fruit."] The name of a tribe or division of *Fungi* which bear their seeds internally.

An-gĭ-og'ra-phy̆. [**Angiogra'phia**; from ἀγγεῖον, a "vessel," and γράφω, to "write."] A description of the vessels of the body.

An-gĭ-o-leū-çi'tis.* [From ἀγγεῖον, a "vessel," and λευκος, "white."] Literally, "inflammation of the white (or lymphatic) vessels." A diseased condition of the lymphatic vessels.

An-gĭ-ol'o-ġy̆. [**Angiolo'gia**; from ἀγγεῖον, a "vessel," and λόγος, a "discourse."] The doctrine or science of the blood-vessels and absorbents.

Angiospermatous, or **Angeiospermatous,** an-jī-o-sper'ma-tus. [**Angiosperm'atus**; from ἀγγεῖον, a "vessel," and σπέρμα, a "seed."] Having seeds in a capsule, or seed-vessel.

Angiospermia,* an-jī'o-sper'me-a. [From ἀγγεῖον, a "vessel," and σπέρμα, a "seed."] The name of an order or division of plants.

An-gi-o-te-lec-ta'sĭ-a,* An-gi-o-te-lec'ta-sis.* [From ἀγγεῖον, a "vessel," τέλος, an "extremity," and ἔκτασις, "extension."] Extension or dilatation of vessels or their terminating capillaries.

An-gĭ-ot'o-my̆. [**Angioto'mia**; from ἀγγεῖον, a "vessel," and τέμνω, to "cut."] Dissection of the blood-vessels and absorbents.

An'gle, Facial (fā'shal). [**An'gulus Facia'lis.**] A straight line from the most prominent part of the forehead to the front edge of the upper jaw, and another from the external auditory foramen to the same point. Some writers attach great importance to the facial angle as a measure of the brain as compared with the rest of the head. If the fore part of the cranium (in which the intellect is supposed to reside) be very full, the facial angle will be large; if that part be very deficient, the facial angle will be proportionably small.

An'gle, Op'tic; An'gle of Viṡ'ion. That formed by two rays of light proceeding from different objects, or opposite extremities of the same object, and meeting in the pupil.

An'glĭ-cus Su'dor.* [*An'glicus*, "English," and *su'dor*, "sweat."] The English sweating-fever, or the *Ephem'era malig'na* of Burserius, described by Dr. Caius as "a contagious pestilential fever of one day." It made its first appearance in London about the year 1480.

An'go-nē.* [From ἄγχω, to "choke."] A sense of strangulation and suffocation. More properly written ANCHONE.

Angor Pectoris. See ANGINA PECTORIS.

Angostura. See ANGUSTURA.

Anguilliformes,* an-gwil'le-for'mēz. [From *anguil'la*, an "eel."] The name of a family of fishes resembling an eel in form.

An-gui'na.* [From *an'guis*, a "serpent."] The name of a family of reptiles.

Anguinidæ,* an-gwin'e-dē. [From *an'guis*, a "serpent."] The name of a family of the *Ophidia* having the *Anguis* for its type.

Angular (ang'gu-lar) **Ar'te-ry̆, An'gular Vein.** Terminations of the facial artery and vein near the inner angle of the eye.

An'gular Proç'ess-es. The orbitary processes of the frontal bone.

An-gu-la'ris Scap'u-læ.* Another name for the muscle called *levator anguli scapulæ*, the "elevator of the angle of the scapula."

Angulate, ang'gu-lāt. [**Angula'tus**; from *an'gulus*, an "angle."] Having angles.

An'gu-lous, or **An'gu-lōse.** [**Angulo'sus**; from *an'gulus*, an "angle."] Full of angles.

An-gus-tĭ-fo'lĭ-āte, or **An-gus-tĭ-fo'lĭ-ous.** [**Angustifo'lius**; from *angus'tus*, "narrow," and *fo'lium*, a "leaf."] Having narrow leaves.

An-gus-tĭ-sep'tus.* [From *angus'tus*, "narrow," and *sep'tum*, a "partition."] Having narrow partitions.

Angustura (an-gŭs-too'rạ, written also **Angostura**) **Bark.** [From *Angostu'ra*, the name of a town of Venezuela.] The bark of *Galipæ'a cuspa'ria* (Lond. Ph.), or *G. officina'lis* (U.S. Ph.).

Angusturin, an-gŭs-too'rin, or **An-gos-tu'rin.** A neutral principle, obtained by submitting the alcoholic tincture of angustura bark to spontaneous evaporation.

An-he-lā'tion. [**Anhela'tio, o'***nis;* from *anhe'lo, anhela'tum*, to "breathe short."] Shortness of breath.

Anhel'itus.* Same as ANHELATION.

An-hȳ'drīte. [From *anhy'drus* (see next article), and λίθος, a "stone."] Anhydrous sulphate of lime; a mineral.

An-hȳ'drous. [**Anhy'drus;** from ἀν (same as *a*), priv., and ὕδωρ, "water."] Without water.

An-ĭ-dro'sis.* [From αν, priv., and ἱδρόω, to "sweat."] Diminution or suppression of the perspiration.

Anil. See INDIGO.

An-il'ic or **In-dĭ-got'ic Aç'id.** An acid formed by the action of nitric acid on indigo.

An'ĭ-līne. [From *an'il*, "indigo."] An oily liquid formed by the action of caustic potash on indigo. Also applied to a greenish substance obtained from nitro-benzole: it forms the base of several beautiful dyes.

An'ĭ-mạ.* [From ἄνεμος, "wind," "breath," or "spirit."] Anciently, any simple volatile substance; also, the purest part of any substance. The vital principle of animals or vegetables.

An'ima Ar-tic-u-lo'rum.* Literally, "life of the limbs;" a name given to colchicum on account of its medicinal virtues in rheumatism and gout. It formed the basis of many popular remedies against gout, such as the *pulvis arthriticus Turneri*, and the Vienna gout decoction.

An'ĭ-mal.* [From *an'ima*, the "spirit," or "life."] An organized body, endowed with life and voluntary motion.

An'imal. [**Anima'lis;** from *an'ima*, "life."] Having life; pertaining to life.

An'imal Aç'id. [**Aç'idum Anima'le.**] An acid existing in animal bodies, or which can be obtained from them, as *Allantoic, Ambreic, Butyric*, etc.

Animal Charcoal, or **Animal Carbon.** See CARBON, ANIMAL.

An'imal E-con'o-mȳ. [**Œcono'mia Anima'lis.**] The system of all matters relating to animal life; physiology. See ECONOMY.

Animal Heat. See CALOR ANIMALIS.

Animal Jelly. See GELATIN.

An'imal King'dom [**Reg'num Anima'le.** Fr. *Règne Animal*, rēñ å'ne'-mål'] denotes, collectively, all those beings possessing animal life, the study of which is called Zoology. See ZOOLOGY.

Animal Magnetism. See MESMERISM.

Animal Temperature. See CALOR ANIMALIS.

Animalcula. See next article.

An-ĭ-mal'cule. [**Animal'culum** (plural **Animal'cula**), which see.] A microscopic animal. These animals doubtless exist in the atmosphere, and in all rivers or ponds. Those best known are—

1. *Infusory Animalcules* (*Animal'cula Infuso'ria*, often called simply *Infusoria*). Observed in nearly all fluids impregnated with any animal or vegetable substance.

2. *Spermatic Animalcules.* Supposed to have been discovered in the semen. See SPERMATOZOA.

An-ĭ-mal'cu-lum,* plural **An-ĭ-mal'cu-lạ.** [The diminutive of *an'imal.*] Literally, a "minute animal." A creature whose true figure cannot be ascertained without a magnifying glass. See ANIMALCULE.

An-ĭ-mal'ĭ-tȳ. [**Animal'itas, a'***tis.*] The assemblage of faculties that distinguish animal organic matter; vital activity of an animal body, considered as unity.

An-ĭ-mal-ĭ-zā'tion. [**Animaliza'tio, o'***nis;* from *an'imal.*] The process by which food is assimilated to the various substances of the body.

An-ĭ-mā'tion. [**Anima'tio, o'***nis;* from *an'imo, anima'tum*, to "give life."] The effect produced by the *vis vitæ* ("power of life"), by which life is begun and maintained.

Animation, Suspended. See ASPHYXIA.

Anime, an'e-me. A resinous substance, improperly called *gum animé*, said to be obtained from the *Hymenæa Courbaril*, and used in perfumes, varnishes, and certain plasters. It resembles copal in appearance, and is often sold under that name.

An'ĭ-mists. [From *an'ima*, the

"soul."] Those physiologists who refer all the phenomena of the living body to the direct agency of the soul or a principle distinct from the body.

An'ĭ-on.* [Gr. ἀνίων, the present participle of ἄνειμι, to "ascend."] A term applied by Dr. Faraday to the body which passes to the positive pole—to the *anode* of the decomposing body—as it is separated by electricity. See KATION.

Anise, an'iss. The PIMPINELLA ANISUM, which see.

An'ĭ-seed, or **An'ise-seed.** The seeds of the *Pimpinel'la ani'sum,* much used as a carminative.

Anisette de Bourdeaux, an'nè'-zet' dẹh boor'dō'. A liqueur made by distilling anise, fennel, and coriander seeds, previously steeped in brandy, with sugar, and one-half water.

Anisi Semina. See ANISEED.

An-ĭ-so-pet'ạ-lous. [**Anisopet'alus;** from ἄνισος, "unequal," and *pet'alum.*] Having unequal petals.

An-ĭ-so-phy̆l'lous. [**Anisophyl'lus;** from ἄνισος, and φύλλον, a "leaf."] Having unequal leaves.

An-ĭ-so-stem'o-nous. [**Anisostem'onis;** from ἄνισος, and στήμον, a "stamen."] Having unequal stamens.

A-ni'sum.* [From ἄνίημι, to "emit."] Anise. The Pharmacopœial name (U.S., Lond., and Ed. Ph.) for the fruit of *Pimpinel'la ani'sum.* See ANISEED.

An'ker. A liquid measure used at Amsterdam, containing about thirty-two gallons English wine-measure.

An-ky̆-lo-bleph'ạ-ron.* [From ἀγκύλη, "noose," and βλέφαρον, the "eyelid."] A preternatural union of the two eyelids.

An-ky̆-lo-glos'sĭ-ạ,* or **An-cy̆-lo-glos'sĭ-ạ.*** [From ἀγκύλη, a "noose" or "bridle," and γλῶσσα, the "tongue."] A natural defect termed *tongue-tie.*

An-ky̆-lo'sis.* [From ἀγκύλη, a "clasp."] The consolidation of the articulating extremities of two or more bones that previously formed a natural joint; stiff-joint.

An-neal'ing. [From the Saxon *on-ælan,* to "set on fire," to "make hot," to "burn."] The process by which substances naturally hard and brittle are rendered tough. It consists in raising the substance (glass or metal) to be annealed, to a high temperature, and then causing it to cool very slowly.

Annelidæ. See ANELLATA.

An-not'to. [Derivation uncertain.] A kind of reddish dye, obtained from the *Bixa Orellana,* or *Orleana;* the *Terra Orleana* of the shops.

An'nu-ens,* plural **An-nu-en'tēs.** [From *an'nuo,* to "nod."] Applied to the muscles called *Recti antici capitis,* because they are employed in nodding the head.

Annular Bone. See Os ANNULARE.

An'nu-lạr Car'tĭ-lage. [**Cartila'go Annula'ris.**] The cricoid cartilage.

An'nular Lig'ạ-ment. [**Ligamen'tum Annula're.**] A strong ligament encircling the ankle; also, the wrist.

An'nular Proç'ess, An'nular Pro-tu'be-rance. [**Proces'sus Annula'ris, Protuberan'tia Annula'ris.**] The *Pons Varolii;* also called *Tuber annulare,* and *Corpus annulare.* See PONS VAROLII.

An'nular Vein. [**Annula'ris Ve'na.**] The vein between the little and ring fingers.

An-nu-la'tus.* [From *an'nulus,* a "ring."] Having rings: an'nulate, or an'nulated. Applied in the neuter plural (*Annula'ta*) to a class of worm-like animals. See ANELLATA.

An'nu-lid-ạ.* The same as ANELLATA, which see.

An'nu-lus.* A Latin word, signifying "ring," forming a part of a number of anatomical names.

Annulus Abdominis. See ABDOMINAL RING.

An'nulus Cil-ĭ-a'ris.* The ciliary circle or ligament; a white ring forming the bond of union between the choroid coat of the eye, the iris, and the corona ciliaris. It is the *annulus gangliformis tunicæ choroïdeæ* of Sœmmering.

An'nulus Lig-ạ-men-to'sus.* The ciliary circle or ligament. See ANNULUS CILIARIS.

An'nulus O-va'lis.* The rounded margin of the septum which occupies the place of the foramen ovale in the fœtus. It is also called the *an'nulus foram'inis.*

An'ode. [From ἀνά, "up," and ὁδός, a "way."] In electro-chemical action, that part of the surface of the decomposing body into which the electric current "ascends" or enters.

A-nod'ic. [**Anod'icus;** from the same.] Used by some writers in the same sense as ANASTALTIC.

An'o-dy̆ne. [**Anod'ynus;** from αν, priv., and ὀδύνη, "pain."] Applied to medicines which assuage pain: antal'gic. See SOPIENS.

A-nom'ạ-lĭ-flo'rous. [**Anomali-**

flo rus; from *anom'alus*, and *flos*, a "flower."] Having anomalous flowers.

A-nom'a-li-pēde. [**Anom'alipes, p'edis;** from *anom'alus*, and *pes*, a "foot."] Having anomalous feet.

A-nom'a-lo-çeph'a-lus.* [From ἀνώμαλος, "irregular," and κεφαλή, the "head."] One whose head is deformed. See ANOMALOUS.

A-nom'a-lous. [**Anom'alus;** from αν, priv., and ὁμαλός, "level," "even," "regular."] Applied to diseases or symptoms out of the regular course.

A-nom-o-çeph'a-lus.* [From α, priv., νομός, a "law" or "rule," and κεφαλή, the "head."] One whose head is deformed; the same as ANOMALOCEPHALUS.

An-om'pha-lous. [**Anom'phalus;** from ἀν, priv., and ὀμφαλός, the "navel."] Having no navel.

A-non'ȳ-mus.* [From αν, priv., and ὄνυμα, a "name."] Literally, *nameless*. A term formerly applied to the cricoid muscle.

An-oph-thăl'mĭ-a.* [From αν, priv., and ὀφθαλμός, the "eye."] The condition of being without eyes.

An-op-lo-the'rĭ-um.* [From αν, priv., ὅπλον, "armor," and θήριον, a "beast."] A fossil animal found in the Paris tertiaries, destitute of horns, tusks, or claws.

An-op'sĭ-a.* [From αν, priv., and ὄψις, "vision."] Defect of sight.

An-or'chous. [**Anor'chus;** from αν, priv., and ὄρχις, a "testicle."] Having no testicles.

An-o-rex'ĭ-a.* [From αν, priv., and ὄρεξις, "desire," "appetite."] Want of appetite: an'orexy. A genus of the order *Dysorexiæ*, class *Locales*, of Cullen's Nosology.

Anormal. See ABNORMAL.

An-os'mĭ-a.* [From αν, priv., and ὄζω, to "smell."] Loss of the sense of smell.

An-os-phre'sĭ-a.* [From αν, priv., and ὄσφρησις, the "sense of smell."] Loss of the sense of smell.

An-o'tus.* [From αν, priv., and οὖς, ὠτός, the "ear."] Without ears.

An'ser.* A goose. In the plural (*An'ser-ēs*) it is applied to an order of birds including all the web-footed waterfowl.

An-ser-i'nus.* [From *an'ser*, a "goose."] Pertaining to a goose: an'serine. See PES ANSERINUS.

Ant-aç'id. [From ἀντί, "against," and *aç'idum*, an "acid."] Destroying or counteracting acidity, by combining with and neutralizing it.

Ant-ac'rid. [**Antac'ridus;** from ἀντί, "against," and *ac'ridus*, "acrid."] Correcting an acrid condition of the secretions.

Ant-ag'o-nism. [**Antagonis'mus;** from ἀντί, "against," and ἀγωνίζω, to "contend."] The action of muscles opposed to each other in their office.

Ant-ag'o-nist. [**Antagonis'ta;** from the same.] Applied to muscles whose function is opposed to that of others, as abductors and adductors, extensors and flexors, etc.

Ant-ăl'gic. [**Antal'gicus;** from ἀντί, "against," and ἄλγος, "pain."] The same as ANODYNE.

Ant-al'ka-line. [**Antalkali'nus;** from ἀντί, "against," and *al'kali*.] Neutralizing alkalies.

Antaphrodisiac, ant'af-ro-dizh'e-ak, **Ant-aph'ro-dit'ic.** [**Antaphrodisi'acus, Antaphrodit'icus;** from ἀντί, and Ἀφροδίτη, the name of "Venus," also "venereal desire."] Tending to subdue amorous desire: anti-venereal.

Ant-arc'tic. [**Antarc'ticus;** from ἀντί, "against," and ἀρκτικός, "pertaining to the north."] Opposite the north; southern.

Antarc'tic Cir'cle. A circle extending 23½ degrees from the South Pole, and marking that portion of the southern hemisphere within which at the winter solstice the sun does not set.

Ant-ar-thrit'ic. [**Antarthrit'icus;** from ἀντί, "against," and ἀρθρῖτις, "gout."] Relieving gout.

Ant-asth-mat'ic. [**Antasthmat'icus;** from ἀντι, "against," and ἄσθμα.] Relieving asthma.

Ant-a-tro'phic. [**Antatroph'icus;** from ἀντί, "against," and ἀτροφία, "atrophy," "defect of aliment."] Overcoming atrophy.

Anteflexio,* an-te-flek'she-o. [From *an'te*, "before," and *flec'to, flex'um*, to "bend."] A bending forward: anteflexion.

Anteflex'io U'ter-i.* Anteflexion of the womb; the fundus sinking forward between its cervix and the neck of the bladder.

An-ten'na,* plural **An-ten'næ.** [A Latin term signifying a "sail-yard," and applied to the horns of insects, because, extending on each side of the head, they are supposed to resemble the yard-arms projecting on each side of the mast of a ship.] Certain articulated filaments inserted in the heads of the *Crustacea* and *Insecta*, peculiarly devoted to a delicate sense of touch. They are popularly called *horns*, or *feelers*.

An-ten'nāte. [**Antenna'tus.**] Having *antennæ.*

An-ten-nif'e-rous. [**Antennif'e-rus;** from *anten'na,* and *fe'ro,* to "bear."] Bearing *antennæ.*

An-ten'nĭ-form. [**Antennifor'-mis;** from *anten'na.*] Having the form of *antennæ;* resembling *antennæ.*

An-te-pec'tus.* [From *an'te,* "before," and *pec'tus,* the "breast."] The anterior segment of the *Pectus,* or inferior surface of the trunk in insects.

Ant-eph-ĭ-ăl'tic. [**Antephial'ti-cus;** from ἀντί, "against," and ἐφιάλτης, "night-mare."] Efficacious against night-mare.

Ant-ep-ĭ-lep'tic. [**Antepilep'ti-cus;** from ἀντί, and ἐπιλεψία, "epilepsy."] Efficacious against epilepsy.

An-te'ri-or.* Before, as applied to muscles and nerves.

An-te-ster'num.* [From *an'te,* "before," and *ster'num,* the "breast-bone."] In Entomology, the first or anterior division of the sternum.

Anteversio,* an-te-ver'she-o. [From *an'te,* "before," and *ver'to, ver'sum,* to "turn."] A turning forward.

Antever'sio U'ter-i.* ("Anteversion of the Womb.") Displacement of the *uterus,* the fundus being thrown forward, so as to compress the neck of the bladder, the mouth being turned to the sacrum.

Ant-hæm-or-rhaġ'ic. [**Anthæm-orrhaġ'icus;** from ἀντί, "against," and αἱμοῤῥαγία, "hæmorrhage."] Checking hæmorrhage.

Ant'he-lix.* [From ἀντί, "against," "opposite to," and ἕλιξ, the "helix."] The inner circular ridge of the external ear.

An-thel-min'tic. [**Anthelmin'-ticus;** from ἀντί, "against," and ἕλμινς, ἕλμινθος, a "worm."] Expelling worms from the intestinal canal: vermifuge.

An'the-mis.* [From ἀνθέω, to "flower."] Chamomile. A Linnæan genus of the class *Syngenesia,* natural order *Compositæ* (sub-order *Corymbiferæ*). The Pharmacopœial name ‖ of the ANTHEMIS NOBILIS, which see.

An'themis Nob'ĭ-lis.* The herb which yields chamomile flowers; called also CHAMÆME'LUM, CHAMÆME'LUM NO'-BILE, and CHAMOMIL'LA ROMA'NA.

An'themis Pȳr'e-thrum.* The pellitory of Spain. The root of this plant, called Pyrethrum by the Pharmacopœias, is a powerful sialagogue. On account of its acrid and stimulating properties, it is used as a masticatory in the toothache, rheumatism of the face, etc.

An'ther. [**Anthe'ra;** from ἄνθος, a "flower."] The part of the flower which contains the pollen, or the male fecundating principle. It is the head and essential part of the stamen.

An-ther-id'ĭ-um.* [The diminutive of *anthe'ra.*] Applied in the nominative plural (*Antherid'ia*) to collections of cells found in cryptogamous plants containing bodies analogous to the *spermatozoa* of animals.

An-ther-if'er-ous. [**Antherif'e-rus;** from *an'ther,* and *fe'ro,* to "bear."] Bearing anthers.

An-the'sis.* [From ἀνθέω, to "flower."] The production of flowers.

Anthiarin, an-the'a-rin. The active principle of a gum resin obtained from the *Anthiaris toxicaria.*

An-thi-a'ris (or **An-ti-a'ris**) **Tox-ĭ-ca'rĭ-ạ.*** The scientific name of the UPAS TREE, which see.

An-tho-car'pous. [**Anthocar'-pus;** from ἄνθος, a "flower," and καρπός, "fruit."] A term applied to fruits produced from masses of flowers adhering to each other, like the pine-apple.

An-tho-çȳ'ạ-num.* [From ἄνθος, a "flower," and κύανος, "blue."] A substance obtained from the blue of flowers.

An-tho'dĭ-um.* [From ἄνθος, a "flower."] A kind of calyx, common to many flowers.

An-thog'rạ-phȳ. [**Anthogra'-phia;** from ἄνθος, a "flower," and γράφω, to "write."] A description of flowers.

An'thoid. [**Anthoi'des;** from ἄνθος, a "flower," and εἶδος, a "form."] Resembling a flower.

An'tho-līte. [**Antholi'tes;** from ἄνθος, a "flower," and λίθος, a "stone."] The fossil impression of a flower.

An-thol'o-ġȳ. [**Antholo'gia;** from ἄνθος, a "flower," and λόγος, a "discourse."] A treatise on flowers, their nature, qualities, appearance, etc.

An'tho-ny's Fire, Saint. [**Ig'nis Sanc'ti Anto'nii.**] Another name for ERYSIPELAS, which see.

An-thoph'ĭ-luṣ.* [From ἄνθος, a "flower," and φίλος, a "lover."] Literally, "loving flowers." Applied in the neuter plural (*Anthoph'ila*) to a family of *hymenopterous* insects: anthoph'ilous.

An-tho-pho'rĭ-um,* **An-thoph'o-rum.*** [From ἄνθος, a "flower," and φέρω, to "bear."] A prolongation of the receptacle, bearing petals, stamen, and pistil: an an′thophore.

An-thox-an′thin. [**Anthoxanthi′na;** from ἄνθος, a "flower," and ξανθός, "yellow."] A substance obtained from the yellow of flowers.

An-thra′ci-a.* [From ἄνθραξ, a "coal."] See FRAMBŒSIA.

Anthra′cia Ru′bu-la.* Dr. Good's term for the disease called "the yaws." See FRAMBŒSIA.

An-thra-cif′er-ous. [**Anthracif′erus;** from ἄνθραξ, "coal" or "carbon," and *fe′ro*, to "bear."] Containing carbon.

An′thra-cite. [**Anthraci′tes;** from ἄνθραξ, a "coal," and λίθος, a "stone."] A species of stone-coal burning without smoke and with little or no effluvia.

Anthraco′des. The same as ANTHRACOI′DES. See ANTHRACOID.

An′thra-coid. [**Anthracoi′des;** from ἄνθραξ, "coal," and εἶδος, a "form."] Resembling carbuncle; having the nature of carbuncle.

An-thra-cok′a-li. The name given to a remedy recently employed in certain herpetic affections. The *simple* preparation consists of a levigated coal-dust and pure potassa; the *sulphurated* preparation is composed of sulphur, levigated coal-dust, and caustic potassa.

An-thra-co-the′ri-um.* [From ἄνθραξ, "coal," and θηρίον, an "animal."] A fossil animal found in coal and in sandstone.

An′thrax, acis.* [Lat. **Carbun′culus,** a "little coal;" Gr. ἄνθραξ, a "coal."] A carbuncle. A hard, circumscribed, inflammatory dark-red or purple tumor, accompanied by a sense of burning, resembling a boil, but having no central core.

An-thro-pog′en-y. [**Anthropoge′nia;** from ἄνθρωπος, a "man," and γένεσις, "generation."] The generation of man.

An-thro-pog′ra-phy. [**Anthropogra′phia;** from ἄνθρωπος, a "man," and γράφω, to "write."] A history or treatise on the structure of man.

An′thro-poid. [**Anthropoi′des;** from ἄνθρωπος, a "man," and εἶδος, a "form."] Resembling man.

An-throp′o-lite. [**Anthropoli′tes;** from ἄνθρωπος, a "man," and λίθος, a "stone."] A petrifaction of human bones.

An-thro-pol′o-gy. [**Anthropolo′gia;** from ἄνθρωπος, a "man," and λόγος, a "discourse."] A treatise on man; a description of man; also, the science which treats of the physical and intellectual nature of man.

An-thro-pom′e-try. [**Anthropome′tria;** from ἄνθρωπος, a "man," and μέτρον, a "measure."] Measurement of the dimensions of man.

An-thro-po-mor′phous. [**Anthropomor′phus;** from ἄνθρωπος, a "man," and μορφή, "shape."] Formed like man; man-shaped.

An-thro-poph′a-gus,* plural **Anthro-poph′a-gi.** [From ἄνθρωπος, a "man," and φαγω, to "eat."] One who eats human flesh; a cannibal.

An-thro-poph′a-gy. [**Anthropopha′gia;** from the same.] The eating of human flesh.

An-thro-pos′co-py. [**Anthroposco′pia;** from ἄνθρωπος, a "man," and σκοπέω, to "observe."] An inspection of the lineaments of man.

An-thro-po-som′a-tol′o-gy. [**Anthroposomatolo′gia;** from ἄνθρωπος, a "man," σῶμα, the "body," and λόγος, a "discourse."] A description of the structure of the human body.

An-thro-pos′o-phy. [**Anthroposo′phia;** from ἄνθρωπος, a "man," and σοφία, "wisdom."] Knowledge of the nature and general character of man.

An-thro-pot′o-my. [**Anthropoto′mia;** from ἄνθρωπος, a "man," and τέμ ω, to "cut."] The dissecting of man; human anatomy.

Ant-hyp-not′ic. [**Anthypnot′icus;** from ἀντί, "against," and ὕπνος, "sleep."] Hindering sleep.

Ant-hyp-o-chon′dri-ac. [**Anthypochondri′acus;** from ἀντί, "against," and υποχονδριακός, "hypochondriac."] Overcoming hypochondriasis.

Ant-hys-ter′ic. [**Anthyster′icus;** from ἀντί, "against," and *hyste′ria*.] Overcoming *hysteria*.

Anti-. [Gr. ἀντί.] A prefix signifying "against," "opposed to," or "corrective of;" as *anti-bilious*, *anti-lithic*, etc.

An-ti′a-des.* [The plural of ἀντιάς, ἀντιάδος, a "tonsil."] Another name for the tonsils.

An-ti-a-di′tis.* [From ἀντιάς, ἀντιάδος, a "tonsil."] Inflammation of the tonsils.

Antiaphrodisiac. See ANTAPHRODISIAC.

Antiaris. See ANTHIARIS.

Antiarthritic. See ANTARTHRITIC.

An′ti-as.* The singular of ANTIADES, which see.

Antiasthmatic. See ANTASTHMATIC.

Antiatrophic. See ANTATROPHIC.

Antibrachial, an-te-brā'ke-al. [**Antibrachia'lis.**] Belonging to the *antibrachium*, or fore-arm.

An-tĭ-bra'chĭ-um.* [From ἀντί, "against," and *bra'chium*, the "arm."] The fore-arm, as opposed to, when bent upon, the proper arm.

An-tĭ-ca-chec'tic. [**Anticachec'ticus;** from ἀντί, "against," and *cachex'ia*, a "bad habit of body."] Opposed to cachectic diseases. See CACHEXIA.

An-tĭ-car'dĭ-um.* [From ἀντί, "against," and καρδία, the "heart."] The *scrobic'ulus cor'dis*, or pit of the stomach.

Anticheir,* an'te-kīr. [From ἀντί, "against," and χείρ, the "hand."] Opposed to the hand. A name sometimes applied to the thumb.

An-tĭ-clī'nal. [**Anticlina'lis;** from ἀντί, "against," and *cli'no*, to "bend."] Bending in opposite directions. Applied in Geology to strata which decline both ways from a longitudinal ridge, called the anticlinal axis.

An-tĭ-din'ic. [**Antidin'icus;** from ἀντί, "against," and δῖνος, "giddiness."] Relieving from giddiness, or vertigo.

An'tĭ-dote. [**Antid'otum, Antid'otus;** from ἀντί, "against," and δίδωμι, to "give."] A medicine given to counteract the effects of poison.

Antidotus. See ANTIDOTE.

An-tĭ-dȳs-en-ter'ic. [**Antidysenter'icus;** from ἀντί, "against," and δυσεντερία, "dysentery."] Preventing or curing dysentery.

Antiephialtic. See ANTEPHIALTIC.

Antiepileptic. See ANTEPILEPTIC.

An-tĭ-feb'rile. [**Antifebri'lis;** from ἀντί, "against," and *fe'bris*, a "fever."] Subduing fever; febrifuge.

An-tĭ-ga-lac'tic. [**Antigalac'ticus;** from ἀντί, "against," and γάλα, "milk."] Lessening the secretion of milk.

An-tĭ-hec'tic. [**Antihec'ticus;** from ἀντί, "against," and ἑκτικός, "hectic."] Assuaging hectic fever.

Antihelix. See ANTHELIX.

Antihelmintic. See ANTHELMINTIC.

An-tĭ-hy-drop'ic. [**Antihydrop'icus;** from ἀντί, "against," and ὕδρωψ, "dropsy."] Curative of dropsy.

Antihypnotic. See ANTHYPNOTIC.

Antihypochondriac. See ANTHYPOCHONDRIAC.

Antihysteric. See ANTHYSTERIC.

An-tĭ-Ic-tĕr'ic. [**Anti-Icter'icus;** from ἀντί, "against," and ἴκτερος, the "jaundice."] Curative of *Icterus*, or jaundice.

An-tĭ-lith'ic. [**Antilith'icus;** from ἀντί, "against," and λίθος, a "stone."] Preventing the formation of stone, or calculus.

An-tĭ-lo'bĭ-um.* [From ἀντί, "against," and λοβός, the "lobe of the ear."] The tragus, or part opposite the lobe of the ear.

An-tĭ-loi'mic, or **An-tĭ-lœ'mic.** [**Antiloi'micus;** from ἀντί, "against," and λοιμός, the "plague."] Curative of plague or pestilence of any kind.

An-tĭ-lȳs'sic. [From ἀντί, "against," and λύσσα, "canine madness."] A remedy against hydrophobia.

An-tĭ-mo'nĭ-al. [**Antimonia'lis;** from *antimo'nium*.] Pertaining to antimony.

Antimo'nial Pow'der. The *Pulvis antimonialis* (Ed. and Dub. Ph.), or *Pulvis antimonii compositus* (Lond. Ph.), used as a substitute for James's Powder.

Antimo'nial Wine. [**Vi'num Antimo'nii.**] A solution of tartar emetic in sherry or other wine; two grains of the tartar emetic being contained in every fluidounce of the preparation.

An-tĭ-mo'nĭ-āte. [**Antimo'nias, a'***tis;* from *antimo'nicum* aç'idum.] A combination of antimonic acid with a base.

An-tĭ-mon'ic Aç'id. [**Antimo'nicum Aç'idum.**] A substance otherwise called peroxide of antimony.

An-tĭ-mo'nĭ-ous Aç'id. Formed by exposing the white hydrate of the peroxide of antimony to a red heat.

An-tim'o-nīte. [**Antim'onis, i'***tis;* from *antimo'nious* acid.] A combination of antimonious acid and an alkaline base.

Antimonium. See ANTIMONY.

An-tĭ-mo'nĭ-um Tar-tar-ĭ-za'tum.* The Pharmacopœial name (Ed. and Dub. Ph.) of emetic tartar, or *antimonii potassio-tartras* (Lond. Ph.), or tartarized antimony. See TARTAR EMETIC.

An'tĭ-mo-nȳ. [**Antimo'nium;** conjectured to be derived from ἀντί, "against," and *min'ium*, "vermilion;" because used in aid of rouge for heightening the complexion.] A metal of which many of the compounds are used in medicine.

An-tĭ-ne-phrit'ic. [**Antinephrit'icus;** from ἀντί, "against," and νεφρῖτις, "disease of the kidneys."] Curative of diseases of the kidneys.

An-tin'ĭ-ad. Applied the same as *antinial* used adverbially. See GLABELLAD.

An-tin'ĭ-al. [From ἀντί, "against," and ἰνιον, the "occiput."] Opposite the occiput. Applied by Dr. Barclay as meaning towards the *glabella*, or space between the eyebrows.

Antiodontalgic. See ANTODONTALGIC.

An-tĭ-or-gas'tic. [**Antiorgas'ticus;** from ἀντί, "against," and ὀργάζω, to "excite."] Allaying excitement; synonymous with sedative.

An'tĭ-par-a-sta-ti'tis.* [From *antiparas'tatæ*, Cowper's glands.] Inflammation of Cowper's glands.

An-tip'a-thy̆. [**Antipathi'a.*** Gr. ἀντιπάθεια; from ἀντί, "against," and πάθος, "feeling," "affection."] Any opposite properties in matter; also, aversion to particular objects.

An-tĭ-pĕr-ĭ-stal'tic. [**Antiperistal'ticus;** from ἀντί, "against," and *peristal'tic*.] Applied to inverted peristaltic motion of the bowels. See PERISTALTIC.

An-tĭ-pes'tĭ-len-tial. [From ἀντί, "against," and *pestilen'tia*, "pestilence."] Same as ANTILOIMIC.

An-tĭ-phar'mic. [From ἀντί, "against," and φάρμακον, a "poison."] The same as ALEXIPHARMIC.

An'tĭ-phlo-ġis'tic. [**Antiphlogis'ticus;** from ἀντί, "against," and φλέγω, to "burn."] Applied to treatment intended to subdue inflammation, or excitement of the system in inflammatory complaints.

Antiphthisic, an-te-tiz'ik. [**Antiphthis'icus;** from ἀντί, "against," and φθίσις, "consumption."] Checking phthisis, or consumption.

An-tĭ-phys'ic. [**Antiphys'icus;** from ἀντί, "against," and φυσάω, to "inflate."] Dispelling flatulency. Also, against nature [from φύσις, "nature"]. For the purpose of distinction it would perhaps be preferable to write *Antiphu'sic* when we mean "dispelling" or "corrective of flatulency."

An-tĭ-plas'tic. [**Antiplas'ticus;** from ἀντί, "against," and πλάσσω, to "form."] Unfavorable to healing, or granulation; disorganizing.

An-tĭ-pleū-rit'ic. [**Antipleurit'icus;** from ἀντί, "against," and πλευρῖτις, "pleurisy."] Curative of pleurisy.

An-tĭ-po-dag'ric. [**Antipodag'ricus;** from ἀντί, "against," and ποδάγρα, the "gout."] Curative of gout.

An-tĭ-pros'ta-tæ Glan'du-læ.* The antiprostate glands; a name for *Cowper's glands;* also called *Antiparas'tatæ*.

An-tĭ-pros-tat'ic. [**Antiprostat'icus;** from ἀντί, "against," and *pros'tata* glan'dula, the "prostate gland."] Opposite the prostate gland.

An-tĭ-pros'ta-tus.* The same as ANTIPROSTATIC.

An-tip-sor'ic. [**Antipsor'icus;** from ἀντί, "against," and ψώρα, the "itch."] Curative of the itch.

An-tĭ-py'ic. [**Antipy'icus;** from ἀντί, "against," and πύον, "pus."] Preventing suppuration.

An-tĭ-py̆-ret'ic. [**Antipyret'icus;** from ἀντί, "against," and πυρετός, "fever."] Curative of fevers. Antifeb'rile: feb'rifuge.

An-tĭ-py̆-rot'ic. [**Antipyrot'icus;** from ἀντί, "against," and πῦρ, "fire."] Curative of burns.

An-tĭ-quar-ta-nā'rĭ-an, An-tĭ-quar'tan. [**Antiquartana'rius;** from ἀντί, "against," and *quarta'na* fe'bris, a "quartan fever or ague."] Curative of quartan ague.

Antirachitic, an-te-ra-kit'ik. [**Antirachit'icus;** from ἀντί, "against," and *rachi'tis*, "rickets."] Corrective of *rachitis*.

Antiscii,* an-tish'e-i, the plural of **Antiscius,** an-tish'e-ŭs. [From ἀντί, "against," and σκιά, a "shade" or "shadow."] Having their shadow in opposite directions at noon, as the people north and south of the equator: antis'cious: antis'cian.

An-tĭ-scol'ic. [**Antiscol'icus;** from ἀντί, "against," and σκώληξ, a "worm."] Against worms; capable of expelling worms: vermifuge; anthelmintic.

An-tĭ-scor-bu'tic. [**Antiscorbu'ticus;** from ἀντί, "against," and *scorbu'tus*, the disease "scurvy."] Corrective of *Scorbutus*, or scurvy.

An-tĭ-scrof'u-lous. [**Antiscrofulo'sus;** from ἀντί, "against," and *scrof'ula*, the "king's evil."] Curative of *Scrofula*.

An-tĭ-sep'tic. [**Antisep'ticus;** from ἀντί, "against," and σήπω, to "putrefy."] Preventing putrefaction.

An-tĭ-spas-mod'ic. [**Antispasmod'icus;** from ἀντί, "against," and σπασμός, a "spasm."] Allaying spasmodic pains.

An-tĭ-spas'tic. [**Antispas'ticus;** from ἀντί, "against," and σπάω, to "draw."] Literally, "drawing against or in an opposite direction." Counteracting a state of spasm. Synonymous with *Antispasmodic.*

An-tĭ-sўph-ĭ-lit'ic. [Antisyphilit'icus; from ἀντί, "against," and *syph'ilis.*] Curative of syphilis.

An-tith'e-nar.* [From ἀντί, "against," and θέναρ, the "hollow of the hand or foot."] Applied in Anatomy to the muscles *Adductor ad indicem* of the hand, and *Adductor* of the great toe.

Antithora. See ANTHORA.

An-tĭ-traġ'ĭ-cus.* Belonging to the *antitragus:* antit'ragic.

An-tit'ra-gus.* [From ἀντί, "against," and *tra'gus.*] The thicker part of the antihelix, opposite the tragus.

An-tit'ro-pous. [Antit'ropus; from ἀντί, "against," and τροπή, a "turning."] Applied, in Botany, to the embryo when the radicle is distant from the *hilum*, the cotyledons being next to the latter; inverted.

An-tĭ-ve-ne're-al. [Antivene'reus; from ἀντί, "against," and *vene'reus*, "venereal."] Curative of venereal disease.

An-tĭ-zўm'ic. [Antizym'icus; from ἀντί, "against," and ζυμόω, to "ferment."] Preventive of fermentation.

Ant'lĭ-a.* [From ἀντλία, a "pump."] The spiral apparatus by which certain insects draw up the juices of plants.

Ant'lia Lac'te-a,* Ant'lia Mamma'rĭ-a.* An instrument for drawing milk from the breast: a milk-pump; a breast-pump.

Ant-o-don-tăl'ġic. [Antodontal'gicus; from ἀντί, "against," and ὀδονταλγία, a "toothache."] Curative of the toothache.

Antonii, Ignis Sancti. See ERYSIPELAS.

Antorgastic. See ANTIORGASTIC.

An-trī'tis.* [From *an'trum*, a "cave" or "cavity."] Inflammation of any cavity of the body.

An'trum.* [From ἄντρον, a "cave."] A cavity. Applied specially to one in the upper maxillary bone, termed *Antrum Highmoria'num.*

An'trum Buccinosum,* bŭk-sin-o'sŭm. [From *buc'cine*, a "trumpet."] The trumpet-like cavity, or *cochlea* of the ear.

An'trum Çe'næ.* According to Quincy, the name given by Casserius to the *Antrum Highmorianum* before Highmore discovered it.

Antrum Highmorianum. See HIGHMORIANUM, ANTRUM.

An'trum Max-il'læ,* An'trum Max-il-la're,* An'trum of High'more. The *Antrum Highmorianum.*

An'trum Pў-lo'ri.* The small extremity of the stomach near the pylorus.

Ants, Acid of. See FORMIC ACID.

An-u'rĭ-a.* [From *a*, priv., and οὖρον, "urine."] Defective secretion of urine: an'ury.

A'nus.* [From *an'nus*, a "circle."] The extremity of the *rectum:* the fundament.

Anus, Artificial. See ARTIFICIAL ANUS.

Anus, Imperforate. See ATRESIA, ATRETUS.

Anx-ī'e-tў. [Anxi'etas, a'tis; from *anx'ius*, "anxious," (from ἄγχω, to "choke," to "distress").] A settled expression of anxiety in the features forming a dangerous symptom in acute diseases.

A-or'ta.* [Gr. ἀορτή, from ἀείρω, to "raise up," to "support," to "suspend;" because it is supported or suspended from the heart.] The large arterial trunk arising from the left ventricle of the heart, and giving origin to every artery except the pulmonary and its ramifications.

Aorteurysma,* or **Aorteurisma,*** a-ort-ū-riz'ma. [From ἀορτή, and ἀνευρύνω, to "dilate."] Aneurism of the aorta.

A-or'tic. [Aor'ticus.] Belonging to the aorta.

A-or-tī'tis, idis.* [From *aor'ta.*] Inflammation of the aorta.

A-paġ'ў-nous. [Apag'ynus; from ἅπαξ, "once," and γυνή, a "woman," "one who brings forth."] Applied to plants which fructify but once and then die. See GYNÆCOLOGY.

Ap'a-thў. [Apathi'a; from *a*, priv., and πάθος, "feeling," "passion."] Absence or privation of all passion, emotion, or excitement.

Ap'a-tite. A phosphate of lime.

A-pep'sĭ-a.* [From *a*, priv., and πέπτω, to "cook," to "digest."] Imperfect digestion. A term formerly used for dyspepsia.

A-pe'rĭ-ent. [Ape'riens; from *ape'rio*, to "open."] Opening. Applied to a medicine which gently opens the bowels.

A-per'tor, o'ris.* [From *ape'rio*, *aper'tum*, to "open."] Literally, "that which opens." The *Levator palpebræ superioris;* otherwise, the *Apertor oculi* ("opener of the eye").

A-pet'a-lous. [**Apeta'leus:** from *a*, priv., and *pet'alum*, a "petal."] Having no petals.

A'pex.* The point or extremity of a cone: hence applied to parts of the body supposed to resemble a cone, as the apex of the heart, of the tongue, etc.

Aphæresis,* a-fĕr'e-sis. [From ἀπό, "from," and αἱρέω, to "take."] A term formerly applied to that branch of Surgery whose business it is to cut off or remove any portion of the body.

Aph-a-nop'te-rus,* or **Aph-a-nip'te-rus.*** [From ἀφανής, "invisible," and πτέρον, a "wing."] In the neuter plural (*Aphanip'tera*, or *Aphanop'tera*) applied to a family of insects apparently without wings: aphanop'terous.

Aph-e'li-on.* [From ἀπό, "from," and ἥλιος, the "sun."] A term used in Astronomy to denote that point of a planet's orbit farthest from the sun.

A-phelx'i-a.* [From ἀφέλκω, to "draw away." See Apo.] *Aphelxia socors*, absence of mind; *Aphelxia intenta*, abstraction; *Aphelxia otiosa*, revery or brown study.

Aphides. See Aphis.

Aph-i-diph'a-gus.* [From *a'phis*, and φαγεῖν, to "eat."] Applied in the plural masculine (*Aphidiph'agi*) to a family of *Coleoptera* which feed on *Aphides:* aphidiph'agous.

A-phid'i-us.* [From *a'phis*.] Belonging to the *Aphides*. In the plural masculine (*Aphid'ii*) applied to a family of hemipterous insects: aphid'ious.

Aph-i-div'o-rous. [**Aphidiv'orus;** from *a'phis*, and *vo'ro*, to "devour."] Eating *aphides*.

A'phis, idis,* plural **Aphides,** af'e-dēz. The plant-louse, the type of a family of *Hemiptera*.

A'phis Vas-ta'tor.* A species of *aphis* remarkable for its destructive powers. See Vastator.

Aph-lo-gis'tic. [**Aphlogis'ticus;** from *a*, priv., and φλόξ, a "flame."] Without flame.

A-pho'ni-a.* [From *a*, priv., and φωνή, the "voice."] Loss of voice: aph'ony. A genus of the order *Dyscinesiæ*, class *Locales*, of Cullen's Nosology. See Anaudia, Vox Abscissa.

A-pho'ri-a.* [From *a*, priv., and φέρω, to "bear."] Barrenness; sterility; inability to conceive offspring.

Aph'o-rism. [From ἀφορίζω, to "limit," to "define."] A maxim. The Aphorisms of Hippocrates, a celebrated work, containing various maxims or short, pithy sentences relating to medicine.

Aph-ro-dis'i-a. [From Ἀφροδίτη, Venus; Ἀφροδίσιος, "pertaining to Venus," "venereal."] Morbid or immoderate desire of venery. The generative act. Also termed Aphrodisiasmus.

Aphrodisiac, af-ro-dizh'e-ak. [**Aphrodisi'acus, Aphrodis'ius;** from the same.] Applied to medicines or food supposed to excite sexual desire or to increase the generative power.

Aphrodisiasmus. Same as Aphrodisia.

Aph'tha,* plural **Aph'thæ.** [From ἅπτω, to "set on fire."] Ulcers of the mouth, beginning with numerous minute vesicles and terminating in white sloughs. *Aphthæ* constitute the characteristic symptoms of "thrush," and also occur in other diseases.

Aph'thoid. [**Aphthoi'des;** from *aph'tha*, and εἶδος, a "form."] Resembling *aphthæ*.

Aph'thous. [**Aphtho'sus;** from *aph'tha*.] Of the appearance or full of *aphthæ*.

A-phyl'lous. [**Aphyl'lus;** from *a*, priv., and φύλλον, a "leaf."] Without leaves.

Apiaceous, ā-pe-ā'shŭs. [**Apia'ceus.**] Having an arrangement as in Apium.

Ap-i-ca'lis.* [From *a'pex, ap'icis*.] Belonging to the *apex:* ap'ical.

Ap-i-ca'tus.* Having a conspicuous *apex:* ap'icated.

A-pic'u-lus.* [The diminutive of *a'pex*.] A term used in Botany to denote the projection of the midrib beyond the end of the leaf; a small, sharp, short point.

A'pis Mel-lif'i-ca.* [*A'pis*, a "bee," *mel*, "honey," and *fa'cio*, to "make."] The honey-bee, affording honey and wax.

A'pi-um.* A genus of the Linnæan class *Pentandria*, natural order *Umbelliferæ*, including the garden-plants celery and parsley.

A'pium Grav'e-o-lens* (or grave'o-lens). The common celery. (Fr. *Ache*, åsh.) When wild, growing in wet places, it is acrid and poisonous; when cultivated in dry ground and partially blanched, it is used as salad. It is slightly aperient and carminative.

A'pium Pe-tro-se-li'num,* otherwise called **Petroseli'num Sa-ti'vum.** Common parsley, the root and seeds of which are diuretic and aperient.

Ap-la-nat'ic. [**Aplanat'icus;** from

a, priv., and πλανάω, to "wander," to "err."] Corrective of the aberrations of the rays of light.

A-plas'tic. [**Aplas'ticus;** from α, priv., and πλάσσω, to "form."] That cannot be organized.

Apleuria,* a-plu're-ą. [From α, priv., and πλευρά, a "rib."] An organic deviation characterized by the absence of ribs.

Ap-neŭ'rĭ-ą.* [From α, priv., and πνεύμων, the "lung."] An organic deviation characterized by the absence of lungs.

Apnœa,* ap-nē'ą, or **Ap-neŭs'tĭ-ą.*** [From α, priv., and πνέω, to "breathe."] Partial privation or entire suspension of the breath.

Apo. [Gr. ἀπό.] A prefix signifying "from," "off," "away." Before a word beginning with *h* the *o* is dropped and the *p* blended with the following letter: thus, *apo-helko* (from ἀπό and ἕλκω), to "draw away," is contracted into *aphelko* (ἀφέλκω).

Ap-o-car'pous. [**Apocar'pus;** from ἀπό, "from," and καρπός, "fruit."] Having capsules distinct from each other.

Ap-o-çe-no'sis,* plural **Ap-o-çe-no'sēs.** [From ἀπό, "from," and κενόω, to "empty out."] Increased discharge, flux, or evacuation.

Apocynaceæ,* ą-pos-se-na'she-ē. An order of dicotyledonous plants in some respects resembling *Asclepiadaceæ*, but of rather more suspicious properties. See APOCYNUM.

Apocynaceous, ą-pos-se-nā'shŭs. [**Apocyna'ceus.**] Applied to plants resembling the *Apocynum*, or dog's bane.

Ap-o-cȳn'e-us.* Same as APOCYNACEUS.

Apocynin, or **Apocynine,** ą-pos'-se-nin. A bitter principle obtained from the *Apocynum cannabinum*, or Indian hemp, or dog's bane.

Apocynum,* ą-pos'se-nŭm. A plant called dog's bane, the root of which is sometimes used as an emetic.

Ap'o-dēs.* [Formed in the plural from α, priv., and πούς, ποδός, a "foot."] Literally, "without feet." A term applied to fishes without ventrals, or fins which correspond to legs and feet.

Ap'o-dus.* [From the same.] Without feet: ap'odous. Applied in the plural neuter (*Ap'oda*) to an order of *Radiata Echinodermata*.

Ap'o-ġee. [**Apogæ'um;** from ἀπό, "from," and γῆ, the "earth."] That point of the orbit of the sun, or of a planet, most distant from the earth.

Ap-o-neŭ-ro'sis.* [From ἀπό, "from," and νεῦρον, a "nerve."] (Fr. *Aponévrose*, å'po'nå'vroz'.) Expansion of a tendon, or tendons, into a fibrous membrane.

A-poph'ȳ-sis,* plural **A-poph'ȳ-sēs.** [From ἀπό, "from," and φύω, to "produce," to "grow."] A process or protuberance of bone. Also applied to excrescences growing from the receptacle of certain mosses.

Ap-o-plec'tic. [**Apoplec'ticus.**] Pertaining to apoplexy.

Ap-o-plex'ĭ-ą Pul-mo-na'ris.* ("Pulmonary Apoplexy.") Extravasation of blood in the lungs from the rupture of vessels.

Ap'o-plex-ȳ. [**Apoplex'ia;** from ἀπό, "from," "away," and πλήσσω, to "strike." Hence αποπλήσσω signifies to "strike *away*,"—*i.e.* to "strike into unconsciousness or insensibility;" so to "faint *away*" means to faint so completely as to become unconscious.] A disease produced by congestion or rupture of the vessels of the brain, and causing a sudden arrest of sense and motion, the person lying as if asleep, respiration and the heart's action continuing.

Ap'oplexy, Cu-tā'ne-ous. A French term (*apoplexie cutanée*, å'po'plĕx'e' kü'-tå'nå') for sudden determination of blood to the skin and adjacent cellular membrane.

Ap-os-te'mą, a*tis*.* [From ἀφίστημι, to "depart from."] An abscess: an ap'osteme. See ABSCESS.

A-poth'e-cą-rȳ. [**Apotheca'rius;** from ἀποθήκη, a "repository" or "store."] One who keeps a store of drugs; one who sells drugs and puts up prescriptions. In Great Britain an apothecary, besides selling and compounding drugs, is entitled to practise medicine, and is in fact a sort of sub-physician.

Ap-o-the'çĭ-ą,* **Ap-o-the'çĭ-um.*** [From ἀποθήκη.] A botanical term applied to the receptacle enclosing the reproductive corpuscles in the lichens.

A-poth'e-mą, a*tis*.* [From ἀπό, and θέμα, a "deposit."] A brown powder deposited when vegetable extract is submitted to prolonged evaporation.

Ap-pą-ra'tus. [From *ap'paro*, *appara'tum*, to "prepare," to "arrange."] Instruments or mechanical arrangements for experimenting, operating, etc. Sometimes applied to organs in animals and plants.

Ap-pen'dĭ-çēs Ep-ĭ-plo'ĭ-çæ.* In Anatomy, a term applied to prolongations of the *peritonæum*, filled with a soft, fatty substance, attached along the large intestines only.

Ap-pen-dic'u-la.* [The diminutive of *appen'dix.*] A little appendage, or appendicle.

Appendicula Vermiformis. See APPENDIX VERMIFORMIS.

Ap-pen-dic'u-lāte. [**Appendicu-la'tus**; from *appendic'ula.*] Having appendicles.

Ap-pen'dix, *icis*,* plural **Ap-pen'-dĭ-çēs.** [From *ad*, "to," and *pen'do*, to "hang" or "join."] A part of or addition to a thing: an appendage.

Appen'dix Ver-mĭ-for'mis,* or **Appen'dix Çæ'ci Ver-mĭ-for'mis.*** (The "worm-shaped appendage of the cæcum.") A small process of the *cæcum*, which hangs into the pelvis. It is often called the *Appendic'ula vermifor'mis.*

Appert's (ap'pairz') **Proç'ess.** A method introduced by M. Appert (ap'-pair') for preserving articles of food unchanged for several years. The articles are enclosed in bottles, which are filled to the top with any liquid, and hermetically closed. They are then placed in kettles filled with cold water, and subjected to heat till the water boils; the boiling temperature is kept up for a considerable time, after which the bottles are suffered to cool gradually. Instead of bottles, tin canisters are sometimes used, and rendered tight by soldering.

Ap'pe-tence or **Ap'pe-ten-cy̆.** [From *ap'peto, appeti'tum*, to "desire."] The disposition of organized beings to acquire and appropriate substances adapted to their support. Also an ardent desire or longing for any object.

Ap'pe-tīte. [**Appeti'tus**; from the same.] The natural desire for food. Also, any natural inclination by which we are incited to act; inordinate desire; lust.

Appetite, Canine. See BULIMIA.

Appetite, Depraved. See PICA.

Appetite, Insatiable. See BULIMIA.

Appetite, Loss of. See ANEPITHYMIA.

Appetite, Voracious. See BULIMIA, ADEPHAGIA.

Ap'ples, Aç'id of. See MALIC ACID.

Ap-po-sĭ'tion. [**Apposi'tio**; from *ad*, "to," or "on," and *po'no, pos'itum*, to "put," or "place."] Literally, "placing or depositing on" or "in addition to." Applied in Surgery to the supplying of deficient parts by placing portions of the adjacent integuments, etc. in contact. Sometimes used synonymously with PROSTHESIS (which see). Also applied to the deposition of matter which takes place in the growth of the non-vascular tissues, such as horn, the nails, etc.

Ap-pres'sus.* [From *ap'primo, appres'sum*, to "press close."] A term in Botany, signifying "pressed close to."

Ap'ter-us.* [From *a*, priv., and πτερόν, a "wing."] Applied in the plural neuter (*Ap'tera*) to a family of insects which have no wings: ap'terous.

A-py̆-ret'ic. [**Apyret'icus**; from *a*, priv., and πυρετός, "fever."] Having no fever or febrile excitement.

Ap-y̆-rex'ĭ-a.* [From *a*, priv., and πύρεξις, a "fever" or "paroxysm."] Absence of fever, or intermission of its paroxysms: ap'yrexy.

Ap'y̆-rous. [From *a*, priv., and πῦρ, "fire."] A term applied to bodies which sustain the action of a strong heat for a long time without change of figure or other properties. It is synonymous with *refractory.*

Aq. = *A'qua*,* "Water," or *A'quæ*, "Of water."

Aq. Bull. = *A'qua bul'liens.** "Boiling water."

Aq. Destil. = *A'quæ destilla'tæ.** "Distilled water."

Aq. Ferv. = *A'qua fer'vens.** "Hot water."

Aq. Font. = *A'quæ fon'tis* or *fonta'-næ.** "Fountain or spring water."

Aq. Marin. = *A'qua mari'na.** "Seawater."

Aq. Pur. = *A'quæ pu'ræ.** "Pure water."

Aqua,* a'kwa, plural **Aquæ**, a'kwē. [As if *æ'qua*, from its equal surface.] Water: the Pharmacopœial name (Lond. and Ed. Ph.) for spring-water. According to the U.S. Pharmacopœia, "natural water in the purest attainable state." The principal varieties of water (not medicated) are the following:—

A'QUA DESTILLA'TA.* [From *destil'lo, destilla'tum*, to "distil."] Distilled water, having a vapid taste from the absence of air, and slightly empyreumatic, in consequence, probably, of the presence of a small quantity of extractive matter which has undergone partial decomposition.

A'QUA EX FLU'MINE.* [From *flu'men, flu'minis*, a "river."] Literally, "water from the river." River-water, generally of considerable purity, but liable to hold in suspension particles of earthy matter, which impair its transparency and sometimes its salubrity.

A'QUA EX LA'CU.* [From *la'cus*, a "lake."] Lake-water. A collection of rain, spring, and river waters, sometimes contaminated with various animal and vegetable bodies, which, from its stagnant nature, have undergone putrefaction in it.

A'QUA EX NI'VE.* [From *nix, ni'vis*, "snow."] Snow-water, differing apparently from rain-water only in being destitute of air, to which water is indebted for its briskness and many of its good effects upon animals and vegetables.

A'QUA EX PALU'DE.* [From *pa'lus, palu'dis*, a "marsh" or "swamp."] Marsh-water; the most impure, as being the most stagnant, of all water, and generally loaded with decomposing vegetable matter.

A'QUA EX PU'TEO.* [From *pu'teus*, a "well."] Well-water; essentially the same as spring-water, being derived from the same source, but more liable to impurity from its stagnation or slow infiltration.

A'QUA FONTA'NA.* [From *fons, fon'tis*, a "fountain."] Spring-water; containing, in addition to carbonic acid and carbonate of lime, a small portion of muriate of soda, and frequently other salts. Spring-water which dissolves soap is termed soft; that which decomposes and curdles it is called hard.

A'QUA MARI'NA.* [From *ma're*, the "sea."] Sea-water; containing sulphate of soda, the muriates of soda, magnesia, and lime, a minute proportion of potash, and various animal and vegetable bodies.

A'QUA PLUVIA'LIS.* [From *a'qua*, "water," and *plu'via*, "rain."] Rain-water; the purest form of natural water, yet holding in solution carbonic acid, a minute portion of carbonate of lime, and traces of muriate of lime.

Aqua Ammoniæ. See LIQUOR AMMONIÆ.

Aqua Amygdalæ Amaræ. See BITTER ALMONDS, WATER OF.

A'qua Bĭ-nel'lĭ.* An Italian quack medicine, supposed to be a solution of creasote, and celebrated at Naples for arresting hæmorrhage.

Aqua Calcis. See LIQUOR CALCIS.

Aqua Camphoræ. See CAMPHOR.

A'qua Cha-lўb-e-a'ta.* An artificial mineral water, consisting of a solution of citrate of iron highly charged with carbonic acid gas and flavored by a little aromatized syrup.

A'qua For'tis.* ("Strong Water.") A name formerly applied to nitric acid, on account of its powerfully corrosive properties. It is distinguished by the terms *double* and *single*, the latter being only half the strength of the former. Concentrated nitric acid, however, is much stronger even than double nitric acid.

A'qua Re'gĭ-a.* ("Royal Water.") A mixture of nitric and muriatic acids.

A'qua Vi'tæ.* ("Water of Life.") Ardent spirits of the first distillation.

Aquæ,* a'kwē, gen. **A-qua'rum,** the plural of **A'qua.** "Water."

A'quæ Min-e-ra'lēs.* [From *minera'lis*, a modern Latin term for our word "mineral."] "Mineral waters;" a term conventionally applied to such waters as are distinguished from spring, lake, river, or other waters by peculiarities of color, taste, smell, or real or supposed medicinal effects. Mineral waters are of four principal kinds:—

ACID'ULOUS. Owing their properties chiefly to carbonic acid: they are tonic and diuretic, and in large doses produce a transient exhilaration.

CHALYB'EATE. Containing iron in the form of sulphate, carbonate, or muriate: they have a styptic, inky taste.

SA-LINE'. Mostly purgative, and advantageously employed in those hypochondriacal and visceral diseases which require continued and moderate relaxation of the bowels.

SULPHU'REOUS. Deriving their character from sulphuretted hydrogen.

Aquæ Stillatitiæ,* a'kwē stil-la-tish'e-ē, also called **A'quæ Destilla'tæ.*** Distilled waters; waters impregnated with the essential oil of vegetables, principally designed as grateful vehicles for the exhibition of more active remedies.

Aq'ue-duct. [**Aquæduc'tus;** from *a'qua*, "water," and *duc'tus*, a "canal" or "passage."] Literally, a "passage for water," though applied in Anatomy to several canals in the body not always containing fluid.

Aq'ueduct of the Coch'le-a. [**Aquæduc'tus Coch'leæ.**] A foramen of the temporal bone, for the transmission of a small vein from the cochlea.

Aq'ueduct of Fal-lo'pĭ-us. [**Aquæduc'tus Fallo'pii.**] The canal by which the portio dura winds through the petrous portion of the temporal bone

Aq'ueduct of Sўl'vĭ-us. [**Aquæduc'tus Syl'vii.**] The canal which extends backwards under the tubercula quadrigemina into the fourth ventricle of the brain.

Aq'ueduct of the Ves-tib'u-lum or **of the Ves'tĭ-būle** [**Aquæduc'tus Vestib'uli**], also called the **Aq'ueduct of Co-tun'nĭ-us** [**Aquæduc'tus Cotun'nii**]. The commencement of a small canal which opens upon the posterior surface of the petrous portion of the temporal bone of the cranium and transmits a small vein.

Aqueous, ā'kwe-ŭs. A term now coming into use for designating definite combinations with water. The term *hydrate* has long been employed for the same purpose. A prefix is used when there is more than one atom, as in *bin*-aqueous, *ter*-hydrate.

Aq'ueous Hu'mor. A colorless fluid in the anterior and posterior chambers of the eye.

Aquila,* ak'wĭ-lạ. Literally, an "eagle." A term which had formerly many epithets joined with it to denote particular substances: thus, *aquila alba*, seu *mitigata*, was one of the fanciful names of calomel.

Aquula,* ak'wul-ạ. [The diminutive of *a'qua*, "water."] Literally, a "small particle of water." Applied to any small aqueous tumor, and sometimes to a fatty tumor under the skin of the eyelid.

Aq'uula A-cous'tĭ-cạ.* The fluid in the cavity of the vestibule of the internal ear.

Ar'ạ-bic, Gum. See GUMMI ACACIÆ. [This word is very often pronounced *a-ră'bic*, a fault to be most carefully avoided by all those who desire to speak correctly.]

Araceæ,* ạ-ra'she-ē, or **Aroideæ,*** ar-o-i'de-ē. The *Arum* tribe of monocotyledonous plants, containing an acrid and in some cases a highly dangerous principle.

A-rach'nĭ-dạ,* **A-rach'nĭ-dēs.*** [From ἀράχνη, a "spider."] The third class of the *Diplo-gangliata* or *Entomoida*, comprising articulated animals, generally with four pairs of legs, without wings or metamorphosis.

A-rach-nĭ'tis, idis.* [From ἀράχνη, a "spider," also a "spider's web."] A faulty term, denoting inflammation of the arachnoid membrane.

A-rach'noid. [**Arachnoi'des;** from ἀράχνη, a "spider's web," and εἶδος, "form" or "resemblance."] Resembling a spider's web. Applied to the second or middle membrane of the brain.

Arachnoid Canal. See BICHAT, CANAL OF.

Arach'noid Mem'brane. *Men'inx media.* The fine *cobweb-like* membrane situated between the dura and pia mater. It is the serous membrane of the cerebro-spinal centres.

A-rach'no-ĭ-dĭ'tis,* or **A-rach-nĭ'-tis.*** Inflammation of the arachnoid membrane.

Arack. See ARRACK.

Ar-æ-om'e-ter, or **Ar-e-om'e-ter.** [From ἀραιός, "thin," "light," and μέτρον, a "measure."] An instrument for determining the specific gravity of liquids into which it is plunged, by the depth to which its weight causes it to sink in them. This instrument is also termed a *hydrom'eter*. The art or process of measuring the density or gravity of liquids is termed *aræom'etry*.

A-ra'lĭ-ạ Can-ạ-den'sis.* Another name for the *Panax Quinquefolium*, or Ginseng.

Ara'lia His'pĭ-dạ,* or Dwarf Elder. A plant sometimes used in dropsy in the form of decoction.

Ara'lia Nu-dĭ-cau'lis,* or Wild Sarsaparilla, is a stimulant tonic and diaphoretic. It is sometimes used as a substitute for the true sarsaparilla. It is known also by the names of American Spikenard (*Nar'dus America'nus*) and Small Spikenard, etc.

Ara'lia Raç-e-mo'sạ,* or American Spikenard, is analogous in its medical properties to the preceding.

Araliaceæ,* a-ra-le-a'she-ē. A natural order of plants of the *Aralia* tribe.

A-rā-lĭ-ā'ceous. [**Aralia'ceus.**] Having an arrangement as in the *Aralia*.

Ar-ạ-ne'ĭ-dæ.* [From *ara'nea*, a "spider."] A family of the *Arachnides Pulmonariæ*.

A-rā'ne-ous. [**Araneo'sus;** from *ara'neum*, a "spider's web."] Of the nature of spider's web.

Arantii (a-ran'she-i), **Cor'pŏ-rạ.*** Small tubercles, one in each semilunar valve of the aorta and pulmonary arteries; called also *Corpora sesamoidea* and *Noduli Arantii*.

Ar'bor, oris.* A "tree." A plant having a single trunk, rising high, durable, woody, and divided into branches which do not perish in winter. In Chemistry it is applied to any crystallization which ramifies like a tree.

Ar'bor Di-a'næ.* A "silver tree." [From *Dia'na*, the "moon," and hence, like *luna*, denoting "silver."] A beautiful arborescent precipitate of silver produced by throwing mercury into a dilute solution of lunar caustic (nitrate of silver).

Ar'bor Ma'ris.* [From *ma're*, gen. *ma'ris*, the "sea."] The "tree of the sea." A name given to coral.

Ar'bor Min-e-ra'lis Phil-o-soph'-ĭ-ca,* Ar'bor Phĭ-los'o-pho'rum.* The *Arbor Dianæ*.

Ar'bor Vi'tæ.* [From *vi'ta*, "life."] Literally, the "tree of life." Applied to the thick mass of white substance in either hemisphere of the *cerebellum*. This mass, when cut parallel to the median line, presents an arborescent or tree-like appearance, caused by the intermixture of the white substance with the cineritious. Also applied to the tree called *Thu'ya Occidenta'lis*.

Ar-bo're-ous. [**Arbo'reus;** from *ar'bor*, a "tree."] Belonging to a tree; dendroid.

Ar-bo-rĕs'çent. [**Arbores'cens;** from *arbores'co*, to "grow like a tree."] Growing like a tree; resembling a tree.

Ar-bus'cu-la.* [The diminutive of *ar'bor*, a "tree."] Applied to the *branchiæ* of certain *Anellata:* an ar'buscule or ar'buscle.

Ar'bu-tus U'va Ur'si.* The trailing arbutus, or bear's whortleberry; now called *Arctostaphylos uva ursi*.

Arc. [**Ar'cus;** see ARCH.] Any part of the circumference of a circle.

Ar'ca Ar-ca-no'rum.* Literally, a "chest of secrets." The alchemical name of the philosopher's stone.

Ar-ca'na,* gen. **Ar-ca-no'rum,** the plural of ARCANUM, which see.

Ar-ca'num.* [From *ar'ca*, a "chest" or "coffer" in which precious things were carefully kept.] A secret. A nostrum or medicine the composition of which is concealed.

Arch. [**Ar'cus.**] Literally, a "bow." A bending in the form of a bow. Any arc, or part of the circumference of a circle.

Arch, Fem'o-ral. [**Ar'cus Femora'lis.**] The name of a considerable arch formed over the concave border of the pelvis. It is bounded above by Poupart's ligament, below by the border of the pubes and ilium. Also termed the crural arch.

Arch of the A-or'ta. The curved parts between the ascending and descending portions.

Archencephalus,* ark-en-sef'a-lŭs. [From ἀρχός, "chief," and ἐγκέφαλον, the "brain."] Applied by Galen to man, because of the intellectual development of his brain: archenceph'alous.

Ar-che-ol'o-ġy̆. [**Archæolo'gia;** from ἀρχαῖος, "ancient," and λόγος, a "discourse."] A discourse or treatise on ancient things or antiquities. The science or knowledge of antiquities.

Ar'che-tȳpe. [**Archet'ypus;** from ἀρχή, "beginning," "origin," and τύπος, a "type."] The original type on which others are formed.

Ar'chil (*ch* as in child). A violet-red paste, prepared from the Lichen Roccella, or Orseille, and other species of lichen, and used in dyeing.

The plant (Lichen Roccella), reduced to a pulp and treated with impure ammoniacal liquor, yields a rich purple tincture, called *litmus*, or turnsole, used in Chemistry as a test.

Ar-chop-to'ma,* or **Ar-chop-to'-sis.*** [From ἀρχός, the "anus," and πτῶμα, or πτῶσις, a "falling."] Prolapsus ani. A descent of the rectum. See PROLAPSUS.

Ar-cho-sy̆r'inx.* [From ἀρχός, the "anus," and σῦριγξ, a "pipe," "fistula."] Another term for *fistula in ano*.

Ar'çĭ-form. [**Arcifor'mis;** from *ar'cus*, a "bow" or "arch."] Formed like an arch.

Ar'ciform Fi'bres. A term applied by Mr. Solly to a set of fibres which proceed from the corpus pyramidale and pass outwards beneath the corpus olivare to the cerebellum. He distinguishes them into two layers, the *superficial cerebellar* and *deep cerebellar fibres*.

Arctatio,* ark-ta'she-o. [From *arc'to*, *arcta'tum*, to "bind closely," to "make narrow."] Constipation of the intestines; also, a preternatural contraction of the vagina.

Arc'tic. [**Arc'ticus;** Gr. ἀρκτικός, "belonging to the north," from Ἄρκτος, the constellation called "The Bear," situated near the North Pole.] North; northern.

Arc'tic Cir'cle. A circle extending $23\frac{1}{2}$ degrees from the North Pole, marking that portion of the northern hemisphere within which the sun at the summer solstice does not set.

Arc'tĭ-um Lap'pa.* The herb called burdock, belonging to the Linnæan class *Syngenesia* and to the natural order

Compositæ. The seeds are cathartic, the root diuretic and diaphoretic. A decoction of the leaves is sometimes used in cutaneous diseases.

Arc-to-staph'ȳ-los.* [From ἄρκτος, a "bear," and σταφυλή, a "grape."] A Linnæan genus of the class *Decandria*, natural order *Ericaceæ* or *Ericineæ*. The term signifies the same as *uva ursi*, *i.e.* "bear-grape."

Arctostaph'ylos U'va Ur'si.* Another name for the *Arbutus uva ursi*. See Uva Ursi.

Ar-cu-a'lis.* [From *ar'cuo*, to "bend like a bow."] Applied to the coronal suture, or *Sutu'ra arcua'lis*, and to the temporal bones, or *Os'sa arcua'lia*.

Arcuatio,* ar-ku-a'she-o. [From *ar'cuo*, *arcua'tum*, to "bend like a bow."] A gibbosity, or curvature, of the dorsal vertebræ, the sternum, or the tibia.

Ar'cus.* A bow, arc, or arch. The periphery of any part of a circle.

Ar'cus Se-ni'lis.* A peculiar arched, or circular, opaque appearance on the eyes of old men, round the margin of the *cornea*.

Ar-de'ĭ-dæ.* [From *ar'dea*, a "heron."] A family having the *Ardea* for their type.

Ar'dent Spir'its. [From *ar'dens*, "burning," a participle of *ar'deo*, to "be hot," to "burn."] A term applied to distilled alcoholic liquors.

Ar'dor, o'ris.* [From *ar'deo*, to "burn."] Intense or morbidly increased sensation of heat.

Ar'dor Fe-bri'lis.* Feverish or febrile heat.

Ar'dor U-ri'næ.* A sensation in the inflamed urethra as if the passing urine were scalding hot.

Ar'dor Ven-tric'u-li.* Heartburn; also called *Ar'dor stom'achi*.

A're-a.* An open space. The internal capacity of any given boundary or limit.

A'rea Dif'fluens [from *dif'fluo*, to "spread"] and A'rea Ser'pens [from *ser'po*, to "creep"] are terms applied by Celsus to different forms of baldness. The latter is the same as Ophiasis, which see.

A'rea Ger-mĭ-na-ti'va.* An opaque spot on the blastodermic vesicle in an egg, opposite to the insertion of the *Mesometrium*.

A'rea O-pa'ca.* A dull circle surrounding the *Area pellucida*, formed by the *Area germinativa* becoming clear in the centre. See preceding article.

A-re'ca.* The betel-nut, the fruit of the *Are'ca Cat'echu*, belonging to the natural order *Palmæ*. It is tonic and astringent, and forms one of the principal ingredients of the *Betel*, so extensively used in the East as a masticatory. See Betel.

Ar-e-fac'tion. [**Arefac'tio, o'nis**; from *a'reo*, "to be dry," and *fa'cio*, to "make."] A mode of drying medicinal substances, by which they may be reduced to dust or powder.

Ar-e-nā'ceous. [**Arena'ceus**; from *are'na*, "sand."] Of the nature of sand; sandy.

Ar-e-nā'rĭ-ous. [**Arena'rius**; from *are'na*, "sand."] Growing in sandy soil.

Ar-e-nic'o-la,* and **Ar-e-nic'o-lus.*** [From *are'na*, "sand," and *co'lo*, to "inhabit."] Inhabiting sandy places.

Ar'e-nose. [**Areno'sus**; from *are'na*, "sand."] Full of sand; sandy.

A-re'o-la.* [The diminutive of *a'rea*.] The halo, or small reddish or brownish circular space, round the nipple of females. Also applied to the circle surrounding certain pustules, such as the vaccine pustule.

Are'ola Pap-ĭl-la'ris.* [From *papil'la*, a "nipple."] The areola round the nipple. See Areola.

A-re'o-læ* (the plural of *are'ola*) is used by anatomists to denote the interstices between the fibres of an organ, or between vessels interlacing with each other.

A-re'o-lar. [**Areola'ris**; from *are'ola*, a "small, open space."] Containing *areolæ*, or small spaces. *Areolar tissue* is the cellular tissue of some writers, named from the interstices which it contains.

A-re'o-lāt-ed. [**Areola'tus.**] Having *areolæ*.

Areometer and **Areometry.** See Aræometer.

Ar'gand Lamp. A name applied to lamps with hollow or circular wicks, first invented by Argand about 1782. The intention of them is to furnish a more rapid supply of air to the flame, and to afford this air to the centre as well as to the outside of the flame.

Ar'ge-ma* or **Ar'ge-mon.*** [From ἀργός, "white."] A small white ulcer of the eye, described by Hippocrates.

Ar-ge-mo'ne.* [From ἄργεμον, a "disease of the eye,"—named from the supposed virtues of one species in curing diseases of the eye.] A genus of plants belonging to the poppy tribe, or *Papaveraceæ.* The *Argemo'ne Mexica'na,* or Thorn Poppy, contains a juice which, when dried, resembles gamboge, and has been used as a hydragogue cathartic. The seeds are sometimes employed as a substitute for ipecacuanha.

Ar'ġen-tāte of Am-mo'nĭ-a. The substance otherwise called FULMINATING SILVER, which see.

Ar-ġen'ti Ni'tras.* "Nitrate of Silver," or lunar caustic; one of the most important and one of the most extensively used of all caustic substances.

Ar-ġen-tif'er-ous. [**Argentif'erus;** from *argen'tum,* "silver," and *fe'ro,* to "bear."] Bearing, or containing silver. Applied to minerals or ores.

Ar'ġen-tīne. [**Argenti'nus;** from *argen'tum,* "silver."] Having the appearance, brightness, or clear sound of silver.

Ar'gentine Flow'ers of An'ti-mo-nȳ. The sesquioxide of antimony, frequently occurring in the form of small, shining needles of silvery whiteness. See ANTIMONY.

Ar-ġen'tum.* [From ἀργός, "white."] Silver; the whitest of metals. It occurs native,—that is, in the metallic state,—and is also obtained from the ores of lead. It is employed in Pharmacy chiefly or solely in the preparation of the nitrate.

Argen'tum Fo-lĭ-a'tum.* [From *fo'lium,* a "leaf."] Silver-leaf; used for covering pills and other substances.

Argen'tum Fu-ġĭ-ti'vum,* Argen'tum Mob'ĭ-le.* The *Argentum vivum,* or quicksilver.

Argentum Musivum. See MOSAIC SILVER.

Argen'tum Vi'vum.* The metal *Hydrar'gyrum,* or mercury; quicksilver.

Ar-ġil'la.* [From ἀργός, "white."] *Alumina,* or pure clay: ar'gil.

Ar-ġil-lā'ceous. [**Argilla'ceus;** from *argil'la,* "clay."] Of the nature of clay.

Ar-ġil-lif'er-ous. [**Argillif'erus;** from *argil'la,* "clay," and *fe'ro,* to "bear."] Containing clay as an accidental ingredient.

Ar'ġil-loid. [**Argilloi'des;** from *argil'la,* "clay," and εἶδος, a "form."] Resembling argil.

Ar'gŏl, or **Ar'gal.** [Fr. *Tartre brut,* tartR brü; "raw" or "coarse tartar."] Wine-stone, or crude tartar; an acidulous concrete salt, deposited by wine, and used by dyers as a mordant.

Ar-ġȳr'ĭ-a.* [From ἄργυρος, "silver."] Disease caused by the use, or abuse, of salts of silver.

Arhythmous, a-rith'mŭs. [**A-rhyth'mus;** from *a,* priv., and ῥυθμός, "number."] Without rhythm or regularity of the pulse.

Ar-ĭ-çi'na.* An alkaloid found in cinchona bark, and very analogous in its properties to cinchonia and quinia. These three alkaloids may be viewed as oxides of the same compound radicle.

Ar'il,* or **A-ril'lus.*** [From *a'reo,* to "be dried up."] A botanical term, signifying a peculiar exterior coat of some seeds; thus the mace is the aril of the nutmeg.

Ar'il-late or **Ar'il-lāt-ed.** [**Arilla'tus.**] Having arils; formed like an aril.

Arillus. See ARIL.

A-ris'ta.* [From *a'reo,* to "be dry."] A term in Botany, denoting the beard of the husk of grasses; the awn.

A-ris'tate. [**Arista'tus;** from *aris'ta.*] Having an awn or long rigid spine; awned; bearded.

A-ris-to-lo'chĭ-a,* or **A-ris'to-lo-chi'a.*** [From ἄριστος, the "best," and λοχεία, or λόχια, "childbirth;" also, "LOCHIA" (which see); because it promotes recovery after childbirth.] Birthwort. A Linnæan genus of the class *Gynandria,* natural order *Aristolochiaceæ.*

Aristolo'chia Ser-pen-ta'rĭ-a.* The *Serpenta'ria Virginia'na,* or Virginia Snake-Root: so named because supposed to be an antidote to the poison of serpents. It is a stimulant and tonic, and is given in cases of debility, and especially in intermittents.

A-ris-to-lo'chĭ-æ,* the plural of **Aristolochia.** The Jussieuan name of a natural order of plants. See ARISTOLOCHIACEÆ.

Aristolochiaceæ,* a-ris-to-lo-ke-a'she-ē, or **A-ris-to-lo'chĭ-æ.*** A natural order of plants resembling the *Aristolochia.* They are tonic and stimulant.

Arm. [**Bra'chium.**] The upper extremity from the shoulder to the wrist, divided by the elbow-joint into the arm proper and the fore-arm.

Ar-ma'rĭ-um.* [From *ar'ma,* "arms" or "implements."] A store of medicines, instruments, &c.

Ar-me'nĭ-an Bole. [**Bo'lus Armе'niæ.**] A pale, red-colored earth, used as a remedy against *aphthæ;* also in tooth-powders, etc.

Ar-mil'la,* plural **Ar-mil'læ.** [From *armil'la,* a "bracelet."] The name of the membranous ligaments confining the tendons of the carpus.

Ar'mil-la-ry. [**Armilla'ris;** from the same.] Applied in Astronomy to an artificial sphere formed of circles, representing orbs of celestial bodies. Also a term applied to plants having leaves like bracelets.

Armora'ciæ (ar-mo-ra'she-ē) **Ra'dix.*** Horseradish-root. See COCHLEARIA ARMORACIA.

Ar'mus.* [From ἀρμός, a "joint."] The shoulder or arm.

Ar-năl'dĭ-a.* A disease formerly known in England, and attended with alopecia, or baldness.

Ar'nĭ-ca.* [From ἄρς, ἀρνός, a "lamb;" from the softness of its leaf.] A Linnæan genus of the class *Syngenesia,* natural order *Compositæ.* Also, the Pharmacopœial name for *Arnica montana.*

Ar'nica Mon-ta'na.* Leopard's bane. This plant is celebrated as a remedy for bruises, and hence has been called *panace'a lapso'rum* (the "panacea of the fallen,"—*i.e.* of those who have had a fall occasioning a severe injury).

Ar'nĭ-çin. [**Arnici'na.**] A bitter resin, the active principle of *Arnica montana.*

A-roi'de-ous. [**Aroi'deus;** from *A'rum,*"Wake-robin," and εἶδος, a "form."] Resembling the Arum, or Wake-robin. The Latin term in the plural feminine (*Aroi'deæ*) forms the name of a natural order of plants. See ARACEÆ.

A-ro'ma,* gen. **A-ro'ma-tis,** plural **A-ro'ma-ta.** [Perhaps from ἀρι, intensive, and ὀδμή, "odor."] The fragrant principle of plants and substances derived from them.

Ar-o-mat'ic. [**Aromat'icus;** from *aro'ma.*] Odoriferous; having an agreeable smell, as spices and such substances.

Ar-o-mat'ĭ-cus Cor'tex.* ("Aromatic bark.") The bark of *Canella alba,* or wild cinnamon.

Arquebusade, Eau d' (Fr.), ō-dark'-bü'zăd'. [From *ar'quebus,* a "hand-gun."] *A'qua Vulnera'ria.* A lotion composed of vinegar, sulphuric acid, honey, alcohol, and various aromatics; originally applied to wounds inflicted by the arquebus.

Ar'rack, or **Ar-rak',** written also **Ar'ack.** An intoxicating beverage made in India by distilling fermented juice of various kinds, but especially from *toddy,* the sweet sap of the palm-tree.

Ar'ra-go-nīte. A species of carbonate of lime, from Aragon, in Spain.

Arrectores Pilorum. See PILORUM ARRECTORES.

Ar-rest'ed. A term used in obstetrics when the head of the child is hindered, *but not impacted,* in the pelvic cavity,—a distinction of the greatest importance.

Ar'row-Root. The fecula or starch from the root of the *Maranta arundinacea* and *M. Indica,* named from its supposed efficacy in poisoned wounds (wounds from poisoned arrows). Arrow-root is also obtained from the root of the *Arum maculatum* and other plants.

Arrow-Shaped. See SAGITTATE and SAGITTALIS.

Ar-se'nĭ-āte. [**Arse'nias, a'***tis;* from *arsen'icum* *aç'idum.*] A combination of arsenious acid with any base.

Ar'sen-ic. [**Arsen'icum;** from ἄρσην, "masculine," "vigorous;" in allusion to its strong and acrimonious properties.] A metal plentifully met with in nature, generally in union with sulphur, or with other metals, or with oxygen, etc. Though arsenic in its metallic state is not dangerous, it is readily converted into a poisonous oxide, and all of its soluble compounds are more or less poisonous. Arsenic is also the common name for arsenious acid, sometimes called white oxide of arsenic, *arsen'icum al'bum* ("white arsenic"), ratsbane, and other names. This is the most common form in which arsenic is found in commerce. The only known antidote for this poison is the hydrated sesquioxide (or peroxide) of iron, which has been found much more efficacious when freshly prepared. This substance produces (by a transfer of a portion of the oxygen from the iron to the acid) an insoluble and therefore inert subarseniate of the protoxide of iron. That this antidote may be perfectly successful, it should be preceded by the use of emetics, or the stomach-pump. See POISONS.

Ar-sen'ĭ-cal. [**Arsenica'lis.**] Belonging to arsenic or arsenious acid.

Arsenical Paste. See PÂTE ARSENICALE.

Arsenicalis Liquor. See LIQUOR ARSENICALIS.

Ar-sen'ĭ-ci Al'bum Ox'ȳd-um Ve-na'le.* (The "white oxide of arsenic of commerce.") The Pharmacopœial name (Dub. Ph.) of arsenious acid, or sublimed oxide of arsenic.

Ar-sen'ĭ-cum Al'bum.* ("White

arsenic") The Pharmacopœial name (Ed. Ph.) of arsenious acid, or sesquioxide of arsenic.

Ar-se'nĭ-ous Aç'id. The *Acidum arseniosum* (U. S. and British Ph.), *Arsenicum album* (Ed. Ph.), or sesquioxide of arsenic, *Arsenici album oxydum venale* (Dub. Ph.). See Arsenic.

Ar'se-nīte. [**Ar'senis, i'**tis.] A combination of arsenious acid with a base.

Arseniuret, ar-sĕn'yu-rĕt. [**Arseniure'tum.**] A combination of arsenic with a metallic or other base.

Ar-sen'o-vin'ic Aç'id. An acid produced by the action of arsenic on alcohol.

Ar-tan'the E-lon-ga'tạ.* A name of the *Matico* plant. See Matico.

Artemisia,* ar-te-mish'e-ạ. [Gr. Ἀρτεμισία, perhaps because sacred to Diana, in Greek Ἄρτεμις.] A Linnæan genus of the natural order *Compositæ.*

Artemis'ia A-brot'ạ-num,* or Southernwood, formerly used as a tonic and anthelmintic.

Artemis'ia Ab-sin'thĭ-um.* Common wormwood, also called *Absinthium commune* and *Absinthium vulgare.*

Artemis'ia Chi-nen'sis.* The Chinese wormwood, or mugwort of China.

Artemis'ia Dra-cunc'u-lus.* Tarragon: a plant which is used to impart a peculiar stimulating flavor to vinegar.

Artemis'ia In'dĭ-cạ.* Indian wormwood, used similarly to *Chinensis.*

Artemis'ia Ju-da'ĭ-cạ.* The same as Artemisia Santonica.

Artemis'ia Lat-ĭ-fo'lĭ-ạ.* The same as Artemisia Chinensis.

Artemis'ia San-ton'ĭ-cạ.* Tartarian southernwood, wormwood, or worm-seed plant.

Ar-tem'ĭ-sin. [**Artemisi'na.**] The bitter principle of *Artemis'a absinthium.*

Artère, ar'tair', the French term for Artery, which see.

Arteria. See Artery.

Ar-te'rĭ-a As'per-ạ.* The "rough artery;" the trachea or windpipe: so called because of the inequalities or roughness of its surface.

Arte'ria In-nom-ĭ-na'tạ.* The "unnamed artery;" the first branch given off from the aorta, dividing into the right carotid and right subclavian arteries.

Arte'ria Mag'nạ.* (The "great artery.") The aorta.

Ar-te'rĭ-ac, or **Ar-te-rī'ạ-cal.** [**Arteri'acus.**] Pertaining to the *Arteria aspera,* or windpipe. Applied to medicines for disorders of the voice or diseases of the windpipe.

Ar-te'rĭ-æ,* gen. **Ar-te-rĭ-a'rum,** the plural of **Arte'ria,** an artery.

Arteriæ Venosæ,* ar-te're-ē veno'sē, the plural of **Arte'ria Veno'sa.** Literally, "venous arteries,"—a name sometimes given to the four pulmonary veins, because they contain arterial blood.

Ar-te'rĭ-al. [**Arteria'lis;** from *arte'ria,* an "artery."] Belonging to an artery.

Arterial Duct. See Ductus Arteriosus.

Ar-te-rĭ-og'rạ-phy̆. [**Arteriogra'phia;** from *arte'ria,* an "artery," and γράφω, to "write."] A description of the arteries.

Ar-te-rĭ-ol'o-ġy̆. [**Arteriolo'gia;** from *arte'ria,* an "artery," and λόγος, a "discourse."] A treatise on the arteries; the science of the arteries.

Ar-te-rĭ-o'sus.* [From *arte'ria,* an "artery."] Having numerous arteries; of the nature of an artery.

Arteriosus, Ductus. See Ductus Arteriosus.

Ar-te-rĭ-ot'o-my̆. [**Arterioto'mia;** from ἀρτηρία, an "artery," and τέμνω, to "cut."] The cutting into, dividing, or opening an artery.

Ar-te-ri'tis.* [From *arte'ria,* an "artery."] Inflammation of an artery.

Ar'ter-y̆. [**Arte'ria,** plural **Arte'riæ;** from ἀήρ, "air or spirit," and τηρέω, to "keep" or "preserve," the arteries having been supposed by the ancients to contain air.] One of the vessels by which the blood is conveyed from the heart towards the various organs and members of the body.

Artesian, ar-te'zhạn. [From *Artois,* Lat. *Arte'sia,* a province of France, in which they were first formed.] A term applied to certain wells or fountains produced by boring through various strata deep enough to reach a subterranean body of water, the sources of which are higher than the mouth of the well.

Ar'thra-grạ.* [From ἄρθρον, a "joint," and ἄγρα, a "seizure."] Same as Arthritis or gout.

Ar-thrăl'ġĭ-ạ.* [From ἄρθρον, a "joint," and ἄλγος, "pain."] Chronic pain of a joint; gout or rheumatism.

Ar-thrit'ic. [**Arthrit'icus.**] Belonging to *Arthritis,* or to gout.

Ar-thri'tis, idis.* [From ἄρθρον, a "joint."] Literally, "inflammation of a joint:" gout. See Podagra.

Arthri'tis Pla-net'ĭ-cạ,* Arthri'tis Rheū-mat'ĭ-cạ,* Arthri'tis

Va'gạ.* Other names for wandering or erratic gout. See PODAGRA.

Ar-thro-c'ạ-ce.* [From ἄρθρον, a "joint," and κάκη, "disease."] An ulcerated condition or caries of the cavity of a bone. Also used as synonymous with *Spina ventosa.*

Ar-thro'dĭ-ạ.* [From ἄρθρον, a "joint."] An articulation admitting of motion on all sides; a variety of *Diarthrosis.*

Ar-thro-dȳn'ĭ-ạ.* [From ἄρθρον, a "joint," and ὀδύνη, "pain."] Pain in a joint, or chronic rheumatism.

Ar-throg'rạ-phȳ. [**Arthrogra'phia;** from ἄρθρον, a "joint," and γράφω, to "write."] A description of the joints.

Ar-throl'o-ġȳ. [**Arthrolo'gia;** from ἄρθρον, a "joint," and λόγος, a "discourse."] A treatise on the joints; the science of joints.

Ar-thron'cus.* [From ἄρθρον, a "joint," and ὄγκος, a "mass," a "swelling."] A distinct cartilaginous body (one or more) which sometimes forms within the knee-joint. Sometimes applied to the tumefaction of a joint.

Ar-thro-pa-thi'ạ.* [From ἄρθρον, a "joint," and πάθος, an "affection."] An affection of the shoulder-joint, with violent pain and swelling of the brachial portion.

Ar-thro-phlo-go'sis.* [From ἄρθρον, a "joint," and φλογόω, to "inflame."] Inflammation of a joint. See ARTHRITIS.

Ar-thro-pu-o'sis.* [From ἄρθρον, a "joint," and πύον, "pus."] Pus in a joint.

Ar-thro'sĭ-ạ.* [From ἄρθρον, a "joint."] Generic name for articular inflammation, according to Dr. Good.

Ar-thro'sis.* [From ἀρθρόω, to "fasten by joints."] Articulation, or connection by joints.

Artichoke. See CYNARA SCOLYMUS.

Ar-tic-u-la'ris.* [From *artic'ulus,* a "joint."] Relating to joints; articular. Applied to arteries, muscles, etc., connected with the joints.

Articula'ris Ġe'nu.* This and the term *subcrurœus* have been applied to a few detached muscular fibres frequently found under the lower part of the cruralis and attached to the capsule of the knee-joint.

Articula'ris Mor'bus.* The same as ARTHRITIS, or gout.

Articulata. See ARTICULATUS.

Ar-tic-u-lā'tion. [**Articula'tio, o'nis;** from *artic'ulus,* a "joint," *artic'ulo, articula'tum,* to "joint," to "make a joint."] The fastening together of the various bones of the skeleton in their natural situation; a joint. Also the distinct utterance of syllables or words.

The articulations of the bones of the body are divided into *synarthroses,* immovable articulations, and *diarthroses,* movable articulations. See DIARTHROSIS, SYNARTHROSIS.

Ar-tic-u-la'tus.* [From the same.] Articulated, jointed, or knotted. Applied in the plural neuter (*Articula'ta*) to the third great division of the animal kingdom, in which articulated rings encircle the body, and frequently the limbs.

Ar-tic'u-li,* gen. **Ar-tiç-u-lo'rum,** plural of **Artic'ulus.**

Ar-tic'u-lus.* [The diminutive of *ar'tus,* a "joint."] A joint, or articulation: a member, or limb. Applied in Botany to that part of the stalk between two knots or joints; also, a knot or joint.

Ar-tĭ-fĭ'çial A'nus. An opening made in the parietes of the abdomen, through which the feces are discharged during life; also an opening made in the natural situation in cases of imperforate anus.

Artifi'cial Eye. A hollow hemisphere, usually made of enamel, so as to present the appearance of the natural eye.

Artifi'cial Joint. A fracture united by the broken ends of the bone becoming rounded and smooth and connected by a fibrous, ligamentous substance; a false joint.

Artifi'cial Pu'pil. The result of an operation for overcoming the effect of adhesions or permanent contraction of the iris.

Ar-to-car'pus.* [From ἄρτος, "bread," and καρπός, "fruit."] A genus of plants growing in Southern India and Polynesia. The *Artocar'pus inci'sa* is the bread-fruit proper; the *Artocar'pus integrifo'lia* has a very coarse fruit, called Jack-fruit, common in the South of India. See BREAD-FRUIT.

Arundinaceus,* a-rŭn-de-na'she-ŭs. [From *arun'do,* a "reed."] Belonging to a reed; resembling a reed. Applied in the feminine plural (*Arundinaceæ,* a-run-de-na'she-ē) to a tribe of plants having the *Arundo* for its type: arundina'ceous.

A-rȳt'æ-no-ĭ-dæ'us.* [See the two following articles.] Belonging to the arytenoid cartilages. The *arytænoidæus* muscle is a muscle extending from one of the arytenoid cartilages to the other.

A-rўt'e-noid. [**Arytænoi'des;** from ἀρύταινα, a "pitcher," and εἶδος, a "form."] Resembling the mouth of a pitcher.

Arўt'enoid Car'tĭ-lag-es. [**Carti-lag'ines Arytænoi'des.**] Two cartilaginous bodies of the larynx, which, in their natural situation, resemble the mouth of a pitcher.

As-a-græ'a Of-fiç'ĭ-na'lis.* The name (Lond. Ph. 1851) of the plant from which *Veratria* is obtained.

A-saph'a-tŭm.* [From ἀσαφής, "obscure," "uncertain;" named in allusion to their deceptive appearance.] A term applied to the collections in the sebaceous follicles of the skin, which, when pressed out, appear like little worms.

A-sa'phĭ-a.* [Gr. ἀσαφής; from α, priv., and σαφής, "clear," "plain."] Defective utterance; a want of clearness of articulation or of speech.

A-sar-a-bac'ca.* The *Asarum Europæum.*

Asari Folia. See ASARUM EUROPÆUM.

Asarin. See ASARI FOLIA.

As'a-rum Can-a-den'se.* Canada snake-root, or Wild Ginger. The root is sometimes used as a substitute for ginger.

As'arum Eu-ro-pæ'um.* The plant *Asarabacca.* The leaves (*As'ari fo'lia*) abound in a bitter principle called *As'arin*, and are used as an errhine.

As-bes'tos.* [From α, priv., and σβέννυμι, to "extinguish."] Literally, "inextinguishable," "that which cannot be extinguished or destroyed." A mineral substance of a fibrous structure from which an incombustible linen is made. The ancients are said to have made use of cloth of asbestos to wrap the bodies of their dead before placing them on the funeral pile.

Ascarides. See ASCARIS.

As'ca-ris,* plural **As-căr'ĭ-dēs.** [Supposed to be derived from ἀσκαρίζω, to "leap," to "kick."] A genus of worms found in the human intestines.

As'caris Lum'brĭ-co-ĭ'dēs.* [From *lumbri'cus*, an "earth-worm."] One of the most common of intestinal worms, resembling the earth-worm.

As'caris Ver-mic-u-la'ris.* The thread-worm, now called OXYURIS.

As-çend'ing Ax'is. Applied to the stem of plants, or that part which grows in an opposite direction from the root (which is the *descending* axis). See AXIS.

As-cen'sus.* [From *ascen'do, ascen'sum*, to "climb," to "ascend."] Literally, an "ascending," or "ascent." Applied in Chemistry to the process of sublimation, formerly termed *Destillatio per ascensum.*

Ascen'sus Mor'bi.* The "ascent or increase of a disease."

Ascia,* ash'e-a. [The Latin term for an "axe" or "hatchet."] A bandage, so called from its shape, and described by Hippocrates.

Ascian. See ASCII.

As-çid'ĭ-āte. [**Ascidia'tus;** from *ascid'ium.*] Shaped like a small bottle or pitcher.

As-çid-ĭ-for'mis.* [From the same.] Formed like a small bottle or pitcher: ascid'iform.

As-çid'ĭ-um.* [From ἀσκίδιον (diminutive of ἀσκός), a "small leathern bag or bottle."] A hollow leaf resembling a small bottle or pitcher, as in the *Nepenthe* (pitcher-plant).

As-çig'ĕr-us.* [From ἀσκός, a "bag," and *ge'ro*, to "bear."] Bearing or containing utricles.

Ascii,* ash'e-i, the plural of **Ascius,** ash'e-ŭs. [From α, priv., and σκία, a "shade" or "shadow."] Literally, "without shadow." A term applied to the people of the Torrid Zone, who have twice in the year the sun perpendicular above their heads, and are without shadow.

As-çi'tēs.* [Gr. ἀσκίτης; from ἀσκός, a "sack of leather," "something swollen or puffed up."] *Hy'drops utricula'rius*, or dropsy of the belly. A genus of the natural order *Intumescentiæ*, class *Cachexiæ*, of Cullen's Nosology. See HYDROXÆLIA.

As-çit'ic. [**Ascit'icus.**] Having or pertaining to *Ascites.*

Asclepiadaceæ,* as-kle'pe-a-da'she-e. A natural order of plants resembling the *Asclepias.* The milky juice formed in plants of this order contains caoutchouc. It is emetic, and is sometimes a dangerous poison.

As-cle'pĭ-as, adis.* [From Ἀσκληπιός, the Greek name of Æsculapius, the god of medicine?] The name of a genus of plants belonging to the Linnæan class *Pentandria*, natural order *Asclepiadaceæ.*

Ascle'pias In-car-na'ta.* The flesh-colored *Asclepias*, a plant whose medical properties appear to be similar to those of the ASCLEPIAS TUBEROSA, which see.

Ascle'pias Sўr-ĭ'a-ca.* The silk-weed; called also milk-weed. Of this plant the bark of the root is given in powder for asthma and other pulmonary affections.

As-cle'pias Tu-be-ro'sa.* Swallow-wort; called also Pleurisy-root. An American plant, the root of which is used as an expectorant and a diaphoretic in catarrh and rheumatism. It is given in powder and decoction or infusion.

A-sep'ta.* [From *a*, priv., and σήπομαι, to "putrefy."] Substances free from the putrefactive process.

Asetiger,* a-set'e-jer. [From *a*, priv., *se'ta*, a "bristle," and *ge'ro*, to "bear."] Without bristles: asetig'erous. Applied in the neuter plural (*Asetig'era*) to a family of *Articulata abranchiata.*

A-sex'u-al. [**Asexua'lis;** from *a*, priv., and *sex'us*, "sex" or "gender."] A botanical term applied to plants having no sexual organs.

Ash. The common name of several trees and shrubs. The true ash includes the various species of the Linnæan genus *Frax'inus*. *Bitter Ash* is the popular name for a species of Quassia growing in the West India islands.

Ash-Color. See CINEREUS.

Ash'es. [**Ci'nis, Cin'eris.**] The residual substance after burning any thing; more usually, the residuum of the combustion of vegetables, containing alkalies and alkaline salts. The common name for the vegetable alkali potash, or *Potassa.*

Asiatic (ā'she-at'ik) **Bâl'sam.** [**Asiat'icum Bal'samum.**] The BALSAMUM GILEADENSE, which see.

Asitia,* a-si'te-a. [From *a*, priv., and σῖτος, "food."] Abstinence from food; also, loss of appetite. See ANOREXIA, FASTIDIUM CIBI.

As-păr'a-gi,* the plural of **Asparagus,** forming the Jussieuan name of a natural order of plants now included in *Liliaceæ.*

As-par'a-gin. [**Asparagi'na.**] A peculiar vegetable principle obtained from the *Asparagus.*

As-par'a-gus (Gr. ἀσπάραγος) **Of-fiç-ĭ-na'lis,*** or Common Asparagus. A plant belonging to the Linnæan class *Hexandria*, natural order *Liliaceæ*. The root and young shoots are diuretic, and are said to exert a sedative, influence on the heart.

As-par'tāte. [**Aspar'tas, a'tis.**] A combination of aspartic acid with a base.

Aspera Arteria. See ARTERIA ASPERA.

As-per-gil'lĭ-form. [**Aspergilliformis;** from *aspergil'lum*, a "brush."] Brush-like; divided into minute ramifications, as the stigmas of grasses, certain hairs of the cuticle, etc.

As'per-ĭ-fo'lĭ-us.* [From *as'per*, "rough," and *fo'lium*, a "leaf."] Rough-leaved: asperifo'lious. Applied by Linnæus, in the plural feminine (*Asperifo'liæ*) to an order of plants now called *Boraginaceous*. See BORAGINACEÆ.

As-per'ma-tous. [**Asper'matus,** or **Asper'mus;** from *a*, priv., and σπέρμα, "seed."] Without seed.

As-per'sion. [**Asper'sio;** from *asper'go, asper'sum*, to "sprinkle."] The sprinkling of the body with a medicinal liquid or powder.

As-phăl'tum.* [From *a*, priv., and σφάλλω, to "slip," to "fail," because when used as a cement it prevented the stones from slipping or giving way.] Native bitumen; a solid, brittle bitumen, found principally on the shores and on the surface of the Dead Sea, which was named Asphaltitis from this substance. A brown-coloring matter is formed from it, which, when dissolved in oil of turpentine, is semi-transparent, and is used as a glaze.

Asphodeleæ,* as-fo-de'le-ē. A subdivision of the natural order *Liliaceæ.*

As-phod'e-li,* the plural of *Asphod'elus*, forming the Jussieuan name of a natural order the same as ASPHODELEÆ, which see.

As-phy̆x'ĭ-a.* [From *a*, priv., and σφύξις, the "pulse."] Literally, the "state of being without pulse:" asphyx'y. Suspended animation; that state in which there is total suspension of the powers of body and mind, usually caused by interrupted respiration, as by hanging or drowning.

Asphyx'ia Al'gĭ-da.* [From *al'geo*, to "be cold."] Asphyxy from intense cold.

Asphyx'ia E-lec'trĭ-ca.* Asphyxy caused by lightning or electricity.

Asphyx'ia Id-ĭ-o-path'ĭ-ca.* ("Idiopathic Asphyxia.") Asphyxy, or sudden death, without any manifest cause. See IDIOPATHIC.

Asphyx'ia Me-phit'ĭ-ca.* Asphyxy by inhalation of some mephitic gas, carbonic acid, or other non-respirable gas.

Asphyx'ia Ne-oph-y̆-to'rum.* [From νέος, "young," "new," and φυτόν, a "plant," also a "child."] Called also **Asphyx'ia Ne-o-na-to'rum.*** [From *na'tus*, "born."] Deficient respiration in new-born children.

Asphyx'ia Suffocatio'nis* (suf-fo-ka·she-o'nis). (The "asphyxy of suffocation.") Asphyxy by hanging or drowning.

As-phyx'i-āt-ed. [**Asphyxia'tus.**] Laboring under asphyxy.

As-pid'i-um.* [From ἀσπίς, a "round shield."] A Linnæan genus of the class *Cryptogamia*, order *Filices*.

Aspid'ium Ath-a-man'ti-cum.* [Etymology uncertain.] A species of fern growing in South Africa, much used as a remedy against worms, especially the tape-worm.

Aspid'ium Fi'lix Mas.* The male fern; called also *Polypodium filix mas*. The root of this plant is considered by many to be an efficacious remedy against the tape-worm.

As-ple'ni-um.* [From *a*, priv., and σπλήν, the "spleen."] A genus of fern called spleenwort and miltwaste, from a belief that it removed disorders or reduced enlargements of the spleen.

Asple'nium Cet'arach*(set'a-rak). A species of fern much used as a remedy in nephritic and calculous diseases, also as a pectoral.

Asple'nium Fi'lix Fœm'i-na.* The female fern, a plant possessing medical properties similar to those of the male fern (*Aspidium filix mas*). The *Asple'nium ru'ta mura'ria*, the *A. scolopen'drium*, and the *A. trichomanoi'des*, have properties similar to those of the *A. cetarach.*

Assafœtida,* as-sa-fet'e-da, written also **Assafetida,*** and **Asafœtida.*** The Pharmacopœial name ‖ for the gum resin, or concrete juice, obtained from the *Narthex assafœtida*, otherwise called *Fer'ula assafœt'ida.* It occurs massive and in tears. It was used by the ancients as a condiment, and at the present day the plant is eaten with relish in some countries of the East. Assafœ'ida is a powerful antispasmodic; it is also a stimulant expectorant and laxative. From its uniting antispasmodic and expectorant virtues, it often proves useful in spasmodic pectoral affections.

As-say'ing. The operation of ascertaining the proportion of any metal in an ore or mixture. See CUPELLATION.

As-sim'i-lāte. [From *ad*, "to," and *sim'ilis*, "like."] Literally, to "make like." In Physiology, to change the food into a substance like the living body; to convert the food into nutriment,—in other words, into chyle and blood.

As-sim-i-lā'tion. [**Assimila'tio,** *o'nis;* from the same.] The act or process of assimilating food. See ALITURA.

As-so'des,* or **A-so'dēs.*** [From ἄση, "disgust," "nausea."] A continual fever, attended with a loathing of food. Sauvages calls it *Trytæophya assodes*, and Cullen arranges it under the tertian remittents.

As-sur'gent. [**Assur'gens;** from *assur'go*, to "rise up."] A botanical term, signifying bent down, then rising erect towards the apex.

A-stat'ic. [**Astat'icus;** from *a*, priv., and ἵστημι, to "stand."] A term applied to a magnetic needle when its directive property is destroyed by the proximity of another needle, of equal magnetic intensity, fixed parallel to it and in a reversed position, each needle having its north pole adjacent to the south pole of the other. In this state, the needles, neutralizing each other, are unaffected by the earth, while they are still subject to the influence of galvanism.

As'ter.* [Gr. ἀστήρ, a "star."] A genus of cryptogamous plants having star-like flowers.

Asteraceæ,* as-ter-a'she-ē. A name given by Lindley to a natural order of plants. See COMPOSITÆ.

A-ster'ni-a.* [From *a*, priv., and *ster'num.*] An organic deviation in the fœtus characterized by absence of the *sternum.*

As'ter-oid. [**Asteroi'des;** from ἀστήρ, a "star" or "planet," and εἶδος, a "form."] Resembling a star. As a noun, the term is applied, in Astronomy, to several small planets, including Ceres, Pallas, Juno, and Vesta.

As-the'ni-a.* [From *a*, priv., and σθένος, "strength."] As'theny. Want or loss of strength: debility.

As-then'ic. [**Asthen'icus:** from *asthe'nia.*] Wanting or deficient in strength; adynamic.

As-the-nol'o-gy. [**Asthenolo'gia;** from *a*, priv., σθένος, "strength," and λόγος, a "discourse."] The consideration (or science) of diseases arising from debility.

Asth'ma, atis.* [Gr. ἄσθμα; from ἀσθμάζω, to "gasp for breath."] A disease attended with difficulty of breathing and a sensation of constriction in the chest, wheezing, cough, and expectoration. A genus of the order *Spasmi*, class *Neuroses*, of Cullen's Nosology.

Asth-mat'ic. [**Asthmat'icus.**] Belonging to, or laboring under, asthma.

A-stig'ma-tism. [**Astigmatis'-**

mus; from *α*, neg., and *στίγμα*, a "point."] A defect in the eye, in which the rays are not brought to one point or focus, but converge at different distances, so as to form two linear images at right angles with each other.—(DUNGLISON.)

As'to-mus.* [From *α*, priv., and *στόμα*, a "mouth."] Having no mouth. Applied to an order of mosses, and to a family of apterous insects.

As-trag'a-loid. [**Astragaloi'des;** from *astrag'alus*, the "ankle-bone," a "die," and *εἶδος*, a "form."] Resembling the *astragalus*.

As'trag-a-loi'dēs Sўph-ĭ-lit'ĭ-ca,* called also **Astrag'alus Es'ca-pus.*** The milk-vetch, a plant the root of which is said to cure syphilis.

As-trag'a-lus.* [Gr. *ἀστράγαλος*.] The ankle-bone.

Astrag'alus Cre'tĭ-cus.* The Cretan milk-vetch, one of the several species of Astragalus which are said to yield the gum tragacanth of commerce.

Astragalus Escapus. See ASTRAGALOIDES SYPHILITICA.

Astrag'alus Trag-a-can'tha.* The plant formerly supposed to yield gum tragacanth, now known to be chiefly obtained from the *Astragalus verus* and the *A. gummifer*.

Astrag'alus Ve'rus.* A plant of the Linnæan class *Diadelphia*, natural order *Leguminosæ*, from which gum tragacanth is principally derived.

As-tric'tion. [**Astric'tio, o'***nis;* from *ad*, "to," and *strin'go*, *stric'tum*, to "bind."] The state produced by astringent medicines.

As-trin'gent. [**Astrin'gens;** from the same.] Producing contraction and condensation in the soft solids, thereby diminishing excessive discharges.

Astrin'gent Prin'cĭ-ple. A vegetable principle found in the bark of many trees and plants. From its use in tanning skins it has obtained the name of TANNIN, which see.

Astrin'gents. A name applied to medicines (such as alum, tannin, etc.) having the power to check discharges, whether of blood, of mucus, or any other secretion. They act by contracting the capillaries and secreting-orifices. See ASTRICTION and ASTRINGENT.

As-trol'o-gў. [From *ἄστρον*, a "star," and *λόγος*, a "discourse."] A description of the heavenly bodies, their nature and distinctions, and, so, like Astronomy; more usually, however, applied to a pretended science which explained the phenomena of nature, and events of human life, by the influence of the stars. Hippocrates considered astrology among the studies necessary for a physician.

As-tron'o-mў. [**Astrono'mia;** from *ἄστρον*, a "star," and *νόμος*, a "law."] Literally, that science which treats of the laws which govern the heavenly bodies; but, more generally, it includes every thing which can be known of those bodies.

A-tax'ĭ-a.* [From *α*, neg., and *τάσσω*, to "order."] Literally, "want of order." Irregularity. A term applied to some diseases.

A-tax'ic. [**Atax'icus;** from *atax'ia*.] Irregular.

At'axy. See ATAXIA.

-Ate. A terminal syllable which, added to the name of an acid ending in *-ic*, expresses a combination of that acid with a base; as, nitr*ate* of silver, or a combination of nitr*ic* acid with the oxide of silver.

At-e-lec'ta-sis,* or **Atelec'tasis Pul-mo'num.*** [From *ἀτελής*, "imperfect," and *ἔκτασις*, "expansion."] Applied to a state of the lungs in new-born children, on account of some obstacle to the complete establishment of respiration. See PULMO.

A-thal'a-mous. [**Athal'amus;** from *α*, priv., and *θάλαμος*, a "marriage-bed."] Applied to plants which have no conceptacles.

Ath-er-ĭ-çe'rus.* [From *ἀθήρ*, the "point of a sword," and *κηρός*, "slender."] Applied in the nominative plural neuter (*Atherice'ra*) to a family of dipterous insects, in which the lower and side pieces of the sucker are linear and pointed, or setaceous: atherice'rous.

A-ther'ma-nous. [**Ather'manus;** from *α*, priv., and *θερμαίνω*, to "make warm."] Not communicating heat.

Ath-er-o'ma, a*tis*.* [From *ἀθάρα*, "gruel."] An encysted tumor containing a soft substance like panada. Beclard observes that this kind of cyst, as well as the varieties termed *meliceris* and *steatoma*, are merely sebaceous follicles enormously dilated.

Ath-er-om'a-tous. [**Atheroma-to'sus.**] Of the nature of *Atheroma*.

Ath-let'ic. [**Athlet'icus;** from *ἀθλητής*, an "athlete," "one who strove for a prize" (from *ἆθλον*, a "prize," a "contest").] Having a strong muscular development, like those who exercised in the ancient games.

At-lan'tad. Same as ATLANTAL used adverbially.

At-lan'tal. Applied by Dr. Barclay as meaning towards the *atlas*.

At'las, an'*tis*.* [From *At'las*, an ancient giant, fabled to bear the heavens upon his shoulders.] The first cervical vertebra, so named, it would seem, because it immediately sustains the head, a burden immensely disproportioned to itself in size.

At-mĭ-dom'e-ter, At-mom'e-ter. [**Atmidom'etrum,** and **Atmom'e-trum.**] [From ἀτμίς, or ἀτμός, "vapor," and μέτρον, a "measure."] An instrument by which the vapor exhaled from a humid surface in a given time may be measured.

At'mo-sphēre. [**Atmosphæ'ra;** from ἀτμός, "vapor," and σφαῖρα, a "globe" or "sphere."] The thin, elastic fluid encompassing the earth to a height judged to be about forty-five miles; the natural air we breathe.

At-mo-sphĕr'ic. [**Atmosphær'i-cus.**] Belonging to the atmosphere.

Atmospher'ic Pres'sure, or weight of the atmosphere, is measured by the length of a column of mercury. A mercurial column thirty inches in length presses on a given surface with the same force as the atmosphere in its ordinary state; and hence the force of a sixty-inch column is equal to the pressure of *two atmospheres*, that of fifteen inches to half an atmosphere, that of one inch to one-thirtieth of the atmospheric pressure.

A-to'çĭ-a,* or **A-to'kĭ-a.*** [From *a*, priv., and τόκος, "offspring."] Sterility.

At'om. [**At'omus;** from *a*, neg., and τέμνω, to "cut," to "divide."] The smallest particle of matter, incapable of farther division.

At'om, Com-po'nent. That which unites with another of different nature to form a third or *compound* atom.

At'om, Com'pound. That formed by two atoms of different nature.

At'om, El-e-men'ta-rȳ. That of a substance not decomposed.

At'om, Or-gan'ic. That of a substance found only in organic bodies.

At'om, Pri'ma-rȳ. Same as ATOM, ELEMENTARY.

At-om'ic. [**Atom'icus.**] Belonging to atoms or particles.

Atom'ic The'o-rȳ. A theory introduced by Dalton for explaining the laws of definite proportions in chemical combinations. It is founded on the supposition that matter consists of ultimate, indivisible particles, called *atoms*, that these are of the same size and shape in the same body, but differ in *weight* in different bodies, and that bodies combine in definite proportions with reference to those weights, which are hence called *atomic weights*. The main features of this theory are briefly stated in the following paragraphs.

In bodies capable of assuming the gaseous form, the weight of the atom is obtained from the *volume:* thus, water being composed of one volume of oxygen united with two volumes (or *one atom*) of hydrogen, the relative weights will be—oxygen, 8, hydrogen, 1, and water, 9.

In bodies which do not assume the gaseous form in their simple state, the weight of the atom is deduced from that of the *compound:* the weight of carbon, for instance, is obtained from that of carbonic acid gas, one volume of which weighs twenty-two times as much as our standard of unity; of the twenty-two parts, sixteen are hydrogen, leaving 6 to represent the primary molecule of carbon.

In the case of bodies which are incapable of assuming a gaseous form, either alone or in combination, the weight must be obtained by *analysis:* thus, marble, or the carbonate of lime, is found to be composed of twenty-two parts of carbonic acid and twenty-eight of lime; 28, therefore, represents the atomic weight of lime.

The atomic weights are generally supposed to be related to one another by *multiple:* hence this law is often called the *law of multiples*, or of combinations in *multiple proportion*. This will be easily seen by referring to the component parts of the following substances:—

	Nitrogen.	Oxygen.
Nitrous oxide	14	8
Nitric oxide	14	16
Hyponitrous acid	14	24
Nitrous acid	14	32
Nitric acid	14	40

When only one combination of any two elementary bodies exists, Dr. Dalton assumes that its elements are united, atom to atom singly, by what he calls *binary* combinations; if several compounds can be obtained from the same elements, they combine, as he supposes, in proportions expressed by some simple multiple of the number of atoms, as in the following table:—

ATOMS—
1 of A + 1 of B = 1 of C, binary.
1 of A + 2 of B = 1 of D, ternary.
2 of A + 1 of B = 1 of E, ternary.
1 of A + 3 of B = 1 of F, quaternary.
3 of A + 1 of B = 1 of G, quaternary.

Atonia. See ATONY.

A-ton'ic. [**Aton'icus;** from *a*, priv., and τόνος, "tone."] Without, or having diminished, tone or power.

At'o-ny. [**Ato'nia;** from the same.] Want or diminution of muscular tone.

Atrabiliary, at-ra-bil'ya-re. [**Atrabilia'rius;** from *atrabi'lis*, "black bile."] Melancholy; atrabilious. Atrabiliary capsules, arteries, and veins, are names applied to the renal or suprarenal glands or capsules, and to the arteries and veins by which they are supplied, because they were formerly supposed to produce black bile. See ATRABILIS.

Atrabilious, at-ra-bil'yŭs. [From the same.] Melancholy, hypochondriac.

At-ra-bi'lis.* [From *a'ter*, "black," and *bi'lis*, "bile."] Black bile; an imaginary fluid, supposed, when existing in excessive quantity, to be the cause of MELANCHOLY, which see.

Atrachelus,* at-ra-ke'lŭs. [From *a*, priv., and τράχηλος, the "neck."] Without a neck; having a very short neck.

At-ra-men'tum.* [From *a'ter*, "black."] A Latin term denoting the coloring matter secreted by the cuttlefish (*Se'pia*); also, ink.

A-tre'si-a.* [From *a*, priv., and τρῆσις, a "boring," a "perforation."] Imperforation; usually applied to the rectum, urethra, etc.

A-tret-o-ceph'a-lus,* **A-tret-o-cor'mus.*** [From *a*, priv., τίτρημι, to "perforate," κεφαλή, the "head," and κορμός, a "trunk."] A monster-fœtus without the natural openings in the head or trunk.

Atriplex Fœtida. See CHENOPODIUM VULVARIA.

A-trip'li-çēs.* The Jussieuan name of a natural order. See CHENOPODIACEÆ.

At'ro-pa.* [From Ἄτροπος, of the three Fates, that one whose special duty it was to cut the thread of life: named on account of its deadly or poisonous qualities.] A Linnæan genus of the class *Pentandria*, natural order *Solanaceæ*.

At'ropa Bel'la-don'na.* The deadly nightshade, or belladonna, a plant belonging to the narcotico-acrid poisons.

A-tro'phi-a.* [From *a*, priv., and τροφή, "nourishment."] Atrophy. A genus of the order *Marcores*, class *Cachexiæ*, of Cullen's Nosology.

At'ro-phy. [**Atro'phia.** See ATROPHIA.] Defect of nutrition; wasting or emaciation, with loss of strength, unaccompanied by fever.

A-tro'pi-a.* A peculiar alkaline principle found in all parts of the *Atropa Belladonna*. It is highly poisonous, and in the most minute proportion has the property of dilating the pupil of the eye.

At'ropin. See ATROPIA.

At'ro-pism. [**Atropis'mus.**] The condition of the system produced by the persevering use of *belladonna*.

Attar Gul, åt'tar gōōl. [From *at'tar*, "essence," and *gul*, a "rose."] A phrase taken from the Persian, and signifying Attar of Roses, or Otto of Roses. See next article.

At'tar of Ro'ses [see preceding etymology], or Oil of Roses. An essence prepared from the petals of the damask rose (and probably from other species) by distillation with water. The oil collects and floats on the surface of the water when it cools.

At-ten'u-ant. [**Atten'uans, an'tis;** from *atten'uo, attenua'tum*, to "make thin."] Applied to medicines supposed to impart to the blood a thinner or more fluid consistence, as water, whey, etc.

At-ten'u-āt-ed. [**Attenua'tus;** from the same.] Become slender; thin.

At'ten-u-ā'tion. [**Attenua'tio;** from the same.] The lessening of weight or of consistency; emaciation. The term is applied to a process by which a fluid becomes of less specific gravity, as when it undergoes fermentation and parts with carbonic acid.

At-tol'lens.* [From *attol'lo*, to "raise up."] Raising up.

Attol'lens Au'rem.* ("Raising the ear.") A muscle whose office is indicated by its name.

Attollens Oculi. See RECTUS SUPERIOR OCULI.

At-tract'. [From *ad*, "to," or "towards," and *tra'ho, trac'tum*, to "draw."] To draw to or towards. See next article.

At-trac'tion. [**Attrac'tio, o'nis;** from the same.] That principle or power in the material universe by which one particle or mass of matter is drawn to or towards another.

ATTRAC'TION OF AFFIN'ITY. The tendency of the atoms of different bodies to combine to form *chemical compounds*. See AFFINITY.

ATTRAC'TION, CAP'ILLARY. The power by which a liquid rises in a fine tube higher than the surface of the liquid which surrounds it. See CAPILLARY.

ATTRAC'TION OF COHE'SION. The tendency of the *molecules* of a body to cohere, to form masses. It is antagonist of AFFINITY.

ATTRAC'TION, ELEC'TRICAL. The property displayed by certain substances of attracting certain others on being rubbed.

ATTRAC'TION OF GRAVITA'TION. The tendencies of *masses* of bodies towards each other. See GRAVITY.

ATTRAC'TION, MAGNET'IC. The tendency of certain bodies, chiefly iron, towards the north pole of the earth, and towards other bodies possessed of the property called magnetism.

Attraction, Double Elective. See AFFINITY, DOUBLE ELECTIVE.

Attraction, Simple Elective. See AFFINITY, SINGLE ELECTIVE.

At'tră-hens.* [The present participle of *at'traho*, to "draw to, or towards." See ATTRACT.] Applied in the neuter plural (*Attrahentia*, at-tra-hen'-she-a) to medicaments which irritate the surface, thereby attracting the fluids to the part, as blisters, sinapisms, etc. See EPISPASTIC.

At'trahens Au'ris.* [*At'trahens*, "drawing" or "drawing to," and *au'ris*, "of the ear."] A muscle which draws the ear forwards and upwards; also called *anterior auris*, and *prior auriculæ*.

Attrahentia. See ATTRAHENS.

Attrition, at-trish'ŭn. [**Attri'tio, O'nis**; from *at'tero, attri'tum*, to "rub against," to "wear away."] An abrasion or solution of continuity of the cuticle; also, a severe kind of *Cardialgia*: sometimes applied in surgery to the violent crushing of a part.

Au'dĭ-to-rў. [**Audito'rius**; from *au'dio, audi'tum*, to "hear."] Belonging to the organ or the sense of hearing. Same as ACOUSTIC.

Au'ditory Nerve. The PORTIO MOLLIS of the seventh pair, which see.

Augite, aw'jīt. [From αὐγή, "brightness," and λιθός, a "stone."] *Pyroxene*. A silicate of lime and magnesia.

Au'ra.* [A Latin word signifying a "breath," a "gentle breeze;" from ἄω, to "breathe."] A subtle vapor, or exhalation.

AU'RA ELEC'TRICA.* Literally, the "electrical breeze." The sensation, as of cold air, experienced when electricity is received from a sharp point.

AU'RA EPILEP'TICA.* The peculiar sensation felt by epileptic patients, as of a cold fluid rising towards the head.

AU'RA HYSTER'ICA.* The sensation as of cold air ascending to the head, said to occur sometimes in *hysteria*.

AU'RA SEMINA'LIS,* AU'RA SEM'INIS.* The supposed vivifying principle of the *Semen virile*, believed to ascend through the Fallopian tubes, thereby impregnating the *ovum* in the *ovarium*.

AU'RA VITA'LIS.* The vital principle.

Aurantia,* au-ran'she-a, the plural of **Auran'tium,** forming the Jussieuan name of a natural order of plants. See AURANTIACEÆ.

Aurantiaceæ,* aw-ran-she-ā'she-ē. [From *auran'tium*, the "orange."] A natural order of exogenous trees and shrubs, natives of the East Indies and other warm climates. It includes the orange, lemon, lime, and citron. The leaves and rind of the fruit abound in a volatile, fragrant, bitter, and exciting oil.

Aurantiaceous, aw-ran-she-ā'shŭs. [**Aurantia'ceus**; from *auran'tium*, an "orange."] Having an arrangement as in the orange-plant. See AURANTIACEÆ.

Aurantium,* aw-ran'she-ŭm. [Supposed to be derived from *au'rum*, "gold."] The orange. The fruit of *Citrus bigaradia* and *C. aurantium* (Lond. Ph.), of *Citrus vulgaris* (Ed. Ph.), or *C. aurantium* (U.S. Ph.).

Au'rāte. [**Au'ras, a'tis.**] A combination of auric acid with a base.

Au'rate of Am-mo'nĭ-a. [**Ammo'niæ Au'ras.**] FULMINATING GOLD, which see.

Au-re'lĭ-a.* [From *au'rum*, "gold."] A term for the chrysalis or pupa of insects, often adorned with golden spots.

Au'ric Açid. [**Au'ricum Açidum**; from *au'rum*, "gold."] A name proposed by Pelletier for the peroxide of gold, on account of its property of forming salts with alkaline bases.

Auricle. See AURICULA.

Au-ric'u-la,* plural **Au-ric'u-læ.** [The diminutive of *au'ris*, the "ear."] The auricle or external portion of the ear.

Auric'ula In'fĭ-ma.* Literally, the "lowest ear." The lobe of the ear.

Au-ric'u-læ Cor'dis.* [From *auric'ula* and *cor, cor'dis*, the "heart."] "Auricles of the heart." A term applied to those cavities of the heart which lead to the ventricles.

Au-ric-u-la'ris.* [From *auric'ula*, an "ear."] Belonging to the ear: auric'ular.

Au-ric'u-late. [**Auricula'tus;** from *auric'ula*, an "ear."] Applied in Botany to a leaf when it has a lobe on each side of its base; eared.

Auricule, ō'rè'kül'. The French term for AURICLE, which see.

Au-ric'u-lo-Ven-tric'u-lar O'pen-ing. The opening between the auricle and ventricle of each side of the heart.

Au-rif'er-ous. [**Aurif'erus;** from *au'rum*, "gold," and *fe'ro*, to "bear."] Bearing or containing gold.

Au'ri-form. [**Aurifor'mis;** from *au'ris*, the "ear."] Formed like the ear.

Au-ri'go,* or **Au-ru'go.*** [From *au'rum*, "gold."] Orange-skin. A term applied to an orange hue diffused over the entire surface of the skin in new-born infants: Sauvages terms it *ephe'lis lu'tea*. Also an old name for jaundice.

Au-rĭ-pig-men'tum.* [From *au'rum*, "gold," and *pig men'tum*, "paint."] Yellow Orpiment. See ORPIMENT.

Au'ris.* The Latin term for the "ear." It is distinguished into the external and the internal.

Au-rĭ-scăl'pum.* [From *scal'po*, to "scrape."] An instrument for cleansing the ear.

Au'rĭ-scōpe. [**Auris'copus;** from *au'ris*, the "ear," and σκοπέω, to "explore."] An instrument for ascertaining the condition of the Eustachian passage.

Aurium, Tinnitus. See TINNITUS AURIUM.

Au'rum.* The Latin for GOLD, which see.

Aurum Fulminans. See FULMINATING GOLD.

Aus-cul-tā'tion. [**Ausculta'tio, o'nis;** from *auscul'to*, *ausculta'tum*, to "listen."] The act of listening to the sound given by particular parts of the body when struck, or to the sounds produced by the functional movements of the lungs or heart.

Ausculta'tion, Im-me'dĭ-ate. That practised directly by the ear of the practitioner without the aid of an instrument.

Ausculta'tion, Me'dĭ-ate. That performed by employing a stethoscope or some similar instrument.

Aus-tra'lis.* [From *Aus'ter*, the "south wind."] Belonging to the south: aus'tral.

Au-to-car'pous. [**Autocar'peus,** or **Autocarpia'nus;** from αὐτός, "itself," and καρπός, "fruit."] Applied to fruit not adherent to the calyx; superior.

Autochthon,* au-tok'thon, plural **Au-toch'tho-nēs.** [From αὐτός, "itself," sometimes "very," and χθών, "land," or "country."] A name given, by those who hold the doctrine that the various races of mankind were originally distinct, to the first inhabitants of a country, supposed to have been produced in the "very country or place itself."

Autochthonous. See THROMBUS.

Au-tog'e-nous. [**Autog'enus;** from αὐτός, "itself," or "one's self," and γένω, to "be born."] Applied in Comparative Anatomy, by Owen, to parts developed from distinct and independent centres.

Au-to-mat'ic. [**Automat'icus;** from αὐτοματίζω, to "act spontaneously."] Applied to functions or motions performed without the will, as digestion, the heart's action, etc.

Au-to-plas'tic. [**Autoplas'ticus.**] Belonging to autoplasty.

Au'to-plas-tȳ. [**Autoplas'tia;** from αὐτός, "one's self," and πλάσσω, to "form."] Operations by which lesions are repaired by means of healthy parts being taken from the neighborhood of the lesion and made to supply the deficiency caused by wounds or disease.

Au-top'so-rin. [From αὐτός, "one's self," and ψώρα, the "itch."] That which is given under the homœopathic doctrine of administering a patient's own virus.

Au'top-sȳ. [**Autop'sia;** from αὐτός, "one's self," and ὄψις, the "act of seeing."] Ocular examination.

A-ve'na.* The oat. The Pharmacopœial name (Ed. Ph.) for the seeds of *Avena sativa*. See AVENÆ SEMINA.

Ave'na Sa-ti'va.* The oat-plant. See AVENÆ SEMINA.

A-ve'næ Fa-ri'na.* ("Meal of Oats.") The Pharmacopœial name (U.S.Ph.) for oatmeal, prepared from the seed of *Avena sativa*. Used for gruels, decoctions, etc.

A-ve'næ Sem'ĭ-na.* [From *se'men*, "seed," plural *sem'ina*.] Literally, the "seeds of the oat." Oats; the fruit of the *Avena sativa*, of the order *Gramineæ*, yielding a flour or meal which forms a common article of food in some parts of Europe. *Groats* are the oats freed from the cuticle, and used in broth and gruels.

A-ve-nā'ceous. [**Avena'ceus.**] Belonging to the *Avena*.

A-ven-ĭ-for'mis.* [From *ave'na*, and *for'ma*.] Like a grain of oats: aven'iform.

A-ve'nĭ-ous. [**Ave'nius;** from *a*, priv., and *ve'na*, a "vein."] Applied to the leaves of plants without veins, or nerves.

A'vēs,* the plural of Avis, which see.

A-vic'u-lar. [**Avicula'ris;** from *avic'ula*, a "little bird."] Pertaining to birds.

A'vis.* A bird. Applied in the plural (*A'ves*) to a class of oviparous *Vertebrata* including all birds proper.

Avoine, å'vwån'. The French for "oats." See Avena.

A-vul'sion. [**Avul'sio;** from *avel'lo, avul'sum*, to "tear asunder."] The forcible separation from each other of parts of the body which were previously more or less intimately united.

Awn. See Arista.

Ax-if'er-ous. [**Axif'erus;** from *ax'is*, and *fe'ro*, to "bear."] Applied to plants having only a stem or axis, variously modified.

Ax-il'la.* The armpit; the cavity under the upper part of the arm and shoulder. Applied in Botany to the angle formed by a branch and the stem, or by a leaf with either of these.

Ax-il-la'ris.* [From *axil'la*, the "armpit;" Fr. *Axillaire*, åx'ė'lain'.] Belonging to the *axilla:* axillary. Applied also to branches and leaves that form an *axilla.*

Ax'il-la-rȳ. Belonging to the armpit. See Axillaris.

Ax'illary Plex'us. [**Plex'us Axilla'ris.**] The brachial plexus formed by the three last cervical and the first dorsal nerves.

Ax'is.* [Perhaps from *a'go*, to "act," to "drive."] Literally, an "axle" about which any revolving body turns. A right line, real or imaginary, passing through the centre of any body. The name of the second vertebra of the neck, its tooth-like process serving as an axis on which the *atlas*, and so the head itself, turns; also termed *Ver'tebra denta'ta.* In Astronomy, the axis of the earth is that diameter about which it performs its diurnal revolution. In Geology, applied to the centre of a mountain-group. In Botany, the stem and root of a plant, termed, respectively, the ascending and descending axis.

Axis, Anticlinal. See Anticlinal.

Axis, Synclinal. See Synclinal Axis.

Ax-ot'o-mous. [**Axot'omus;** from ἄξων, the "axis," and τέμνω, to "cut."] Applied to minerals which are cleavable in one direction, perpendicular to the axis.

Ax-un'gi-a.* [From *ax'is*, an "axletree," and *un'guo*, to "anoint," to "smear;" Fr. *Axonge*, åx'ôɴzh'.] Hog's lard. The Pharmacopœial name (Ed. Ph.) of the fat of the *Sus scrofa*, the *Adeps* (U. S. Ph.), or *Adeps suillus* (Dub. Ph.). See Adeps.

Axun'gia Porci'na.* The same as Adeps Suillus, which see.

Az-e-tā'ic Aç'id. An acid obtained by treating oleic with nitric acid. It closely resembles suberic acid. Another acid, the *Azoleic*, is procured by the same process. The terms are derived from the words *azote* and *oleic.*

Az-o-ben'zide. A new substance obtained by heating a mixture of nitrobenzide with an alcoholic solution of potassa.

Az-o-lit'mạn. A pure coloring material, of a deep blood-red color, obtained from litmus.

Az'ote. [**Azo'tum;** from α, priv., and ζάω, to "live;" because unfit for sustaining life.] Nitrogen gas.

A-zōt'ic Aç'id. Another name for Nitric Acid, which see.

Az-o'tous Aç'id. Another name for nitrous acid; the hyponitrous acid of Turner. See Nitrous Acid.

Az-ōt-u'rĭ-ạ.* [From *azo'tum*, and οὖρον, the "urine."] A class of diseases characterized by a great increase of *urea* in the urine.

Az-ul'mic Aç'id. The name given by Boullay to the black matter deposited during the decomposition of prussic acid. It is very similar to ulmic acid. See Ulmin.

Azure, a'zhūr. A fine blue pigment, commonly called *smalt*, consisting of glass colored with oxide of cobalt and ground to an impalpable powder.

Az'ure Stone. [**La'pis Laz'uli.**] An azure-blue mineral from which the unchangeable blue color *ultramarine* is prepared.

Azygos Uvulæ. See Azygous Muscle.

Az'ȳ-gous. [**Az'ygos;** from α, priv., and ζυγός, a "yoke."] Without a fellow, or corresponding part.

Az'ygous Mus'cle. A muscle of the uvula.

Az'ygous Proç'ess. [**Proces'sus Az'ygos.**] A process of the sphenoid bone.

Az'ygous Vein. [**Ve'na Az'ygos.**] A vein formed by the union of the lower intercostal veins of the left side, and ascending in front of the spine on the right side of the aorta.

B.

B. A. = *Bal'neum Are'næ.** A sand-bath.

Bab'lah. The rind or shell which surrounds the fruit of the *Mimosa cineraria.* It is brought from the East Indies, under the name of *nebneb*, and is employed as a dye-stuff.

Bac'ca.* A berry; an inferior, indehiscent, pulpy fruit, as the gooseberry. The term is often otherwise applied by botanists.

Bac'cate. [**Bacca'tus;** from *bac'ca*, a "berry."] Resembling a berry.

Bacchia,* bak-ki'a. [From *Bac'chus*, the "god of wine."] *Gutta Rosacea.* The pimpled condition of the face consequent on hard drinking. See ACNE ROSACEA.

Bacciferous, bak-sif'er-ŭs. [**Bac'cifer,** or **Baccif'erus;** from *bac'ca*, a "berry," and *fe'ro*, to "bear."] Bearing berries.

Bacciform, bak'se-form. [**Bacci-for'mis;** from *bac'ca*, a "berry."] Having the form of a berry.

Baccivorous, bak-siv'o-rŭs. [**Bac-civ'orus;** from *bac'ca*, a "berry," and *vo'ro*, to "devour."] Eating or living on berries.

Băch'e-lor's But'tons. A name sometimes applied to NUX VOMICA, which see.

Bach'er's Ton'ic Pills. Extract of hellebore and myrrh, of each ℥j, with ʒiij of powdered *carduus benedictus*, to be divided into pills of one grain each: dose, two to six three times a day.

Backbone. See SPINE.

Bac'u-lus.* Literally, a "stick" or "staff," and hence the name of a lozenge, shaped into a little, short roll.

Baignoire. See BAPTISTERIUM.

Bain, băng. The French word for BATH, which see.

Ba'ker's Itch. A species of *Psori'asis diffu'sa*, resulting from the irritating qualities of yeast.

Bā'ker's Salt. A name given to the subcarbonate of ammonia, or smelling-salts, from its being used by bakers as a substitute for yeast in the manufacture of some of the finer kinds of bread.

Ba-læ'na Mac-ro-çeph'a-lus.* A species of PHYSETER MACROCEPHALUS, which see.

Balænidæ,* ba-len'e-dē. [From *balæ'na*, a "whale."] A family of the *Cetacea.*

Bal'ance E-lec-trom'e-ter. An instrument, constructed on the application of the common balance and weights, to estimate the mutual attraction of oppositely-electrified surfaces.

Bal-a-nif'er-ous. [**Balanif'erus;** from βάλανος, an "acorn," and *fe'ro*, to "bear."] Bearing acorns.

Bal'a-nism. [**Balanis'mus;** from βαλανίς, a "pessary."] The application of a pessary.

Bal-a-ni'tis.* [From βάλανος, the "*glans penis.*"] Inflammation of the *glans penis* and prepuce, commonly complicated with phymosis; otherwise termed *Gonorrhœ'a bal'ani, Bal'ano-posthi'tis,* and *Posthitis.*

Bal'a-noid. [**Balanoi'des;** from βάλανος, an "acorn."] Resembling an acorn.

Balanophoraceæ,* bal'a-no-fo-ra'-she-ē. [Named from *Balanoph'ora*, one of the genera.] A natural order of fungus-like parasitical plants. They belong to the class of *Rhizogens.*

Bal'a-no-Pos-thi'tis, idis.* [From βάλανος, the "*glans penis,*" and πόσθη, the "prepuce."] The same as BALANITIS.

Bal'a-nus.* [Gr. βάλανος, an "acorn," a "gland."] The *Glans penis* and *Glans clitoridis.*

Ba-laus'ti-um.* [From βαλίος, "various."] The flower of the pomegranate-tree.

Balbuties,* băl-bu'she-ēz. [From *balbu'tio*, to "stammer."] Hesitation of speech; stammering. See STAMMERING.

Ball-and-Socket Joint. See ENARTHROSIS.

Bal-lis'mus.* [From βαλλίζω, to "dance."] A name for *Chorea*, or St. Vitus's dance.

Bal-loon'. [Fr. *Ballon*, bal'lōng'.] A spherical glass receiver, with one or two necks for adaptation to a retort or other vessel.

Bal-lo'ta La-na'ta.* A plant indigenous in Siberia, recommended by Brera in rheumatic and gouty affections.

Ballottement, bal'lott'mōng'. [From the French *ballotter*, bal'lot'tā', to "toss as a ball," to "shake about."] The passive movements of the fœtus in the *liquor amnii*, felt by applying the finger to the *cervix uteri* and raising it suddenly upwards, when the fœtus will strike on the finger in its descent.

Balm, bâm. [From *bal'samum*, "balsam."] A soothing or healing medicine.

Balm of Gilead. See BALSAM OF MECCA.

Balm Tea. An infusion of the leaves of *Melis'sa officina'lis*, or common balm.

Băl-ne-og'ra-phy̆. [**Balneogra'phia;** from *bal'neum*, a "bath," and γράφω, to "write."] A description of baths.

Băl-ne-ol'o-gy̆. [**Balneolo'gia;** from *bal'neum*, a "bath," and λόγος, a "discourse."] A treatise on baths; the science of baths.

Băl'ne-o-thĕr-a-pi'a.* [From *bal'neum*, a "bath," and θεραπεία, "attendance."] The proper employment of baths.

Băl'ne-um.* [Gr. βαλανεῖον.] The Latin term for BATH, which see.

Bal'neum An-i-ma'le.* Any part of a newly-killed animal, wrapped round the body or a limb.

Bal'neum Ar-e'næ.* ("Bath of sand.") See BATH.

Bal'neum Ma-ri'æ,* Bal'neum Ma'ris.* A water-bath, a vessel being put into another containing water, which is placed on the fire; heat is thus gradually communicated.

Bal'neum Med-i-ca'tum.* A medicated bath; a bath impregnated with medicinal substances.

Bal'neum Sic'cum.* ("Dry bath.") Immersion in any dry substance, as ashes, salt, sand, etc.

Bal'neum Sul-phu're-um.* A bath containing sulphur.

Bals. Abbreviation for *Balsamum.** "Balsam."

Balsam. See BALSAMUM.

BAL'SAM (baul'sam) OF THE AU'GIA SINEN'SIS, or CHINESE' VAR'NISH: it dries into a smooth, shining lac, used for lacquering and varnishing.

BALSAM OF COPAIBA. See COPAIBA.

BAL'SAM OF LIQUIDAM'BAR. Balsam which flows from incisions made into the trunk of the *Liquidambar styraciflua:* it dries up readily, and thus occurs in the solid form.

BAL'SAM OF MEC'CA ("Mecca Balsam"), or O'POBALSAM. Balsam obtained by incisions of, and by boiling, the branches and leaves of the *Amyris Gileadensis* (otherwise called *Balsamomendron Gileadense*), and the *A. Opobalsamum.* It becomes eventually solid.

BAL'SAM OF PERU'. (*Bal'samum Peruvia'num.**) A balsam procured from the *Myrospermum Peruiferum.* There are two kinds: the *brown* balsam, extracted by incision, very rare, imported in the husk of the cocoanut, and hence called balsam *en coque;* and the *black* balsam, obtained by evaporating the decoction of the bark and branches of the tree. These are semi-fluid balsams.

BAL'SAM OF STO'RAX. Balsam said to be procured from the *Liquidambar attina* and *Orientale.* The substance sold as *strained storax* is prepared from an impure variety of liquid storax.

BAL'SAM OF TO'LU. (*Bal'samum Toluta'num.**) A balsam which flows spontaneously from the trunk of the *Myrospermum toluiferum* and dries into a reddish resinous mass.

The following artificial balsams may be named:—

BAL'SAM OF HORE'HOUND. An aqueous infusion of horehound and liquorice-root, with double the proportion of proof spirit, or brandy, to which are then added opium, camphor, benzoin, squills, oil of aniseed, and honey.

BAL'SAM OF LIQ'UORICE. This consists principally of paregoric elixir, very strongly impregnated with the oil of aniseed.

BAL'SAM OF SUL'PHUR. A solution of sulphur in volatile oils.

Balsamaceæ,* băl-sa-ma'she-ē, or **Băl-sa-mif'lu-æ.*** A natural order of balsamiferous trees, consisting of one genus, the *Liquidambar.* This order is termed by Lindley *Altingiaceæ.*

Balsamatio (băl-sa-ma'she-o), **o'nis.*** [From *bal'samum.*] The process of embalming dead bodies. See EMBALMING.

Băl-sa'me-us.* Of the nature of a balsam. Also the specific name of a tree which produces balsam.

Băl-sam'ic. [**Balsam'icus.**] Pertaining to balsam; of the nature of balsam.

Băl-sam'ic-a.* Balsamics. A term generally applied to substances of a smooth and oily consistence, possessing emollient and generally aromatic properties.

Băl-sa-mif'e-ra Bra-zil-i-en'sis.* An ther name for the *Copaifera officinalis.*

Băl-sa-mif'er-ous. [**Balsamif'erus;** from *bal'samum*, a "balsam," and *fe'ro*, to "bear."] Bearing or yielding balsam.

Balsaminaceæ,* băl-sam-in-a'she-ē. [From *Balsami'na*, one of the genera.]

A natural order of herbaceous plants including the *Impatiens noli-tangere.* They are prized for their showy flowers.

Băl-sa-mo-den'dron.* [From βάλσαμον, a "balsam," and δένδρον, a "tree."] A Linnæan genus of the class *Octandria.* See AMYRIS.

Balsamoden'dron Mỹr'rha.* The tree supposed to yield myrrh.

Băl'sa-mum.* [Gr. βάλσαμον; from Heb. *baal samen*, the "prince of oils."] A balsam. A vegetable juice, liquid, or semifluid, or spontaneously becoming concrete.

Bal'samum Can-a-den'se.* Canadian balsam: obtained from the *Pinus balsamea.*

Bal'samum Co-pai'bæ.* Balsam of copaiba or copaiva; vulgarly, *capivi,* and *capivi oil.* See COPAIBA.

Balsamum Gileadense. See BALSAM OF MECCA.

Bal'samum Ju-da'ĭ-cum.* Another term for the *Balsamum Gileadense.*

Balsamum Peruvianum. See BALSAM OF PERU.

Bal'samum Sapona'ceum*(sap-o-na'she-ŭm). The camphorated soap liniment, or opodeldoc.

Bal'samum Sỹr-i'a-cum.* The *Balsamum Gileadense.*

Balsamum Tolutanum. See BALSAM OF TOLU.

Bal'samum Ve'rum.* ("True Balsam.") The *Balsamum Gileadense.*

Ban'dage. [**Fas'cia, Deliga'tio, o'***nis*, and **Des'ma.**] One or more pieces of cotton, linen, or flannel, for wrapping round any part of the body: they are simple, as the circular, spiral, uniting, etc., or compound, as the T bandage, the suspensory, eighteen-tailed, etc. etc.

Ban-dan'a. A style of calico-printing practised in India, in which white or brightly-colored spots are produced upon a red or dark ground.

Ban'dỹ-Legged. [*Bandy* is a corruption of the French participle *bandé,* "bent," from *bander,* to "bend."] Having legs the bones of which are curved outwards, or otherwise. See DEVALGATUS.

Bang, or **Bangue.** See CANNABIS INDICA, and BHANG.

Ban'yer's Oint'ment. An ointment consisting of half a pound of litharge, two ounces of burnt alum, one ounce and a half of calomel, half a pound of Venice turpentine, and two pounds of lard well rubbed together. It is used in Porrigo.

Baobab, bå'o-båb'. The African name of the *Adanso'nia digita'ta,* a tree growing native in West Africa and cultivated in Egypt and Abyssinia. The trunk is said to attain, in some instances, the enormous thickness of ten yards. The leaves, in the form of powder, are sometimes used in African cookery. The fruit has a subacid juice, which renders it valuable in fevers. The bark of the Baobab abounds in mucilage. It is said to have sometimes been given in fevers as a substitute for cinchona.

Baphicus Coccus, or **Baphicum Coccum.** See KERMES BERRY.

Bap-tis-te'rĭ-um.* [From βαπτίζω, to "dip," to "bathe;" Fr. *Baignoire,* bĕñ'-wåR'.] A bathing-place.

Baptorrhœa,* bap-to-re'a. [From βαπτός, "infected," and ῥέω, to "flow."] A term intended to designate *Gonorrhœa, Blennorrhœa, Blennorrhagia,* etc.

Bar-bā'does Leg. A disease of hot climates; the *Elephantiasis Arabum.*

Barba'does Nuts. [**Nu'ces Barbaden'ses.**] The fruit of the *Jatropha curcas.* The seeds are called *physic nuts.* See JATROPHA.

Barba'does Tar. The *Bitumen Barbadense, Bitumen petroleum,* or *Petroleum Barbadense.*

Bar'ba-rỹ Gum, or **Mo-roc'co Gum.** A variety of gum Arabic said to be produced by the *Acacia gummifera.*

Bar'bate. [**Barba'tus;** from *bar'ba,* a "beard."] Bearded.

Bar'bel-late. [**Barbella'tus;** from *barbel'la,* a "little beard."] Having barbels.

Bar'biērs. A disease of India and the Malabar coast; a peculiar species of palsy.

Bar-big'er-ous. [**Barbig'erus;** from *bar'ba,* a "beard," and *ge'ro,* to "bear."] Having a beard; hairy.

Barége, bå'råzh', written also **Barrége.** A village situated on the French side of the Pyrenees, celebrated for its thermal waters. A peculiar substance has been obtained from these and other waters and termed *baregin,* băr'å-zhin.

Ba-ril'la. [From the Spanish *barilla,* bar-rēl'yå, a plant called "salt-wort."] Impure carbonate of soda imported from Spain and the Levant. British barilla, obtained by burning sea-weeds, is called kelp.

Ba'rĭ-um.* [From βαρύς, "heavy."] The metallic basis of the earth *baryta,* so named from the great density of its compounds.

Bark. [**Cor'tex.**] In the plural, a popular term for Peruvian bark, or that of any species of cinchona. See CINCHONA.

Bark, Car-i-be'an, or **Saint Luci'a Bark,** sometimes improperly called **Cin-cho'na Caribæ'a.*** The bark of the *Exostem'ma Caribæ'um*, and perhaps of some other trees. It is a useful substitute for cinchona, and, though containing neither quinia nor cinchonia, is one of the most valuable of the spurious barks.

Bark, Es-sen'tial Salt of. This is merely an extract, prepared by macerating the bruised substance of bark in cold water, and submitting the infusion to a very slow evaporation.

Bar'ley. [**Hor'deum.**] The seeds of *Hordeum distichon* or *vulgare*.

Bar'ley, Caus'tic. The seeds of *Veratrum sabadilla*.

Barm. See FERMENTUM CEREVISIÆ.

Bar-o-mac-rom'e-ter. [**Baromac-rom'etrum;** from βάρος, "weight," μάκρος, "length," and μέτρον, a "measure."] An instrument for ascertaining the weight and length of new-born infants.

Ba-rom'e-ter. [Lat. **Barom'etrum;** Fr. *Baromètre*, bå'ro'mĕtr'; from βάρος, "weight," and μέτρον, a "measure."] An instrument for ascertaining the weight or pressure of the atmosphere; a weather-glass.

Bar'o-scope. [**Barosco'pium;** from βάρος, "weight," and σκοπέω, to "observe."] A barometer sensible to the slightest atmospheric variations.

Ba-ros'ma.* [From βαρύς, "heavy," and ὀσμή, "odor."] A genus of plants of the order *Rutaceæ*. The leaves of several species constitute *buchu*. Formerly called *Diosma*.

Bar'ras (French pron., bå'rå'). An oleo-resinous substance. See GALIPOT.

Barrenness. See STERILITY.

Barringtoniaceæ,* băr'ring-to-ne-a'she-ē. A natural order of trees or shrubs, found in the tropics.

Bartholinianæ, Glandulæ,* glan'-du-lē bar'to-le-ne-a'nē. The sublingual glands, named after Bartholin.

Bar'wood. A red dye-wood brought from Africa, and used with sulphate of iron for producing the dark red upon British bandana handkerchiefs.

Baryecoia,* bar'e-e-ko'ya. [From βαρύς, "heavy," and ἀκοή, "hearing."] Dulness of hearing; deafness.

Ba-rўph'o-nў. [**Barypho'nia;** from βαρύς, "heavy," and φωνή, the "voice."] Difficulty of speech.

Ba-rў'ta,* or **Ba-rў'tēs.*** [From βαρύς, "heavy;" on account of its weight.] An alkaline earth, the heaviest of all the earths. It is a virulent poison. The native sulphate of baryta is termed *heavy spar*.

Basalt, ba-sault'. [From the Latin *basal'tes*, described by Pliny as a kind of marble very hard and of an iron color.] A common species of trap rock, essentially composed of feldspar and augite. It is of a compact texture and of a dark-green, gray, or black color. It is often found in regular columns, of which the Giants' Causeway and the island of Staffa furnish magnificent examples.

Ba-sal'tĭ-form. [**Basaltifor'mis;** from *basalt'*.] Formed like basalt.

Ba-sal'toid. [**Basaltoi'des;** from *basalt'*, and εἶδος, a "form."] Resembling basalt.

Bas'a-nīte. [From βάσανος, a Lydian stone.] A sort of touchstone by which the purity of gold was tried, and of which medical mortars were made. It consists of silica, lime, magnesia, carbon, and iron.

Bas-cu-lā'tion. [From the French *basculer*, to "see-saw."] A term used in examinations of the uterus in retroversion: the fundus is pressed upwards, the cervix downwards. It is half the *see-saw* movement.

Base. [**Ba'sis;** Gr. βάσις, a "foundation."] The earth, alkali, or metallic oxide which, combined with an acid, forms a salt. In Pharmacy it denotes the principal ingredient of any compound preparation.

Basellaceæ,* băs-el-la'she-ē. A natural order of herbaceous plants, found in tropical regions.

Ba-sĭ-a'tor, o'ris.* [From *ba'sio, basia'tum*, to "kiss."] A muscle whose office it is to contract the mouth. See ORBICULARIS ORIS.

Bas-ĭ-bran'chĭ-al. [**Basibranchi-a'lis;** from *ba'sis* and *branchia'lis*.] Applied by Owen to certain parts of the branchial arch in fishes.

Bā'sic. [**Bas'icus.**] Belonging to, or like, a base.

Bas-ĭ-hў'al. [**Basihya'lis;** from *ba'sis*, "base," and *hyoi'des*, "hyoid."] A term in Comparative Anatomy applied to the two small subcubical bones on each side, forming the body of the inverted hyoid arch.

Bas'ĭ-lad. The same as BASILAR used adverbially.

Bas'ĭ-lar. Applied by Dr. Barclay

as meaning "towards the base of the skull."

Ba-sil'ic. [**Basil'icus;** from *βασιλεύς*, a "king."] Kingly, royal; sometimes applied by the ancients to parts supposed to hold an important place in the animal economy.

Basil'ic Vein. A large vein situated at the fold of the elbow, in front of the humeral artery. It was important because often opened in cases of bloodletting.

Ba-sil'i-con Oint'ment, sometimes written **Basil'icum.** [From the Greek *βασιλικός*, Lat. *basil'icus*, "royal;" so named on account of its great virtues.] The *Cera'tum resi'næ* (U.S. and Lond. Ph.), composed of five parts of resin, eight of lard, and two of yellow wax. It is much used as a stimulating application to blistered surfaces, indolent ulcers, burns, etc.

Bā'sin. [From the French *bas'sin*, a "wet dock."] A geological term denoting the sloping of strata in several directions towards a centre.

Ba'si-o-. A prefix denoting connection with the basilar process of the occipital bone.

Basio-Chondro-Cerato-Glossus. See HYOGLOSSUS.

Ba'sio-Glos'sus.* [From *ba'sis*, and *γλῶσσα*, the "tongue."] A muscle running from the base of the os hyoïdes to the tongue.

Basioccipital, bas'e-ok-sip'e-tal. [**Basioccipita'lis;** from *ba'sis*, "base," and *occipita'le* os, the "occipital bone."] Applied in Comparative Anatomy, by Owen, to a bone homologous with the basilar process of the occipital bone.

Ba'sis.* [Gr. *βάσις*, from *βαίνω*, to "go," to "step," hence, "that on which one steps or stands," a "foundation."] The substance with which an acid is combined in a salt. See BASE. A *mordant*, or substance used in dyeing, which has an affinity both for the cloth and the coloring matter. Also, the principal medicine in a prescription.

Ba'sis Cor'dis.* [*Cor, cor'dis*, the "heart."] The "base of the heart." The broad part of the heart is thus called, as distinguished from the *apex* or point.

Bas-i-sphe'noid. [**Basisphenoi'des.**] Applied in Anatomy and Comparative Anatomy, by Owen, to a bone homologous with the base of the sphenoid bone.

Bas'tard. [**No'thus.**] Applied to a plant or a disease closely resembling but not really what it appears to be.

Bas'tard Dit'ta-ny. The root of the *Dictamus fraxinella*, now fallen into disuse.

Bā'sȳle. [From *βάσις*, a "base," and *ὕλη*, "stuff," "substance."] A term proposed by Mr. Graham to denote the metallic radical of a salt. Thus, sodium is the *basyle* of sulphate of soda.

Bate'man's Pec'to-ral Drops. These consist principally of the tincture of castor, with portions of camphor and opium, flavored with aniseed and colored by cochineal. Used in coughs or lung-affections.

Bates's Al'um Wat'er. The *Li'quor Alu'minis compos'itus* of the London Pharmacopœia; a powerful astringent solution employed for stimulating and cleansing foul ulcers.

Bath. [**Bal'neum,** plural **Bal'nea.**] A term applied to any yielding medium, such as water, sand, etc., in which a body is immersed. Baths are commonly divided into *general* and *partial:* they may consist of simple water, or be *medicated*. As the physiological and therapeutic effects of baths are modified by their temperature, they may be arranged under the following heads:—

GENERAL BATHS.

ARTIFIC'IAL SEA-WA'TER BATH. (*Bal'neum ma'ris facti'tium.**) A solution of one part of common salt in thirty parts of water.

COLD BATH. (*Bal'neum frig'idum.**) The temperature ranges from 33° to 60° Fahr. Below 50° it is considered very cold.

COOL BATH. (*Bal'neum frig'idum.**) Temperature from 60° to 75° Fahr.

HOT-AIR BATH. (*Bal'neum sudato'rium.**) The "sweating bath." Temperature from 100° to 130° Fahr.

HOT BATH. (*Bal'neum cal'idum.**) Temperature from 98° to 112° Fahr.

TEM'PERATE BATH. (*Bal'neum tempera'tum.**) Temperature from 75° to 85° Fahr.

TEP'ID BATH. (*Bal'neum tep'idum.**) Temperature from 85° to 92° Fahr.

VA'POR BATH. (*Bal'neum vapo'ris;** *bal'neum lacon'icum.**) Temperature from 122° to 144–5° Fahr. When a vapor bath is applied only to a particular part of the body, it is called a *fumigation*, or vapor douche.

WARM BATH. (*Bal'neum cal'idum.**) Temperature from 92° to 98° Fahr.; that is, about that of the body.

SAND BATH. (*Bal'neum are'næ.**) This consists of an iron dish, containing fine sand, placed on a fire. A glass vessel may be immersed in this and gradually heated without danger of breaking.

Batrachia. See BATRACHIUS.

Bat'ra-chite. [**Batrachi'tes;** from βάτραχος, a "frog," and λίθος, a "stone."] A stone like a frog; the toad-stone.

Ba-tra'chi-us.* [From βάτραχος, a "frog."] Applied in the plural neuter (*Batra'chia*) to an order of *Reptilia*: batra'chian.

Bat'ra-choid. [**Batrachoi'des;** from βάτραχος, a "frog," and εἶδος, a "form."] Resembling a frog.

Bat'ra-chus.* [Gr. βάτραχος, a "frog."] The same as RANULA, which see.

Bat'te-ry, E-lec'tric-al. A series of coated jars, or of pieces of copper and zinc, for producing electrical or electro-chemical action.

Bat'tery, Gal-van'ic. A combination of several pairs of zinc and copper plates soldered together, and so arranged that the same metal shall always be on the same side of the compound plate.

Bauhin (bō'ăNº'), **Văl'vule of.** A valve in the cæcum, whose office it is to prevent the return of the excrementitious matters from the cæcum into the small intestine. The extremities of its two lips form rugæ in the straight part of the cæcum, called by Morgagni *fræna of the valvule of Bauhin.*

Baume, bōme. The French for BALSAM, which see.

Baume de Vie, bōm dẹh vè. ("Balm of life.") The compound decoction of aloes.

Bay Ber'ries. [**Bac'cæ Lau'ri.**] The berries of the *Laurus nobilis*, or Sweet Bay. A solid substance is extracted from them, called *laurin*, or camphor of the bay berry.

Bay Cher'ry̆, Bay Lau'rel. The *Prunus lauroceramus.*

Bay Salt. Chloride of sodium, or common salt, as obtained by solar evaporation on the shores of the Mediterranean.

Bdella. See HIRUDO.

Bdel'li-um.* A name applied to two gum-resinous substances. One of these is the *Indian bdellium*, or *false myrrh*, procured from the *Am'yris commiph'ora.* The other is called *African bdellium*, and is obtained from the *Hendelo'tia Africa'na.*

Bdellometer, del-lom'e-tẹr. [**Bdellom'etrum;** from βδέλλα, a "leech," and μέτρον, a "measure."] An instrument intended as a substitute for the leech.

Bead'ed. [**Granula'tus.**] Applied to roots knotted, like beads strung closely together.

Bead'-Proof. A term denoting the strength of spirituous liquors, as shown by the continuance of the bubbles or beads on the surface.

Beak. [**Ros'trum.**] The tubular portion of a retort. In Ornithology, the prolongation of the mouth, or substance investing the mandibles, almost always horny, and of various forms, according to the kind of food used by each species; the bill.

Bean of St. Ignatius. See STRYCHNOS IGNATIA.

Beard'ed. [**Barba'tus.**] Having a beard, or some beard-like appendage.

Bear's Ber'ry̆, Bear's Bil'ber-ry̆, Bear's Whor'tle-ber-ry̆. The *Arctostaphylos uva ursi,* formerly called *Arbutus uva ursi.*

Be-bee-rin'. [**Bebeeri'na.**] A vegetable alkali discovered in the *Bebeeru*, or green-heart tree, of British Guiana.

Bebeeru, or **Bibiru,** be-bē'roo. A tree of British Guiana, the timber of which is known to wood-merchants by the name of Green-heart. It yields a substance, called *bebeerin*, of antiperiodic properties.

Bec'ca-bun'ga.* [From the German *Bachbungen*, "water-herb."] Specific name of *Veron'ica Beccabun'ga.*

Bec de Cuiller (Fr.), bĕk dẹh kwè'yå'. An instrument for extracting balls.

Bec de Lièvre. See HARE-LIP.

Bechic, bĕk'ik. [**Bech'icus;** from βήξ, βηχός, "cough."] Belonging to, or relieving, a cough.

Bechica,* bĕk'e-kạ. [See preceding article.] A general term for medicines tending to relieve cough of any kind.

Bedegar, or **Bedeguar,** bed'ẹ-gar. A remarkable gall, termed *sweet-brier sponge*, found on various species of *Rosa*, and produced by the puncture of several species of insects, more especially the *Cynips Rosæ.*

Beer. [**Cerevi'sia;** Fr. *Cervoise*, sĕR'vwåz'.] The fermented infusion of malted barley, flavored with hops. The term "beer" is also applied to beverages consisting of a saccharine liquor partially advanced into the vinous fermentation and flavored with peculiar substances, as spruce-beer, ginger-beer, etc.

Bees'tings. The first milk taken from the cow after calving.

Bees' Wax. [**Ce'ra.**] Wax obtained from the comb of the *Apis mellifica.* See CERA.

Begoniaceæ,* be-go-ne-a'she-ē. A natural order of plants, mostly herbaceous, found in the tropics, including the *Begonia.* They are prized for their showy flowers.

Be-lem'nite. [**Belemni'tes;** from βέλεμνον, a "dart."] The arrow-stone, or fossil thunder-bolt; the petrified remains of certain sea-animals belonging to the same class with the *Nautilus.* They are slender, straight, and conical or sharp at one end. Often found in chalk.

Bel-la-don'na.* [It. a "handsome lady;" the juice being used as a cosmetic.] The Pharmacopœial name (Br. Ph.) for the leaves of *At'ropa belladon'na.* It is a powerful narcotic. When applied to the eye, it has the remarkable property of greatly dilating the pupil.

Bel-la-don'næ Fo'li-um* ("Leaf of Belladonna"), and **Belladon'næ Ra'dix*** ("Root of Belladonna"). See BELLADONNA.

Bell-Met'al. An alloy of copper, zinc, and tin, used for bells, mortars, etc.

Bellows'-Sound. See BRUIT DE SOUFFLET.

Belly. See ABDOMEN, ALVUS, VENTER.

Bel'o-noid. [**Belonoi'des;** from βελόνη, a "bodkin," and εἶδος, a "form."] Resembling a bodkin. Applied to processes of bone: styloid.

Belvisiaceæ,* bel-vis-e-a'she-ē. [From *Belvis'ia,* one of the genera.] A natural order of exogenous plants, found only in Africa. It includes the *Napoleona imperialis.*

Belvisieæ. See BELVISIACEÆ.

Ben, Oil of. The expressed oil of Ben-nut, or the *Morynga pterygo-sperma,* remarkable for not becoming rancid for many years.

Ben-e-dic'tus.* [From *benedi'co, benedic'tum,* to "bless."] Literally, "blessed." A term prefixed to compositions and herbs on account of their supposed good qualities: thus, antimonial wine was termed *benedictum vinum,* etc.

Ben'ja-min. A corruption of *Benzoin.* See BENZOINUM.

Ben'jamin Flow'ers. Benzoic acid.

Benne Leaves. See SESAMUM.

Benzine. See MINERAL TURPENTINE.

Ben'zo-āte. [**Ben'zoas,** *atis.*] A combination of benzoic acid with a base.

Ben-zo'ic. [**Benzo'icus.**] Applied to an acid obtained from gum benzoin.

Ben-zo-if'e-ra.* [From *benzo'inum,* and *fe'ro,* to "bear."] A name applied to the tree commonly known as the *Styrax benzoin.*

Benzoin. See BENZOINUM.

Ben'zo-in, Ben'zo-ine. [**Benzoi'na.**] A compound obtained from oil of bitter almonds.

Ben-zo'ĭ-num.* [Arab. *Benzo'ah.*] The Pharmacopœial name of gum benzoin; obtained from the *Styrax benzoin.* It is a stimulant and expectorant. The inhalation of the vapor of benzoin has been recommended in chronic laryngitis.

Berberaceæ. See BERBERIDACEÆ.

Berberidaceæ,* ber-bĕr-e-da'she-ē, or **Ber-ber-id'e-æ.*** A natural order of plants, named after the *Berberis* (Barberry, or Berberry), which is the most important genus it contains.

Ber'ber-in. [**Berberi'na.**] An alkaline substance obtained from the *Berberis vulgaris.*

Ber'ga-mot. An essence prepared from the rind of the *Citrus bergamia,* otherwise called *Citrus mella rosa.*

Bergmehl (Ger.), bĕrg'māl. Literally, "mountain meal;" an earth, found in Sweden, resembling fine flour, and celebrated for its nutritious qualities. It is found to be composed entirely of the shells of microscopic animalcules.

Beriberi, bā-re-bā'rē. A spasmodic rigidity of the lower limbs, etc.; an acute disease occurring in India, and commonly considered the same as *Barbiers,*—but the latter is a chronic disease. The word *beriberi* is, in all probability, derived from the reduplication of the Hindoo word *beri,* signifying irons or fetters fastened to the legs of criminals, elephants, etc. A person afflicted with this disease is literally "fettered."

Berlin Blue. See PRUSSIAN BLUE.

Ber'rў. A pulpy, indehiscent pericarp, having the seeds scattered loosely in the pulp; as the grape, gooseberry, etc.

Bertin (bĕr'tăng'), **Spon'gў Bones of.** Two small, triangular, turbinated bones, often found beneath the small opening of the sphenoidal sinus.

Bĕr'ўl. [Gr. βήρυλλος.] A variety of the *emerald,* a mineral or gem usually of a green color of various shades, passing into honey-yellow and sky-blue. When colored green by oxide of chromium, it forms the true emerald, and when colorless and transparent, *aquamarina.*

Bē'tel. A famous masticatory employed in the East, consisting chiefly of the *areca, betel,* or *pinang nut,* the produce of the *Areca Catechu,* or Catechu Palm. A portion of the nut is rolled up with a little lime in the leaf of the Piper betel, and the whole chewed.

Betulaceæ,* bet-u-la'she-ē, **Bet-u-lin'e-æ.*** [From *bet'ula,* a "birch-tree."] A natural order of trees, consisting of the various kinds of Birch and Alder. These trees formed part of the Jussieuan order *Amentaceæ.*

Betulaceous, bet-u-lā'shŭs, or **Bet-u-lin'e-ous.** [**Betula'ceus, Betulin'eus;** from *bet'ula,* the "birch-tree."] Having an arrangement as in the *Betula.* See BETULACEÆ.

Be-zo'ar, or **Be-zo'ard.** [Pers. *Pazahar;* from *pa,* "against," and *zahar,* a "poison."] A calculous concretion sometimes found in the stomach, intestines, and bladder of certain land-animals, such as the ox, horse, deer. These concretions were formerly considered to possess wonderful medicinal virtues, and to be completely efficacious not only against poisons, but also against pestilential and other diseases.

Bez'o-ar'dics. A class of medicines supposed to possess virtues similar to those of the bezoar.

Bhang, b'hăng, or băng. The *Can'nabis In'dica,* or Indian Hemp. A plant common in India, containing powerful narcotic properties. It is used in various forms by the people of India for the purpose of intoxication. The tops and tender parts of the plant, when dried, constitute the hashish (hå-sheesh') of the Arabs. See CANNABIS INDICA.

Bi-. [From *bis,* "twice."] A prefix in certain compound names, signifying two, or twice; as *biceps,* "two-headed."

Bib. = *Bibe.** "Drink" (imperative mood of the verb *bibo*).

Bī-bā'sic. [**Bibas'icus;** from *bi-,* "two," and *ba'sis,* a "base."] Having two bases, as the tartrate of potash and soda.

Bib-ĭ-to'rĭ-us.* [From *bi'bo, bib'itum,* to "drink."] A former name of the *rectus internus oculi,* from its drawing the eye inwards towards the nose, and thus directing it into the cup in drinking.

Bib'u-lous. [**Bib'ulus;** from *bi'bo,* to "drink."] Attracting moisture; absorbing.

Bī-cap'su-lar. [**Bicapsula'ris;** from *bi-,* "two," and *cap'sula,* a "capsule."] Having two capsules.

Bī-car'bo-nate. [**Bicarbo'nas, a'tis;** from *bi-,* "two," and *carbo'nas,* a "carbonate."] Two equivalents of carbonic acid combined with one of base.

Bī-cau'dal. [**Bicauda'lis;** from *bi-,* "two," and *cau'da,* a "tail."] Having two tails. Applied to a muscle.

Bī-çe-pha'lĭ-um.* [From *bis,* "twice" or "twofold," and κεφαλή, the "head."] A large *sarcoma* on the head, as if another were grown upon it.

Bī-çeph'a-lous. [**Biceph'alus;** from the same.] Having two heads.

Bī'ceps,* gen. **Bi-cip'ĭ-tis.** [From *bi-,* "two," and *ca'put,* the "head."] Having two heads. Applied to a muscle of the arm, and to one of the thigh.

Bichat (bē'shå'), **Ca-năl' of.** A small round hole above the pineal gland, opening into the third ventricle of the brain: called also the arachnoid canal.

Bī-chlo'rīde of Mer'cu-rȳ. Corrosive sublimate.

Bī-cip'ĭ-tal. [**Bicipita'lis.**] Belonging to the *biceps* muscle.

Bī-con'ju-gate. [**Biconjuga'tus;** from *bi-,* "two," and *con'jugo,* to "yoke together."] In pairs.

Bī-cor'nous. [**Bicor'nis;** from *bi-,* "two," and *cor'nu,* a "horn."] Two-horned.

Bī-cus'pid, or **Bī-cus'pĭ-dāte.** [**Bicus'pis, Bicuspida'tus;** from *bi-,* "two," and *cus'pis,* the "point of a spear."] Having two points. See TOOTH.

Bī-den'tal. [**Bi'dens, en'tis, Bidenta'lis;** from *bi-,* "two," and *dens,* a "tooth."] Having two teeth.

Bī-den'tate. [**Bidenta'tus;** from the same.] Having two teeth.

Bī-dig'ĭ-tate. [**Bidigita'tus;** from *bi-,* "two," and *dig'itus,* a "finger."] Having two fingers.

Bī-dig-ĭ'ti-Pin-na'tus.* [From the same, and *pinna'tus,* "pinnate."] Applied to a pinnate leaf with two leaflets at the end of the common petiole.

Bī-en'nĭ-al. [**Bien'nis;** from *bien'nium* (*bi-,* "two," and *an'nus,* a "year"), the "space of two years."] Of two years' duration.

Bī-fā'rĭ-ous. [**Bifa'rius;** from *bi-,* "two," and *fa'ri,* to "speak."] Having a double meaning; pointing two ways.

Bif'er-ous. [**Bi'fer, Bif'erus;** from *bi-* for *bis,* "twice," and *fe'ro,* to "bear."] Bearing twice in the year.

Bī'fid. [**Bif'idus;** from *bi-,* "two," and *fin'do,* to "cleave."] Divided into two: cleft.

Bī-flo'rous, or **Bī-flo'rate.** [**Biflo'rus;** from *bi-,* "two," and *flos,* a "flower."] Having two flowers.

Bi-fo'rate, or **Bi-fo'rous.** [**Bifora'tus, Bif'orus;** from *bi-*, "two," and *fo'res*, a "door."] Having two entries or apertures.

Bi-fur'cate. [**Bifurca'tus;** from *bi-*, "two," and *fur'ca*, a "fork."] Divided into two, like a fork.

Bi-fur-cā'tion. [**Bifurca'tio, o'nis;** from the same.] A dividing into two, as a fork into its prongs.

Bi-gas'ter.* [From *bi-*, "two," and γαστήρ, the "belly."] The same as BIVENTER.

Bi-ġem'i-nate. [**Bigemina'tus;** from *bi-*, and *gem'ini*, "twins."] Applied in Botany to leaves having two secondary petioles, each of which has a pair of leaflets.

Bignoniaceæ,* big-no-ne-a'she-ē. A natural order of plants, including the *Bigno'nia* (trumpet-flower) and Catalpa. Many of them are trees or twining plants remarkable for the beauty of their flowers.

Bignoniaceous, big-no-ne-ā'shŭs. [**Bignonia'ceus;** from *Bigno'nia*, the "trumpet-flower."] Having an arrangement as in the *Bignonia*. See BIGNONIACEÆ.

Bignoniæ,* big-no'ne-ē, the plural of **Bigno'nia,** forming the Jussieuan name of a natural order of plants. See BIGNONIACEÆ.

Bi-ho'rĭ-us.* [From *bi-*, "two," and *ho'ra*, an "hour."] Enduring two hours.

Bi'ju-gate. [**Bijuga'tus,** or **Bij'ugus;** from *bi-*, "two," and *ju'gum*, a "yoke."] Double-yoked; in two pairs.

Bi'labe. [*Bila'bium?* probably from *bis*, "twice," or "two," and *la'bium*, a "lip."] An instrument for extracting foreign bodies of sufficiently moderate size from the bladder through the urethra.

Bi-lā'bi-ate. [**Bilabia'tus;** from *bi-*, and *la'bium*, a "lip."] Having two lips.

Bi-la-cin'ĭ-ate. [**Bilacinia'tus;** from *bi-*, and *lacinia'tus*, "fringed."] Double-fringed.

Bi-lam'el-late. [**Bilamella'tus;** from *bi-*, and *lamella'tus*, "having little plates."] Having two layers of little plates.

Bi-lat'er-al. [**Bilatera'lis;** from *bi-*, and *latera'lis*, "pertaining to the side."] Applied to leaves proceeding from different points as well as different sides, and so somewhat distinct from opposite.

Bile. [**Bi'lis,** or **Fel;** Gr. χολή; Fr. *Bile*, bēl, and *Fiel*, fe-ĕl'.] The gall, or peculiar secretion of the liver. It is a viscid fluid, of a greenish-yellow color, and exceedingly bitter, whence the proverb "bitter as gall." The bile or gall of the ox (*bi'lis bovi'na*) has often been used medicinally as a tonic and anthelmintic, and as a laxative in cases of deficient biliary secretion. It has also been supposed to possess great healing virtues when applied externally to bruises and other sores.

Bil'ia-rȳ. [**Bilia'ris.**] Belonging to the bile.

Bi'lin, or **Bi'line.** [**Bili'na;** from *bi'lis*.] A gummy, pale-yellow mass, considered to be the principal constituent of the bile.

Bilious, bil'yŭs. [**Bilio'sus;** from *bi'lis*.] Having much bile, full of bile, or relating to the bile.

Bil-ĭ-phe'in. [**Biliphæi'na;** from *bi'lis*, and φαιός, "of a brown color."] The most important coloring matter of the bile.

Bilis. See BILE.

Bilis Atra. See MELANCHOLIA.

Bi'lis Bo-vi'na.* The Latin term for ox's gall. See BILIS.

Bil-ĭ-ver'din. [**Biliverdi'na;** Fr. *Bile*, and *vert*, "green-color."] A green substance obtained from the yellowish coloring matter of bile.

Bi-lo'bate. [From *bi-*, "two," and λοβός, a "lobe."] Having two lobes.

Bi-loc'u-lar. [**Bilocula'ris;** from *bi-*, "two," and *loc'ulus*, a "little cell."] Having two cells.

Bim'a-nous. [**Bim'anus;** from *bi-*, "two," and *ma'nus*, a "hand,"] Having two hands. Applied in the plural neuter to an order of *Mammalia*, of which man constitutes the only genus.

Bi-mes'tris.* [From *bi-*, "two," and *men'sis*, a "month."] Of two months; two months old.

Bin-. The same as *Bi-*, the *n* being added for the sake of euphony before a vowel; as, bi*n*oxalate, etc.

Bi'na-rȳ. [**Bina'rius;** from *bi'nus*, "by couples."] Consisting of two, as two elements, two measures, etc.

Bi'nate. [**Bina'tus;** from *bi-*, "two," and *na'tus*, "born," "produced."] Growing in pairs or couples.

Bi-ner'vate, Bi-ner'vĭ-ous. [**Biner'vatus, Biner'vius;** from *bi-*, and *nerva'tus*, "nerved."] Having two nerves.

Bi-noc'u-lar. [**Binocula'ris;** from *bin-*, "two," and *oc'ulus*, the "eye."] Having the use of both eyes.

Bi-noc'u-lus.* [From *bin-*, and *oc'-*

ulus, the "eye."] Applied in Surgery to a bandage for maintaining dressings on both eyes. Also the name of an animal resembling the king-crab.

Bī-nox'a-lāte. [**Binox'alas, a'tis**; from *bin-*, "two," or "twice," and *ox'alas*, an "oxalate."] A combination of an excess of oxalic acid with a base.

Bī-o-dȳn-am'ics. [**Biodynam'ica**; from *βίος*, "life," and *δύναμις*, "power."] The doctrine or science of the vital forces.

Bī-ol'o-ġȳ. [**Biolo'gia**; from *βίος*, "life," and *λόγος*, a "discourse."] The doctrine or science of life.

Bi-ol'ȳ-sis.* [From *βίος*, "life," and *λύω*, to "dissolve," to "destroy."] The destruction of life.

Bī-o-lȳt'ic. [**Biolyt'icus**; from the same.] Destroying or impairing life. Applied to agents of a deleterious quality, as the more powerful acids, narcotics, etc.

Bi-o-mag-ne-tis'mus.* [From *βίος*, "life," and *magnetis'mus*, "magnetism."] Another name for animal magnetism.

Bī-par'tīte. [**Biparti'tus**; from *bi-*, "two," and *par'tio*, to "divide."] Divided deeply into two.

Bī-pel'tate. [**Bipel'tatus**; from *bi-*, "two," and *pel'ta*, a "target" or "buckler."] Having two shields. Applied to a family of the *Crusta'cea Stomap'oda.*

Bi'pes,* gen. **Bip'ed-is.** [From *bi-*, "two," and *pes*, a "foot."] Having two feet: bi'ped.

Bī-pin'nate. [**Bipinna'tus**; from *bi-*, "two," and *pin'na*, a "leaflet."] Having double leaflets.

Bī-pin-nat'ĭ-fid. [**Bipinnatif'idus**; from *bi-*, "two," and *pinnatif'idus.*] Doubly pinnatifid.

Bird'līme. [**Vis'cus.**] A glutinous substance prepared from the bark of the holly. It contains resin, which has been called *viscina.*

Bi-ros'trate. [**Birostra'tus, Biros'tris**; from *bi-*, and *ros'trum*, a "beak."] Having two beaks.

Bī-sex'u-al. [**Bisexua'lis**; from *bi-*, and *sexua'lis.*] Of both sexes.

Bis. ind. = *Bis in di'es.** "Twice daily."

Bis'muth. [**Bismu'thum.** Ger. *Bis'mut.*] A yellowish-white metal, found generally native or in the metallic state.

Bis-mu'thi Subni'tras. See next article.

Bis-mu'thum Al'bum.* The Pharmacopœial name (Br. Ph.) of the trisnitrate of bismuth: flake-white, or pearl-white, sometimes called the subnitrate of bismuth (*Bismuthi subnitras*).

Bis-tor'ta,* or **Bis'tort.** [From *bis*, "twice," and *tor'queo*, to "twist:" so named from the form of the root.] See next article.

Bis-tor'tæ Ra'dix.* The root of the *Polygonum bistorta*, Great Bistort or Snake-Weed.

Bistoury, bis'tŭr-e. [Fr. *Bistouri*; from *Pistori*, a town where it was manufactured.] A small knife, or scalpel, for surgical purposes. There are the *straight*, the *curved*, and the *probe-pointed*, which is also curved.

Bis'tre. A brown color, made of wood-soot boiled and evaporated. Beech-soot is said to make the best.

Bī-sul'phāte. [**Bisul'phas, a'tis**; from *bi-*, "two," and *sul'phas.*] A combination of two equivalents of sulphuric acid with one of the base.

Bī-sul'phīte. [**Bisul'phis, i'tis**; from *bi-*, "two," and *sul'phis.*] A combination of two equivalents of sulphurous acid with one of the base.

Bī-tar'trāte. [**Bitar'tras, a'tis**; from *bi-*, and *tar'tras.*] A supersalt with twice as much tartaric acid as the corresponding neutral salt.

Bī-ter'nate. [**Biterna'tus**; from *bis*, "twice," and *terna'tus.*] Twice ternate, or doubly threefold.

Bit'ter Alm'onds, Wat'er of, or **Bit'ter Alm'ond Wat'er.** [**A'qua Amyg'dalæ Ama'ræ,** or **A'qua Amygdala'rum Ama'rum.**] In this preparation there are sixteen minims of the oil of bitter almonds to two pints of water, or half a minim to a fluidounce. It is employed as a vehicle for other medicines in nervous coughs and spasmodic affections.

Bit'ter Ap'ple, Bit'ter Cu'cumber, Bit'ter Gourd. The plant and fruit of *Cucumis colocynthis.*

Bit'ter Prin'cĭ-ple. A peculiar principle, on the presence of which the bitter quality of certain vegetables depends; as in the wood of quassia, gentian root, the hop, etc.

Bit'ter-Sweet. The SOLANUM DULCAMARA, which see.

Bit'ter-ing. Corruptly called *Bittern.* A preparation for adulterating beer, composed of Cocculus Indicus, liquorice, tobacco, quassia, and sulphate of iron or copperas. A similar preparation is sold under the name of "bitter balls."

Bit'tern. The water remaining after

the crystallization of common salt from sea-water or salt springs.

Bit'ters. [**Ama'ra.**] A term applied to several medicinal substances, expressing their quality as particularly perceptible to the taste, and which are further distinguished into aromatic, pure, and styptic bitters.

Bi-tu'men, minis.* [As if *pittu'men;* from πίττα, "pitch."] A name for certain inflammable mineral substances, of different consistencies ranging from fluid to solid.

Bitu'men Bar-ba-den'se.* The *Petroleum* of the Pharmacopœias (Lond. and Ed.), or "Barbadoes Tar."

Bi-tu'min-i-zā'tion. [**Bituminiza'tio, o'nis.**] The transformation of organic matter into *bitumen,* as wood into coal, and the remains of vegetable substances into peat.

Bi-tu'min-ous. [**Bitumino'sus;** from *bitu'men.*] Of the nature of bitumen.

Bi'valve. [**Bival'vis;** from *bi-,* and *val'va,* a "valve."] Having two valves.

Bi-ven'ter.* [From *bi-,* and *ven'ter,* the "belly."] Double-belly. A faulty term used for *Digastricus;* also called *Bigaster.*

Bixaceæ,* bix-a'she-ē. A natural order of tropical trees and shrubs, including the Bixa, which produces *arnotto* or *annotto,* used to color cheese.

Black Death. [Lat. **Mors Ni'gra,** or **Pes'tis Ni'gra;** Fr. *Peste Noir,* pĕst nwår.] The name given in Germany and the North of Europe to an Oriental plague which occurred in the fourteenth century, characterized by inflammatory boils and black spots on the skin, indicating putrid decomposition. In Italy it was called *la mortalega grande,* "the great mortality." In many of its characters this pestilence resembled the present bubo plague, complicated with pneumonia and hæmorrhages.

Black Draught. A popular purgative, consisting of the infusion of senna with sulphate of magnesia.

Black Drop. [**Gut'tæ Ni'græ.** Literally, "black drops."] A solution of opium in verjuice, corresponding nearly in its medicinal properties to the *Acetum Opii* of the U. S. Pharmacopœia. One drop of this solution is equal to about three of laudanum. It is less apt to disturb or excite the nervous system than the latter preparation. See U. S. Pharmacopœia, page 67.

Black Flux. A mixture of charcoal and carbonate of potash, obtained by deflagrating tartar with half its weight of nitre.

Black Lead. See PLUMBAGO.

Black Vom'it. [**Vom'itus Ni'ger.**] The throwing up, in certain fevers, of a dark-colored fluid resembling coffee-grounds. This fluid consists chiefly of blood changed by the morbid secretions of the stomach. It is one of the most fatal symptoms attending yellow fever, which in Spanish is often called simply *El vom'ito* ("the vomit"), or *El vom'ito ne'gro* ("the black vomit").

Black Wash. [**Lo'tio Ni'gra,** or **Lo'tio Hydrar'gyri Ni'gra.**] A lotion made with calomel in lime-water, much used for syphilitic sores.

Blad'der. [**Vesi'ca.**] Generally, the receptacle of the urine in man and other animals. Applied in Botany and Natural History to various objects and productions of similar appearance, as those of sea-wrack, the air-bag of fishes, etc.

Blad'der-Fu'cus, Blad'der-Wrack. The *Fucus vesiculosus.*

Blad'der, Gall. See GALL-BLADDER.

Bladder, Urinary. See URINARY BLADDER.

Bladdery Fever. [**Fe'bris Bullo'sa.**] See PEMPHIGUS.

Blæs'i-tas, a'tis.* [From βλαισός, "one who has crooked legs;" also "one who stammers."] The defect of speech termed stuttering or stammering. Some writers understand by it the substitution of soft consonants for hard,—as *d* for *t, b* for *p,* etc. See PSELLISMUS.

Blain. A pustule, blotch, or sore. See CHILBLAIN.

Blanc de Troyes, blŏng dẹh trwå. Spanish White, prepared chalk, or the *Cre'ta præpara'ta* of the Pharmacopœias.

Blas-te'ma, atis.* [From βλαστάνω, to "germinate."] A term applied to the rudimental mass of an organ in the process of formation.

Blas'to-derm. [**Blastoder'ma, atis;** from βλαστάνω, to "germinate," and δέρμα, the "skin."] A minute, thin membrane on that surface of the yolk which, whatever be the position of the egg, is, by a peculiar arrangement, always uppermost; the germinal membrane, or *Cicatricula.*

Blas-to-der'mic. [**Blastoder'micus.**] Belonging to the blastoderm.

Blastoder'mic Ves'i-cle. [**Vesic'ula Blastoder'mica.**] A distinct envelope immediately surrounding the yelk, and covered by the vitelline membrane; afterwards called the umbilical vesicle.

Blas-to-gen'e-sis.* [From βλαστός, a "sprout," and γένεσις, "generation."] The multiplication of plants by means of buds.

Bleach. [From the German *blei'chen*, to "whiten."] To whiten by the removal of, or by changing the nature of, the coloring matter in any substance. See next article.

Bleach'ing. [**Dealba'tio;** from *de*, intensive, and *al'bus*, "white."] The chemical process of *whitening* linen or woollen stuffs. Linen is usually bleached by means of chlorine or a solution of chloride of lime. Woollen stuffs are bleached by exposure to the vapor of sulphurous acid.

BLEACH'ING POW'DER. Chloride of lime, formerly called oxymuriate of lime; prepared by exposing hydrate of lime gradually to chlorine gas.

BLEACH'ING LIQ'UID. [Fr. *Eau de Javelle*, ō dẹh zhå'vĕll'.] This is the preceding compound obtained in solution by transmitting a stream of chlorine gas through hydrate of lime suspended in water.

Blear'-Eye. A chronic catarrhal inflammation of the eyelids.

Bleb. See BULLA.

Bleeding. See BLOOD-LETTING, HÆMORRHAGE.

Blende, blĕnd. [Perhaps from the Saxon *blen'dan*, to "mix together."] The native sulphuret of zinc in black crystals, and called by miners *black jack*. The term is sometimes applied to other ores, as *manganese blende*, etc.

Blen'nad-e-ni'tis, idis.* [From βλέννα, "mucus," and *adeni'tis*.] Inflammation of mucous glands.

Blen'ne-lỹt'rĭ-ạ.* [From βλέννα, "mucus," and ἔλυτρον, a "sheath."] Same as LEUCORRHŒA.

Blen'nen-te'rĭ-ạ.* [From βλέννα, "mucus," and ἔντερον, an "intestine."] Mucous flow from the intestines.

Blen'no-gen'ic. [**Blen'nogen'icus;** from βλέννα, "mucus," and γεννάω, to "generate."] Generating mucus; muciparous.

Blen-nog'e-nus.* The same as BLENNOGENIC, which see.

Blen'no-me-tri'tis, idis.* [From βλέννα, "mucus," and *metri'tis*.] Mucous flow accompanying *Metritis*.

Blen'noph-thăl'mĭ-ạ.* [From βλέννα, "mucus," and *ophthal'mia*.] Inflammation of the mucous membrane of the eye.

Blen-nor-rha'ġĭ-ạ.* [From βλέννα, "mucus," and ῥήγνυμι, to "break" or "burst."] Literally, a "bursting forth of mucus:" hence, an excessive discharge of mucus, or muco-purulent matter, more especially from the genital organs.

Blennorrhœa,* blen-no-rē'ạ. [From βλέννα, "mucus," and ῥέω, to "flow."] A flowing, or excessive secretion, from mucous glands in any situation; sometimes applied to the increased secretion in the urethra and vagina of an infectious purulent or muco-purulent discharge, and called *Gonorrhœa*. See BAPTORRHŒA.

Blennorrhœ'a Chron'ĭ-cạ.* Gleet; also named *Catarrhus urethralis*.

Blennorrhœ'a Sim'plex.* Increased secretion of mucus from the urethra.

Blen-ny'men, enis.* [From βλέννα, "mucus," and ὑμήν, a "membrane."] A mucous membrane.

Blen-ny'me-ni'tis, idis.* [From βλέννα, "mucus."] Inflammation of a mucous membrane.

Bleph'ạr-ad'e-ni'tis, idis.* [From βλέφαρον, the "eyelid," and ἀδήν, a "gland."] Inflammation of the Meibomian glands.

Bleph'ạr-i'tis, idis.* [From βλέφαρον, the "eyelid."] Inflammation of the eyelids.

Bleph'ạr-on'cus.* [From βλέφαρον, the "eyelid," and ὄγκος, a "tumor."] A tumor on the eyelid.

Bleph'ạr-oph-thăl'mĭ-ạ.* [From βλέφαρον, the "eyelid," and ὀφθαλμία, "inflammation of the eye."] Inflammation of the eye and eyelids coexisting.

Bleph'ạr-oph-thăl'mic. [**Blepharophthal'micus.**] Belonging to *Blepharophthalmia*.

Bleph'ạr-o-plas'tic. [**Bleph'aroplas'ticus.**] Belonging to blepharoplasty.

Bleph'ạr-o-plas-tỹ. [**Bleph'aroplas'tia;** from βλέφαρον, the "eyelid," and πλάσσω, to "form."] An operation for repairing any lesion of the eyelids, by taking a flap from the sound parts contiguous.

Bleph'ạr-o-ple'ġĭ-ạ.* [From βλέφαρον, the "eyelid," and πληγή, a "stroke."] The falling down of the upper eyelid from paralysis.

Bleph'ạ-rop-to'sis.* [From βλέφαρον, the "eyelid," and πτῶσις, a "falling."] The same as BLEPHAROPLEGIA.

Blessed. See BENEDICTUS.

Blight, blīt. The popular name of a slight palsy, caused by sudden cold or damp. "Blight in the eye" is another term for catarrhal ophthalmia.

Blindness, Day. See NYCTALOPIA.

Blindness, Night; Blindness, Nocturnal. See HEMERALOPIA.

Blis'ter. [Lat. **Vesic'ula;** Fr. *Vessie,* vĕs'sē'.] A collection of serous fluid beneath the cuticle. In common language, the plaster itself [Lat. **Vesicato'rium;** Fr. *Vésicatoire,* vā'sē'kā'twăʀ'] which produces the blis'er. See BULLA.

Blister-Bee'tle, Blister-Fly. See CANTHARIS.

Blis'tered. See BULLATUS.

Blis'ters, Fly'ing. [Fr. *Vésicatoires volants,* vā'zē'kā'twăʀ' vo'lŏɴᵍ'.] A mode of treatment employed by the continental practitioners for the purpose of insuring a more diffusive counter-irritation. According to this plan, the blister remains only till it produces a rubefacient effect; a second blister is then applied to some other part, and so on in succession.

Blood. [Lat. **San'guis, inis**; Gr. *αἷμα*; Fr. *Sang,* sŏɴᵍ.] The red fluid which circulates through the cavities of the heart, the arteries and veins. Every organ of the body, and every tissue, is nourished by the blood, which is also the source of every secretion. It is red and usually warm in vertebrated animals, but cold and white for the most part in the *Invertebrata.*

Blood contains albumen in three states of modification:—viz., *albumen* properly so called, *fibrin,* and *red particles.* On coagulation it separates into—

SE'RUM.* A yellowish liquid, containing albumen and various saline matters suspended in water; and

CRASSAMEN'TUM,* called also CRU'OR.* A red solid, consisting of fibrin and red particles.

Blood'-Let-ting. [**Mis'sio San'guinis,** or **Detrac'tio San'guinis.**] A term embracing every artificial discharge of blood for the cure or prevention of disease. It is *general,* as in venesection and arteriotomy, or *topical,* as in the application of leeches, cupping-glasses, or by scarification.

Blood'-Shot. A distension or preternatural fulness of the blood-vessels of the eye, from inflammation or other cause. See HYPERÆMIA.

Blood'stone. [**Hæmati'tes.**] A species of chalcedony supposed to be useful in stopping a bleeding from the nose.

Blood-Stroke. See COUP DE SANG.

Bloody Flux. See DYSENTERY

Blossom. See COROLLA.

Blow'-Pipe. A simple, tapering, tube-like instrument of silver or brass, used for the purpose of inflation; also for directing a stream of air into the flame of a lamp, which thus assumes a conical form, at the point of which the heat is equal to that of a powerful furnace.

The *oxy-hydrogen blow-pipe* is an apparatus for producing intense heat, by supplying a stream of hydrogen with pure oxygen, so that the two gases issue together in the form of a jet from the nozzle of the blow-pipe. The heat produced by this apparatus (which is also called the *compound blow-pipe*) is so intense as to quickly fuse substances completely infusible by any other means except a powerful galvanic battery or a very large burning lens.

Blue Black. Another name for ivory-black, or the *ebur ustum;* from its bluish hue.

Blue Disease. [**Mor'bus Cæru'leus.**] See CYANOSIS.

Blue John. A name given by miners to fluor spar; also called Derbyshire spar.

Blue Mass. [**Mas'sa de Hydrar'gyro.**] A substance formed by rubbing metallic mercury with conserve of roses until all the globules disappear. Of this mass blue pills are made. This is regarded as one of the mildest preparations of mercury. See PILULÆ HYDRARGYRI.

Blue Oint'ment. The *Unguentum hydrargyri.*

Blue Pills. The *Pilulæ hydrargyri.* See BLUE MASS.

Blue Pot. Another term for a black-lead crucible, made of a mixture of coarse plumbago and clay.

Blue, Prussian. See PRUSSIAN BLUE.

Blue Stone, Blue Vit'ri-ol. [**Cæru'leus La'pis.**] The sulphate of copper (*Sulphas cupri*).

Blunt Hook. [**Embryul'cus.**] An instrument used in Obstetrical Surgery.

B. M. = *Bal'neum mari'æ.** A "water-bath."

Boat'-Shaped. See NAVICULAR and SCAPHOID.

Bod'y̆. [Lat. **Cor'pus, Cor'poris;** Gr. *σῶμα*; Fr. *Corps,* koʀ.] Any mass or portion of matter. In a more restricted sense, the material part of man or of any animal, considered separately from the soul or life. The term is often employed synonymously with "trunk."

Bog-Bean'. The common name for *Menyan'thes trifolia'ta.*

Bo-hēa'. The *The'a ni'gra,* or black tea.

Bo'hun U'pas. A bitter gum-resin which exudes from incisions in the bark of a large tree, in Java and the neighboring islands, called *Antiar,* or *Antikar,* by the Javanese; the *Antiaris toxicaria,* or *Ipo toxicaria,* of botanists. It is a deadly poison.

Boil. See FURUNCULUS.

Boil'ing Point of Wa'ter, near the level of the sea, is 212° of Fahrenheit; *in vacuo,* 67°; under sufficient pressure, water may be raised almost to a red heat. According to the Centigrade thermometer, the boiling point is 100°; according to Reaumur's, 80°.

Bois, bwå, the French word for "wood:" hence **Bois Amer,** bwåz å'-maiʀ' ("bitter wood"), another name for QUASSIA, which see.

Bois de Campêche, bwå dęh kŏɴ'-pĕsh'. ("Campeachy Wood.") A name for Logwood. See HÆMATOXYLUM.

Bol. = *Bolus.** See BOLUS.

Bole. See BOLUS.

Bo-le'tāte. [**Bole'tas, a'***tis.*] A combination of boletic acid with a base.

Bo-let'ic Aç'id. An acid discovered in the *Boletus pseudo-igniarius.*

Bo-le'tus.* [From βῶλος, a "mass."] A kind of fungus referred to the genus *Lycoperdon.*

Bole'tus Ig-nĭ-a'rĭ-us.* [From *ig'nis,* "fire;" because often used as tinder.] The agaric of the oak, or touchwood. See AGARICUS QUERCUS.

Bole'tus Pur'gans.* Larch agaric; formerly employed as a drastic purgative.

Bo'lus.* [Gr. βῶλος, a "lump" or "mass."] Any roundly-formed medicine, larger than an ordinary-sized pill, yet small enough to be swallowed. A kind of argillaceous earth: bole.

Bolus Armeniæ. See ARMENIAN BOLE.

Bombaceæ,* bom-ba'she-ē. [From *Bom'bax,* the "cotton-tree."] A natural order of trees, including the gigantic *Baobab* and cotton-tree of India. They grow in tropical countries. The cotton of the *Bombax* is too short for textile tissues. This order is called *Sterculiaceæ* by Lindley.

Bom'bax, a'*cis.** A Linnæan genus of the class *Monadelphia,* natural order *Bombaceæ.* The cotton-tree.

Bom'bĭ-āte. [**Bom'bias, a'***tis.*] A combination of bombic acid with a base.

Bom'bic. [**Bom'bicus;** from βόμβυξ, a "silk-worm."] Pertaining to the *Bombyx.*

Bom'bic Aç'id. An acid obtained from the silk-worm chrysalis.

Bom'bus.* [Gr. βόμβος, the "buzzing of bees."] A ringing noise in the ears; also, the sound of flatus moving through the intestines. See TINNITUS AURIUM, and BORBORYGMUS.

Bone. [Lat. **Os, Os'sis;** Gr. ὀστέον; Fr. *Os,* ō.] A substance consisting chiefly of phosphate of lime and gelatine, forming the solid frame-work or skeleton in vertebrated animals. See OSTEOLOGY, and SKELETON.

Bone'-Bind-er. The *Osteocolla.*

Bone Earth. Phosphate of lime; the earthy basis of the bones of animals.

Bone Spir'it. A brown, ammoniacal liquor, obtained in the process of manufacturing animal charcoal from bones.

Bon-plan'dĭ-a Trĭ-fo-lĭ-a'ta.* [Named from *M. Bonpland,* the discoverer.] The former name of the tree affording *Angustura bark,* now referred to the *Galipea cusparia.*

Bo-raç'ic Aç'id. An acid obtained from borax.

Boraginaceæ,* bo-raj-e-na'she-ē. A natural order of plants, comprising the Borage (*Bora'go, Bora'ginis*), and possessing mucilaginous and emollient properties.

Bo-ra-gin'e-æ.* The Jussieuan name of an order of plants. See BORAGINACEÆ.

Bo'rāte. [**Bo'ras, a'***tis;* from *bo-raç'icum aç'idum.*] A combination of boracic acid with a base.

Bo'rax, a'*cis.** The Pharmacopœial name (Br. Ph.) for the borate of soda (*So'dæ Bo'ras*), otherwise called biborate of soda (*So'dæ Bibo'ras*). Borax is a mild refrigerant and diuretic; in the form of powder mixed with sugar, it is often used as a remedy for aphthæ in children.

Bor-bo-rȳg'mus.* [From βορβορύζω, to "produce a rumbling in the bowels."] The gurgling noise produced by the movements of flatus in the intestines.

Bor'ne-ĕn. The name given to a

compound of carbon and hydrogen found in valeric acid, and which, on exposure to moisture, acquires the properties of *Borneo camphor:* it is supposed to be identical with liquid camphor. The camphor itself has been named *borneol;* and it is converted by the action of nitric acid into laurel camphor.

Bor'ne-o Cam'phor, called also Sumatra Camphor. A crystalline solid found in crevices of the wood of the *Dryobal'anops aromat'ica.*

Bo'ron. [**Bo'rium.**] The base of boracic acid.

Bōr'ū-ret. [**Borure'tum;** from *bo'ron.*] A combination of boron with a simple body.

Bos-op'ric Aç'id. A strong, colorless acid, procured from fresh cow-dung, of great efficacy in purifying mordanted cotton. A better term would be *bucopric acid.*

Boṡ-wel'lĭ-ạ Ser-ra'tạ.* The tree believed to afford *Olibanum.*

Botal's Hole. [**Fora'men Bota'le.**] See FORAMEN OVALE.

Bot-an-ol'o-ġȳ. [**Botanolo'gia;** from βοτανή, an "herb," and λόγος, a "discourse."] The science of plants; the same as BOTANY.

Bot'ạ-nȳ. [**Botan'ica;** from βοτανή, an "herb."] That branch of Natural History which treats of plants, or of the vegetable kingdom.

Both-rĭ-o-çeph'ạ-lus.* [From βοθρίον, a "little pit," and κεφαλή, the "head."] Another name for the TÆNIA LATA, which see.

Bot'rȳ-oid. [**Botryoi'des;** from βότρυς, a "cluster of grapes."] Resembling a cluster of grapes.

Bot-rȳ-oid'ạl. The same as BOTRYOID, which see.

Bottle-Shaped. See LAGENÆFORMIS.

Botts. Small worms which breed in the intestines of horses: they are the larvæ of the *Œstrus*, or gadfly, which deposits its eggs on the hair of the horse, and by the licking of the animal they are swallowed.

Bot-u-lin'ic [from *bot'ulus*, a "sausage"] **Aç'id.** An acid found in putrid sausages, supposed to be the same principle as ALLANTOTOXICUM.

Bougie (Fr.), boo'zhē'. [A "wax candle," from their having formerly been sometimes made of wax.] A slender instrument for introduction into the *urethra;* also, stronger, for the *rectum, vagina,* and *œsophagus.*

Bougie', Armed, or **Bougie', Caus'tic.** A bougie with a piece of lunar caustic fixed in its extremity.

Bouillon (Fr.), boo'yòɴɢ'. A broth or soup made by boiling the flesh of animals in water.

Bo-vi'nạ Fa'mēṡ.* The disease BULIMIA, which see.

Brac'cate. [**Bracca'tus;** from *brac'ca*, "breeches."] Having breeches.

Bra-che'rĭ-um.* [From *bra'chium*, the "arm."] See SUBLIGAMEN.

Brach-ĭ-æ'us.* Same as BRACHIAL.

Bra'chĭ-al. [**Brachia'lis;** from *bra'chium*, the "arm."] Belonging to the arm.

Brach-ĭ-ăl'ġĭ-ạ.* [From *bra'chium*, the "arm," and ἄλγος, "pain."] Pain of the arm, or of any part of it.

Bra'chĭ-ate. [**Brachia'tus;** from *bra'chium*, the "arm."] Having branches in pairs at right angles with those above and below.

Bra'chĭ-o-. [From the same.] A prefix in compound names of vessels, ligaments, etc., connected with the arm.

Brachiopoda. See BRACHIOPODOUS.

Bra-chĭ-op'o-dous. [**Brachiop'odus;** from βραχίων, an "arm," and πούς, a "foot."] Applied in the plural neuter (*Brachiop'oda*) to a class of *Mollusca* with two fleshy arms instead of feet.

Bra'chĭ-um.* [Gr. βραχίων; Fr. *Bras*, brâ.] The arm, from shoulder to wrist; strictly, from the shoulder to the elbow, forming the proper arm.

Brạ-chȳp'ter-us.* [From βραχύς, "short," and πτερόν, a "wing."] Brachyp'terous. Applied in the neuter plural (*Brachyp'tera*) to a family of birds with small wings.

Brach-ȳ-u'rus.* [From βραχύς, and οὐρά, a "tail."] Having a short tail; brachyu'rous. Applied in the plural neuter (*Brachiu'ra*) to a family of *Crustacea Decapoda.*

Brac'te-ạ,* plural **Brac'te-æ.** A Latin term, denoting a thin leaf or plate of any metal. It is applied in Botany to all those modifications of leaves which are found upon the inflorescence and are situated between the true leaves and the calyx of the flower. They compose the *involucrum* of Compositæ, the *glumes* of Gramineæ, the *spathes* of Arum, etc.

Brac'te-ate. [**Bractea'tus;** from *brac'tea.*] Having floral leaves.

Brac-te'ĭ-form. [**Bracteifor'mis;** from *brac'tea.*] Resembling a floral leaf.

Brac'te-ole. [**Bracte'ola;** diminutive of *brac'tea.*] A little floral leaf.

Brac-te'o-late. [**Bracteola'tus.**] Having *bracteoles.*

Brad-y̆-sper-ma-tis'mus.* [From βραδύς, "slow," and σπέρμα, "seed."] Too slow emission of the semen: bradysper'-matism.

Brain. A word generally denoting the whole nervous mass within the *cranium,* or skull. See CEREBRUM.

Brain, Little. See CEREBELLUM.

Bran. See FURFUR TRITICI.

Branch. [Lat. **Ra'mus;** Fr. *Branche,* brŏnsh.] In Anatomy, applied to the several portions of blood-vessels, etc., as they divide, like the branches of a tree.

Branched. See RAMOSUS.

Branchia. See next article.

Branchiæ,* brank'e-ē. [Gr. βράγχια.] The gills, or breathing apparatus, in fishes, analogous to the lungs of land-animals. Also, the organs of respiration in *Mollusca, Crustacea,* and some *Reptilia.*

Branchiopoda. See BRANCHIOPODUS.

Branch-ĭ-op'o-dus.* [From βράγχια, "gills," and πούς, a "foot."] Applied in Zoology to an order (*Branchiopoda,* brank'e-op'o-da) of *Crustacea Entomostraca,* in which the *branchiæ* constitute part of their feet.

Branch-ĭ-os'te-gal. [**Branchiostega'lis;** from βράγχια, "gills," and στέγω, to "cover."] Covering the gills. Applied in Comparative Anatomy to appendages of the hyoid and scapular arches.

Branch-ĭ-os'te-ous. [**Branchios'teus;** from βράγχια, "gills," and ὀστεόν, a "bone."] Having gills wiih bony rays.

Bran'dy̆. [Lat. **Vi'num Adus'tum,** or **A'qua Vi'tæ;** Fr. *Eau de Vie,* ō dẹh vê; Ger. *Branntwein,* brânt'wīn, literally, "burnt wine."] The spirit distilled from wine; one of the most popular forms in which alcoholic spirit is administered.

Bras. See BRACHIUM.

Brasque, brask. A French term used by metallurgists to denote the lining of a crucible or a furnace with charcoal.

Brass. [Lat. **Æs, Æ'ris;** Fr. *Airain,* â'răNG'.] An alloy of copper and zinc. Common brass consists of three parts of copper and one of zinc.

Brassicaceæ,* bras-se-ka'she-ē. A name given by Lindley to an order of plants, including mustard, cabbage, etc.

Brayera. See KOUSSO.

Bra-zil'-Nut. A triangular nut growing in Brazil; the fruit of the *Bertholle'tia excel'sa,* or cream-nut.

Brazil'-Root. [**Radix Brazilien'sis.**] A name sometimes given to the root of the *Ipecacuanha.*

Brazil'-Wood. The wood of the *Cæsalpi'na Brazilien'sis,* which yields a red coloring matter used by dyers.

Braz-ĭ-let'to. An inferior species of Brazil-wood, brought from Jamaica. It is one of the cheapest and least esteemed of the red dye-woods.

Bread-Fruit Tree. The *Artocarpus incisa,* a tree of the order *Urticaceæ.* It has broad, lobed leaves and large, globular heads of fruit. "This fruit is to the inhabitants of Polynesia what corn is to the inhabitants of other parts of the world."—(HOBLYN.)

Break-Bone Fever. See DENGUE.

Breast. The *mamma* of females; the *mammilla* of males; also, popularly, the thorax, or chest. See PECTUS.

Breast-Bone. See STERNUM.

Breast-Pump. The same as ANTLIA MAMMARIA.

Breath. [**Hal'itus** and **Spir'itus.**] The air received and discharged by expansion and contraction of the lungs.

Breccia, brĕt'châ. [It. a "fragment."] Rock with fragmentary structure, the agglomerated grains of which are angulous fragments with sharp edges.

Brecciolar, brĕtch'o-lar. [**Brecciola'ris.**] Applied to rocks having various bodies in their paste or substance.

Bredouillement (Fr.), brẹh-dool'-mŏNG'. A defective utterance, in which only a part of the words is pronounced. It differs from stammering in being produced solely by a too great rapidity of speech.

Breg'ma, atis.* [From βρέχω, to "moisten:" so named because it was deemed to cover the most humid part of the brain.] An anatomical term for the sinciput, or top of the head. See SINCIPUT.

Breph-o-tro'phĭ-um.* [From βρέφος, an "infant," and τρέφω, to "nourish."] A foundling-hospital.

Bres'lau Fe'ver. An epidemic which broke out in the Prussian army at Breslau in the middle of the last century, and which has been named by Sauvages *Tritæophia Vratislaviensis.*

Brev-ĭ-pen'nate. [**Brevipen'nis;** from *bre'vis,* "short," and *pen'na,* a "wing."] Short-winged. A term applied to certain birds.

Bre-vis'sĭ-mus Oc'u-li.* [From *bre'vis,* "short," and *oc'ulus,* the "eye."] A synonym of the *obliquus inferior,* from its being the "shortest [muscle] of the eye."

Brexiaceæ,* brex-e-a'she-ē. A natural order of trees, allied to the Saxifrages, with coriaceous leaves and green flowers. It includes the genus *Brex'ia,* which is a native of Madagascar.

Brez'ĭ-lin. The name applied to the coloring matter of Brazil-wood obtained from several species of *Cæsalpinia.*

Brick'lay-er's Itch. A species of local tetter, or impetigo, produced on the hands of bricklayers by the contact of lime.

Bright's Dis-ease'. [**Mor'bus Brigh'tii.**] A genus or group of diseases of the kidney, first described by Dr. Bright. See NEPHRITIS.

Brim'stone. [Perhaps a corruption of Brenstone, or Burnstone, referring to its great combustibility.] A name for sulphur. The sublimed sulphur of the Pharmacopœia is termed *flowers of brimstone* or *of sulphur.*

Brise-pierre, brēz' pe-aiR'. [From the French *briser,* to "break," and *pierre,* a "stone."] An instrument for breaking stones in the bladder. See LITHOTRITY.

Brit'ish Gum. A term applied to starch when reduced to a *gum-like* state by exposure to heat. It then becomes of a brown color, and in that state is employed by calico-printers.

Brit'ish Oil. An artificial preparation, composed as follows:—camphor, one ounce; rectified spirits of wine, four ounces; sweet oil, twelve ounces; oil of hartshorn, five ounces: boiled together. This name is also given to the *O'leum Pe'træ Vulga're,* or common oil of petre, a variety of petroleum.

Bro'dĭ-um.* A term synonymous in Pharmacy with *jusculum,* or broth, the liquor in which any thing is boiled; as *bro'dium sa'lis,* a decoction of salt.

Bro'ma.* [From βιβρώσκω, to "eat."] Food; any thing that is masticated.

Bro'māte. [**Bro'mas, a'tis.**] A combination of bromic acid with a base.

Brom-a-tog'ra-phy̆. [**Bromatogra'phia;** from βρῶμα, "food," and γράφω, to "describe."] A treatise on foods; or a description of different kinds of food.

Brom-a-tol'o-ġy̆. [**Bromatolo'gia;** from βρῶμα, "food," and λόγος, a "discourse."] The consideration of food, its nature, quality, and uses; the science of food.

Brōme, or **Bro'mīne.** [**Bro'mium,** or **Bromin'ium;** from βρῶμος, a "stench."] An elementary body usually obtained from the residue of sea-water, called Bittern; named on account of its powerful, suffocating odor. It is a liquid of a deep-red color, and is very poisonous.

Bromeliaceæ,* bro-me-le-a'she-ē. [From *Brome'lia,* one of the genera.] A natural order of endogenous plants, found in tropical regions, and capable of growing in air without contact with the earth. It includes the Ananas, or Pine-Apple, and other plants prized for their flowers.

Bromeliæ,* bro-me'le-ē, the plural of **Brome'lia,** forming the Jussieuan name of an order of plants. See BROMELIACEÆ.

Bro'mic. [**Brom'icus.**] Belonging to brome.

Bro'mic Aç'id. A compound of bromine and oxygen.

Bro'mīde. [**Bro'mis, i'dis;** from *bro'mium.*] A combination of bromine with a metallic base.

Bro-min'ĭ-um.* The Pharmacopœial name (U. S. Ph.) of BROME, or BROMINE, which see.

Bromium. See BROME.

Bro'mo-form. [From *bro'mium,* and *for'myle.*] A peculiar substance compounded of bromine and formic acid, somewhat analogous in its effects to chloroform and sodoform.

Bro'mu-ret. [**Bromure'tum;** from *bro'mium.*] A combination of brome with a base.

Bronches. The French term for BRONCHIA, which see.

Bronchi,* bronk'ī (the plural of **Bronch'us**). The same as BRONCHIA, which see.

Bronchia,* brŏnk'e-a, gen. **Bron-chĭ-o'rum** (found only in the plural). Fr. *Bronches,* brŏNsh. [From βρόγχος, the "windpipe."] The first two branches of the *bronchus,* or windpipe; otherwise called *bronchi.*

Bronch'ĭ-al. [**Bronchia'lis;** from *bron'chia.*] Belonging to the *bronchia,* or *bronchi.*

Bronch'ial Tubes. The minute ramifications of the bronchi, terminating in the *bronchial cells,* or air-cells of the lungs.

Bronchitis,* bronk-i'tis. [From *bron'chia.*] Inflammation of the *bronchia.*

Bronch-lem-mi'tis.* A membrane-like inflammation of the *bronchia.*

Bronch'o-çēle.* [From βρόγχος, the "windpipe," and κήλη, a "tumor."] An indolent swelling of the thyroid gland; goître; tracheocele. Called also Derbyshire neck.

Bronchohæmorrhagia,* bronk'o-hem'o-ra'je-ą. [From *bron'chus,* and *hæmorrha'gia,* "hæmorrhage."] A term recently proposed by Andral to designate the exhalation of blood from the lining membrane of the bronchial tubes, commonly called bronchial hæmorrhage.

Bronch-oph'o-nĭsm, Bronch-oph'o-nȳ. [**Bronchophonis'mus, Bronchopho'nia;** from βρόγχος, and φωνή, the "voice."] The sound of the voice, heard by means of the stethoscope, in the *bronchia.*

Bronchorrhœa,* bronk-o-rē'ą. [From *bron'chi,* and ῥέω, to "flow."] Increased discharge of mucus from the *bronchia.*

Bronch-ot'o-mȳ. [**Bronchoto'-mia;** from βρόγχος, the "windpipe" or "bronchia," and τέμνω, to "cut."] The operation of cutting into the *bronchus,* or windpipe.

Bron'chus.* [Gr. βρόγχος, the "windpipe."] Same as TRACHEA. In the plural, *bronchi* is used synonymously with *bronchia.*

Bron'to-līte, or **Bron'to-lĭth.** [**Brontoli'tes;** from βροντή, "thunder," and λίθος, a "stone."] A thunder-stone; another name for *Aërolite,* or meteoric stone.

Brŏnze. A compound metal, consisting of copper with a small proportion of tin; similar to bell-metal.

Brook'lime. The *Veron'ica beccabun'ga.*

Broom. The *Spar'tium scopa'rium.*

Brown'ing. A preparation of sugar, port-wine, spices, etc., for coloring and flavoring meat, etc.

Brown'ĭsm. The theory or doctrines of John Brown. See BRUNONIAN THEORY.

Bru'çin, or **Brucine,** broo'sin. [**Bru'cia,** or **Bruci'na.**] A vegetable alkali discovered in the false Angustura bark and in the *Nux vomica.* It is of a pearly-white color, very bitter and styptic: it is poisonous, but less active than strychnine.

Bruissement (Fr.), bʀwėss'mŏɴɢ'. Corvisart's term for the *purring tremor,* or *frémissement cataire,* of Laennec.

Bruit, bʀwė. A French term, signifying "noise." Applied to the different conditions of the sound perceived by means of the stethoscope, according as the thorax or its organs are affected.

Bruit de Craquement, bʀwė dẹh krak'mŏɴɢ' ("crackling sound"), or **Bruit de Cuir Neuf,** bʀwė dẹh kwėʀ nŭf ("sound of new leather"). A sound caused by friction of the pericardium in certain diseased conditions.

Bruit de Soufflet, bʀwė dẹh soo'flȧ' ("bellows-sound"). A sound sometimes heard during the contraction of the auricles and ventricles of the heart. It is also termed *Bruit de Souffle,* bʀwė dẹh soofl, or "blowing sound."

Bruit Tympanique, bʀwė tăᴍ'pȧ'-nėk' ("tympanic sound"). See TYMPANITIS.

Bruniaceæ,* broo-ne-a'she-ē. A natural order of exogenous shrubs, found at the Cape of Good Hope. Their properties are unknown.—(LINDLEY.)

Brun'ner's Glands. [**Glan'dulæ Brunne'rii.**] The *Glan'dulæ solita'riæ,* or mucous follicles discovered by Brunner in the mucous membrane of the small intestines.

Brunoniaceæ,* broo-no-ne-a'she-ē. A natural order of herbaceous plants, found in New Holland. It consists of one genus,—*Bruno'nia.*

Bru-no'nĭ-an The'o-rȳ. A theory or system founded by John Brown, who maintained that all diseases are the result either of an excess or deficiency of *excitability* in the animal system.

Bruns'wick Green. An ammoniaco-muriate of copper, used for oil-painting.

Brȳg'mus.* [Gr. βρυγμός; from βρύχω, to "gnash with the teeth."] Gnashing or grating with the teeth; one of the symptoms occurring in certain diseases.

Brȳ'o-nȳ. [**Bryo'nia;** from βρύω, to "abound."] A Linnæan genus of the class *Monœcia,* natural order *Cucurbitaceæ.*

Bry-o'nĭ-ą Al'bą.* The *Bryonia diöica.*

Bryo'nia Dĭ-oi'cą.* The wild vine; also called *Bryonia alba,* wild hops, and tetter-berry.

Bu'bo, o'nis,* Bu'bon, o'nis.* [From βουβών, the "groin."] The inflammatory swelling of a lymphatic gland, particularly in the groin or axilla. A genus of the order *Tumores,* class *Locales,* of Cullen's Nosology. Adeni'tis. In Botany, a Linnæan genus of the class *Pentandria* natural order *Umbelliferæ.*

Bu'bōn Gal'ba-num.* The former name of the plant which yields galbanum; now called *Galbanum officinale.*

Bu-bo-năl'gĭ-a.* [From βουβών, the "groin," and ἄλγος, "pain."] Pain in the groin: bubonal'gy.

Bu-bon'o-çēle.* [From βουβών, the "groin," and κήλη, a "tumor."] A species of hernia in which part of the bowels protrudes at the abdominal ring; synonymous with inguinal hernia.

Buc'cal. [**Bucca'lis;** from *buc'ca,* the "cheek."] Belonging to the cheek.

Buc'cal Glands. The name of numerous follicles situated beneath the mucous layer of the cheek.

Buc'cal Nerve, called also the **Buc'-co-Lab-ĭ-a'lis.*** A nerve generally arising from the inferior maxillary: it sends its branches to the buccinator muscle.

Buc-çĭ-na'tor, o'ris.* [From *buc'-cino, buccina'tum,* to "sound a trumpet."] The trumpeter's muscle. A flat muscle which forms the wall of the cheek: so called from its being much used in blowing the trumpet.

Buccinoidæ,* bŭk-se-no'ĭ-dē. [From *buc'cinum,* a shell-fish like a trumpet or horn.] A name in Zoology given to a family of the *Mollus'ca Gasterop'oda Pectinibranchia'ta,* having the *Buccinum* for its type.

Bucco-Labialis Nerve. See BUCCAL NERVE.

Buc'cu-la.* [The diminutive of *buc'-ca,* the "cheek."] The fleshy part under the chin.

Buchu,* boo'koo. The Pharmacopœial name (U.S. Ph.) of the *Baros'ma crena'ta,* and other species of *Baros'ma;* the *Bucco* of the British Pharmacopœia.

Buck-Bean. A plant of the natural order *Gentianaceæ,* used by brewers in some parts of Germany as a substitute for hops. See MENYANTHES TRIFOLIATA.

Buck'-Thorn. The common name of the *Rham'nus cathar'ticus.* The berries yield a delicate green, named by painters *verdevis'sa.*

Buck'u.* The Pharmacopœial name (Ed. Ph.) for the leaves of several species of *Barosma.* See BUCHU.

Buc-ne'mĭ-a.* [From βοῦ, a particle of increase, and κνήμη, the "leg."] A disease of the leg, distinguished by tense, diffuse, inflammatory swelling.

Bucopric Acid. See BOSOPRIC ACID.

Bud. [Lat. **Gem'ma;** Fr. *Bouton,* boo'tôNᵍ'.] The rudiments of a plant in a latent state, till evolved at the proper season and by the influence of other circumstances.

Bŭf'fȳ Coat. [**Co'rium Phlogis'-ticum.**] The inflammatory crust or buff-colored substance on the surface of the *crassamentum* of blood taken from persons laboring under inflammation, when coagulation is completed.

Bu-lam' Fe'ver. A name given by the natives on the African coast to the yellow fever.

Bŭlb. [Lat. **Bul'bus;** Gr. βολβός.] In Botany, a globular, coated body, solid, or composed of fleshy scales or layers, constituting the lower part of some plants, and sending off radicles from the flattened basis. Also applied in Anatomy to portions of the body resembling a bulb.

Bulb of the U-re'thra. The bulb-like commencement of the corpus spongiosum penis: hence the included urethra is called the *bulbous portion.*

Bul-bif'er-ous. [**Bulbif'erus;** from *bul'bus,* a "bulb," and *fe'ro,* to "bear."] Bearing bulbs.

Bul'bil. [**Bulbil'lus,** or **Bul'bu-lus;** the diminutive of *bul'bus.*] A small, solid, or scaly bud, which being detached from a plant becomes developed and perfectly similar to it.

Bul'bo-Cav-er-no'sus.* [Named from its connection with the bulb of the urethra and the corpus cavernosum.] A muscle of the urethra. The same as ACCELERATOR URINÆ, which see.

Bul'bous. [**Bulbo'sus;** from *bul'-bus,* a "bulb."] Having bulbs, or full of bulbs.

Bulbulus. See BULBIL.

Bul'bus Ar-te-rĭ-o'sus.* ("Arterial Bulb.") The name of the anterior of the three cavities of the heart in all Vertebrata, as exhibited in the early period of their development.

Bul'bus Ol-fac-to'rĭ-us.* ("Olfactory Bulb.") That portion of the olfactory nerve which expands into a bulb-like form and rests upon the cribriform plate of the ethmoid bone.

Bu-lim'ĭ-a,* Bu-lĭ-mi'a-sis,* Bu-lĭ'mus.* [From βοῦ, a particle of increase, and λιμός, "hunger."] A disease causing great voracity or insatiable hunger; canine hunger. A genus of the order *Dysorexiæ,* class *Locales,* of Cullen's Nosology.

Bu'lith-um.* [From βοῦς, an "ox," and λίθος, a "stone."] A bezoar stone found in the kidneys, the gall, or urinary bladder of the ox. See BEZOAR.

Bull. = *Bul'liat.** "Let it boil."

Bul'la.* Literally, a "bubble." A transparent vesicle caused by burns, scalds, or otherwise; a bleb; a blister.

Bul'late. [**Bulla'tus, Bullo'sus;** from *bul'la*, a "blister."] Having *bullæ*, or full of *bullæ*,—an appearance produced by the surface of a leaf being raised above its veins.

Bunion, or **Bunyon,** bŭn'yạn. [From βούνιον, the "earth-nut."] Inflammation (or rather its effects) of the *bursa mucosa*, at the ball of the great toe, induration of adjacent parts, enlargement of the joint, etc.

Bu'nĭ-um.* [From the same.] The generic name of the plant producing the earth-nut. It has a tuberous root, which is eaten roasted or raw.

Buphthalmia,* būf-thăl'me-ạ, or **Bu-oph-thăl'mĭ-ạ,*** or **Buph-thăl'mus.*** [From βοῦς, an "ox," and ὀφθαλμός, the "eye."] The first stage of *Hydrophthalmia*, or ox-eye.

Bur'dock. The common English name of the *Arc'tium lap'pa*, and *Lap'pa mi'nor*.

Bur'gun-dȳ Pitch. The *Pix Burgun'dica* of the Pharmacopœias.

Burmanniaceæ,* bŭr-man-ne-a'-she-ē. A natural order of endogenous plants related to the *Orchids*.

Burn. [**Us'tio** and **Ambus'tio, o'***nis*.] A lesion caused by the application of heat.

Burnt Alum. See ALUMEN EXSICCATUM.

Burnt Sponge. [**Spon'gia Us'ta.**] This substance is prepared by cutting sponge into small pieces, and burning it in a covered vessel until it becomes black and friable, when it is rubbed into a fine powder. It is employed as a remedy in goître and scrofulous swellings.

Bur'sạ,* plural **Bur'sæ.** [Gr. βύρσα, a "leathern bottle."] A sac, or purse.

Bur'sa Mu-co'sạ,* plural **Bur'sæ Muco'sæ.** A membranous sac for secreting a substance (*syno'via*) to lubricate tendons and joints, rendering their motion easy.

Bur-sa'lis.* [From *bur'sa*.] Belonging to a purse or bag: bur'sal.

Bur-sal'o-ġȳ. [**Bursalo'gia;** from βύρσα, a "bag," and λόγος, a "discourse."] The consideration (or science) of the *bursæ mucosæ*.

Bu'te-ạ Gum. A gum procured from natural fissures and wounds made in the bark of the *Bu'tea frondo'sa*, a leguminous plant of India.

Butomaceæ,* bu-to-ma'she-ē. A natural order of aquatic plants, including the *Bu'tomus*.

But'ter. [Lat. **Bu'tyrum;** Gr. βούτυρον.] An oil, more or less concrete, obtained from the milk of animals. It can be separated from milk or cream by almost any kind of violent and continued agitation. This process of separation is popularly termed "churning."

But'ter of Ca-ca'o. An oily, concrete, white matter, of a firmer consistence than suet, obtained from the *Cacao*, or Cocoanut, of which chocolate is made.

But'ter-flȳ-Shaped. See PAPILIONACEUS.

Butua. See PAREIRA BRAVA.

Bu-tȳ-rā'ceous. [**Butyra'ceus;** from *bu'tyrum*, "butter."] Of the appearance or consistence of butter.

Bu'tȳ-rāte. [**Bu'tyras, a'***tis*.] A combination of butyric acid with a base.

Bu-tȳr'ic Aç'id. A volatile acid obtained from butter.

Bu'tȳ-rin. [**Butyri'na;** from *bu-ty'rum*, "butter."] The essential fatty matter of butter: the butyrate of glycerin.

Bux'in. [**Buxi'na.**] An alkaline substance obtained from the common box-tree (*Bux'us sempervi'rens*).

B. V. = *Bal'neum Vapo'ris.** A "vapor-bath."

Bȳs'sum,* **Bȳs'sus.*** [Gr. βύσσος, a kind of fine flax.] In Anatomy, the *Pudendum muliebre*. Applied in Botany to a genus of lichens. Also, the hairy appendage by which the *Mollusca* attach themselves to rocks, etc.

Byttneriaceæ,* bit-ne-re-a'she-ē. A natural order of exogenous trees or shrubs, including the *Byttne'ria* and *Theobro'ma Ca'cao*, which produces chocolate or cocoa.

C.

C. An abbreviation for *Congius,** a "gallon;" also for "compound," or "composite," *Carbonium,** *compositi,** or *compositæ.**

Cab'al-line. [**Caballi'nus;** from *cabal'lus,* a "horse."] Applied to a coarse kind of aloes fit only for horses.

Cab'bage-Tree. The *Geoffræa inermis,* or *Andira inermis.*

Cabombaceæ,* kab-om-ba'she-ē, or **Ca-bom'be-æ.*** [From *Cabom'ba,* the name of one of the genera.] A natural order, including aquatic plants with floating peltate leaves. It is also called *Hydropeltideæ.*

Cacao. See COCOA.

Cachectic, kạ-kek'tik. [**Cachec'ticus;** from *cachex'ia.*] Pertaining to *Cachexia.*

Cach-el-co'mạ, *atis.** [From κακός, "bad," and ἕλκος, an "ulcer."] A malignant ulcer.

Cạ-chex'ĭ-ạ.* [From κακός, "bad," "evil," and ἕξις, a "habit."] A depraved habit of body. Applied in the plural to a class of Cullen's Nosology. Cachex'y.

Cac-o-chȳm'ĭ-ạ.* [From κακός, "bad," and χυμός, "juice," "humor."] A depraved condition of the humors.

Cac-o-col'pĭ-ạ.* [From κακός, "bad," and κόλπος, a "sinus," also, the "womb," or "vulva."] A putrid condition of the vulva and vaginal entrance.

Cac'o-dȳl. [From κακώδης, "fetid."] A limpid liquid, of fetid odor, derived from acetyl. *Cacodylic acid* is formed from cacodyl by oxygenation.

Cac-o-e'thēs.* [From κακός, "bad," and ἦθος, "manner" or "disposition."] A bad habit or disposition.

Cac-o-so'mĭ-um.* [From κακός, "bad," and σῶμα, a "body," also, "state of body."] A lazaretto for leprosy and other incurable diseases.

Cactaceæ,* kak-ta'she-ē. A natural order of plants of the Cactus tribe, remarkable for their large and gay flowers. They are succulent shrubs, found wild in hot, dry countries.

Cac'ti,* the plural of *Cac'tus* (a "prickly pear"), the Jussieuan name of an order of plants. See CACTACEÆ.

Ca-cu'men,* plural **Ca-cu'mĭ-nạ.** The "top" of any thing. In Pharmacopœial language, the tops of plants.

Cạ-dav'er-ic. [**Cadaver'icus;** from *cada'ver,* a "corpse."] Belonging to a dead body.

Cạ-dav'er-ous. [From the same.] Having the appearance of a dead body; pertaining to a dead body.

Cadet', Liq'uor of. A liquid obtained by distilling acetate of potash and arsenious acid, and remarkable for its insupportable odor and spontaneous inflammability in air.

Cad'mĭ-ạ,* or **Cad-mi'a.** [Gr. καδμία, or καδμεία, "calamine," or "cadmia."] A name applied to several metallic substances, or ores,—calamine, cobalt, tutty, etc.

Cad'mĭ-um,* or **Cad-mi'um.** [From *cad'mia,* "calamine" or "tutty," in which it was first observed.] The name for a metal, resembling tin, found in several of the ores of zinc. A dilute solution of the sulphate of cadmium has been used as a collyrium for spots on the cornea, and for chronic inflammation of the conjunctiva. See preceding article.

Cạ-du'cạ.* [See next article.] A name sometimes given to the deciduous membrane of the uterus.

Cạ-du'cus.* [From *ca'do,* to "fall."] Falling off: cadu'cous.

Caduque (Fr.), kå'dük'. The same as CADUCA, which see.

Cæ'cal, or **Ce'cal.** [**Cæca'lis;** from *cæ'cum,* the "blind gut."] Belonging to the *Cæcum.*

Cæcitas (sĕs'e-tas), ***a'tis.**** [From *cæ'cus,* "blind."] Blindness.

Cæ-ci'tis.* [From *cæ'cum.*] Inflammation of the cecum.

Cæ'cum.* [Neuter singular of *cæ'cus,* "blind."] The blind gut (*intes'tinum* being understood), or first portion of the large intestine; the *Ca'put co'li.*

Cæ-ru'le-us Mor'bus.* (The "blue disease.") See CYANOSIS.

Cærulina. See CERULIN.

Cæsalpinia,* ses-al-pin'e-ạ. [Named from *Cæsalpi'nus.*] A genus of trees of the order *Leguminosæ.* See BRAZIL WOOD.

Cæ-sā're-an Op-er-ā'tion, Cæsa'rean Sec'tion. [**Opera'tio Cæsa'rea, Sec'tio Cæsa'rea;** from *Julius Cæsar,*—said to have been born thus; more probably from *cæ'do, cæ'sum,* to "cut."] In Obstetrics, the operation of cutting into the womb through the parietes of the abdomen when natural delivery is impracticable: hysterotomy. According to Pliny, persons thus born were called *Cæso'nes.*

Café Citrin (Fr.), kå'få' se'trăNG'. An infusion of unroasted coffee; so named on account of its yellow or citrine color.

Caf'fe-a.* The Pharmacopœial name (U.S. Ph.) of the seed of the *Caf'fea Arab'ica* (the coffee-plant). See COFFEE.

Caf'fe-in. [**Caffei'na;** from the French *Café,* "coffee."] A bitter principle obtained from coffee. The same as THEIN.

Ca-in'ca,* or **Ca-hin'ca,*** called also **Chi-o-coc'ca,*** a plant of the order *Rubiaceæ,* the root of which has recently been employed as a tonic and diuretic.

Cajeput, kăj'e-pŏŏt, written also **Cai'eput** and **Caj'uput.** [**Cajupu'tum.**] See CAJUPUTI OLEUM.

Caj-u-pu'ti O'le-um.* ("Oil of Cajeput.") The Pharmacopœial name (Ed. Ph.) for Cajuput or Cajeput oil, obtained from the *Melaleu'ca cajupu'ti.* It is stimulant and aromatic, and is considered very efficacious in some forms of rheumatism.

Cal-a-bar' Bean. A medicinal substance having the remarkable property of causing contraction of the pupil of the eye,

Cal-a-mi'na.* [From *cad'mia lapido'sa,* an ore of zinc.] The Pharmacopœial name of a native impure carbonate of zinc.

Ca-lam-i-na'ris.* Belonging to calamine, or *Lapis calaminaris.*

Cal'a-mi Ra'dix.* ("Root of Calamus.") See CALAMUS.

Cal'a-mus.* [From the Arabic *Ka'lam,* the "stalk of a plant," a "reed."] A Latin word signifying a "reed," and hence a "pen." The name of a Linnæan genus of the class *Hexandria,* natural order *Aroideæ;* also the Pharmacopœial name (U.S. Ph.) of the rhizoma of *Ac'orus cal'amus.*

Cal'amus Ro'tang,* or **Cal'amus Dra'co.*** A plant generally supposed to yield the substance known as dragon's blood, said likewise to be obtained from the *Pterocar'pus dra'co.*

Cal'amus Scrip-to'ri-us.* A "writing-pen." Applied in Anatomy to a narrow fissure on the back and in the median line of the *Pons Varolii.*

Ca-lap'pite. [From the Malay *Calap'pa,* the "cocoa-tree."] A stony concretion sometimes found in the inside of the cocoanut; also called a *vegetable bezoar.*

Cal-a-thid'i-um.* [From καλαθίς, a "little basket."] A kind of inflorescence composed of sessile flowers thickly placed upon a common involucre.

Cal-ca'ne-um.* [From *calx,* the "heel."] The largest bone of the tarsus; the heel-bone, or *os calcis.*

Căl'ca-rate. [**Calcara'tus;** from *cal'car,* a "spur."] Having spurs; like the flower of the larkspur.

Cal-cā're-ous. [**Calca'rius;** from *calx, cal'cis,* "lime."] Belonging to lime; containing lime.

Calca'reous Earth. Lime.

Calca'reous Spar. Crystallized carbonate of lime. Iceland spar is one of its purest varieties.

Căl'ce-i-form. [**Calceifor'mis;** from *cal'ceus,* a "shoe."] Like a shoe.

Căl-cif'er-ous. [**Calcif'erus;** from *calx,* "lime," and *fe'ro,* to "bear."] Containing lime or carbonate of lime.

Calcification. See PETRIFACTION.

Căl-cig'e-nous. [**Calcig'enus;** from *calx,* "lime," and γεννάω, to "generate."] Applied to metals which with oxygen form a calx or earthy-looking substance.

Căl-ci-nā'tion. [**Calcina'tio, o'nis.** See CALCINE.] The application of heat to saline, metallic, or other substances, to deprive them of moisture, etc.

Căl-ci-na'tus.* Reduced to powder by heat; calcined. See CALCINATION.

Căl'cine. [**Cal'cino, Calcina'tum;** from *calx, cal'cis,* "lime."] To burn as lime; to reduce to a powder, or to an oxide, by heat. See CALCINATION.

Calcium,* kăl'she-ŭm. [From *calx,* "lime."] The metallic base of lime.

Cal'cu-li,* the plural of CALCULUS, which see.

Căl-cu-lif'ra-gus.* [From *cal'culus,* and *fran'go,* to "break."] Breaking or reducing *calculi:* calculif'ragous. See LITHOTRIPTIC. As a noun, *Calculif'ragus* forms the name of a surgical instrument for breaking down calculi in the bladder. See LITHOTRIPTOR.

Căl'cu-lous. [**Calculo'sus;** from *cal'culus.*] Of the nature of stone or calculus. Having a calculus, or full of *calculi.* Applied to those afflicted with stone in the bladder.

Căl'cu-lus,* plural **Cal'cu-li.** [The diminutive of *calx,* "limestone," or "chalk." See CALX.] Fr. *Calcul,* kål'kül', and *Pierre,* pe-aiR'. A stone-like concretion in the urinary bladder, kidney, gall-bladder, intestines, or in and about the joints.

URINARY CALCULI, commonly called "stone," or "gravel," vary in composition according to the *diathesis* of the patient. Sometimes they are of a reddish or brick color, consisting usually of lithate of ammonia, or of crystals of lithic and uric acid. At others, they are white, or whitish, and are for the most part composed of the phosphates of magnesia and ammonia, occasionally mixed with the phosphate of lime. Urate of ammonia and oxalate of lime sometimes occur in a crystalline form.

BILIARY CALCULI (*Cal'culi Bilio'si* or *Bilia'rii*) are usually found in the gall-bladder, and are then termed *cystic;* sometimes they occur in the substance of the liver, in which case they are called *hepatic* calculi. In many instances they seem to be little more than bile in a concrete state: many of them are composed chiefly of Cholesterin.

CALCULOUS CONCRETIONS, called *arthritic* calculi (*Cal'culi arthrit'ici, Cal'culi podag'rici,* or *Tuber'cula arthrit'ica*), are found in the ligaments, and within the capsules of the joints, in persons afflicted with the gout. These are for the most part composed of uric acid and soda combined with a small portion of animal matter; sometimes of urate of lime.

CALCULI found in the intestines of animals are called BEZOARS, which see.

Cal-e-fā'cient. [**Calefa'ciens;** from *cal'idus,* "warm," and *fa'cio,* to "make."] Exciting warmth; making warm. Applied to medicines or external applications causing a sense of warmth.

Cal-e-fac'tion. [**Calefac'tio, o'***nis;* from the same.] The act of applying heat.

Cal'en-tūre. [Sp. *Calentura,* kå-lĕn-too'rå.] A violent fever, attended with delirium, incident to persons in hot countries. Under its influence it is said that sailors imagine the sea to be green fields, and will throw themselves into it if not restrained.

Ca-li'go, ģ'*inis.** [Fr. *Brouillard,* broo'yaR'.] Dimness of sight sometimes coming on without apparent cause; blindness. A genus of the order *Dysæsthesiæ,* class *Locales,* of Cullen's Nosology.

Cali'go Cor'ne-æ.* ("Obscurity of the Cornea.") Dimness of sight arising from opacity of the cornea, or sometimes a mere speck on the cornea.

Cali'go Hu-mo'rum.* ("Obscurity of the Humors.") Obscurity of vision, or blindness, arising from a defect in the humors of the eye. See GLAUCOMA.

Cali'go Len'tis.* ("Obscurity of the Lens.") The true CATARACT, which see.

Cal-i-sa'ya Bark. The *Cinchona flava.*

Cal-is-then'ics. [**Calisthen'ica** and **Calisthe'nia;** from καλός, "beautiful," and σθένος, "strength."] An exercise for strengthening the body and giving ease and elegance to the movements of the limbs.

Callitrichaceæ,* kal'le-tre-ka'she-ē. [From κάλλος, "beauty," and θρίξ, gen. τριχός, "hair."] A natural order or family of aquatic plants. By some they are considered allies of *Urticaceæ,* by others, Monocotyledons.

Cal-los'ĭ-tў. [**Callos'itas, a'***tis;* from *cal'lus.*] A preternatural hardness in the skin or naturally soft parts.

Cal'lus.* The osseous substance deposited between the divided portions of a fractured bone. Also, unnatural hardness or induration of any soft part, or a thickening of the cuticle, caused by pressure or friction.

Calomel. See next article.

Ca-lom'e-las, a*nos.** [From καλός, "beautiful," "good," and μέλας, "black;" conjectured to have been so named because it was good for black bile.] Calomel. The Pharmacopœial name (Br. Ph.) for the protochloride or mild chloride of mercury. See HYDRARGYRI CHLORIDUM MITE.

Ca'lor.* The Latin term for heat. *Calor fervens* denotes boiling heat, or 212° Fahr.; *Calor lenis,* gentle heat, between 90° and 100° Fahr.

Ca'lor An-ĭ-ma'lis.* Animal caloric, or animal heat. The term applied to the caloric constantly generated in the bodies of living mammalia and birds, by means of which the animal is kept at nearly a uniform temperature. That of the mammalia varies from about 96° to 106° or 107°,—the Arctic fox, the Arctic wolf, and the whale being among those that have the highest temperature. The animal heat of birds ranges somewhat higher than that of the mammalia, the temperature of several species being above 108°, while that of the Arctic finch (*Fringilla Arctica*), the redbreast (*Rubecula*), and some others is said to reach 111°.

The temperature of those animals even which are commonly termed cold-blooded, is often found to be considerably above that of the surrounding medium; among fishes, the most highly organized, such as the tunny-fish (*Thynnus*) and the shark, have usually the warmest blood.

Ca'lor Mor'dĭ-cans.* Literally, a

"biting heat." A term applied to a dangerous symptom in typhus, in which there is a biting and pungent heat upon the skin, leaving a smarting sensation on the fingers for several minutes after touching it.

Ca-lor'ic. [**Calor'icum;** from *ca'lor*, "heat."] The matter or cause of the sensation of heat; igneous fluid.

SENSIBLE or FREE CALORIC is that which produces the sensation of heat or affects the thermometer.

INSENSIBLE or LATENT CALORIC, formerly supposed to be in a state of combination, is that which passes into bodies during a change of form. Thus, it may pass into ice at 32°, changing it to water, *but not increasing the temperature* (it has hence been termed the *caloric of fluidity*), or into water at 212°, converting it to vapor (and termed, in consequence, the *caloric of evaporation*).

SPECIFIC CALORIC denotes the unequal quantities of caloric required by the same quantity of different bodies to heat them to a given temperature. Thus, if equal weights of water at 40° and mercury at 160° be mixed together, the resulting temperature is 45°, showing that, computing by weight, water has twenty-three times as great a capacity for caloric as mercury.

Cal-o-riç'ĭ-tȳ. [**Caloriç'itas, a'***tis;* from *ca'lor*, "heat."] The faculty of generating the heat necessary to life, and maintaining the proper temperature of the body in all situations.

Cal-o-rif'ic. [**Calorif'icus;** from *ca'lor*, and *fa'cio*, to "make."] Heat-producing; heat-creating.

Cal-o-rim'e-ter. [**Calorim'etrum;** from *ca'lor*, and μέτρον, a "measure."] An instrument for ascertaining the quantity of caloric disengaged from any substance.

Ca-lor-ĭ-mo'tor, o'r*is*.* [From *ca'lor*, and *mo'tor*, a "mover."] An electric apparatus which produces by its discharge highly elevated temperatures.

Cal-ot'ro-pis Ģi-gan-te'a.* An asclepiadaceous plant introduced from India under the name of *mudar*, or *madar*, as an alterative and sudorific.

Ca-lum'ba.* [From *Colom'bo*, in Ceylon, whence the drug was once supposed to be derived.] The Pharmacopœial name ‖ for the root of *Coc'culus palma'tus*, or *Menisper'mum palma'tum:* the *Colombæ Radix* (Dub. Ph.). The name is often written *Colomba*. See COLUMBO.

Cal-va'rĭ-a.* [From *cal'veo*, "to be bald."] That portion of the *cranium* above the orbits, temples, ears, and occipital protuberance.

Calvities,* kăl-vish'e-ēz. [From *cal'vus*, "bald."] Want or loss of hair, particularly on the sinciput; baldness.

Călx,* gen. **Căl'cis.** The heel.

Călx,* gen. **Căl'cis.** [From χάλιξ, a "small stone," "rubbish."] Literally, "chalk," or "limestone." The Pharmacopœial name for lime, or calcined carbonate of lime.

Calx Chlo-rĭ-na'ta.* ("Chlorinated Lime.") The Pharmacopœial name for the preparation popularly known as chloride of lime. See LIME, CHLORIDE OF.

Calx Vi'va.* Quicklime.

Calycanthaceæ,* kal-e-kan-tha'-she-ē, or **Cal-ȳ-can'the-æ.*** [From *Calycan'thus*, one of the genera.] A natural order of exogenous shrubs, found in Japan and North America. The flowers have an aromatic odor.

Calyceraceæ,* kal-e-se-ra'she-ē. A small natural order of exogenous herbaceous plants, including the genus *Calycera.*

Calyces,* kal'e-sēz. [The plural of *ca'lyx*, a "cup."] Small, membranous, *cup-like* pouches, which invest the points of the papillæ of the kidney. Their union forms the *infundibula.*

Cal'ȳ-cĭ-flo'ræ.* [From *ca'lyx*, a "flower-cup," and *flos*, a "flower."] Plants which have their flowers furnished with both a calyx and a corolla, the latter consisting of distinct petals and their stamens perigynous.

Cal'ȳ-cĭ-flo'rate. [**Calyciflo'rus;** from *ca'lyx*, and *flos*, a "flower."] Having the stamens inserted into the calyx.

Cal'ȳ-cĭ-form. [**Calycifor'mis;** from *ca'lyx*, and *for'ma.*] Formed like a calyx.

Cal'ȳ-cine. [**Calyci'nus;** from *ca'lyx.*] Belonging to a calyx.

Cal'ȳ-coid. [**Calycoi'des;** from *ca'lyx*, and εἶδος, a "form."] Resembling a calyx.

Ca-lȳc'u-late. [**Calycula'tus;** from *calyc'ulus.*] Having *calyculi.*

Ca-lȳc'u-lus,* plural **Ca-lȳc'u-li.** [The diminutive of *ca'lyx.*] The membranous margin surrounding the apex of a seed; also, a little calyx exterior to a proper one.

Ca-lȳp'tra,* plural **Ca-lȳp'træ.** [Gr. καλύπτρα, a "veil;" from καλύπτω, to "cover."] A membranous covering over the *antheræ* in mosses; also, the proper covering or coat of the seed, which falls off spontaneously.

Ca-lўp-tra'tus.* [From *calyp'tra*, the "veil of mosses."] Having *calyptræ:* calyp'trate.

Ca'lўx,* plural **Cal'ў-çēs.** [Gr. κάλυξ, a "covering," the "cup of a flower."] A membranous cup or sac surrounding one or two of the *papillæ* of the kidney. See CALYCES. Applied in Botany to the flower-cup, or empalements which cover the flower, for the most part green and surrounding the *corolla.* Also the Physiological name of the very vascular capsule enclosing the vesicle, or yelk, formed of the three layers of the *ovarium.*

Cam'bĭ-um.* [Probably from *cam'bio*, to "change."] A glutinous fluid between the bark and *alburnum* of trees, supposed by some physiologists to furnish the material out of which the new wood is formed.

Cam-bo'gĭ-a.* The Pharmacopœial name (British Ph.) of gamboge (*gambogia*), obtained from an undetermined tree.

Cam'e-ra,* plural **Cam'e-ræ.** [From καμάρα, an "upper gallery."] In the plural, the anterior and posterior chambers of the eye.

Cam-pa'na.* [From *Campa'nia*, in Italy, where they were first used in churches.] A bell. Applied in Chemistry to a dish or cover shaped like a bell, employed in making sulphuric acid.

Campanaceus,* kam-pa-na'she-ŭs. [From *campa'na.*] Like a bell. Applied in the plural feminine (*Campanaceæ*, kam-pa-na'she-ē) to an order in Linnæus's Natural method: campana'ceous.

Cam-pan'ĭ-form. [**Campanifor'mis;** from *campa'na*, a "bell."] Formed like a bell.

Campanulaceæ,* kam-pan'u-la'she-ē, or **Cam-pan'u-læ.*** [From *Campan'ula*, the name of one of the genera.] A natural order of herbaceous plants, found in temperate climates, and prized for the beauty of the flowers.

Cam-pan-u-lā'ceous. [**Campanula'ceus;** from *campan'ula*, a "little bell;" also the "bell-flower."] Having an arrangement as in the *Campanula.* See CAMPANULACEÆ.

Cam-pan'u-late. [**Campanula'tus;** from *campan'ula*, a "little bell."] Like a little bell.

Campeachy Wood. See HÆMATOXYLUM.

Camphene, or **Camphine,** kamfēn'. [From *cam'phora.*] A substance procured from common turpentine; with an equivalent of oxygen it forms camphor; also called *Cam'phogen* (*i.e.* "producing camphor").

Cam'pho-ra.* [Gr. καμφουρά, "camphor."] The Pharmacopœial name ‖ of "a peculiar concrete substance derived from *Camphora officinarum* and purified by sublimation" (U.S. Ph., 1860). The effect of camphor in moderate doses is to allay nervous irritation; but in overdoses it is poisonous and may produce death.

Cam'phora Of-fiç-ĭ-na'rum.* The plant which yields the officinal camphor.

Cam'pho-ræ Flo'rēs.* ("Flowers of Camphor.") A name sometimes given to sublimated camphor.

Cam'pho-rāte. [**Cam'phoras,a'***tis.*] A combination of camphoric acid with a base.

Cam'pho-rāt-ed. [**Camphora'tus;** from *cam'phora.*] Having camphor, or combined with camphor.

Cam-phor'ic. [**Camphor'icus;** from *cam'phora*, "camphor."] Belonging to camphor. Applied to an acid obtained from camphor.

Camp-Vin'e-gar is prepared as follows. Steep in the best vinegar for a month one drachm of cayenne pepper, two tablespoonfuls of soy, and four of walnut ketchup, six anchovies chopped, and a small clove of garlic minced fine. Shake it frequently, strain through a tamis, and keep it well corked in small bottles.

Cam-pў-lot'ro-pous. [From καμπύλος, "curved," and τρέπω, to "turn."] A term applied to the ovule of plants, when its axis, instead of remaining rectilinear, is curved down upon itself, the base of the nucleus still continuing to be contiguous to the hilum.

Cam'wood. A red dye-wood, principally obtained from the vicinity of Sierra Leone.

Ca-năl'. [From *cana'lis*, a "channel," or "pipe."] Applied in Anatomy to any passage in the body.

CANAL OF FONTA'NA. A minute vascular canal situated within the ciliary ligament, and so named from its discoverer. It is also termed the ciliary canal.

CANAL OF PETIT (peh-tē'). A triangular canal situated immediately around the circumference of the crystalline lens: so named from its discoverer. When distended with air or size-injection, it presents a plaited appearance, and has hence been called by the French *canal godronné.*

Can-a-lic-u-la'tus.* [From *canalic'ulus.*] Having a little canal or channel: channelled; canalic'ulated.

Can-a-lic'u-li,* the plural of **Can-a-lic'u-lus.** The name given by Morgagni to some large lacunæ which secrete mucus in the canal of the urethra.

Can-a-lic'u-lus.* [The diminutive of *cana'lis.*] A small channel or vessel.

Ca-na'lis,* plural **Ca-na'lēs.** [From *can'na,* a "hollow reed."] A canal, or channel. Applied to blood-vessels, cavities, etc. See ALVEUS.

Cana'lis Ar-te-ri-o'sus.* ("Arterial Canal.") A blood-vessel which unites the pulmonary artery and aorta in the fœtus.

Cana'lis Ve-no'sus.* ("Venous Canal.") A canal which conveys the blood from the *venæ portæ* of the liver to the ascending *vena cava* in the fœtus.

Can-cel-la'tus.* [From *cancel'li.*] Having a latticed appearance: cancel'-lated.

Can-cel'li,* gen. **Cancello'rum.** Lattices: minute divisions in the reticulated structure of bones.

Can'cer,* gen. **Can'cri,** or **Can'-cer-is.** A crab. A genus of *Crustacea Malacostraca.*

Can'çer.* [Literally, a "crab," the turgid veins around it being supposed to resemble a crab's claws.] A painful scirrhous tumor, terminating in a fatal ulcer. See CARCINOMA.

Can'cer As'ta-cus.* The craw-fish, affording the *Lapilli cancrorum,* or crabs' eyes.

Can'cer Mun-di-to'rum.* ("Chimney-Sweeper's Cancer.") See CANCER SCROTI.

Can'cer Pa-gu'rus.* The crab-fish, affording the *Chelæ cancrorum,* or crabs' claws.

Can'cer Scro'ti.* ("Cancer of the Scrotum"), called also Chimney-Sweeper's Cancer (*Can'cer Mundito'rum*). A form of cancer to which chimney-sweepers are especially exposed, on account of the irritating effects of soot.

Can'cri,* gen. **Can-cro'rum.** The plural of *can'cer,* a "crab."

Can'croid. [**Cancroi'des;** from *can'cer,* and εἶδος, a "form."] Resembling cancer.

Cancroïde, kŏNᵍ'kro'ēd'. The French form of the preceding term.

Can-cro'rum [see CANCRI] **Che'læ.*** ("Crabs' Claws.") The claws of the *Cancer pagurus,* the black-clawed, or large, edible crab: these, when prepared by grinding, constitute the prepared crabs' claws of the shops, formerly used to correct acidity in the stomach and bowels.

Cancro'rum La-pil'li* ("Crabs' Stones"), and **Cancro'rum Oc'u-li*** ("Crabs' Eyes"), are used for the same purposes as the preceding.

Can'crum.* Low Latin for "canker." It appears to be used only in the following phrase.

Can'crum O'ris.* ("Canker of the Mouth.") A deep, foul, fetid, irregular ulcer inside the lips and cheeks: often attended with a discharge of blood.

Can'dle-Tree Oil. A solid oil obtained from the seed of the *Croton sebiferum,* or Candle-tree, a native of China. It is used by the Chinese for making candles.

Ca-nel'la.* [From *can'na,* a "reed."] A Linnæan genus of the class *Dodecandria,* natural order *Meliaceæ.* The Pharmacopœial name for the bark of *Canella alba;* the *Canellæ albæ cortex* of the Dublin Pharmacopœia.

Canel'la Al'ba.* ("White Canella.") The laurel-leaved canella, yielding a bark somewhat resembling cinnamon.

Ca-nic-u-la'ris.* [From *canic'ula,* a "little dog," the "dog-star."] Applied to the hottest days of the year, the *Di'es canicula'res,* or dog-days.

Can'īne. [**Cani'nus;** from *ca'nis,* a "dog."] Belonging to the dog.

Canine Appetite. See BULIMIA.

Canine Madness. See HYDROPHOBIA.

Can'ine Teeth. [**Den'tes Cani'ni** or **Cuspida'ti.**] Eye-teeth; the four teeth which immediately adjoin the incisors.

Ca-ni'nus Mus'cu-lus,* or **Can'ine Mus'cle.** The *Levator anguli oris.*

Cani'nus Ri'sus.* ("Canine laugh.") An involuntary or spasmodic contraction of the canine muscle, causing what is popularly known as a sardonic laugh.

Cani'nus Spas'mus.* The *Spasmus cynicus.*

Canities,* ka-nish'e-ēz. [From *ca'-nus,* "gray-haired."] Grayness of the hair.

Can'na, or **Can'na Starch.** The fecula prepared from the rhizoma of an undetermined species of canna, and used for the same purpose as arrow-root.

Cannabinaceæ,* kan-na-be-na'she-ē, or **Can-na-bin'e-æ.*** [From *Can'nabis,* "hemp."] A natural order of herbaceous plants, including the hemp and hop, which have narcotic and intoxicating properties.

Can'na-bĭne. [**Cannabi'na;** from *Can'nabis,* "hemp."] A resin extracted from the *Cannabis Indica.*

Can'na-bis.* [Gr. κάνναβις.] A Linnæan genus of the class *Diœcia,* natural order *Cannabinaceæ* (formerly assigned to *Urticaceæ*). Hemp.

Can'nabis In'dĭ-ca.* ("Indian Hemp.") A kind of hemp well known in South America, Turkey, Asia Minor, India, etc., the leaves of which furnish an intoxicating drug called *Bhang,* or *Bang,* or *Bangue,* among the Hindoos, *Hashish* by the Arabs, *Maslach* by the Turks, and among the Hottentots *Dacha.* It is supposed to be merely a variety of the common hemp, or *Cannabis sativa.*

Can'nabis Sa-ti'va.* (Fr. *Chanvre,* shŏNvr.) The systematic name of common hemp. See preceding article.

Can'næ,* the plural of *Can'na,* a "reed," forming the Jussieuan name of an order of plants. See ZINGIBERACEÆ or MARANTACEÆ.

Can'nel Coal. A bituminous substance which yields on combustion a bright flame without smoke. The term is probably a corruption of *candle coal,* in allusion to its illuminating properties.

Can'nu-la.* [The diminutive of *can'na,* a "reed."] A tubular surgical instrument, introduced by means of a *stilette* into a cavity or tumor, for drawing off fluid.

Can-thăr'ĭ-dēs.* The plural of CANTHARIS, which see.

Can-thăr'ĭ-din. [**Cantharidi'na;** from *can'tharis,* the "Spanish fly."] A peculiar substance in *Cantharides,* on which their vesicating quality depends.

Can'tha-ris,* plural **Can-thăr'ĭ-dēs.** [From κάνθαρος, a "beetle."] The Pharmacopœial name ‖ of the blistering-fly; the *Can'tharis vesicato'ria;* called also the *Mus'ca Hispanio'la* ("Spanish fly"), *Lyt'ta vesicato'ria,* and *Mel'öe vesicato'rius.*

Cantharis Vesicatoria. See preceding article.

Can-thi'tis.* [From *can'thus.*] Inflammation of one or both *canthi.*

Can'tho-plas-tÿ. [**Canthoplas'tia;** from κανθός, the "angle of the eye," and πλάσσω, to "form."] The operation of transplanting a portion of the *conjunctiva* of the eyeball to the external *canthus* of the eyelids.

Can'thus,* plural **Can'thi.** [Gr. κανθός.] The angle formed by the junction of the eyelids; the internal being the *greater,* the external the *lesser, canthus.*

Can'ton's Phos'pho-rus. A substance made by exposing calcined oyster-shells and sulphur to a red heat. On exposure to the air it acquires the property of shining in the dark.

Canula. See CANNULA.

Caoutchouc,* koo'chŏŏk, or ka-oo'-chŏŏk. Elastic gum, or India rubber; the concrete juice of the *Hævea Caoutchouc, Jatropa elastica, Ficus Indica,* and *Artocarpus integrifolia.*

Caoutchoucin, koo'chŏŏ-sin. [**Caoutchouci'na.**] The principle on which the properties of caoutchouc depend.

Cap. = *Ca'pe,** "take," or *Ca'piat,* "let him take."

Că'pers. The pickled buds of the *Cap'paris spino'sa,* a low shrub growing out of the joints of old walls and the fissures of rocks in Southern Europe and in Syria.

Capillaire, kå'pēl'lair'. [From *Capil'lus Ven'eris,* "Venus's hair."] A syrup made with sugar or honey from the fern termed *Adian'tum capil'lus Ven'eris* (popularly known as "Maiden's-hair"). The name is also sometimes given to other syrups made in imitation of the above. Capillaire is employed as a demulcent in coughs.

Cap'il-la-rÿ. [**Capilla'ris;** from *capil'lus,* "hair."] Resembling a hair in size. Applied to the minute ramifications of arteries terminating on the surfaces of the body, etc.,—in other words, to the vessels which intervene between the minute arteries and veins; often called *capillaries.*

Cap-il-lic'u-lus,* plural **Cap-il-lic'-u-li.** [Diminutive of *capil'lus,* the "hair."] Applied in Anatomy to the arterial and venous radicles pervading, more minutely than the capillaries, the ultimate elements of every organ.

Cap-il-lĭ-fo'lĭ-ous. [**Capillifo'lius;** from *capil'lus,* "hair," and *fo'lium,* a "leaf."] Having hair-like leaves.

Ca-pil'lĭ-form. [**Capillifor'mis;** from *capil'lus,* "hair."] Formed like hair.

Ca-pis'trum.* [From *ca'pio,* to "take."] Literally, a "bridle." The single split-cloth bandage; so called from its being used to support the lower jaw like a bridle.

Cap'ĭ-ta,* gen. **Cap'ĭ-tum,** the plural of CAPUT, which see.

Cap'ĭ-tal. [**Capita'lis;** from *ca'put,* the "head" or "life."] Belonging to the head or life,—and, hence, of great or vital importance. The upper part of an alembic. Applied in the plural neuter to medicines for the head,—*Capita'lia medicamen'ta.* Also applied in Surgery to the more important operations.

Cap'ĭ-tate. [**Capita'tus;** from *ca'put,* a "head."] Growing in heads; a term used in Botany.

Capitellatus. The same as CAPITULATE.

Cap'ĭ-tĭ-lu'vĭ-um.* [From *ca'put,* the "head," and *lu'o,* to "wash."] A bath for the head.

Cap'ĭ-tis,* the genitive of *Ca'put,* the "head."

Ca-pit'u-late, or **Ca-pit'u-lāt-ed.** [**Capitula'tus.**] Having a *capitulum,* or knob on the top.

Ca-pit'u-lum.* [The diminutive of *ca'put.*] A little head, or knob. A protuberance of bone received into a hollow portion of another bone. A kind of inflorescence consisting of a number of flowers in a globular form on a common peduncle. An alembic.

Capivi Oil. See COPAIBA.

Cap'no-mor.* [From καπνός, "smoke," and μοῖρα, "part;" so called from its being one of the ingredients of smoke.] A colorless, transparent liquid,—the oily ingredient in tar which can dissolve caoutchouc. It occurs along with creasote in the heavy oil of tar.

Capparidaceæ,* kap-păr-e-da'she-ē. A natural order of plants, including the *Cap'paris* (caper). They have all a strong pungent, or even acrid, taste, and have been used as a substitute for mustard. Some of them are poisonous.

Cap-pa-rid'e-æ,* the Jussieuan name of a natural order of plants. See CAPPARIDACEÆ.

Cap'rāte. [**Ca'pras, a'tis.**] A combination of capric acid with a base.

Ca-pre'o-late, Ca-pre'o-la-rȳ. [**Capreola'tus, Capreola'ris;** from *capre'olus,* a "tendril."] Applied to the spermatic vessels, or *Vasa capreolaria,* from their twisted appearance.

Cap'ric Aç'id. [From *cap'ra,* a "she-goat."] A volatile acid, a constituent of butter from the milk of the goat or cow.

Cap'rĭ-dæ.* [From *ca'per,* a "goat."] A family of animals of which the goat is the type.

Cap-rĭ-fo'lĭ-a,* the plural of *Caprifo'lium,* the "honeysuckle," forming the Jussieuan name of a natural order of plants. See CAPRIFOLIACEÆ.

Caprifoliaceæ,* kap-re-fo-le-a'-she-ē. [From *Caprifo'lium,* the "honeysuckle."] A natural order of plants, comprising the honeysuckle, elder and viburnum. The leaves of the elder are emetic and cathartic; and these properties are possessed in some degree by most of the genera of this order.

Cap'ro-āte. [**Cap'roas, a'tis.**] A combination of caproic acid with a base.

Ca-pro'ic Aç'id. [**Capro'icum Aç'idum;** probably from *cap'ra,* a "she-goat," the milk of which is often used in making butter.] An oily, limpid liquid, obtained from the caproate of baryta, and entering into the constitution of butter.

Cap'sĭ-çin. An acrid, soft resin, obtained by digesting the alcoholic extract of the *Capsicum annuum* in ether and evaporating the etherial solution.

Cap'sĭ-cum.* [From κάπτω, to "devour," to "bite."] A Linnæan genus of the class *Pentandria,* natural order *Solanaceæ.* Also, the Pharmacopœial name || of the capsules and seeds of *Capsicum annuum,* and other species of capsicum.

Capsicum is a powerful stimulant without any narcotic effect. Whether taken into the stomach or applied externally, it causes a decided sense of heat or burning; but its influence upon the general system bears no proportion to its local action. Capsicum is chiefly used in medicine as a stomachic and rubefacient.

Cap'sicum An'nu-um.* The Capsicum, Cayenne, or Guinea-pepper plant.

Cap'sicum Fru-tēs'çens.* The species which yields the capsules mostly sold as *Guinea pepper* and *bird pepper.*

Cap'su-la.* [Diminutive of *cap'sa,* a "box."] A capsule. A membranous bag, containing some part, or organ, or the extremities of bones forming a joint. A membranous pericarp which splits in a determinate manner.

Cap'su-lar Lig'a-ment. [**Ligamen'tum Capsula're.**] A kind of ligamentous bag surrounding every movable articulation, and containing the *synovia.*

Capsule of Glisson. See GLISSON, CAPSULE OF.

Cap'sule, Re'nal. The Renal Capsules (*Cap'sulæ rena'les*) are two yellowish, triangular and flattened bodies, lying over the kidneys in the fœtus, in which they are as large as the kidneys themselves. In the adult they are two lobes. Called, also, supra-renal capsules.

Cap-su-lif'er-ous. [**Capsulif'erus**; from *cap'sula*, a "capsule," and *fe'ro*, to "bear."] Containing capsules.

Cap-su-li'tis, *idis*.* [From *cap'sula*, a "capsule."] Inflammation of the capsule of the eye.

Ca'put,* gen. **Cap'i-tis.** The head, consisting of the *cranium*, or skull, and the face. Also applied to any prominent object like a head.

Ca'put Co'li.* The "head of the colon,"—that is, the *Cæcum*.

Ca'put Gal-li-nag'i-nis.* The *Veru monta'num*, or prominent fold of the lining membrane in the prostatic portion of the urethra.

Caramel, kä'rä'měl'. The French name for sugar partly decomposed by the action of heat.

Căr'a-pāce. Applied in Zoology to the hard covering or shell on the upper part of the body of the *Chelonia*.

Căr'a-way. The *Carum carui*.

Car'bo Anima'lis.* ("Animal Charcoal.") The Pharmacopœial name (U.S. Ph.) for animal charcoal prepared from bone. See CARBON, ANIMAL.

Car'bo Lig'ni.* ("Charcoal of Wood.") The Pharmacopœial name ‖ of charcoal.

Car'bon. [**Carbo'nium**; from *car'bo*, a "coal."] The basis of charcoal; also, charcoal itself. Carbon is found pure in the diamond.

Car'bon, An'i-mal. Animal charcoal, bone charcoal, and ivory-black, are names applied to bones calcined or converted into charcoal in a close vessel. Animal charcoal is also prepared by calcining dried blood, horns, hoofs, clippings of hides, etc., in contact with carbonate of potash, and washing the calcined mass afterwards with water. Animal charcoal is principally used to decolorize vegetable principles, such as gallic acid, quinia, veratria, etc.

Car'bon, Min'e-ral. A term applied to charcoal with various proportions of earth and iron, without bitumen. It has a silky lustre, and the fibrous texture of wood. It occurs stratified with various kinds of coal.

Car-bo-nā'ceous. [**Carbona'ceus**; from *car'bo*, "coal," "carbon."] Of the nature of carbon.

Car'bo-nāte. [**Carbo'nas, a'***tis*; from the same.] A combination of carbonic acid with a base.

Car-bon'ic Aç'id. [**Carbon'icum Aç'idum**; from *car'bo*, "coal."] An acid formed in the burning of charcoal, and very abundant in nature, composing 0.44 of the weight of limestone, marble, etc. In the form of *carbonic acid gas* it constitutes a small proportion of atmospheric air. It is often found in mines, dry wells, etc. When unmixed or nearly so (as it frequently is in mines, and in ill-ventilated rooms where charcoal is burning), breathing it proves extremely deleterious, and often fatal to animal life. See CHOKE-DAMP, and POISONS.

Carbon'ic Ox'ide. A colorless gas, formed when carbon is burned with an imperfect supply of oxygen.

Car-bo-nif'er-ous. [**Carbonif'erus**; from *car'bo*, "coal," and *fe'ro*, to "bear."] Having or containing coal.

Car-bon-i-zā'tion. [**Carboniza'tio, o'***nis*; from *car'bon*.] The process of converting organic substances into charcoal.

Car'bun-cle. [**Carbun'culus**; the diminutive of *car'bo*, "coal."] The name of a gem of a deep bright-red color. Applied in Surgery to an inflammation of a gangrenous nature attended with a severe sense of burning. The same as ANTHRAX.

Car'bu-ret. [**Carbure'tum**; from *car'bon*.] The combination of carbon with another substance.

Car'bu-ret-ted. [From *carbure'tum*, a "carburet."] Of the nature of a *carburet*.

Car'buretted Hy'dro-gen. A colorless, inflammable gas, abundantly formed in nature in stagnant pools, wherever vegetables are undergoing the process of putrefaction: it also forms the greater part of the gas obtained from coal. Of this gas there are two kinds: the one termed light carburetted hydrogen is found abundantly in some coal-mines, where, under the name of fire-damp, it was the cause of those terrible explosions which were so common before the invention of the safety-lamp by Davy. The other kind, called heavy carburetted hydrogen or olefiant gas, forms the essential part of the gas used to light our streets.

Car-çi-no'ma, a'*tis*.* [From καρκίνος, an "eating ulcer."] A name for cancer.

Car-çi-nom'a-tous. [**Carcinom'atus**; from *carcino'ma*.] Belonging to *carcinoma*.

Car-dam'i-ne Pra-ten'sis.* The cuckoo flower, which yields cardamine flowers; the *Nastur'tium aquat'icum*.

Car'da-mom. [**Cardamo'mum.**] The fruit of several species of *Elettaria* and *Amomum*, the capsules of which furnish a warm and pleasant aromatic.

Car'dĭ-a.* [Gr. *καρδία.*] The heart; also the superior opening of the stomach.

Car'dĭ-ac. [**Cardi'acus;** from *car'-dia.*] Belonging to the heart. Applied to the superior opening of the stomach. Also applied to invigorating medicines.

Car'dĭ-ac Plex'us. [**Plex'us Car-di'acus.**] The principal cardiac plexus is situated on the bifurcation of the trachea. It is formed by the meeting of the middle and inferior cardiac nerves. There are two other cardiac plexuses,—the one termed *anterior*, and the other *posterior*,—situated respectively before and behind the ascending aorta, near its origin.

Car-di'a-gra.* [From *καρδία*, and *ἄγρα*, a "seizure."] Pain or gout of the heart.

Car-dĭ-ăl'gĭ-a.* [From *καρδία*, the "heart," and *ἄλγος*, "pain."] An uneasy or painful sensation in the stomach; heart-burn: car'dialgy.

Cardianastrophe. See ECTOPIA CORDIS.

Car-dĭ-ec'ta-sis.* [From *καρδία*, the "heart," and *ἔκτασις*, "extension" or "dilatation."] Dilatation of the heart.

Car'dĭ-o-çēle.* [From *καρδία*, and *κήλη*, a "tumor."] The protrusion of the heart through a wound of the diaphragm.

Car'dĭ-o-dy̆n'ĭ-a.* [From *car'dia*, and *ὀδύνη*, "pain."] Pain in the heart. See CARDIAGRA.

Car-dĭ-og'mus,* or **Kar-dĭ-og'-mos.*** Another term for cardialgia. Sometimes applied to palpitation of the heart and to *Angi'na pec'toris.*

Car-dĭ-o-păl'mus.* [From *καρδία*, the "heart," and *παλμός*, "palpitation."] See CARDIOTROMUS.

Car'dĭ-o-pĕr-ĭ-car-dī'tis, *idis.** [From *car'dia*, and *pericardi'tis.*] Inflammation of the heart and *pericardium.*

Cardiorhexis,*kar'de-o-rex'is. [From *καρδία*, the "heart," and *ῥῆξις*, a "breaking" or "laceration."] Rupture of the heart.

Car-dĭ-ot'ro-mus.* [From *καρδία*, the "heart," and *τρόμος*, a "trembling."] Fluttering of the heart.

Car-dī'tis.* [From *καρδία*, the "heart."] Inflammation of the heart. A genus of the order *Phlegmasiæ*, class *Pyrexiæ*, of Cullen's Nosology.

Car'do,* gen. **Car'dĭ-nis.** A hinge. Applied in Anatomy to the articulation called *Ginglymus.*

Caribean Bark. See BARK, CARIBEAN.

Căr'ĭ-ca Pa-pa'ya.* The Papaw-tree; the milky juice of which contains an abundance of fibrin resembling animal matter.

Car'ĭ-çæ Fruc'tus.* The preserved fruit of the fig. See FICUS CARICA.

Cā'rĭ-ēs.* (Literally, "rottenness.") A disease of bones, analogous to ulceration of the soft parts.

Ca-rī'na.* (Literally, the "keel of a ship.") Applied in Botany to the lower petal of the papilionaceous corolla.

Căr'ĭ-nate, or **Căr'ĭ-nāt-ed.** [**Carina'tus;** from *cari'na.*] Keel-shaped. Applied to leaves, petals, etc.

Cā'rĭ-ous. [**Cario'sus;** from *ca'ries.*] Having, or affected with, *caries.*

Car-mĭn'a-tĭve. [**Carminati'vus;** from *car'men*, a "song" or "charm."] Applied to medicines which assuage pain and relieve flatulence.

Car'mīne. A most beautiful coloring matter or pigment, prepared from cochineal combined with alumina and the oxide of tin; also called *Coccinellin.*

Carneæ Columnæ. See COLUMNÆ CARNEÆ.

Car'ne-us.* [From *ca'ro, car'nis*, "flesh," "fleshy."] Belonging to flesh: car'neous. See CARNOSUS.

Car-nĭ-fĭ-cā'tion. [**Carnifica'tio,** *o'nis;* from *ca'ro*, "flesh," and *fi'o*, to "become."] The change of any texture of the animal body into flesh. The term has been applied by Laennec to a diseased condition of the lungs when they have become converted into a substance resembling muscular flesh.

Car-nĭ-for'mis.* [From *ca'ro*, "flesh."] Resembling flesh.

Car-nĭv'o-ra.* [From *ca'ro*, "flesh," and *vo'ro*, to "devour."] A term applied to animals which feed upon flesh; more especially to that tribe of the *Mammalia*, such as the wolf, lion, etc., whose teeth are peculiarly adapted for seizing and destroying living animals.

Car-nĭv'o-rous. [**Carniv'orus;** from the same.] Flesh-devouring, or feeding on flesh.

Car-no'sus.* [From *ca'ro*, "flesh."] Fleshy; full of flesh: car'nose. Applied in the plural to an order of *Polypi.*

Ca'ro,* gen. **Car'nis.** The red fibrous part, or belly, of muscles; the flesh. Also the soft portion of fruits.

Căr-o-lī'na Pink. The *Spigelia Marilandica.*

Caroncule, kå'rôɴº'kül'. The French term for CARUNCULA, which see.

Ca-ro'ta.* The Pharmacopœial name (Lond. and U.S. Ph.) for the root of the carrot (*Dau'cus caro'ta*).

Ca-rot'i-cus.* [From καρόω, to "stupefy."] Having power to stupefy: carot'id. Applied in the plural neuter (*Carot'ica*) to narcotics.

Ca-rot'id. [**Caro'tis,** *idis;* from καρόω, to "stupefy."] Applied to an artery on each side of the neck, carrying blood to the head. They were so named from an idea that tying them would produce coma.

Car'o-tin. [**Carot'ina;** from *caro'ta.*] A peculiar crystalline principle of the carrot, or *Daucus carota.*

Car'pal. [**Carpa'lis.**] Belonging to the *carpus,* or wrist.

Car'pel. [**Carpel'lium,** or **Carpel'lum;** from καρπός, "fruit."] Applied in Botany to a simple pistil, or to one of the elements of a compound pistil. —(GRAY.)

Car-phol'o-gy. [**Carpholo'gia;** from κάρφος, "chaff," and λέγω, to "collect."] The movements of delirious patients in searching for or grasping at imaginary objects, picking the bed-clothes, etc.: floccilation. It is considered a very unfavorable symptom in fevers.

Car-pol'o-gy. [**Carpolo'gia;** from καρπός, "fruit," and λόγος, a "discourse."] A description of fruits or seeds; that part of Botany which treats of the fruits or seeds of plants.

Car-pot'i-cus.* [From καρπός, "fruit," "offspring."] Applied in the plural neuter (*Carpot'ica*) to an order of Dr. Good's class *Genetica,* or diseases affecting impregnation: carpot'ic.

Car'pus.* [Gr. καρπός.] The Latin term for the WRIST, which see.

Căr'ra-gēēn Moss, Căr'ra-ghēēn Moss. A species of moss, or sea-weed, found on the rocks and shores of Northern Europe, and in Carragheen, near Waterford, Ireland.

Car-ra-gēē'nin. The name given by Dr. Pereira to the mucilaginous matter called by some writers *vegetable jelly,* by others *pectin.*

Carrara (kar-rå'rå) **Wa'ter.** The name of a liquid prepared in imitation of the qualities of certain springs of Carrara, in Italy, famous for its marble-quarries.

Car'ron Oil. So called because used at the Carron Iron-Works, in Scotland. The *Linimentum Aquæ Calcis,* or LINIMENTUM CALCIS, which see.

Car'tha-min, Car'tha-mine, or **Car'tham-ic Aç'id.** A red coloring matter obtained from safflower.

Car'tha-mus Tinc-to'ri-us.* The safflower, or *bastard* saffron. A plant of the order *Compositæ;* the flowers are used by dyers. The seeds are cathartic and diuretic.

Car'ti-lage. [**Cartila'go,** *inis.* As if *Carnilage,* from *ca'ro,* "flesh," and *a'go,* to "yield."] A pearly white, glistening, elastic, uniform substance, adhering to articular surfaces of bones.

Car-ti-lag'i-nous, or **Car-ti-la-gin'e-ous.** [**Cartilagin'eus,** or **Cartilagino'sus.**] Of the nature of cartilage. Applied in Botany to leaves having a hard margin of different substance from the disk.

Căr'u-i.* The Pharmacopœial name (British Ph.) for the fruit of the *Ca'rum car'ui.*

Ca'rum.* [From the Arabic *Carvi,* or *Carvia.*] A Linnæan genus of the class *Pentandria,* natural order *Umbelliferæ.* Also the Pharmacopœial name (U.S. Ph.) for the fruit of the *Carum carui.*

Ca'rum Căr'u-i.* The caraway plant.

Ca-run'cu-la,* plural **Ca-run'cu-læ.** [Diminutive of *ca'ro,* "flesh."] A little fleshy excrescence: a car'uncle.

Carun'cula Lach-ry-ma'lis.* [Fr. *Caroncule lacrymale,* kå'rôɴº'kül' lå'kre'-mål'.] The small, red body situated in the inner angle of the eye.

Ca-run'cu-læ Myr-ti-for'mēs.* The remnants of the lacerated *hymen,* two, three, or four in number.

Ca'rus.* [Gr. κάρος.] A deep, heavy sleep; lethargy.

Caryophyllaceæ,* kar-e-of-il-la'-she-ē. A natural order of plants, including the *Dianthus,* carnation, and pink, and many weeds. Named from *Caryophyllus,* the specific name of the carnation or clove-pink.

Caryophyllata.* [From *caryo-phyl'lus,* the "clove-tree."] See GEUM URBANUM.

Căr-y-o-phyl'le-æ.* The Jussieuan name of an order of plants. See CARYOPHYLLACEÆ.

Căr-y-o-phyl'lic Aç'id. [From the same.] Eugenic acid; clove acid, or heavy oil of cloves; one of the two oils composing oil of cloves: the other is light oil, called *clove hydro-carbon.*

Căr-ȳ-o-phȳl'lin. [From the same.] Clove sub-resin; a crystalline substance extracted from cloves by alcohol.

Căr-ȳ-o-phȳl'lum.* [From the same.] The Pharmacopœial name (Brit. Ph.) for the unexpanded flower of *Caryophyllus aromaticus.* See CLOVE.

Căr-ȳ-o-phȳl'lus.* [From κάρυον, a "nut," and φύλλον, a "leaf," because supposed to be the leaf of the Indian nut plant.] A Linnæan genus of the class *Polyandria,* natural order *Myrtaceæ.* Also the Pharmacopœial name (Ed. and U.S. Ph.) of the CLOVE, which see.

Caryophyl'lus Ar-o-mat'ĭ-cus.* The systematic name of the clove-tree. Also the Pharmacopœial name (Dub. Ph.) for the clove. See CLOVE.

Căr-ȳ-op'sis.* [From κάρυον, a "nut," and ὄψις, an "appearance."] In Botany, a one-seeded pericarp, adhering closely to the integument of the seed, as in oats, rice, etc.

Cas-ca-ril'la.* [Diminutive of *cas'cara,* the Spanish word for "bark."] The Pharmacopœial name ‖ of the bark of the *Cro'ton eleuthe'ria.*

Cascarillæ Cortex.* ("Bark of Cascarilla.") See CASCARILLA.

Că'se-in, Că'se-ĭne, or **Ca'se-um.*** [From *ca'seus,* "cheese."] The albumen of milk; the curd separated from milk by the addition of an acid or rennet, constituting the basis of cheese in a state of purity.

Caseous, kā'she-ŭs, or kā'se-ŭs. [**Caseo'sus;** from *ca'seus,* "cheese."] Having, or full of, cheese: cheesy.

Ca-shew'-Tree. The *Anacar'dium Occidenta'le,* a tree belonging to the natural order *Anacardiaceæ,* found in the West Indies. It produces a kidney-shaped nut, yielding a caustic oil, which is used as a marking-ink, and also as a remedy for warts, etc.

Cassava,* kås-så'vå. A fecula separated from the juice of the root of the *Janipha Manihot,* and exposed to heat; a principal article of diet in South America. The same substance differently prepared and granulated constitutes *tapioca.*

Casserian (Ganglion). See GASSERIAN.

Cassia,* kash'e-a. [Gr. κασία, or κασσία.] A Linnæan genus of the class *Decandria,* natural order *Leguminosæ.* The Pharmacopœial name (Brit. Ph.) of the fruit of *Cas'sia fis'tula.* Several species of the genus *Cassia*—e.g. *C. acutifolia, C. elongata,* and *C. obovata*—produce the senna of commerce. See SENNA.

Cas'sia Fis'tu-la.* The purging cassia-tree. The Pharmacopœial name (U.S. Ph.) for the fruit of the *Cassia fistula.*

Cassia Lignea. See LAURUS CASSIA.

Cas'sia Măr-ĭ-lan'di-ca.* The Pharmacopœial name (U.S. Ph.) for the leaves of *Cassia Marilandica,* or American Senna.

Cas'sia Oil. The common oil of cinnamon, procured from cassia.

Cassiæ (kash'e-ē) **Pul'pa.*** ("Pulp of Cassia.") The Pharmacopœial name (Ed. Ph.) for the fruit of *Cas'sia fis'tula.*

Cassius (kash'e-ŭs), **Pur'ple of.** A purple-colored precipitate, obtained by mixing the proto-chloride of tin with a dilute solution of gold.

Cassonade (Fr.), kas'so'nåd'. Raw sugar; the crystallized and dried portion of sugar.

Cassythaceæ,* kas-se-tha'she-ē. A natural order of exogenous parasitical plants, consisting of one genus, the *Cassy'tha.*

Castaneæ,* kas-ta'ne-ē, the plural of **Cas-ta'nĭ-a,** a "chesnut." A name given by some botanists to a natural order including the chesnut, oak, etc. See CUPULIFERÆ.

Cas'tor. Another name for CASTOREUM, which see.

Cas'tor Oil. [**O'leum Riç'ini.**] An oil extracted from the seeds of the *Riç'inus commu'nis;* one of the most valuable of purgatives, being at the same time mild and speedy in its operation.

Cas-to're-um.* [From *cas'tor,* the "beaver."] The Pharmacopœial name ‖ of a peculiar concrete substance obtained from the follicles of the prepuce of the *Castor fiber,* or beaver. It is a moderate stimulant and antispasmodic.

Cas-tor'ĭ-dæ.* [From *cas'tor,* the "beaver."] A family of animals, of which the *Castor* is the type.

Cas'to-rin, or **Cas'to-rĭne.** [**Castori'na;** from *casto'reum.*] The active matter of *castoreum.*

Cas-trā'tion. [**Castra'tio, o'nis;** from *cas'tro, castra'tum,* to "cut off," to "emasculate."] The removal of a testicle, or both; orchotomy; emasculation. Applied in Botany to the removal of the anthers of a flower.

Cas-tren'sis.* [From *cas'tra,* a "camp."] Applied to diseases which soldiers encamped under unhealthy circumstances are particularly liable to, as *Febris castrensis,* "camp-fever."

Casuarinaceæ,* kas-u-ăr-ĭ-na'she-ē. [From *Casuari'na*, the name of one of the genera.] A curious natural order of exogenous trees without leaves, found in Australia. They are prized for their hard and heavy timber.

Cat. = *Cataplas'ma.** A "cataplasm."

Ca'ta (κατά). A Greek preposition signifying, in composition, "against," "according to," but most frequently "down," as in *catarrh* (from καταῤῥέω), literally, a "flowing down." It is often an intensive, as in CATACAUSIS, CATACLYSM, and CATALEPSY, which see. Before a vowel and before *h* the final *a* is dropped. See CATION, CATHODE, etc.

Cat-a-cau'sis.* [From κατακαίω, to "burn completely up."] A term denoting the phenomenon called preternatural or spontaneous combustion.

Cat'a-clȳsm. [**Cataclys'mus;** from κατακλύζω, to "inundate."] A deluge, or inundation. An affusion.

Cat-a-cous'tĭ-ca* (for pronunciation see ACOUSTIC). [From κατά, "against," and ἀκούω, to "hear."] That branch of Acoustics which treats of reflected sounds: catacous'tics.

Cat'a-lep-sȳ. [**Catalep'sia,** and **Catalep'sis;** from καταλαμβάνω, to "seize."] A total suspension of sensibility and voluntary motion, and, for the most part, of mental power, the action of the heart and lungs continuing: trance.

Cat-a-lep'tic. [**Catalep'ticus.**] Belonging to catalepsy.

Ca-tal'ȳ-sis.* [From καταλύω, to "dissolve."] A force or power which decomposes a compound body by mere contact: thus, peroxide of hydrogen is decomposed by contact with platinum, which is termed, in consequence, the *catalytic* agent.

Cat-a-lȳt'ic, Cat-a-lȳt'ĭ-cal. [**Catalyt'icus.**] Belonging to, or causing, *Catalysis*. Sometimes applied to a medicine supposed to destroy a morbific agency in the blood. See preceding article.

Cat-a-me'nĭ-a,* gen. **Cat-a-me-nĭ-o'rum,** found only in the plural. [From κατά, "according to," and μήν, a "month."] The monthly discharge from the uterus; otherwise called the menses, menstrual discharge, or courses, etc. See MENSES.

Cat-a-phon'ĭ-ca.* [From κατά, "against," and φωνή, "sound."] That branch of Acoustics which treats of the reflection of sound: cataphon'ics.

Ca-taph'o-ra.* [From καταφέρομαι, to "be weighed down," to "fall asleep."] The *co'ma somnolen'tum* of many writers; a variety of lethargy, attended with short remissions, or intervals of imperfect waking, sensation, and speech.

Cat'a-plaṡm. [**Cataplas'ma,** *atis;* from καταπλάσσω, to "overlay with plaster."] A soft application or poultice of bread, linseed-meal, oat-meal, etc., medicated or not.

Catapotium,* kat-a-po'she-ŭm. [From καταπίνω, to "drink," to "gulp," to "swallow down."] A pill or medicine to be swallowed without chewing. Written also *Catapotion.*

Cat'a-ract. [**Catarac'ta;** from καταῤῥάσσω, to "confound."] Obstructed sight, produced by opacity of the crystalline lens or its capsule.

Ca-ta'rĭ-a.* The Pharmacopœial name (U.S. Ph.) for the leaves of the *Nep'eta cata'ria*, or catnep.

Ca-tarrh'. [**Catar'rhus;** from καταῤῥέω, to "flow down."] A common cold in the head or chest; also, *Influenza;* likewise the mucous fluid poured out by the bladder under disease or catarrh of that organ, the discharge in *Leucorrhœa*, or catarrh of the vagina.

Ca-tarrh'al. [**Catarrha'lis.**] Belonging to catarrh.

Cat-a-stag'mus.* [From κατά, "down," and στάζω, to "drop," to "flow by drops."] A term applied by some medical writers to a defluxion from the fauces, etc. The same as CATARRH.

Cat-a-stăl'tic. [**Catastal'ticus;** from καταστέλλω, to "restrain."] Having power to restrain, check, or astringe. Applied to medicines that check evacuations, as astringent and styptic substances; the same as ANASTALTIC. Applied by M. Hall to the action of the *Vis nervosa*, from above downwards.

Catechu, kat'e-kū. [Said to be derived from the Japanese *Kate*, a "tree," and *chu*, "juice."] The Pharmacopœial name for an extract obtained chiefly from the wood of *Acacia catechu*. The term is applied to a variety of astringent extracts, which are imported under the names of *terra japonica* (Japan earth), *cutch*, and *gambir*.

Cat-e-chu'ic Aç'id. An acid (somewhat resembling gallic acid) obtained by Buchner from catechu.

Cath. = *Cathar'ticus.** "Cathartic."

Cath-æ-ret'ic, or **Cath-e-ret'ic.** [**Cathæret'icus;** from καθαιρέω, to "remove."] Mildly caustic, as nitrate of silver.

Ca-thar'sis.* [From καθαίρω, to

"purge."] Purgation of the excrements, medically or naturally.

Ca-thar'tic. [**Cathar'ticus;** from the same.] Applied to a medicine which quickens or increases evacuation from the intestines, or produces purging.

Ca-thar'tin. [**Catharti'na;** from καθαίρω, to "purge."] A peculiar principle obtained from jalap and senna leaves, on which their purging quality depends.

Ca-thar'to-car'pus Fis'tu-la.* Another name for the tree producing cassia. See Cassia Fistula.

Căth'e-ter.* [Gr. καθετήρ; from καθίημι, to "thrust into."] A surgical instrument like a tube, closed, but with several small perforations towards the extremity, which is introduced into the bladder through the urethra for the purpose of drawing off the urine in cases of retention, etc.

Cath'e-ter-is'mus.* [From *cath'eter.*] The operation of introducing the catheter: cath'eterism.

Cath'ōde. [From κατά, "down," and ὁδός, a "way."] In electro-chemical action, that part of the decomposing body which the electric current leaves.

Cath-od'ic. [**Cathod'icus;** from κατά, "downwards," and ὁδός, a "way."] Proceeding downwards. Applied by M. Hall to the course of action of the nervous influence. See Catastalticus.

Ca-thol'ĭ-con.* [From καθολικός, "universal," "unchanging."] A panacea, or universal medicine.

Ca'tĭ-on.* [Gr. κατιόν, the present participle of κάτειμι, to "go down," to "descend."] Literally, "descending," or "passing down." A term in electro-chemical action for a body that passes to the cathode of the decomposing body.

Cat'kin. The same as Amentum, which see.

Cat'ling. A double-edged, sharp-pointed, straight knife for amputations.

Catnep. See Cataria.

Cat'o-che,* or **Cat'o-chus.*** [From κατέχω, to "restrain," to "retain," to "keep."] A kind of catalepsy in which the body is kept rigidly in an erect posture.

Cat-op'tric, Cat-op'trĭ-cal. [**Catop'tricus;** from κάτοπτρον, a "mirror."] Belonging to a mirror, or to Catoptrics.

Cat-op'trics. [**Catop'trica;** from the same.] That branch of Optics which treats of the reflection of light.

Cat's Eye. A mineral brought from Ceylon: so called from a peculiar play of light arising from white fibres interspersed. The French call this appearance *chatoyant* (shå'twå'yŏnᵍ').

Cat's Purr. A characteristic sound of the chest, heard by means of the stethoscope.

Cat's Tail. The common name for the *Typha.*

Cau'da E-qui'na.* ("Horse-tail.") The termination of the spinal marrow, giving off a large number of nerves, which, when unravelled, resemble a horse's tail.

Cau'dal. [**Cauda'lis;** from *cau'da,* a "tail."] Belonging to the tail.

Cau'date. [**Cauda'tus;** from the same.] Having a tail.

Cau'dex.* The trunk of a tree. In Botany, the stem, or ascending axis of growth, is termed *caudex ascendens;* the root, or descending axis, *caudex descendens.*

Cau-dic'u-la.* [Diminutive of *cau'da,* a "tail."] A prolongation in certain plants in the form of a filament, which bears the masses of pollen: a cau'dicule, or cau'dicle.

Caul. The epiplöon, or omentum. Sometimes applied to a portion of the amnion which occasionally envelops the child's head at birth.

Cau-lĕs'çent. [**Caules'cens;** from *cau'lis,* a "stem," and *-esco,* a Latin termination signifying to "grow."] Growing to a stem.

Cau-lic'u-lus.* [Diminutive of *cau'lis,* a "stem."] The intermediary part of the embryo which has germinated between the cotyledons and the root; a cau'licule, or cau'licle.

Cau-lĭ-flo'rous. [**Cauliflo'rus;** from *cau'lis,* a "stem," and *flos,* a "flower."] Having flowers on the stem.

Cau'lĭ-flow-er Ex-crĕs'çence. A disease of the os uteri, supposed by Gooch to be encephalosis.

Cau'lĭ-form. [**Caulifor'mis;** from *cau'lis,* a "stem."] Formed like a stem.

Cau'līne. [**Cauli'nus;** from *cau'lis,* a "stem."] Belonging to a stalk or stem. Applied to leaves which arise directly from the stem.

Cau-lo-car'pous. [**Caulocar'peus;** from *cau'lis,* a "stem," and καρπός, "fruit."] Having persistent stems, frequently bearing fruit.

Cau'ma, a*tis. [From καίω, to "burn."] The burning heat of fever.

Caus'tic. [**Caus'ticus;** from καίω, to "burn."] Possessing causticity. As a noun (Lat. *Caus'ticum*) it denotes a substance which, by its chemical properties, destroys the texture of organized bodies: such are the pure alkalies, the concentrated mineral acids, lunar caustic, etc.

Caus'tic Al'ka-li. An alkali comparatively pure, or one which has not lost its caustic properties by combination with another substance, as, for example, with carbonic acid, or with oil.

Caustic, Lunar. See LUNAR CAUSTIC.

Caustic Potash. See POTASSA.

Caus-tiç'i-ty. [**Caustiç'itas, a'***tis;* from *caus'ticus.*] The quality which distinguishes caustic substances. See CAUSTIC.

Caus'ti-cum A-cer'ri-mum* (the superlative degree of *a'cer,* "sharp"). The old name for caustic potash,—the strongest common caustic.

Cau'sus.* [Gr. καῦσος, a "burning heat."] A variety of malignant remittent fever: so named on account of its excessive heat. It has been termed *fe'bris ar'dens,* "ardent" or "burning fever."

Cau-ter-i-zā'tion. [**Cauteriza'tio, o'***nis.*] The act of applying the cautery.

Cau'ter-y. [**Caute'rium;** from καίω, to "burn," or more directly from καυτήριον, a "red-hot iron" or "branding-iron."] The application of a caustic substance, or of a hot iron; also, the hot iron or substance thus applied.

Cau'tery, Ac'tu-al. [**Caute'rium Actua'le.**] The employment of actual burning (*i.e.* heated iron, fire, etc.) for the cure or removal of a diseased part. See ACTUAL CAUTERY.

Cau'tery, Po-ten'tial. [**Caute'rium Potentia'lis.**] The application of caustic substances, as potassa, lunar caustic, etc.

Cav'er-nous. [**Caverno'sus;** from *caver'na,* a "cavern."] Having cells or caverns.

Cav'ernous Si'nus. A sinus on the base of the cranium.

Cawk. A name sometimes given to the sulphate of barytes, or heavy spar.

Cayenne (kā-yĕn') **Pep'per.** The ground pods and seeds of the *Capsicum annuum;* Guinea pepper.

C. C. = *Cucurbit'ula Cruen'ta.** A cupping-glass.

C. C. = *Cor'nu Cer'vi.** Hartshorn.

C. C. U. = *Cor'nu Cer'vi Us'tum.** Burnt hartshorn.

Ceanothus. See RED ROOT.

Cebadilla (Sp.), sȧ-BA-DEEL'yȧ. The seeds of the *Asagrea officinalis,* a plant of the order *Melanthaceæ.* See VERATRIA.

Ce'cal. [**Cæca'lis.**] Belonging to the *Cæcum.* See CÆCAL.

Cecum. See CÆCUM.

Cedrelaceæ,* sed-re-la'she-ē. An important natural order of trees (including *Cedrela* and Mahogany) found in the tropics of America and India. In general the bark is a powerful astringent, and the wood fragrant. The bark of the *Cedre'la too'na* and of Mahogany is febrifugal; the former is astringent, and a tolerably good substitute for Peruvian bark in intermittent fevers.

Ce'dron. The common name of the *Sima'ba Ce'dron,* a tree growing in South and Central America. The seeds are considered to be a remedy for snake-bites and other animal poisons. The raspings of the wood have been used in intermittents as a substitute for quinine.

Celandine. See CHELIDONIUM.

Celastraceæ,* sel-as-tra'she-ē. [From *Celas'trus,* one of the genera.] A natural order of shrubs, which have acrid properties, sometimes stimulant. The *Euonymus* (Spindle-Tree, or Burning Bush) is an example.

Ce-las'trus.* The name of a genus of plants of the class *Pentandria,* natural order *Celastraceæ.*

Celas'trus Scan'dens* (the "Climbing Celastrus"), sometimes called the Climbing Staff-tree and False Bittersweet. A climbing shrub common in the United States: the bark is said to possess narcotic as well as emetic and diaphoretic properties.

Çe'lē.* [Gr. κήλη.] A word formerly used for *hernia;* now, added as a suffix to another word, it signifies a tumor caused by protrusion of some soft part or parts denoted by the first portion of the term, as *Enterocele, Epiplocele,* etc.; also, swelling of a part, as *Sarcocele;* or its enlargement by the presence of fluid, as *Hydrocele.*

Cel'es-tine. [From *cæ'lum,* the "sky."] Sulphate of strontian; so named from its frequently presenting a blue color.

Cell. [**Cel'la;** supposed to be derived from *ce'lo,* to "conceal."] Literally, a "cellar" or "cavity," hence, any hollow space. In Botany the term is applied to the cavity or cavities of a pericarp in which the seeds are lodged. According to the number of these cavities, a pericarp is termed *one-celled, two-celled,* etc. It also denotes the cavity of an anther, ovary, etc. In Physiology, a cell or cellule constitutes the origin or commencement of every plant and animal, and the elementary form of every tissue. In fact, the entire organized body, whether animal or vegetable, may be considered to be made up of a congeries of cells, each set having its own appropriate endowment or function, as nutrition, secretion, absorption, etc.

Cell-Nucleus. See CYTOBLAST.

Cell-The'o-rȳ. The theory or proposition that there exists one general principle for the formation of all organic productions,—*i.e.* the formation of cells; also, the conclusions drawn from this proposition.

Cell'u-lar. [**Cellula'ris;** from *cel'lula.*] Having, or consisting of, cells. See CELLULAR TISSUE.

Cell'ular Plants [termed in Latin **Cellula'res**]. A name sometimes applied to cryptogamous plants.

Cell'ular Tis'sue. [**Te'la Cellula'ris** and **Te'la Cellulo'sa;** Fr. *Tissu cellulaire,* tè'sü' sĕl'ü'laiR'.] Called also **Cell'ular Mem'brane.** The most common of all the organic tissues, constituting the net-work which connects the minute parts of most of the structures of the body. It has also been called **Are'olar Tis'sue,** on account of the *areolæ,* or interstices, with which it abounds. See AREOLAR.

Cell'ūle. [**Cel'lula,** the diminutive of *cel'la,* a "cell."] A little cell. See CELL.

Cell'u-lōse. [From *cel'lula.*] The substance of which the cellular tissue of plants is chiefly composed.

Ce-lot'o-mȳ. [**Celoto'mia;** from κήλη, a "tumor," "hernia," and τέμνω, to "cut."] The operation for hernia.

Ce'ment. [**Cæmen'tum.**] Any substance used for cementing together what may have been broken, as lute, solder, etc. Also, a composition by which metals are changed. See TOOTH.

Cem-en-tā'tion. [**Cæmenta'tio, o'nis;** from *cæmen'tum.*] A process by which metals are purified or changed in their qualities by heat without fusion, by means of a composition, called a cement, with which they are covered.

Çe-not'ĭ-ça.* [From κένωσις, "evacuation."] Morbid [fluid] evacuations or discharges. The name of an order in Dr. Good's class GENETICA.

Cen-tau'rĭ-i Ca-cu'mĭ-na.* The tops of the *Erythræa centaurium;* directed for use by the Colleges of London and Edinburgh. See ERYTHRÆA.

Cen-tau'rĭ-um.* [From κένταυρος, a "centaur."] The Pharmacopœial name (Ed. Ph.) of *Erythræa centaurium,* the medicinal properties of which are similar to those of Gentian.

Cen-tĭ-fo'lĭ-ous. [**Centifo'lius;** from *cen'tum,* a "hundred," and *fo'lium,* a "leaf."] Having a hundred leaves.

Cen'tĭ-grāde. [**Centig'radus;** from *cen'tum,* a "hundred," and *gra'dus,* a "grade."] Having a hundred grades or degrees. Applied to a French thermometer thus divided.

Centigramme, sen'te-grăm. French pronunciation, sŏNº'tè'grâmm'. [From *cen'tum,* a "hundred," and *gram'ma,* a "gramme."] The hundredth of a gramme, equal to 0.154 of a grain avoirdupois, or one-sixth of a grain troy.

Centilitre, sŏN'te-lètr'. [Fr. *cent,* a "hundred," and *li'tre.*] The one-hundredth part of a litre; equal to 0.6102 of an English cubic inch.

Centimetre, sĕn-te-me'tr, or sŏN'te-mêtR'. [Fr. *cent,* a "hundred," and *mètre.*] The one-hundredth part of a metre; equal to 0.394, or two-fifths, of an English inch.

Cen'tĭ-pēde. [**Cen'tipes, p'edis;** from *cen'tum,* a "hundred," and *pes,* a "foot."] Having a hundred feet, or many feet. The name of an animal (or insect) having many feet.

Cen'trad. [From *ad,* "to" or "towards," and *cen'trum,* the "centre."] Applied the same as *Central* used adverbially.

Cen'tral. [**Centra'lis;** from *cen'trum,* the "centre."] Applied by Dr. Barclay to the body and organs generally, as meaning towards the centre.

Cen'tre of Grav'ĭ-tȳ. That point in a body about which all the parts exactly balance one another, so that, if that point be supported, every part would be *in æquilibrio* and the whole body be at rest.

Cen'tres, Ner'vous. The brain, spinal cord, and sympathetic ganglia.

Cen-trif'u-gal. [**Centrif'ugus;** from *cen'trum,* the "centre," and *fu'gio,* to "fly."] Flying from the centre.

Centrif'ugal Force. That force by which a body moving in a circular orbit, and striving (according to the laws of forces) to proceed in a straight course, tends to fly off from the centre in a tangent to the orbit.

Cen-trip'e-tal. [**Centrip'etus;** from *cen'trum,* the "centre," and *pe'to,* to "seek."] Tending towards the centre.

Centrip'etal Force. That force by

which a body moving round another tends or is impelled to the centre.

Cen-tro-stăl'tic. [**Centrostal'ticus;** from *cen'trum*, the "centre," and *stal'ticus*, "staltic."] Applied by M. Hall to the action of the *Vis nervosa* in the spinal centre.

Cen'trum.* [Gr. κέντρον; from κεντέω, to "prick" or "pierce."] Literally, a "centre." Applied by Owen, in Comparative Anatomy, to the homologues of the body of a *vertebra*.

Cen'trum Com-mu'ne.* Literally, the "common centre" [of nerves or of ganglia]. The solar plexus.

Centrum Ovale (of Vicq D'Azyr). See Vicq D'Azyr, etc.

Centrum Ovale* (of Vieussens). See Vieussens, etc.

Ceph-a-e'lis.* A Linnæan genus of the class *Pentandria*, natural order *Cinchonaceæ*.

Cephaë'lis Ip-e-cac-u-an'ha.* The plant from which ipecacuanha is obtained.

Çeph-a-læ'a.* [From κεφαλή, the "head."] A term for diseases of the head.

Çeph'a-læ-ma-to'ma,* or **Ceph'a-lo-hæ-ma-to'ma.*** [From κεφαλή, the "head," and αἷμα, "blood."] A sanguineous tumor, sometimes occurring in new-born children.

Çeph-a-læ'mi-a.* [From κεφαλή, the "head," and αἷμα, "blood."] Congestion of the head or of the brain.

Çe-phal'a-gra.* [From κεφαλή, the "head," and ἄγρα, a "seizure."] Chronic pain of the head, gouty or rheumatic.

Çeph-a-lăl'ġi-a.* [From κεφαλή, the "head," and ἄλγος, "pain."] Headache, or pain in the head: ceph'alalgy.

Çe-phal'ic. [**Cephal'icus;** from κεφαλή, the "head."] Belonging to the head.

Çephal'ic Vein. The anterior vein of the arm: formerly opened in disorders of the head.

Cephalitis. See Encephalitis.

Çeph'a-lo-. [From κεφαλή, the "head."] This, in compound names of muscles, etc., denotes connection with the head.

Çeph'a-lo-dy̆n'i-a.* [From κεφαλή, the "head," and ὀδύνη, "pain."] Headache; pain in the head.

Çeph'al-o-ġen'e-sis.* [From κεφαλή, the "head," and γένεσις, "generation," or "creation."] The doctrine of the formation of the brain.

Çeph-a-log'ra-phy̆. [**Cephalogra'phia;** from κεφαλή, the "head," and γράφω, to "write."] A description of heads.

Cephalohæmatoma. See Cephalæmatoma.

Çeph'a-loid. [**Cephaloi'des;** from κεφαλή, the "head."] Resembling the head.

Çeph-a-lol'o-ġy̆. [**Cephalolo'gia;** from κεφαλή, the "head," and λόγος, a "discourse."] A treatise on the head; the science of the head considered in its anatomical and physiological aspects.

Çeph-a-lo'ma.* [From κεφαλή, the "head."] A medullary tumor; a morbid product resembling brain, sometimes called *encephaloid*, or cerebriform tumor, medullary sarcoma, etc.

Çeph-a-lom'e-ter. [**Cephalom'etrum;** from κεφαλή, the "head," and μέτρον, a "measure."] An instrument for ascertaining the size of the fœtal head during parturition.

Çeph'a-lo-phăr-y̆n-ġæ'us.* [From κεφαλή, the "head," and φάρυγξ, the "pharynx."] A designation of the *constrictor superior pharyngis* muscle.

Çeph-a-loph'o-ra.* [From κεφαλή, the "head," and φέρω, to "bear;" because supported by their heads.] See Cephalopoda.

Cephalop'oda, or **Ceph'alopods.** See Cephalopodus.

Çeph'a-lop'o-dus.* [From κεφαλή, the "head," and πούς, a "foot."] Cephalop'odous. Applied in the neuter plural (*Cephalop'oda*, or Ceph'alopods) to a class of *Mollusca* in which the strong fleshy members by means of which they crawl proceed from the head,—in other words, the head is situated between the body and the feet.

Çeph'a-lot.* [From κεφαλή, the "head."] A peculiar fat found in the brain, containing phosphorus and sulphur.

Çeph'a-lo-tho'rax.* [From κεφαλή, the "head," and θώραξ, the "chest."] The first segment of the *Arachnida* and *Crustacea*, including in one what in insects is divided into head and thorax.

Çeph'a-lo-tōme. [**Cephalot'omus;** from κεφαλή, the "head," and τέμνω, to "cut."] An instrument for cutting or breaking down the head of the fœtus. There are various forms and adaptations of it.

Çeph-a-lot'o-my̆. [**Cephaloto'mia;** from κεφαλή, the "head," and τέμνω, to "cut."] Dissection of the head; also, the cutting or breaking down of the fœtal head.

Çeph'a-lo-trībe.* [From κεφαλή, the "head," and τρίβω, to "break down."] An instrument intended to supersede the crotchet and perforator in the operation of craniotomy.

Ce'ra.* [Gr. κηρός, "wax; Fr. *Cire*, sĕr.] Wax. The Pharmacopœial name (Brit. Ph.) of bleached yellow wax. A membrane covering the base of the beak of birds in which the nostrils are pierced.

Ce'ra Al'ba.* ("White Wax.") Yellow wax bleached.

Ce'ra Fla'va.* ("Yellow Wax.") Bees'-wax in its natural state; "a peculiar concrete substance prepared by *Apis mellifica*" (U.S. Ph.).

Ce-rā'ceous. [**Cera'ceus;** from *ce'ra*, "wax."] Of the appearance or consistence of wax.

Ceramiaceæ,* se-ram-e-a'she-ē. [From *Cera'mium*, one of the genera.] A natural order of cryptogamous plants, consisting of sea-weeds (*Algæ*). It includes several species which are gelatinous and valuable for food. Among these are the Dulse of the Scots, and Carrageen moss. The esculent nests of the Chinese swallow are supposed to derive their value from a plant of this order.—(LINDLEY.)

Cérat, sā'rā'. The French term for CERATE. See CERATUM.

Ce-ra'ta,* the plural of CERATUM, which see.

Cerate. See CERATUM.

Çer-a-ti'tis.* [From κέρας, a "horn."] The same as CORNEITIS, which see.

Çe-ra'to-. [From κέρας, a "horn."] A prefix denoting connection with the *cornu* or horn of the hyoid bone, or with the cornea.

Çe-rat'o-bran'chĭ-al. [**Cerato-branchia'lis;** from *cera'to*, and βράγχια, the "gills."] Applied in Comparative Anatomy to the longer bent pieces, supported by the bones which form the lower extremities of the branchial arches in fishes.

Çe-rat'o-çēle.* [From κέρας, a "horn," and κήλη, a "tumor."] A hernia of the cornea.

Çe-rat'o-glos'sus.* [From *cera'to*, and γλῶσσα, the "tongue."] A name for the *Hyo-glossus* muscle, from its appearance and insertion: cerat'oglossal.

Çe-rat'o-hȳ'al. [**Ceratohya'lis;** from κέρας, a "horn," and *hyoi'des*, "hyoid."] Applied by Owen to the lower and larger of the two principal parts of the *cornu* of the hyoid bone.

Çĕr'a-toid. [**Ceratoi'des;** from κέρας, a "horn," and εἶδος, a "form."] Resembling a horn.

Ceratoma. See KERATOMA.

Ceratonyxis. See KERATONYXIS.

Çeratophyllaceæ,* se-rat'o-fil-la'-she-ē, or **Çe-rat'o-phȳl'le-æ.*** A natural order of plants, consisting of one genus, *Ceratophyllum*, a weed found in ditches and constantly submerged.

Çe-rat'o-plas'tĭ-ca.* [From κέρας, a "horn," and πλάσσω, to "form."] The artificial formation of the *cornea*: cer'-atoplasty.

Çĕr-a-to'sus.* [From κέρας, a "horn."] Having, or containing, horn; full of horn.

Çe-rat'o-tōme. [**Ceratot'omus;** from κέρας, a "horn," and τέμνω, to "cut."] A knife for dividing the cornea.

Çĕr-a-tot'o-mȳ. [**Ceratoto'mia;** from κέρας, a "horn," and τέμνω, to "cut."] Cutting of the cornea.

Ce-ra'tum,* plural **Çe-ra'ta.** [From *ce'ra*, "wax."] Ce'rate. A compound ointment in which wax predominates as an ingredient, and which is, therefore, of a somewhat firmer consistency than common ointments. Also applied to compounds of a similar consistency, though not containing wax.

Cera'tum Ad'ĭ-pis.* ("Cerate of Lard.") The Pharmacopœial name (U.S. Ph., 1860) for simple cerate. See CERATUM SIMPLEX.

Cera'tum Can-thăr'ĭ-dis.* ("Cerate of Cantharides.") The common blistering plaster (or salve) of the shops. It is composed of twelve parts of powdered cantharides, of yellow wax and resin each seven parts, and of lard ten parts.

Cera'tum Plum'bi Sub-aç-e-ta'-tis.* ("Cerate of Subacetate of Lead.") The Pharmacopœial name for what is commonly called GOULARD'S CERATE, which see.

Cera'tum Re-si'næ.* ("Cerate of Resin.") The Pharmacopœial name for what is popularly known as Basilicon Ointment. See BASILICON.

Cera'tum Sim'plex* ("Simple Cerate") is prepared by melting together eight parts of lard and four of white wax, and stirring the mixture until it is cool. Used as a mild and emollient application to inflamed surfaces.

Cerchnus,* serk'nŭs. [Gr. κέρχνος; from κέρχω, to "render hoarse."] A noisy respiration: wheezing.

Ce're-al. [**Cerea'lis;** from *Ceres*, the goddess of Corn.] Pertaining to corn.

Ce-re-a'lĭ-a.* [From *cerea'lis*, "belonging to *Ceres*."] All sorts of corn, of which bread or any nutritious substance is made.

Ce're-a-lin. [**Cereali'na;** from *Ceres,* the goddess of Corn.] The nutritious principle of flour.

Cĕr-e-bel-li'tis.* [From *cerebel'lum.*] Inflammation of the *cerebellum.*

Cĕr-e-bel'lum.* [Diminutive of *cer'ebrum,* the "brain."] (Fr. *Cervelet,* sĕʀv'lȧ'.) The little brain, situated at the lower and back part of the cranium. It was considered by Gall to be the seat of venereal desire; but this view is contradicted by many facts.

Cĕr'e-bral. [**Cerebra'lis;** from *cer'ebrum,* the "brain."] Belonging to the brain; brain-like.

Cer-e'bric. [**Cereb'ricus;** from *cer'ebrum,* the "brain."] Applied to a fatty acid existing in the brain in combination with soda.

Cer-e'bri-form. [**Cerebrifor'mis;** from *cer'ebrum,* the "brain."] Like the form or substance of the brain; encephaloid.

Cĕr'e-brin, or **Cĕr'e-brine.** [**Cerebri'na;** from *cer'ebrum,* the "brain."] A reddish, fatty substance found in the brain.

Cĕr-e-bri'tis.* [From *cer'ebrum,* the "brain."] Inflammation of the brain. See Encephalitis.

Cĕr'e-bro-. A prefix in compound terms denoting connection with the *cerebrum.*

Cĕr'e-broid. [**Cerebroi'des;** from *cer'ebrum,* the "brain."] Resembling brain.

Cĕr'e-brot.* [From *cer'ebrum,* the "brain."] The same as Cephalot.

Cĕr'e-brum.* [From κάρα, the "head;" Fr. *Cerveau,* sĕʀ'vō', and *Cervelle,* sĕʀ'-vĕll'.] The brain proper, occupying the entire upper portion of the cranium, and separated from the cerebellum by the *tentorium.* It is divided on its upper surface, by a deep median cleft, into two equal portions, called hemispheres, which are united at the base by a hard body, called the *corpus callosum,* or *commissura magna.* The lower surface of the cerebrum is divided into three lobes, called anterior, middle, and posterior.

The brain is primarily composed of two substances, the one white, medullary, and fibrous, constituting the interior portion, the other gray, or cineritious, situated chiefly on the surface.

Cerevisia,* sĕr-e-vish'e-a. [As if *Cereris vis in aqua,* the "strength of corn in water."] Any liquor brewed from corn; ale; beer.

Cerevis'iæ Fer-men'tum.* ("Leaven or Yeast of Beer.") Yeast, or barm.

Cĕr'ic Aç'id. [From *ce'ra,* "wax."] An acid produced by the action of the fixed alkalies on wax.

Ce'rin, or **Ce'rine.** [**Ceri'na;** from *ce'ra,* "wax."] A component of common wax which dissolves in sixteen times its weight of boiling alcohol, and has properties almost exactly the same as those of wax.

Ce'ri-um.* A white metal found in a Swedish mineral called *cerite,* also in *allanite.* See Tellurium.

Cer'nu-ous. [**Cer'nuus;** from *cer'nuo,* to "bow downward."] Nodding, or stooping.

Ce-ro'ma.* [From κηρός, "wax."] Another name for Cerate. Sometimes applied to an adipose tumor of the brain, from its waxy appearance; called also *lardaceous degeneration.*

Cĕr'u-lin. [**Cæruli'na;** from *cæru'lus,* "blue."] The name given to the coloring matter of a peculiar substance obtained from indigo by the action of sulphuric acid.

Ce-ru'men,* gen. **Ce-ru'min-is.** [From *ce'ra,* "wax."] Ear-wax. The wax-like secretion of the ear given out by follicles of the inner surface of the *Meatus auditorius externus.*

Ce-ru'mi-nous. [**Cerumino'sus;** from *ceru'men.*] Belonging to the cerumen; of the nature of cerumen.

Ce'rūse, or **Ce'russe.** [**Cerus'sa;** from κήρ, a "plague," "death," or "poison;" from its poisonous qualities.] The subcarbonate of lead; white lead.

Cerveau, Cervelle. See Cerebrum.

Cervelet. See Cerebellum.

Cer'vi-cal. [**Cervica'lis;** from *cer'vix,* the "neck."] Belonging to the neck.

Cer'vi-dæ.* [From *cer'vus,* a "stag."] A family of animals having the *Cervus* for their type.

Cer'vix, i'cis.* The neck, more particularly the back part. Also applied to those parts of organs that are narrowed like a neck.

Cervoise, sĕʀ'vwȧz'. The French term for beer. See Cerevisia.

Cer'vus.* [From κέρας, a "horn."] A "stag." Also the name of a genus of *Mammalia Ruminantia.*

Cer'vus El'e-phas.* The systematic name of the stag, the horns of which afford some valuable medicines. See Cornu.

Ces'pi-tōse. [**Cespito'sus;** from *ces'pes, ces'pitis,* a "turf."] Producing many stems from one root, forming a surface of turf or sod.

Cetacea,* se-ta'she-ạ, or **Cetaceans,** se-tā'shŭns. [From *ce'tus,* a "whale."] An order of Mammalia living in the sea, including the whale,dolphin,porpoise,etc. They breathe air, have warm blood, and can remain but a limited time under water. As they are often compelled to come to the surface for air, to facilitate their ascent and descent, they are furnished with a horizontal tail-fin, and are thus obviously distinguished from the true fishes, in which the tail-fin is vertical.

Ce-tā'ceous. [**Ceta'ceus;** from *ce'tus,* a "whale."] Belonging to the whale; of the nature of the whale.

Cetaceum,* se-ta'she-ŭm. [From *ce'tus,* a "whale."] The Pharmacopœial name ‖ of spermaceti, an oily, concrete, crystalline, semi-transparent matter obtained from several species of whale, but chiefly the *Physe'ter macroceph'alus.*

Ce'tic Aç'id. A supposed peculiar acid resulting from the saponification of *cetin,* found to be only a mixture of margaric acid and *cetin.*

Ce'tin. [**Ceti'na;** from *ce'tus,* a "whale."] Another name for spermaceti.

Ce-tra'ri-ạ.* The Pharmacopœial name ‖ of the *Cetraria Islandica,* or Iceland moss.

Cetra'ria Is-lan'dĭ-cạ.* The systematic name of Iceland moss, otherwise called *Lichen Islandicus* and *Lichen Cetraria.*

Ce-trā'rin. [**Cetrari'na.**] The bitter principle of the *Cetraria Islandica.*

Ce-vad'ic Aç'id. An acid produced by the saponification of the oil of the *Veratrum Sabadilla* or *Cevadilla,* sometimes called *Sabadilic acid.*

Ceylon Moss. See JAFNA MOSS.

Chaff. See PALEA.

Chailletiaceæ,* kĭl-le-te-a'she-ē. [From *Chaille'tia,* the name of one of the genera.] A natural order of exogenous trees or shrubs, found in hot climates.

Cha-la'sis.* The name given by Sauvages to the porcine species of scrofula.

Cha-la'zạ.* [Gr. χάλαζα, a "hailstone."] A small tumor or tubercle found chiefly on the eyelid. See CHALAZION. In Botany, applied to an enlargement of the *raphe,* where it joins the base of the nucleus. In the plural (*Chalazæ*) it denotes two spiral bodies, situated one at each end of the egg, the apex of each adhering to the yelk.

Cha-la'zĭ-on,* **Cha-la'zĭ-um.*** [From the same.] A small, transparent tubercle on the edge of the eyelid; called also *Chalaza.*

Cha-lạ-zo'sis.* [Gr. χαλάζωσις.] The same as CHALAZA and CHALAZION.

Chăl-can'thum.* [From χαλκός, "brass," and ἄνθος, a "flower."] The "flowers of brass," or the sulphate of zinc; Pliny's term for copperas, or the sulphate of iron.

Chăl-çed'o-nous, or **Chăl-çe-do'nĭ-ous.** [**Chalced'onus, Chalcedon'icus.**] Having the external characters or appearance of chalcedony.

Chăl-çed'o-nȳ (or kăl'se-do-ne). [From *Chalce'don,* a town of Asia Minor where it was originally found.] A siliceous stone, much used in jewelry.

Chaleur, shå'lᴜʀ'. The French word for "caloric" or "heat." See CALORIC.

Chalk, chawk. [Lat. **Cre'ta;** Fr. *Craie,* ᴋʀå.] Carbonate of lime; whitening.

Chalk, Black. Drawing-slate; a bluish-black clay, containing about twelve per cent. of carbon.

Chalk, Red. A species of argillaceous iron ore.

Chalk, Span'ish. Steatite, or soapstone.

Chalk-Stone. [**Cal'culus Arthrit'icus,** or **Cal'culus Podag'ricus.**] A concretion deposited in the hands and feet of those afflicted with gout, resembling chalk, though chemically different; gout-stone. They consist chiefly of uric acid and soda, sometimes, though rarely, of urate of lime.

Cha-lȳb'e-ate. [**Chalybea'tus;** from χάλυψ, gen. χάλυβος, "iron" or "steel."] Containing iron; impregnated with iron.

Chalyb'eate Wa'ters. Mineral waters whose predominating or active principle is iron. There are two kinds: the *carbonated,* containing carbonate of the protoxide of iron; and the *sulphurated,* containing sulphate of iron. Some of the latter contain sulphate of alumina, and are called *aluminous sulphated chalybeates.*

Chamaceæ,* kạ-ma'she-ē, or **Chamaceans,** kạ-mā'shạns. [From *cha'ma,* a "clam."] A family of acephalous mollusks, of which the common clam is the type.

Cha-mæ'le-on.* A name given to certain thistles, from the variety and uncertainty of their colors, like the changing hues of the chameleon.

Cha-mæ'le-on'ĭ-dæ.* [From *chamæ'leon.*] A family of *Reptilia Sauria,* having the chameleon for its type.

Chamælianciaceæ,* kạ-me-le-an-se-a'she-ē. A natural order of plants, allied to the Myrtleblooms, found in Australia. They are bushes with fragrant leaves.

Cham-æ-me'lum.* [From χαμαί, "on the ground," and μῆλον, an "apple;" so named, probably, on account of its globe-like flowers, or perhaps from its fragrance being supposed to resemble that of apples.] Literally, "ground-apple;" one of the names of the *An'themis nob'ilis*, or chamomile.

Chamæme'lum Nob'ĭ-le.* The *Anthemis nobilis*.

Chambers of the Eye. See CAMERA.

Cha-me'le-on Min'e-ral. A combination of black oxide of manganese and potash, which gives a green color to water, passes gradually through all the shades of the prism, and at last becomes colorless.

Cham'o-mile. [See CHAMÆMELUM.] The popular name for the *An'themis nob'ilis*. An infusion of the flowers of this plant forms an excellent bitter tonic.

Cham-o-mil'la Ro-ma'na.* Another name for the *Anthemis nobilis*.

Chancre, shank'ẹr; Fr. pronunciation, shŏNKR. [A French corruption of the Latin *cancer*.] A sore or ulcer arising from the direct application of the syphilitic poison.

Chan'doo'. An extract of opium prepared by the Chinese for smoking.

Change of Life. In popular language, the constitutional disturbance often attending the cessation of the menstrual discharge in females.

Chanvre. See CANNABIS SATIVA.

Characeæ,* ka-ra'she-ē. [From *Cha'ra*, one of the genera.] A natural order of cryptogamous, aquatic plants, remarkable for the distinctness with which the rotation of their fluids may be seen under a microscope. See CHARA HISPIDA.

Chăr'ac-ters, Chem'ĭ-cal. Various systems of these have been introduced, but are now almost entirely discarded from use. Abbreviations and contractions are employed instead. See Appendix.

Cha'ra His'pĭ-da.* A submersed, leafless, aquatic plant, interesting to the physiologist as displaying the special circulation in plants, and as being analogous in Botany to the frog in Zoology.

Char'coal commonly denotes coal from burnt wood (or *carbo ligni*), but is often used indefinitely for the residue of any animal or vegetable and of many mineral substances when heated to redness in close vessels. There are several varieties of charcoal, termed gas-carbon, lamp-black, wood-charcoal, coke, and ivory-black.

Charpie (Fr.), shar-pee'. A substance composed of a collection of filaments separated from morsels of old linen rag, used as lint.

Chartreux, Poudre de, poodR dẹh shaR'truh'. See KERMES MINERAL.

Chāy Root, or **Cha'ya Root.** The root of the *Oldenlan'dia umbella'ta*, used for giving the beautiful red of the Madras cottons.

Cheek. See BUCCA, GENA, MALA.

Cheek'-Bone. The *Os juga'le, Os ma'læ*, or *Os zygomat'icum*.

Cheese. [Lat. **Ca'seus;** Fr. *Fromage*, fro'mâzh'.] A substance prepared from milk, composed chiefly of *casein* mixed with a small but variable proportion of oil (butter). See CASEIN.

Cheese Ren'net. The popular name for GALIUM VERUM, which see.

Cheiloplastic, kī-lo-plas'tik. [**Cheiloplas'ticus.**] Belonging to the operation of cheiloplasty.

Cheiloplasty, kī'lo-plas-te. [**Cheiloplas'tice;** from χεῖλος, the "lip," and πλάσσω, to "form."] The operation of supplying deficiencies of the lips by appropriating a sufficient portion of the neighboring healthy substance to that purpose.

Cheiroptera. See CHEIROPTERUS.

Cheiropterus,* kī-rop'ter-ŭs. [From χείρ, the "hand," and πτερόν, a "wing."] Literally, "hand-winged,"—that is, having both wings and hands. Applied in the plural neuter (*Cheirop'tera*) to a family of *Mammalia* that have a fold of skin extending from the neck between their fore-feet and toes, enabling certain of them to fly, as the bat-tribe: cheirop'terous.

Che'la.* [Gr. χηλή.] A Latin word signifying "claw," but found in the Roman writers only in the plural, **Che'læ.** It is applied in Natural History especially to the claws of the crab, lobster, and other Crustaceans.

Chelæ Cancrorum. See CANCRORUM, LAPILLI et CHELÆ.

Che-liç'e-ra.* [From *che'la*, a "claw," and κέρας, a "horn."] In the plural (*Cheliç'eræ*) applied to the prehensile organs of certain *Arachnides*, terminated by two fingers, or a single one resembling a hook or claw.

Chel-ĭ-do'nĭ-um.* [From χελιδών, a

"swallow," because its flowering coincides in time with the appearance of the swallow.] The *Celandine* (sel'ạn-dīn), a genus of plants belonging to the Linnæan class *Polyandria,* natural order *Papaveraceæ.*

Chelido'nium Ma'jus.* (The "Greater Celandine.") An herb, the yellow juice of which has been employed as an escharotic to destroy warts.

Che-lif'er-ous. [**Chelif'erus;** from *che'la,* a "claw," and *fe'ro,* to "bear."] Bearing, or having, claws, or pincers.

Chel'ĭ-form. [**Chelifor'mis;** from *che'la,* a "claw."] Formed like a claw.

Che'loid. [**Cheloi'des;** from χέλυς, a "tortoise," and εἶδος, a "form."] Applied to a skin-disease; resembling the tortoise.

Che-lo'nĭ-ạ.* [From χελώνη, a "tortoise."] An order of *Reptilia,* including the several varieties of the tortoise. See TESTUDO.

Chem'ĭ-cal. [**Chem'icus;** from *che'mia.*] Of, or belonging to, chemistry.

Chem'is-trỹ. [Lat. **Che'mia, Chi'mia,** or **Chy'mia;** supposed by some to be derived from the Greek χύω, to "pour out," or to "melt;" others derive it from the Arabic. Fr. *Chimie,* shè'mè'.] "The science which investigates the composition of natural substances, and the permanent changes of constitution which their mutual actions produce."

Che-mo'sis,* or **Chy-mo'sis.*** [From χυμός, a "humor," or χήμη, an "aperture."] Inflammation of the *conjunctiva,* with lymph or blood effused in the cellular substance connecting it with the eyeball, so that it is greatly elevated and the cornea seems to form the bottom of a cavity.

Chêne (Fr.), shàn. See QUERCUS.

Chenopodiaceæ,* ke-no-po-de-a'-she-ē. [From *Chenopo'dium,* one of the genera.] The *Atrip'lices* of Jussieu, a natural order of plants, comprising spinage, beet, and many weeds found in nearly all parts of the world.

Che-no-po'dĭ-um.* [From χήν, a "goose," and πούς, ποδός, a "foot."] A plant called Goosefoot, belonging to the Linnæan class *Pentandria,* natural order *Chenopodiaceæ.* Several species of this genus possess anthelmintic properties.

Chenopo'dium An-thel-min'tĭ-cum.* Wormseed; a plant growing in different parts of the United States. The seeds are given in powder, as a remedy for worms, in the dose of one or two teaspoonfuls to a child three or four years old. Of the oil, the dose is from four to eight drops.

Cher'rỹ-Lau'rel, or **Cherry, Bay.** The *Pru'nus laurocer'asus.*

Chevestre, shẹ-vĕs'tr (Fr. pronunciation, shẹh-vêtR'). [Lat. *Capis'trum, i.e.* a "halter."] A double roller applied to the head in cases of fracture or luxation of the lower jaw.

Chew'ing Balls. Masticatories used in farriery, composed of the wood of the bay and juniper trees, assafœtida, liver of antimony, and pellitory of Spain.

Chewing the Cud. See RUMINATION.

Chī-aś'mạ, atis.* [From χιάζω, to "make the letter X."] Chi'asm. The crossing of the fibres of the optic nerve. See INTRICATURA.

Chiaster,* ke-as'tẹr. A bandage for stopping hæmorrhage from the temporal artery, and named from its being shaped like a cross or the Greek letter X (chi). Written also *Kiaster.*

Chick'en Pox. The popular English name for *Varicella.*

Chigre, chig'ger, **Chigo,** chee'go. (Fr. *Chique,* shèk.) A small sand-flea of the West Indies, which insinuates itself into the soft and tender parts of the fingers and toes.

Chil'blain. [**Per'nio, o'***nis.*] See BLAIN. A painful inflammatory swelling on the fingers, toes, or heels, consequent on exposure to severe cold; a kibe.

Child-Bed Fever. See PUERPERAL FEVER.

Chī-maph'ĭ-lạ.* [From χεῖμα, "winter," and φιλέω, to "love."] The Pharmacopœial name for the *Chimaph'ila corymbo'sa.* A Linnæan genus of the class *Decandria,* natural order *Pyrolaceæ.* See PYROLA.

Chimaph'ila Cor-ỹm-bo'sạ,* Chimaph'ila Um-bel-la'tạ.* The *Pyr'ola umbella'ta,* or American winter-green.

Chimie, shè'mè'. The French term for CHEMISTRY, which see.

Chim'ney-Sweep'er's Can'cer. [**Can'cer Mundito'rum.**] See CANCER SCROTI.

Chī'nạ Glaze. A preparation for printing blue frit, made from ten parts of glass, two parts of lead, and three or more of blue calx.

China Nova,* KE'nå no'vå. The name given in Germany to the red bark known in France as *Quinquina nova* (or *Quinquina rouge*); it is the produce of the *Cinchona oblongifolia.* It is very different from the red bark of English commerce, though they have been confounded by the London College.—(HOBLYN.)

Chinchina,* kin-kee'na. Cinchona, or Peruvian bark.

Chinchona. See CINCHONA.

Chin-Cough. See PERTUSSIS.

Chi-nese' Worm'wood. The *Artemisia Chinensis.*

Chi-noi'din. [**Chinoidi'na;** from *chi'na,* "Peruvian bark," and εἶδος, "likeness."] A substance containing a small portion of amorphous quinine.

Chī'ra-gra,* or **Cheir'a-gra.*** [From χείρ, the "hand," and ἄγρα, a "seizure."] Gout in the joints of the hand.

Chi-ret'ta.* The Pharmacopœial name (U.S. and Ed. Ph.) for the herb and root of the *Agathotes chirayta,* or GENTIANA CHIRAYTA, which see.

Chī-ro'ni-a.* [From *Chi'ron,* the "centaur," fabled to have been a skilful physician.] A Linnæan genus of the class *Pentandria,* natural order *Gentianaceæ.*

Chiro'nia Cen-tau'ri-um.* An herb called the Lesser Centaury. (Fr. *Centaurée petite,* sŏNG'to'rā' peh-tēt'.) The tops (*Centau'rii cacu'mina*) are aromatic and tonic.

Chī-rur'geon. See SURGEON.

Chī-rur'ger-y. [**Chirur'gia;** from χείρ, the "hand," and ἔργον, a "work."] Literally, a "manual operation:" hence, that part of medicine which heals with the hand, without, however, excluding other remedies. See SURGERY.

Chī-rur'gi-cal. [**Chirur'gicus;** from *chirur'gia.*] Belonging to surgery; surgical.

Chī-rur'gus.* [From χείρ, the "hand," and ἔργον, a "work."] A surgeon, or chirurgeon.

Chi-ti'na.* [From χιτών, a "doublet."] The hard crust forming the outward integument,—especially the *elytra* of certain insects; the chitine.

Chlænaceæ,* kle-na'she-ē. [From χλαῖνα, a "cloak," and, hence, an "involucrum," all plants of this order having involucra.] A natural order of exogenous trees and shrubs, found in Madagascar: many of them have showy flowers. Sometimes written *Chlenaceæ.*

Chlo-as'ma, atis.* [From χλοάζω, to "be green."] A cutaneous affection exhibiting spots and patches of a yellowish-brown color, sometimes called *Mac'ulæ hepat'icæ* ("liver spots"), from a supposition that they are caused by disease of the liver. The *Pityriasis versicolor* of Willan.

Chlor-a-cet'ic Aç'id. A remarkable acid, in which the three atoms of the hydrogen of acetic acid are replaced by three atoms of chlorine.

Chlo'ral. This term, derived from the first syllable of the words *chlorine* and *alcohol,* has been applied by Liebig to a new compound of chlorine, carbon, and oxygen, prepared by the mutual action of alcohol and chlorine.

Chloranthaceæ,* klo-ran-tha'she-ē. [From *Chloran'thus,* one of the genera.] A natural order of plants, found in the hot parts of India and America. They have stimulating properties of great importance. The root of *Chloran'thus officina'lis* is prized in Java as a remedy for typhus fever.

Chlo'rāte. [**Chlo'ras, a'tis;** from *chlor'icum* aç'idum.] A combination of chloric acid with a base.

Chlo'ric. [**Chlo'ricus;** from *chlo'rium,* "chlorine."] Derived from chlorine; of the nature of chlorine.

Chlo'ric E'ther. Under this name two compounds have been confounded. One of these results from the action of chlorine on olefiant gas, and is generally known as the *oil of the Dutch chemists.* The other is obtained by passing hydrochloric acid gas into alcohol to saturation and distilling the product; this is generally called hydrochloric ether.

Chlo'ride. [**Chlo'ridum;** from *chlo'rium.* Fr. *Chlorure,* klo'rür'.] A combination of chlorine with different substances.

Chloride of Mercury. See HYDRARGYRI CHLORIDUM.

Chlo'rine. [**Chlo'rium;** from χλωρός, "green."] An elementary body, formerly called oxy-muriatic acid, also *dephlogisticated marine acid.*

Chlo-ri'o-dāte. [**Chlori'odas, a'tis;** from *chloriod'icum* açidum.] A combination of chloriodic acid with a base.

Chlo-ri-od'ic. [**Chloriod'icus;** from *chlo'rium,* "chlorine," and *iodin'ium,* "iodine."] Belonging to chlorine and iodine. Applied to an acid obtained from this compound.

Chlo'ro-. A prefix in compound terms, meaning that chlorine is one of the components of the substance denoted, or is employed in its preparation.

Chlo-ro-car-bon'ic. [**Chlorocarbon'icus;** from *chloro-,* and *carbo'nium.*] Applied to an acid obtained from chlorine and carbon. See PHOSGENE GAS.

Chlo'ro-form, or **Chlo-ro-for'-**

myle. [**Chlorofor'mum;** from *chlo'rine,* and *for'myle.*] A colorless volatile liquid varying in specific gravity from 1.45 to 1.49, obtained by distilling a mixture of chloride of lime and alcohol. It is a powerful anæsthetic agent. It is usually administered in the form of vapor, being inhaled into the lungs. It is sometimes taken into the stomach, as an anodyne or soporific, in which case a fluidrachm is equivalent to about thirty-five drops of laudanum.

Chlo-ro-for'mum Ve-na'le.* ("Commercial Chloroform.") The Pharmacopœial name (U.S. Ph.) of the terchloride of formyle. See preceding article.

Chlo-rom'e-ter. [**Chlorom'e-trum;** from *chlo'rium,* and μέτρον, a "measure."] An apparatus for estimating the quantity of chlorine in combination with water, or a base; but especially for ascertaining the bleaching power of a solution of chlorine, or chloride of lime, etc. See next article.

Chlo-rom'e-trÿ, or **Chlo-rim'e-trÿ.** [From the same.] The process of estimating the bleaching power of chloride of lime, by the quantity of a solution of sulphate of indigo which a known weight of chloride can discolor or render yellow.

Chlo'ro-phÿll, written also **Chlorophylle.** [From χλωρός, "green," and φύλλον, a "leaf."] The green coloring matter of leaves.

Chlo-ro'sis.* [From χλωρός, "green."] A disease peculiar to young females under retention or suppression of the menstrual discharge; green-sickness. A genus of the order *Adynamiæ,* class *Neuroses,* of Cullen's Nosology.

Chlo-rot'ic. [**Chlorot'icus.**] Belonging to *chlorosis.*

Chlo'rous Aç'id. The peroxide of chlorine, because approaching to an acid in its nature.

Chlōr'ū-ret. [**Chlorure'tum;** from *chlo'rium.* Fr. *Chlorure,* klo'rüʀ'.] A combination of chlorine with a metal, or inflammable body. See Chloride.

Chlōr-ÿ'dric Aç'id. The name given by Thénard to muriatic, now called hydrochloric, acid.

Choke'-Damp. (Ger. *Dampf,* a "vapor.") A name applied by miners to all irrespirable gases, but more especially to carbonic acid gas.

Cho-læ'mĭ-a.* [From χολή, "bile," and αἷμα, "blood."] The presence of bile-pigment in the blood: chole'my.

Chol'a-gŏgue. [**Cholago'gus;** from χολή, "bile," and ἄγω, to "lead or carry off."] Applied to a medicine which has the property of increasing the evacuation of bile.

Cho'le.* [Gr. χολή.] Bile. See Bilis.

Cho'le-āte. [**Cho'leas, a'tis.**] A combination of choleic acid with a base.

Cho-le-çÿs-ti'tis, idis.* [From *cholecys'tis,* the "gall-bladder."] Inflammation of the gall-bladder.

Chol'edoch. See Choledochus.

Cho-led'o-chus.* [From χολή, and δέχομαι, to "receive."] (Fr. *Cholédoque,* ko'lā'dok'.) Receiving gall or bile. See Ductus Communis Choledochus.

Cho-le'ic. [**Chole'icus;** from χολή, "bile."] Relating to bile. Applied to an acid obtained from bile.

Cho-le'in. [**Cholei'na;** from χολή, "bile."] The peculiar principle of bile.

Chol-e-pÿr'rhin. [**Cholepyrrhi'na;** from χολή, "bile," and πυῤῥός, "yellow."] A term synonymous with *Biliphein.*

Chol'e-ra.* [From χολή, "bile," and ῥέω, to "flow;" or χολάς, the "intestines," and ῥέω, to "flow."] A vomiting and purging of bile (this is true at least respecting European Cholera), with painful griping, and spasm of the muscles of the abdomen and calves of the legs, etc. A genus of the order *Spasmi,* class *Neuroses,* of Cullen's Nosology.

Chol'era, Asiat'ic. [*Chol'era Asiat'ica.*] A remarkable epidemic disease, consisting in a malignant form of cholera, in which all the symptoms are much more severe and rapid in their progress to a too generally fatal issue.

Chol'era Bilio'sa.* ("Bilious Cholera.") Copious and frequent vomiting, at first of the alimentary and fecal matters, with redundancy of bile, and spasms of the legs and thighs. This is nothing more than a form or variety of European Cholera.

Chol'era, Europe'an. [*Chol'era Europæ'a.*] A name given to cholera as it usually appears in Europe when not epidemic, to distinguish it from the epidemic and malignant form of the disease known as Asiatic Cholera.

Chol'era Infan'tum.* ("Cholera of Infants.") A name applied to a disease common among children in the United States during the summer months, and hence called the "summer-complaint." It is attended with vomiting and purging of green or yellow matter often mixed with slime or blood.

CHOL'ERA MOR'BUS.* A common name of non-epidemic cholera. See CHOLERA, EUROPEAN.

Chol-e-ră'ic. [**Cholera'icus.**] The same as CHOLERICUS.

Cho-lĕr'ĭ-cus.* (Fr. *Cholérique*, ko'-lȧ'rěk'.) Belonging to cholera. Also, bilious.

Chol'er-oid. [**Choleroi'des**; from *chol'era*, and εἶδος, a "form."] Resembling cholera. Applied to diseases of this character.

Chol'er-o-pho'bĭ-ạ.* [From *chol'era*, and φόβος, "fear."] A dread of cholera.

Chol'er-o-pho'ne.* [From *chol'era*, and φωνή, the "voice."] The *Vox chol-er'ica*, or faint whispering voice of choleraic patients.

Chol'e-ste-ạ-to'mạ, a*tis*.* [From χολή, "bile," and *steato'ma*.] A fatty tumor, laminated and pearly, principally composed of crystals of cholesterin.

Chol-es-ter-æ'mĭ-ạ.* [From *choles'-terin*, and αἷμα, "blood."] Applied to a morbid excess of cholesterin in the blood, resulting from non-excretion.

Chol-es-tĕr'ic Aç'id. An acid formed by the action of nitric acid on cholesterin.

Cho-lĕs'ter-in, or **Cho-lĕs'ter-ĭne.** [**Cholesteri'na**; from χολή, "bile," and στερεός, "firm," or "solid."] A pearl-like, fatty substance, of which human biliary calculi are chiefly composed.

Chol'ic. [**Chol'icus**; from χολή, "bile."] Belonging to bile; bilious.

Chol'ic Aç'id. [**Aç'idum Chol'i-cum.**] A peculiar acid obtained from bile.

Chol'ĭ-nāte. [**Chol'inas, a'***tis*.] Cholinic acid combined with a base.

Cho-lin'ic Aç'id. [**Aç'idum Cho-lin'icum.**] A peculiar substance obtained from bile.

Chololic. See CHOLIC.

Chol-o-lith'ic. [**Chololith'icus**; from *cholol'ithus*.] Belonging to a gall-stone.

Cho-lol'ĭ-thus.* [From χολή, "bile," and λίθος, a "stone."] A gall-stone, or biliary calculus.

Cho-lo'sis.* [From χολή, "bile."] In the plural (*Cholo'ses*), biliary diseases.

Chon-drăl'ġĭ-ạ.* [From χόνδρος, "cartilage," and ἄλγος, "pain."] Pain (rheumatic, arthritic, or inflammatory) of the cartilages.

Chon'drin, or **Chon'drĭne.** [**Chon-dri'na**; from χόνδρος, "cartilage."] Gelatin obtained from the permanent cartilages, cornea, etc. See **Chondrogen.**

Chon'dro-ġen. [From χόνδρος, "cartilage," and γεννάω, to "produce."] The base of true cartilage and of the cornea. By boiling it is resolved into CHONDRIN.

Chon-dro-ġen'e-sis.* [From the same.] The formation of cartilage.

Chon-dro-glos'sus.* A small muscle, or rather fasciculus of muscular fibres, running from the cartilage of the *os hyoides* to the tongue. It may be considered as a part of the *hyoglossus*.

Chon-drog'rạ-phȳ. [**Chondro-gra'phia**; from χόνδρος, "cartilage," and γράφω, to "write."] A history or description of the cartilages.

Chon'droid. [**Chondroi'des**; from χόνδρος, "cartilage," and εἶδος, a "form."] Resembling cartilage.

Chon-drol'o-ġȳ. [**Chondrolo'gia**; from χόνδρος, "cartilage," and λόγος, a "discourse."] A dissertation on the nature and structure of cartilages; the science of cartilages.

Chon-dro'mạ, a*tis*.* [From χόνδρος, "cartilage."] A cartilaginous growth.

Chon-drop-te-rȳġ'ĭ-us.* [From χόνδρος, "cartilage," and πτερύγιον, a "little wing."] "Cartilage-finned." Applied in the plural masculine (*Chondropte-ryġ'ii*) to a tribe or series of fishes.

Chondros. See CARTILAGE.

Chon-dro'sis.* The progress of *Chondroma*. The formation of cartilage.

Chon-drot'o-mȳ. [**Chondroto'-mia**; from χόνδρος, "cartilage," and τέμνω, to "cut."] Dissection or division of cartilage.

Chon'drus Crisp'us.* Carrageen, or Irish moss. A plant belonging to the natural order *Algaceæ*.

Chor'dạ.* [Gr. χορδή, an "intestine," a "chord."] A chord; originally the string of a harp: hence, any string; a sinew, or nerve. Applied in Geometry to a right line extending from one extremity of an arch to another.

Chor'da Mag'nạ.* (The "Great Cord, or Sinew.") The *Tendo Achillis*.

Chor'da Tym'pan-i.* (The "Cord of the Tympanum.") A branch of the seventh pair of nerves.

Chor'da Ven-tric'u-li.* ("Nerve of the Stomach.") A designation of the gastric plexus of the *par vagum*.

Chor'dæ Ten-din'e-æ.* ("Tendinous Cords.") Attachments connecting the *Carneæ columnæ* of the ventricles to the auricular valves of the heart.

Chor'dæ Vo-ca'lēs.* ("Vocal Chords.") The thyro-arytenoid ligaments of the larynx, or the inferior ligaments of the glottis: so named because they were supposed to produce the voice.

Chordæ Willisii. See WILLIS, CHORDS OF.

Chor-dap'sus.* [From χορδή, "intestine," and ἅπτω, to "bind," to "seize," to "attack."] A kind of violent spasmodic cholic, in which the large intestines seem as it were twisted into knots.

Chor-dee'. [Lat. **Chorda'ta;** Fr. *Chordé,* kor'dà'; literally, "corded," or "twisted"?] A painful tension and downward curvature of the penis, experienced in *Gonorrhœa.*

Cho-re'a,* or **St. Vi'tus' Dance.** [From χορεία, a "dancing."] A convulsive disease, characterized by irregular and involuntary movements of the limbs.

Cho-re'ic. Pertaining to CHOREA.

Cho'ri-on.* [Gr. χορίον, "skin," "leather."] The second or most external membrane involving the fœtus. Also the *Membra'na putam'inis,* or membrane of the shell of the egg.

Cho'ri-um,* or **Cho'ri-on.*** [From the same.] The dermis, or innermost layer of the skin; the true skin.

Cho'roid. [**Choroi'des;** from *cho'rion,* and εἶδος, a "form."] Resembling the chorion.

Cho'roid Mem'brane. [**Membra'na Choroi'des.**] The second membrane of the eyeball, immediately beneath the sclerotic coat. Also, the *Ve'lum interpos'itum,* or choroid membrane of the brain.

Cho'roid Plex'us. [**Plex'us Choroi'des.**] A plexus of vessels, or fold of thin vascular membrane, derived from the *Pia mater,* situated in the lateral ventricles of the brain.

Christ'mas Rose. The *Helleborus niger.*

Chro'māte. [**Chro'mas, a'tis.**] A combination of chromic acid with a base.

Chro-mat'ic. [**Chromat'icus;** from χρῶμα, χρώματος, "color."] Relating to color, or colors; having color. See ACHROMATIC.

Chro'ma-tism. [**Chromatis'mus;** from the same.] The prismatic aberration of the rays of light,—or, in other words, the aberration of refrangibility,—caused by the different kinds of rays being refracted unequally.

Chro'ma-tog'e-nous. [**Chromatog'enus;** from χρῶμα, "color," and γεννάω, to "generate."] Generating or forming color. Applied chiefly to the functions of the *derma.*

Chro-ma-tol'o-gy̆. [**Chromatolo'gia;** from χρῶμα, "color," and λόγος, a "discourse."] The science of colors.

Chro'ma-top'sy̆. [**Chromatop'sia;** from χρῶμα, "color," and ὄψις, "vision."] Colored vision.

Chro'ma-trōpe. [**Chromat'ropus,** or **Chromatro'pium;** from χρῶμα, "color," and τρέπω, to "turn."] An instrument for exhibiting, on the principle of the magic lantern, a variety of colors producing, by a rapid revolving motion, beautiful and highly pleasing figures.

Chrōme. A metal. See CHROMIUM.

Chrome Al'um. A crystallizable, double salt, formed of the sulphates of chromium and of potash.

Chrome Yel'low. The chromate of lead, much used as a pigment.

Chro'mic. [**Chro'micus.**] Belonging to *Chromium.* See CHROMIC ACID.

Chro'mic Aç'id. [**Aç'idum Chro'micum.**] A teroxide of chromium forming a valuable escharotic for the removal of morbid growths, especially those of syphilitic origin. It has been assigned a place on the primary list of the Materia Medica in the U.S. Pharmacopœia for 1860.

Chro-mi-dro'sis.* [From χρῶμα, a "color," and ἱδρόω, to "sweat."] Abnormal coloration of the perspiration.

Chro'mi-um,* or **Chrōme.** [From χρῶμα, a "color."] A metal extracted from native chromate of lead or of iron. It is whitish, brittle, and very difficult to fuse. The specific gravity is 5.5.

Chro'mo-gen. [**Chromoge'nium;** from χρῶμα, a "color," and γεννάω, to "generate."] Vegetable coloring matter, which, acted on by acids and alkalies, produces red, yellow, or green tints.

Chromopsy. See CHROMATOPSY.

Chro'mule, or, better, **Chro'my̆le.** [From χρῶμα, "color," and ὕλη, "material," "substance."] Other names for *chlorophyll,* or the coloring matter of plants.

Chron'ic. [**Chron'icus;** from χρόνος, "time."] Long-continued; opposed to *acute.*

Chron'o-ther'mal. [**Chronotherma'lis;** from χρόνος, "time," and θέρμη, "heat."] Relating to time and temperature. Applied to a theory that all diseases have periodic intermissions, with alternate chills and heats.

Chro-op'si-a,* written also **Chrup'sia** (by a contraction of the Greek χροοψία into χρουψία, which in Latin becomes *Chrupsia*). The same as CHROMATOPSIA. See CHROMATOPSY.

Chrot'ic. [**Chrot'icus;** from χρώς, "skin."] Of or belonging to the skin.

Chrys'a-lis, idis.* [From χρυσός, "gold."] The second stage in the metamorphosis of insects. See AURELIA.

Chrysobalanaceæ,* kris-o-bal-a-na'she-ē. [From *Chrysobal'anus*, one of the genera.] A natural order of shrubs and trees, related to *Rosaceæ*. Several species produce esculent stone-fruits.

Chrys'o-bal'a-nus.* [From χρυσός, "gold," and βάλανος, a "corn."] Literally, the "golden acorn" or "nut." A name sometimes given to the nutmeg.

Chrys'o-bĕr'yl. [From χρυσός, "gold," and βήρυλλος, "beryl."] A beautiful gem of a pale yellow or green color, consisting of glucina and alumina.

Chrys'o-col'la.* [From χρυσός, "gold," and κόλλα, a "glue."] "Glue for Gold." The Greek name for borax. But it does not appear that borax was known to the ancients: their chrysocolla is said to have been a very different substance, composed of the rust of copper triturated with urine. The name *chrysocolla* is now applied to a mineral composed chiefly of silica and oxide of iron.

Chrys'o-lite. [From χρυσός, "gold," and λίθος, a "stone."] A mineral composed chiefly of silicate of magnesia and iron. It is often of a golden-yellow color, and is used in jewelry.

Chry-som'e-la.* [From χρυσός, "gold," and μέλας, "black."] A genus of coleopterous insects, named from the brilliant metallic hues, mostly of green and gold, with which their wing-covers are adorned.

Chrys'o-me'li-a.* [From χρυσός, "gold," and μῆλον, an "apple."] The Seville orange, or the *Aurantii Bacca*.

Chrys'o-mel'i-dæ.* A family of coleopterous insects, of which the *Chrysom'ela* is the type.

Chthonophagia,* tho'no-fa'je-a. [From χθών, "earth," and φάγω, to "eat."] A disease not uncommon among the negroes of the South, accompanied by a strong desire to eat dirt or earthy matter. Also called *Cachex'ia Africa'na*.

Chŭr'rus. An extract obtained from Indian hemp. See CANNABIS INDICA.

Chyle. [**Chy'lus;** from χυλός, "juice."] The milk-like liquor from which the blood is formed, occupying the lacteal vessels and thoracic duct.

Chy-lif'er-ous. [**Chylif'erus;** from *chy'lus*, "chyle," and *fe'ro*, to "bear," to "carry," to "convey."] Bearing or conveying chyle.

Chy-li-fi-cā'tion. [**Chylifica'tio, o'nis;** from *chy'lus*, "chyle," and *fa'cio*, to "make."] The process by which the chyle is separated from the chyme.

Chy-lo-poi-et'ic. [**Chylopoiet'icus;** from *chy'lus*, "chyle," and ποιέω, to "make."] Connected with the formation of chyle.

Chy-lo'sis.* [From χυλός, "juice."] The same as CHYLIFICATION.

Chy-lu'ri-a.* [From *chy'lus*, "chyle," and οὖρον, "urine."] A discharge of chyle with the urine.

Chyme. [Lat. **Chy'mus;** Gr. χυμός, "juice."] The pulpy mass formed by the food in its first great change in the process of digestion.

Chymia and **Chymie.** See CHEMISTRY.

Chym-i-fi-cā'tion. [**Chymifica'tio, o'nis;** from *chy'mus*, and *fa'cio*, to "make."] The conversion of the food into chyme.

Chymistry. See CHEMISTRY.

Cibatio,* se-ba'she-o. [From *ci'bus*, "food."] The act of taking food.

Cic-a-tric'u-la.* [Diminutive of *cica'trix*.] The blastoderm.

Ci-ca'trix, i'cis.* [From *cicatri'co*, to "heal, leaving a scar."] The scar or seam of a healed wound, sore, or ulcer.

Cic-a-tri-zā'tion. [**Cicatriza'tio, o'nis;** from the same.] The process by which a cicatrix is formed.

Cic-a-tri-za'tus.* [From the same.] Cicatrized; scarred. In Botany, having a scar, or the appearance of a scar.

Cic'a-trize. [From the same.] Literally, to "form a scar;" hence, to heal, or skin over.

Cichoraceæ,* sik-o-ra'she-ē. The Jussieuan name of a natural order of plants, or of a section of the order *Compositæ*. It includes lettuce, endive, etc.

Ci-cu'ta.* A Latin name for the CONIUM MACULATUM. The *Cicu'ta macula'ta*, however, of modern botanists, is a different plant.

Cicutin. See CONEIN.

Cil'i-a.* (The plural of **Cil'i-um,** which see.) The eyelashes, or hairs on the eyelids. Sometimes applied to minute, slender objects attached to certain animals, that have a vibratile motion.

Cil'i-a-ry. [**Cilia'ris;** from *cil'ium*, the "eyelash."] Belonging to the *cilium*, or eyelash. Also applied to several parts corresponding to the junction of the cornea to the sclerotic coat.

Cil'ĭ-ate. [**Cilia'tus;** from *cil'ium,* the "eyelash."] Having hairs, or a species of pubescence, on the margin of a leaf or petal; having *cilia.*

Cil'ĭ-um.* [From *cil'leo,* to "stir," to "twinkle."] A Latin term denoting the eyelid, or rather the edge of the eyelid out of which the hairs grow; also the eyelash. Used mostly in the plural. See CILIA.

Cil-lo'sis.* [From the same.] Spasmodic trembling or agitation of the eyelids.

Cim-ĭ-cif'u-ga.* [From *ci'mex, cim'icis,* a "bug," or "louse," and *fu'go,* to "put to flight."] The Pharmacopœial name (U.S. Ph.) of the root of the *Cimicif'uga racemo'sa,* otherwise called *Actæ'a cimicif'uga* and *Actæ'a racemo'sa,* a plant belonging to the natural order *Ranunculaceæ,* and common in the United States. It is a tonic and powerful antispasmodic, and has been employed with great success in cases of chorea and uterine convulsions.

Cĭ-mo'lĭ-a Ter'ra.* ("Cimolian Earth.") The same as CIMOLITE, which see.

Cim'o-līte [from *Cimo'lus,* an island where it was found, and λίθος, a "stone"], or **Cĭ-mo'lĭ-an Earth.** A celebrated variety of fuller's earth, consisting, it is said, of silex, alumina, oxide of iron, and water.

Cin-cho'na.* [Named from the Countess *del Chinchon* or *Cinchon,* signally cured by its use.] A Linnæan genus of the class *Pentandria,* natural order *Cinchonaceæ.* Some recent writers insist that the proper spelling of the word is *Chinchona.* Also, a general term for the various species of Peruvian bark; including the following kinds:—

CINCHO'NA FLA'VA.* ("Yellow Cinchona.") The bark *Cincho'na Calisa'ya,* called in commerce "Calisaya Bark," and containing not less than two per cent. of alkaloids yielding crystallizable salts.

CINCHO'NA PAL'LIDA.* ("Pale Cinchona.") The bark of *Cincho'na Condamin'ea* and of *C. Micran'tha.*

CINCHO'NA RU'BRA.* ("Red Cinchona.") The bark of an undetermined species of cinchona, called in commerce "Red Bark," and containing not less than two per cent. of alkaloids yielding crystallizable salts. (See U.S. Pharmacopœia for 1860.)

To which may be added the

CINCHO'NA PURPU'REA,* the produce of which is termed in commerce "Brown Bark" and "Huamilies Bark."

The virtues of Peruvian bark, the discovery of which forms an era in the science of medicine, are due to a number of different principles, among which the alkaloids *quinia* and *cinchonia* are the most important. Both of these are in a high degree tonic and febrifuge; but they are especially remarkable for their efficacy against diseases of a periodical character, as tertians, quartans, etc. Hence those alkaloids, as well as the bark in substance, have been termed *antiperiodics.*

Cinchonaceæ,* sin-ko-na'she-ē. [From *Cincho'na,* the most important of the genera.] A large natural order of exogenous plants, mostly trees or shrubs, found in hot climates, including, besides the Cinchona, the Coffee-tree, the Cephaëlis Ipecacuanha, and other important plants. Powerful febrifugal properties in the bark, or emetic in the roots, are the great features of this order, the most valuable products of which are cinchona and ipecacuanha. The beauty or fragrance of the flowers of some plants of this order (for example, the *Gardenias* and *Ixoras*) is unsurpassed in the vegetable kingdom.

Cin-cho-nā'ceous. [**Cinchona'ceus.**] Having an arrangement as in the *Cinchona.* See CINCHONACEÆ.

Cin-chon'ic. [**Cinchon'icus;** from *Cincho'na.*] Belonging to *Cinchona.* Applied to an acid obtained from all the species. See KINIC ACID.

Cin'cho-nin, or **Cin'cho-nīne.** [**Cinchoni'na;** from *Cincho'na.*] A peculiar vegetable principle, or alkali, discovered in the *Cinchona Condaminea.*

Cin'er-ēs,* the plural of **Ci'nis,** signifying "ashes." Usually applied to pot- or pearl-ashes.

Cin'eres Clav-el-la'ti.* [From *ci'nis,* plural *cin'eres,* and *cla'vus,* a "nail," a "wedge."] Pearl-ash, or the *Potassa impura.* The name is derived from the little wedges or billets into which the wood was cut to make potash.

Ci-ne're-us.* The same as CINERITIOUS, which see.

Cineritious, sin-e-rish'ŭs. [**Cineri'tius;** from *ci'nis, cin'eris,* the ashes of any burnt substance.] Belonging to or resembling ashes in color. Applied to the cortical substance of the brain, etc.

Çi-net'ĭ-cus.* [From κινέω, to "move."] Cinet'ic. Applied in the plural neuter (*Cinet'ica*) to an order of the *Neurotica* of Dr. Good, including diseases which affect the muscles.

Ci'nis,* gen. **Cin'er-is.** The Latin term for "ash" or "ashes." See CINERES.

Çin'na-bar. [Lat. **Cinnab'aris;** Gr. κιννάβαρι.] The red sulphuret or bisulphuret of mercury. Also applied to a resinous substance of a bright red color obtained from the juice of an Indian tree.

Cin'na-bar-ine. [**Cinnabari'nus.**] Belonging to cinnabar; containing cinnabar.

Cinnabre, sin'nâbr'. The French for CINNABAR, which see.

Cin-nam'ic Aç'id. An acid procured from the oil of cinnamon.

Cin-na-mo'mum,* or **Cin'na-mon.** [From the Arabic *Kinamon.*] The Pharmacopœial name ‖ for the bark of the *Cinnamo'mum Zeylan'icum;* otherwise called the *Lau'rus cinnamo'mum.* The U.S. Pharmacopœia embraces under the name of *Cinnamomum,* or Cinnamon, the bark of the *C. aromaticum* as well as the *C. Zeylanicum.* Cinnamon is a most grateful and efficient aromatic. It is warm and cordial to the stomach, carminative and astringent, and is well adapted to relieve nausea and flatulence.

Cinnamon. See CINNAMOMUM.

Cin'na-mon Su'et. A production of the cinnamon-tree, used in Ceylon for making candles. According to Dr. Christison, it contains eight per cent. of a fluid oil not unlike olive oil; the remainder is a waxy principle, which answers very nearly to *cerin.*

Cin'namon-Tree. The *Cinnamo'mum Zeylan'icum.*

Cin'namon-Tree, Wild. The *Laurus cassia.*

Çi-o-ni'tis, idis.* [From κιονίς, the "uvula."] Inflammation of the uvula.

Çi-o-nor-rha'phi-a.* [From κιονίς, the "uvula," and ῥάφη, a "seam."] The same as STAPHYLORRHAPHY, which see.

Çi-o-not'o-my. [**Cionoto'mia;** from κιονίς, the "uvula," and τέμνω, to "cut."] Cutting off of a part of the uvula when too long.

Cip'o-lin. [From *cipol'la,* the Italian word for "onion;" named in allusion to the zones, supposed to resemble the layers of an onion.] A green marble, with white zones, brought from Rome. It gives fire with steel, though with difficulty.

Ci-prin'i-dæ.* [From *cypri'nus,* a "carp-fish."] A family of *Malacopterygii Abdominales,* having the *Cyprinus* for its type.

Cir-ci-na'lis.* The same as CIRCINATE.

Cir'ci-nate. [**Circina'tus;** from *cir'cino, circina'tum,* to "compass about," to "make into a circle."] Literally, "made into a circle." Applied in Botany to leaves rolled inwards from the point to the base.

Cir'cle. [From *cir'culus,* a "ring."] A plane figure bounded by a curved line, to which all the right lines that can be drawn from a point in the middle of it, called the centre, are equal.

Cir-cu-lā'tion. [**Circula'tio;** from *cir'culus,* a "circle;" *cir'culo, circula'tum,* to "move round," to "move in a circle," to "circulate."] That vital action by which the blood is sent from the heart through the arteries, diminishing in calibre till they end in minute ramifications on the entire surface, where they are connected to correspondingly minute veins, which, increasing in size, return the blood to the heart.

Cir'cu-lus.* A circle, or ring. Applied to any part of the body which is round or circular,—e.g. *cir'culus oc'uli,* the "orb of the eye." It is sometimes used to denote a connection of parts through which there is a circulation; as the *Cir'culus Willis'ii* ("Circle of Willis"), an anastomotic circle formed by the anterior and posterior cerebral arteries connected by the arteries of Willis.

Cir'culus Ar-te-ri-o'sus Ir'i-dis.* ("Arterial Circle of the Iris.") An artery of the eye which encircles the iris.

Cir'cum. A Latin preposition signifying "round," or "about," and forming the prefix of a number of compound words.

Cir'cum-a-gen'tēs.* [The present participle of *cir'cuma'go,* to "drive" or "move round."] A term applied to the oblique muscles of the eye.

Cir-cum-cis'ion. [**Circumci'sio, o'nis;** from *circumci'do, circumci'sum,* to "cut about."] The operation of cutting off a circular piece of the prepuce.

Cir-cum-duc'tion. [**Circumduc'tio, o'nis;** from *cir'cum,* "about," and *du'co, duc'tum,* to "lead."] Circular movement of a limb.

Cir'cum-flex. [**Circumflex'us;** from *cir'cum,* "about," and *flec'to, flex'um,* to "bend."] Bent about; curved like a bow or part of a circle. Applied in Anatomy to various arteries, veins, etc.

It is also used to designate a particular accent represented in Latin and French by this sign [^], as *musâ, tempête,* the term denoting that the accent, instead of being straight like the other accents, is bent over or around the letter.

Cir-cum-ġȳ-rā'tion. [**Circumgyra'tio, o'**nis; from *cir'cum,* "about," and *gy'rus,* a "circle."] Movement in a circle.

Cir-cum-sçis'sĭle. [**Circumscis'silis;** from *cir'cum,* "about," "around," and *scin'do, scis'sum,* to "cleave," to "divide."] Applied to dehiscent fruits, the upper part of which opens like a lid.

Cir-cum-sçis'sus.* [From the same.] "Cleft, or cut around." Applied in Botany to parts having a circular cut or fissure.

Cire, sēr. The French term for "wax." See Cera.

Çir-rhon'o-sus.* [From κιῤῥός, "tawny," and νόσος, a "disease."] A golden-yellow appearance of the pleura, peritonæum, etc., in the fœtus.

Cirrhopoda. See Cirropoda.

Çĭr-rho'sis.* [From κιῤῥός, "reddish-yellow," or "tawny."] A name proposed for granulated or tuberculated liver, as designative of the appearance of the organ in that diseased state. Also applied to a disease of the kidney.

Cir'ri,* the plural of Cirrus, which see.

Cĭr-rif'er-ous, or **Cĭr-riġ'er-ous.** [**Cirrif'erus,** or **Cirriġ'erus;** from *cir'rus,* and *fe'ro, ge'ro,* to "bear."] Bearing or producing *cirri.*

Cĭr'rĭ-grāde. [**Cirrig'radus;** from *cir'rus,* and *gra'dior,* to "walk."] Progressing by means of *cirri.*

Cĭr-rĭ-pe'dĭ-ạ,* or **Cĭr'rĭ-peds.** [From *cir'ri,* and *pes, pe'dis,* a "foot."] The same as Cirropoda, which see.

Cĭr'rĭ-pēs, p'*edis,** or **Cĭr'rĭ-ped.** [From *cir'rus,* and *pes,* a "foot."] The same as Cirropodus.

Cĭr-rop'o-dạ,* or **Cĭr'rĭ-pods.** [See Cirrop'odus.] A class of the *Diploneura* (or *Mollusca?*) consisting of aquatic animals, having multivalve shells, and furnished with a number of long, curled, articulated, setigerous processes (called *cirri*) analogous to the feet of the Crustacea. These animals are popularly called barnacles, and acorn-shells.

Cĭr-rop'o-dus.* [From *cir'rus,* and ποῦς, a "foot."] Cirrop'odous. Fringe-footed. Applied to a class of animals having *cirri* instead of feet. See preceding article.

Cĭr'rous, or **Cĭr'rōse.** Sometimes improperly written *Cirrhous* and *Cirrhose.* [**Cirro'sus;** from *cir'rus.*] Having *cirri,* or full of *cirri.*

Cĭr'rus,* plural **Cĭr'ri.** [A Latin term signifying a "lock of curled hair," a "fringe."] In Botany, a clasper or tendril, one of the *fulcra* of plants; also termed *Clavicula.* Applied to a peculiar set of organs found in certain aquatic animals. (See Cirropoda.) The term *cirrus* is also applied to thin, fleecy clouds, floating in the atmosphere at a great elevation.

Çir'so-çēle.* [From κιρσός, a "varicose vein," and κήλη, a "tumor."] A varicose enlargement of the spermatic vein.

Çir'soid. [**Cirsoi'des;** from κιρσός, a "varicose vein," and εἶδος, a "form."] Resembling a varix.

Çir-som'phạ-los.* [From κιρσός, a "varicose vein," and ὀμφαλός, the "navel."] A varicose condition around the navel.

Çir-soph-thăl'mĭ-ạ.* [From κιρσός, a "varicose vein," and ὀφθαλμός, the "eye."] A varicose condition of the eye: cirsophthal'my.

Çir'sos* (κιρσός). The Greek term for a varix, or dilated vein.

Çir-sot'o-mȳ. [**Cirsoto'mia;** from κιρσός, a "varicose vein," and τέμνω, to "cut."] Extirpation of a varix.

Çis-sam'pe-los.* [From κισσός, "ivy," and ἄμπελος, the "vine."] The wild vine. A Linnæan genus of the class *Diœcia,* natural order *Menispermaceæ.*

Cissam'pelos Cạ-pen'sis.* A species found in Cape Colony. The root is used by the inhabitants as a cathartic and emetic.

Cissam'pelos Pareira* (pạ-rā'rạ). The *Pareira brava,* or American wild vine. See Pareira.

Cistaceæ,* sis-ta'she-ē. A natural order of shrubs or herbaceous plants, including the rock-rose. The *Cistus Creticus* produces a resinous balsamic substance called *Lada'num.*

Cis'ti,* the plural of **Cis'tus,** forming the Jussieuan name of a natural order of plants. See Cistaceæ.

Cis'tus.* A genus of the natural order *Cistaceæ.*

Cis'tus Cre'tĭ-cus.* The name of the plant which produces a sort of gum-resin called *Lada'num* or *Labda'num.* This substance has a warm and bitter taste and an agreeable odor. It is sometimes used as an ingredient in plasters.

Cit'rāte. [**Ci'tras, a'**_tis._] A combination of citric acid with a base.

Cit'ric Aç'id. [**Aç'idum Cit'ricum;** from _Ci'trus._] An acid obtained from lemon-juice.

Cit'rïne Oint'ment. [Named from its fine yellow or citrine color.] The common name of the _Unguentum hydrargyri nitrātis_ of the Pharmacopœias. Used as a stimulant and alterative application in _psoriasis_ and other cutaneous affections.

Cit'ron. [**Ci'tro, o'**_nis;_ **Cedrom'ela.**] The fruit of the _Citreum,_ or citron-tree, a variety of the _Citrus medica._

Ci-trul'lus Cŏl-ŏ-çÿn'this.* A name of the _Cucumis Colocynthis._

Ci'trus.* [From κιτρία, the "lemon" or "citron."] A Linnæan genus of the class _Polyadelphia,_ natural order _Aurantiaceæ._

Ci'trus Auran'tium* (au-ran'she-ŭm). The systematic name of the orange-tree.

Ci'trus Big-a-ra'dĭ-a.* Another name for the _Citrus aurantium,_ or orange-tree.

Ci'trus Li-met'ta Ber-găm'ĭ-um.* The tree from the rind of whose fruit oil of bergamot is obtained.

Ci'trus Li-mo'num,* Ci'trus Med'ĭ-ca.* Names of the plants which bear the _Limones_ (lemons, or limes) of the Pharmacopœias.

Citrus Vulgaris. See Citrus Aurantium.

Civ'et. [**Civet'ta.**] An unctuous substance collected in a bag under the tail of the civet-cat, and used as a perfume.

Clāir-voy'ance. [See Clairvoyant.] Literally, "clearsightedness," or "clear vision." Applied to a condition of the mind or the "mind's eye," usually induced by mesmeric influence, in which, it is alleged, the mesmerized person can see not only in the dark, but the most intricate internal arrangements of his own or of another's body, and even the remotest objects, though separated from the clairvoyant by interposing walls or mountains.

Clāir-voy'ant. [Fr. _clair,_ "clear," and _voyant,_ "seeing," from _voir,_ to "see."] Literally, "seeing clearly;" hence, having the power of clairvoyance. As a noun, it signifies one who is endowed with clairvoyance.

Clammy. See Viscosus.

Clap. [Old Fr. _Clapises,_ public shops of infamous character.] A term for _Gonorrhœ'a impu'ra._

Clăr-ĭ-fĭ-cā'tion. [**Clarifica'tio, o'**_nis;_ from _cla'rus,_ "clear," and _fa'cio,_ to "make."] The purifying or freeing a fluid from heterogeneous matter or impurities.

Clasper. See Cirrus, Clavicle.

Class. [**Clas'sis.**] A primary division of bodies having some general resemblance to each other, but further divisible into distinctive orders.

Clas-sĭ-fĭ-cā'tion. [From _clas'sis,_ and _fa'cio,_ to "make."] The systematic arrangement into classes of natural productions and phenomena, including the diseases of the animal body.

Clav'ate. [**Clava'tus;** from _cla'va,_ a "club."] Club-shaped; clubbed.

Clavatio,* kla-va'she-o. [From _cla'vus,_ a "nail."] The same as Gomphosis.

Clav'el-late. [**Clavella'tus** and **Clavello'sus;** from _cla'va,_ a "club."] Having, or formed like, clubs.

Clav'ĭ-cle. [**Clavic'ula,** or **Clavic'ulus;** the diminutive of _cla'vis,_ a "key."] The collar-bone. In Botany, a tendril, clasper, or _cirrus._

Clav-ĭ-cor'nate. [**Clavicor'nis;** from _cla'va,_ a "club," and _cor'nu,_ a "horn."] Applied to a family of coleopterous insects, in which the _antennæ_ are thick at the extremity, frequently forming a solid club.

Cla-vic'u-lar. [**Clavicula'ris;** from _clavic'ula,_ the "collar-bone."] Belonging to the clavicle, or collar-bone.

Cla-vic'u-late. [**Clavicula'tus;** from _clavic'ula._] Having clavicles, as man and the _Simiæ._

Clav'ĭ-form. [**Clavifor'mis;** from _cla'va,_ a "club."] Club-shaped.

Clavo, klå'vo. The Spanish term for Clove, which see.

Cla'vus.* Literally, a "nail" or "spike." Applied to a corn, or horny round cutaneous formation, the effect of continued pressure generally on the prominent parts of the toes. Also, a very acute pain confined to a small part of the head, as if a nail were being driven into it,—called _Cla'vus hyster'icus._ Also, condyloma of the uterus. Likewise, a tubercle on the white of the eye.

Claw. [**Un'guis.**] The nail or talon of birds and other animals. The lower, narrow part of a petal.

Clay. _Argil'la,_ or argillaceous earth.

Clay, Pure. The earth called _Alumina._

Cleans'ings. The same as Lochia, which see.

Clēav'age. The property of splitting

or of being split in certain determinate directions, as minerals: foliated fracture.

Clĕi'do- [from κλείς, κλειδός, a "key," the "clavicle"], in compound names of muscles, etc., denotes attachment to or connection with the clavicle.

Cleis'a-gra.* [From κλείς, "clavicle," and ἄγρα, a "seizure" or "attack."] The gout in the articulation of the clavicles.

Clep-sy̆'dra.* [From κλέπτω, to "steal," and ὕδωρ, "water,"—named in allusion to the water stealing away so gradually as to be almost unperceived.] An instrument for measuring time, by allowing water to drop through a small hole from one vessel to another.

Clĭ-mac'ter,* plural **Cli-mac-te'-rēs.** [Gr. κλιμακτήρ; from κλιμάζω, to "proceed by degrees."] Literally, the "step of a stair" or a "ladder;" hence, applied to the stages of human life, reckoned by periods of seven years.

Clĭ-mac'ter-ic, or klim-ak-tĕr'ik. [**Climacter'icus;** from the same.] Applied to a particular epoch of the ordinary term of life, marked by periods of seven years, at which the body was by the ancients supposed to be peculiarly affected and to suffer considerable change. The ninth period, or sixty-third year, at which the most decided change takes place, was regarded as the "grand climacteric."

Climac'teric Dis-ease'. That sudden change which occurs in many instances of advanced life, generally at the grand climacteric, that is, about the end of the sixty-third year, sixty-three being nine times seven. See CLIMACTERIC.

Climac'teric Teeth'ing. The production of teeth at a very late period of life, after the loss of the permanent teeth by accident or natural decay,—commonly between the sixty-third and eighty-first year, or the interval which fills up the two grand climacteric years of the Greek physiologists.

Climat, klē'mâ'. The French for CLIMATE, which see.

Clī'mate. [Lat. **Cli'ma, Clim'a-tis;** Gr. κλίμα, a "region," "clime," or "climate."] In a hygienic point of view, the term denotes peculiarities in temperature, quality of air, etc., with respect to which different countries or regions differ from each other in their effects upon the health of those who inhabit them. Among the various influences which tend to promote health or produce disease, there is perhaps none more deserving the attention of the medical student than the peculiarities and varieties of climate. But the limits of the present volume will permit only a few general remarks; for a thorough consideration of the subject in all its details, the reader is referred to more extensive and elaborate works.

In recommending a change of residence on account of ill health, the judicious physician will take into consideration not only the character of the disease, but the peculiarities of the patient's constitution. In general terms, it may be stated that diseases of the lungs or pleura require a mild or warm climate; and fevers, especially when complicated with visceral derangement, a cool or cold one: yet it will often be found that persons laboring under lung-complaints are more injured than benefited by a warm climate; for, though a mild air and unchecked perspiration are very decided advantages in themselves, the debility resulting from a less bracing atmosphere will frequently prove more than a counterbalance to those advantages. Mountain air, which is generally pure, light, and exhilarating, will be found beneficial in certain cases, while sea air, which is less rarefied and less dry, will be better adapted to others. The air of a small island completely surrounded by a wide expanse of sea, like Madeira or the Bermudas, possesses the great advantage of having a more equable and uniform temperature than can ever be found on a continent or on any extensive tract of land. It is scarcely necessary to remark that the purity or impurity of the air must, in an especial manner, never be overlooked. Yet it is said that the impure air of certain districts where tertians are common, has been found eminently beneficial in some forms of pulmonary disease.

Clī-ma-tog'ra-phy̆. [**Climatogra'-phia;** from *cli'ma*, "climate," and γράφω, to "write," to "describe."] A description of climates.

Clī-ma-tol'o-gy̆. [**Climatolo'gia;** from *cli'ma*, and λόγος, a "discourse."] A treatise on climate; the science of climates.

Clī-nan'drĭ-um.* [From κλίνη, a "bed," and ἀνήρ, a "male."] The part of the column of fructification of the *Orchideæ* in which the anther is fixed.

Clin'ĭ-cal. [Lat. **Clin'icus;** from κλίνη. Fr. *Clinique*, klē'nēk'.] Pertaining to a bed; as clinical lectures, which are those delivered by medical attendants at the bedside.

Clinique, klē'nēk'. The French term for CLINICAL, which see. As a noun, it is used for a clinical school, thus: *La Clinique de la Charité* (lå klē'nēk' dęh lå shå'rē'tå') signifies "The Clinical School of [the Hospital] La Charité."

Clī'noid. [Clinoi'des; from κλίνη, and εἶδος, a "form."] Resembling a bed. Applied to four processes of the sphenoid bone.

Clī-nom'e-ter. [Clinom'etrum; from κλίνω, to "incline," and μέτρον, a "measure."] An apparatus for measuring the inclination of a line in relation to a horizontal plane. Used for ascertaining the *dip* of geological strata.

Clis-e-om'e-ter. [Cliseom'etrum; from κλίσις, "inclination," and μέτρον, a "measure."] An instrument for measuring the angle which the axis of the female pelvis makes with that of the body.

Clit-Bur. The *Arctium lappa;* also called Clot-bur.

Clit'o-ris,* gen. **Clī-tŏr'ĭ-dis.** [Gr. κλειτορίς; from κλείω, to "shut up," to "enclose;" because concealed by the *labia pudendi.*] A small, elongated, glandiform body at the anterior part of the vulva, resembling in its internal structure the *corpus cavernosum* of the penis.

Clit-o-ris'mus.* Morbid swelling of the *clitoris.*

Clit-o-ri'tis, idis.* [From *clit'oris.*] Inflammation of the *clitoris.*

Clo-a'ca.* [From *clu'o,* an antique form for *col'luo,* to "wash," to "scour," or "make clean."] Literally, a "sink" or "sewer." Applied in Zoology to a cavity in birds and certain other animals, in which the oviducts terminate. In the plural (*Cloa'cæ*), the openings through the new bony shell (in cases of necrosis of a long cylindrical bone) into the *sequestrum,* or enclosed dead bone, by which the matter formed in the interior is discharged.

Cloaque, klo'åk'. The French for CLOACA, which see.

Clon'ic. [Clon'icus; from κλόνος, "commotion."] Belonging to an agitated or irregular movement. Applied to spasms in which contractions and relaxations are alternate, as in epilepsy.

Clot. [From the Belgian *Klot,* a "mass of thickened fluid."] The *Crassamentum* of the blood.

Clot-Bur. See CLIT-BUR.

Clou. See CLOVE.

Clōve. [From the Latin *Cla'vus,* a "nail" or "spike;" Fr. *Clou,* kloo, Sp. *Clavo,* klå'vo, both signifying originally a nail or spike; so called from its resemblance to a nail.] The calyx, or unexpanded flower, of the *Caryophyl'lus aromat'icus,* otherwise called *Euge'nia caryophylla'ta.* The clove is a warm, pungent, and highly-stimulating aromatic. It is sometimes employed to relieve nausea or vomiting; but it is chiefly used to assist or modify the action of other medicines.

Clove-Ġil'lī-flow-er, Clove-Pink. The *Dian'thus caryophyl'lus.*

Clove-Tree. The *Caryophyl'lus aromat'icus* (or *Euge'nia caryophylla'ta*).

Clo'ven Spine. The same as SCHISTORRHACHIS, which see.

Club-Foot. See TALIPES.

Clu-pe'ĭ-dæ.* [From *Clu'pea,* a small fish of the herring kind.] A family of fishes having the *Clupea* for their type.

Clusiaceæ,* klu-ze-a'she-ē, or **Gut-tif'er-æ.*** A natural order of trees and shrubs, found in the tropics, including the *Clu'sia,* the Mangosteen, and other excellent fruits. Many species of this order secrete an acrid, purgative gum-resin, as gamboge.

Cluster. See RACEMUS, and THYRSUS.

Clўp'e-al. [Clypea'lis; from *cly'-peus,* a "shield."] Belonging to a shield.

Clўp'e-ate. [Clypea'tus; from the same.] Bearing a shield, or formed like a shield.

Clўs'sus.* [From κλύζω, to "dash," to "wash."] A term formerly used to denote the vapor produced by the detonation of nitre with any inflammable substance.

Clўs'ter.* [Gr. κλυστήρ; from κλύζω, to "wash away."] An injection into the *rectum;* an *en'ema;* a glyster.

C. M. = *Cras ma'ne.** "To-morrow morning."

C. N. = *Cras noc'te.** "To-morrow night."

Cni'cus Ben-e-dic'tus,* or **Cen-tau're-a Ben-e-dic'ta.*** ("Blessed Thistle.") A composite plant, regarded as "blessed" on account of its medicinal virtues. It contains a brown, bitter principle, called *cnicin.*

Co. See CON.

Co-ad'u-nate. [Coaduna'tus; from

coadu'no, to "join together."] Clustered.

Co-ag'u-la-ble. [**Coagulabi'lis;** from *coag'ulo, coagula'tum*, to "curdle."] Having the property of coagulation.

Coag'ulable Lymph. A term applied to the fibrin of the blood.

Co-ag-u-lā'tion. [**Coagula'tio, o'***nis;* from the same.] The thickened state of the albuminous portion of certain animal and vegetable fluids on applying acids or heat.

Co-ag'u-lum.* [From the same.] The jelly-like consistence assumed by albuminous substances, blood, etc., when acted on by heat.

Coal (Min'e-ral). A combustible mineral, consisting of two principal varieties,—*anthracite* and *bituminous coal.* The former burns with little or no smoke or flame; in the latter, as its name implies, bitumen is an important ingredient, producing vapor and gas when exposed to heat.

Co-a-lĕs'çent. [**Coales'cens;** from *coales'co*, to "grow together."] Growing together.

Co-ap-tā'tion. [**Coapta'tio, o'***nis;* from *co* for *con*, "together," and *ap'to, apta'tum*, to "fit."] The fitting together of the ends of a fractured bone.

Co-arc'tate. [**Coarcta'tus;** from *coarc'to, coarcta'tum*, to "straighten."] Pressed close together.

Co-arc-tā'tion. [**Coarcta'tio, o'***nis;* from the same.] A straightening, or pressing together. Applied to strictures of the intestine or urethra.

Coat. See Tunica.

Coat'ed. (Fr. *Enduit*, ŏNᵍ'dwẻ'.) Applied to the condition of the tongue, as indicative of visceral disturbance.

Cobalt, ko'bault. [Lat. **Cobal'tum;** from the German *Ko'bold*, a "goblin" or "demon;" so called because its discovery was regarded by miners as an ill omen, —*i.e.* as unfavorable to the presence of more valuable metals.] A metal generally found in combination with arsenic. The salts of cobalt are irritant poisons. The oxide is employed to impart a blue color to porcelain and glass.

Co-bâl'tic. [**Cobal'ticus.**] Belonging to cobalt.

Co-ba'lus.* The same as *Kobold*, the demon of miners, from which cobalt is said to have been named.

Cobra de Capello, ko'brå då kå-pĕl'lo. ("Snake with a Hood.") The Portuguese name for the hooded snake, the *Na'ja vulga'ris* (otherwise called the *Na'ja tripu'dians*), a very poisonous serpent common in India.

Cob'web. [**Ara'neum.**] The web of the *Aranea*, or spider.

Co'ca,* called also **Ypada,** e-på'då. The leaf of the *Erythrox'ylon co'ca*, a plant in extensive use among the Indians of the Andes, as a stimulant. See Erythroxylon Coca.

Coc'çi,* the plural of **Coc'cus.** The Pharmacopœial name (Ed. Ph.) for cochineal insects.

Cocciferous, kok-sif'er-ŭs. [**Coccif'erus;** from *coc'cus*, a "berry," and *fe'ro*, to "bear."] Bearing berries, or objects like them.

Coccinella,* kok-se-nel'la. [Diminutive of *coc'cus*, a "berry."] The cochineal insect: cochineal. (See Coccus Cacti.) A genus of coleopterous insects; the lady-bird, or lady-bug.

Coccinel'la Sep-tem-punc-ta'ta* (*i.e.* "having seven points or spots"), or Lady-bug. This insect, if bruised upon an aching tooth, is said to cure it.

Coc-cĭ-nel'lin. [**Coccinelli'na.**] The coloring principle of cochineal; carmine.

Coc'cu-lus.* [Diminutive of *coc'cus*, a "berry."] A genus of the class *Diœcia*, natural order *Menispermaceæ.* The Pharmacopœial name (Br. Ph.) for the fruit of the *Anamirta cocculus*, or *Cocculus Indicus.*

Coc'culus, An-a-mir'ta.* The plant which produces the *Cocculus Indicus*, sometimes termed *Levantnut*, or *Bac'ca Orienta'lis* ("Oriental Berry").

Coc'culus In'di Ar-o-mat'ĭ-cus,* or (plural) **Coc'cu-li In'di Ar-o-mat'ĭ-çi.** Other names for the *Myrtus pimenta*, or Jamaica pepper.

Coc'culus In'dĭ-cus.* The berries of the *Anamir'ta coc'culus* (the *Menispermum cocculus* of Linnæus). The kernels of these berries are whitish and oily, and have an intensely bitter taste. They contain a peculiar bitter principle called *picrotoxin*, which is very poisonous. The *Cocculus Indicus* belongs to the acronarcotic class of poisons. As a medicine it is never administered internally. In India it is employed to stupefy fish in order that they may be more easily caught. It is said that the fish thus taken are not poisonous. An ointment made of the powdered berries is sometimes used in certain cutaneous diseases.

Coc'culus Pal-ma'tus.* The plant which affords Calumba, Colomba, or Columbo root; called, also, *Menispermum palmatum.*

Coc'cum.* (See Coccus.) A kind of seed-vessel distinguished from a capsule, the sides of which, being elastic, project the seeds with great force, as in the *Euphorbiæ.*

Coc'cum Baph'ĭ-cum.* The kermes berry.

Coc'cus.* [From κόκκος, a "grain" or "kernel;" also, an "insect."] The Pharmacopœial name (Brit. and U.S. Ph.) for the *Coccus cacti.* In Botany, a cell or capsule. Also the name of a genus of hemipterous insects.

Coc'cus Cac'ti.* ("Coccus of the Cactus.") The *Coccinella,* or cochineal insect.

Coc'cus In-fec-to'rĭ-us.* The insect which produces the kermes grains or berries.

Coc'cus Lac'ca.* The insect which produces *Lac.*

Coc-çȳġ'e-us,* or kok-se-je'ŭs. [From *coc'cyx.*] Belonging to the coccyx: coc-çȳġ'eal.

Coc-çȳ-o-dȳn'ĭ-a.* [From *coc'cyx,* and ὀδύνη, "pain."] Pain in the coccyx, occurring especially in women.

Coc'çȳx,* gen. **Coc-çy'ġis.** [From κόκκυξ, the "cuckoo;" because like its bill.] The small triangular bone appended to the point of the *sacrum.*

Coch'ĭ-nēal. [**Coccinel'la;** from *coccinel'la,* probably derived through the Italian *cocciniglia,* pronounced kot-che-nēl'yå.] The *Coccus cacti, Coccinella,* or cochineal insect, brought from South America as a reddish grain. Cochineal is thought by some to possess anodyne and antispasmodic properties, and has been recommended for the hooping-cough and other nervous affections. In Pharmacy it is used to color tinctures, ointments, etc.

Cochinilin, kotch'e-nil'in. (See Cochineal.) A coloring matter obtained from cochineal. It is a constituent of *carmine.*

Cochl. Ampl., Cochl. Mag. Abbreviations for *Cochlea're am'plum** or *mag'num,** a "tablespoon."

Cochl. Med. = *Cochlea're me'dium.** A "dessert-spoon."

Cochl. Min. = *Cochlea're min'imum.** A "teaspoon."

Coch'le-a.* Literally, a "shell," a "snail-shell;" hence, any thing of a spiral form. A conical cavity of the internal ear.

Coch-le-a're.* [From *coch'lea,* a "shell," more especially a "snail-shell."] The Latin word for "spoon;" so named from its resemblance to a shell. It is commonly used in medical prescriptions for "spoonful."

Coch-le-a'rĭ-a.* [From *cochlea're,* a "spoon."] A Linnæan genus of the class *Tetradynamia,* natural order *Cruciferæ.*

Cochlea'ria Armora'cia* (ar-mo-ra'she-a). The horse-radish plant; called, also, the *Raph'anus rustica'nus.* The root of this plant (*Armoraciæ Radix*) is pungent and powerfully stimulant. Its virtues depend on an essential oil which is dissipated by drying.

Coch-le-ăr'ĭ-form. [**Cochleariformis;** from *cochlea're,* a "spoon."] Formed like a spoon.

Coch'le-ate. [**Cochlea'tus;** from *coch'lea,* a "snail-shell."] In Botany, spiral, or having a spiral form.

Co-co'a. The fruit of *Theobroma cacao.*

Co-coon'. [Etymology uncertain.] The silken case of certain *Arachnides,* etc., in which they deposit their eggs, change their teguments, or retire for the winter.

Coc'tion. [**Coc'tio;** from *co'quo, coc'tum,* to "cook," to "digest."] The process of reducing the aliment to chyle.

Codaga-Pala Bark. See Nerium Antidysentericum.

Co'de-āte. [**Co'deas, a'tis;** from *code'icum* aç'idum.] A combination of codeic acid with a base.

Co-de'ic. [**Code'icus.**] Applied to an acid obtained from codein.

Co'de-in, Co'de-ĭne, or **Co-de'ĭa.*** [From κωδία, or κωδεία, a "poppy-head."] An alkaloid discovered by Robiquet in opium. As a soporific it is considered to possess about half the strength of morphia.

Cod'-Liv'er Oil, or **Cod'fish Oil.** [**Mor'rhuæ O'leum.**] Obtained from the liver of the *Ga'dus mor'rhua,* or codfish. See Oleum Morrhuæ.

Coecum. See Cæcum.

Cœlia,* sē'le-a. [Gr. κοιλία, the "belly;" from κοῖλος, "hollow."] The belly, especially the lower portion; also, the stomach.

Çœ'lĭ-ac. [**Cœli'acus;** from *cœ'lia,* the "belly."] Belonging to the belly.

Cœ'liac Pas'sion. [**Pas'sio Cœli'aca.**] A chronic flux, in which the aliment is discharged half digested; the *Diarrhœ'a cœli'aca* of Cullen.

Çœ'liac Plex'us. A name for the Solar Plexus, which see.

Çœ-li'a-ca.* [Neuter plural of *cœli'-acus.* See Cœliac.] The first class of Dr. Good's Nosology, embracing diseases of the digestive organs. Sometimes applied to medicines which act on those organs.

Cœliacus. See Cœliac.

Çœ-li-ăl'gi-a.* [From *cœ'lia,* the "belly," and ἄλγος, "pain."] Pain in the belly.

Cœnæsthesis,* sĕn-ĕs-the'sis. [From κοινός, "common," and αἴσθησις, "perception," "feeling," or "sensibility."] A term expressive of the general feeling or consciousness in the entire body; consciousness of existence. Some writers have termed it a sixth sense, not limited, like the other senses, to one particular part, but common to the whole system.

Çœ-nu'rus.* [From κοινός, "common," and οὐρά, a "tail" or "hinder part."] A *cœ'nure,* or hydatid, containing several animals (*Entozoa*) grouped together and adhering to its sides, which thus form a common base or termination of many heads and bodies.

Cœruleus Lapis. See Blue-Stone.

Cœruleus Morbus. See Cyanosis.

Cœur, kur. The French word for "heart." See Cor, and Heart.

Cof'fe-a.* (See Caffea.) A Linnæan genus of the class *Pentandria,* natural order *Cinchonaceæ* (according to Lindley, though formerly ranked with the *Rubiaceæ*).

Cof'fea A-rab'ĭ-ca.* The plant which affords coffee. See Caffea Arabica.

Cof'fee. [Lat. **Caf'fea,** or **Cof'fea;** Fr. *Café,* kȧ'fȧ'.] The seed of the *Caf'fea Arab'ica,* a tree from fifteen to thirty feet in height, growing native in Southern Arabia and Abyssinia, and cultivated extensively in Java, Ceylon, and other parts of the East Indies; also in South America and the West India islands. The infusion of the roasted seeds is exhilarating and tonic, and has been used, it is said, with the most beneficial results in cases of poisoning with opium, and chronic asthma. Coffee (*Caffea*) has been assigned a place on the Primary List of the Materia Medica in the last edition of the U.S. Pharmacopœia (1860). See Caffein.

Co-hab-ĭ-tā'tion. [**Cohabita'tio, o'nis;** from *co* for *con,* "together," and *hab'ito, habita'tum,* to "dwell."] In Medical Jurisprudence, the dwelling together of two persons of opposite sex, including the habit of venereal congress, without the sanction of marriage.

Co-he'sion. [**Cohe'sio, o'nis;** from *co* for *con,* "together," and *hæ'reo, hæ'sum,* to "stick."] The power by which the particles of bodies adhere to each other.

Co-ho-bā'tion. [**Cohoba'tio, o'nis;** from *co'hob,* used by Paracelsus to signify *repetition.*] The pouring of a fluid again and again on the matter from which it was distilled, and as often distilling it, to render it more efficacious.

Coitio,* ko-ish'e-o, or **Co-ĭ'tion.** The same as Coitus, which see.

Co'ĭ-tus.* [From *co* for *con,* "together," and *e'o, i'tum,* to "go" or "come."] The coming together of male and female in the act of procreation. In Chemistry, the union of substances by incorporation or mixture.

Coke. The charcoal obtained by heating bituminous coal with the imperfect access of air, or by its distillation. The former is usually called *oven coke,* the latter *gas coke,* being abundantly produced in gas-works. The weight of coke usually amounts to between sixty and seventy per cent. of the coal employed. Coke is a valuable fuel for many purposes in the arts.

Col. A French word signifying "the neck." See Collum.

Col'a-to'ri-um.* [From *co'lo, cola'tum,* to "strain."] A strainer of any kind; a sieve.

Col-a-tu'ra.* [From the same.] Any filtered or strained liquor.

Col'chĭ-çi Cor'mus.* The Pharmacopœial name (Brit. Ph.) for the bulbs of *Colchicum autumnale.*

Col'chici Ra'dix.* ("Root of Colchicum.") The cormus of *Col'chicum autumna'le* (U.S. Ph.).

Col'chici Se'men.* ("Seed of Colchicum.") The seed of *Col'chicum autumna'le* (U.S. and Brit. Ph.).

Col'chici Sem'ĭ-na.* ("Seeds of Colchicum.") The Pharmacopœial name (Ed. Ph.) for the seeds of the *Col'chicum autumna'le.*

Colchicia,* kol-chish'e-a. The same as Colchicin.

Col'chĭ-cin, or **Col'chĭ-cine.** [**Colchici'na.**] An alkaloid substance obtained from *Col'chicum autumna'le,* of which it is believed to be the active principle.

Colchicum,* kŏl'che-kŭm. [From *Col'chis,* a country of Asia.] A Linnæan genus of the class *Hexandria*, natural order *Melanthaceæ*. The name is often used as synonymous with *Col'chicum autumna'le*, including the various preparations of the root and seeds.

Col'chĭ-cum Au-tum-na'le.* The meadow saffron. The root and the seeds appear to possess similar medicinal properties. The former is narcotic, diuretic, and cathartic. From its sedative effects, it has often proved very useful in gout and rheumatism. In an over-dose, however, it sometimes produces excessive nausea, vomiting and purging, sinking of the pulse, attended with extreme prostration, and may prove fatal.

Col'co-thar. A mixture of red oxide of iron and the persulphate, used as a paint, etc.

Cold. [Fri'gus, *go'ris*, **Catar'rhus.]** Properly, the privation of heat. In popular language, it denotes a catarrh, cough, or other effects from exposure to cold.

Co-le-op'ter-a.* An order of insects. See next article.

Co-le-op'ter-us.* [From κολεός, a "sheath," and πτέρον, a "wing."] Applied in the neuter plural (*Coleop'tera*) to an order of insects in which the inferior wings are covered by others like sheaths or cases: coleop'terous.

Co-le-o-rhi'za.* [From κολεός, a "sheath," and ῥίζα, a "root."] Applied in Botany to a kind of case which envelops certain radicles.

Co'lĕs.* [Essentially the same word as *Cau'lis*: both are derived from καυλός, a "stalk," or "stem."] Originally, a stalk; but used by Celsus as a designation of the penis.

Col'ic. (Fr. *Colique*, ko'lēk'.) (See Col'ica.) Acute pain in the abdomen, aggravated at intervals. So named from its having been supposed to have its seat in the colon.

Col'ĭ-ca.* [From *col'icus*, "pertaining to the colon," *pas'sio*, "suffering," or "pain," being usually understood. See Colica Passio.] Literally, pain in the colon, or large intestine. The colic, or belly-ache. A genus of the order *Spasmi*, class *Adynamiæ*, of Cullen's Nosology.

Col'ica Accidenta'lis.* Colic induced by particular articles of diet. This may also be flatulent colic. See Colica Flatulenta.

Col'ica Bilio'sa.* Bilious colic, occasioned by an excess of bile in the intestines.

Col'ica Calculo'sa.* [From *cal'culus*.] Colic caused by intestinal calculi.

Col'ica Flatulen'ta.* [From *fla'tus*, "wind."] Flatulent colic, caused by wind in the intestines.

Col'ica Meconia'lis.* Colic resulting from retention of the meconium in infants.

Col'ica Pas'sio* (pash'e-o). Another name for colic. See Colica.

Col'ica Pic'tonum.* The "colic of the Pictones," a name for the people of Poitou, where it is said to have been an endemic. Otherwise called dry belly-ache; Devonshire colic; painter's colic (*Col'ica picto'rum*); also *Col'ica saturni'na*, as being produced by the poison of lead.

Col'ica Picto'rum.* [From *pic'tor*, a "painter."] "Painter's Colic." See Colica Pictonum.

Col'ica Sterco'rea.* [From *ster'cus*, *ster'coris*, "fæces."] Colic arising from an excessive accumulation of the contents of the bowels.

Col'ĭ-cus.* Belonging to the *colon*.

Col-ĭ-for'mis.* [From *co'lum*, a "colander," or "strainer," a "sieve."] Col'iform. Resembling a sieve, or sieve-like. Applied to the ethmoid bone (*os colifor'me*).

Colique. See Colic.

Co-li'tis.* [From *co'lon*.] Inflammation of the mucous coat of the *colon*.

Col'la Pis'cium* (pish'e-ŭm). "Glue of Fishes." See Ichthyocolla.

Col'la-gen. [From κολλά, "glue," and γεννάω, to "produce."] The chief constituent of bone, cartilage, ligaments, tendons, etc. By boiling it forms glue or gelatin.

Col-lapse'. [Collap'sus; from *col'labor*, *collap'sus*, to "fall down."] A state of extreme depression or complete prostration of the vital powers, as occurs in Asiatic cholera, etc.

Col'lar. [Colla're; from *col'lum*, the "neck."] The *prothorax*, or anterior segment of the trunk, in insects.

Col'lar-Bone. The clavicle.

Col-le'sis.* [From κολλάω, to "glue."] An old term for Agglutination.

Collet, kol'lā'. A French term signifying "a collar." See Neck.

Col-lic'u-lus.* [Diminutive of *col'lis*, a "hill," or "elevation."] A little hill, or eminence. Applied in Anatomy to various small elevations or protuberances.

Collic'ulus Ner'vi Æth-moi-da'lis.* ("Protuberance of the Ethmoid

Nerve.") The same as the CORPUS STRIATUM, which see.

Collic'ulus Ner'vi Op'ti-ci.* ("Protuberance of the Optic Nerve.") The optic *thalamus*.

Collic'ulus Sem-i-na'lis.* ("Seminal Protuberance.") A small elevation in the prostate gland.

Col-liq-ua-men'tum.* [From *colliq'ueo*, to "melt;" so called, probably, in allusion to its exceeding softness, or want of firm consistency.] A term applied by Harvey to the first rudiments of the embryo in generation.

Col-liq'ua-tive. [Colliquati'vus; from *colliq'ueo*, to "melt."] Applied to any excessive discharge or evacuation.

Col-lo'di-um,* or **Col-lo'di-on.*** [From κόλλα, "glue."] A peculiar substance prepared by dissolving gun-cotton in sulphuric ether. For particular directions in its preparation, see U.S. Pharmacopœia, 1860, page 125. It is much used as an application to abraded surfaces and superficial wounds. When applied to a part, the ether evaporates, and a solid adhesive material is left, which acts like adhesive plaster, keeping the parts together and excluding the air.

Collo'dium cum Can-thăr'i-de.* ("Collodion with Cantharides," U.S. Ph., 1860.) A preparation of collodion and cantharides, used as a blistering application. It produces a blister in about the same time as the ordinary cerate, and has the great advantage of being easily applied to uneven surfaces.

Col'loid. [Colloi'des; from κόλλα, "glue," and εἶδος, a "form."] Resembling glue.

Col-lo-ne'ma, atis.* [From κόλλα, "glue."] A very soft tumor, containing a clear, grayish-yellow substance like gelatine, or fresh glue.

Col'lum.* [Diminutive of *colum'na*, a "pillar"?] (Fr. *Col*, kol, and *Cou*, koo.) The neck. Applied to any part which, from its situation, form, or connection, resembles a neck.

Col-lu-to'ri-um.* [From *col'luo*, *collu'tum*, to "wash."] A gargle; a liquid applied to the mouth or throat for local purposes.

Col-lyr'i-um.* [Gr. κολλύριον, a "little cake;" diminutive of κολλύρα, a "small loaf" or "roll of bread."] Originally, an eye-salve made up in small cakes; or, any salve. Now usually applied to a wash or lotion for the eyes.

Co-lo-bo'ma, atis.* [From κολοβόω, to "mutilate."] A mutilation, or defect.

Colobo'ma Ir'i-dis.* ("Mutilation of the Iris.") A name applied to fissures of the lower portion of the iris with a prolongation of the pupil to the edge of the cornea.

Colocynth. See COLOCYNTHIS.

Col-o-cyn'this, idis.* [From κολόκυνθα, a "gourd."] Col'ocynth. The Pharmacopœial name ‖ of the dried pulp of the bitter cucumber; also called *Coloquin'tida*. The pulp of colocynth is a powerful hydragogue cathartic, and, as such, is sometimes given in dropsy. In large doses, however, it is a dangerous poison. It is most frequently administered in combination with other medicines.

Co-lom'ba.* The former Pharmacopœial name (U.S. Ph.) of the root of the *Coc'culus palma'tus*. See CALUMBA, and COLUMBO.

Co'lon.* [Gr. κῶλον.] That portion of the large intestine extending from the *cæcum* to the *rectum*.

Co-loph'o-ny. [Colopho'nia; from *Col'ophon*, a city of Ionia, whence it was originally obtained.] A dark-colored resin, prepared from the distillation of rough turpentine without water.

Coloquinte, ko'lo'kăNT'. The French term for colocynth. See COLOCYNTHIS.

Coloquintida. See COLOCYNTHIS.

Col'ored. [Colora'tus; from *colo'ro*, *colora'tum*, to "color."] Applied in Botany to objects of any other color than green.

Col-o-rif'ic. [Colorif'icus; from *co'lor*, and *fa'cio*, to "make."] Making or producing colors. Applied to the luminous rays.

Col'or-ing Mat'ter. A coloring principle existing in vegetable substances. Colors are termed *substantive* when they adhere to the cloth without a basis; *adjective*, when they require a basis or mordant.

Col-os-trā'tion. [Colostra'tio, o'nis.] A term for the diseases of new born infants, caused by the *colostrum*.

Co-los'tric. [Colos'tricus.] Belonging to the *colostrum*.

Colos'tric Flu'id. The imperfect secretion of milk ere the mother has recovered from delivery, on account of the presence of *colostrum;* popularly, "green milk."

Co-los'trous. [Colostro'sus; from *colos'trum*.] Having *colostrum*, or full of *colostrum*.

Co-los'trum.* [Perhaps from κολόν, "food."] A substance in the first milk after delivery, giving to it a greenish or yellowish color.

Co-lot'o-my̆. [**Coloto'mia;** from *co'lon*, and τέμνω, to "cut."] Cutting into the colon.

Col'po-çēle.* [From κόλπος, the "womb," or "vagina," and κήλη, a "tumor."] *Her'nia vagina'lis*, or hernia in the vagina.

Col-pop-to'sis.* [From κόλπος, the "womb," or "vagina," and πτῶσις, a "falling."] Falling down, or *prolapsus*, of the vagina.

Colt's Foot. See TUSSILAGO FARFARA.

Col'u-ber Be'rus.* The systematic name for the viper, a poisonous snake common in Europe.

Co-lum'bic Aç'id. An acid obtained by fusing the ore of *Columbium* with the carbonate or the bisulphate of potassa; a soluble columbate of potass is obtained, and the acid is precipitated in the form of a white hydrate.

Co-lum'bĭ-um.* [From *Colum'bia*, one of the names of America.] A metal first found (in 1801) in a mineral discovered in Massachusetts. It has since been found in a Swedish mineral called Tantalite; but its ores are extremely rare.

Co-lum'bo.* The common name for the root of the *Coc'culus palma'tus*. (See CALUMBA.) This root is one of the most valuable of the mild tonics. Being without astringency, it is generally acceptable to the stomach, and is an excellent remedy in cases of simple debility of the digestive organs or of the alimentary canal, resulting from whatever cause.

Columella. See COLUMNELLA.

Columelliaceæ,* kol-u-mel-le-a'-she-ē. [From *Columel'lia*, one of the genera.] An obscure natural order of exogenous shrubs and trees, found in Mexico and Peru. Allied to the Jasminaceæ.

Co-lum'na̤,* plural **Co-lum'næ.** [Fr. *Colonne*, ko'lonn'.] Literally, a "column," or "pillar." Often applied in Anatomy to parts supposed to resemble a column, as those of the *ve'lum pala'ti*, and the *columnæ carneæ*, or muscular fasciculi of the internal walls of the heart.

Colum'na Na'si.* ("Column of the Nose.") The fleshy termination of the septum of the nose.

Colum'na O'ris.* ("Column of the Mouth.") The uvula.

Colum'na Ver-te-bra'lis.* ("Vertebral Column.") The spinal column.

Col-um'næ Car'ne-æ.* ("Fleshy Columns.") (Fr. *Colonnes Charnues*, ko'lonn' shaʀ'nü'.) The muscular projections in the ventricles of the heart.

Co-lum'nar. [**Columna'ris;** from *colum'na*, a "pillar."] Belonging to a pillar or column; pillar-like.

Col-um-nel'la̤,* or **Col-u-mel'la̤.*** [Diminutive of *colum'na*.] Applied in Botany to a substance passing through the capsule, connecting the several partitions and seeds.

Col-um-nif'er-ous. [**Columnif'erus;** from *colum'na*, a "column," and *fe'ro*, to "bear."] Applied in Botany to plants that have the stamens and pistil like a column in the middle of the flower.

Co-lum'nu-la̤.* [Diminutive of *colum'na*.] The filament which passes through the middle of the capsule of frondose mosses.

Coluvrine de Virginie, ko'lü'vrėn' dẹh vėʀ'zhė'nė'. The French for Virginia Snake-root. See ARISTOLOCHIA.

Col'za̤ Oil. A liquid extracted from the grain of the *Bras'sica Arven'sis*, used in making soft soap.

Co'ma̤, atis,* plural **Co'ma̤-ta̤.** [Gr. κῶμα, "deep sleep."] A state of lethargic drowsiness, produced by compression of the brain and other causes.

Co'ma.* [Gr. κόμη, the "hair of the head."] Literally, a "head of hair." Applied in Botany to a bush or head of leaves terminating a stem.

Co'ma-Vig'il.* ("Watchful Coma.") The lethargic condition of the patient in bad cases of typhus, in which he is watchful and muttering in delirium.

Co'ma̤-ta̤,* the plural of **Co'ma.** Applied to soporose diseases. An order of the class *Neuroses* of Cullen's Nosology.

Co'ma̤-tōse. [**Comato'sus;** from *co'ma*.] Having a constant propensity to sleep: full of sleep.

Com-bĭ-nā'tion. [**Combina'tio, o'nis;** from *com'bino, combina'tum*, to "set in couples together" (from *con*, "together," and *bi'nus*, "two by two").] A true chemical union of two or more substances, as opposed to mere mechanical mixture.

Combretaceæ,* kom-bre-ta'she-ē. [From *Combre'tum*, one of the genera.] A natural order of exogenous shrubs and trees, all natives of the tropics, mostly astringents. Some species of it produce valuable dyestuffs.

Com-bus'tion. [**Combus'tio, o'***nis;* from *combu'ro, combus'tum,* to "burn."] Burning. The evolution of heat and light during chemical action, by absorbing oxygen from atmospheric air.

Combustion, Preternatural, Combustion, Spontaneous. See SPONTANEOUS COMBUSTION.

Com'et. [**Come'ta,** or **Come'tes;** from the Greek κομήτης, "long-haired;" from the stream of light usually appended to them, like a tail.] The name of a heavenly body, supposed to be planetary, forming a part of our system.

Commander's Balsam. See TINCTURA BENZOINI.

Commelynaceæ,* or **Commelinaceæ,*** kom-me-le-na'she-ē. [From *Commely'na,* one of the genera.] A natural order of endogenous herbaceous plants, including the Spider-wort, *Tradescantia.*

Com'mĭ-nūt-ed. [**Comminu'tus;** from *commin'uo, comminu'tum,* to "break" or "crush into small pieces."] Applied to fractures in which the bone is broken into several pieces.

Com-mis-su'ra.* [From *con,* "together," and *mit'to, mis'sum,* to "put."] A joining together; something which joins together: a com'missure.

Commissu'ra Mag'na.* ("Great Commissure.") The *Corpus callosum.*

Commissu'ra Mol'lis.* ("Soft Commissure.") The name of the gray mass uniting the thalami of the brain.

Commissure. See COMMISSURA.

Common Integuments. See INTEGUMENTS.

Com-mu'nĭ-cans,* plural **Com-mu-nĭ-can'tēs.** [The present participle of *commu'nico, communica'tum,* to "communicate."] Communicating; that which establishes communication.

Commu'nicans Tib'ĭ-æ.* ("Communicating [Nerve] of the Tibia.") Applied to the external saphenal branch of the tibial nerve.

Commu'nicans Wil-lis'ĭ-i.* ("Communicating [Artery] of Willis.") A branch of the internal carotid artery, passing to the posterior cerebral artery.

Com-mu-nĭ-can'tēs Ar-te'rĭ-æ.* ("Communicating Arteries.") Of these, there are two within the cranium, the principal of which is the COMMUNICANS WILLISII.

Comparative Anatomy. See ANATOMY, COMPARATIVE.

Com-plex'us.* [From *con,* "together," and *plec'to, plex'um,* to "plait," to "weave."] Literally, "woven together." Applied to a muscle situated at the back part of the neck. It is so named from the intricate mixture of its muscular and tendinous parts. It is attached to the occipital bone, and to the cervical and upper dorsal vertebræ.

Com'plĭ-cāt-ed. [**Complica'tus;** from *con,* "together," and *pli'co, plica'tum,* to "fold," to "knit."] Applied to fractures that are combined with other circumstances that make their treatment difficult; as a wounded artery, dislocation, injury of the viscera, etc.

Com-plĭ-cā'tion. [**Complica'tio, o'***nis;* from the same.] The coexistence of two or more diseases, which modify each other, without being in their nature inseparable.

Compositæ,* kom-poz'e-tē. [From *con,* "together," and *po'no, pos'itum,* to "put."] The largest of all known natural groups of plants, and so called because the old botanists who invented the name regarded the flower-heads as compound flowers. It answers to the *Syngenesia polygamia* of Linnæus. It is characterized by having capitate flowers, syngenesious anthers, and an inferior ovary, with a single erect ovule. This order includes about nine hundred genera and eight thousand species.

Com-pos'ĭ-tus.* [From *con,* "together," and *po'no, pos'itum,* to "put."] Compound; opposed to "simple." Applied in the plural feminine to a natural order of plants. See COMPOSITÆ.

Compôte (Fr.), kom'pōt'. (A contraction of COMPOSITUS, which see.) Fruits preserved with sugar; generally stone fruits.

Com'pound. [**Compos'itus;** a corruption of *componed,* passive participle, from the obsolete verb *compone,* to "put together," to "arrange." See COMPOSITUS.] Applied in Mineralogy to a form contained under planes not homologous, or equal, similar, and equally disposed to each other. In Pharmacy and Chemistry, applied to a mixture or substance composed of two or more ingredients or elements.

Compound Blowpipe. See BLOWPIPE.

Com'pound Frac'ture. A term in Surgery denoting a case wherein the fracture of the bone is accompanied with laceration of the integuments, causing an external wound. See FRACTURE.

Com'press. [**Compres'sus;** from *con,* "together," and *pre'mo, pres'sum,* to "press."] Literally, "something pressed together." A portion of folded linen, lint, or other material, made into a kind of pad to be placed over parts which require particular pressure.

Com-pressed'. [**Compres'sus;** from the same.] Flattened in a lateral direction.

Com-pres-sĭ-bil'ĭ-tȳ. [From the same.] A property of masses of matter, by which their particles are capable of being brought nearer together. Bodies which recover their former bulk on removal of the compressing cause are called *elastic.*

Com-pres'sion. [**Compres'sio, o'***nis;* from the same.] The act of compressing, or pressing together. Applied to an abnormal state of a part produced by something pressing upon it: generally used in reference to the brain.

Com-pres'sor, o'r*is.** [From the same.] That which compresses. Applied to a muscle which presses upon any part. In Surgery, it denotes a certain instrument.

Compressor of Dupuytren. See DUPUYTREN, COMPRESSOR OF.

Compres'sor Pros'ta-tæ.* ("The Compressor of the Prostate [Gland].") The anterior fibres of the *Levator ani,* which embrace the prostate gland.

Con. A Latin particle signifying "together," and sometimes "with." It is usually changed to *com* before *b, m,* and *p,* and to *co* before a vowel, or *h.* Hence we have *combine, compress,* instead of *conbine* and *conpress; coagulate* and *cohabit,* instead of *conagulate* and *conhabit.* Sometimes *con* is intensive, as *concu'tio, concus'sum,* to "shake violently."

Co-na'rĭ-um.* [From κῶνος, a "cone."] Another name for the pineal gland; so called on account of its conical form.

Con-cat'e-nate. [From *con,* "together," and *cate'na,* a "chain."] "Chained together." A term applied to the glands of the neck, presenting in children a kind of knotty cord, extending from behind the ear to the collar-bone.

Con-cau'sa.* [From *con,* "together," and *cau'sa,* a "cause."] A cause combined with another: a concause.

Con'cāve. [From *con,* intensive, and *ca'vus,* "hollow."] Regularly hollowed out, like the inside of a hollow sphere.

Con-cā'vo-con'cāve. [**Con'cavo-con'cavus.**] Having two concave faces.

Con-cā'vo-con'vex. [**Con'cavo-convex'us.**] Having one face concave, the other convex.

Con-cen'trāte. [From *con,* "together," and *cen'trum,* a "centre."] Literally, to "bring together [as an army] towards a common centre:" hence, to condense, to strengthen.

Con-cen-trā'tion. [**Concentra'tio, o'***nis;* from the same.] Applied in Chemistry to the operation of rendering a fluid stronger by evaporating a portion of the water it contains.

Con-cen'tric. [**Concen'tricus;** from *con,* "together" or "with," and *cen'trum,* a "centre."] Having one common centre.

Con-çep'ta-cle. [**Conceptac'u-lum;** from *concip'io, concep'tum,* to "conceive."] Applied in Botany to the case or vessel containing the reproductive corpuscles in cryptogamous plants. The conceptacles are also termed *capsules, thecæ,* and *sporangiæ.*

Con-cep'tion. [From the same.] The impregnation of the female *ovulum* in the *ovarium* by the semen of the male, whence results a new being.

Concep'tion, False. An imperfect impregnation or blighted ovum.

Concha,* konk'a. [Gr. κόγχη, a "shell."] Literally, a "shell." Applied in Anatomy to the hollow portion of the external ear, etc.

Con'chæ Na'rĭ-um.* (The "Shells of the Nostrils.") The turbinated portion of the ethmoid bone, and the inferior spongy bones.

Con-chif'er-a.* [From *con'cha,* a "shell," and *fe'ro,* to "bear," to "carry."] The second class of the *Cyclo-gangliata,* or *Mollusca,* comprising acephalous aquatic animals covered with a bivalve or multivalve shell.

Con-chif'er-ous. [**Conchif'erus;** from the same.] Bearing, or having, shells.

Conch'oid. [**Conchoi'des;** from κόγχη, a "shell," and εἶδος, a "form."] Resembling a shell.

Con-choi'dal. The same as CONCHOID.

Con-chol'o-ġȳ. [**Concholo'gia;** from κόγχη, a "shell," and λόγος, a "discourse."] The science of shells; that branch of Natural History which treats of the form, structure, and peculiarities of shells.

Conch'us.* [From κόγχη, a "shell."] The cranium. In the plural (*Con'chi*) it is applied to the cavities of the eye.

Con-chȳl-e-om'e-ter. [**Conchyli-om'etrum;** from κογχύλιον, a "shell," and μέτρον, a "measure."] An instrument for measuring shells.

Con-chȳl-ĭ-o-lo'gĭ-a.* [From κογχύλιον, a "shell," and λόγος, a "discourse."] The same as CONCHOLOGY.

Con-coc'tion. [**Concoc'tio, o'nis;** from *con*, intensive, and *co'quo, coc'tum*, to "cook," to "digest."] The changing process which the food undergoes in the stomach and bowels: the same as *Digestion*, though the latter is by some medical writers limited to the process in the stomach.

Con-crēte', or kong'krēt. [**Con-cre'tus;** from *con*, "together," and *cres'co, cre'tum*, to "grow."] Applied to substances converted from a fluid to a more solid consistence.

Con-cre'tion. [**Concre'tio, o'nis;** from the same.] The growing together of parts naturally separate, as the fingers or toes. Applied in Chemistry to the condensation of a fluid, or other substance, into a more solid consistence.

Con-cu'bĭ-tus.* [From *con*, "together," and *cu'bo, cu'bitum*, to "lie."] The same as COITUS.

Con-cus'sion. [**Concus'sio, o'nis;** from *concu'tio, concus'sum*, to "shake," to "shake violently."] A diseased state, producing alarming symptoms, caused by great violence offered to the head, though no fissure, fracture, or extravasation can be discovered.

Con-den-sā'tion. [**Condensa'tio, o'nis;** from *con*, "together," and *den'so, densa'tum*, to "thicken," to "make thick."] The process of bringing the component parts of vapor or gas nearer to each other by pressure or cold. Applied to increased density or solidity of the blood or tissues.

Con-den'ser, or **Con-den-sā'tor.*** [From the same.] A vessel or apparatus for condensing gas, vapor, or air. Also an instrument for rendering sensible the weakest quantities of electricity.

Con-dĭ-men'ta.* [The plural of *condimen'tum*, a "sauce" or "seasoning;" from *con'dio*, to "season."] Condiments: substances taken with the food to improve its flavor, to promote its digestion, or to correct its injurious qualities.

Con-duc'tion. [**Conduc'tio, o'nis;** from *condu'co, conduc'tum*, to "lead together," to "conduct."] The passing of caloric or electricity from one particle of matter to another, as in an iron rod heated at one end, in which case the caloric is conducted gradually along the particles of the iron.

Con-duc'tor, o'ris.* [From the same.] Applied to a body which readily transmits electricity or caloric.

Con-du'plĭ-cate. [**Conduplica'tus;** from *con*, "together," and *duplica'tus*, "doubled."] Folded together.

Con'dȳle. [**Con'dylus;** from κόνδυλος, a "knuckle," a "knob."] The round eminence at the end of a bone in a joint.

Con'dȳ-loid. [**Condyloi'des;** from κόνδυλος, a "knob," a "condyle," and εἶδος, a "form."] Resembling a condyle.

Con-dȳ-lo'ma, atis.* [From κόνδυλος, a "knob" or "tubercle."] A small, hard tumor, or wart-like excrescence, about the anus and pudendum of both sexes.

Cone. [Lat. **Co'nus;** Gr. κῶνος.] A solid formed by the rotation of a right-angled triangle about its perpendicular, called the axis of the cone.

Cone-Shaped. See CONICAL.

Co-ne'in, or **Co-ne'ĭne.** [**Coni'a**, or **Coneia**, ko-nī'a; from *coni'um*, "hemlock."] The active principle of *Coni'um macula'tum;* also termed **Cicutin.**

Conf. = *Confec'tio.** A "confection."

Confectio,* kon-fek'she-o, plural **Confectiones**, kon-fek-she-o'nēz. (Fr. *Confit*, kôNᵍ'fè'.) A confection. Under this title the London College and U.S. Pharmacopœia comprehend the *conserves* and *electuaries* of its former Pharmacopœias.

Confec'tio Ar-o-mat'ĭ-ca.* ("Aromatic Confection.") Take of aromatic powder, four troyounces; clarified honey, four troyounces, or a sufficient quantity. Rub the aromatic powder with clarified honey until a uniform mass is obtained of the proper consistence. (U.S.Ph., 1860.)

Confec'tio Auran'tii (au-ran'she-i) **Cor'tĭ-çis.*** ("Confection of Orange-peel.") Take of sweet orange-peel, recently separated from the fruit by grating, twelve troyounces; sugar, thirty-six troyounces. Beat the orange-peel with the sugar, gradually added, until they are thoroughly mixed. (U.S. Ph., 1860.)

Confec'tio O'pĭ-i.* ("Confection of Opium.") Take of opium, in fine powder, two hundred and seventy grains; aromatic powder, six troyounces; clarified honey, fourteen troyounces. Rub the opium with the aromatic powder, then add the honey, and beat the whole together until thoroughly mixed. (U.S. Ph., 1860.)

Confec'tio Ro'sæ.* ("Confection

of Rose.") Take of red rose, in fine powder, four troyounces; sugar, in fine powder, thirty troyounces; clarified honey, six troyounces; rose-water, eight fluidounces. Rub the rose with the rose-water heated to 150°, then gradually add the sugar and honey, and beat the whole together until thoroughly mixed. (U.S. Ph., 1860.)

Confec'tio Sen'næ* ("Confection of Senna") is composed of eight parts of senna, four of coriander, sixteen of purging cassia, ten of tamarind, seven of prune, twelve of figs, thirty of sugar, and of water a sufficient quantity. (For particular directions in the preparation, see U.S. Pharmacopœia, 1860, pp. 129 and 130.)

Confectiones. See CONFECTIO.

Con-fer'va.* [From *confer'veo,* to "boil together," to "boil up;" so named, perhaps, in allusion to its floating like scum on the surface of the water.] The *Confervæ* are chiefly fresh-water plants, composed of jointed capillary tubes, the joints containing granules variously arranged.

Confervaceæ,* kon-fer-va'she-ē. [From *Confer'va,* a genus of aquatic plants.] A natural order of flowerless aquatic plants, common in fresh water. At one period of their existence they have the power of rapid and quasi-voluntary motion.

Con-flā'tion. [**Confla'tio;** from *con'flo, confla'tum,* to "blow together," to "forge," to "melt."] The casting or melting of metal.

Con'flu-ent. [**Con'fluens;** from *con,* "together," and *flu'o,* to "flow," to "run."] Applied in Botany to leaves connected at their base. Applied also to the eruption in *Variola,* and some other exanthematous diseases, when the pustules are so thick as to run together, appearing like one mass of inflammation.

Con-for-mā'tion. [**Conforma'tio, o'***nis;* from *confor'mo,* to "shape" or "form together," to "adapt one thing or part to another."] The natural form of a part.

Cong. = *Con'gius.** A "gallon."

Con-ge-lā'tion. [**Congela'tio, o'***nis;* from *con,* intensive, and *ge'lo, gela'tum,* to "freeze."] The process whereby the change of a liquid to a solid body is produced by the losing of its caloric.

Con'ge-ner, er*is.** [From *con,* "together," and *ge'nus,* a "kind" or "race."] (Fr. *Congénère,* kôNᴳ'zhā'nair'.) Literally, "of the same kind with another." Applied to muscles which perform the same action. Applied to *genera* nearly allied, or to species of the same *genus.*

Con-gen'i-tal. [**Congen'itus;** from *con,* "together," or "with," and *gen'itus,* "born."] (Fr. *Congénial,* kôNᴳ'zhā'-ne-ăl'.) Born with a person; existing from birth: connate.

Con-ge'ri-ēs.* [From *conge'ro,* to "carry together," to "heap up."] A collection of a number of particles into one mass.

Con-ges'tion. [**Conges'tio, o'***nis;* from *conge'ro, conges'tum,* to "carry or heap together."] An excessive accumulation of the contents of any of the blood-vessels or ducts.

Con-ges'tive. [**Congesti'vus;** from the same.] Capable of producing, or tending to produce, congestion.

Con'gi-us.* A gallon.

Con'glo-bate. [**Congloba'tus;** from *conglo'bo, congloba'tum,* to "gather into a ball."] Formed into a ball.

Con'globate Gland [from *con,* "together," and *glo'bus,* a "ball"], or Simple. A gland subsisting by itself; as those of the absorbent system.

Con-glom'er-ate. [**Conglomera'tus;** from *conglom'ero, conglomera'tum,* to "wind," as on a ball, to "heap together." See AGGLOMERATE.] Irregularly crowded together.

Conglom'erate Gland [from *con,* "together," and *glo'mus, glom'eris,* a "heap"], or Compound. A gland composed of various glands; as the salivary, parotid, pancreatic, etc.

Conglutinantia,* kon-glu-te-nan'-she-a. [From *conglu'tino,* to "glue together."] The same as AGGLUTINANTIA. See AGGLUTINANT.

Con-gres'sus,* or **Con'gress.** [From *congre'dior, congres'sus,* to "meet together."] The meeting of the male and female in the act of procreation. The same as COITUS.

Co'ni,* the plural of CONUS, which see.

Co'ni Vas-cu-lo'si.* ("Vascular Cones.") The conical convolutions of the *vasa efferentia* of the testis. They constitute the *epididymis.*

Co-ni'a.* The same as CONEIN, which see.

Conic. See CONICAL.

Con'i-cal. [**Con'icus.**] Belonging to a cone; shaped like a cone.

Con'i-cin. [**Conici'na.**] The same as CONEIN, which see.

Co-nif'er-æ* [from *co'nus*, a "cone," and *fe'ro*, to "bear"], or **Pinaceæ,*** pi-na'she-ē. A natural order of exogenous trees and shrubs, found in nearly all parts of the world, and usually evergreen. It includes the pine, cedar, spruce, cypress, juniper, and other trees of great value for timber. No order can be named of more universal importance to man, whether we view it with reference to its timber or its secretions, among which are turpentine, resin, balsam, and pitch.

Co-nif'er-ous. [Conif'erus; from *co'nus*, a "cone," and *fe'ro*, to "bear."] Bearing cones. See CONIFERÆ.

Coniform. See CONOID.

Co-ni'i Fo'li-a.* ("Leaves of Conium.") See CONIUM.

Co-ni-ros'tris.* [From *co'nus*, a "cone," and *ros'trum*, a "beak."] Applied in the plural feminine to a family of birds having a strong conical beak: coniros'trate.

Co-ni'um.* [Gr. *κώνειον*.] Called in English *Hemlock*. (Fr. *Ciguë*, sē'gü'.) A Linnæan genus of the class *Pentandria*, natural order *Umbelliferæ*. The Pharmacopœial name ‖ of the fresh-dried leaves of *Conium maculatum*. Hemlock is narcotic and sedative. In large doses it causes vertigo, dimness of vision, nausea, numbness in the limbs, convulsions, and death. Sometimes death ensues from paralysis without coma or convulsions. It is employed medicinally as a palliative in cancerous ulcers, painful scrofulous tumors, etc.; also in chronic rheumatism, neuralgia, asthma, and phthisis.

Coni'um Mac-u-la'tum.* The systematic name of the hemlock, termed *Cicu'ta* by the Latin authors; but it is quite distinct from the *Cicuta maculata* of modern botanists.

Conjonctive, kōnᵍ'zhōnk'tēv'. The French for *Conjunctiva*. See CONJUNCTIVUS.

Con'ju-gate. [Conjuga'tus; from *con*, "together," and *ju'go*, *juga'tum*, to "yoke," to "join."] Yoked; joined in pairs. Applied to the leaves of plants.

Conjunctiva. See CONJUNCTIVUS.

Con-junc-ti-vi'tis, idis.* Inflammation of the *conjunctiva*.

Con-junc-ti'vus.* [From *con*, "together," and *jun'go*, *junc'tum*, to "join."] Applied to a delicate mucous membrane (*Membra'na Conjuncti'va*) which lines both eyelids and covers the external portion of the eyeball.

Connaraceæ,* kon-na-ra'she-ē. [From *Con'narus*, one of the genera.] A natural order of trees and shrubs, found in the tropics. One species produces the beautiful zebra-wood of the cabinet-makers.

Con'nate. [Conna'tus; from *con*, "together," and *nas'cor*, *na'tus*, to "be born," to "grow."] Born with one; congenital. In Botany, grown together.

Con-nec'tive [see next article] **Tis'sue.** The same as CELLULAR TISSUE.

Con-nec-ti'vum.* [From *con*, "together," and *nec'to*, to "knit" or "tie."] In Botany, the transverse body by which the lobes of the anther are united.

Con-ni'vens,* plural **Con-ni-ven'tēs.** [From *con*, "together," and *ni'veo*, to "wink."] Converging, as the eyelids in winking, etc. See VALVULÆ CONNIVENTES.

Co'noid. [Conoi'des; from *κῶνος*, a "cone," and *εἶδος*, a "form."] Resembling a cone; coniform.

Co'noid Lig'a-ment. [Ligamen'tum Conoi'des.] The ligament which passes from the root of the coracoid process to the clavicle.

Conque, kōnk (Fr.). See CONCHA.

Con-ser'van-cy. [From *conser'vo*, *conserva'tum*, to "preserve."] Preservation. Applied in medicine to the prevention of decay in excreta, etc., with a view to promoting health.

Con-ser-va'trix, i'cis.* [From the same.] Preserving. (Used only in the feminine.) See VIS CONSERVATRIX.

Con'serve. [Conser'va.] A composition of some vegetable substance and sugar, beaten into a uniform mass.

Consommé (Fr.), kōnᵍ'som'mā', *i.e.* "complete," "perfect." [From *consommer;* literally, to "sum up;" hence, to "finish," to "perfect."] A rich broth or soup containing a large proportion of gelatine. Named, it would seem, on account of its summing up, or containing in a concentrated form, all the richest and best ingredients of the meat.

Con-stel-lā'tion. [Constella'tio, o'nis; from *con*, "together," and *stel'la*, a "star."] A collection of fixed stars representing an animal or other figure, according to their arrangement.

Con-sti-pā'tion. [Constipa'tio, o'nis; from *con*, "together," and *sti'po*, *stipa'tum*, to "stuff," to "cram close."] (Fr. *Échauffement*, ā'shōf'mōnᵍ'.) Costiveness; tardiness in evacuating the bowels.

Con-stit'u-ens.* [Present participle

of *constit'uo*, to "constitute," to "compose," to "make," or "form."] Literally, "that which constitutes" or helps to constitute or form any compound. The vehicle; a constituent part of a medicinal formula, commonly signifying that which furnishes a convenient and agreeable form. See PRESCRIPTION.

Con-sti-tu'tion. [**Constitu'tio, o'***nis;* from *constit'uo, constitu'tum*, to "form," to "constitute" (from *con*, "together," and *stat'uo*, to "set" or "place").] The general habit or temperament of the body. See DIATHESIS.

Constitu'tion of the Air. That peculiar condition of the air which causes epidemics, or which impresses upon epidemic or sporadic diseases their peculiar character.

Con-sti-tu'tion-al. Belonging to, or dependent upon, the constitution.

Con-stric'tor,* plural **Con-stric-to'rēs.** [From *con*, "together," and *strin'go, stric'tum*, to "draw," to "bind."] Applied to a muscle that draws together or contracts any opening of the body, such as the pharynx.

Constrictor Ani. See SPHINCTER ANI.

Constrictor Oris. See ORBICULARIS ORIS.

Con-stric-to'rēs Pha-ryn'gis.* ("Constrictors of the Pharynx.") These are muscles forming a part of the parietes of the pharynx, which they contract.

Constringentia,* kon-strin-jen'-she-a. [The neuter plural of the present participle of *constrin'go*, to "bind together."] Applied to medicines which contract the tissues and check the secretions, etc. The same as ASTRINGENTS, which see.

Con-sump'tion. [**Consump'tio, o'***nis;* from *consu'mo, consump'tum*, to "consume" or "waste away."] Any wasting away of the body, but usually applied to *Phthisis pulmonalis*. See PHTHISIS and TABES.

Contabescentia,* kon-tab-ĕs-sen'-she-a. [From *con*, intensive, and *tabes'-co*, to "waste away."] Atrophy, or consumption; wasting away of the whole body. See TABES.

Con-tā'gion. [**Conta'gio, o'***nis;* from *contin'go*, to "touch," to "affect."] The communication of a disease by contact, or by inhaling the effluvia from one already affected; often used as synonymous with INFECTION, which see.

Con-tā'gious. [**Contagio'sus;** from the same.] Applied to diseases which are spread by CONTAGION.

Con-tin'ūed Fe'ver. [**Fe'bris Contin'ua.**] A fever in which the symptoms do not intermit till its termination.

Con-tĭ-nu'ĭ-tȳ. [**Continu'itas;** from *contin'eo*, to "hold" or "keep together."] A union of parts so complete that they cannot be separated without laceration or fracture.

Continu'ity, So-lu'tion of. The separation by fracture or laceration of parts previously continuous.

Contorsio, or **Contortio** (kon-tor'-she-o), **o'***nis.** [From *con*, intensive, and *tor'queo, tor'sum* or *tor'tum*, to "twist."] A twisting or contortion.

Con-tort'. [From the same.] To twist, or twist together: thus, the leaves or petals of certain plants, and sometimes arteries and veins, are said to be *contorted*.

Con'tra. A Latin preposition, signifying "against," "over against," or "opposite to."

CON'TRA-APERTU'RA.* [From *con'tra*, "opposite," and *apertu'ra*, an "aperture."] A counter-opening. An opening made in an abscess opposite to one already existing in it, to facilitate the discharge of matter.

CON'TRA-EXTEN'SIO* (ex-ten'she-o). Counter-extension. The holding of the upper part of a broken limb or a dislocated joint towards the trunk, while extension is being employed with the lower part.

CON'TRA-FISSU'RA.* (Fr. *Contrecoup*, kôNt'r'koo', and *Contrefente*, kôNt'r'fŏNt'.) A fracture in a part opposite or distant from that in which the blow is received. See FISSURA.

CON'TRA-IN'DICATE. [From *con'tra*, and *indi'co*, to "indicate," to "show."] To prohibit or prevent the use of a particular remedy. See next article.

CON'TRA-INDICA'TION. [*Con'tra-indica'tio, o'nis;* from the same.] That which forbids the use of a particular remedy which otherwise it would be proper to exhibit.

Con-trac'tile. [**Contrac'tilis;** from *con*, "together," and *tra'ho, trac'tum*, to "draw."] Possessing CONTRACTILITY, which see.

Contractilité. See CONTRACTILITY.

Con-trac-til'ĭ-tȳ. [**Contractil'itas, a'***tis;* from the same. Fr. *Contractilité*, kôN'trâk'tè'lè'tà'.] A property by which the particles of bodies resume their original position when the power applied to separate them is withdrawn. Also, that vital property which gives to certain parts (muscles, for example) the power of contracting, by means of which all the various tribes of animals perform their motions.

Contractility is *voluntary* in what are termed the organs of *animal* life (such as the hands, feet, tongue, etc.), and *involuntary* in those of *organic* life (as the heart, the stomach, etc.). Contractility is sometimes used as synonymous with IRRITABILITY, which see.

Con-trac'tion. [**Contrac'tio, o**'*nis;* from the same.] The shortening of living fibre on the application of stimulus. Also, the shortening of a muscle from some morbid cause.

Con-trac-tu'ra.* [From the same.] Literally, "contraction." The name of a genus of the order *Dyscinesiæ*, class *Locales*, of Cullen's Nosology. A disease attended with permanent rigidity of the flexor muscles. It is sometimes the result of rheumatism, *colica pictonum*, and other diseases.

Con-tra-jer'va,* or **Con-tra-yer'va.*** A former name for the root of the *Dorste'nia contrayer'va.* See DORSTENIA.

Contre-coup, Contre-fente, Contre-fracture. (Fr.) The same as CONTRA-FISSURA, which see.

Con-tu'sion. [**Contu'sio, o**'*nis;* from *contun'do, contu'sum,* to "bruise."] (Fr. *Meurtrissure,* mur'trè'sür'.) Injury by an obtuse weapon, or violent collision against a hard body, without breach of the integuments: a bruise.

Co'nus.* [Gr. κῶνος.] A cone. Applied in Botany to a particular kind of fructification, as the fir-top. See STROBILUS.

Con-va-lĕs'çence. [**Convalescen'tia;** from *convales'co,* to "grow strong" or "well."] The state or period between the removal of actual disease and the full recovery of the strength.

Con-va-lĕs'çent. [**Convales'cens;** the present participle of the same.] Literally, "growing strong" or "well." Returning to full health after a disease is removed.

Con-val-la'rĭ-a.* [From *conval'lis,* a "valley;" named from its abounding in valleys.] A genus of plants, of which several species were formerly used in medicine. The flowers and root of the *Convalla'ria maia'lis* (or *maja'lis*) have been employed as an errhine, and the former as a cathartic.

Con'vex. [**Convex'us;** from *con,* "together," and *ve'ho, vec'tum* or *vex'um,* to "carry."] Literally, "brought together;" hence, heaped up, swelling up like a heap of grain or like the part of a sphere.

Convexo-Concavus. See CONCAVO-CONVEX.

Con-vex'o-Con'vex. [**Convex'o-Convex'us.**] Having both surfaces convex.

Con-vo-lu'ta Os'sa.* ("Convoluted Bones.") A term applied to the upper and lower turbinated bones of the nose. See CONVOLUTUS.

Con-vo-lu'tion. [**Convolu'tio, o**'*nis;* from *con,* "together," and *vol'vo, volu'tum,* to "roll," to "wrap."] Any thing which is rolled together or upon itself. Hence the term is applied to the tortuous eminences of the *cerebrum;* also, to the irregular foldings of the intestines.

Con-vo-lu'tus.* [From the same.] Rolled up; con'voluted.

Convolvulaceæ,* kon-vol-vu-la'-she-ē, or **Con-vol'vu-li.*** [From *Convol'vulus,* one of the genera.] A natural order of herbaceous or shrubby twining plants, yielding a milky juice when wounded. They are abundant in the tropics, and possess purgative qualities in their roots, depending upon a peculiar resin, of which scammony and jalap may be taken as examples.

Con-vol-vu-lā'ceous. [**Convolvula'ceus.**] Having an arrangement like the *Convolvulus.*

Con-vol'vu-li,* the plural of **Convol'vulus,** forming the Jussieuan name of a natural order of plants. See CONVOLVULACEÆ.

Con-vol'vu-lus.* [From *convol'vo,* to "wrap together," to "entwine."] Bindweed. A Linnæan genus of the class *Pentandria,* natural order *Convolvulaceæ.*

Convol'vulus Ja-la'pa.* The name given by Linnæus to the jalap-plant; now referred to the genus *Ipomœa.* See IPOMŒA JALAPA.

Convol'vulus Scam-mo'nĭ-a.* The systematic name of the scammony-plant.

Convulsio. See CONVULSION.

Convulsio Canina. See RISUS SARDONICUS.

Convul'sio (kon-vŭl'she-o) **Ha-bit-u-a'lis.*** ("Habitual Convulsion.") One of the names of *Chorea,* or St. Vitus's Dance.

Con-vul'sion. [**Convul'sio, o**'*nis;*

from *convel'lo, convul'sum,* to "pull together."] Violent agitation of the limbs or body, generally marked by clonic spasms. See SPASMUS.

Copahu, ko'på'ü'. The French term for COPAIBA, which see.

Co-pāi'ba* (Spanish pronunciation ko-pī'BÅ, almost ko-pī'vå). [From *Co'pal,* an odoriferous gum, and *i'ba* or *i'va,* a "tree."] A resinous juice, or oleo-resin, obtained from the *Copaifera multijuga* and other species of *Copaifera.* The Pharmacopœial name ‖ of balsam of copaiba.

Copaiba is gently stimulant, diuretic, and laxative, and in large doses sometimes actively purgative. It is much used as a remedy in gonorrhœa and other diseases of the mucous membranes, especially those of a chronic character.

Copai'bæ O'le-um.* ("Oil of Copaiba.") An oil distilled from the oleo-resin of copaiba (Lond. Ph., 1851).

Co-pa-if'er-a.* [From *copai'ba,* and *fe'ro,* to "bear."] A Linnæan genus of the class *Decandria,* natural order *Leguminosæ.*

Copaif'era Mul-tij'u-ga.* The systematic name of the tree which produces copaiba, growing native in Venezuela, also found in some of the West India islands, particularly Trinidad and Martinique. It is a handsome tree, with a lofty stem much branched at the top and crowned with a thick canopy of foliage.

Copaif'era Of-fiç-ĭ-na'lis.* One of the plants which afford copaiba.

Co-pāi'va. The same as COPAIBA, which see.

Co'pal. (Sp. *Copal,* ko-pål'.) A resinous substance obtained from the *Hymenæa Courbaril* and other species of *Hymenæa.* Dissolved in alcohol, it has been used as a remedy for spongy gums. It is at present chiefly or solely employed as a varnish.

Co-pho'sis.* [From κωφός, "deaf."] Deafness.

Copper. See CUPRUM.

Cop'per-as. A name for the sulphates of copper, iron, and zinc; also respectively called blue, green, and white vitriol.

Cop'per-nick'el. A native arseniuret of nickel, a copper-colored mineral found in Westphalia.

Cop-ra-go'gus.* [From κόπρος, "excrement," and ἄγω, to "carry" or "bring away."] Applied in the plural neuter (*Coprago'ga*) to purgatives,—that is, medicines which bring away the fæces: cop'ragogue.

Cop'ro-lite, Cop'ro-lith. [**Coprol'ithus;** from κόπρος, "excrement," and λίθος, a "stone."] A ball of hardened fæces or other mass in the bowels.

Co-pros'ta-sis.* [From κόπρος, "fæces," and ἵστημι, to "stand," to "be stationary."] Costiveness; undue retention of the fæces in the intestines. Hence the terms *Copragoga* or *Eccoprotica,* denoting purgatives.

Cop-u-lā'tion. [**Copula'tio, o'nis;** from *cop'ulo, copula'tum,* to "couple together."] The same as CONGRESSUS, which see.

Cor,* gen. **Cor'dis.** [Gr. καρδία; Fr. *Cœur,* KUR.] The Latin term for the heart, the central organ of circulation. See HEART.

Cŏr'a-co-. A prefix denoting attachment to the coracoid process of the scapula.

Cŏr'a-coid. [**Coracoi'des;** from κόραξ, κόρακος, a "raven" or "crow," and εἶδος, a "form."] Resembling a crow's beak. Applied to a process of the scapula; also applied by Owen to the homologues of the coracoid process of the scapula.

Cor'acoid Lig-a-ment. [**Ligamen'tum Coracoi'deum.**] A small ligament extending from the coracoid process across the notch of the scapula, converting the notch into a foramen.

Cor'acoid Proç'ess. [**Proces'sus Coracoi'deus.**] A projection or process on the anterior and upper margin of the scapula, supposed to resemble the beak of a crow.

Cor-a-co-i'de-us.* [From *coracoi'des.*] Belonging to the coracoid process of the scapula. See CORACOID LIGAMENT and CORACOID PROCESS.

Cŏr'al. [Lat. **Coral'lium** or **Coral'lum;** Gr. κοράλλιον; supposed to be derived from κόρη, a "daughter," and ἅλς, the "sea."] A stony or horny substance growing in the sea, once supposed to be a plant, but now regarded as the skeleton or shell of a congeries of small *Polypi.*

Cor-al-lif'er-ous. [**Corallif'erus;** from *coral'lum,* and *fe'ro,* to "bear."] Coral-bearing. Applied in the plural masculine (*Corallif'eri*) to an order of *Polypi.*

Cor-al'li-form. [**Corallifor'mis;** from *coral'lium* or *coral'lum.*] Formed like coral.

Cor-al-lig'er-us.* [From *coral'-*

lum, and *ge'ro*, to "bear."] The same as CORALLIFEROUS.

Cŏr'al-loid. [**Coralloi'des;** from *coral'lum*, and εἶδος, a "form."] Resembling coral.

Coralloidal. See CORALLOID.

Cor'cu-lum.* [Diminutive of *cor*, the "heart."] The heart and essence of the seed; the embryo, or germ.

Cor'date. [**Corda'tus;** from *cor*, *cor'dis*, the "heart."] Heart-shaped.

Cordiaceæ,* kor-de-a'she-ē. [From *Cor'dia*, one of the genera.] A natural order of exogenous trees, natives of the tropics. They are the Sebestens of the European Materia Medica.

Cordial, kord'yal. [**Cordia'lis;** from *cor*, the "heart."] Any stimulating medicine which raises the spirits.

Cor'dĭ-form. [**Cordifor'mis;** from *cor*, the "heart."] Formed like a heart.

Cordon Ombilicale, kor'dōng' ōm'-bē'lē'kâl'. The French term for FUNICULUS, which see.

Core. [From *cor*, the "heart."] The hard portion of sloughy or purulent matter found in boils.

Cor-ec-to'mĭ-a.* [From κόρη, the "pupil," and ἐκτέμνω, to "cut out."] The operation for artificial pupil by removal of a part of the iris: corec'tomy. See CORETOMIA and IRIDECTOMY.

Cor-e-dĭ-al'ȳ-sis.* [From κόρη, the "pupil," and διάλυσις.] The operation for artificial pupil, separating part of the external margin of the iris from the *Corpus ciliare*. See IRIDODIALYSIS.

Cor-e-mor-pho'sis.* [From κόρη, the "pupil," and μόρφωσις, "formation."] An operation for forming an artificial pupil. See CORECTOMIA, IRIDECTOMY.

Cor-en-cleï'sis.* [From κόρη, the "pupil," and ἐγκλείω, to "include."] An operation for artificial pupil by drawing a portion of the iris through an incision in the cornea, and cutting it off.

Co-re-on'çĭ-on,* Co-re-on'cĭ-um,* or ko-re-on'she-ŭm. [From κόρη, the "pupil," and ὄγκος, a "hook."] A kind of hook for the operation for artificial pupil.

Cor'e-plas'tĭ-ca,* Cor'e-plas'tĭ-çe.* [From κόρη, the "pupil," and πλαστική, the "art of making images."] Operation for artificial pupil in general: cor'eplasty.

Cor-e-to'mĭ-a.* [From κόρη, the "pupil," and τέμνω, to "cut."] Operation for artificial pupil by simply cutting through the iris: coret'omy. See IRIDITOMIA.

Co-rĭ-ā'ceous. [**Coria'ceus;** from *co'rium*, "leather."] Of the nature of leather; leathery.

Co-rĭ-an'drum.* [From κόρις, a "bug;" from the smell.] A Linnæan genus of the class *Pentandria*, natural order *Umbelliferæ*. Also the Pharmacopœial name ‖ for the fruit of *Coriandrum sativum*.

Corian'drum Sa-ti'vum.* The coriander-plant.

Co'rĭ-um.* [Gr. χόριον.] Literally, the "skin or hide of animals." The *Cutis*, or true skin.

Cor'mus.* [Gr. κορμός, a "trunk" or a "tail."] A corm. The body, or trunk of a tree; also the bulb of bulbous plants.

Corn. [From *cor'nu*, a "horn. Fr. *Cor*, kor.] A horny hardness of the skin, occurring chiefly on the joints of the toes, and caused by continued pressure or friction.

Cornaceæ,* kor-na'she-ē, or **Cor'-ne-æ.*** A natural order of trees and shrubs, found in temperate climates, including the *Cornus*, or Dog-Wood, the bark of which is said to rank among the best tonics in North America.

Corne. See CORNU.

Cor'ne-a.* [From *cor'nu*, a "horn."] A transparent, convexo-concave, nearly circular substance, forming the anterior part of the eyeball. It is often termed the *Cornea lu'cida*, or *C. transpa'rens*, or the "transparent cornea."

Cor'nea O-pa'ca.* The sclerotic coat of the eye.

Cor-ne-i'tis, *idis*.* [From *cor'nea*.] Inflammation of the cornea. The same as CERATITIS.

Cor'ne-ous. [**Cor'neus;** from *cor'-nu*.] Belonging to horn; horny.

Cornicle. See CORNICULUM.

Cor-nic'u-late. [**Cornicula'tus;** from *cornic'ulum*, a "little horn."] Having horns or parts resembling them.

Cor-nic'u-lum* [diminutive of *cor'-nu*, a "horn"], or **Cornic'ulum La-rȳn'ġis*** ("Cornicle of the Larynx"). A small cartilaginous body surmounting the arytenoid cartilage.

Cor'nĭ-form. [**Cornifor'mis;** from *cor'nu*, a "horn."] Horn-shaped.

Cor-niġ'er-ous. [**Cornig'erus;** from *cor'nu*, and *ge'ro*, to "bear."] Having horns.

Cor'nin, or **Cor'nĭne.** A term applied to a peculiar bitter principle said to have been found in the bark of the *Cornus Florida:* its properties resemble those of quinine.

Cor'nu,* plural **Cor'nu-ạ.** (Fr. *Corne*, KORN.) A Latin word signifying a "horn." Applied to a certain kind of warts, on account of their horny hardness. Also the Pharmacopœial name (Lond. and Ed. Ph.) of hartshorn. See CORNU CERVI.

COR'NUA U'TERI* ("Horns of the Uterus.") The angles of the uterus where the Fallopian tubes are given off.

Cor'nu Am-mo'nis,* Cor'nu A-ri'e-tis.* The appearance like a ram's horn presented by the cortical substance of the *cerebrum* when the *pes hippocampi* is cut transversely through.

Cor'nu Cer'vi.* ("Horn of the Stag.") The horn of the *Cervus elephas;* hartshorn. An impure carbonate of ammonia was formerly obtained from burning the shavings of hartshorn; while the residue, called *Cornu ustum* ("burnt horn"), consisting chiefly of phosphate of lime with a small proportion of free lime, was used as an antacid.

Cor'nu Us'tum.* [From *u'ro, us'tum*, to "burn."] A name for the phosphate of lime prepared from horn by fire. See CORNU CERVI.

Cor'nus Cir-ci-na'tạ,* and **Cor'nus Seriç'eạ.*** Small trees or shrubs found in the Northern and Middle United States. Their bark possesses medical virtues similar to those of CORNUS FLORIDA.

Cor'nus Flŏr'ĭ-dạ.* A small tree of the Linnæan class *Tetrandria*, natural order *Cornaceæ*. It grows in all the United States east of the Mississippi, but most abundantly in the Middle States. Also the Pharmacopœial name (U.S. Ph.) of the bark of the *Cornus Florida*, which appears to possess, though in an inferior degree, the tonic and antiperiodic virtues of cinchona.

Cornus Sericea (se-rish'e-ạ). See CORNUS CIRCINATA.

Cor'nute. [**Cornu'tus;** from *cor'nu*, a "horn."] Having horns; horned.

Co-rol'lạ.* [Diminutive of *coro'na*, a "crown."] Literally, a "little crown." Usually the most beautiful portion of the flower (the separate pieces of which are called petals), situated between the calyx and internal organs.

Cor'ol-lạ-rӯ. [**Corolla'rium;** from *corol'la.*] Applied to a tendril formed by a petal or segment of a *corolla*. Also, a truth necessarily following from some preceding truth or demonstration.

Cor'ol-late. Having a corolla.

Cor-ol-lif'er-ous. [**Corollif'erus;** from *corol'la*, and *fe'ro*, to "bear."] Bearing a corolla.

Cor-ol'lĭ-form. [**Corollifor'mis;** from *corol'la.*] Having the appearance of a corolla.

Co-rol'lu-lạ.* [Diminutive of *corol'la.*] The partial floret of a compound flower.

Co-ro'nạ.* [From κορώνη, the "crest" or "summit" of any thing.] A crown. Applied in Anatomy and Natural History to eminences of bone, or any objects or parts bearing resemblance to a crown.

Coro'na Glan'dis.* ("Crown of the Glans.") The ring or rim running round the base of the *Glans penis.*

Coro'na Ven'e-ris.* ("Crown of Venus.") (Fr. *Couronne de Vénus*, koo'-ronn' dẹh vȧ'nüs'.) Syphilitic blotches which often extend around the forehead, like a crown.

Co-ro'nad. Applied the same as CORONAL used adverbially.

Cor-o'nal, or kor'o-nal. [**Corona'lis;** from *coro'na*, a "crown."] Applied by Dr. Barclay in reference to the aspects of the head; towards the crown of the head.

Coro'nal Su'ture. [**Sutu'ra Corona'lis.**] The suture formed by the union of the frontal with the two parietal bones.

Cor'o-na-rӯ. [**Corona'rius;** from *coro'na*, a "crown."] (Fr. *Coronaire*, ko'ro'nêʀ'.) Applied to vessels, ligaments, and nerves which encircle parts like a crown, as the "coronary arteries of the heart," the "coronary artery of the stomach," etc.

Cor-o-na'tus.* [From *coro'na*, *corona'tum*, to "crown."] Literally, "crowned." Applied in the plural feminine (*Corona'tæ*) to a class or division of plants having the seed-bud crowned by the flower-cup.

Co-ro'ne.* [Gr. κορώνη, a "crow," any thing curved like a crow's beak.] The acute process of the lower jawbone,—so named from its supposed resemblance to a crow's bill.

Cor'o-ner. [From *coro'na*, a "crown."] Originally an officer who had authority from the Crown to make inquest before a jury of twelve, as to the true cause of death, in every case of sudden decease. The word was formerly written *Crowner.*

Cor'o-noid. [**Coronoi'des;** from κορώνη, a "crow," and εἶδος, a "form."] Applied to processes of bones in any way like a crow's beak. Applied by

Owen to the subdivision in the mandible of reptiles, into which the crotaphite muscle is always more or less inserted.

Co-ron'u-la.* [Diminutive of *coro'na*, a "crown."] A coronet or downy tuft surrounding the seeds of certain flowers. A cor'onule.

Cor'po-ra,* gen. **Cor'po-rum,** the plural of CORPUS, which see.

Cor'pora Albican'tia* (ăl-be-kan'-she-a). (The "Whitish Bodies." See ALBICANS.) Two small protuberances on the base of the brain. Called also Mammillary Tubercles or Mammillary Bodies, from their resemblance to a nipple.

Corpora Amylacea. See NEUROGLIA.

Cor'pora Cav-er-no'sa.* ("Cavernous Bodies;" so called from the cavities or cells found in them.) The *crura* of the penis. Also, the same part or parts of the *Clitoris*. As the *Corpora cavernosa* are only partially separated, it is more correct to call this portion of the organ the *Corpus cavernosum* ("Cavernous Body").

Cor'pora Gen-ic-u-la'ta.* [From *genicula'tus*, "jointed" or "bent like a knee."] Two tubercles, *internum* and *externum*, on the inferior part of the optic *thalami*.

Cor'pora Lu'te-a.* ("Yellow Bodies.") Yellow spots found in the *ovaria*, in place of *ova*, removed by impregnation or otherwise.

Cor'pora Mam-mil-la'ri-a.* The CORPORA ALBICANTIA, which see.

Cor'pora Ol-ĭ-va'ri-a* ("Olive-shaped Bodies"), **Cor'pora O-va'ta*** ("Oval Bodies"). The two external oval prominences on the *Medulla oblongata*.

Cor'pora Pўr-am'ĭ-da'lĭ-a.* ("Pyramidal Bodies.") The two anterior eminences of the *Medulla oblongata*.

Corpora Quadrigemina. See TUBERCULA QUADRIGEMINA.

Cor'pora Res-tĭ-for'mĭ-a.*("Rope-like Bodies.") The two posterior oval eminences on the *Medulla oblongata*.

Corpora Sesamoidea. See ARANTII, CORPORA.

Cor'pora Stri-a'ta.* ("Striated Bodies.") Two smooth cineritious convexities, one on the fore part of each lateral ventricle of the brain. When cut, a mixture of gray and white matter in alternate layers is exhibited, causing a striated appearance.

Corpulency. See POLYSARCIA.

Cor'pus,* gen. **Cor'po-ris.** (Fr. *Corps*, KOR.) A Latin word signifying BODY, which see.

Cor'pus An-nu-la're.* The *Pons Varolii*.

Cor'pus Cal-lo'sum.* ("Callous Body" or Substance.) The white medullary substance joining the hemispheres of the brain; the *Commissura magna*.

Corpus Cavernosum. See CORPORA CAVERNOSA.

Cor'pus Ci-ne're-um* ("Ash-colored Body"), or **Cor'pus Den-ta'tum*** ("Dentated Body"). A small oval mass of gray substance seen on a section of either hemisphere of the *cerebellum*, about an inch from the median line. On its circumference are a number of indentations.

Cor'pus Fim-bri-a'tum.* ("Fringed Body.") A narrow white band along the concave edge of the inferior *cornu* of the lateral ventricle of the brain; the *Tænia hippocampi*.

Cor'pus Glan-du-lo'sum.* ("Glandulous Body.") A spongy eminence surrounding the orifice of the female urethra; sometimes called the "female prostate gland" (*Glan'dula pros'tata mulie'bris*).

Corpus Mucosum. See RETE MUCOSUM.

Cor'pus Pam-pĭn-ĭ-for'me.* ("Tendril-like Body.") A plexus formed by the spermatic veins, above the *testis*.

Corpus Psaloides.* The *Fornix*. See FORNIX.

Corpus Pyramidale. See CORPUS PAMPINIFORME.

Corpus Reticulare, or **Corpus Reticulare Malpighi.** See RETE MUCOSUM.

Corpus Rhomboideum. See CORPUS DENTATUM.

Corpus Spongiosum Penis. See next article.

Cor'pus Spon-gĭ-o'sum U-re'-thræ.* ("Spongy Body [or Substance] of the Urethra.") A cellular, vascular, dark-red, or purple substance, which covers the urethra.

Cor'pus Văr-ĭ-co'sum.* ("Varicose Body.") The spermatic plexus.

Cor'pus-çle. [**Corpus'culum;** diminutive of *cor'pus*.] A small body; an atom.

Cor-pus'cu-lar. [**Corpuscula'ris;** from *corpus'culum*, a "corpuscle" or "minute body."] Belonging to a corpuscle, or to the doctrine of atoms.

Cor'ri-gens.* [The present participle of *cor'rigo, correc'tum*, to "correct."] A constituent part of a medicinal formula; "that which corrects its operation." See PRESCRIPTION.

Cor-rob'o-rant. [**Corrob'orans;** from *corrob'oro*, to "strengthen."] Strengthening, or giving strength.

Cor-ro'sive. [**Corrosi'vus;** from *cor* for *con*, intensive, and *ro'do, ro'sum*, to "gnaw," to "eat away."] Literally, "eating away." Destroying the texture or substance of a body, more especially of a living body.

Corrosive Sublimate. See HYDRARGYRI CHLORIDUM CORROSIVUM.

Cor'ru-găt-ed. [**Corruga'tus;** from *cor* for *con*, "together," or intensive, and *ru'go, ruga'tum*, to "wrinkle."] Wrinkled.

Cor-ru-gā'tion. [**Corruga'tio;** from the same.] The contraction of the surface of a body into wrinkles.

Cor-ru-ga'tor, o'ris.* [From the same.] Literally, a "wrinkler." Applied to a muscle which contracts the skin into wrinkles.

Corruga'tor Su-per-cil'ĭ-i.* ("Wrinkler of the Brow.") The muscle which knits or contracts the brow into wrinkles.

Corselet, kors'lęt. In Entomology, the *Prothorax*, collar, or anterior segment of the trunk.

Cort. = *Cor'tex.** "Bark."

Cor'tex,* gen. **Cor'tĭ-çis.** [As if *Con'tex;* from *con'tego*, to "cover over."] (Fr. *Écorce*, à'korss'.) The outermost covering of the stem and branches of all plants, analogous to the skin of animals.

Cor'tex Cĕr'e-bri.* (The "Cortex, or Cortical Substance, of the Brain.") The gray or cineritious substance found on the exterior of the cerebrum and cerebellum, covering the whitish medullary matter beneath as the bark of a tree covers the alburnum.

Cor'tex Cu-lĭ-la'wan.* The name for the bark of the *Laurus culilawan.*

Cor'tex E-leŭ-the'rĭ-æ. The bark of the *Croton cascarilla.*

Cor'tĭ-cal. [**Cortica'lis;** from *cor'tex, cor'ticis*, "bark."] Belonging to bark; of the nature of bark. Applied to that which covers a part, as the cortical portion of the brain or the kidneys.

Cor'tĭ-cate. [**Cortica'tus;** from *cor'tex*, "bark."] Having bark; barked.

Cor-tĭ-çif'er-ous. [**Corticif'erus;** from *cor'tex*, "bark," and *fe'ro*, to "bear."] Bearing, or producing, bark.

Cor-tiç'ĭ-form. [**Corticifor'mis;** from *cor'tex*, "bark."] Appearing like bark.

Cor'tĭ-cōse. [**Cortico'sus;** from *cor'tex*, "bark."] Having bark, or full of bark.

Corylaceæ,* kŏr-e-la'she-ē. [From *Cor'ylus*, the "hazel-tree."] A name given by Lindley to a natural order of plants. See CUPULIFERÆ.

Cŏr'y̆mb. [**Corym'bus;** from κόρυς, the "crown of the head."] A kind of spike, the partial flower-stalks of which are gradually longer, so that all the flowers are nearly on a level at the top.

Cor'y̆m-bif'er-æ.* [From *corym'bus*, a "corymb," and *fe'ro*, to "bear."] A name given by Jussieu to a division of the order *Compositæ*, including the Aster.

Cor-y̆m-bif'er-ous. [**Corymbif'erus;** from *corym'bus*, a "corymb," and *fe'ro*, to "bear."] Bearing corymbs.

Co-ry'za.* [Supposed to be derived from κάρα, the "head," and ζέω, to "boil."] A limpid, ropy, mucous defluxion from the nostrils.

Co-se'cant. The secant of the complement of an arc. See SECANT.

Cos-met'ic. [**Cosmet'icus;** from κοσμέω, to "adorn."] Applied to medicines supposed to have the power of removing freckles and blotches. Many substances used as cosmetics—such as lead, bismuth, and arsenic—sometimes give rise to cutaneous affections, and often cause a permanent deterioration in the texture of the skin.

Cos-mog'o-ny̆. [**Cosmogo'nia;** from κόσμος, the "universe," and γονή, "birth," "origin."] That science which treats of the origin of the universe.

Cos-mog'ra-phy̆. [**Cosmogra'phia;** from κόσμος, the "universe," and γράφω, to "write."] A description of the universe.

Cos-mol'o-gy̆. [**Cosmolo'gia;** from κόσμος, the "universe," and λόγος, a "discourse."] The doctrine or science of the universe, its formation and arrangement.

Cos'ta.* A rib. (Fr. *Côte*, kōt.) The ribs are twenty-four in number,—twelve on each side. The spaces between them are called intercostal spaces. The ribs are divided into—

1. The *true*, or *sterno-vertebral.* The first seven pairs; so called because they are united by their cartilages to the sternum: these are called *custo'des*, or preservers of the heart.

2. The *false*, or *vertebral*. The remaining five pairs, which are successively united to the lowest true rib and to each other.

The vertebral extremity of a rib is called the *head;* the contracted part which adjoins it forms the *neck;* at the back of the rib is the *tubercle;* farther outward the bone bends forward, producing the *angle,* from which proceeds the *body,* which passes forwards and downwards to the sternal extremity.

The term *costa,* or rib, is applied in Botany to the tapering, nerve-like substance extending from the base to the apex of a leaf.

Cos'tal. [**Costa'lis;** from *cos'ta,* a "rib."] Belonging to a rib or ribs.

Cos'tate. [**Costa'tus;** from *cos'ta,* a "rib."] Furnished with nerves or ribs.

Costiveness. See CONSTIPATION.

Cos'to-. [From *cos'ta,* a "rib."] A prefix in compound names, denoting connection with a rib or ribs.

Cotangent. See TANGENT.

Côte. See COSTA.

Cotton-Plant. See GOSSYPIUM.

Cotton-Tree. See BOMBAX.

Cotula. See MAYWEED.

Cotunnii Aquæductus, or **Cotunnius, Aqueduct of.** See AQUEDUCT OF THE VESTIBULUM.

Co-tun'nĭ-us, Nerve of. The nasopalatine nerve.

Cotun'nius, Wa'ter of. A fluid within the membrane lining the vestibule and semicircular canals of the internal ear.

Cot-y̆-le'don, o'n*is.** [Gr. κοτυληδών; from κοτύλη, a "cavity."] In Botany, the seed-lobe, or seminal leaf, of a young plant, perishing as the plant grows up. In *dicotyledonous* plants (in the *bean,* for example) the cotyledon consists of one-half of the seed, which, on germinating, divides into two equal parts.

Cot-y̆-led'on-ous. [**Cotyledo'neus, Cotyle'donus;** from *cotyle'don.*] Belonging to cotyledons; having cotyledons.

Cot'y̆-loid. [**Cotyloi'des;** from κοτύλη, a "small drinking-cup."] Resembling an ancient drinking-cup.

Cot'yloid Cav'ĭ-ty̆. The same as ACETABULUM, which see.

Cou, koo. A French word signifying "neck." See COLLUM.

Couche, koosh. [From *coucher,* to "lie down," to "go to bed;" also, to "put to bed."] A French term signifying "child-bed," "confinement," or "delivery:" e.g. *une couche heureuse,* ün koosh uh'ruz', "a happy delivery."

Couch'ing. (Fr. *Coucher,* to "put to bed," to "cause to lie down;" because the lens is pushed down from its upright position.) The operation of putting down or displacing the opaque lens in cataract.

Couch'ing-Nee'dle. The instrument used in couching.

Cough, kof, or kawf. [Lat. **Tus'sis;** Fr. *Toux,* too.] A sonorous and violent expulsion of air from the lungs.

Couleur, koo'lur'. The French word for COLOR, which see.

Coumarin, or **Coumarine,** koo'-mą-rin. The odoriferous principle of the Tonka bean, the produce of the *Coumarou'na odora'ta.*

Counter-Extension. See CONTRA-EXTENSIO.

Counter-Fissure. See CONTRA-FISSURA.

Counter-Indication. See CONTRA-INDICATIO.

Coun'ter-Ir-rĭ-tā'tion. [**Con'tra-Irrita'tio.**] The application of a blister or other irritating substance to one part for the purpose of relieving pain in another part, usually beneath or adjacent to the irritated surface.

Counter-Opening. See CONTRA-APERTURA.

Counter-Stroke. See CONTRE-COUP.

Coup de Sang, koo dẹh sŏnᵍ. Blood-stroke. A term used by some French physicians to designate an instantaneous and universal congestion without any escape of blood from the vessels. (See APOPLEXY.) Some authors have applied this name to hæmorrhages occurring in different parts of the body.

Coup de Soleil (Fr.), koo dẹh so'lēl (or so'lāl'). A stroke of the sun; generally, any affection produced by a scorching sun.

Coup de Vent (Fr.), koo dẹh vŏnᵍ. A stroke of the wind; an affection caused by exposure to a keen wind, extremely cold, or with rain or sleet.

Couperosé (Fr.), koop'ro'zā'. ("Copper-colored.") A term applied to the *Acne rosacea* (or carbuncled face); so named from the redness of the spots.

Courap, koo'răp'. A form of impetigo peculiar to India, described by Sauvages under the term *Scabies Indica.*

Couronne, koo'ronn'. The French

word for "crown." See CORONA, and CROWN.

Cours'es. A popular English term for the *menses*, or *catamenia*.

Couvrechef (Fr.), koov'R'shĕf'. (Literally, "head-cover.") A name given to certain forms of bandage applied to the head.

Cow'hage, Cow'-Itch. The down covering the pods of the *Dol'ichos pru'riens*, now called *Mucu'na pru'riens*. See MUCUNA.

Cow'-Pox. [**Vacci'nia.**] Pustules of a peculiar character on the teats of the cow, from which the vaccine fluid derives its origin.

Cowper's Glands. See ANTIPROSTATÆ GLANDULÆ.

Cox'a,* plural **Cox'æ.** (Fr. *Hanche*, hŏNsh.) The hip, haunch, or hip-joint; also, the *Ischium* and *Coccyx*. Applied in Zoology to the first articulation of the feet of the *Crustacea*, *Arachnides*, and *Insecta*.

Cox-æ-lu'vĭ-um.* [From *cox'a*, the "hip," and *la'vo*, or *lu'o*, to "wash."] A bath for the lower portion of the body; a hip-bath.

Cox-ăl'ġĭ-a.* [From *cox'a*, the "hip," and ἄλγος, "pain."] Pain in the hip-joint; hip-joint disease, or *Mor'bus coxa'rius*.

Cox-a'rĭ-us.* [From *cox'a*, the "hip."] Belonging to the hip-joint.

Cox-a'rum,* the genitive plural of COXA, which see.

COXA'RUM MOR'BUS.* ("Disease of the Hips.") A caries of the head of the os femoris, causing a permanent shortening of the limb, and often accompanied with spontaneous luxation of the bone.

Cox'o-. A prefix denoting connection with the *Ischium*.

Crab's Claws and **Crab's Stones.** See CANCRORUM LAPILLI ET CHELÆ.

Crab-Louse. See PEDICULUS PUBIS.

Crack Wil'low. See SALIX FRAGILIS.

Cra'dle. [**Ar'culus.**] A kind of frame for keeping the bedclothes off a wounded or fractured limb.

Cramp. [Low Latin **Cram'pus;** Ger. *Krampf*.] Spasmodic and involuntary contraction of muscles. See SPASMUS.

Crā'nĭ-al. [**Crania'lis.**] Belonging to the *cranium*.

Crā-nĭ-og'ra-phy̆. [**Craniogra'phia;** from *cra'nium*, and γράφω, to "write."] A description of the skull.

Crā-nĭ-ol'o-ġy̆. [**Craniolo'gia;** from *cra'nium*, and λόγος, a "discourse."] The science which treats of skulls in regard to their variety of shape, size, proportions, etc.

Crā-nĭ-om'e-ter. [**Craniom'etrum;** from *cra'nium*, and μέτρον, a "measure."] An instrument for measuring the *cranium*.

Crā-nĭ-ot'o-my̆. [**Cranioto'mia;** from *cra'nium*, and τέμνω, to "cut."] The opening of the fœtal head, where necessary, to effect delivery.

Cra'nĭ-um.* [Gr. κρανίον; from κάρα, or κάρηνον, the "head."] The skull, or upper part of the head, containing the brain and its connections, and consisting of eight bones.

Craquement Pulmonaire (Fr.), kråk'mōN' pül'mo'nêR'. A crackling sound often heard at the top of the lungs in the early stage of phthisis.

Cras. = *Cras'tinum,** or *Cras'tinus.** "For to-morrow."

Cras-sa-men'tum.* [From *cras'sus*, "thick."] The soft, almost solid, mass, of a deep brownish red, formed by venous blood soon after it has been extracted.

Crassulaceæ,* kras-su-la'she-ē [from *Cras'sula*, one of the genera], or **Semper-vi'væ.*** A natural order of plants, growing in hot and dry situations, remarkable for the succulent nature of their stems and leaves. The *Sedum majus*, or *Semper vivum* ("Live-forever"), is a good example of this order.

Cra'ter, e'ris.* [Gr. κρατήρ, a "bowl."] Literally, a "cup" or "bowl;" usually applied to the mouth of a volcano.

Cra-tĕr'ĭ-form. [**Craterifor'mis;** from the same.] Formed like a bowl.

Craw. The crop of a bird. See CROP.

Craw'-Fish, or **Cray'-Fish.** The *Cancer astacus*, or *C. fluviatilis*.

Crēam of Lime. A mixture of lime and water used for purifying coal gas, by its property of absorbing or combining with the contaminating gases.

Cream of Tar'tar. [**Cre'mor Tar'tari.**] Bitartrate, or supertartrate, of potash. See POTASSÆ BITARTRAS.

Cre'a-sōte, or **Kre'a-sōte.** [**Creaso'tum;** from κρέας, "flesh," and σώζω, to "preserve."] A colorless, brilliantly transparent liquid, obtained from crude pyroligneous acid, and from wood tar. It is irritant, narcotic, styptic, powerfully antiseptic, and somewhat escharotic. Its use internally has been recommended in cholera, sea-sickness, and other affections of the stomach and bowels. In large doses, it is a dangerous poison. It has been employed externally with great advantage in some cutaneous affections, and especially in malignant ulcers. The editor of this work has used it with the happiest effects in indolent and malignant ulcers resulting from chilblain, after all the other remedies usually recommended in such cases had failed.

Cre'asote Wa'ter. [**A'qua Creaso'ti.**] Take of creasote a fluidrachm; distilled water a pint. Mix them, and agitate the mixture till the creasote is dissolved. (U.S. Ph., 1860.)

Cre'a-tin, or **Cre'a-tine.** [**Creati'na;** from κρέας, κρέατος, "flesh."] A nitrogenized crystallizable substance. A neutral body obtained from a fluid produced by mixing chopped animal muscle with an equal bulk of water, and subjecting this, in a bag, to strong pressure. It does not combine with either acids or alkalies. Also spelled *Kreatin.*

Cre-at'i-nin, or **Cre-at'i-nine.** [**Creatini'na.**] An alkaline base into which *Creatin* is changed by heating with hydrochloric or other acids. Also spelled *Kreatinin.*

Creep'ing Sick'ness. (Ger. *Kriebelkrankheit,* krē'bel-krånk'hīt.) The name by which the gangrenous form of Ergotism is known in Germany. See ERGOTISM.

Cre-mas'ter.* [From κρεμάω, to "suspend."] A muscle which supports and compresses the testicle and spermatic vessels. See SPERMATIC CORD.

Cre'mor, o'ris.* [From κρίμνον, the "thick juice of barley."] Cream; any substance skimmed from the surface of a fluid; also, a thick decoction of barley.

Cre'nate. [**Crena'tus;** from *cre'na,* a "notch."] Notched; scolloped.

Cren'u-lāt-ed. [**Crenula'tus;** from *cren'ula,* a "little notch."] Having small notches.

Crep'i-tant. [**Crep'itans.** See next article.] Crackling, or rattling.

Crep-i-tā'tion. [**Crepita'tio, o'nis;** from *crep'ito, crepita'tum,* to "crackle."] The sound caused by pressing any portion of cellular tissue, in which air is collected, between the fingers. Also, the noise produced by the act of grating the ends of a fractured bone together. See CREPITUS.

Crep'i-tus.* [From *cre'po, crep'itum,* to "make a noise."] The discharge of gas or flatus from the bowels. The crackling noise occasioned by pressing a part when air is collected in the cellular tissue. The grating sensation produced by the ends of a fractured bone being rubbed against each other.

Crescentiaceæ,* krĕs-sen-she-a'-she-ē or krĕs-sen-te-a'she-ē, or **Crĕs-çen-tin'e-æ.*** A natural order of exogenous trees, natives of the tropical regions of Asia, Africa, and America. The chief plant of this order is the Calabash-tree, *Crescen'tia* (krĕs-sen'she-a) *cuje'te,* producing an esculent fruit in a shell which is used as a bottle.

Crest. [**Cris'ta.**] Applied to several objects which surmount others.

Crest'ed. [**Crista'tus.**] Having a crest.

Cre'ta.* [From *Cre'ta,* the island of Crete.] (Fr. *Craie,* krå.) Chalk. The Pharmacopœial name (Ed. and U.S. Ph.) for native friable carbonate of lime.

Cre'ta Præp-a-ra'ta.* ("Prepared Chalk.") The Pharmacopœial name (Br. Ph.) for chalk finely pulverized by levigation.

Cre-tā'ceous. [**Creta'ceus;** from *cre'ta,* "chalk."] Of the nature of chalk; chalky.

Cre'ti-nism. [**Cretinis'mus;** etymology uncertain.] An endemic disease common in Switzerland and other mountainous countries, characterized by *goître,* stinted growth, swelled abdomen, wrinkled skin, wan complexion, vacant and stupid countenance, misshapen cranium, idiocy, and comparative insensibility.

Crī-brā'tion. [**Cribra'tio, o'nis;** from *cri'bro, cribra'tum,* to "sift" (from *crib'rum,* a "sieve").] The act or process of sifting, or passing through a sieve.

Crib'rĭ-form. [**Cribrifor'mis;** from *crib'rum,* a "sieve."] Perforated like a sieve.

Cri'co-. A prefix denoting attachment to the cricoid cartilage.

Crī'coid. [**Cricoi'des** and **Cricoi'deus;** from κρίκος, a "ring," and εἶδος, a "form."] Resembling a ring.

Crī'coid Car'tĭ-lage. [**Cartila'go Cricoi'des.**] The name given to one of the cartilages of the larynx.

Criminal Abortion. See FŒTICIDE.

Crī'nate. [**Crina'tus;** from *cri'nis.*] Having hair.

Crī'nis.* [From κρίνω, to "distinguish"?] The hair of the head, especially of the back part. See CAPILLUS.

Crī'noid. [**Crinoi'des;** from κρίνον, a "lily," and εἶδος, a "form."] Resembling a lily.

Crinones. See MALIS GORDII.

Cri'sis.* [Gr. κρίσις; from κρίνω, to "distinguish," to "judge," to "decide."] Literally, a "judgment," "decision," or "determination." In the course of a disease, that point or period which determines its favorable or unfavorable termination, or, in common language, its "turning-point."

Cris-pa'tus,* Cris'pus.* [From *cris'po, crispa'tum,* to "curl."] Curled; crisp.

Cris'ta.* A crest. Applied in Anatomy to parts or processes of bones resembling a crest. In Botany it denotes a peculiar organ of the *Gramineæ.* Applied in Surgery to an excrescence about the *anus* and *pudenda.*

Cris'ta Gal'li.* ("Cock's Crest.") The peculiar process on the ethmoid bone to which the *falx cerebri* is attached.

Cris'tate. [**Crista'tus;** from *cris'ta.*] Having a crest; crested.

Crit'i-cal. [**Crit'icus;** from *cri'sis,* "decision" or "determination."] Determining the issue of a disease. Also applied to periods of life as decisive of certain changes of constitution, habits, etc. See CRISIS.

Crit'ical Age. [**Æ'tas Crit'ica.**] That period of female life when the *catamenia* become irregular, and ultimately cease. It is often attended with serious constitutional disturbance, and is sometimes the commencement of fatal diseases. See CHANGE OF LIFE.

Croc-o-dil'i-dæ.* [From κροκόδειλος, the "crocodile."] A family of Saurian reptiles, having the crocodile for their type.

Cro'cus.* [Gr. κρόκος, "saffron."] A Linnæan genus of the class *Triandria,* natural order *Iridaceæ* or *Irideæ.* The Pharmacopœial name ‖ for the prepared stigmas of the *Crocus sativus.*

Cro'cus Sa-ti'vus.* The systematic name of the saffron-plant; also called *Crocus officinalis.*

Crop. [**Inglu'vies.**] An enlargement of the *œsophagus* in birds; the craw.

Cross Birth. [**Parodyn'ia Perver'sa.**] In popular language, preternatural labor of any kind.

Crot'a-lus.* [From κρόταλον, a "rattle."] The rattlesnake; a genus of poisonous snakes found in North America.

Crot'a-phe,* or **Cro-ta'phi-um.*** [From κρόταφος, the "temple of the head."] A painful pulsation or throbbing in the temple, accompanied with drumming in the ears.

Crot'chet. (Fr. *Crochet,* kro'shà', a "hook.") A curved instrument for extracting the fœtus.

Cro'ton, o'nis.* [Gr. κρότων, the "dog-tick," which the seeds of some plants of this genus are fancied to resemble.] A Linnæan genus of the class *Monœcia,* natural order *Euphorbiaceæ.*

CRO'TON CASCARIL'LA,* or CRO'TON ELEUTHE'RIA* (or ELEUTE'RIA*). The plant believed to afford Cascarilla bark.

CRO'TON TIG'LIUM.* The plant from the seeds of which croton oil is obtained. It is a small tree or shrub, growing native in Hindostan and the East India islands. See OLEUM TIGLII.

Cro'ton-āte. [**Croto'nas, a'tis.**] A combination of crotonic acid with a base.

Cro-to'ne.* [Gr. κροτώνη; from κροτών, a "kind of tick."] Originally, a fungous excrescence on trees, caused by an insect (κροτών). Now usually applied to small fungous excrescences on the periosteum.

Cro-ton'ic Aç'id. An acid obtained from the acrid matter of croton oil.

Croton Oil. See OLEUM TIGLII.

Crotophus. See CROTAPHE.

Croup, kroop. [**Cynan'che Trachea'lis.**] A disease marked by laborious and suffocative breathing, with a stridulous noise, short, dry cough, and expectoration of a concrete membranous sputum.

Cru'cial. [**Crucia'lis;** from *crux,* a "cross."] Belonging to a cross.

Cru'cial In-cis'ion. Two incisions made to cross each other.

Cru'ci-ble. [**Crucib'ulum;** from *cru'cio,* to "torture."] A vessel made of baked earth, or metal, used as a receptacle for substances to be fused or exposed to a great heat.

Cru-cif'er-æ.* [From *crux, cru'cis,* a "cross," and *fe'ro,* to "bear." See next article.] A natural order of Exogens: they are said to possess universally antiscorbutic and stimulant properties, and their seeds abound in a fixed oil. Mustard may be taken as a representative of this order.

Cru-cif'er-us.* [From *crux, cru'cis,* a "cross," and *fe'ro,* to "bear."] Crucif'erous. Literally, "bearing a cross." Applied to plants whose flowers are in the form of a cross. See CRUCIFERÆ.

Cru'ci-form. [**Crucifor'mis;** from *crux, cru'cis,* a "cross."] Like a cross.

Cru'di-tÿ. [**Cru'ditas, a'tis;** from *cru'dus,* "raw."] Bad digestion; rawness.

Cru'els. (Fr. *Écrouelles*, ȧ'kroo'ĕll', "scrofula.") Popularly, scrofulous swellings of the glands of the neck.

Cru'or, o'ris.* The red or purplish colored portion of the blood.

Cru'ra,* gen. **Cru'rum,** the plural of Crus, which see.

Cru'ra Cĕr-e-bel'li.* (The "Legs or Limbs of the Cerebellum.") Two white cords, extending one along the circumference of each hemisphere of the *cerebellum.*

Cru'ra Cĕr'e-bri.* (The "Legs or Limbs of the Cerebrum.") Two thick white *fasciculi,* one from the inferior surface of each hemisphere of the *cerebrum.*

Cru'ra Di-a-phrag'ma-tis.* ("Legs of the Diaphragm.") Two appendices situated behind and below the central tendon of the diaphragm.

Cru-ræ'us.* [From *crus, cru'ris,* a "leg."] Belonging to the leg. The name of a muscle of the leg.

Cru'ral. [**Crura'lis;** from *crus, cru'ris,* a "leg."] Belonging to the leg; applied also to the cruræus muscle.

Cru'ral Arch. Otherwise called Fallopius' or Poupart's ligament. See Poupart's Ligament.

Crural Hernia. See Hernia Cruralis.

Crus,* gen. **Cru'ris,** plural **Cru'ra.** [From κρούω, to "kick."] (Fr. *Jambe,* zhŏmb, and *Cuisse,* kwèss.) The leg. Applied to symmetrical projections or appendages, as the *Crus* of either hemisphere; in other words, the *Crura* of the cerebrum.

Crŭs'ta.* (Literally, a "crust.") The external cover or shell in the *Mollusca, Crustacea,* and in certain insects. Also, a scab.

Crustacea, krŭs-ta'she-a, or **Crustaceans,** krŭs-tā'shŭnz. See next article.

Crustaceus,* krŭs-ta'she-ŭs. [From *crus'ta,* a "crust."] Crusta'ceous. Having a hard shell. Applied in the plural neuter (*Crusta'cea*) to a class of *Articulata* in which the envelop, or crust, is usually solid and more or less calcareous.

Cry-oph'o-rus.* [From κρύος, "cold," and φέρω, to "bear," to "produce."] Literally, "cold-producing." An instrument in which water is made to freeze by the cold produced by its own evaporation.

Crȳp'ta,* plural **Crȳp'tæ.** [From κρύπτω, to "hide."] Small round points at the end of the minute arteries of the cortical substance of the kidneys: also, a follicle, or follicular gland.

Crȳp-to-çeph'a-lus.* [From κρυπτός, "concealed," "obscure," and κεφαλή, a "head."] A monster-fœtus, in which the head is very small and does not project from the trunk.

Crȳp-to-ga'mĭ-a.* [See next article.] The twenty-fourth class of plants in the system of Linnæus. It comprises all flowerless plants. (See Cryptogamius.) All other plants are included under a second grand division, called Phanerogamia.

Crȳp-to-ga'mĭ-us.* [From κρυπτός, "hidden," or "obscure" (from κρύπτω, to "hide"), and γάμος, "nuptials."] Literally, denoting plants "whose marriage is obscure or doubtful." Applied by Linnæus to a class whose parts of fructification have not been sufficiently ascertained to refer them to any class according to the sexual system.

Crȳp-tor'chis.* [From κρυπτός, "concealed," and ὄρχις, a "testicle."] One whose testicles have not descended into the scrotum.

Crȳp'tous. [**Cryp'tus;** from κρύπτω, to "hide."] Hidden, or concealed.

Crȳs'tal. [Lat. **Crystal'lum,** or **Crystal'lus;** Gr. κρύσταλλος, "ice;" properly, "clear ice."] A hard, bright, transparent substance, like ice or the clearest glass. The geometrical figures assumed by crystallizable bodies when they pass from a fluid to a solid state.

Crȳs'tal-lin, or **Crȳs'tal-line.** [**Crystalli'na;** from *crystal'lum,* "crystal."] A peculiar substance forming the basis of the crystalline lens of the eye. Also, one of the products of the distillation of indigo.

Crȳs'tal-line. [**Crystalli'nus;** from the same.] Belonging to crystal; like crystal.

Crys'talline Lens. A transparent, double convex lens situated in the fore part of the vitreous humor of the eye. It was formerly often called the *crystalline humor* of the eye.

Crȳs-tal-lĭ-zā'tion. [**Crystalliza'tio, o'nis;** from *crystal'lum,* "crystal."] A property by which crystallizable substances pass from a fluid to a solid state, assuming certain determinate geometrical figures.

Crystalliza'tion, Wa'ter of. That portion of water which combines with salts in the act of crystallizing, and which cannot be removed without destroying their crystalline structure.

Crȳs-tal-log'ra-phȳ. [**Crystallogra'phia;** from *crystal'lum,* a "crystal," and γράφω, to "write."] A description of crystals.

Crys'tal-loid. [**Crystalloi'des;** from *crystal'lum,* a "crystal," and εἶδος, a "form."] Resembling crystal.

Ctenoid, te'noid. [**Ctenoi'des;** from κτείς, κτενός, a "comb," and εἶδος, a "form."] Resembling a comb. Applied to an order of fishes with dentated scales.

Cu (Fr.), kü. See ALULA.

Cūbe. [Lat. **Cu'bus;** Gr. κύβος.] A solid bounded by six equal squares at right angles with each other.

Cu-be'ba.* [From the Arabic *Cuba'-bah.*] Cubeb, or Cubebs. The Pharmacopœial name for the berries of the *Piper cubeba.*

Cu-be'bæ* ("Cubebs"), the plural of CUBEBA, which see.

Cu-be'bin. [**Cubebi'na;** from *Cube'ba.*] A crystalline substance obtained from cubebs.

Cu'bebs. In the plural, the English term for the berries of the *Piper cubeba.* See CUBEBA.

Cu-bĭ-for'mis.* [From *cu'bus.*] Having the form of a cube: cu'biform.

Cu-bĭ-tæ'us.* Pertaining to the *Cubit,* or fore-arm.

Cu'bĭ-tal. [**Cubita'lis;** from *cu'-bitus.*] Belonging to the fore-arm.

Cu'bĭ-tus.* [From *cu'bo,* to "lie down."] (Fr. *Coude,* kood.) The fore-arm, extending between the elbow and wrist; also, the *ulna,* or *Os cubiti.*

Cu'boid. [**Cuboi'des;** from κύβος, a "cube," and εἶδος, a "form."] Like a cube.

Cuc'koo-Flow'er. The *Cardamine pratensis.*

Cu-cul-la'ris.* [From *cucul'lus,* a "hood."] Like a hood.

Cu'cul-late. [**Cuculla'tus;** from *cucul'lus,* a "hood."] Hooded.

Cu'cum-ber. The fruit of different species of *Cucumis.*

Cu'cumber, Bit'ter. The fruit of the *Citrullus colocynthis.* See COLOCYNTHIS.

Cu'cumber, Squirt'ing, Cu'cumber, Wild. The *Momordica elaterium.*

Cu'cu-mer,* Cu'cu-mis.* A Linnæan genus of the class *Monœcia,* natural order *Cucurbitaceæ.*

Cu'cumis A-gres'tis,* Cu'cumis As-ĭ-ni'nus.* The *Momordica elaterium.*

Cu'cumis Col-o-çy̆n'this.* The former name of the plant which yields colocynth: now called *Citrullus colocynthis.*

Cucurb. cruent. = CUCURBITULA CRUENTA, which see.

Cu-cur'bĭ-ta.* [From *cur'vo,* to "curve," or "bend."] Literally, a "gourd." A distilling vessel shaped like a gourd: a cu'curbit. Also, a cupping-glass. See CUCURBITULA.

Cucurbitaceæ,* ku-kŭr-be-ta'she-ē. [From *cucur'bita,* a "gourd."] A natural order, comprising the melon, cucumber, gourd, and other valuable plants. They are most abundant in hot and tropical climates. The fruits of many species of *cucumis* are powerfully cathartic. The *colocynth* is one of the most valuable medicines derived from this order.

Cu-cur-bĭ-tā'ceous. [**Cucurbita'-ceus;** from *cucur'bita,* a "gourd."] Having an arrangement as in the *Cucurbita.* See CUCURBITACEÆ.

Cu-cur-bit'u-la.* [Diminutive of *cucur'bita,* a "gourd."] A cupping-glass. (Fr. *Ventouse,* vŏnᴳ'tooz'.)

Cucurbit'ula Cru-en'ta* (a "Bloody Cupping-Glass," or one intended to draw blood), **Cucurbit'ula cum Fer'-ro*** ("Cupping-Glass [armed] with Iron"). A cupping-glass, with scarification. Names applied to the common cupping-glasses used for drawing blood, as distinguished from those employed in *dry* cupping.

Cucurbit'ula Sic'ca.* (A "Dry Cupping-Glass.") One used for dry cupping without scarification.

Cuisse (Fr.), kwėss. See FEMUR.

Cuivre (Fr.), kwėvr. See CUPRUM.

Cuj. = *Cu'jus.** "Of which."

Cujusl. = *Cujus'libet.** "Of any," or "of which you please."

Cul-de-Sac (Fr.), kül dęh sȧk. A tube or cavity closed at one end.

Cŭlm. [**Cul'mus;** from κάλαμος, a "reed."] A reed, or straw; the proper stem or trunk of grasses, rushes, etc.

Cŭl-mif'er-ous. [**Culmif'erus;** from *cul'mus,* "straw," a "culm," and *fe'ro,* to "bear."] Bearing or having culms.

Cul'mĭ-nāt-ing. [**Cul'minans;** from *cul'mino,* to "arrive at the top, or highest point."] Applied particularly to stars when at their highest point in the heavens.

Cul-trĭ-for'mis.* [From *cul'ter,* a "knife."] Formed like a knife: cul'-triform.

Cu-mi'num.* [Gr. κύμινον.] A Linnæan genus of the class *Pentandria,* natural order *Umbelliferæ.*

Cumi'num Çy-mi'num.* The plant *Cumin*, or *Fœnic'ulum Orienta'le.*

Cu'ne-al. [**Cunea'lis**; from *cu'neus*, a "wedge."] Belonging to a wedge.

Cu'ne-ate. [**Cunea'tus**; from *cu'neus*, a "wedge."] Wedge-shaped.

Cu'ne-ĭ-form. [**Cuneifor'mis**; from the same, and *for'ma*, "likeness."] Formed like a wedge.

Cunoniaceæ,* ku-no-ne-a'she-ē. [From *Cuno'nia*, one of the genera.] A natural order of exogenous trees and shrubs, found in India, South America, etc.

Cu'pel. [From *cupel'la*, a "cup."] A small vessel in which gold and silver are refined by melting them with lead.

Cu-pel-lā'tion. [**Cupella'tio, o**'*nis;* from the same.] The process of refining gold and silver by melting them in a cupel with lead.

Cu'po-lạ. The dome-like extremity of the canal of the cochlea. See COCHLEA.

Cup'ped. Applied to the hollowed surface of the *Crassamentum* of blood caused by inflammation.

Cup'ping. Application of *Cucurbitulæ*, or cupping-glasses.

Cupping Glass. See CUCURBITULA.

Cu-prif'er-ous. [**Cuprif'erus**; from *cu'prum*, "copper," and *fe'ro*, to "bear."] Bearing or containing copper.

Cu'prum,* gen. **Cu'pri.** [From Κύπρος, the island of Cyprus, where the ancients procured the best copper.] (Fr. *Cuivre*, kwėvr.) Copper, a red metal, malleable and ductile. Specific gravity 8.6.

CU'PRI ACE'TAS.* Acetate of copper, improperly called *distilled* or *crystallized verdigris.*

CU'PRI SUBACE'TAS.* ("Subacetate of Copper.") Verdigris. The *ærugo* of the London Pharmacopœia. It is sometimes used as an application to malignant ulcers, and as an escharotic for venereal warts.

CU'PRI SUL'PHAS.* The Pharmacopœial name ‖ of sulphate of copper, or blue *vitriol.* Its use in small doses has been recommended in diarrhœa; but it is chiefly employed as an external application for ill-conditioned ulcers, and as a styptic for bleeding surfaces.

Cu'pu-lạ.* (Literally, a "cup.") Applied in Botany to the cup or husk of certain plants,—*e.g.* the cup of an acorn, or husk of the hazel-nut. Also called a cu'pule.

Cu-pu-lif'er-æ.* [See next article.] A natural order of arborescent or shrubby Exogens, producing fruit enclosed in a cup or husk. It comprises the oak, beech, chestnut, hazel, etc. They abound in all, or nearly all, temperate climates. An astringent principle pervades all the order. This order is called *Corylaceæ* by Lindley.

Cu-pu-lif'er-us.* [From *cu'pula*, and *fe'ro*, to "bear."] Bearing *cupulæ:* cupulif'erous.

Cu-ra're Poi'son. A most deadly poison, obtained, it is said, from a plant belonging to the family *Strychniæ*. The South American Indians use it to poison their arrows.

Curatio,* ku-ra'she-o. [From *cu'ro, cura'tum*, to "take care" of, to "cure."] The *treatment* of a disease, or wound.

Cur-cu'mạ.* A Linnæan genus of the class *Monandria*, natural order *Zingiberaceæ*. The root is a stimulant aromatic, somewhat resembling ginger. It is much used in India as a condiment, and is one of the ingredients in curry. Also the Pharmacopœial name for the rhizoma of the *Curcu'ma lon'ga.*

Cur-cu'mạ Lon'gạ.* The turmeric-plant.

Curcu'ma Pa'per. Paper stained with a decoction of TURMERIC, which see.

Cur-cu'min. [From *Curcu'ma lon'ga*, the "turmeric-plant."] The coloring matter of turmeric obtained in a state of purity by separating it from its combination with oxide of lead.

Curd. The coagulum which separates from milk upon the addition of acid, rennet, or wine.

Cur'sor,* plural **Cur-so'rēs.** [From *cur'ro, cur'sum*, to "run."] Applied to a family of birds which run along the ground.

Cur-so'rĭ-us.* [From the same.] Applied in the plural neuter (*Curso'ria*) to a family of orthopterous insects with legs solely adapted for running.

Cuscutaceæ,* kŭs-ku-ta'she-ē. A natural order of exogenous parasitical plants, consisting of one genus, *Cuscu'ta.* It includes the common Dodder.

Cus-pa'rĭ-ạ.* A Linnæan genus of the class *Pentandria*, natural order *Diosmeæ.* Also the Pharmacopœial name (Brit. Ph.) of the bark of *Galipea cusparia*, or *G. officinalis.* See GALIPEA.

Cuspa'ria Fe-brif'u-gạ.* The tree supposed by some to yield Angustura bark, now called *Bonplandia trifoliata;* some refer it to the *Galipea cusparia*, or *G. officinalis.*

Cus-pĭ-da'tus.* [From *cus'pis, cus'pidis*, a "point."] Cus'pidate. Having a pointed extremity. Applied in the plural masculine (*Cuspida'ti*) to certain teeth (see DENTES CUSPIDATI).

Cu-ta'ne-ous. [**Cuta'neus;** from *cu'tis*, the "skin."] Belonging to the skin.

Cuta'neous Ab-sorp'tion. A function of the skin by which certain preparations rubbed into the skin have the same action as when given internally, only in a less degree. Thus, mercury, applied in this manner, cures syphilis and excites salivation, tartrate of antimony is said to occasion vomiting, and arsenic produces poisonous effects.

Cu-ta'ne-us Mus'cu-lus.* The *Platysma-myodes*, a muscle of the neck having the appearance of a very thin fleshy membrane.

Cu'tĭ-cle. [**Cutic'ula;** diminutive of *cu'tis*, the "skin."] The *Epidermis*, or scarf-skin.

Cu'tis.* [From σκυτίς or σκῦτος, a "skin" or "hide."] The skin consisting of the *Cutis vera*, *Rete mucosum*, and *Cuticula*.

Cu'tis An-ser-i'na.* ("Goose-skin.") That condition of the skin, produced by cold and other causes, in which the *papillæ* become rigid and erect, resembling the skin of a plucked goose.

Çȳ'a-nāte. [**Cy'anas, a'tis.**] A combination of cyanic acid with a base.

Çȳ-an'ic. [**Cyan'icus.**] Applied to an acid composed of cyanogen and oxygen.

Çȳ-an'o-gen. [From κύανος, "blue," and γεννάω, to "generate."] A peculiar principle composed of nitrogen and carbon, obtained by decomposing the cyanuret of mercury by heat. It is sometimes called *Prussin*, or *Prussine*.

Çy'a-no-pa-thi'a.* [From κύανος, "blue," and παθός, "affection," "disease."] "Blue disease;" another term for *Cyanosis*.

Çy-a-no'sis.* [From κύανος, "blue."] (Fr. *Cyanose*, sē'ā'nōz'.) A blue color of the skin, resulting from congenital malformation of the heart, by which venous and arterial blood are mixed so as to be not wholly oxygenated: the *Morbus cœruleus*.

Çȳ-an'ū-ret. [**Cyanure'tum;** from *cyanoge'nium*.] A combination of cyanogen with a base.

Çy-a-nu'ric. [**Cyanu'ricus.**] Belonging to cyanogen and urine; applied to an acid.

Çy-an'u-rin. [**Cyanuri'na;** from κύανος, "blue," and οὖρον, the "urine."] A very rare substance deposited as a blue powder by the urine.

Çy-ath-ĭ-for'mis.* [From *cy'athus*, a "cup."] Shaped like a cup: cy'athiform.

Çy'a-thus.* [From κύαθος, a "drinking-cup."] In prescriptions, it signifies a wine-glass.

Cycadaceæ,* sik-a-da'she-ē, or **Cyca'deæ.*** [From *Cy'cas*, *Cyc'adis*, one of the genera.] A small natural order of exogenous trees and shrubs, found in the tropics. Several plants of this order furnish starch and sago which are used for food. The Cycads were formerly classed with the Palms.

Cy'cas Cir-ci-na'lis.* An East Indian palm-tree, the central portion of which yields a kind of sago.

Çȳ'cle. [**Cy'clus;** from κύκλος, a "circle."] Applied to a revolution of the sun of twenty-eight years, and of the moon of nineteen years. A continual revolution of numbers which go on without interruption to the last, and then return to the first.

Çȳc'lĭ-cus.* [From κύκλος, a "circle."] Belonging to a cycle or circle: cyc'lic. Applied in the plural neuter (*Cyc'lica*) to a family of coleopterous insects in which the body is generally orbicular or oval.

Çȳc-lo-branch-ĭ-a'tus,* **Çȳc-lo-branch'ĭ-us.*** [From *cy'clus*, and *branchia'tus*, "having *branchiæ*."] Applied in the plural neuter (*Cyclobranchia'ta*) to an order of *Mollusca Gasteropoda*, in which the *branchiæ* form a circle: cyclobranch'iate, cyclobranch'ious.

Çȳc-lo-gan-glĭ-a'ta.* [From κύκλος, a "circle," and *ganglia'tus*, "furnished with ganglia," or "having ganglia."] A term applied by some naturalists to the fourth sub-kingdom of animals, or *Mollusca*, comprising animals mostly aquatic, slow-moving or fixed, without internal skeleton, covered with a permanent calcareous or cartilaginous shell, and distinguished by the high development of the cerebral ganglia and their circular distribution around the œsophagus. The classes are the *Tunicata*, *Conchifera*, *Gasteropoda*, *Pteropoda*, and *Cephalopoda*. See MOLLUSCA.

Çȳ'cloid. [**Cycloi'des;** from κύκλος, a "circle," and εἶδος, a "form."] Resembling a circle.

Çȳc-lo-neū'ra.* [From κύκλος, a "circle," and νεῦρον, a "nerve."] A term applied by some writers to the first sub-kingdom of animals, or *Radiata*, on account of the *circular* form of the nervous axis in this division.

Çȳc-lo-neū'rus.* [From the same.] Having a circular nervous arrangement. See preceding article.

Çȳc-los'to-mus.* [From κύκλος, and στόμα, a "mouth."] ("Round-mouthed.") Applied in the plural masculine (*Cyclos'-tomi*) to a family of fishes. Also named *Suctorii.*

Çy-do'nĭ-a.* [From *Cy'don*, in Crete, where it is said to be native.] A Linnæan genus of the class *Icosandria*, natural order *Rosaceæ.*

Çȳdo'nia Vul-ga'ris,* The *Pyrus Cydonia*, or quince-tree.

Çy-do'nĭ-um.* The Pharmacopœial name for quince-seeds, which are sometimes used in medicine for their mucilage.

Çydo'nium Ma'lum.* ("Cydonian Apple.") The quince: the fruit of the *Pyrus Cydonia.*

Cȳ-lin'drĭ-cal. [**Cylin'dricus.**] Shaped like a cylinder.

Cȳ-lin-drĭ-for'mis.* [From *cylin'-drus*, a "cylinder."] Shaped like a cylinder.

Cȳl'in-droid. [**Cylindroi'des;** from *cylin'drus*, a "cylinder," and εἶδος, a "form."] Resembling a cylinder.

Cȳm'bĭ-form. [**Cymbifor'mis;** from *cym'ba*, a "boat."] Shaped like a boat. See NAVICULARIS, SCAPHOID.

Çȳme, or **Çȳ'ma.*** [Gr. κῦμα, a "stem of colewort."] A kind of inflorescence, like that of the elder, resembling a corymb, and consisting of several flower-stalks springing from one centre, each irregularly subdivided.

Çȳ-mi'num.* The Pharmacopœial name (Lond. Ph.) for the fruit of *Cuminum cyminum.*

Çȳ-nan'che.* [From κύων, a "dog," and ἄγχω, to "strangle."] (Fr. *Angine*, ŏnᵍ'zhēn'.) Inflammation of the throat; sore throat. A genus of the order *Phlegmasiæ*, class *Pyrexiæ*, of Cullen's Nosology.

Cynanche Laryngea. See CROUP.

Çynan'che Ma-lig'na.* Putrid sore throat, often an attendant on scarlatina.

Çynan'che Par-o-tid'e-a.* The same as PAROTITIS.

Cynanche Pharyngea. See PHARYNGITIS.

Çynan'che Strep-ĭ-to'rĭ-a,* Cynan'che Strid'ŭ-la,* Cynan'che Suf-fo-ca-ti'va.* Names for *Croup.*

Çynan'che Ton-sil-la'ris.* *Tonsilli'tis phlegmono'des*, or quinsy.

Çynan'che Trach-e-a'lis.* The croup; otherwise called *Cynanche laryngea.* See CROUP.

Cynanche Ulcerosa. See TONSILLITIS MALIGNA.

Çȳn-an-thro'pĭ-a.* [From κύων, a "dog," and ἄνθρωπος, a "man."] A kind of *Melancholia*, in which the patient fancies himself changed into a dog, and imitates its bark and actions.

Çȳn'a-ra Scol'ȳ-mus.* The botanical name of the garden artichoke, a thistle-like plant growing in the south of Europe and cultivated for the fleshy sweet receptacle of its flowers. It belongs to the Linnæan class *Syngenesia*, natural order *Compositæ.* The juice of the leaves mixed with wine is sometimes given in dropsies. (For fuller information see BRANDE'S "Dictionary of Science.")

Çȳn'ĭ-cus.* [From κύων.] Like a dog: cyn'ic. See CANINE.

Çy'nips Quer-cĭ-fo'lĭ-i.* A hymenopterous insect found in the gall of the oak. The gall itself is called *Cyni'phis ni'dus*, or the "nest of the cynips."

Çȳn-o-lis'sa.* [From κύων, a "dog," and λύσσα, "madness."] Canine madness. See HYDROPHOBIA.

Çȳn-o-rex'ĭ-a.* [From κύων, a "dog," and ὄρεξις, "appetite."] Canine appetite.

Cyperaceæ,* sip-er-a'she-ē, **Cyp'er-o-i'de-æ.*** [From *Cype'rus*, one of the genera.] Sedges. A natural order of endogenous grass-like plants, found in marshes, ditches, meadows, heaths, etc., from the Arctic to the Antarctic Circle. Some species of it are used as food. The Egyptian *Papyrus* belongs to this order.

Cyperoi'deæ.* The Jussieuan name of a natural order of plants. See CYPERACEÆ.

Çy-prĭ-pe'dĭ-um.* [From Κύπρις, a name of Venus, and πέδιον, a "slipper."] "Venus's Slipper." The Pharmacopœial name (U.S. Ph.) of the root of the *Cypripe'dium pubes'cens.*

Cyprus Powder. See ABELMOSCHUS.

Cȳ'prus Tur'pen-tīne. A limpid, fragrant substance obtained from the *Pistacia terebinthinus.*

Cyrillaceæ,* sĭr-il-la'she-ē. A natural order of evergreen shrubs, natives of North America, including the *Cyrilla* and two other genera.

Çyr-to'sis.* [From κυρτός, "curved."] A term denoting among the ancients a recurvation of the spine, or posterior crookedness. It has more recently been termed *Cyrton'osus* or *mor'bus incur'vus.*

Çȳs-tăl'ġĭ-ạ.* [From κύστις, the "bladder," and ἄλγος, "pain."] Painful spasmodic affection of the bladder.

Cystectasy. See LITHECTASY.

Çys'tic. [**Cys'ticus;** from κύστις, the "bladder."] Belonging to the urinary or gall bladder.

Çys'tic Duct. [**Duc'tus Cys'ticus.**] The duct which proceeds from the gall-bladder and, uniting with the hepatic duct, forms the *ductus communis choledochus.*

Cystic Oxide. See CYSTIN.

Çȳs-tĭ-çer'cus.* [From κύστις, a "bladder," and κέρκος, a "tail."] The tailed bladder-worm. Applied to a genus of *Entozoa Parenchymata,* otherwise termed *Hydatids.*

Çȳs-tĭ-fel-le-ot'o-my̆. [**Cystifelleoto'mia;** from κύστις, a "bladder," *fel,* the "gall," and τέμνω, to "cut."] Operation by which a gall-stone is extracted from the gall-bladder.

Çȳs'tin. [**Cysti'na;** from κύστις, the "bladder."] A peculiar substance, very rare, in a urinary calculus; also termed *Cystic Oxide.*

Çȳs-tir-rha'ġĭ-ạ.* [From κύστις, the "bladder," and ῥήγνυμι, to "burst forth."] A discharge from the bladder, whether of blood or mucus.

Çȳs-tir-rhœ'ạ.* [From κύστις, the "bladder," and ῥέω, to "flow."] A mucous discharge from the bladder; vesical catarrh. See CYSTORRHŒA.

Çȳs'tis.* [Gr. κύστις, the "bladder."] A bladder, or sac; specially, the *Vesica urinaria.* The membranous bag in which any morbid substance is contained: a cyst.

Çȳs-tī'tis, *idis.** [From κύστις, the "bladder."] Inflammation of the bladder. A genus of the order *Phlegmasiæ,* class *Pyrexiæ,* of Cullen's Nosology.

Çȳs'tĭ-tōme. [**Cystit'omus;** from κύστις, a "bladder," or "sac," and τέμνω, to "cut."] An instrument for opening the capsule or sac of the crystalline lens.

Çȳs'to-bu-bon'o-çēle.* [From κύστις, the "bladder," βουβών, the "groin," and κήλη, a "tumor."] A rare kind of *Hernia,* in which the urinary bladder protrudes through the inguinal opening.

Çȳs'to-çēle.* [From κύστις, the "bladder," and κήλη, a "tumor."] Hernia in which the urinary bladder is protruded; *Hernia vesicalis.*

Çȳs-to-dȳn'ĭ-ạ.* [From κύστις, the "bladder," and ὀδύνη, "pain."] Pain in the bladder.

Çȳs'toid. [**Cystoi'des;** from κύστις, the "bladder," and εἶδος, a "form."] Resembling a cyst or bladder.

Çȳs-to-lĭ-thi'ạ-sis.* [From κύστις, the "bladder," and λίθος, a "stone."] Urinary calculous disease.

Çȳs-tol'ĭ-thus.* [From the same.] A urinary calculus: a cys'tolith.

Çȳs-to-plas'tic. [**Cystoplas'ticus.**] Belonging to cystoplasty.

Çȳs'to-plas-tȳ. [**Cystoplas'tia;** from κύστις, the "bladder," and πλάσσω, to "fabricate."] Operation for vesico-vaginal fistula, consisting in uniting a flap taken from the external *labium,* by suture, to the newly-pared edges of the sore.

Çȳs-to-ple'ġĭ-ạ,* Çȳs-to-plex'ĭ-ạ.* [From κύστις, the "bladder," and πλήσσω, to "strike."] Paralysis of the bladder.

Çȳs-top-to'sis.* [From κύστις, the "bladder," and πίπτω, to "fall."] Relaxation of the internal coat of the bladder, which protrudes into the urethra.

Çȳs-tor-rhœ'ạ.* The same as CYSTIRRHŒA.

Çȳs-to-spas'tic. [**Cystospas'ticus;** from κύστις, the "bladder," and σπάω, to "draw."] Belonging to spasm of the bladder.

Çȳs'to-tōme. [**Cystot'omus;** from κύστις, the "bladder," and τέμνω, to "cut."] A knife or instrument employed in *Cystotomy.*

Çȳs-tot'o-my̆. [**Cystoto'mia;** from κύστις, the "bladder," and τέμνω, to "cut."] Operation of cutting into the bladder. See LITHOTOMY.

Cytinaceæ,* sit-e-na'she-ē. [From *Cyt'inus,* one of the genera.] A natural order of parasitical plants (Rhizogens), found in Southern Europe and at the Cape of Good Hope.

Çȳt'ĭ-sin. [**Cytisi'na.**] A bitter principle found in the seeds of the *Cytisus laburnum.*

Çȳt'ĭ-sus.* [Gr. κύτισος.] A Linnæan genus of the class *Diadelphia,* natural order *Papilionaceæ.*

Çȳt'isus Sco-pa'rĭ-us.* One of the names of the broom-plant.

Çȳt'o-blast. [**Cytoblas'ta;** from κύτος, a "cavity," and βλαστάνω, to "bud" or "burst forth," to "produce."] The nucleus of cellular or elementary corpuscles in all vegetable and animal tissues; the *Areola,* or cell-nucleus. Also, the nucleus of those cells, growing within cells by a generative power of their own, which constitute the parenchyma or substance of morbid growths.

Çȳt-o-blas-te'ma, a'tis.* The fluid or mother liquid in which the cells containing the nucleus, or *cytoblast*, originate.

Çȳt-o-ġen'e-sis.* [From κύτος, a "cavity," or "cell," and γίνομαι, to "be produced."] The generation of cavities or cells; cell-development.

D.

D. = *Do'sis.** A "dose."

Dac'rȳ-o-. [From δάκρυον, a "tear."] A prefix denoting connection with the lachrymal apparatus.

Dac'rȳ-o-ad'en-i'tis, idis.* [From *dac'ryo*, and *adeni'tis*, "inflammation of a gland."] Inflammation of the lachrymal gland.

Dac'rȳ-o-çȳst. [**Dacryocys'tis;** from δάκρυον, a "tear," and *cys'tis*, a "bag" or "sac."] The lachrymal sac.

Dac-rȳ-o-çȳs-ti'tis, idis.* [From the same.] Inflammation of the lachrymal sac.

Dac-rȳ-o-çȳs-to-blen-nor-rhœ'a.* [From δάκρυον, a "tear," and *blennorrhœ'a*, a "flow of mucus."] A discharge of mucus from the lachrymal sac.

Dac-rȳ-o-hæm-or-rhœ'a.* [From δάκρυον, a "tear," and *hæmorrhœ'a*, a "flow of blood."] Sanguineous lachrymation, or a flow of tears mingled with blood.

Dac'rȳ-o-līte. [**Dacryoli'tes;** from *dacryo-*, and λίθος, a "stone."] A calculous concretion in the lachrymal passage.

Dac-rȳ-o'ma, atis.* [From δακρύω, to "weep."] An obstruction in one or both of the *puncta lachrymalia*, causing an overflow of tears.

Dac-tȳ-lif'er-us.* Bearing dates. See next article.

Dac'tȳ-lus.* [From δάκτυλος, a "finger;" a "date," from its resemblance to a small finger.] The same as Digitus. Also, the date, or fruit of *Phœnix dactylifera.*

Dæ'mo-no-ma'nĭ-a.* [From δαίμων, the "devil," and μανία, "madness."] A variety of *Melancholia* in which the patient fancies himself possessed by devils.

Daguerreotype, da-gĕr'ro-tīp. [From *M. Daguerre*, dȧ'gair', the discoverer, and *ty'pus*, a "likeness," or "figure" of any thing.] The system or process of producing pictures by the action of light on certain prepared metallic plates, introduced into France by M. Daguerre. See Photography.

Dah'līne. A vegetable principle discovered in the dahlia, similar to starch.

Dalby's (dawl'bēz) **Car-min'a-tīve.** A popular empirical carminative for children, composed of the carbonate of magnesia, with a small quantity of the tincture of assafœtida, tincture of opium, oil of peppermint, aniseed, and other aromatic oils.

Dal'ton-ĭsm. [**Daltonis'mus.**] Inability to distinguish colors, which Dalton, the celebrated chemist, labored under.

Dam'ask-Rose. The *Rosa centifolia.*

Damp. (Ger. *Dampf*, "vapor.") A term applied to noxious gases found in mines. See Choke-Damp and Fire-Damp.

Dam'son. [A corruption of *Damasce'num*, "belonging to Damascus."] The fruit of a variety of the *Prunus domestica.*

Dan-de-lī'on. (Fr. *Dent-de-lion*, dŏɴᴳ'dẹh'lè'ŏɴᴳ', like *leontodon*, signifying "Lion's-Tooth.") The *Leon'todon tarax'acum.* See Taraxacum.

Dan'driff. [**Fur'fur, ur**is.] The disease *Pityriasis capitis.*

Danse de Saint Guy, dŏɴs dẹh sȧɴᴳ ġè. The French name for *Chorea.*

Daph'ne.* [Gr. Δάφνη.] A Linnæan genus of the class *Octandria*, natural order *Thymelaceæ.*

Daph'ne Al-pi'na.* A dwarf species of *Daphne*, from which has been obtained an acrid alkaline principle called Daphnin, which see.

Daph'ne Gnid'ium* (nid'e-ŭm). The bark of this tree is employed in France as a vesicatory under the name of *Daphné Garou* (dâf'nȧ' gȧ'roo').

Daphne Mezereon. See next article.

Daph'ne Me-ze're-um (or **Me-ze-re'um**).* Spurge-olive. The plant which affords mezereon bark. See Mezereon.

Daph'nin, or **Daph'nine.** [**Daphni'na.**] An acrid, volatile, alkaline principle, obtained from the bark of the *Daph'ne Alpi'na.* It is this principle (as is supposed) to which the different species of *Daphne* owe their vesicating power.

Dar'tos.* [Gr. δαρτός, "skinned," or, perhaps, "made like skin," "resembling skin;" from δέρας, a "skin."] The cellular tissue subjacent to the skin of the *scrotum*, by the contractility of which, during life, the latter is corrugated.

Dartre (Fr.), dartr. Often indefinitely applied by French authors to different cutaneous diseases: it seems, however, to agree pretty nearly with *Herpes*.

Dāte. [Lat. **Dac'tylus;** Fr. *Datte*, dått.] The fruit of the date palm, or *Phœ'nix dactylif'era*.

Datiscaceæ,* dat-is-ka'she-ē. A small natural order of exogenous plants, found in Europe, India, and North America. It includes the *Datis'ca*, which is used as a purgative in fevers.

Datte. See DATE.

Da-tu'ra.* A Linnæan genus of the class *Pentandria*, natural order *Solanaceæ*.

Datu'ra Stra-mo'nĭ-um.* The thorn-apple, or Jamestown weed. See STRAMONIUM.

Dat-u'rin. [**Datu'ria.**] An alkaline principle discovered in *Datura stramonium*.

Dau'ci Ra'dix.* ("Root of the Carrot.") See DAUCUS CAROTA.

Dau'cus.* [Gr. δαῦκος.] A Linnæan genus of the class *Pentandria*, natural order *Umbelliferæ*.

Dau'cus Ca-ro'ta.* The systematic name of the common garden-carrot (variety *sati'vus*).

Day-Blindness. See NYCTALOPIA.

Day'-Mare. [**In'cubus Vigilan'tium.**] A species of incubus occurring during wakefulness, and attended with that distressing pressure on the chest which characterizes nightmare.

Day-Sight. See HEMERALOPIA.

D. D. = *De'tur ad.** "Let it be given to."

De. A Latin particle usually signifying "down," or "from;" frequently it is *intensive*, and occasionally *privative*, or *negative*, having sometimes nearly the force of the English particle *un:* e.g. *decoquo*, to "boil down," to "boil thoroughly;" *deform* [from *for'ma*, "form," "grace," "beauty"], to "deprive of grace or beauty;" *decompose*, to "uncompound."

Dead'ly Night'shade. The *At'ropa belladon'na*.

Deaf. See SURDUS.

Deaf-Dumb'ness. Dumbness arising from congenital or early deafness.

Dealbatio, or **Dealbation.** See BLEACHING.

Deaur. pil. = *Deaur'etur pil'ula.** "Let the pill be gilded."

De-bil'ĭ-tў. [**Debil'itas;** from *deb'ilis*, "weak."] (Fr. *Faiblesse*, få'-blĕss'.) Weakness, or feebleness; decay of strength either of mind or body.

Deb. Spiss. = *Deb'ita Spissitu'do,** "a due thickness or consistency," or *Deb'itæ Spissitu'dinis*, "of a due consistency."

Dec. = *Decan'ta.** "Pour off."

Dec'a-gon. [**Decago'num;** from δέκα, "ten," and γωνία, an "angle."] A figure having ten equal angles and sides.

Dec-ag'o-nal. [**Decago'nus.**] Belonging to a decagon; having the form of a decagon.

Decagramme, dek'a-grăm. [**Decagram'ma,** *atis;* from δέκα, "ten," and (Fr.) *gramme.*] Ten grammes, equal to 154.34 grains Troy.

Decagynia. See DECAGYNIUS.

Dec-a-ġўn'ĭ-us.* [From δέκα, "ten," and γυνή, a "woman" or "female."] Having ten pistils. Applied to a Linnæan order comprising plants with ten pistils.

Decalitre, dĕk'å-lètr'. [From δέκα, "ten," and (Fr.) *litre.*] Ten litres, equal to 610.28 English cubic inches.

Decametre, dĕk'a-mē't'r (French pronunciation, då'kå'mêtr'). [From δέκα, "ten," and (Fr.) *mètre.*] Ten metres, equal to 393.71 English inches, or about thirty-two and three-quarters English feet.

De-can'drĭ-a.* [From δέκα, "ten," and ἀνήρ, "man" or "male."] A class of plants in the Linnæan system, characterized by having ten stamens.

De-can'drĭ-ous. [**Decan'drius.**] Having ten stamens. See DECANDRIA.

De-can-tā'tion. [**Decanta'tio.**] The pouring off of clear fluid from sediments.

Dec-a-phўl'lous. [**Decaphyl'lus;** from δέκα, "ten," and φύλλον, a "leaf."] Having ten leaves.

Decapitation. See DECOLLATION.

De-cap'o-da,* or **Dec'a-pods.** [From δέκα, "ten," and πούς, ποδός, a "foot."] A name given by Cuvier to an order of Crustaceans having ten thoracic feet. Also applied to a tribe of Cephalopods having ten locomotive and prehensile appendages proceeding from the head, two of which, called *tentacles*, are always longer than the rest.

De-cap'o-dous. [**Decap'odus;** from δέκα, "ten," and πούς, ποδός, a "foot."] Literally, "having ten feet." See DECAPODA.

De-cem'fĭ-dus.* [From *de'cem*, "ten," and *fin'do*, to "cleave."] Cleft into ten parts: decem'fidous.

De-cem-loc'u-lar. [**Decemlocu-la'ris;** from *de'cem*, "ten," and *loc'ulus*, a "little pocket."] Having ten little compartments.

De-cid'u-a.* [See DECIDUUS.] A spongy membrane, or *chorion*, produced at the period of conception, and thrown off from the uterus after parturition.

Decid'ua Mem-bra'na (or **Tu'ni-ca**) **Re-flex'a.*** The same as DECIDUA REFLEXA, which see.

Decid'ua Membra'na (or **Tu'nica**) **U'te-ri.*** ("Deciduous Membrane of the Uterus.") The same as DECIDUA VERA.

Decid'ua Re-flex'a.* That portion of the decidua which is reflected over, and surrounds, the ovum.

Decid'ua Ve'ra.* That portion of the decidua which lines the interior of the uterus.

De-cid'u-us.* [From *deç'ido*, to "fall down," to "fall off."] Falling off: decid'uous.

Decigramme, des'se-grăm. (Fr. *Décigramme*, dà'sè'grâmm'. [From *deç'-imus*, "tenth," and (Fr.) *gramme*.] The tenth part of a gramme, equal to 1.544 grains avoirdupois, or one and a half grains troy.

Decilitre, dess'e-lètr'. [From *deç'-imus*, "tenth," and (Fr.) *litre*.] The tenth part of a litre, equal to 6.1028 English cubic inches.

Decimetre, dess'e-mē't'r (French pronunciation, dà'sè'mêtr'). [From *deç'-imus*, "tenth," and (Fr.) *mètre*.] The tenth part of a metre, equal to 3.937, or nearly four, English inches.

De-cli'nal. [From *decli'no*, to "bend downwards."] Applied to the slope of *strata* from an axis.

Dec'li-nate. [**Declina'tus;** from the same.] Bending down.

De-cli'vis.* [From *de*, "down," and *cli'vus*, the "descent of a hill."] Descending.

Decoct. = *Decoc'tum.** "A decoction."

De-coc'ta,* the plural of DECOCTUM.

Decocté, dà'kok'tà'. The French for DECOCTUM, which see.

De-coc'tion. [**Decoc'tum,** or **De-coc'tio, o'nis;** from *de*, "down," and *co'quo, coc'tum*, to "boil."] A continued ebullition with water, to separate such parts of bodies as are soluble only at that degree of heat. A medicine made by boiling some medicinal substance in a watery fluid. In this latter signification it corresponds to DECOCTUM, which see.

De-coc'tum,* plural **De-coc'ta.** [From the same.] A decoction. The Pharmacopœial term for a medicinal preparation made by boiling some vegetable substance in water for the purpose of extracting the soluble ingredients.

Decoc'tum Ce-tra'ri-æ.* ("Decoction of Iceland Moss.") Take of Iceland Moss half a troyounce; water, a sufficient quantity. Boil the Iceland Moss in a pint of water for fifteen minutes, strain with compression, and add sufficient water through the strainer to make the decoction measure a pint.

Decoc'tum Chi-maph'i-læ.* ("Decoction of Pipsissewa.") Take of pipsissewa, bruised, a troyounce; water, a sufficient quantity. Boil the pipsissewa in a pint of water fifteen minutes, strain, and add sufficient water through the strainer to make the decoction measure a pint.

Decoc'tum Cin-cho'næ Fla'væ.* ("Decoction of Yellow Cinchona.") Take of yellow cinchona, bruised, a troyounce; water, a sufficient quantity. Boil the yellow cinchona in a pint of water for fifteen minutes, strain, and add sufficient water through the strainer to make the decoction measure a pint.

Decoc'tum Cin-cho'næ Ru'bræ.* ("Decoction of Red Cinchona.") Take of red cinchona, bruised, a troyounce; water, a sufficient quantity. Boil the red cinchona in a pint of water for fifteen minutes, strain, and add sufficient water through the strainer to make the decoction measure a pint.

Decoc'tum Cor'nûs Flor'i-dæ.* ("Decoction of Dogwood.") Take of dogwood, bruised, a troyounce; water, a sufficient quantity. Boil the dogwood in a pint of water for fifteen minutes, strain, and add sufficient water through the strainer to make the decoction measure a pint.

Decoc'tum Dul-ca-ma'ræ.* ("Decoction of Bittersweet.") Take of bittersweet, bruised, a troyounce; water, a sufficient quantity. Boil the bittersweet in a pint of water for fifteen minutes, strain, and add sufficient water through the strainer to make the decoction measure a pint.

Decoc'tum Hæm-a-tox'y̆-li.* ("Decoction of Logwood.") Take of logwood, rasped, a troyounce; water, a sufficient quantity. Boil the logwood in a pint of water for fifteen minutes, strain, and add sufficient water through the strainer to make the decoction measure a pint.

Decoc'tum Hor'de-i.* ("Decoction of Barley.") Take of barley two troyounces; water, a sufficient quantity. Having washed away the extraneous matters which adhere to the barley, boil it with half a pint of water for a short time, and throw away the resulting liquid. Then, having poured on it four pints of boiling water, boil down to two pints, and strain.

Decoc'tum Quer'cûs Al'bæ.* ("Decoction of White-Oak Bark.") Take of white-oak bark, bruised, a troyounce; water, a sufficient quantity. Boil the white-oak bark in a pint of water for fifteen minutes, strain, and add sufficient water through the strainer to make the decoction measure a pint.

Decoc'tum Sar-sa-pa-ril'læ Com-pos'ĭ-tum.* ("Compound Decoction of Sarsaparilla.") Take of Sarsaparilla, sliced and bruised, six troyounces; bark of sassafras-root, sliced, guaiacum-wood, rasped, liquorice-root, bruised, each a troyounce; mezereon, sliced, one hundred and eighty grains; water, a sufficient quantity. Macerate with four pints of water for twelve hours; then boil for a quarter of an hour, strain, and add sufficient water through the strainer to make the decoction measure four pints.

Decoc'tum Sen'e-gæ.* ("Decoction of Seneka.") Take of seneka, bruised, a troyounce; water, a sufficient quantity. Boil the seneka in a pint of water for fifteen minutes, strain, and add sufficient water through the strainer to make the decoction measure a pint.

Decoc'tum U'væ Ur'si.* ("Decoction of Uva Ursi.") Take of uva ursi a troyounce; water, a sufficient quantity. Boil the uva ursi in a pint of water for fifteen minutes, strain, and add sufficient water through the strainer to make the decoction measure a pint.

De-col-lā'tion. [From *de*, privative, and *col'lum*, the "neck."] Applied to the removal of the head of the child in cases of difficult parturition.

De-com-po-sĭ'tion. [**Decomposi'tio, o'**_nis;_ from *de*, negative, or "from," and *compo'no, compos'itum,* to "put together."] The separation of compound bodies into their constituent parts or principles; analysis.

De-com-pos'ĭ-tus.* [From the same.] Applied in the feminine plural (*Decompos'itæ*) to a class or division of plants having a common foot-stalk supporting a number of lesser leaves, each of which is compounded.

De-cor-tĭ-cā'tion. [**Decortica'tio, o'**_nis;_ from *de*, priv., or "from," and *cor'tex*, "bark."] The removal of bark, husk, or shell.

Dec're-ment. [**Decremen'tum;** from *decres'co*, to "grow less."] The decrease or proportion in which any thing is lessened.

De-crep-ĭ-tā'tion. [**Decrepita'tio, o'**_nis;_ from *decrep'ito, decrepita'tum,* to "crackle" or "explode."] The crackling noise produced by certain bodies when heated, as common salt, etc.

Decub. = *Decu'bitus,** or *Decu'bitu.** "Lying down," or "On lying down" (*i.e.* going to bed).

De-cu'bĭ-tus.* [From *decum'bo, decu'bitum,* to "lie down."] A lying down, or reclining in the horizontal position. An important symptom in certain diseases is to be observed from the manner of lying in bed.

De-cum'bens.* [From the same.] Lying down: decum'bent.

De-cur'rens.* [From *decur'ro, decur'sum,* to "run down."] Applied to leaves which run down the stem in a leafy border or wing: decur'rent.

De-cur'sĭve. [**Decursi'vus;** from the same.] Applied to leaves that run down the stem, attached by their middle nerve only.

De-cus'sāte. [From *decus'so, decussa'tum,* to "cross" (from *decus'sis*, the number "ten," represented by a cross, X).] To cross each other. See next article.

Dec-us-sā'tion. [**Decussa'tio, o'**_nis;_ from the same.] The crossing or running of one portion athwart another, as in the case of the optic nerves, which cross each other within the cranium.

De-cus-so'rĭ-um.* An instrument for depressing the dura mater after trephining.

De D. in D. = *De Di'e in Di'em.** "From day to day."

Défaillance, dā'fā'yōnss'. The French term for "fainting." Like the Latin *defectio*, its primary signification is a "failing" of the strength.

Def-e-cā'tion. [**Defæca'tio, o'**_nis;_ from *defæ'co, defæca'tum,* to "deprive of the dregs" (fæces), to "strain through a sieve."] The removal of fæces, lees, or sediment from any thing. The act of discharging the fæces.

Defectio,* de-fek'she-o. [From *defi'cio*, to "lack" or "fail."] A failing; a failing of heart, strength, or courage.

Defec'tio An'ĭ-mi.* Literally, the

"failing of the mind;" hence, fainting. The same as DELIQUIUM ANIMI.

Def'er-ens,* plural neuter **Deferentia,** def-er-en'she-ạ. [From *def'ero,* to "carry down," to "convey."] Conveying: def'erent. See VAS DEFERENS.

Def'lạ-grā'tion. [**Deflagra'tio, o'***nis;* from *defla'gro, deflagra'tum,* to be "set on fire," to "be utterly consumed."] The burning of an inflammable substance or metal with nitre, chlorate of potash, etc.

De'flex. [**Deflex'us;** from *deflec'to,* to "bend down."] Bending a little downwards.

De-flo'rate. [**Deflora'tus;** from *deflo'ro, deflora'tum,* to "deflower."] Applied to anthers that have shed their pollen, and plants, their flowers.

Def-lo-rā'tion. [**Defloratio, o'***nis;* from the same.] In Medical Jurisprudence, connection without violence, in contradistinction from rape. Loss of the marks of virginity by connection with a male.

Defluxion, de-flŭk'shŭn. [**Deflux'io, o'***nis;* from *de,* "down," and *flu'o, flux'um* or *fluc'tum,* to "flow."] A flowing of humors downwards.

De-fo-lĭ-ā'tion. [**Defolia'tio, o'***nis;* from *de,* priv., and *fo'lium,* a "leaf."] The fall of leaves, as contradistinguished from frondescence, or their renovation.

De-for-mā'tion. [**Deforma'tio, o'***nis;* from *defor'mo, deforma'tum,* to "mar" or "disfigure."] Distortion of any part, or general deformity of the body.

De-ġen-er-ā'tion. [Lat. **Degenera'tio, o'***nis;* from *degen'ero, degenera'tum,* to be "worse than one's ancestors;" Fr. *Dégénérescence,* dȧ'zhȧ'nȧ'rĕs'sŏɴss'.] Deterioration. Applied in Pathology to a morbid change in the structure of parts: such as LARDACEOUS DEGENERATION.

Deg-lu-tĭ'tion. [**Degluti'tio, o'***nis;* from *deglu'tio, degluti'tum,* to "swallow down."] The act of swallowing.

De-gree'. [Lat. **Gra'dus,** a "step," or "rank."] The 360th part of a circle. Also, the rank or title of Bachelor, Master, or Doctor, conferred by the Faculty of a university or college. See DOCTOR.

De-his'çence. [**Dehiscen'tia;** from *dehis'co,* to "gape" or "burst open."] A bursting open. Applied to capsules.

De-his'çent. [From the same.] Opening or splitting, as the capsules of certain plants.

Dej. Alv. = *Dejectio'nes Alvi'næ.** "Alvine dejections."

De-jec'tion. [**Dejec'tio, o'***nis;* from *deji'cio, dejec'tum,* to "throw down."] The discharge of any excrementitious matter; also, the matter discharged; a stool, or evacuation of the bowels. Also, depression, exhaustion, or prostration.

Délayant, dȧ'lȧ'yŏɴɢ'. The French term for DILUENT, which see.

Del-e-te'rĭ-ous. [**Delete'rius;** from *de'leo, dele'tum,* to "destroy."] Literally, "destroying." Injurious; poisonous.

Del-ĭ-gā'tion. [**Deliga'tio, o'***nis;* from *del'igo, deliga'tum,* to "bind up."] The act of applying a bandage.

Del-ĭ-quĕs'çence. [From *deliques'co,* to "grow moist" or "liquid."] The liquescent state assumed by certain saline bodies in consequence of their attracting water from the air.

Deliquium,* de-lik'we-ŭm. [From *delin'quo,* to "fail."] A failing; a fainting or swooning.

Deliq'uium An'ĭ-mi.* ("Failing of the Mind.") Swooning or fainting; syn'cope; also called *Defectio animi.*

De-lĭr'ĭ-um.* [From *deli'ro,* to "rave."] A symptom consisting in being fitful and wandering in talk.

Delir'ium Tre'mens.* ("Trembling Delirium.") (Fr. *Délire Tremblant,* dȧ'lēʀ' trŏɴ'blŏɴɢ'.) An affection resulting from an excessive indulgence in strong liquors, or opium. See MANIA A POTU.

Del-ĭ-tĕs'çence. [From *delites'co,* to "lie hid."] A term used principally by the French physiologists to express a more sudden disappearance of the symptoms of inflammation than occurs in resolution.

De-liv'er-ў. (Fr. *Délivrer,* dȧ'lē'vʀȧ', to "free.") The expulsion of a child by the mother, or its extraction by the obstetrical practitioner. The expulsion of the placenta and membranes, however, is necessary to complete the delivery.

Del-phin'ic Aç'id. An acid procured from the oil of the *Delphi'nus del'phis,* or dolphin.

Del-phin'ĭ-um.* [From δελφίν, the "dolphin."] A Linnæan genus of the class *Polyandria,* natural order *Ranunculaceæ.* Also the Pharmacopœial name (U.S. Ph., 1860) for the seed of the *Delphinium consolida.* As a diuretic, it is sometimes given in dropsy.

Delphin'ium Staph-ĭ-sa'grĭ-ạ.* The plant stavesacre.

Del'toid. [**Deltoi'des;** from Δ, the Greek triangular letter, and εἶδος, a "form."] Shaped like the Greek letter

Δ (*delta*). The name of a large triangular muscle covering the shoulder-joint.

Del-to-i'de-us.* [From *deltoi'des.*] Belonging to the deltoid muscle.

Dementia,* de-men'she-ạ. [From *de*, priv., and *mens*, the "mind."] (Fr. *Démence*, dȧ'mŏnss'.) Want of intellect; a species of insanity.

De-mer'sus.* [From *demer'go*, *demer'sum*, to "dip in water."] Growing beneath the surface of water. Applied to leaves naturally so situated.

Demi-Bain, dmė băng. ("Half-Bath.") The French term for a hip-bath.

De-mul'çents. [**Demulcentia,** de-mŭl-sen'she-ạ; from *demul'ceo*, to "soothe."] (Fr. *Adoucissants*, ȧ'doo'sė'-sŏng'.) "Soothing [medicines]." Applied to medicines of a mucilaginous or oily consistence.

Den'drĭ-form. [**Dendrifor'mis;** from δένδρον, a "tree."] Formed like a tree.

Den'drīte. [**Dendri'tes;** from δένδρον, a "tree," and λίθος, a "stone."] Any figure of a tree or shrub observed in fossils and minerals.

Den-drit'ic. [**Dendrit'icus;** from δένδρον.] Belonging to a tree or shrub.

Den-drog'rạ-phȳ. [**Dendrogra'phia;** from δένδρον, a "tree," and γράφω, to "write."] A history of trees and shrubs.

Den'droid. [**Dendroi'des;** from δένδρον, a "tree," and εἶδος, a "form."] Resembling a tree or shrub.

Den'dro-līte. [**Dendroli'tes;** from δένδρον, a "tree," and λίθος, a "stone."] A petrified tree or shrub.

Den-drol'o-ġȳ. [**Dendrolo'gia;** from δένδρον, a "tree," and λόγος, a "discourse."] A treatise on trees; the science of trees.

Den-drom'e-ter. [**Dendrom'etrum;** from δένδρον, a "tree," and μέτρον, a "measure."] An instrument for measuring trees.

Dèngue (Sp.), dĕn'gȧ. A fever of America, characterized by sharp pains down the thighs and legs, and general soreness of the flesh and bones.

Den-ĭ-grā'tion. [**Denigra'tio;** from *deni'gro*, *denigra'tum*, to "blacken."] Another term for *Melanosis*, derived from its black appearance. See Melanosis.

Dens,* gen. **Den'tis.** [Sanscrit *Dântâ*: Gr. ὀδούς, ὀδόντος.] A tooth. See Tooth.

Dens Le-o'nis.* ("Lion's Tooth.") The same as dandelion, or *Leon'todon tarax'acum.*

Dent, dŏng'. The French for "tooth." See Dens.

Den'ta-grạ.* [From *dens*, and ἄγρα, a "seizure."] The same as Odontalgia. Also, a kind of forceps, or tooth-key, for extracting teeth.

Dentaire. See Dental.

Den'tal. [**Denta'lis;** from *dens*, *den'tis*, a "tooth."] (Fr. *Dentaire*, dŏng'-têr'.) Pertaining to teeth.

Den-ta'tạ.* The name of the second vertebra, so called from its projecting tooth-like process.

Den'tate. [**Denta'tus;** from *dens.*] Toothed.

Den'tēs,* gen. **Dentium,** den'she-ŭm, the plural of Dens, a "tooth." See Teeth.

Den'tes Cus-pĭ-da'ti,* or simply **Cuspida'ti.*** Four pointed teeth, two in each jaw, situated adjoining and posterior to the lateral incisors. The two cuspidati of the upper jaw are in popular language called eye-teeth.

Den'tes Sapien'tiæ* (sap-e-en'she-ē). The "Teeth of Wisdom," or wisdom-teeth. A name given to the last grinder teeth, because they come in mature years.

Den-tic'u-late, or **Den-tic'u-lāt-ed.** [**Denticula'tus;** from *dentic'ulus*, diminutive of *dens.*] Having little teeth.

Den'tĭ-frice. [**Dentifri'cium;** from *dens*, a "tooth," and *fri'co*, to "rub."] A medicinal powder for the teeth; tooth-powder.

Den'tine, or **Den'tin.** [**Denti'na;** from *dens*, a "tooth."] The bone-like substance forming the inner part of the body, neck, and roots of the teeth.

Den-tĭ-ros'tris,* plural **Den-tĭ-ros'trēs.** [From *dens*, a "tooth," and *ros'trum*, a "beak."] Applied in the plural to a family of birds having a tooth-like beak: dentiros'trate.

Den-tĭ-scăl'pĭ-um.* [From *dens*, a "tooth," and *scal'po*, to "scrape."] An instrument for scaling teeth.

Dentist. See Surgeon Dentist.

Den-tĭ'tion. [**Denti'tio, o'nis;** from *den'tio*, *denti'tum*, to "breed or produce teeth."] The first appearing of the teeth in infancy; teething.

Dentium. See Dentes.

Den'tium Cor'tex.* ("Bark or Rind of the Teeth.") A name applied to the enamel which forms the most important part of the covering of the teeth. See Enamel.

Den'tium Do'lor.* ("Pain of the Teeth.") See Odontalgia.

Den'toid. [**Dentoi'des;** from *dens*,

a "tooth," and εἶδος, a "form."] Resembling a tooth.

De-nu'date. [**Denuda'tus;** from *denu'do, denuda'tum,* to "make bare."] Made bare.

Den-u-dā'tion. [**Denuda'tio, o'***nis;* from the same.] The laying bare of any part.

De-ob'stru-ent. [**Deob'struens;** from *de,* "from," and *ob'struo,* to "obstruct."] Applied to medicines for removing obstructions.

De-o-do-rĭ-zā'tion. [**Deodoriza'tio, o'***nis;* from *de,* priv., and *o'dor,* a "smell."] The correcting of any foul or unwholesome effluvia, through the operation of chemical substances.

De-ox-ĭ-dā'tion. [**Deoxyda'tio, o'***nis;* from *de,* priv., and *ox'ygen.*] The driving off of oxygen from any substance.

Dep. = *Depura'tus.** "Purified."

De-pau'per-āt-ed. [From *de,* intensive, and *pau'per,* "poor."] In Botany, imperfectly developed; shrivelled as from scanty nutriment.

De-phleg-mā'tion. [**Dephlegma'tio, o'***nis;* from *de,* priv., and *phleg'ma,* "phlegm" or "humor."] The separating of the water from chemical liquors.

Deph-lo-ġis'tĭ-cāt-ed. [From *de,* priv., and *phlogis'ton.*] Deprived of phlogiston; in other words, oxidized. See Phlogiston.

Dephlogisticated Air. Oxygen gas.

Dephlogis'ticated Ma-rine' Aç'id. The name given by Scheele to chlorine.

De-pil'a-to-rȳ. [**Depilato'rius;** from *de,* priv., and *pi'lus,* the "hair."] Removing hair from any part.

Déplétif. See Depletory.

De-ple'tion. [**Deple'tio, o'***nis;* from *dep'leo, deple'tum,* to "empty."] The act of emptying or lightening the blood-vessels by means of venesection, cathartics, etc.

Dep'le-to-rȳ. [From the same. Fr. *Déplétif,* dȧ'plȧ'tēf'.] Causing or promoting depletion.

Dep-lu-mā'tion. [From *deplu'mis,* "without feathers," "callow;" from *de,* priv., and *plu'ma,* a "feather."] Literally, "plucking of the feathers." Applied to a disease of the eyelids in which the hair falls off.

De-poŝ'it. [**Depos'itum;** from *de,* "down," and *po'no, pos'itum,* to "put," "place," or "throw."] What is thrown down from a liquid in which it has been suspended.

Dep-ra-vā'tion. [**Deprava'tio, o'***nis;* from *depra'vo, deprava'tum,* to "vitiate" or "deprave."] Deterioration or change for the worse.

De-pressed'. [**Depres'sus.** See Depression.] A botanical term signifying "pressed down."

De-pres'sion. [**Depres'sio, o'***nis;* from *dep'rimo, depres'sum,* to "press down."] Lowness of spirits. The state of a part which is pressed down. Also, a term for one of the operations for cataract.

De-pres'sor, o'*ris.** [From the same.] Applied to a muscle which draws or presses down.

De-pres'sor An'gu-li O'ris.* ("Depressor of the Corner of the Mouth.") A muscle whose office is indicated by its name.

Dep'rĭ-mens.* [See Depression.] Pressing down.

Dep'rimens Oc'u-li.* (The "Depressing [Muscle] of the Eye.") A name given to the *rectus inferior,* from the action of this muscle in drawing down the eyeball.

De-pu'rans.* [From *depu'ro, depura'tum,* to "purify."] Purifying.

Depurantia,* de-pu-ran'she-a (the neuter plural of Depurans, which see). Applied to medicines supposed to have the power of purifying the blood.

Dep-u-rā'tion. [**Depura'tio, o'***nis;* from the same.] The clarifying of a liquid: defecation. The removal of impurities from the fluids of the body.

Der-ad-en-i'tis.* [From δερή, or δειρή, the "neck," and ἀδήν, a "gland."] Inflammation of a gland of the neck.

Der'bȳ-shire Neck. Another name for Bronchocele.

Derbyshire Spar. See Fluor Spar.

De-riv'a-tĭve. [**Derivati'vus;** from *de,* "from," and *ri'vus,* a "stream;" *deri'vo, deriva'tum,* to "draw off water," as from a large stream or river.] Diverting from one part to another: applied to blisters, rubefacients, epispastics, etc.

Der'ma, a*tis.** [Gr. δέρμα.] The skin, or *Cu'tis ve'ra.*

Der'mad. Applied the same as Dermal used adverbially.

Der'mal. [From *der'ma.*] Applied by Dr. Barclay as meaning "towards the skin."

Der-ma-tăl'ġĭ-a.* [From δέρμα, δέρματος, the "skin," and ἄλγος, "pain."] *Neuralgia* of the skin; pain of the skin.

Der-ma-tog'ra-phȳ. [**Dermatogra'phia;** from δέρμα, the "skin," and γράφω, to "write."] A description of the skin.

Der-ma-tol'o-ġy̆. [**Dermatolo'gia;** from δέρμα, the "skin," and λόγος, a "discourse."] The consideration (or science) of the skin, its nature and qualities.

Der-ma-tot'o-my̆. [**Dermatoto'mia;** from δέρμα, the "skin," and τέμνω, to "cut."] Dissection or cutting of the skin.

Dermography. See DERMATOGRAPHY.

Der'moid, or **Der'ma-toid.** [**Dermoi'des,** or **Dermatoi'des;** from δέρμα, the "skin," and εἶδος, a "form."] Resembling the skin.

Dermology. See DERMATOLOGY.

Der-mo-skel'e-ton. [**Dermoscel'eton;** from δέρμα, the "skin," and σκελετόν, a "skeleton."] The outward covering of many invertebrate animals, such as the lobster, the beetle, etc.; also in certain vertebrated animals, as the tortoise, the armadillo, etc.

Derosne's Salt. See NARCOTINE.

De-sçen-so'rĭ-um.* [From *descen'do, descen'sum,* to "move downwards."] The apparatus in which distillation by descent is performed.

De-sçen'sus,* accusative **De-sçen'sum.** [From the same.] Distillation *per descensum* is performed by placing the fire upon and around the vessel or apparatus (*descensorium*), the orifice of which is at the bottom.

Descriptive Anatomy. See ANATOMY, DESCRIPTIVE.

Des-ic-cā'tion. [**Desicca'tio, o'nis;** from *de,* intensive, and *sic'co, sicca'tum,* to "dry."] The act of drying.

De-sic'ca-tĭve. [**Desiccati'vus;** from the same.] Applied to substances that dry or lessen the moisture of a wound or sore.

Des-mi'tis, idis.* [From δεσμός, a "ligament."] Inflammation of a ligament.

Des-mo-dy̆n'ĭ-a.* [From δεσμός, a "ligament," and ὀδύνη, "pain."] Pain in a ligament, or in the ligaments: desmod'yny.

Des-mog'ra-phy̆. [**Desmogra'phia;** from δεσμός, a "ligament," and γράφω, to "write."] A history or description of the ligaments.

Des'moid. [**Desmoi'des;** from δέσμη, a "bundle," and εἶδος, a "form."] Applied to certain fibrous tumors which on section present numerous white fibres arranged in bundles. Also, resembling a ligament. (From δεσμός, a "ligament.")

Des-mol'o-ġy̆. [**Desmolo'gia;** from δεσμός, a "ligament," and λόγος, a "discourse."] A treatise on the ligaments; the science of the ligaments.

Des-pu-mā'tion. [**Despuma'tio, o'nis;** from *despu'mo, despuma'tum,* to "clarify."] The process of clarifying any fluid; defecation; depuration.

Des-pu-ma'tus.* Freed from impurities.

Des-qua-mā'tion. [**Desquama'tio, o'nis;** from *desqua'mo,* to "scale fishes."] The separation of *laminæ* or scales from the skin or bones; exfoliation.

Desquamative Nephritis. See NEPHRITIS.

Dest. = *Destil'la.** "Distil."

Destillatio. See DISTILLATION.

Desudatio (de-su-da'she-o), **o'nis.*** [From *de,* intensive, and *su'do, suda'tum,* to "sweat."] Excessive sweating; also, an eruption in children. See SUDAMEN.

Desvauxiaceæ,* då-vo-ze-a'she-ē. A natural order of endogenous herbaceous plants, found in Australia and the South Sea islands.

Det. = *De'tur.** "Let it be given."

De-ter'ġent. [**Deter'gens;** from *de,* intensive, and *ter'geo, ter'sum,* to "wipe," to "cleanse."] Applied to medicines which cleanse wounds and ulcers.

De-ter'mĭ-nate. [**Determina'tus;** from *deter'mino, determina'tum,* to "terminate," to "limit."] Applied to branches and stems that commence or end abruptly.

De-ter-mĭ-nā'tion. [**Determina'tio, o'nis;** from the same.] A flowing or rushing to a particular part, as blood to the head.

Det-o-nā'tion. [**Detona'tio, o'nis;** from *det'ono, detona'tum,* to "thunder."] Instantaneous combustion with loud explosion. See FULMINATION.

Det'ra-hens.* [From *det'raho,* to "draw away," to "draw from."] Drawing away.

De-tri'tal. [**Detri'tus;** from *det'ero, detri'tum,* to "wear away."] Relating to DETRITUS.

De-tri'tus.* [From the same.] The waste substance formed by the action of frost or rains on the sides of ruts, the action of rivers on their banks, etc.

De-tru'sor, o'ris.* [From *detru'do, detru'sum,* to "thrust down" or "force out."] Applied to the muscular coat of the bladder, by the contractile power of which the urine is expelled.

Detru'sor U-ri'næ.* ("Expeller of the Urine.") The aggregate of the muscular fibres of the bladder which expel the urine.

Deū-ter-o-path'ic. [**Deutero-path'icus.**] Belonging to deuteropathy.

Deū-ter-op'a-thy̆. [**Deuteropa'-thia;** from δεύτερος, "second," and πάθος, "disease."] A sympathetic affection, or one consequent upon another.

Deū-tox'ide. [**Deutox'ydum;** from δεύτερος, "second," and *ox'ydum*, an "oxide."] A term applied to a substance which is in the *second degree* of oxidation. This term is often used to denote a compound o^f three atoms of oxygen with two of metal, as in deutoxide of manganese, of lead, etc.

De-văl'gate. [**Devalga'tus;** from *de*, intensive, and *val'gus*, "bow-legged."] Having bowed legs; bandy-legged.

De-vel'op-ment. (Fr. *Développer*, to "unfold.") The organic change from the embryo state to maturity; growth.

De-vel-op-men'tal. [**Metamor'phicus.**] Belonging to, or connected with, development. Applied to certain diseases.

Devonshire Colic. See COLICA PICTONUM.

Dew. [Lat. **Ros, Ro'ris;** Fr. *Rosée*, ro'zā'.] Moisture precipitated at night from the atmosphere upon the surface of bodies whose temperature has been diminished by the absence of the sun. Clouds prevent the fall of dew, because the radiation of heat, by which bodies become colder than the surrounding air, does not take place to any great extent unless the sky is clear. Though dew may fall on a windy night, it is soon absorbed by the fresh dry air continually coming in contact with the moist surface of bodies.

Dew'ber-ry̆. The common name of the *Rubus trivialis.*

Dew'berry Plant. The common name of the *Rubus cæsius*, or heath-bramble.

Dewlap. See PALEAR LAXUM.

Dew'point. The temperature of the atmosphere at which the moisture begins to condense and deposit itself as dew.

Dex'trin. [**Dextri'na.**] Mucilaginous starch, prepared by boiling a solution of starch with a few drops of sulphuric acid. Its name is derived from its property of turning the plane of the polarization of light to the right hand.

Di. The same as DIS, which see.

Di'a (διά). A Greek particle signifying "through," "by means of," and sometimes "apart," "between." Words compounded with διά often imply separation.

Dī-a-be'tēs.* [From διά, "through," and βαίνω, to "go."] An immoderate and morbid flow of urine. It is termed *insip'idus* ("tasteless") where the urine retains its usual taste, and *melli'tus* ("honeyed") where the saccharine state is the characteristic symptom. A genus of the order *Spasmi*, class *Neuroses*, of Cullen's Nosology.

Dī-a-bet'ic. [**Diabet'icus.**] Belonging to *Diabetes.*

Diabetic Sugar. See GLUCOSE.

Dī-a-caus'tic. [**Diacaus'ticus;** from διακαίω, to "burn."] Applied to a double convex lens used to cauterize parts of the body.

Dī-aç'e-tate of Cop'per. *Ærugo*, or verdigris.

Di-a-chy'lon.* [From διά, "by means of," and χυλός, "juice."] A name formerly given to plasters prepared from expressed *juices*, now applied to the *Emplastrum plumbi* (Lond. Ph.), or *Emplastrum lithargyri* (Ed. and Dub. Ph.).

Di-a-co'dī-um.* [From κωδία, a "poppy-head."] The old name of the *Syrupus Papaveris*, or syrup of poppies.

Di-ac'rī-sis.* [From διακρίνω, to "distinguish."] The distinguishing of diseases by a consideration of their symptoms. See DIAGNOSIS.

Di-a-del'phi-a.* [From δίς, "twice," and ἀδέλφος, a "brother."] The seventeenth class of plants in Linnæus's system, in which the filaments of the stamens are united into two parcels or brotherhoods.

Diæresis,* dī-ĕr'e-sis. [Gr. διαίρεσις; from διαιρέω, to "take apart," to "divide."] A division of parts resulting from a wound, ulcer, or burn, or the like: a solution of continuity.

Diæretic, dī-e-ret'ik. [**Diæret'icus;** from the same.] Having power to divide, dissolve, or corrode; escharotic; corrosive.

Diæta. See DIET.

Dī-ag-no'sis.* [From διαγινώσκω, to "discern."] The science of signs or symptoms, by which one disease is distinguished from another.

Diagno'sis, Dif-fer-en'tial. The determining of the distinguishing features of a malady when nearly the same symptoms belong to two different classes of disease, as rheumatism and gout, etc.

Di-ag'o-nal. [**Diagona'lis;** from διά, "through," and γωνία, an "angle."] Applied to a right line drawn between any two opposite angles of a four-sided figure.

Diagrydium. See SCAMMONY.

Di-a-grȳd'ĭ-um,* or **Diagryd'ium Cy-do-nĭ-a'tum.*** One part of quince juice and two parts of scammony; formerly used as a purgative.

Di-al'ȳ-sēs,* the plural of DIALYSIS. Solutions of continuity. An order of the class *Locales* of Cullen's Nosology.

Di-al'ȳ-sis.* [From διαλύω, to "dissolve."] Weakness of the limbs, as if from a dissolving of their firmer parts. Applied to *analysis by liquid diffusion*, advantage being taken of the different degrees of diffusibility of different substances in solution to produce separation.

Dī-a-mag'net-ism. [**Diamagnetis'mus.**] A term employed by Faraday for a force or influence discovered by him in magnetic bodies.

Di-am'e-ter. [**Diam'eter,** or **Diam'etrus;** from διά, "through," and μέτρον, a "measure."] A right line drawn through the centre of a circle and terminated on both sides by the circumference. The central and shortest dimension of a sphere or cylinder.

Dī'a-mond. (Fr. *Diamant*, a corruption of ADAMANT, which see.) A precious stone; the crystallized and pure state of carbon; the hardest and most brilliant of all substances.

Di-an'drĭ-a.* [From δίς, "twice" or "two," and ἀνήρ, ἀνδρός, a "man" or "male."] The name of a Linnæan class having flowers with two stamens.

Di-an'thus.* [From δίς, "twice," and ἄνθος, a "flower."] A Linnæan genus of the class *Decandria*, natural order *Caryophyllaceæ.*

Dian'thus Car-ȳ-o-phȳl'lus.* The clove-pink, or clove-gilliflower. The flowers of this plant are used for flavoring syrup employed as a vehicle for other medicines.

Diapensiaceæ,* di-a-pen-she-a'-she-ē. [From *Diapen'sia*, one of the genera.] A small natural order of exogenous under-shrubs, found in Europe and North America.

Dī-aph'a-nous. [Gr. διαφανής; from διά, "through," and φαίνω, to "shine."] Transparent; shining through.

Dī-a-pho-re'sis.* [From διαφορέω, to "carry through," to "carry off."] Literally, a "carrying off through [the pores]" or by perspiration. A state of perspiration.

Dī-a-pho-ret'ic. [**Diaphoret'icus.**] Applied to medicines having power to produce diaphoresis. When they are so powerful as to occasion sweating, they have been called *Sudorifics.*

Diaphragm, dī'a-frăm. [**Diaphrag'ma,** *atis;* from διαφράσσω, to "divide in the middle by a partition."] A large muscle separating the thorax and abdomen: the midriff.

Di-a-phrag-măl'gȳ. [**Diaphragmal'gia;** from *diaphrag'ma*, the "diaphragm," and ἄλγος, "pain."] Pain in the diaphragm.

Di-a-phrag-mat'ic. [**Diaphragmat'icus.**] Belonging to the diaphragm.

Diaphragmat'ic Gout. A term applied to *Angina Pectoris.*

Di-a-phrag-ma-ti'tis, *idis.** [From *diaphrag'ma.*] Inflammation of the diaphragm. A term sometimes applied to that variety of partial pleurisy in which the effused fluid exists between the base of the lung and the diaphragm.

Di-a-phrag-mat'o-çēle.* [From *diaphrag'ma*, and κήλη, a "tumor."] Hernia, or tumor, from some portion of the *viscera* escaping through the diaphragm.

Di-aph'ȳ-sis,* plural **Di-aph'ȳ-sēs.** [From διαφύω, to "be produced between."] The cylindrical or prismatic shaft of the long bones between the *epiphyses.* Also, a fissure.

Di-a-poph'ȳ-sis.* [From διά, "between," and ἀποφύω, to "arise from."] Applied by Owen to the homologue of the upper transverse process of a *vertebra.*

Di-a'rĭ-us.* [From *di'es*, a "day."] Lasting one day; ephemeral.

Di-ar-rhœ'a.* [From διά, "through," and ῥέω, to "flow."] A purging, looseness, or too frequent passing of the fæces. A genus of the order *Spasmi*, class *Neuroses*, of Cullen's Nosology.

Diarrhœ'a Car-no'sa.* Dysentery in which flesh-like portions are voided.

Diarrhœ'a Chy-lo'sa.* The *Ileac passion.*

Di-ar-thro'dĭ-al. [**Diarthrodia'lis.**] Belonging to *Diarthrosis.*

Di-ar-thro'sis,* plural **Di-ar-thro'sēs.** [From διά, "through," as implying no impediment, and ἄρθρον, a "joint."] An articulation, permitting the bones to move freely on each other in every direction, like the shoulder and hip joints.

Diary Fever. [**Fe'bris Dia'ria.**] See EPHEMERA.

Di-as-cor'dĭ-um.* [From διά, "by means of," and σκόρδιον, the "water germander."] An electuary so named because this plant forms one of the ingredients.

Di-a-stăl'tic. [**Diastal'ticus;** from *διά*, and *στέλλω*, to "contract" or "dispose."] Applied by M. Hall to the reflex action of the excito-motory system of nerves, because performed through the spinal marrow.

Diastal'tic Arc. Applied by M. Hall to the course of the *Vis nervosa*, in complete or uninterrupted reflex or diastaltic action. Also called *Reflex arc.*

Diastal'tic Ner'vous Sȳs'tem. A term substituted by M. Hall for his former one of the *Spinal System.*

Di'a-stāse. [From *διΐστημι*, to "set apart," to "cause division or separation."] Literally, that which produces separation or decomposition. A substance produced during the germinating of seeds and buds, having the property of converting starch into sugar.

Di-as'ta-sis.* [From the same.] A forcible separation of bones without fracture.

Di-a-ste'ma, a*tis*.* [From the same.] A space or cleft. Applied in many terms like the following.

Di-as-tem-a-te-lȳt'rĭ-a.* [From *diaste'ma*, and *ἔλυτρον*, the "vagina."] A malformation consisting in a longitudinal fissure of the vagina.

Di-as'to-le.* [From *διαστέλλω*, to "dilate."] The dilatation of the heart, by which, with its alternate contraction (*Systole*), the circulation of the blood is carried on.

Di-a-ther'ma-nous. [From *διαθερμαίνω*, to "warm through."] A term denoting free permeability to heat.

Di-a-ther-man'sis.* [From the same.] The transit of the rays of heat.

Di-ath'e-sis.* [From *διατίθημι*, to "arrange," to "dispose."] A particular habit or disposition of the body; thus, we say, "an inflammatory diathesis," *i.e.* a habit or disposition of body peculiarly susceptible to inflammatory diseases.

Di-a-thet'ic. Belonging to diathesis.

Diatomaceæ,* di-a-to-ma'she-ē. [From *Diat'oma*, one of the genera.] A natural order of cryptogamous plants, found in still waters and oozy places. The green mucous slime seen on stones and walls which are always damp consists of these plants.

Di-at'o-mous. [**Diat'omus;** from *διά*, "through," and *τέμνω*, to "cut."] Cleavable throughout. Applied to *cleavage.*

Di-chlam-ȳd'e-us.* [From *δίς*, "twice" or "two," and *χλαμύς*, a "short cloak."] Applied to plants in the flowers of which there are two whorls.

Di-chot'o-mous. [**Dichot'omus;** from *δίχα*, "double," and *τέμνω*, to "cut."] Twice divided. A term applied to stems or branches which bifurcate, or are continually divided into pairs.

Dī'chro-ism. [**Dichrois'mus;** from *δίς*, "twice" or "two," and *χρία*, "color."] The property by which some minerals, when examined by transmitted light, exhibit different colors, according to the direction in which the rays of light pass through them.

Di-coc'cous. [**Dicoc'cus;** from *δίς*, "twice" or "two," and *κόκκος*, a "berry."] Having two capsules united, one cell in each.

Di-cot-ȳ-le'don,* plural **Di-cot-ȳ-le'do-nēs.** [From *δίς*, "twice" or "two," and *κοτυληδών*, a "cotyledon."] One of a class of plants having two cotyledons, or seed-lobes. Applied to a Jussieuan division of plants.

Dī-cot-ȳl-ed'o-nous. [**Dicotyle'donus, Dicotyledo'neus;** from the same.] Belonging to the division of plants termed *Dicotyledones.*

Di-cræ'us.* [From *δίς*, "twice," or "two," and *κραάς*, a "head."] Having two heads; also, bifid; cloven.

Dī-crot'ic. [**Dicrot'icus;** from *δίς*, "twice," and *κροτέω*, to "strike."] Applied to the pulse when there is a rebounding like a double pulsation.

Dic'ro-tous. [**Dic'rotus.**] The same as DICROTIC, which see.

Dic-tam'nus.* [From *Dic'te*, a mountain of Crete.] A genus of the class *Decandria*, natural order *Rutaceæ.*

Did'ȳ-mi,* the plural of DIDYMUS. Applied to the testicles.

Di-dȳm'ĭ-um.* [From *δίδυμος*, "twin."] The name of a metal recently discovered united with oxide of cerium, and so called from its being as it were the twin brother of lantanium, which was previously found in the same substance.

Did'ȳ-mus.* [From *δίδυμος*, "double," "twin."] By two and two: did'ymous. As a noun it denotes the *testis.*

Did-ȳ-na'mĭ-a.* [From *δίς*, "twice," or "twofold," probably meaning "of two kinds," and *δύναμις*, "power."] The fourteenth class of Linnæus's system of plants, characterized by the presence of four stamens, of which two are long and two short.

Dieb. alt. = *Die'bus alter'nis.** "On alternate days."

Dieb. tert. = *Die'bus ter'tiis.** "Every third day."

Di'ēs.* A Latin word signifying "day." It is often used in giving directions for taking medicines. The cases most used are the accusative singular, *Di'em*, ablative singular, *Di'e*, nominative plural, *Di'es*, ablative plural, *Die'bus*. See Appendix.

Di'et. [**Diæ'ta**; from δίαιτα, "regimen."] The food proper for invalids. *La Diète*, lå dè'ĕt', as used by French physicians, signifies extreme abstinence.

Di'et Drink. The *Decoct. Sarsaparillæ Comp.* of the Pharmacopœias.

Di-e-tet'ic. [**Diætet'icus**; from διαιτάω, to "feed."] Belonging to the taking of proper food, or to diet.

Di-e-tet'ics. [**Diætet'ica**; from the same.] The consideration (or science) of regulating the food or diet.

Differential Diagnosis. See DIAGNOSIS, DIFFERENTIAL.

Differential Thermometer. See THERMOMETER, DIFFERENTIAL.

Difficulty of Breathing. See DYSPNŒA.

Dif-for'mis.* [From *di* for *dis*, implying "difference," and *for'ma*, "shape."] Of different shapes; irregularly formed.

Dif-frac'tion. [**Diffrac'tio, o'nis**; from *dis*, "apart" or "aside," and *fran'go, frac'tum*, to "break."] The breaking of rays of light from their right course. See REFRACTION.

Dif-fu'sĭ-ble. [**Diffusib'ilis**; from *diffun'do, diffu'sum*, to "pour about," to "spread."] That which may be spread in all directions.

Dif-fu'sion Tube. An instrument for determining the rate of diffusion for different gases. It is simply a graduated tube closed at one end by plaster of Paris, a substance, when moderately dry, possessed of the requisite porosity.

Diffu'sion Vol'ume. A term used to express the different dispositions or tendencies of gases to interchange particles; the diffusion volume of air being 1, that of hydrogen is 3.33.

Dif-fu'sus.* [From *diffun'do, diffu'sum*, to "spread."] Widely spread: diffused.

Dig. = *Digera'tur.** "Let it be digested."

Dī-gas'tric. [**Digas'tricus**; from δίς, and γαστήρ, a "belly."] Having two bellies: the name of a muscle attached to the *os hyoïdes*; it is sometimes called *biven'ter maxil'læ inferio'ris*. The term is also applied to one of the interior *profundi* of Meckel, given off by the facial nerve; the other is called the *stylo-hyoïdeus*.

Digas'tric Groove. [See DIGASTRIC.] A longitudinal depression of the mastoïd process, so called from its giving attachment to the muscle of that name.

Diġ'er-ens.* [From *diġ'ero, diges'tum*, to "digest."] Digesting; digestive. Applied in the neuter plural (*Digerentia*, dij-e-ren'she-ạ) to medicines which promote the secretion of healthy pus.

Dĭ-ġes'ter. [From the same.] A strong iron or copper kettle, with a safety-valve, for subjecting bodies to vapor at a high temperature and under great pressure.

Dĭ-ġes'tion. [**Diges'tio, o'nis**; from the same.] The slow action of matters on each other, by subjection to heat. The conversion of food into chyle in the stomach.

Dĭ-ġes'tĭve. [**Digesti'vus**; from the same.] Belonging to digestion. Also applied to substances which promote suppuration; as cerates, poultices, etc.

Diges'tive Salt of Sȳl'vĭ-us. A salt discovered by Sylvius, since named muriate of potash, and now chloride of potassium.

Diġ'it. [From *diġ'itus*, a "finger."] The twelfth part of the sun's or moon's diameter, employed to denote the extent of an eclipse.

Digital. See DIGITALIS.

Diġ'ĭt-ạ-lin, or **Diġ'ĭt-ạ-lĭne.** [**Digitali'na**; from *Digita'lis*, the "foxglove."] A substance erroneously supposed to be the active principle of the *Digitalis purpurea*.

Diġ-ĭ-ta'lis.* [From *diġ'itus*, a "finger."] Belonging to a finger: diġ'ital.

Digita'lis.* [From *digita'le*, the "finger of a glove."] Foxglove. A Linnæan genus of the class *Didynamia*, natural order *Scrofulanaceæ*. Also, the Pharmacopœial name ‖ of the recent and dried leaves and stem of the *Digitalis purpurea*. According to the U.S. Pharmacopœia, "The leaves of the *D. purpurea* from plants of the second year's growth."

Digitalis is narcotic, sedative, and diuretic. It has a remarkable sedative effect on the heart, reducing the force, and especially the frequency, of the pulse: hence it is frequently given to moderate the action of the heart and arteries in phthisis, and especially in cases of hæmorrhage. As a diuretic, it is sometimes found very useful in dropsy. In large doses, it is poisonous, producing vertigo, nausea, and vomiting, syncope, convulsions, and death. For dose, see Appendix.

Digita'lis Pur-pu're-a.* The systematic name of the plant called foxglove.

Diġ-i-tate. [**Digita'tus;** from *dig'itus,* a "finger."] Having fingers. Applied to the leaves of plants so divided as to have the appearance of fingers.

Diġ-i-ta'to-Pin-na'tus.* Applied to a digitated leaf having pinnated leaflets.

Diġ'i-ti,* gen. **Diġ-i-to'rum.** The plural of DIGITUS, which see.

Diġ'iti Pe'dis,* gen. **Digito'rum Pe'dis.** The plural of DIGITUS PEDIS, which see.

Diġ'it-i-form. [**Digitifor'mis;** from *dig'itus,* a "finger, and *for'ma,* "likeness."] Formed like a finger.

Diġ'it-i-grāde. [**Digitig'radus;** from *dig'itus,* a "toe," and *gra'dus,* a "step."] Applied to carnivorous Mammals, which when standing or walking have the heel elevated.

Diġ'i-tus,* plural **Diġ'i-ti.** (Fr. *Doigt,* dwå.) A finger (or a toe). The fingers of the hand are the *in'dex,* or fore-finger; the *me'dius,* or middle finger; the *annula'ris,* or ring-finger; and the *auricula'ris,* or little finger. The bones of the fingers are called phalanges. See PHALANX, and FINGER.

Diġ'itus Ma'nus.* ("Finger of the Hand.") A finger.

Diġ'itus Pe'dis.* (Literally, "Finger of the Foot.") A toe.

Di-glos'sum.* [From δίς, "double," and γλῶσσα, a "tongue;" because a small leaf grows above the ordinary one, looking like two tongues.] A Botanical name of the *Prunus lauro-cerasus.*

Dī-ġy̆n'i-a.* [See next article.] A Linnæan order of plants having two styles.

Dī-ġy̆n'i-ous, or **Diġ'y̆-nous.** [**Digyn'ius;** from δίς, "two," and γυνή, a "woman" or "female."] Having two styles. Applied to a Linnæan order. See DIGYNIA.

Dil. = *Dil'ue,** "dilute," or *Dilu'tus,** "diluted."

Dil-a-tā'tion. [**Dilata'tio, o'nis;** from *dila'to, dilata'tum,* to "enlarge."] An enlargement or expansion, as of the heart, etc.

Di-la-ta'tor, o'ris.* [From the same.] The same as DILATOR, which see.

Di-lāt'ed. [**Dilata'tus;** from the same.] Enlarged.

Di-la'tor.* [From *di,* "apart," and *fe'ro, la'tum,* to "carry."] Literally, "that which carries or draws apart." A term applied to muscles whose office is to dilate certain parts, such as the inspiratory muscles, which dilate or expand the chest; also, to instruments used for dilating wounds, canals, etc.

Dill. The English name of the *Ane'thum grav'eolens.*

Dilleniaceæ,* dil-le-ne-a'she-ē. [From *Dille'nia,* one of the genera.] A natural order of exogenous plants, mostly trees, found in hot climates. Some species of this order are remarkable for the beauty of their flowers. Their properties are generally astringent.

Diluc. = *Dilu'culo.** "At daybreak."

Dil'u-ent. [**Dil'uens, en'tis;** from *dil'uo, dilu'tum,* to "dilute."] (Fr. *Délayant,* dà'là'yŏnᴳ'.) Applied to substances that increase the fluidity of the blood.

Dī-lūt'ed. [**Dilu'tus;** from the same.] Mixed.

Dī-lu'vi-al. [**Diluvia'lis;** from *dilu'vium,* a "flood."] Belonging to a flood, or to the Deluge.

Dim. = *Dimid'ius.** "One-half."

Dim'e-rous. [From δίς, "two," and μέρος, a "part."] Having two parts in each whorl. See TRIMEROUS.

Dī-mid'i-ate. [**Dimidia'tus;** from *dimid'ius,* the "half."] Divided into two.

Dimness of Sight. See CALIGO.

Dī-mor'phism. [**Dimorphis'mus;** from δίς, "twice," or "two," and μορφή, a "form."] The property of many solid bodies to assume two distinct crystalline forms; as sulphur, carbon, etc.

Dī-mor'phous. [From the same.] Having two forms. See DIMORPHISM.

Dim-y̆-a'ri-a.* [From δίς, "twice" or "two," and μῦς, μυός, a "muscle."] An order of bivalve Mollusks having shells marked by two impressions or indentations for the attachment of muscles.

Din'i-cal. [**Din'icus;** from δῖνος, "giddiness."] Belonging to giddiness. Applied to medicines that remove giddiness.

Di'nus.* [Gr. δῖνος; from δινεύω, to "whirl round."] Vertigo; dizziness; giddiness.

Di-o-don-çeph'a-lous. [**Diodon-ceph'alus;** from δίς, "twice," "double," ὀδούς, a "tooth," and κεφαλή, a "head."] A monster with double rows of teeth.

Diœcia,* di-ē'shẹ-ạ. The name of a Linnæan class of plants having diœcious flowers. See DIŒCIOUS.

Diœcious, di-e'shŭs. [**Diœ'cius;** from δίς, "twice" or "two," and οἰκία, a "house" or "habitation."] Literally, "having two houses," because the male and female, instead of forming one family, occupy separate habitations. A term applied by Linnæus to plants having male flowers on one and female flowers on another plant of the same species.

Dī-oġ'en-ēṡ' Cup. A name applied to the cup-like cavity of the hand formed or occasioned by bending the metacarpal bone of the little finger; so called because Diogenes is said to have thrown away his drinking-cup and used only his hand, for the sake of greater simplicity.

Di-op'trạ.* [From διόπτομαι, to "see through."] An instrument for measuring the height and distance of objects.

Di-op'tric, Di-op'tric-al. [**Diop'tricus;** from the same.] Belonging to Dioptrics.

Di-op'trics. [**Diop'trica;** from the same.] The branch of Optics which treats of refracted light, as contradistinguished from Catoptrics, which treats of reflected light.

Di-or-tho'sis.* [From διορθόω, to "regulate."] The restoration of parts to their proper situation; one of the ancient divisions of surgery.

Dioscorea. See YAM.

Dioscoreaceæ,* de-os-ko-re-a'she-ē, or **Di-os-co're-æ.*** A natural order of endogenous plants, found in the tropics. It includes the *Dioscorea* (Yam), the farinaceous tuber of which forms an important article of food.

Di-os'mạ.* [From Διός, "of Jove," and ὀσμή, an "odor," the compound signifying "divine odor or fragrance."] A Linnæan genus of the class *Pentandria*, natural order *Rutaceæ*. The former Pharmacopœial name (Lond. Ph., 1836) of *Buchu* leaves; but (Lond. Ph., 1851) said to be from the *Barosma crenata, B. crenulata*, and *B. serratifolia*.

Dios'ma Cre-na'tạ.* The plant the leaves of which were called buchu.

Di-os'me-æ.* The former name of a tribe of dicotyledonous plants. See RUTACEÆ.

Di-os'pȳ-ros.* [From Διός, "of Jove," and *py'rus*, a "pear-tree."] The persimmon; the Pharmacopœial name (U.S. Ph.) of the unripe fruit of the *Dios'pyros Virginia'na.*

Di-ox'ide. [From δίς, "twice" or "two," and *ox'ide.*] According to the electro-chemical theory, the elements of a compound may in relation to each other be considered oppositely electric; the equivalents of the *negative* element may then be distinguished by Latin numerals, those of the *positive* by Greek: thus, a *bin*-oxide denotes a compound which contains two equivalents of the negative element oxygen, whereas a *di*-oxide indicates that one equivalent of oxygen is combined with two of some *positive* body. And so of the *bi*-chloride, *di*-chloride, etc.

Dī-pet'ạ-lous. [**Dipet'alus;** from δίς, "twice" or "two," and πέταλον, a "petal."] Having two petals.

Diph-the'rĭ-ạ.* [From διφθέρα, "skin," "leather," or "membrane."] Inflammatory disease of the throat and glands, in which false membranes are formed.

Diph-the-ri'tis, *idis*.* [From the same.] A variety of *Pharyngitis*, in which a false membrane is formed, and for which the word *Diphtheria* has of late been very generally substituted.

Dī-phȳl'lous. [**Diphyl'lus;** from δίς, "twice" or "two," and φύλλον, a "leaf."] Having two leaves.

Dip'lo-Car'dĭ-ac. [From διπλόος, "double," and καρδία, a "heart."] Having a double heart, pulmonic and systemic, like mammals and birds.

Dip'lo-e.* [From διπλόω, to "double."] The cellular osseous tissue between the two tables of the skull.

Dip'lo-Gang-lĭ-a'tạ.* [From διπλόος, "double," and γαγγλίον, a "nerve-knot."] A term applied by Dr. Grant to the third sub-kingdom of animals, or *Entomoïda*, consisting chiefly of articulated animals with articulated members, the *Insects* of Linnæus, having their nervous columns arranged in the same relative position as the diplo-neura, with the ganglia increased in size, corresponding to their higher development. See INSECTS.

Dĭ-plo'mạ, *atis*.* [From διπλόω, to "fold," to "double."] Literally, a "folding" or "doubling," "something doubled." A double vessel; a water-bath. The charter (originally a folded letter) by which the physician or surgeon is declared qualified to practise his profession. Also, a certificate of graduation given to every one who has successfully passed through a university or collegiate course.

Dip-lo-my-e'li-a.* [From διπλόος, "double," and μυελός, "marrow."] Congenital division of the spinal marrow lengthwise.

Dip'lo-Neū'ra.* A term applied by Dr. Grant to the second sub-kingdom of animals, or *Helminthoïda*, comprising the various forms of worms in which the nervous columns have their ganglionic enlargements very slightly developed, and are marked by a greater lateral separation from each other along the median line than is observed in the DIPLO-GANGLIATA.

Dip-lo'pi-a.* [From διπλόος, "double," and ὄπτομαι, to "see."] An affection consisting in double vision: dip'lopy.

Dip-lop'ter-ous. [**Diplop'terus;** from διπλόος, "double," and πτέρον, a "wing."] Applied to insects having doubled or folded wings.

Dip'pel's Oil. An animal oil procured by the destructive distillation of animal matter, especially of albuminous and gelatinous substances.

Dipsacaceæ,* dip-sa-ka'she-ē, or **Dipsaceæ,*** dip-sa'she-ē. A natural order of herbaceous plants, including *Dip'sacus* (Teasel), used by fullers.

Dip'sa-cus.* [From δίψα, "thirst."] A name formerly given to diabetes, from the thirst accompanying that affection.

Dip-so'sis.* [From δίψα, "thirst."] Morbid thirst; excessive or impaired desire to drink.

Dip'ter-a.* An order of insects. See DIPTERUS.

Dipteraceæ,* dip-ter-a'she-ē. [From *Dipterocar'pus*, one of the genera.] A natural order consisting mostly of gigantic trees, found in India, and abounding in resinous juice. It includes the *Dryobalanops camphora*, which yields the hard camphor of Sumatra. A species of this order produces the *Saul*, or *Sal*, the best and most extensively used timber of India.

Dipterocarpeæ. See DIPTERACEÆ.

Dip'ter-us.* [From δίς, "twice" or "two," and πτέρον, a "wing."] Having two wings: dip'terous. Applied in the plural neuter (*Dip'tera*) to an order of two-winged insects, such as the common fly, mosquito, etc.

Di-rec'tor, o'ris.* [From *dir'igo, direc'tum*, to "guide."] A grooved instrument for guiding a bistoury, etc., in certain surgical operations.

Dir'i-gens.* [From the same.] An ancient constituent in a prescription, meaning that which directs the operation of the associated substances: thus, *nitre* in conjunction with *squill* is diuretic; with *guaiacum* it is diaphoretic.

Dir. Prop. = *Directio'ne Pro'pria.** "With a proper direction."

Dirt-Eating. See CHTHONOPHAGIA.

Dis, or **Di.** A Latin particle usually signifying "apart," implying separation or division, as in *divellent*. It is sometimes negative or privative, as in *displease* (Lat. *displi'ceo*).

Dis'çi-form. [**Discifor'mis;** from *dis'cus*, a "disk."] Resembling a disk; discoid.

Dis'coid. [**Discoi'des;** from δίσκος, a "quoit," and εἶδος, a "form."] Resembling a quoit, or disk; quoit-shaped: disciform.

Discus. See DISK.

Dis-cuss'. [From *discu'tio, discus'sum*, literally, to "strike apart;" hence, to "scatter," to "dissipate."] To promote or effect the resolution of tumors, etc.

Discutient, dis-ku'shent. [**Discu'tiens;** from the same.] Applied to substances having the property of promoting the resolution of tumors.

Dis-ease'. [From the French *dés*, negative, and *aise*, "ease." Lat. **Mor'bus;** Fr. *Maladie*, mâ'lâ'dè'.] Any departure from the state of health.

Dis-in-fect'ants. [From *dis*, negative, and *infi'cio, infec'tum*, to "corrupt," to "infect."] Applied to agents which destroy the causes of infection. Among these agents, chlorine is one of the most efficient.

Dis-in-fect'ing. [**Disinfi'ciens;** from the same.] Purifying the atmosphere from contagious influences.

Dis-in-fec'tion. [**Disinfec'tio, o'nis;** from the same.] The act of purifying the atmosphere from contagious influences by renewing the air, or by chemical action.

Disk. [**Dis'cus;** from δίσκος, a "quoit."] The round, central part of a compound flower; also, the whole surface within the margin of a leaf.

Dis-lo-cā'tion. [**Disloca'tio, o'nis;** from *dis*, "division," and *lo'co*, to "place."] Displacement of a bone of a movable articulation from its natural situation; luxation.

Dispensaire. See DISPENSARY, and DISPENSATORY.

Dis-pen'sa-rȳ. [Lat. **Dispensa'rium;** Fr. *Dispensaire*, dè'spŏng'saiR'; from *dispen'so, dispensa'tum*, to "dispense," to "distribute."] A place where medicines are prepared and dispensed. Generally applied to a charitable institution for the sick poor of large communities.

Dis-pen'sa-to-ry̆. [Lat. **Dispensa-to'rium;** Fr. *Dispensaire*, dĕ'spŏNG'saiR'; from the same.] A book which describes the various articles of the Materia Medica and gives directions for preparing and compounding medicines.

Dis-plāce'ment. A process applied to pharmaceutical preparations, and founded on the long-known fact that any quantity of liquid with which a powder may be saturated, when put into a proper apparatus, may be displaced by an additional quantity of that or of another liquid.

Dis-sect'ed. [**Dissec'tus.** See DISSECTION.] Incised; cut.

Dis-sec'tion. [**Dissec'tio,** *o'nis;* from *dis*, "apart," and *se'co, sec'tum*, to "cut."] The cutting up of an animal or vegetable in order to ascertain its structure.

Dī-sper'ma-tous, or **Di-sper'-mous.** [**Disper'matus;** from δίς, "twice" or "two," and σπέρμα, a "seed."] Having two seeds.

Dis-sep'ĭ-ment. [**Dissepimen'-tum;** from *disse'pio*, to "separate."] A separation, or partition, that divides the cells of a capsule.

Dis-ten'tion. [**Disten'tio;** from *dis*, "apart," and *ten'do, ten'tum* or *ten'sum*, to "stretch."] The dilatation of a hollow viscus by too great accumulation of its contents.

Dis-tich'ĭ-a,* **Dis-tĭ-chi'a-sis.*** [From δίς, "twice" or "two," and στίχος, a "row."] An affection in which the *tarsus* has a double row of eyelashes, one inwards against the eye, the other outwards.

Dis'tĭ-chous. [**Dis'tichus;** from the same.] Double ranked; ranged in two rows, like the leaves of certain grasses.

Distillatio per Descensum. See DESCENSUS.

Dis-til-lā'tion. [**Distilla'tio,** or, more correctly, **Destilla'tio;** from *distil'lo, distilla'tum*, to "drop by little and little," or *destil'lo, destilla'tum*, to "drop down" or "fall in drops."] The process of separating the volatile from the more fixed parts by heat.

Distilla'tion, De-struc'tĭve. The decomposition of bodies by strong heat in one vessel, and collection of the products in another.

Dis'to-ma He-pat'ĭ-cum.* [From δίς, "twice" or "two," στόμα, a "mouth," and ἡπατικός, "belonging to the liver."] The fluke (Fr. *Douve*, doov), a worm sometimes found in the liver and gall-bladder of man, but more commonly in those of sheep, goats, etc. It is an obovate flat worm, nearly an inch in length and about the third of an inch broad. From the gall-bladder it occasionally passes into the intestinal canal.

Dis-tor'tion. [**Distor'tio,** *o'nis;* from *dis*, "apart" or "awry," and *tor'-queo, tor'tum*, to "twist."] Unnatural direction or disposition of parts, as curvature of the spine, etc.

Dis-tor'tor.* [From the same.] That which distorts. See next article.

Distor'tor O'ris.* ("Distorter of the Mouth.") A name given to one of the zygomatic muscles, from its action in distorting the mouth in rage, grinning, etc.

Dis-trich'ĭ-a. The same as DISTICHIA.

Dis'trix.* [From δίς, "twice," or "double," and θρίξ, the "hair."] Forky hair; a disease of the hair in which it splits at the end.

Dī-u-re'sis.* [From διά, "through," and οὐρέω, to "pass water."] Increased discharge of urine, from whatever cause.

Dī-u-ret'ic. [**Diuret'icus;** from the same.] Belonging to *diuresis;* causing *diuresis*.

Di-ur'nal. [**Diur'nus;** from *di'es*, a "day."] Belonging to the daytime. Applied to a family of rapacious birds which fly chiefly by day, to distinguish them from others, such as owls, that fly by night. Also applied to a family of insects.

Di-ur-nā'tion. [From *diur'nus*, "daily."] A term introduced by M. Hall to express the state of some animals, the bat, for example, during the day, contrasted with their activity at night.

Div. = *Div'ide.** "Divide."

Dī-văr'ĭ-cate. [**Divarica'tus;** from *divar'ico, divarica'tum*, to "stride" or "straddle."] Straddling; diverging at an obtuse angle.

Dī-văr-ĭ-cā'tion. [From the same.] The bifurcation, or separating into two, of an artery, a nerve, etc.

Di-vel'lent. [**Divel'lens;** from *dis*, "apart," and *vel'lo, vul'sum*, to "pluck," to "pull."] Pulling asunder, or separating.

Divellent Affinity. See AFFINITY, DIVELLENT.

Di-ver-sĭ-flo'rus.* [From *diver'sus,* "different," and *flos,* a "flower."] Having different flowers: diversiflo'rate.

Di-ver-tic'u-lum.* [From *diver'to,* to "turn aside."] A variation or departure from the natural conditions; a malformation.

Di-vul'sion, or **Divulsio,*** di-vul'-she-o. [See DIVELLENT.] Applied in Surgery to the forcible separation or laceration of a part.

Dizziness. See DINUS, and VERTIGO.

Dobereiner's (do'be-rī'nerz) **Lamp.** A method of producing an instantaneous light by throwing a jet of hydrogen gas upon recently prepared spongy platinum; the metal instantly becomes red-hot, and then sets fire to the gas. This discovery was made by Professor Dobereiner, of Jena, in 1824.

Doç-i-ma'sĭ-ạ.* [From δοκιμάζω, to "test," to "examine," to "prove."] Doç'imacy. The art of examining fossils or metals to ascertain their composition.

Docima'sia Pul-mo'num,* or **Docima'sia Pul-mo-na'lis.*** ("Testing of the Lungs.") In Medical Jurisprudence, the testing of the lungs of a dead new-born child, in order to ascertain whether it has ever respired; in other words, whether it was born alive or dead.

Doç-i-mas'tic. [**Docimas'ticus.**] Belonging to *Docimasia.*

Docimas'tic Art. The art of assaying.

Dock, Sour. The *Ru'mex aceto'sa.*

Dock, Wa'ter. The common name for the *Rumex hydrolapathum.*

Doc'tor, o'ris.* [From *do'ceo, doc'tum,* to "teach."] Literally, a "teacher" or "instructor." A degree or title conferred by the Medical Faculty of a university, or college, on "those who have *successfully undergone previous examination and trial,*" constituting them physicians; also, a title conferred on those who have received the highest degree in law or divinity. The appellation originally implied that he who bore it was so thoroughly conversant with his art or profession as to be qualified to teach it.

Do-dec'ạ-gon. [**Dodecago'num;** from δώδεκα, "twelve," and γωνία, an "angle."] A figure having twelve sides and angles.

Do-dec-ag'o-nạl. [**Dodecago'nus.**] Belonging to a dodecagon.

Do'dec-ạ-he'drạl. [**Dodecahe'drus.**] Belonging to a dodecahedron.

Do'dec-ạ-he'dron. [From δώδεκα, and ἕδρα, a "base."] A solid figure of twelve equal bases or sides.

Do-de-can'drĭ-ạ.* [From δώδεκα, "twelve," and ἀνήρ, a "man" or "male."] The eleventh class of plants in the Linnæan system, characterized by the presence of from twelve to nineteen stamens.

Do-de-can'drĭ-ous. [**Dodecan'drius;** from δώδεκα, and ἀνήρ, ἀνδρός, a "man" or "male."] Having twelve stamens. See DODECANDRIA.

Dog-Rose. The *Rosa canina,* or hip-tree.

Do-lab'rĭ-form. [**Dolabrifor'mis;** from *dolab'ra,* a "hatchet" or "axe."] Having the form of a hatchet.

Do'li Ca'pax.* ("Capable of Deceit.") Applied in Medical Jurisprudence to a criminal for whom insanity is pleaded in excuse, when inquiry is made as to his mental capacity when the crime was committed.

Dol'ĭ-chos.* [Gr. δολιχός, "long."] A Linnæan genus of the class *Diadelphia,* natural order *Leguminosæ.*

Dol'ichos Pru'rĭ-ens.* ("Itching Dolichos.") The cowhage, or cow-itch, now called *Mucu'na pru'riens.*

Dol'o-mīte. A species of magnesian limestone.

Do'lor,* plural **Do-lo'rēs.** [From *do'leo,* to "be in pain," to "ache;" Fr. *Douleur,* doo'lur'.] Pain.

Do'lor Cap'ĭ-tis.* ("Pain of the Head.") See CEPHALALGIA.

Do'lor Den'tium.* ("Pain of the Teeth.") See ODONTALGIA.

Do'lor Fa-cĭe'i.* ("Pain of the Face.") See NEURALGIA.

Dom-bey'ạ Ex-çel'sạ.* A tree growing in South America, and yielding the glutinous, milk-like fluid known as Dombeya Turpentine.

Do-re'mạ, atis.* [Gr. δώρημα, a "gift."] A Linnæan genus of the class *Pentandria,* natural order *Umbelliferæ.*

Dore'ma Am-mo-ni'ạ-cum.* The systematic name of the plant which produces *Ammoniacum:* gum-ammoniac.

Do-ron'ĭ-cum Mon-ta'num.* Another name for ARNICA MONTANA.

Dor'sad. DORSAL (used adverbially).

Dor'sal. [**Dorsa'lis;** from *dor'sum,* the "back."] Belonging to the back. Applied by Dr. Barclay as meaning "towards the back."

Dor'si,* the genitive of DORSUM, which see.

Dor'sĭ-branch-ĭ-a'tus.* [From

dor'sum, the "back," and *bran'chiæ*, "lungs."] Dorsibran'chiate. Applied in the plural neuter (*Dorsibranchia'ta*) to an order of *Articulata* having *branchiæ* equally distributed along the body.

Dor'so-. A prefix denoting connection with the back; as, *Dor'so-Cos'tal*, having connection with the back and ribs.

Dor-ste'ni-a.* A genus of urticaceous plants, in which the flowers are arranged upon a fleshy receptacle, usually flat and of a very variable form.

Dor'sum,* gen. **Dor'si.** [Gr. νῶτος; Fr. *Dos*, dō.] The back of man or beast. The superior surface of other parts, as of the foot, hand, etc.

Dōse. [**Do'sis;** from δίδωμι, to "give."] Literally, "any thing given" or "administered." The determinate quantity of a medicine prescribed or given to patients at one time. It is obvious that the same quantity of any medicine should not be given to an infant as to an adult. The difference of sex, peculiarities of constitution, and the previous habits of the patient must also be taken into consideration by the judicious physician. It may be stated, in a general way, that the dose for an infant one year old should not be more than about one-twelfth part of a dose for a grown person; for a child three years of age, one-sixth; for one seven years old, one-third; and for one of twelve years, one-half as much as for an adult. Women usually require smaller doses of medicine than men. For a table of doses, see Appendix.

Dos'sil. A small roll or pledget of lint for introduction into wounds, etc.

Doth-in-en-ter-i'tis,* or, more properly, **Do-thi-en-en-ter-i'tis.*** [From δοθιήν, a "boil," and ἔντερον, an "intestine."] Enlargement and inflammation of the glandular follicles of the intestinal canal.

Doŭb'ler. An instrument used in electrical experiments, and so contrived that, by executing certain movements, very small quantities of electricity communicated to part of the apparatus, may be continually doubled until it becomes perceptible by means of an electroscope.

Douce-Amère, dooss å'mêR'. [From *doux*, "sweet," and *amer*, "bitter."] The French for DULCAMARA, which see.

Douche (Fr.), doosh. Literally, a "pumping, as at the bath." The sudden descent of a stream or column of water, usually cold, on the head, or other part. The *douche* is often found to be an excellent means of taming a furious maniac.

Douleur. See DOLOR.

Douve, doov. The French name for the *Fluke*, an intestinal worm. See DISTOMA HEPATICUM.

Do'ver's Pow'der. The *Pulvis Ipecacuanhæ compositus.*

Dove'tail Joint. The suture or serrated articulation, as of the bones of the head.

Drach. = *Drach'ma.** A "drachm."

Drachm, drăm. [**Drach'ma;** from δραχμή, a Greek weight of about sixty-six grains avoirdupois.] In Pharmacy, a weight of sixty grains, or three scruples, or the eighth part of an ounce.

Draçine. [From *dra'co*, a "dragon."] A precipitate formed by mixing cold water with a concentrated alcoholic solution of dragon's blood.

Dracontium,* dra-kon'she-ŭm. A genus of plants of the Linnæan class *Tetrandria*, natural order *Araceæ*. Also, the Pharmacopœial name (U.S. Ph.) of the root of the *Dracontium fœtidum.* It is stimulant, antispasmodic, and narcotic; and it has been highly recommended in asthma.

Dracon'tium Fœt'idum* (fet'e-dŭm). The systematic name of the skunk-cabbage, a plant growing abundantly in many parts of the Northern and Middle United States. See preceding article.

Dra-cunc'u-lus.* [Diminutive of *dra'co*, a "dragon;" Gr. δράκων.] The Guinea-Worm, which breeds under the skin, and is common among the natives of Guinea. It is also termed the *Dracunculus gordius.* See GUINEA-WORM.

Dra-gan'tin, or **Dra-gan'tine.** A mucilage obtained from gum tragacanth.

Drag'on's Blood. [**San'guis Draco'nis.**] The dark, concrete, resinous substance obtained from the *Calamus Rotang*, or, according to some writers, the *Dracæna draco*, *Pterocarpus draco*, and the *Pterocarpus santalinus*, etc.

Dras'tic. [**Dras'ticus;** from δραστικός, "working," "active," "efficacious."] A term applied to purgative medicines which are powerful or violent in their operation.

Draught, drăft. [**Haus'tus.**] A potion, or what a person drinks at once.

Drench. A form of medicine used in farriery, analogous to a draught.

Dri'mўs.* [From δριμύς, "pungent."]

A Linnæan genus of the class *Dodecandria*, natural order *Magnoliaceæ*.

Dri'mys Win-te'ri,* called also **Dri'mys Ar-o-mat'i-ca.*** The systematic name of the tree which produces the Winter's bark. See WINTERA.

Driv'el-ling. Involuntary flow of the saliva, as in old age, infancy, and idiocy; slavering.

Droit, drwå ("right," or "straight"). The French term for *Rectus*, applied to various muscles of the body.

Drop. [**Gut'ta.**] The smallest quantity of a liquid. See MINIM.

Drop, Serene. See GUTTA SERENA.

Drop'sy̆. [Lat. **Hy'drops;** Gr. ὕδρωψ, from ὕδωρ, "water."] The disease *Hydrops*, variously distinguished according to the part affected.

Dropsy of the Belly. See ASCITES.

Dropsy of the Brain. See HYDROCEPHALUS.

Dropsy of the Chest. See HYDROTHORAX.

Dropsy of the Flesh. See ANASARCA.

Dropsy of the Joint. See HYDROPS ARTICULI.

Dropsy of the Spine. See HYDRORACHITIS.

Dropsy of the Testicle. See HYDROCELE.

Dropsy of the Uterus. See HYDROMETRA.

Droseraceæ,* dros-er-a'she-ē. [From *Dros'era*, one of the genera.] Sundews. A natural order of exogenous herbaceous plants, found in nearly all parts of the world where there are marshes. It includes the *Dionea* (Fly-Catcher), remarkable for the irritability of the hairs with which its leaves are bordered.

Drowning. See SUBMERSIO.

Drowsiness. See LETHARGY, SOMNOLENTIA.

Drug. (Fr. *Drogue*, drog.) [Probably from the Anglo-Saxon *Drugan*, to "dry," or from essentially the same root in some cognate language, as a large majority of drugs are vegetable substances that have been dried in order to preserve them.] A term originally, and still most frequently, applied to medicines in their simple form, but also used to include all substances which are employed as medicines.

Drum of the Ear. See TYMPANUM.

Drunkenness. See TEMULENTIA.

Drupaceæ,* dru-pa'she-ē. [See next article.] A natural order of exogenous trees and shrubs, found in cold and temperate climates, including the peach, plum, almond, and cherry. Prussic or hydrocyanic acid abounds in the leaves and kernels of the fruit.

Dru-pā'ceous. [**Drupa'ceus;** from *dru'pa*, a "drupe."] Having drupes. See DRUPACEÆ.

Drupe. [**Dru'pa;** from δρύππα, a "ripe olive."] A fleshy fruit containing a stone or nut, as the cherry, etc.

Dru'sy̆. Applied in Mineralogy to a surface coated with a number of minute crystals.

Dry Bel'ly-Ache. The *Colica Pictonum*.

Dry Cup'ping. The application of the cupping-glass *without scarification*, in order to produce revulsion of blood from any part of the body.

Dry Pile. The name of a galvanic apparatus, formed without any acid or liquid, usually constructed with pairs of metallic plates separated by layers of farinaceous paste mixed with common salt.

Dry Rot. A species of decay to which wood is subject. The wood loses all its cohesion, and becomes friable, and fungi generally appear on it. The first destructive change is probably of a chemical kind.

Dry-o-băl'a-nops Ar-o-mat'i-ca.* A tree of the order *Dipteraceæ*, yielding a liquid called *camphor oil* and a crystalline solid termed *Sumatra* or *Borneo Camphor*.

Dryobal'anops Cam'pho-ra.* The tree which affords camphor in greatest quantity.

Du-al'i-ty̆. [**Dual'itas, a'***tis;* from *dua'lis*, "pertaining to two."] A term used in reference to a theory that the two hemispheres of the brain are capable of acting independently of each other.

Duct of Ste'no. The excretory duct of the parotid gland.

Duct of Whar'ton. [**Duc'tus Whartonia'nus; Duc'tus Saliva'ris Infe'rior.**] The excretory duct of the submaxillary gland. These two last, with the sublingual, constitute the *salivary* ducts.

Duc-til'i-ty̆. [**Ductil'itas, a'***tis;* from *du'co, duc'tum*, to "draw."] A property by which bodies can be drawn out as into wire.

Ducts of Bellini (bel-lee'ne). [**Duc'tus Bellinia'ni.**] The orifices of the uriniferous canals of the kidneys.

Duc'tus,* plural **Duc'tus.** [From *du'co, duc'tum,* to "lead."] A canal, or duct.

Duc'tus ad Na'sum* ("Duct [leading] to the Nose"), otherwise called **Lach'rỹ-mal Duct.** A duct extending from the lachrymal sac and opening into the inferior meatus of the nose.

Duc'tus A-quo'si.* ("Watery Ducts.") Lymphatic vessels; the aqueous ducts.

Duc'tus Ar-te-rĭ-o'sus.* ("Arterial Duct.") A blood-vessel peculiar to the fœtus, communicating directly between the pulmonary artery and the aorta.

Duc'tus Com-mu'nis Chol-ed'o-chus.* ("Common Bile-receiving Duct.") The bile-duct formed by the junction of the cystic and hepatic ducts. It conveys the bile from the liver into the duodenum.

Duc'tus Çỹs'tĭ-cus.* ("Cystic Duct.") The excretory duct which leads from the neck of the gall-bladder to join the hepatic, forming with it the *Ductus communis choledochus.*

Duc'tus Def'er-ens.* Another name for the VAS DEFERENS, which see.

Duc'tus E-jac-u-la-to'rĭ-us* ("Ejaculatory Duct"), plural **Duc'tus E-jac-u-la-to'rĭ-i.** A duct within the prostate gland, opening into the urethra, into which it conveys the semen: it is about three-fourths of an inch long.

Duc'tus Gal-ac-tof'er-i or **Lac-tif'er-i.*** ("Milk-bearing or Milk-conveying Ducts.") Milk-ducts arising from the glandular grains of the mamma and terminating in sinuses near the base of the nipple.

Duc'tus He-pat'ĭ-cus.* ("Hepatic Duct.") The duct which is formed by the union of the proper ducts of the liver. See DUCTUS COMMUNIS CHOLEDOCHUS.

Duc'tus In-ci-so'rĭ-us.* A continuation of the *fora'men incisi'vum* between the palatine processes into the nose.

Ductus Lachrymalis. See DUCTUS AD NASUM.

Duc'tus Lỹm-phat'ĭ-cus Dex'ter.* ("Right Lymphatic Duct.") A duct formed by the lymphatics of the right side of the thorax, etc., and opening into the junction of the right jugular and subclavian veins.

Duc'tus Pan-cre-at'ĭ-cus.* ("Pancreatic Duct.") The pancreatic duct, which joins the gall-duct at its entrance into the duodenum. Near the duodenum this duct is joined by a smaller one, called *Ductus Pancreaticus Minor* ("Lesser Pancreatic Duct").

Duc'tus Pro-stat'ĭ-ci.* ("Prostatic Ducts.") The ducts of the prostate gland, from twenty to twenty-five in number, opening into the prostatic urethra on each side of the *veru montanum.*

Duc'tus Sal-ĭ-va'ris In-fe'rĭ-or.* ("Inferior Salivary Duct.") See DUCT OF WHARTON.

Ductus Thoracicus. See THORACIC DUCT.

Duc'tus Tho-raç'ĭ-cus Dex'ter.* ("Right Thoracic Duct.") A designation of the right great lymphatic vein, formed of lymphatic vessels arising from the axillary ganglia of the right side.

Duc'tus Ve-no'sus.* ("Venous Duct.") A blood-vessel peculiar to the fœtus, communicating from the *Vena cava ascendens* to the *Vena portæ.*

Duelech, dü'lĕk. A term employed by Van Helmont to denote the state in which the spirit of urine is precipitated when it forms calculous concretions.

Dul-ca-ma'ra.* [From *dul'cis,* "sweet," and *ama'rus,* "bitter."] (Fr. *Douce-Amère,* dooss â'mêr'.) Bitter-sweet. The Pharmacopœial name ‖ of the stalks of the *Solanum dulcamara.* Dulcamara possesses narcotic, diuretic, and diaphoretic properties. It is chiefly employed as a remedy in diseases of the skin, such as *psoriasis, lepra,* etc.

Dul-çe'do.* [From *dul'cis,* "sweet."] Sweetness. See next article.

Dulce'do Spu-to'rum.* [See SPUTA.] Literally, "sweetness of the sputa, or spittle." The name given by Frank to that form of ptyalism in which the saliva has a sweet or mawkish taste.

Dumb. See MUTE.

Dumbness. See APHONIA.

Du-mōse'. [From *du'mus,* a "bush."] Bushy or shrubby.

Du-o-de'num.* [From *duode'ni,* "twelve."] The first portion of the small intestine, its length being about twelve fingers' breadth.

Du'plĭ-cate. [**Duplica'tus;** from *du'plico, duplica'tum,* to "double."] Doubled.

Du'plum.* [From *du'o,* "two," and *pli'ca,* a "fold."] The double of any thing. As a prefix, *duplo* signifies "twofold:" as, *duplo*-carburet, twofold carburet.

Dupuytren (dü'pwē'trŏNᵍ'), **Compres'sor of.** An instrument invented by Dupuytren, for compressing the femoral artery.

Du'ra Ma'ter.* (The "Hard Mother." Fr. *Dure Mère,* dür mêr.) The tough external membrane of the brain, once supposed to give origin to all the other membranes of the body.

Du-ra'men.* [From *du'ro, dura'tum,* to "harden," or *du'rus,* "hard."] The interior, more deeply-colored, and harder portion of the trunk and branches of trees, commonly called *heart-wood,* as distinguished from the exterior portion, alburnum or sap-wood.

Dutch Gold. An alloy of copper and zinc, in which the zinc is in greater proportion than it exists in brass. It is allied to *tombac* and *pinchbeck.*

Dutch Liq'uid. The chloride of olefiant gas; also called *Dutch oil.*

Dutch Min'e-ral. Metallic copper beaten out in very thin leaves.

Dutch Oil. See DUTCH LIQUID.

Dutch Pink. Chalk, or whiting, dyed yellow with a decoction of birch-leaves, French berries, and alum.

Dye. See DYES.

Dyers' Alkanet. See ANCHUSA TINCTORIA.

Dyers' Broom, or **Dyers' Weed.** See GENISTA TINCTORIA.

Dyers' Oak. See QUERCUS TINCTORIA.

Dyes. Coloring matters, whether vegetable, animal, or mineral, used to impart to cloth, yarn, etc., a color different from that which they already possess.

Dy̆-na'mĭ-a.* [From δύναμις, "power."] Vital power, or strength.

Dy̆-nam'ic. [**Dynam'icus;** from the same.] Belonging to the vital power, or strength.

Dy̆-nam'ics. [**Dynam'ica;** from the same.] The science of the forces of bodies in relation to each other. *Vital Dynamics* is the science which treats of vital forces.

Dy̆-nam-om'e-ter. [**Dynamom'etrum;** from δύναμις, "power," and μέτρον, a "measure."] An instrument by which to measure strength and power.

Dys. [Gr. δύς.] A Greek particle signifying "difficult," or "with difficulty," "bad," or "badly," "painfully," etc.

Dy̆s-æs-the'sĭ-a.* [From δύς, "difficult," and αἰσθάνομαι, to "perceive."] Dulness of any of the senses, particularly touch. Applied to an order of the class *Locales* of Cullen's Nosology.

Dy̆s-cat-a-po'sĭ-a.* [From δύς, "difficult," and κατάποσις, the "act of swallowing."] Difficulty of swallowing liquids. A term applied by Dr. Mead to hydrophobia.

Dy̆s-çĭ-ne'sĭ-a.* [From δύς, "difficult," and κινέω, to "move."] Diminution of the power of motion. Applied in the plural (*Dyscine'siæ*) to an order of the class *Locales* of Cullen's Nosology.

Dy̆s-cra'sĭ-a.* [From δύς, "bad," and κρᾶσις, a "tempering" or "temperament."] A faulty state of the constitution: dys'crasy.

Dy̆s-e-co'ĭ-a.* [From δύς, "difficult," and ἀκοή, "hearing."] Diminished or impaired hearing; deafness. A genus of the order *Dysæsthesiæ,* class *Locales,* of Cullen's Nosology.

Dy̆s'en-tĕr-y̆. [**Dysente'ria;** from δύς, "difficult," or "painful," and ἔντερον, a "bowel."] A disease marked by much griping, tenesmus, and stools consisting chiefly of mucus, often mixed with blood.

Dy̆s'ly̆s-in. [From δύς, "difficult," and λύσις, "solution."] Literally, "difficult of solution." Applied to an ingredient of bilin which remains undissolved as a resinous mass during the solution and digestion of bilin in dilute hydrochloric acid.

Dy̆s-men-or-rhœ'a.* [From δύς, "difficult," μήν, a "month," and ῥέω, to "flow."] (Fr. *Dysménorrhée,* dės'mà'-no'rà'.) Difficult menstruation.

Dy̆s-o'dēs.* [From δύς, "bad," and ὄζω, to "smell."] Having a bad smell. A term applied by Hippocrates to a fetid disorder of the small intestines.

Dy̆s-op'sĭ-a.* [From δύς, "difficult," or "painful," and ὄψις, "vision."] Painful or defective vision. A genus of the order *Dysæsthesiæ,* class *Locales,* of Cullen's Nosology.

Dy̆s-o-rex'ĭ-a.* [From δύς, "bad," or "difficult," and ὄρεξις, "appetite."] Depraved appetite. Applied in the plural to an order of the class *Locales* of Cullen's Nosology.

Dy̆s-os-phre'sĭ-a.* [From δύς, "difficult," and ὄσφρησις, "smell."] Impaired condition of the sense of smell.

Dy̆s-pep'sĭ-a.* [From δύς, "difficult," and πέπτω, to "concoct."] Indigestion: dyspep'sy. A genus of the order *Adynamiæ,* class *Neuroses,* of Cullen's Nosology.

Dy̆s-pha'ġĭ-a.* [From δύς, "difficult," and φάγω, to "eat."] Dys'phagy; difficulty in swallowing. A genus of the order *Dyscinesiæ,* class *Locales,* of Cullen's Nosology. See ACATAPOSIS.

Dy̆s-pho'nĭ-a.* [From δύς, "difficult," and φωνή, "voice."] Difficulty of speaking.

Dy̆s-pho'rĭ-ạ.* [From δύς, "difficult," and φέρω, to "bear."] Inquietude: a difficulty of enduring one's self. It embraces the affections of *anxiety* and *fidgets*.

Dyspnœa,* dĭsp-nē'ạ. [From δύς, "difficult," and πνέω, to "breathe."] (Fr. *Dyspnée*, dĕs'pnå'.) Difficult or labored breathing. A genus of the order *Spasmi*, class *Neuroses*, of Cullen's Nosology.

Dy̆s-sper-ma'sĭ-ạ,* **Dy̆s-sper-mạ-tis'mus.*** [From δύς, "difficult," and σπέρμα, "seed."] Difficult or imperfect discharge of semen: dyssper'matism. A genus of the order *Epischeses*, class *Locales*, of Cullen's Nosology.

Dy̆s-thet'ĭ-cạ.* [From δύς, "bad," and τίθημι, to "place," to "make," to "constitute."] The name of an order in Dr. Good's Nosology, denoting diseases dependent upon a bad habit or constitution of the body.

Dy̆s-u'rĭ-ạ.* [From δύς, "difficult," and οὖρον, the "urine."] Difficult or painful and incomplete discharge of urine. A genus of the order *Epischeses*, class *Locales*, of Cullen's Nosology.

Dy̆s'u-ry̆. The same as DYSURIA.

E.

E, or **Ex.** A Latin particle signifying "out," "out of." It is sometimes privative. See Ex.

Ear. [Lat. **Au'ris;** Fr. *Oreille*, o'rēl.] The organ of hearing, comprehending the external, middle, and internal ear.

Ear, Inflammation of. See OTITIS.

Ear-Ache. See OTALGIA.

Ear-Wax. See CERUMEN.

Eared. See AURICULATE.

Earth [Ter'ra], in popular language denotes the friable matter or soil on the surface of the globe which we inhabit. In Chemistry, the *earths* are solid, incombustible substances, entering largely into the composition of the mineral strata, and not convertible into metals by any of the ordinary methods of reduction. Many of them, such as lime, magnesia, baryta, and strontia, like alkalies combine with acids to form what in Chemistry are termed salts. The four here named are called alkaline earths, as they have both an alkaline taste and change vegetable blues to green.

Earth-Bath. [Arena'tio.] A remedy consisting literally of a bath of earth or sand (usually hot) with which the patient is covered.

Earth, Japan. See ACACIA CATECHU.

Earth of Alum. A preparation used in making paints, and procured by precipitating the alumina from alum dissolved in water, by adding ammonia or potassa.

Earth of Bone, or **Bone-Earth.** A phosphate of lime, sometimes called *bone phosphate*, existing in bones after calcination.

Eau, ō. The French term for "water;" the name of a distilled water.

Eau de Bababe, ō dẹh bå'båb'. A liquor manufactured in Barbadoes from lemon-peel.

Eau de Cologne, ō dẹh ko-lōn' (or ko'loñ'). **[A'qua Colonien'sis.]** Cologne-water; a perfume, and an evaporating lotion often used in headache, fever, etc.

Eau de Javelle, ō dẹh zhå'vĕl'. Bleaching liquid, or the *A'qua Alkali'na Oxymuriat'ica* of the Dublin Pharmacopœia.

Eau de Luce, ō dẹh lüss'. The *Tinctura Ammoniæ Composita* of the Pharmacopœias. The French name is derived from that of an apothecary of Lille.

Eau de Naphre, ō dẹh nåfʀ'. A bitter aromatic water, prepared by distilling the leaves of the Seville orange with water.

Eau de Rabel, ō dẹh rå'bĕl'. **[A'qua Rabellia'na.]** So named from its inventor, the empiric Rabel. It consists of one part of sulphuric acid and three of rectified spirit of wine, constituting a sort of sulphuric ether.

Eau de Vie. [A'qua Vi'tæ.] See BRANDY.

Eau Médicinale d' Husson, ō må'dē'sē'nål' düs'sôɴᵍ'. A celebrated remedy for gout, prepared as follows. Macerate two ounces of the root of colchicum, cut in slices, in four fluidounces of Spanish white wine, and filter.

Ebenaceæ,* eb-e-na'she-ē. [From *Eb'enum*, "ebony."] A natural order of exogenous trees and shrubs, mostly Indian and tropical. Some species are remarkable for the hardness and blackness of the wood, as ebony and ironwood. The Jussieuan name of this order is *Guaiacanæ*.

Eb'la-nin, or **Eb'la-nine.** *Pyroxanthin*, a substance obtained from raw pyroxylic spirit.

E-brac'te-ate. [**Ebractea'tus;** from *e*, priv., and *brac'tea*, a "floral leaf."] Without a floral leaf.

Eb-ul-li'tion. [**Ebulli'tio, o'nis;** from *ebul'lio*, to "bubble up" or "boil up."] The act or state of boiling.

Eb-ur-nā'tion. [From *e'bor*, "ivory."] A state of the osseous system in which there is an increased and morbid deposit of phosphate of lime, especially on the cartilages of the joints.

Eburnification. See EBURNATION.

E'bur Us'tum Ni'grum* ("Ivory Burnt Black"), called Cologne-black, or Ivory-black. Charcoal prepared from charred ivory shavings.

Ec (ἐκ), and **Ex** (ἐξ) before a vowel. A Greek preposition signifying "out," "out of," "from," etc.

Écaille, à'kăl'. The French term for SCALE, which see.

E-căl-ca-ra'tus.* [From *e*, priv., and *cal'car*, a "spur."] Without a spur, or horn.

E-cau'date. [**Ecauda'tus;** from *e*, priv., and *cau'da*, a "tail."] Without a tail.

Ec-ba'li-um Of-fiç-i-na'le.* Another name for *Momor'dica Elate'rium*, or wild cucumber.

Ec-bol'ic. [**Ecbol'icus;** from ἐκβάλλω, to "cast out."] Applied to medicines which induce abortion.

Ec-cen'tric. [**Eccen'tricus;** from ἐκ, "out of," "from," and *cen'trum*, the "centre."] Away from the centre.

Ec-cen-triç'i-tȳ. [**Eccentriç'itas, a'tis;** from the same.] In Astronomy, the distance between the centre of a planet's orbit and the centre of the sun.

Ec-chȳ-mo'ma, a'tis.* [From ἐκχυμόω, to "pour out."] A soft blue swelling from a bruise; extravasation of blood into the cellular tissue. A genus of the order *Tumores*, class *Locales*, of Cullen's Nosology.

Ec-chȳ-mo'sis.* The same as ECCHYMOMA, which see.

Ec-co-prot'ic. [**Eccoprot'icus;** from ἐκ, "out," and κόπρος, "dung."] Evacuating the contents of the bowels.

Ec-cri-nol'o-gȳ. [**Eccrinolo'gia;** from ἐκκρίνω, to "secrete," and λόγος, a "discourse."] The doctrine or science of the secretions.

Ec-crit'i-ca.* [From ἐκκρίνω, to "strain off."] Diseases of the excernent function. The name of a class in Dr. Good's Nosology.

Ec-çȳ-e'sis.* [From ἐκ, "out" or "without," and κύησις, "gestation."] Extra-uterine fœtation.

Échancrure, à'shŏNG'krür'. A French term denoting a depression or notch in the bones. See NOTCH.

Écharpe, à'sharp'. The French for the surgical apparatus called a SLING, which see.

Ech'i-nate, or **E-chī'nate.** [**Echina'tus;** from ἐχῖνος, the "hedge-hog."] Beset with prickles.

Échine, à'shēn'. See SPINE.

E-chin-o-coc'cus.* [From ἐχῖνος, the "hedge-hog," and κόκκος, a "berry."] A species of hydatid.

E-chin'o-der'ma-ta.* [See ECHINODERMATUS.] The fourth class of the *Cycloneura*, or *Radiata*, consisting of simple aquatic animals covered with a spiny shell or a coriaceous skin.

E-chin'o-der'ma-tus.* [From ἐχῖνος, the "hedge-hog," and δέρμα, the "skin."] Echinoder'matous. Having a skin like the *Echinus*. Applied to a class of *Radiata*. See ECHINODERMATA.

E-chin-o-rhȳn'chus.* [From ἐχῖνος, the "hedge-hog," and ῥύγχος, a "beak."] The name for a genus of *Entozoa*, order *Acanthocephalæ* of Rudolphi.

E-chi'nus.* [From ἐχῖνος, the "sea-urchin."] A term applied to a calcareous petrifaction of the sea-urchin.

Ec-lamp'sȳ. [**Eclamp'sia, Eclamp'sis;** from ἐκλάμπω, to "shine."] Literally, "flashing of light;" "effulgence." A convulsive disease of infancy; also, epilepsy, and the appearance of flashes of light, forming one of its symptoms. Sometimes applied to a form of puerperal convulsions resembling epilepsy in severity.

Ec-lec'tic. [**Eclec'ticus;** from ἐκ, "out," and λέγω, to "gather" or "choose."] Selected, or chosen from among others. Applied to an ancient sect of physicians (as well as to a school of philosophy), who held that we ought not to confine ourselves to one single system or school, but to select what is best from all the different systems. It was at its acme about the beginning of the second century. The name is also applied to a modern school of recent origin.

Ec-leg'ma,* or **Ec-leig'ma.*** [Gr

ἐκλείγμα; from ἐκλείχω, to "lick up."] (Fr. *Looch*, lōk.) A pharmaceutical preparation of a certain consistence and of a sweet flavor. See LINCTUS.

E-clipse'. [Lat. **Eclip'sis;** Gr. ἔκλειψις, from ἐκλείπω, to "fail."] In Astronomy, the obscuration of the light of one heavenly body by the intervention of another.

E-clip'tic. [**Eclip'ticus.**] Belonging to an eclipse. Applied to an imaginary circle in the heavens, which the sun appears to describe in the course of the year; so named because eclipses only happen when the moon is in the same plane or very near it.

Éclisse, à'klèss'. The French for SPLINT, which see.

E-con'o-mȳ. [**Œcono'mia;** from οἶκος, a "house," and νέμω, to "distribute," to "arrange."] Literally, "household order or arrangement." Applied to order or proper management in doing any thing.

ANIMAL ECONOMY denotes collectively all the laws or arrangements which are necessary to the animal system.

Écorce, à'korss'. The French term for "bark." See CORTEX.

Ec-phly'sis.* [From εκφλύζω, to "bubble up."] Vesicular eruption confined in its action to the surface. This term comprehends the several species of *pompholyx, herpes, rhypia,* and *eczema.* Compare EMPHLYSIS.

Ec-phro'nĭ-a.* [From ἔκφρων, "out of one's mind."] Insanity; craziness; a term comprising melancholy and madness.

Ec-phy'ma.* [From ἐκφύω, to "spring out."] A cutaneous excrescence, including the several species *verruca, caruncula, clavus, callus.*

Ec-pȳ-e'sis.* [From ἐκπυέω, to "suppurate."] Humid scall, including the species *impetigo, porrigo, ecthyma,* and *scabies.* Compare EMPYESIS.

Écraseur, à'krâ'zur'. [Fr. *Écraser*, to "crush."] Literally, a "crusher." A kind of steel chain tightened by a screw, used for removing piles, *polypi,* or malignant growths.

Écrouelles, à'kroo'ěll'. The French term for SCROFULA, which see.

Ecstasis. See ECSTASY.

Ec'sta-sȳ. [**Ec'stasis;** from ἐξίσταμαι, to "be out of one's senses."] A total suspension of sensibility, voluntary motion, and for the most part of mental power,—the body erect and inflexible, the pulsation and breathing not affected.

Ec'ta-sis.* [From ἐκ, "out," and τείνω, to "stretch."] Extension or expansion.

Ec-thy'ma, atis.* [From ἐκθύω, to "break out."] An eruption of phlyzacious pustules, without fever.

Ec-to'pĭ-a.* [From ἔκτοπος, "out of place."] Protrusion, or displacement. Applied in the plural to an order of the class *Locales* of Cullen's Nosology.

Ecto'pia Cor'dis.* ("Displacement of the Heart.") Applied to any case where the heart is out of its proper place or in an unnatural position.

Ec-top-tĕr'ȳ-goid. [**Ectopterygoi'des;** from ἐκτός, "without," and πτερυγοειδής, "pterygoid."] A term proposed by Owen for the *transverse* bone of Cuvier in reptiles.

Ec-to-zo'on,* plural **Ec-to-zo'a.** [From ἐκτός, "without," and ζῶον, an "animal."] Those parasitic insects (such as lice) that infest the surface of the body, in contradistinction from the *Entozoa,* which are found within the body.

Ec-tro'pĭ-um.* [From ἐκ, "out," and τρέπω, to "turn."] Eversion of the eyelid or eyelids.

Ec-trot'ic. [**Ectrot'icus;** from ἐκτιτρώσκω, to "cause a miscarriage."] Applied to the treatment by which the development of disease is hindered.

Ec'ze-ma, atis.* [From ἐκζέω, to "boil up."] A smarting eruption of small pustules, generally crowded together, without fever, and not contagious.

Ec-zem'a-tous. [**Eczem'atus.**] Belonging to *Eczema.*

E-den-ta'ta.* [See next article.] Toothless animals; quadrupeds without front teeth, as the armadillo.

E-den-ta'tus.* [From *e*, priv., and *dens*, a "tooth."] Without teeth: eden'tate. Applied to an order of *Mammalia.* See EDENTATA.

E-dul-co-rā'tion. [From *dul'cis*, "sweet."] The sweetening of any medicinal preparation. Also, the process of freeing an easily soluble substance from one that is soluble with difficulty, by means of distilled water.

E-dul-co-rā'tor. [From the same.] A dropping-bottle. An instrument for supplying small quantities of sweetened liquid, water, etc., to any mixture, or to test-tubes, watch-glasses, etc.

Eel Oil. An oil procured from eels by roasting: employed as an ointment for stiff joints, and by ironmongers for preserving steel from rust.

Ef'fer-ens, en'*tis*.* [From *ef'fero*, to "carry out."] Ef'ferent. Carrying or conveying out. Applied in the plural to certain vessels of the *testis*. See VASA EFFERENTIA.

Ef-fer-vĕs'çence. [Effervescen'tia; from *efferves'co*, to "boil over."] The agitation produced on mixing certain substances, caused by the sudden escape of a gas.

Ef-fer-ves'çing Draught. Dissolve a scruple of carbonate of soda or potassa in an ounce of water; mix two drachms of cinnamon water with a drachm and a half of syrup of orange-peel; add to these a tablespoonful of fresh lemon-juice, and drink the mixture immediately.

Ef-flo-rĕs'çence. [Efflorescen'tia; from *efflores'co*, to "flower," to "flourish."] The blooming of flowers; the time of flowering. In Chemistry, the spontaneous conversion of crystals to powder in consequence of the loss of their water of crystallization. Also, a morbid redness of the skin.

Ef-flu'vĭ-a,* the plural of EFFLUVIUM, which see.

Ef-flu'vĭ-um,* plural **Ef-flu'vĭ-a.** [From *ef'fluo*, to "flow out."] A term applied to exhalations or vapors (especially those of a morbific character) proceeding from any body. It is also frequently applied to animal or vegetab e odors.

Ef-fu'sion. [Effu'sio, o'*nis*; from *effun'do*, *effu'sum*, to "pour out."] The escape of any fluid out of its natural vessel, or viscus, into another cavity, or into the cellular texture or substance of parts.

Egesta. See EGESTUS.

E-ġes'tus.* [From *eġ'ero*, *eges'tum*, to "carry out," or "cast out."] Applied in the plural neuter (*Eges'ta*) to the natural excretions or evacuations of the body, such as the urine, fæces, etc.

Egg. See OVUM.

Egg-Shaped. See OVAL, OVATE, and OVOID.

E-gland'u-lous. [Eglandulo'sus; from *e*, priv., and *glans*, a "gland."] Deprived of glands.

Egophony. See ÆGOPHONY.

Ehretiaceæ,* ā-re-te-a'she-ē. [From *Ehre'tia*, one of the genera.] A natural order of exogenous plants, mostly tropical trees or shrubs. It includes the Peruvian Heliotrope.

Eighth Pair of Nerves. See PNEUMO-GASTRIC.

E-jac'u-lans.* [From *e*, "out," and *jac'ulor*, *jacula'tus*, to "throw" or "cast."] Throwing forth, or casting out. See EJACULATORY.

E-jac-u-la'tor, o'*ris*.* [From the same.] Applied to a muscle of the penis. See ACCELERATOR.

E-jac'u-la-to-rȳ. [Ejaculato'rius; from the same.] Ejecting, or having power to eject.

Ejaculatory Ducts. See DUCTUS EJACULATORIUS.

E-jec'tion. [Ejec'tio, o'*nis*; from *eji'cio*, *ejec'tum*, to "throw or thrust out."] The act or process of discharging any thing from the body.

Ek. See EC.

Elæagnaceæ,* el-ē-ag-na'she-ē, or **El-æ-ag'ni.*** A natural order of exogenous trees and shrubs. dispersed through the whole Northern hemisphere. It includes the *Elæagnus*, or Oleaster.

El-æ-ag'ni,* the plural of **El-æ-ag'nus** ("Oleaster"), forming the Jussieuan name of a natural order of plants. See ELÆAGNACEÆ.

El-æ-op'ten. [From ἔλαιον, "oil," and πτηνός, "flying" or "fleeting," hence "volatile."] The liquid portion of a volatile oil. The concrete portion is called *stearopten*. The volatile oils when exposed to cold generally separate into a solid and liquid portion, showing that they are mixtures of two oils differing in fluidity.

El-æ-o-sac'cha-ra.* [From ἔλαιον, "oil," and *sac'charum*, "sugar."] The mixtures or compounds of volatile oils and sugar.

El'a-in. [Elai'na; from ἔλαιον, "oil."] The oily principle of solid fats.

El-ai-om'e-ter. [Elaiom'etrum.] An instrument for detecting the adulteration of olive oil.

El'a-is Guineen'sis* (ġin-e-ĕn'sis). The Guinea palm-tree, which yields the palm-oil, and, it is said, the best kind of palm-wine.

Elaopten. See ELÆOPTEN.

E-las'tic. [Elas'ticus. See ELASTICITY.] Having the property of elasticity, or springiness.

Elastic Gum, or **Indian Rubber.** See CAOUTCHOUC.

E-las'tĭ-cin. [Elastici'na; from *elas'ticus*, "elastic."] The peculiar solid material of the elastic tissue. It is remarkable for its insolubility in all ordinary menstrua.

El-as-tiç'ĭ-tȳ. [From ἐλαύνω, to "drive," to "strike" or "impel," as the string of a bow impels the arrow.] A property by which bodies return forcibly and of themselves to the same form or dimensions they possessed before their displacement or compression by external force.

E-lat'er-in. [**Elateri'na.**] A crystallizable matter, distinct from *Elatin,* found in the juice of *Elaterium.*

El-a-te'ri-um.* [From ἐλαύνω, to "drive," to "drive through," referring to its violent action on the alimentary canal.] The Pharmacopœial name ‖ of the fecula of the *Momor'dica elate'rium,* otherwise called the *Ecba'lium officina'rum* (or *officina'le*).

Elaterium is a powerful hydragogue cathartic. In over-doses, it operates with extreme violence both on the stomach and bowels, and sometimes causes death.

El'a-tin. [**Elati'na.**] The active principle of *Elaterium.*

Elatinaceæ,* el-a-tin-a'she-ē. A natural order of annual plants, found in marshes in the four quarters of the globe. It includes *Elati'ne* (Water-Pepper).

Elatio,* e-la'she-o. [From *ef'fero, ela'tum,* to "carry out," to "carry beyond bounds," to "transport."] Quixotism; a species of mental extravagance.

El'a-ȳl. [From ἔλαιον, "oil," and ὕλη, "material."] The name given by Berzelius to hydruret of acetyl, otherwise called olefiant gas and etherine.

El'bōw. [Lat. **Cu'bitus;** Fr. *Coude,* kood.] Originally, the angle formed by the arm when bent on the fore-arm. Commonly applied to the articulation of the arm with the fore-arm. More particularly it denotes the projection of the olecranon. See ANCON, and OLECRANON.

El'der-Tree. The *Sambucus nigra.*

El-e-cam-pane'. The *Inula Helenium.*

Elect. = *Electua'rium.** An "electuary."

E-lec-triç'i-tȳ. [**Electriç'itas,** *a'tis;* from ἤλεκτρον, "amber," in which it was first observed.] A subtile fluid or principle produced by the friction of certain substances, such as glass, amber, sealing-wax, etc. Electricity has been highly recommended as a stimulant in cases of paralysis, rheumatism, amaurosis, etc., and has sometimes proved very useful in such affections.

Electricity, Galvanic, or **Voltaic.** See GALVANISM.

E-lec'tro-Chem'i-cal Ac'tion. Chemical action induced by electrical arrangements.

Elec'tro-Dȳ-nam'ics. The science which treats of the effects or phenomena of electricity in motion.

Elec'tro-Mag'net-ism. Magnetism excited or produced by electricity,—usually by galvanic electricity.

E-lec'trode. [From ἤλεκτρον, "amber," and ὁδός, a "way."] In electro-chemical action the electrodes are the surfaces by which the electricity passes into or out from other media, they being regarded as the roads or ways along which the electric fluid travels.

E-lec-tro-ġen'e-sis.* [From ἤλεκτρον, "amber," and γένω, to "be born."] The production of electricity.

E-lec-tro-ġen'ic. [**Electrogen'icus.**] Belonging to *electrogenesis.*

E-lec-tro-ge'ni-um.* [From ἤλεκτρον, "amber," and γεννάω, to "beget."] The unknown cause of the phenomena of electricity: elec'trogen.

E-lec-trol'o-ġȳ. [**Electrolo'gia;** from ἤλεκτρον, "amber," and λόγος, a "discourse."] A treatise on electricity; the science of electricity.

E-lec-trol'ȳ-sis.* [From ἤλεκτρον, "amber," and λύω, to "loosen," to "dissolve."] Decomposition by electricity.

E-lec'tro-lȳtes. [From the same.] Applied to bodies which can be decomposed directly by electricity.

E-lec-trom'e-ter. [**Electrom'etrum;** from ἤλεκτρον, "amber," and μέτρον, a "measure."] An instrument for ascertaining the quality and quantity of electricity in an electrified body.

E-lec-troph'o-rus.* [From ἤλεκτρον, "amber," and φορέω, to "bear."] (An "electricity-bearer.") An apparatus employed in electric experiments.

E-lec'tro-scope. [**Electros'copus,** or **Electrosco'pium;** from ἤλεκτρον, "amber," and σκοπέω, to "spy."] An instrument for ascertaining the presence of electricity.

E-lec'tro-tȳpe. [From ἤλεκτρον, "amber," or "electricity," and τύπος, a "model" or "mould."] The process by which *fac-simile* medals are executed in copper by means of electricity. It consists in preparing for a negative plate models or moulds of objects to be copied, and in so arranging a battery or apparatus which generates the voltaic current as to deposit the metals in a compact form on the surface of the mould. Electrotype is also used as a verb.

E-lec'tro-Vi'tal (or **Neū'ro E-lec'-**

tric) Cur'rents. The name of two electric currents supposed to exist in animals,—the one external and cutaneous, moving from the extremities to the cerebro-spinal axis; the other internal, going from the cerebro-spinal axis to the internal organs.

E-lec'trum.* [Gr. ἤλεκτρον.] A term used by the ancients for *amber;* also, for a mixture of four parts of gold and one of silver.

Electuarium Aromaticum. See CONFECTIO AROMATICA.

Electuarium Opii. See CONFECTIO OPII.

Electuarium Sennæ. See CONFECTIO SENNÆ.

E-lec'tu-a-rў. [**Electua'rium;** from *el'igo, elec'tum,* to "choose" or "pick out," because some agreeable substance is chosen as a vehicle for the medicine.] (Fr. *Électuaire,* à'lêk'tü'êr'.) A confection, or conserve. See LINCTUS.

El'e-ments. [**Elemen'ta.**] Rudiments, or first principles; substances which cannot be further decomposed.

El-e-men'tum,* plural **El-e-men'-ta.** See ELEMENTS.

El'e-mi.* The Pharmacopœial name (Br. Ph.) of a concrete resinous exudation, probably from the *Canarium commune:* chiefly imported from Manilla.

El-e-phan-ti'a-sis.* [From ἐλέφας, ἐλέφαντος, an "elephant."] Applied to two distinct diseases of quite different character, now designated as *Elephantiasis Arabum* and *Elephantiasis Græcorum.*

ELEPHANTI'ASIS AR'ABUM* (the "Elephantiasis of the Arabians"), otherwise called BUCNE'MIA, BARBA'DOES LEG, and EL'EPHANT-LEG. A disease characterized by the leg being much swollen and misshapen, and thus supposed to resemble that of an elephant.

ELEPHANTI'ASIS GRÆCO'RUM.* ("Elephantiasis of the Greeks.") An affection nearly allied to leprosy, if not the same disease. It is said to be characterized by shining tubercles on the face, ears, and extremities, with a thickened, rugous state of the skin, whence it has been termed *Elephant-skin;* also, *Le'pra Ar'abum.*

El-et-ta'ri-a.* [From the Malay *Elettari,* the "lesser cardamom."] The name of a new genus of plants, of the class *Monandria,* natural order *Zingiberaceæ.*

Eletta'ria Car-dă-mo'mum.* The lesser cardamom-plant, formerly referred to the genus *Alpinia.*

Elévateur, à'là'vâ'tuR'. ("Elevator.") The French for LEVATOR, which see.

El-e-vā'tor. [**Elevato'rium;** from *el'evo, eleva'tum,* to "lift or raise up."] (Fr. *Élévatoire,* à'là'vâ'twåR'.) An instrument for raising depressed portions of bone.

E-lim'ĭ-nāte. [From *e,* "out of," or "out from," and *li'men,* a "threshold."] Literally, to "put out" or "expel:" hence, to "send forth," to "throw off," to "set free."

El-ĭ-quā'tion. [**Eliqua'tio, o'nis;** from *el'iquo, eliqua'tum,* to "melt down" or "melt out."] The process by which one substance more fusible than another is separated from it by applying heat in a sufficient degree.

E-lix'ir. [Said to be derived from the Arabic *El-ekser,* or *Al-eksir,* "quintessence."] A preparation similar to a compound tincture. Also, an extract, or quintessence.

Elix'ir, Păr-e-gŏr'ic. The *Tinctu'ra cam'phoræ compos'ita.* See PAREGORIC.

E-lu-trĭ-ā'tion. [**Elutria'tio, o'nis;** from *elu'trio, elutria'tum,* to "wash out," to "pour off."] The process of pulverizing metallic ores or other substances, and mixing them with water, so that the lighter parts are separated from the heavier.

Elytra. See ELYTRON.

El-ў-tri'tis, idis.* [From ἔλυτρον, a "sheath," the "vagina."] Inflammation of the vagina.

El'ў-tron,* plural **El'ў-tra.** [Gr. ἔλυτρον; from ἐλύω, to "wrap up," to "cover" or "conceal."] A sheath; the hard case or shell which covers the wings of coleopterous insects. Also, the vagina.

El'ў-tro-plas'tic. [**Elytroplas'ticus.**] Belonging to elytroplasty.

El'ў-tro-plas-tў. [**Elytroplas'tia;** from ἔλυτρον, and πλάσσω, to "form."] The operation of closing a vesico-vaginal fistulous opening by borrowing a flap from the *labia,* or *nates.*

El-ў-trop-to'sis.* [From ἔλυτρον, and πτῶσις, a "falling down."] Inversion of the vagina.

El'ў-trum,* plural **El'ў-tra.** The same as ELYTRON, which see.

Emaciation, e-mā-she-ā'shŭn. [**Emacia'tio, o'nis;** from *ema'cio, emacia'tum,* to "make lean."] The state of being or becoming lean. See ATROPIA, and MARASMUS.

Email, ā'mäl'. The French term for Enamel, which see.

Em-a-nā'tion. [**Emana'tio, o'**nis; from *e*, "out" or "from," and *ma'no*, *mana'tum*, to "flow."] That which flows or proceeds from any substance.

Emansio,* e-man'she-o. [From *ema'-neo*, *eman'sum*, to "remain out" or "absent."] Literally, "absence" or "staying away." See next article.

Eman'sio Men'sium* (men'she-ŭm). Retention of the *catamenia*. See Amenorrhœa.

E-mar'gin-ate. [**Emargina'tus;** from *emar'gino*, to "take away the edge."] Having a notch at the margin.

E-mas'cu-late. [**Emascula'tus;** from *emas'culo*, *emascula'tum*, to "make impotent." See Mas.] Deprived of virility; incapable of generating.

E-mas-cu-lā'tion. [**Emascula'tio, o'**nis; from the same.] The act of rendering impotent by injury or removal of the generative organs.

Em-balm'ing. [From *en*, "in," and *balm*, a word used somewhat vaguely for any "fragrant ointment" or "aromatic substance."] A process by which a dead body is preserved against putrefaction. This process originally consisted in impregnating the body with balsams or spices.

Emboîtement (Fr.), ŏm'bwåt'mŏng'. [From *boîte*, a "box."] The situation of one box within another. A term used by Bonnet to designate that theory of generation by which thousands of individuals are supposed to lie one within the other, each possessing a complete series of organized parts.

Em-bo'lĭ-a.* [From ἐν, "in" or "into," and βάλλω, to "throw," to "thrust."] A term employed by Virchow to denote the obstruction of an artery or vein in consequence of a piece or clot of coagulated blood being lodged in it. See Embolus, and Thrombosis.

Em-bol'ic. [**Embol'icus.**] Pertaining to Embolia.

Em'bo-lism. [**Embolis'mus.**] The same as Embolia, which see.

Em'bo-lus.* [See Embolia.] Literally, "any thing thrown or thrust in," as a wedge or stopper. Applied to a piece of coagulum, which has been formed in the large vessels in certain morbid conditions, and has afterwards been forced into one of the smaller arteries so as to obstruct the circulation. See Thrombus.

Embonpoint (Fr.), ŏm'bŏng'pwăng'. Plumpness or fulness of flesh.

Em-bro-cā'tion. [**Embroca'tio, o'**nis; from ἐμβρέχω, to "soak."] A fluid application for rubbing on any part.

Em'bry̆-o, o'nis.* [Gr. ἔμβρυον; from ἐν, "within," and βρύω, to "swell as buds," to "grow."] Literally, "that which grows within." The *fœtus in utero*, before the fifth month of pregnancy. Also, the germ of a plant: the *corculum*.

Em-bry̆-oc'to-ny̆. [From ἔμβρυον, a "fœtus," and κτείνω, to "kill."] The same as Embryotomy.

Em-bry̆-oġ'e-ny̆. [From *em'bryo*, and γένω, to "be born or produced."] The formation or production of an embryo.

Em-bry̆-og'ra-phy̆. [**Embryogra'phia;** from ἔμβρυον, a "fœtus," and γράφω, to "write."] A description of the fœtus.

Em-bry̆-ol'o-ġy̆. [**Embryolo'gia;** from ἔμβρυον, a "fœtus," and λόγος, a "discourse."] A treatise on the fœtus.

Em'bry̆-o-nate. [**Embryona'tus;** from *em'bryo*.] Having an embryo, germ, or *corculum*.

Em-bry̆-ot'o-my̆. [**Embryoto'mia;** from ἔμβρυον, a "fœtus," and τέμνω, to "cut."] The destruction or separation of any part or parts of the fœtus *in utero*, where circumstances exist to prevent delivery in the natural way.

Em-bry̆-ul'cĭ-a.* [From ἔμβρυον, a "fœtus," and ἕλκω, to "draw."] The drawing or extracting of the fœtus, generally by destructive instruments, in order to effect delivery: embryul'cy.

E-mer'sus.* [From *emer'go*, *emer'sum*, to "rise out," as from water.] Applied to leaves and flowers that are above the surface of the water.

Em'er-y̆. A variety of *Corundum*. The powder, attached to brown paper, called *emery-paper*, is used for polishing, for preparing razor-strops, etc.

Em'e-sis,* or **E-me'sĭ-a.*** [From ἐμέω, to "vomit."] The act of vomiting.

E-met'ic. [**Emet'icus;** from the same.] (Fr. *Émétique*, ā'mā'tēk'.) Having power to excite vomiting. Also, a medicine which causes vomiting.

E-met-ĭ-co-lo'ġĭ-a.* [From *emet'icus*, "emetic," and λόγος, a "discourse."] A treatise on emetics.

Em'e-tin, or **Em'e-tĭne.** [**Emeti'na;** from *emet'icus*, "emetic."] The principle on which the emetic virtues of ipecacuan depend.

Emétique. See Emetic.

Em-et-ol'o-ġy̆. The doctrine or science of emetics.

E-mis'sion. [**Emis'sio, o'**nis; from

e, "out" or "forth," and *mit'to, mis'sum*, to "send" or "throw."] A sending forth.

Em-men'a-gogue. [**Emmenago'gus;** from ἐμμήνια, the "menses," and ἄγω, to "lead or carry away."] Having power to excite the discharge of the *catamenia*.

Em-me'nĭ-a.* [Gr. ἐμμήνια; from ἐν, "in," "at," "by," and μήν, a "month."] The menses, or catamenial discharge.

Em-me-nol'o-ġȳ. [**Emmenolo'gia;** from ἐμμήνια, the "menses," and λόγος, a "discourse."] That branch of Physiology which treats of menstruation.

E-mol'lĭ-ent. [**Emol'liens,** plural **Emollien'tia;** from *emol'lio*, to "soften."] Softening or soothing an irritated surface, or one harsh from dryness. Emollient applications consist chiefly of oils, fomentations, poultices, etc.

Em-pa-the'ma, atis.* [From εμπαθής, "in a passion or violent emotion."] Ungovernable passion; including excitement, depression, and hair-brained passion, or the *manie sans délire* of Pinel.

Empetraceæ,* em-pe-tra'she-ē. A small natural order of exogenous shrubs, found in Europe and America.

Em'phlȳ-sis.* [From ἐν, "in" or "on," and φλύσις, an "eruption."] A vesicular tumor or eruption on the skin.

Em-phy'ma, atis.* [From ἐν, "in" or "within," and φύω, to "produce," to "grow."] A tumor originating below the integuments.

Em-phȳ-se'ma, atis.* [From ἐμφυσάω, to "inflate."] A collection of air in the cellular texture under the skin, or beneath the pleural and interlobicular cellular tissue of the lungs.

Em-phȳ-sem'a-tous. [**Emphysemato'sus;** from *emphyse'ma*.] Of the nature of emphysema.

Em-pĭr'ic. [**Empir'icus;** from ἐμπειρικός, "experienced," "experimental."] A practitioner whose skill is the result of mere experience. Generally used synonymously for a "quack."

Em-pĭr'ĭ-cal. [**Empir'icus.**] Belonging to an empiric, or to a quack.

Em-pĭr'ĭ-çism. [**Empiricis'mus;** from ἐμπειρία, "experience."] (Fr. *Empirisme*, ŏm'pè'rèzm'.) The knowledge of physic acquired by experience alone, as contradistinguished from that in which a thorough acquaintance with general principles (such as the great laws of physiology, chemistry, etc.) is combined with the knowledge derived from experience; commonly applied, however, to quackery.

Em-plas'trum,* plural **Em-plas'tra.** [Gr. ἔμπλαστρον; from ἐν, "on," and πλάσσω, to "form," to "mould," to "spread."] (Fr. *Emplâtre*, ŏm'plåtr'.) A plaster of any kind: usually formed of a solid tenacious compound, adhesive at the ordinary temperature of the human body.

☞ The limits of the present work forbid the insertion of all the *Emplastra* of the U.S. Pharmacopœia. Only a few, the directions for the preparation of which are comparatively simple and brief, are here given. For the others the inquirer is referred to pp. 135–142 of the Pharmacopœia.

Emplas'trum Ad-hæ-si'vum.* The Emplastrum Resinæ, which see.

Emplas'trum Ar'nĭ-çæ.* ("Plaster of Arnica.") Take of alcoholic extract of arnica, a troyounce and a half, resin plaster, three troyounces. Add the extract to the plaster, previously melted by means of a water-bath, and mix them.

Emplas'trum Pi'cis Bur-gun'dĭ-çæ.* ("Plaster of Burgundy Pitch.") Take of Burgundy Pitch, seventy-two troyounces; yellow wax, six troyounces. Melt them together, strain, and stir constantly until they thicken on cooling.

Emplas'trum Pi'cis Can-a-den'sis.* ("Plaster of Canada Pitch, or Hemlock Pitch.") The directions for preparing this plaster, and the proportion of the ingredients, are the same as the preceding, with the single exception that Canada Pitch is substituted for Burgundy Pitch.

Emplas'trum Re-si'næ* ("Plaster of Resin"), commonly called Adhesive Plaster, or Resin Plaster. Take of resin in fine powder, six troyounces; plaster of lead, thirty-six troyounces. To the plaster, melted over a gentle fire, add the resin, and mix them.

Emplâtre, ŏm'plâtr'. The French word for "plaster." See Emplastrum.

Em-pres'ma, atis.* [From ἐν, "within," and πρήθω, to "burn."] Internal inflammation; a term employed in its simple sense by Hippocrates, and revived by Dr. Good as a generic term for all those visceral inflammations generally distinguished by the suffix *-itis*.

Em-pros-thot'o-nos.* [From ἔμπροσθεν, "forwards," and τείνω, to "stretch."] Literally, "a stretching or bending forwards." A variety of *Tetanus*.

Em-pȳ-e'ma, atis.* [From ἐν, "within," and πύον, "pus."] A collection of pus in the cavity of the chest.

Em-pȳ-e'sis.* [From ἐμπυέω, to "suppurate."] A genus of diseases characterized by phlegmonous pimples, which gradually fill with purulent fluid: as *Variola, Varicella*, etc.

Em'pȳ-o-çēle.* [From ἐν, "in," πύον, "pus," and κήλη, a "tumor."] A collection of pus within the *scrotum*.

Em-pȳ-om'pha-lus.* [From ἐν, "in," πύον, "pus," and ὀμφαλός, the "navel."] A collection of pus about the navel.

Em-pȳ-reū'mą, atis.* [From ἐμπυρεύω, to "kindle."] A peculiar disagreeable smell of animal and vegetable matter when burned in close vessels.

Em-pȳ-reū-mat'ic. [**Empyreumat'icus.**] Belonging to *empyreuma*.

E-mul'ġent. [**Emul'gens, en'tis**; from *emul'geo, emul'sum*, to "milk out."] Straining through. Applied to the vessels of the kidneys, supposed to strain the serum through the kidneys.

E-mul'sin, or **E-mul'sine.** The same as AMYGDALIN, which see.

E-mul'sion. [**Emul'sio, o'nis**; from the same.] The expressed oil of seeds, or kernels, diffused through water by the medium of the sugar, mucilage, and fecula which they contain.

E-munc'to-rȳ. [**Emuncto'rius**; from *emun'go, emunc'tum*, to "carry off."] Applied to the excretory ducts of the body.

En (ἐν). A Greek preposition signifying "in," or "within." Before *b, m*, and *p*, it is changed to *m*; as, *Embolus*, something which is "thrown into" the arteries, veins, etc.

En-æ-o-re'mą, atis.* [From ἐναιωρέομαι, to "float."] The *nubecula* which floats, or is suspended, in the middle of the urine.

En-am'el. (Fr. *Email*, ā'măl'.) A very hard, compact, white substance, investing the crown of the teeth. See TOOTH.

En-an-the'sis.* [From ἐν, and ἀνθέω, to "blossom."] Rash exanthem, including scarlet fever, measles, and nettle-rash.

En-ar-thro'sis.* [From ἐν, "in," and ἄρθρον, a "joint."] The ball-and-socket joint. A variety of the class *Diarthroses*.

En-can'this.* [From ἐν, "in," and κάνθος, the "angle of the eye."] A small red excrescence on the *Caruncula lachrymalis* and semilunar fold of the *Conjunctiva*.

Encanthus. See ENCANTHIS.

En-çeph-ą-la'tą.* [From *enceph'alon*, the "brain."] A name sometimes applied to the *Vertebrata*, or highest of the grand divisions of animals, comprising such as have a brain enclosed in a case of bone.

En-çeph-ą-li'tis, idis.* [From ἐγκέφαλος, the "brain."] Inflammation of the brain and its membranes.

En-çeph'ą-lo-çēle.* [From ἐγκέφαλος, the "brain," and κήλη, a "tumor."] Protrusion of a portion of the brain through a preternatural opening in the skull: *Hernia cerebri*.

En-çeph'ą-loid. [**Encephaloi'des**; from ἐγκέφαλος, the "brain."] Resembling the substance of the brain.

En-çeph-ą-lo-lo'ġĭ-ą.* [From ἐγκέφαλος, the "brain," and λόγος, a "discourse."] A description of the brain; also, the science of the brain: encephalol'ogy.

En-çeph-ą-lo'mą, atis.* [From ἐγκέφαλος, the "brain."] The *Hernia cerebri*.

En-çeph'ą-lon.* [Gr. ἐγκέφαλον; from ἐγκέφαλος, the "brain."] The brain; the contents of the skull, consisting of the *cerebrum, cerebellum, medulla oblongata*, and membranes.

En-çeph-ą-lo'sis.* The progress of *Encephaloma*.

En-chon-dro'mą, atis.* [From ἐν, "in" or "within," and χόνδρος, a "cartilage."] A cartilaginous tumor or growth proceeding from the bones, and, therefore, deep "within."

En-chon'drus.* [From ἐν, "in," and χόνδρος, a "cartilage;" also, a "grain."] Cartilaginous: enchon'drous. Also, having grains; granular.

En-çȳst'ed. [From ἐν, "in," and κύστις, a "bag."] Enclosed in a cyst, or sac.

En-dem'ic, En-de'mĭ-ąl. [**Endem'icus,** or **Ende'mius**; from ἐν, "in," and δῆμος, a "people," a "district."] Belonging to a particular district.

En-der'mic, En-der-mat'ic. [**Ender'micus,** or **Endermat'icus**; from ἐν, "in" or "on," and δέρμα, the "skin."] Applied to the method of rubbing medicines into the skin, or sprinkling them on the denuded surface where a blister has previously been formed.

En-do-bran-chĭ-a'tus.* [From ἔνδον, "within," and βραγχία, "gills."] Endobran'chiate. Applied in the plural neuter (*Endobranchia'ta*) to a family of *Anellata* which have no external *branchiæ*.

En-do-car'dĭ-ąl. [**Endocardia'lis**; from ἔνδον, "within," and καρδία, the "heart."] Within the heart.

En-do-car-di'tis, idis.* [From the same.] Inflammation of the lining membrane of the heart.

En-do-car'di-um.* [From the same.] The lining membrane of the heart.

En'do-carp. [**Endocar'pus;** from ἔνδον, "within," and καρπός, "fruit."] Applied in Botany to the inner membrane of a pericarp; the *putamen.*

En-do-gas-tri'tis, idis.* [From ἔνδον, "within," and γαστήρ, the "stomach."] Inflammation of the lining membrane of the stomach.

En'do-gen. An endogenous plant.

En-dog'e-nous. [**Endog'enus;** from ἔνδον, "within," and γένω, to "be born," to "grow."] Applied to stems in which the new matter by which they increase in diameter is added at the centre. The palm-tree is an example of an endogenous plant.

En-do-lym'pha.* [From ἔνδον, "within," and *lym'pha,* "water."] The small portion of fluid in the labyrinth of the ear: en'dolymph.

En'do-plast. [**Endoplas'ta;** from ἔνδον, "within," and πλάσσω, to "form."] The contents of animal and vegetable cells, consisting of vesicular bodies, into which much nitrogen enters.

En-do-pleu'ra.* [From ἔνδον, "within," and πλευρά, the "side."] Collectively, the three coats of the seed, which in the ovule were the Tercine, Quartine, and Quintine.

En-do-rhi'zous. [**Endorhi'zus;** from ἔνδον, "within," and ῥιζόω, to "take root."] Having the radicle enclosed in a sheath.

En'do-Skel'e-ton. [From ἔνδον, "within," and σκελετόν, a "skeleton."] The ordinary skeleton of *Vertebrata.*

En-dos'mic. [**Endos'micus.**] Belonging to *endosmose.*

En-dos-mom'e-ter. [**Endosmom'etrum;** from *endosmo'sis,* and μέτρον, a "measure."] An instrument for showing the gradual progress of *endosmose.*

En-dos-mose'. [**Endosmo'sis;** from ἔνδον, "in" or "within," and ὠσμός, "impulsion."] A peculiar movement in liquids separated by a membrane, by which the rarer fluid passes through the membranous partition into the cavity containing the denser fluid. This term is given to the action of the liquid absorbed internally.

En'do-sperm. [**Endosper'ma, a**tis; from ἔνδον, "within," and σπέρμα, a "seed."] The albumen between the integuments and the embryo.

En'dos-tome. [**Endos'toma, a**tis; from ἔνδον, "within," and στόμα, a "mouth."] The inner opening of the ovula.

En'dos-tome. [**Endosto'ma, a**tis; from ἔνδον, "within," and *osteo'ma.*] A chronic tumor within a bone.

Enduit. See COATED.

Enecia,* e-ne'she-a. [From ἠνεκής, "continuous."] A generic term employed by Dr. Good to denote continued fever.

En'e-ma, atis.* [From ἐνίημι, to "inject."] A medicine thrown into the rectum; a clyster, or glyster; an injection.

En-ep-i-der'mic. [From ἐν, "on," and *epider'mis,* the "cuticle."] A term denoting the application of medicines, such as plasters, blisters, etc., to the skin. See ENDERMIC.

En'er-gy. [**Ener'gia;** from ἐνεργέω, to "be active."] The force exercised by any power: as, nervous energy, vital energy, etc.

E-ner'vāt-ing (or en'er-vāt-ing). [**Ener'vans;** from *ener'vo, enerva'tum,* to "weaken."] Destroying the energy of the nervous system.

E-ner'vis,* E-ner'vi-us.* [From *e,* negative, and *ner'vus,* a "nerve."] Having no rib, or nerve: ener'vious.

Enfant, Enfance. See INFANT, and INFANCY.

Engelure, ŏɴzh'lüʀ'. The French term for CHILBLAIN, which see.

En-gorge'ment. [From the French *engorger,* to "choke up."] A state of vascular congestion.

En-ne-a-gyn'i-ous, or **En-ne-ag'y-nous.** [**Enneagyn'ius;** from ἐννέα, "nine," and γυνή, a "woman" or "female."] Applied to an order of plants having nine pistils.

En-ne-an'dri-a.* [From ἐννέα, "nine," and ἀνήρ, "man" or "male."] The ninth class of plants in Linnæus's system, comprising those which have nine stamens.

En-ne-a-pet'a-lous. [**Enneapet'alus;** from ἐννέα, "nine," and πέταλον, a "petal."] Having nine petals.

Ennui (Fr.), ŏn'wē'. Weariness; irksomeness; languor of mind from the lack of occupation.

E-node'. [**Eno'dis;** from *e,* negative, and *no'dus,* a "knot."] Having no knots, or joints.

En-os-to'sis.* [From ἐν, "in," and ὀστέον, a "bone."] A tumor occurring in the medullary canal of a bone.

Ens. [The present participle of *es'se,* to "be."] A term in Chemistry denoting a substance supposed to contain in a small compass all the virtues of the ingredients from which it is extracted.

En'sate. [**Ensa'tus;** from *en'sis*, a "sword."] Having the form of a sword. Applied to an order or division of plants.

En'sĭ-form. [**Ensifor'mis;** from *en'sis*, a "sword."] Like a sword. See XIPHOID.

En'siform Car'tĭ-lage. The cartilaginous extremity of the *sternum*, or breast-bone.

Ens Mar'tis,* Fer'rum Am-mo-nĭ-a'tum.* Ammoniated iron, or martial flowers of the muriate of ammonia and iron.

Ens-pri'mum.* A name given by the alchemists to a tincture which they supposed to have the power of transmuting the metals.

Ens Ven'e-ris.* [From *Ve'nus*, an alchemical name for "copper."] The ancient designation of the muriate of ammonia and copper.

En-ta'sĭ-a.* [From ἔντασις, a "violent straining."] Applied by Good as a generic name for trismus, tetanus, etc.

En'ta-sis.* [From ἐντείνω, to "stretch."] A term denoting tension, and applied by Good to constrictive spasm, cramp, locked-jaw, etc.

En'ter-a.* [From ἔντερα, the plural of ἔντερον, an "intestine."] The bowels, or intestines.

En-ter-ăl'ğĭ-a.* [From ἔντερον, an "intestine," and ἄλγος, "pain."] En'teralgy. Nervous pain in the bowels.

En-tĕr'ic. [**Enter'icus;** from ἔντερον, an "intestine."] (Fr. *Entérique*, ôNᵒ'tà'rèk'.) Belonging to the intestines.

En-tĕr'ĭ-ca.* [From the same.] An order in Good's Nosology, comprising diseases of the alimentary canal.

En-ter-i'tis, *idis*.* [From the same.] Inflammation of the bowels. A genus of the order *Phlegmasiæ*, class *Pyrexiæ*, of Cullen's Nosology.

En'ter-o-çēle.* [From ἔντερον, an "intestine," and κήλη, a "tumor."] Hernia in which a portion of intestine is protruded.

En-ter-og'ra-phy̆. [**Enterogra'phia;** from ἔντερον, an "intestine," and γράφω, to "describe."] A description of the intestines.

En-ter-o-lĭ-thi'a-sis.* [From ἔντερον, an "intestine," and λιθίασις, "formation of stone."] The formation of intestinal concretions.

En-ter-ol'ĭ-thus.* [From ἔντερον, an "intestine," and λίθος, a "stone."] Any kind of concretion generated in the stomach and bowels.

En-ter-ol'o-ğy̆. [**Enterolo'gia;** from ἔντερον, an "intestine," and λόγος, a "discourse."] That branch of science (anatomical or physiological) which treats of the intestines.

En-ter-or'a-phy̆. [**Enterora'phia;** from ἔντερον, an "intestine," and ῥαφή, a "suture."] The stitching or sewing together of the divided edges of the intestine.

En'ter-or-rha'ğĭ-a.* [From ἔντερον, an "intestine," and ῥήγνυμι, to "burst forth."] Intestinal hæmorrhage.

En'ter-or-rhœ'a.* [From ἔντερον, an "intestine," and ῥέω, to "flow."] Undue increase of the mucous secretion of the intestines.

En-ter-os'che-o-çēle.* [From ἔντερον, an "intestine," ὄσχεον, the "scrotum," and κήλη, a "tumor."] Scrotal hernia.

En-ter-ot'o-my̆. [**Enteroto'mia;** from ἔντερον, an "intestine," and τέμνω, to "cut."] Any cutting operation on the intestines.

En-ter-o-zo'on.* [From ἔντερον, an "intestine," and ζῶον, an "animal."] An animal living in the intestines.

En-thet'ic. [**Enthet'icus;** from ἐν, "in," and τίθημι, to "place."] Applied to diseases arising from a morbific virus being placed or implanted in the system, as syphilis, leprosy, etc.

En-to-mog'ra-phy̆. [**Entomogra'phia;** from ἔντομον, an "insect," and γράφω, to "write."] A description of insects.

En'to-moid. [**Entomoi'des;** from ἔντομον, an "insect," and εἶδος, a "form."] Resembling an insect.

Entomoline. See CHITINA.

En-to-mol'o-ğy̆. [**Entomolo'gia;** from ἔντομον, an "insect," and λόγος, a "discourse."] The science of insects.

En-to-mom'e-ter. [**Entomom'etrum;** from ἔντομον, an "insect," and μέτρον, a "measure."] An instrument for measuring the parts of insects.

En-to-moph'a-gous. [**Entomoph'agus;** from ἔντομον, an "insect," and φάγω, to "eat."] Eating, or feeding on, insects.

En-to-mos'tra-cous. [**Entomos'tracus;** from ἔντομον, an "insect," and ὄστρακον, a "shell."] Insects with shells. Applied to a class or division of *Crustacea*.

En-to-mot'o-my̆. [**Entomoto'mia** from ἔντομον, an "insect," and τέμνω, to "cut."] The dissection of insects.

En-toph'y̆-tous. [**Entoph'ytus**

from ἐντός, "within," and φυτόν, a "plant."] Growing within a plant. Applied to parasitical fungi.

En-top-tĕr'ÿ-goid. [**Entoptery-goi'des;** from ἐντός, "within," and *pterygoi'des.*] Applied by Owen to the internal pterygoid process of the sphenoid bone.

En-to-zo'a,* the plural of ENTOZOON.

En-to-zo'on.* [From ἐντός, "within," and ζῶον, an "animal."] An animal that lives within another. Applied in the plural (*Entozo'a*) to a class or division of radiated animals. Among the most important and common Entozoa are the *Tæ'nia so'lium* (the ordinary tape-worm), the *As'caris lumbricoi'des,* the *As'caris vermicula'ris* (or thread-worm), and the *Dis'toma hepat'icum.*

En-tro'pĭ-um.* [From ἐν, "in," and τρέπω, to "turn."] A disease in which the eyelash and eyelid are turned in towards the eyeball.

E-nu'cle-ate. [**Enuclea'tus;** from *e,* "out of," and *nu'cleus,* a "kernel."] Applied to tumors taken from the substance in which they were imbedded, like a kernel from its shell.

En-u-re'sis.* [From ἐνουρέω, to "be incontinent of urine."] Incontinency of urine. A genus of the order *Apocenoses,* class *Locales,* of Cullen's Nosology.

E'o-cēne. [From ἠώς, the "dawn," and καινός, "recent."] The lower tertiary strata, regarded as the beginning or dawn of the existing (or recent) condition of creation, on account of the small proportion of living species of animals found in them.

Epacridaceæ,* e-pak-re-da'she-ē. A natural order of Exogens, mostly shrubs, found in Australia and Polynesia. They are remarkable for the beauty of the flowers.

Ep-an'e-tus.* [From ἐπανίημι, to "relax," to "remit."] A term denoting "remittent," and applied by Dr. Good to remittent fever, including the mild form, the malignant form, and hectic fever.

Ep-en-çe-phal'ic. [**Epencephal'icus;** from ἐπι, "upon," and ἐγκέφαλος, the "brain."] Situated on or over the contents of the head or the brain. Applied the same as NEUROCCIPITAL.

Ep-en'dÿ-ma, *atis.** [From ἐπενδύω, to "clothe upon," to "cover."] Literally, an "upper garment." The lining membrane of the ventricles of the brain; also, that of the cerebro-spinal axis.

Eph'e-lis,* plural **E-phel'ĭ-dēs.** [From ἐπί, "upon," and ἥλιος, the "sun."] Freckles. See ÆSTATES.

E-phem'e-ra.* [From ἐπί, "for," and ἡμέρα, a "day."] A fever which runs its course of the cold, hot, and sweating stages in twelve hours.

Ephemera is also the name of a genus of insects (popularly called the "day-fly"), the entire period of whose existence, in their perfect state, is only about twenty-four hours.

E-phem'e-ral. [**Ephem'erus;** from the same.] Enduring one day. See EPHEMERA.

Eph-ĭ-al'tēs.* [From ἐφάλλομαι, to "leap upon."] Nightmare, or incubus: a distressing state of feeling during sleep, as of fright, and inability to call for help: *Oneirodyn'ia gra'vans.*

Eph-ĭ-dro'sis.* [From ἐπί, intensive, and ἱδρόω, to "sweat."] Violent, morbid perspiration. A genus of the order *Apocenoses,* class *Locales,* of Cullen's Nosology.

Ephippium. See SELLA TURCICA.

Ep'ĭ. A Greek preposition signifying "on" or "upon," "over," "at," "by," "for," "after." It is sometimes intensive. The final *i* is generally dropped before a word beginning with a vowel or with *h,* as *Epencephalic* for *Epiencephalic; Ephidrosis* for *Ephihidrosis,* etc.

Ep'ĭ-an. The same as FRAMBŒSIA, which see.

Ep-ĭ-bran'chĭ-al. [**Epibranchia'lis;** from ἐπί, "upon," and *branchia'lis,* "branchial."] Applied by Owen to the upper portion of the branchial arch.

Ep-ĭ-can'thus.* [From ἐπί, "upon," and κανθός, the "corner of the eye."] A fold of skin covering the inner canthus.

Ep'ĭ-carp. [**Epicar'pus;** from ἐπί, "upon," and καρπός, "fruit."] The external covering of the pericarp, commonly called the skin of fruits.

Ep-ĭ-car'pĭ-um.* The same as EPICARP, which see.

Ep-ĭ-chro'sis.* [From ἐπί, "upon," and χρώζω, to "paint."] A macular or spotted state of the skin, or a simple discoloration of its surface.

Ep-ĭ-col'ic. [**Epicol'icus;** from ἐπί, "upon," and κῶλον, the "colon."] Over the course of the colon on each side.

Ep-ĭ-con'dÿle. [**Epicon'dylus;** from ἐπί, "upon," and κόνδυλος, a "condyle."] The external protuberance of the inferior end of the *Os humeri.*

Ep-ĭ-co-rol'le-us.* [From ἐπί, "upon," and *corol'la,* a "corol."] Applied to monopetalous, dicotyledonous plants, in which the stamens are epigynous, or inserted above the ovary.

Ep-ĭ-crā'nĭ-al. [**Epicra'nius.**] Situated on the cranium; belonging to the *epicranium*.

Ep-ĭ-cra'nĭ-um.* [From ἐπί, "upon," and κρανίον, the "cranium."] The integuments, aponeurosis, and muscular expansion upon the cranium; the scalp.

Ep-ĭ-cra'nĭ-us.* A name sometimes given to the *occipito-frontalis* muscle, from its covering the cranium.

Ep-ĭ-dem'ic. [**Epidem'icus;** from ἐπί, "upon," and δῆμος, a "people."] Applied to any disease which seems to be upon the entire population of a country at one time, as distinguished, on the one hand, from *sporadic* disease (or that which occurs in insulated cases), and, on the other, from *endemic* disease, or that which is limited to a particular district.

Ep-ĭ-dem-ĭ-og'ra-phy̆. [**Epidemiogra'phia;** from *epide'mia*, "epidemic diseases," and γράφω, to "write."] A description of epidemic diseases.

Ep-ĭ-dem-ĭ-ol'o-ġy̆. [**Epidemiolo'gia;** from *epide'mia*, "epidemic diseases," and λόγος, a "discourse."] A dissertation on epidemic diseases; the science of epidemic diseases.

Ep'ĭ-dem-y̆. [**Epide'mia;** from ἐπί, "upon," and δῆμος, a "people."] An epidemic disease.

Ep-ĭ-der'mic. [**Epider'micus.**] Belonging to the epidermis.

Epidermidoid. See EPIDERMOID.

Ep-ĭ-der'mis, idis.* [From ἐπί, "upon," and δέρμα, the "skin."] The external covering of the body; the cuticle, or scarf-skin. Applied in Botany to a thin membrane covering every part of the plant; also, the outer covering of grasses.

Ep-ĭ-der'moid. [**Epidermoi'des;** from *epider'mis*, and εἶδος, a "form."] Resembling the epidermis.

Ep-ĭ-did'y̆-mis, idis.* [From ἐπί, "upon," and δίδυμοι, the "testicles."] An oblong substance formed by numerous convolutions of the *Vas deferens*, attached to the upper part of the testicle by vessels, and the reflected layer of the *tunica vaginalis*.

Ep-ĭ-gas-trăl'ġĭ-a.* [From *epigas'trium*, and ἄλγος, "pain."] Pain in the epigastrium.

Ep-ĭ-gas'tric. [**Epigas'tricus.**] Belonging to the epigastrium.

Ep-ĭ-gas'trĭ-um.* [From ἐπί, "upon," and γαστήρ, the "stomach."] That part of the abdomen immediately over the stomach.

Ep-ĭ-ġe'an, or **Ep-ĭ-ġe'al.** [**Epige'us;** from ἐπί, "upon" or "above," and γῆ, the "earth."] Applied to cotyledons that make their way above ground, and appear like leaves.

Ep-ĭ-ġen'e-sis.* [From ἐπί, "at," "on," or "after," and γίνομαι, to "be born," implying that the existence of the new being commences at or after the act of conception; while the pre-existence of the germ is implied in the other theories stated below.] The theory that the embryo is the joint production of both sexes, as distinguished either from the doctrine that the male parent furnishes the germ and the female simply the *nidus*, or resting-place, in which it is nourished; or from the theory that the female furnishes the germ, which is merely quickened by the influence of the male. See GENERATION.

Ep-ĭ-glot'tic. [**Epiglot'ticus.**] Belonging to the epiglottis.

Ep-ĭ-glot-tĭd'e-us.* [From *epiglot'tis*.] The same as EPIGLOTTIC, which see.

Ep-ĭ-glot'tis, idis.* [From ἐπί, "upon," and γλωττίς, the "glottis," or "entrance to the windpipe."] The cartilage at the root of the tongue which forms a lid or cover for the aperture of the windpipe.

Ep-iġ'y̆-nous. [**Epiġ'ynus;** from ἐπί, "above," and γυνή, a "female;" referring to the female portion of the flower.] Applied to stamens when inserted above the ovary.

Ep-ĭ-hy̆'al. [From ἐπί, "upon" or "above," and *hyoi'des*, "hyoid."] Applied by Owen to a triangular piece of bone, pretty constant in fishes, which articulates above to the *Stylohyal*.

Epilampsis, or **Epilampsia.** See ECLAMPSIA.

Ep-ĭ-lep'sy̆. [**Epilep'sia;** from ἐπιλάμβανω, to "seize upon."] A disease which attacks persons suddenly, consisting of convulsions, with coma, and generally frothing at the mouth; the falling sickness. A genus of the order *Spasmi*, class *Neuroses*, of Cullen's Nosology.

Ep-ĭ-lep'tic. [**Epilep'ticus.**] Belonging to epilepsy.

Epilepticæ Auræ. See AURA EPILEPTICA.

Ep-ĭ-lep-tĭ-for'mis.* [From *epilep'sia*.] Like epilepsy: epilep'tiform.

Ep-ĭ-lep'toid. [**Epileptoi'des;** from *epilep'sia*, and εἶδος, a "form."] Resembling epilepsy.

Ep-ĭ-me'rus.* [From ἐπί, "upon," and μήρος, the "thigh."] One of the lateral pieces of the thorax in insects.

Épine (Fr.), à'pèn'. See SPINE.

Ep-ĭ-nўc'tis,* plural **Ep-ĭ-nўc'tĭ-dēs.** [From ἐπί, "on," "at," or "by."] Eruptions which appear on the skin by night and disappear during the day.

Ep-ĭ-pet'a-lous. [**Epipeta'leus, Epipet'alus;** from ἐπί, "upon," and πέταλον, a "petal."] Situated on the petals.

Ep-ĭ-phlœ'um.* [From ἐπί, "upon," and φλοιός, "bark."] The layer of bark next the epidermis.

E-piph'o-ra.* [From ἐπιφέρομαι, to "be borne upon," to "rush upon as a flood."] A superabundant secretion of tears. A genus of the order *Apocenoses*, class *Locales*, of Cullen's Nosology. Also, an overflowing of tears in consequence of an obstruction of the lachrymal duct.

Ep-ĭ-phrag'ma, a*tis*.* [From ἐπί, "upon," and φράγμα, a "partition."] The slender membrane which sometimes shuts the *peristoma* of mosses.

Ep-ĭ-phўl-lo-sper'mous. [**Epiphyllosper'mus;** from ἐπί, "upon," φύλλον, a "leaf," and σπέρμα, a "seed."] Having seeds on the leaves.

Ep-ĭ-phўl'lous. [**Epiphyl'lus;** from ἐπί, "upon," and φύλλον, a "leaf."] Applied to flowers which grow on the surface of a leaf, and also to parasitical *fungi* on the leaves of other plants.

E-piph'ў-sis,* plural **E-piph-ў-sēs.** [From ἐπί, "upon," and φύω, to "produce," to "grow."] A piece of bone growing upon another, as the bulky extremities of long bones, which exist, for a time, separate from the shaft.

Ep'ĭ-phyte. [**Epiph'yton;** from ἐπί, "upon," and φυτόν, a "plant" or "germen."] A parasitic plant or fungus, which grows on the leaves of other plants.

Ep-ip'lo-çēle.* [From ἐπίπλοον, the "omentum," and κήλη, a "tumor."] Hernia in which a portion of the omentum is protruded.

Ep-ĭ-plo'ic. [**Epiplo'icus.**] Belonging to the epiplöon, or omentum.

E-pip-lo-is'chĭ-o-çēle.* [From ἐπίπλοον, the "omentum," ἰσχίον, the "ischium," and κήλη, "hernia."] Hernia in which the omentum protrudes through the ischiadic foramen.

Ep-ĭ-plo-ī'tis, i*dis*.* [From ἐπίπλοον, the "omentum."] Inflammation of the epiplöon; also termed *Omentitis*.

Ep-ĭ-plo-mĕr'o-çēle.* [From ἐπίπλοον, the "omentum," μηρός, the "thigh," and κήλη, "hernia."] Femoral hernia, with protrusion of the omentum.

Ep-ip-lom'pha-lo-çēle.* [From ἐπίπλοον, the "omentum," ὀμφαλός, the "navel," and κήλη, "hernia."] Hernia, with protrusion of the omentum, at the navel.

Ep-ĭp'lo-on.* [Gr. ἐπίπλοον, "that which is *folded upon* the intestines;" allied to ἅπλοος, "without fold," and διπλόος, "twofold."] The omentum, or epiplöon. See OMENTUM.

Ep-ĭ-plos'che-o-çēle.* [From ἐπίπλοον, the "omentum," ὄσχεον, the "scrotum," and κήλη, "hernia."] Hernia, with a portion of omentum, in the scrotum.

E-pis'che-sis,* plural **E-pis'che-sēs.** [Gr. ἐπίσχεσις; from ἐπέχω, to "hold up," to "check," to "restrain."] A suppression of excretions. An order of the class *Locales* of Cullen's Nosology.

Ep-ĭ-spa'dĭ-as.* [From ἐπί, "upon," and σπάζω, to "pierce through."] An unnatural perforation of the penis, the urethra terminating on the upper part of it.

Ep-ĭ-spas'tic. [**Epispas'ticus;** from ἐπισπάω, to "draw upon," or simply to "draw."] (Fr. *Epispastique*, à'pè-spås'tèk'.) Literally, "drawing." Producing a serous or puriform discharge, by exciting previous inflammation; on the principle of derivation or revulsion.

Épispastique. See EPISPASTIC.

Ep'ĭ-sperm. [**Episper'ma, a***tis;* from ἐπί, "upon," and σπέρμα, a "seed."] The whole integuments of a seed taken together.

Ep-ĭ-staph-ў-lī'nus.* [From ἐπί, "upon," and σταφυλή, the "uvula."] Belonging to the uvula: epistaph'yline.

Ep-ĭ-stax'is.* [From ἐπιστάζω, to "distil."] Bleeding at the nose. A genus of the order *Hæmorrhagiæ*, class *Pyrexiæ*, of Cullen's Nosology.

Ep-ĭ-ster'nal. [**Episterna'lis;** from ἐπί, "upon," and *ster'num*, the "breast-bone."] Upon or above the *sternum*.

Ep-ĭ-the'lĭ-al. [**Epithe'lius.**] Belonging to the *epithelium*.

Ep-ĭ-the'lĭ-um.* [From ἐπί, "upon," and θηλή, the "nipple."] The cuticle covering the nipple, or any mucous membrane.

Ep'ĭ-them. [**Epith'ema, a***tis;* from ἐπί, "upon," and τίθημι, to "place."] A term applied to any kind of external application not comprised under the head of ointments or blisters, such as poultices, fomentations, etc.

Ep-ĭ-tўm'pa-nic. [**Epitympan'icus;** from ἐπί, "upon," and *tym'panum*.] Applied by Owen to the uppermost subdivision of the tympanic pedicle which supports the mandible in fishes.

Ep-ĭ-zo'on,* plural **Ep-ĭ-zo'a.** The same as Ectozoon, which see.

Ep-ĭ-zo-ot'ic. [**Epizoot'icus;** from *ἐπί*, "upon" or "against," and *ζῶον*, an "animal."] Applied to contagious disease attacking numbers of cattle at the same time and place.

Ep-ĭ-zo'o-tў. [**Epizöo'tia.**] Epizöotic disease.

Éponge, å'pòNzh'. The French term for Sponge, which see.

Ep'som Salts. The sulphate of magnesia. See Magnesiæ Sulphas.

Ep-u'lis, *idis.** [From *ἐπί*, "upon," and *οὖλα*, the "gums."] A small swelling on the gums.

Ep-u-lot'ic. [**Epulot'icus;** from *ἐπουλόω*, to "cicatrize."] Having power to cicatrize.

Épurge, å'pürzh'. The French term for Euphorbia Lathyris, which see.

E-quā'tor. [**Æqua'tor, o'ris;** from *æ'quo, æqua'tum*, to "make equal."] A great circle of the earth, equidistant from the two poles, and separating the globe into northern and southern hemispheres.

Eq'uĭ-dæ.* [From *e'quus*, a "horse."] Applied to a family of Mammals having the horse for its type.

E-quĭ-lib'rĭ-um. [**Æquilib'rium;** from *æ'què*, "equally," and *li'bro*, to "balance."] Equipoise. Often applied to the equality of temperature which all bodies on the earth are constantly tending to attain (see Caloric), and to the equal distribution of the electric fluid in its natural undisturbed state.

E-qui'nĭ-a.* [From *e'quus*, a "horse."] (Fr. *Morve*, morv.) A disease of horses called Farcy, or Glanders. See Farcy.

E-quĭ-noc'tial. [**Æquinoctia'lis.**] Belonging to the equinox.

E'quĭ-nox. [**Æquinoc'tium;** from *æqu'us*, "equal," and *nox*, "night."] The time when the days and nights are of equal length all over the earth.

Equisetaceæ,* ek-we-se-ta'she-ē. A natural order of cryptogamous plants (or *Gymnosperms*), found in ditches and moist places. It includes the *Equise'tum* (Horse-tail), which is rendered useful for polishing furniture, by a large quantity of silex in the cuticle.

Eq-uĭ-se-tā'ceous. [**Equiseta'ceus.**] Resembling the *Equisetum*. See Equisetaceæ.

Eq'uĭ-tant. [**Eq'uitans;** from *eq'uito, equita'tum*, to "ride."] Laminated; riding, or folded one upon another.

Eq-uĭ-tā'tion. [**Equita'tio, o'nis;** from the same.] Exercise on horseback; riding.

E-quiv'a-lents. [**Æquivalen'tia;** from *æquiva'leo*, to "be of like value."] The system of definite ratios in which elements always combine, referred to a common standard reckoned unity. Thus, 1 is the equivalent number of hydrogen, 8 of oxygen, 28 of lime, 20 of magnesia, 48 of potash, 54 of nitric acid, and 40 of sulphuric acid: hence, if hydrogen combines with oxygen, it is always in the proportion of 1 to 8; so if nitric acid is saturated with lime, the compound (nitrate of lime) will be in the proportion of 54 of the acid to 28 of lime; the nitrate of magnesia, in the proportion of 54 of the acid to 20 of magnesia, etc.; so likewise when sulphuric acid combines with magnesia, it is always in the proportion of 40 to 20; if with potash, of 40 to 48, etc.

Er'bĭ-um.* A newly-discovered metal, occurring along with yttria.

E-rec'tile Tis'sue. [**Te'la Erec'tilis.** See next article.] A peculiar tissue, susceptible of erection, or rapid turgescence, by an increased flow of blood to the part. It is chiefly composed of arteries and veins, the latter greatly predominating, with cells or minute cavities communicating with each other.

E-rec'tor, o'ris.* [From *er'igo, erec'tum*, to "erect."] Applied to certain muscles.

Er-e-ma-cau'sis.* [From *ἠρέμα*, by "degrees," and *καῦσις*, a "burning."] The slow combustion, or oxidation, to which organic bodies are liable.

Er'e-thism. [**Erethis'mus;** from *ἐρεθίζω*, to "irritate."] The state of increased sensibility and irritability attending the early stage of acute diseases, or the excessive use of mercury.

Er-e-this'mus Trop'ĭ-cus.* ("Tropical Erethism.") A name applied by recent writers to that morbid condition of the system which results from a sunstroke.

Ergot. See Ergota.

Er-go'ta.* [From the French *Ergot*, ĕR'go', "spurred rye."] Er'got. The Pharmacopœial name ‖ of the seed, diseased by a parasitic fungus, of *Seca'le cerea'le*, or rye. Ergot has the remarkable property of exciting powerfully the contractile force of the uterus, and it is chiefly employed for this purpose. Its long-continued use, however, is highly dangerous. Bread made of flour containing ergot, has not unfrequently occasioned, in Europe, fatal epidemics, usually attended with dry gangrene.

Er'go-tism. [**Ergotis'mus.**] The poisonous effects of ergot of rye.

Ericaceæ,* ĕr-e-ka'she-ē, or **Er'i-cæ.*** A natural order of exogenous shrubs or under-shrubs, found in Europe, Asia, America, and South Africa. It includes the *Arbutus*, *Azalea*, *Erica* (Heath), *Kalmia*, *Rhododendron*, and other genera prized for the beauty of their flowers. The plants of this order are generally astringent and diuretic.

E-rig'er-on.* [From ἦρ, "spring," and γέρων, an "old man;" because it is hoary in spring.] Fleabane. The Pharmacopœial name (U.S. Ph.) for the herb of *Erig'eron heterophyl'lum*, and of *Erig'eron Philadel'phicum*.

Erig'eron Can-a-den'se.* Canada Fleabane. The Pharmacopœial name (U.S. Ph.) for the herb of *Erigeron Canadense*.

Eriocaulaceæ,* e-re-o-kau-la'she-ē, or **E-ri-o-cau-lo'ne-æ.*** [From *Eriocau'lon*, one of the genera.] A natural order of endogenous plants, found in marshes in Australia and tropical America.

E-ro'ded. [**Ero'sus;** from *e*, "out," and *ro'do*, *ro'sum*, to "gnaw."] A botanical term signifying "notched."

E-ro'dent. [**Ero'dens;** from the same.] Eating out, or eating away.

E-ro'sion. [**Ero'sio, o'nis;** from the same.] An eating or gnawing away. Similar to ULCERATION.

E-rot'ic. [**Erot'icus;** from ἔρως, ἔρωτος, "love."] Pertaining to love; arising from love.

E-ro-to-ma'ni-a.* [From ἔρως, "love," and μανία, "madness."] Melancholy, or madness, caused by love.

Er-rat'ic. [**Errat'icus;** from *er'ro*, *erra'tum*, to "wander."] Wandering; moving from one place to another.

Erreur de Lieu. See ERROR LOCI.

Er'rhine. [**Errhi'nus;** from ἐν, "in," and ῥίν, the "nose."] A medicine which increases the natural secretion of the membrane lining the nose: sternutatory.

Er'ror Lo'ci.* ("Mistake of Place or Position.") (Fr. *Erreur de Lieu*, ĕr'RUR' deh le-uh'.) A term formerly applied to certain derangements in the capillary circulation. Boerhaave conceived that the vessels for the circulation of blood, lymph, and serum, were of different sizes; and that when the larger-sized globules passed into the smaller vessels the obstruction caused inflammation.

E-ruc-tā'tion. [**Eructa'tio, o'nis;** from *eruc'to*, *eructa'tum*, to "belch."] Any sudden burst of wind, or liquid, from the stomach, by the mouth.

E-rupt'. [See next article.] To burst through; as a tooth through the gum.

E-rup'tion. [**Erup'tio, o'nis;** from *e*, "out," and *rum'po*, *rup'tum*, to "burst" or "break."] A discoloration, or breaking out of pimples on the skin.

E-rup'tive Fe'vers. A designation applied by Dr. Good to diseases belonging to his order *Exanthematica*.

Er-va-len'ta.* A powder of farina obtained from *Ervum lens*, or common lentil. The dietetical use of it is said to prevent constipation.

Ervum Lens. See ERVALENTA.

E-ryn'go. The candied root of the *Eryn'gium Campes'tre*, regarded by Boerhaave as the first of aperient diuretic roots. It is now but little used.

Er-y-sip'e-las, atis.* [From ἐρυθρός, "red," and πέλος, or πέλλα, a "skin."] (Fr. *Érysipèle*, à'rè'zè'pĕl' or à'rè'zè'pål'.) Redness or inflammation of some part of the skin, with fever, inflammatory or typhoid, and, generally, vesications on the affected part, and symptomatic fever. It is also called St. Anthony's Fire, *Ig'nis Sa'cer* ("Sacred Fire"), the Rose, and other names.

Er-y-sip-e-la-to-i'dēs.* [From *erysip'elas*, and εἶδος, a "form."] Resembling erysipelas: erysip'elatoid.

Érysipèle. See ERYSIPELAS.

Er-y-the'ma, atis.* [From ἐρυθαίνω, to "redden."] (Fr. *Érythème*, à'rè'tĕm'.) Redness of a part; a mere rash or efflorescence not accompanied by swelling, vesication, or fever.

Érythème. See ERYTHEMA.

Er-y-thræ'a.* [From ἐρυθραῖος, "red."] A genus of plants of the class *Pentandria*, natural order *Gentianaceæ*.

Erythræ'a Cen-tau'ri-um.* The common centuary, or *Chironia centaurium*.

E-ryth'ric Açid. [From ἐρυθρός, "red."] An acid obtained by the action of nitric acid on lithic acid, yellow at first, but becoming red by being exposed to the sun's rays.

Er'yth-rin, or **Er'yth-rine.** [**Erythri'na;** from ἐρυθρός, "red."] The coloring matter of the *Lichen roccella*. See ARCHIL.

Er-ȳth'ro-ḡen. [**Erythroge'nium;** from ἐρυθρός, "red," and γεννάω, to "generate."] Literally, "that which produces red." Applied to a peculiar animal principle, considered as the base of the coloring matter of the blood. Also, a variety of *Chromogen* (the coloring matter of vegetables); because it produces a red color with acids.

Er'ȳ-throid. [**Erythroi'des;** from ἐρυθρός, "red," and εἶδος, a "form," "resemblance."] Of a red color: reddish.

Er'ythroid Coat. The vaginal coat of the testis.

Er'ythroid Ves'ĭ-cle. An enlargement of the (future) umbilical cord in the embryo of most of the *Ruminantia*, and of the pig.

E-rȳth'ro-phȳll, or **Er'ȳ-thro-phȳlle,** called also **Er'ȳ-thro-phȳl'lin.** [From ἐρυθρός, "red," and φύλλον, a "leaf."] A term applied by Berzelius to the red coloring matter of fruits and leaves in autumn.

Er-ȳ-thro'sis.* [From ἐρυθρός, "red."] *Pletho'ra arterio'sa.* A form of plethora in which the blood is rich in fibrin and in bright red pigment; a state corresponding in some measure with what has been termed the "arterial constitution."

Erythroxylaceæ,* ĕr-e-throx-e-la'she-ē. [From *Erythrox'ylon,* one of the genera.] A natural order of exogenous trees and shrubs, found in South America and the West Indies.

Er-ȳ-throx'ȳ-lon Co'ca.* A shrub growing in South America, the leaves of which (known by the name of *coca*) are a powerful nervous stimulant; so that those who chew them can work or travel a whole day without food.

Escalloniaceæ,* es-kal lo-ne-a'she-ē. [From *Escallo'nia,* one of the genera.] A natural order of exogenous shrubs, found in temperate climates.

Es'char. [**Es'chara;** from ἐσχαρόω, to "scab over."] The hard, black, or gray slough caused by caustic or cautery.

Es-char-ot'ic. [**Escharot'icus.**] Applied to a substance which forms an eschar.

Es'cu-lent. [**Esculentus;** from *es'co,* to "feed upon a thing."] Fit for food.

Esculin. See ÆSCULIN.

Es'o-en-ter-i'tis.* [From ἔσω, "within," and *enteri'tis.*] Inflammation of the mucous membrane of the intestines.

Es'o-gas-tri'tis.* [From ἔσω, "within," and *gastri'tis.*] Inflammation of the mucous membrane of the stomach.

Es-o-tĕr'ic. [**Esoter'icus;** from ἐσώτερος, "within."] Applied to a series of phenomena or changes, resulting from causes internal and proper to the organism.

Esprit, es'prè'. The French term for "spirit" or "essence." Any subtile and volatile product of distillation.

Es'sence. [**Essen'tia;** from *es'se,* to "be."] The chief properties or virtues extracted from any substance.

Es'sence of Su'gar. Oxalic acid.

Essen'tia (es-sen'she-a) **Ab-i'e-tis.*** Essence of Spruce; prepared by boiling in water the young tops of some coniferous plant, as the *Abies nigra,* or Black Spruce, and concentrating the decoction by evaporation.

Essen'tia Bi'na.* A substance used to color brandy, porter, etc.; prepared by boiling coarse sugar till it is black and bitter; it is then made into a syrup with lime-water.

Es-sen'tial Oils. Oils obtained by distillation from odoriferous vegetable substances. They are also called volatile oils.

Essen'tial Salt of Lem'ons. A mixture of cream of tartar and binoxalate of potash.

Es'se-ra.* [From the Arabic.] Another name for Nettle-Rash, or the *Urticaria* of Willan.

Estivation. See ÆSTIVATIO.

Estomac, ĕs'to'mâ' or ĕs'to'mâk'. The French term for STOMACH, which see.

Étage, à'tâzh'. The French term for STAGE, which see.

Étain, à'tăNᵍ'. The French term for TIN (or pewter), which see.

E'thal. A peculiar oily substance obtained from spermaceti; also termed *hydrate of oxide of cetyl.* The term is formed of the first syllables of *ether* and *alcohol.*

E'ther. [**Æ'ther, eris;** from αἰθήρ, "air."] A volatile liquor obtained from alcohol and a concentrated acid.

E'ther, Ni'trous. [**Æ'ther Nitro'sus.**] The ether obtained by distilling equal weights of alcohol and concentrated nitric acid.

E'ther, Rec'tĭ-fied. [**Æ'ther Rectifica'tus.**] Sulphuric ether freed from the small portion of alcohol and sulphurous acid which it contains, by the process of rectification.

E'ther, Sul-phu'ric, or **Æ'ther Sul-phu'rĭ-cus.*** The Pharmacopœial name (Ed. and Dub. Ph.) of ether obtained from a mixture of rectified spirit and sulphuric acid; also called *Æther vitriolicus*. See SPIRITUS ÆTHERIS SULPHURICI.

Éthéré. See ETHEREAL.

E-the're-al. [**Æthe'reus,** or **Æ-the'rius;** from *æ'ther*.] (Fr. *Ethéré*, à'tà'rà'.) Applied to any highly rectified essential oil or spirit.

Ethe'real Oil. The *Oleum vini* found in the residuum of sulphuric ether, and forming the basis of Hoffman's celebrated anodyne.

Eth'er-in, or **Eth'er-ïne.** A term synonymous with olefiant gas, elayl, or hydruret of acetyl.

E-ther-ĭ-zā'tion. [**Ætheriza'tio, o'***nis*.] The inhaling the fumes of eth'er, to produce insensibility to pain.

Eth'er-ole. A carbo-hydrogen, commonly known as *light oil of wine*.

E-thĭ-on'ic Aç'id. An acid formed by the action of sulphuric acid on ether and alcohol.

Ethiops Mineral. See ÆTHIOPS MINERAL.

Eth'moid. [**Ethmoi'des;** from ἠθμός, a "sieve," and εἶδος, a "form."] Resembling a sieve; cribriform.

Eth'moid Bone. [Lat. **Os Ethmoi'deum;** Fr. *Os Cribleux*, ō krè'-bluh'.] One of the bones composing the cranium; so named because its upper plate is pierced with a number of small holes, through which pass the filaments of the olfactory nerves. In Comparative Anatomy, the term is restricted by Owen to the part of the bone directly concerned in supporting the membrane and cells of the olfactory organ.

Eth-moi'dal. [**Ethmoida'lis.**] Belonging to the ethmoid bone.

Eth-nog'ra-phȳ. [**Ethnogra'phia;** from ἔθνος, a "nation," and γράφω, to "write."] The history of the manners, customs, origin, etc., of nations.

Eth-nol'o-ġȳ. [**Ethnolo'gia;** from ἔθνος, a "nation," and λόγος, a "discourse."] The science which treats of the different nations and races of men, their correlation, their anatomical, physiological, and mental peculiarities, etc.

Eth'ȳle. [From αἰθήρ, "ether," and ὕλη, "material."] A hypothetical substance composed of hydrogen and etherin, and considered to be the radical of ethers and their compounds.

E-tĭ-o-lā'tion. [**Etiola'tio, o'***nis*.] (Fr. *Etiolement*, à'tè'ol'mŏNᴳ'; from *étiolé*, "blanched.") The state of being blanched. Applied to certain plants from which the light is excluded as much as possible.

Étiolement. See ETIOLATION.

Etiology. See ÆTIOLOGY.

Étouffement, à'toof'mŏNᴳ'. The French term for SUFFOCATION, which see.

Étourdissement, à'tooR'dèss'mŏNᴳ'. The French term for VERTIGO, which see.

Étranglement, à'trŏNᴳ'g'l'mŏNᴳ'. The French term for STRANGULATION, which see.

Et'ȳ-mon.* [From ἔτυμον, the neuter of ἔτυμος, "true."] The true origin of a word; the radical word or root: hence, ETYMOLOGY, the science which explains or treats of the derivation of words.

Eū'chlo-rïne. [From εὖ, "fine," and χλωρός, "green."] The name given by Davy to the protoxide of chlorine, on account of its deep yellow-green color.

Eū-chron'ic Aç'id. [From εὖ, "fine," and χρόα, "color."] An acid procured by the decomposition of the neutral mellitate of ammonia by heat. It forms a blue compound with zinc, called *Euchrone*.

Eū-dĭ-om'e-ter. [**Eudiom'etrum;** from εὐδία, "fine weather," also "goodness of the air," and μετρέω, to "measure."] An instrument to measure the purity of the air or of any gaseous compound, or the quantity of oxygen contained in it.

Eū-dĭ-om'e-trȳ. [**Eudiome'tria;** from the same.] The method by which the purity of atmospheric air is ascertained.

Eū-ġe'nĭ-a.* [From Prince *Eugene* of Savoy.] A Linnæan genus of the class *Icosandria*, natural order *Myrtaceæ*. The name of the tree affording pimento.

Euge'nia Car-ȳ-o-phȳl-la'ta.* The tree which produces the clove; otherwise called the *Caryophyl'lus aromat'icus*.

Euge'nia Pi-men'ta.* The name of the tree which yields pimento.

Eū-ġen'ic Aç'id. [**Aç'idum Eugen'icum;** from *Euge'nia caryophylla'ta*, one of the names of the clove-tree.] Called also CARYOPHYLLIC ACID, and HEAVY OIL OF CLOVES. An acid found in cloves, along with a neutral salt. *Eu'genin* is a crystallizable compound, found also in cloves, and said to be isomeric with eugenic acid. *Caryophyl'lin* is another of these compounds.

Eū'nuch. [**Eunu'chus;** from εὐνή, a "couch," and ἔχω, to "keep," to "guard."] (Fr. *Eunuque*, uh'nük'.) A man in whom the spermato-poietic, or entire genital organs have been removed. So named because commonly employed in the East, from a remote antiquity, to guard the harem of princes.

Eunuque. See EUNUCH.

Eū-on'ȳ-mus.* Wahoo. The Pharmacopœial name (U.S. Ph., 1860) for the bark of *Euon'ymus atropurpu'reus.* It is recommended as a remedy in dropsy, and is said to combine the virtues of a tonic with those of a hydragogue cathartic and diuretic.

Eupatoire. See EUPATORIUM.

Eū-pa-to'rĭ-um.* (Fr. *Eupatoire,* uh'på'twåR'.) Thoroughwort. The Pharmacopœial name (U.S. Ph.) for the tops and leaves of the *Eupato'rium perfolia'tum.*

Euphorbe. See EUPHORBIA.

Eū-phor'bĭ-a.* [From *Euphor'bus,* the name of a noted physician.] (Fr. *Épurge,* å'püRzh', or *Euphorbe,* uh'foRb'.) A Linnæan genus of the class *Dodecandria,* natural order *Euphorbiaceæ.*

Euphor'bia Cor-ol-la'ta.* Large-flowering Spurge. The Pharmacopœial name (U.S. Ph.) for the root of *Euphorbia corollata.*

Euphor'bia Ip-e-cac-u-an'ha.* Ipecacuanha Spurge. The Pharmacopœial name (U.S. Ph.) for the root of *Euphorbia Ipecacuanha.*

Euphor'bia Of-fiç-ĭ-na'lis,* Euphor'bia Of-fiç-ĭ-na'rum.* ("Euphorbia of the Shops.") The plant which produces *Euphorbium.*

Euphorbiaceæ,* ū-for-be-a'she-ē. [From *Euphor'bia,* one of the genera.] A very large natural order of exogenous plants, found in nearly all parts of the globe. It includes the *Ricinus* (castor-oil plant), *Siphonia* (the Caoutchouc, or India-Rubber tree), and *Croton,* which yields croton oil. A large proportion of the plants of this order are poisonous. The stem of *Jatropha Manihot,* or Cassava, which when raw is a violent poison, becomes a wholesome nutritious food when roasted. This order is nearly allied to the *Malvaceæ* and *Rhamnaceæ.*

Eū-phor-bĭ-ā'ceous. [Euphorbia'ceus.] Resembling *Euphorbia.* See EUPHORBIACEÆ.

Eū-phor'bĭ-um.* A resinous substance obtained from the *Euphorbia officinarum,* and of undetermined species of *Euphorbia;* called, also, the *Euphorbiæ gummi-resina.*

Eu'pĭ-on.* [From εὖ, "well," or "fine," and πίων, "fat."] A colorless liquid, obtained by distillation from the tar of animal matters, and so named from its great limpidity.

Eu-plas'tic. [From εὖ, "well," and πλάσις, "formation."] A term applied by Lobstein to the elaborated organizable matter by which the tissues of the body are renewed. The same writer speaks of another animal matter, the tendency of which is softening and disorganization: this he terms *cacoplastic.*

Eu-pȳr'ĭ-on.* [From εὖ, "easily," and πῦρ, "fire."] Any contrivance for obtaining an instantaneous light, as the phosphorus-bottle, etc.

Eū-stā'chĭ-an Tube. (Fr. *Trompe* [or *Conduit,* kòNᵍ'dwè'] *d'Eustache,* tròMp dus'tåsh'.) A tube or canal extending from behind the soft palate to the tympanum of the ear, first described by Eustachius.

Eusta'chian Valve. The semilunar fold of the lining membrane of the heart, anterior to the opening of the inferior *vena cava.*

E-vac'u-ant. [Evac'uans; from *evac'uo, evacua'tum,* to "empty."] Having the property of increasing evacuations from the bowels, etc.

E-vac-u-ā'tion. [Evacua'tio, o'nis; from the same.] The act of discharging the contents of the bowels, or defecation; also, the discharge itself; a dejection or stool.

Évanouissement, å'vå'nwèss'mòNᵍ'. The French term for SYNCOPE, which see.

E-vap-o-rā'tion. [Evapora'tio, o'nis; from *e,* "out," and *vapo'ro, vapora'tum,* to "steam," to "send out vapor."] The conversion of a liquid into vapor. In Medicine, the transformation of a liquid into vapor in order to obtain the fixed matters contained in it in a dry and separate state.

E-ven-trā'tion. [Eventra'tio, o'nis; from *e,* "out of," and *ven'ter,* the "belly."] The condition of a monster-fœtus, in which the abdominal viscera are extruded from the natural cavity, and enclosed in a projecting membranous sac.

E-ven-tu-al'ĭ-tȳ. The phrenological term for the faculty of observing and recollecting events, occurrences, etc.

Eversion of Eyelid. See ECTROPIUM.

Ev-o-lu'tion. [Evolu'tio, o'nis; from *e,* "out," and *vol'vo, volu'tum,* to "roll;" whence, *evol'vo,* to "roll out," or "unfold."] Synonymous, generally, with DEVELOPMENT, which see.

Evolu'tion, Spon-ta'ne-ous. A term applied to obstetrical cases where, in the presentation or protrusion of the arm and shoulder, spontaneous turning takes place, and the case thus becomes one of breech-presentation.

E-vul'sion. [**Evul sio, o**'*nis;* from *e,* "out," and *vel'lo, vul'sum,* to "pluck," to "pull."] The act or process of drawing out forcibly.

Ex, or **E.** A Latin preposition signifying "out," or "forth," "out of," "from," "beyond." It often has the force of "up;" as *Exsiccation,* a "drying up." Sometimes it is privative. *Ex* is usually changed to *f* before a word beginning with *f;* as *efferens* for *ex ferens.* Before the liquids, *l, m, n, r,* and also before *b* and *v, e* is used instead of *ex.*

Ex (ἐξ). A Greek preposition, signifying "out." See Ec.

Ex-aç-er-bā'tion. [**Exacerba'tio, o**'*nis;* from *exacer'bo, exacerba'tum,* to "become severe or sharp."] An increased force or severity of the symptoms of a disease.

Exæresis,* ex-ĕr'e-sis. [From ἐξαιρέω, to "take away," to "remove."] One of the old divisions of Surgery, implying the removal of parts.

Ex-al-bu'mi-nous. [**Exalbu'minus;** from *ex,* "without," and *albu'men.*] Without albumen or perisperm.

Ex-an-ġeī'ạ,* or **Ex-an-ġi'ạ.*** [From ἐξ, "out," and ἀγγεῖον, a "vessel."] A term sometimes applied to diseases in which the large vessels are ruptured, or unnaturally distended.

Ex-a'nĭ-ạ.* [From *ex,* "out," and *a'nus.*] A prolapsus, or falling down, of the anus. See Archoptosis.

Ex-an-the'mạ,* plural **Ex-an-them'ạ-tạ.** [From ἐξανθέω, to "burst forth as flowers," to "bloom," to "break out in pustules."] (Fr. *Exanthème,* ĕx'-ǎnᴳ'tĕm', or *Élevure,* à'là'vüʀ'.) A rash, or eruption on the skin; also called *Exanthisma.* Applied in the plural to an order of the class *Pyrexiæ* of Cullen's Nosology.

Ex-an-the-mat'ic. [**Exanthemat'icus.**] Belonging to exanthema; eruptive.

Ex-an-the-mat'ĭ-cạ.* [The neuter plural of **Exanthemat'icus.** See Exanthematic.] A name given by Dr. Good to an order comprising all eruptive fevers.

Ex-an-them-ạ-tol'o-ġȳ. [**Exanthematolo'gia;** from *exanthe'ma,* "eruption," and λόγος, a "discourse."] The consideration of the exanthemata.

Ex-an-them'ạ-tous. [**Exanthemato'sus;** from *exanthe'ma,* "eruption."] Pertaining to exanthemata; having exanthemata.

Exanthème. See Exanthema.

Ex-an-the'sis,* and **Ex-an-this'-mạ.*** Nearly the same as Exanthema, which see.

Ex-ar-thro'sis,* or **Ex-ar-thro'-mạ.*** [From ἐξ, "out," and ἄρθρον, a "joint."] The same as Luxation.

Ex-cip'ĭ-ent. [**Excip'iens;** from *excip'io,* to "receive."] Applied to the substance used for receiving medicines, or hiding their nauseous qualities in its more pleasant taste, as the confections, conserves, etc.

Ex-ciṡ'ion. [**Exci'sio, o**'*nis;* from *ex,* "out" or "off," and *scin'do, scis'sum,* to "cut."] The cutting out, or cutting off, of any part.

Ex-cī-tạ-bil'ĭ-tȳ. [**Excitabil'itas, a**'*tis;* from *ex'cito, excita'tum,* to "call forth," to "raise up."] The capacity of organized beings to be affected by certain agents termed *stimuli,* excitants, or exciting powers.

Ex-cī'tant. [**Ex'citans;** from the same.] Exciting; stimulating.

Ex-cĭ-tā'tion. [**Excita'tio, o**'*nis;* from the same.] The act of rousing, or quickening into active exercise, some power or susceptibility.

Ex-cīte'ment. [From the same.] The state of being excited.

Ex-cī'ting Cause. That which excites, or is the immediate cause of, a disease.

Ex-cī'to-Mo'tor-ȳ (or **Ex-cī'to-Mo'tor**) **Pow'er.** A peculiar power or property seated in the spinal system of nerves, by which, if their extremities be excited, the impression is conveyed to the spinal marrow, and reflected from it to the part or limb excited.

Ex-co-rĭ-ā'tion. [**Excoria'tio, o**'*nis;* from *ex,* "from," and *co'rium,* the "skin."] Abrasion or removal, partial or complete, of the skin.

Ex'cre-ment. [**Excremen'tum;** from *excer'no, excre'tum,* to "excrete," to "void by stool."] The alvine fæces, or waste matter discharged from the bowels; dung; ordure.

Excrementitious, ex-kre-men-tish'-ŭs. [**Excrementi'tius.**] Belonging to excrement.

Ex-crĕs-çence. [**Excrescen'tia;** from *excres'co,* to "grow out of."] (Fr. *Excroissance,* ĕx'kʀwå'sŏɴss'.) Any preternatural formation on any part of the body.

Ex-cre'tion. [**Excre'tio, o**'*nis;* from *excer'no, excre'tum,* to "sift out," to "separate."] The separation of those fluids from the blood which are supposed to be useless, as urine, perspiration, etc.; also, any such fluid itself.

Excrétoire. See EXCRETORY.

Ex'cre-to-rў. [Excreto'rius; from the same.] (Fr. *Excrétoire*, ĕx'kRȧ'twåR'.) Having the power of separating and throwing off what is superfluous; belonging to excretion.

Ex'cretory Ducts. [Duc'tus Excreto'rii.] Small vessels that conduct the secretion out of a gland.

Ex-cre'tus.* [See EXCRETION.] Thrown off as superfluous or useless.

Excroissance. See EXCRESCENCE.

Ex'e-dens.* [From *ex'edo*, to "eat out," to "eat as a worm or sore."] Eating; consuming.

Ex-em-brў-o-na'tus.* [From *ex*, priv., and *em'bryo*, the "germ of a plant."] Having no embryo. Applied in the plural feminine (*Exembryona'tæ*) to the *Cryptogamia*.

Ex-fœ-tā'tion. [From *ex*, "out" or "without," and *fœ'tus*.] Extra-uterine fœtation, or imperfect fœtation in some organ exterior to the uterus. See ECCYESIS.

Ex-fo-lĭ-ā'tion. [Exfolia'tio, o'nis; from *ex*, "from," or "off," and *fo'lium*, a "leaf;" whence *exfo'lio*, *exfolia'tum*, to "shed the leaf."] The separation or scaling off of a dead piece of bone from the living; also, the separation of scales or laminæ from any substance.

Exhalaison. See EXHALATION.

Ex-hā'lant. [Exha'lans; from *exha'lo*, *exhala'tum*, to "send forth a breath."] Giving off fumes; exhaling.

Ex-ha-lā'tion. [Exhala'tio, o'nis; from the same.] (Fr. *Exhalaison*, ĕx'ȧ'lā'zōNᵍ'.) A vapor, fume, or steam. A subtile spirit or vapor, from the surface of the body. Evaporation of moisture or water by the sun's heat, etc.

Ex-hib'it. [From *exhib'eo*, *exhib'itum*, to "show" or "exhibit," to "give."] To administer or give to a patient some medicine, or medicinal substance.

Exo (ἔξω). A Greek particle, signifying "without."

Ex-o-car'dĭ-al. [Exocardia'lis; from ἔξω, "without," and καρδία, the "heart."] External to the heart.

Ex-oc-cip'ĭ-tal. [Exoccipita'lis; from ἔξω, "without," and *occipita'lis*, "occipital."] Applied by Owen to the lateral part of the occipital bone.

Exoccip'ital Bone. In Anthropotomy, the condyloid process of the occipital bone: its homologue in the archetypal skeleton is called the "neurapophysis." See VERTEBRA.

Ex-od'ic. [Exod'icus; from ἔξω, "without," and ὁδός, a "way."] Proceeding out of the spinal marrow. A term proposed by Dr. M. Hall as preferable to *Reflex motor*.

Ex'o-ġen. An exogenous plant.

Ex-oġ'en-ous. [Exog'enus; from ἔξω, "without," and γένω, to "be born," to "grow."] Applied to stems of plants in which the new matter, whereby they increase in diameter, is added at the external surface. Applied by Owen to those parts, properly called processes, of bone, which shoot out as continuations of preceding elements. See AUTOGENOUS.

Ex-og'o-num Pur'ga.* One of the names of the jalap-plant. See JALAP.

Ex-om'pha-los,* Ex-om'pha-lus.* [From ἐξ, "out," and ὀμφαλός, the "navel."] (Fr. *Hernie ombilicale*, ĕR'nè' ōM'bè'lè'kål'.) Umbilical hernia. See OMPHALOCELE.

Ex-oph-thăl'mĭ-a.* [From ἐξ, "out," and ὀφθαλμός, the "eye."] A swelling and protrusion of the eyeball; the same as OPHTHALMOPTOMA.

Ex-or'mĭ-a.* [From ἐξ, "out," and ὁρμή, "rushing."] Literally, a "rushing or breaking out." A term used by the Greeks as synonymous with ecthyma, or papulous skin, comprising gum-rash, etc.

Ex-or-rhi'zous. [Exorrhi'zus; from ἔξω, "without," and ῥίζα, a "root."] Applied to plants having the radicle free and naked, that is, not enclosed in any sheath.

Ex'o-Skel'e-ton. [Exoscel'eton; from ἔξω, "without," and σκελετόν, a "skeleton."] The skeleton in such animals as have a hard or bony case, or external skeleton. See DERMOSKELETON.

Ex-os'mic. [Exos'micus.] Belonging to *exosmose*.

Ex-os-mose'. [Exosmo'sis; from ἔξω, "without," and ὠσμός, "impulsion."] A movement in liquids separated by a membranous partition, by which their principles are interchanged. This term is given to the liquid passing outwards. See ENDOSMOSE.

Exostemma Caribeum. See BARK, CARIBEAN.

Ex-os'to-ma.* [From ἔξω, "without," and στόμα, a "mouth."] See MICROPYLE.

Exosto'ma.* Nearly the same as EXOSTOSIS, which see.

Ex-os-to'sis.* [From ἔξω, "without," and ὀστεόν, a "bone."] An exuberant growth of bony matter on the surface of a bone; the enlargement of a part or the whole of a bone.

Ex-o-tĕr'ic. [**Exoter'icus;** from ἐξώτερος, the comparative degree of ἔξω.] Applied to a series of periodic, vital phenomena, being such as result from causes external to the organism.

Exothecium,* ex-o-the'she-ŭm. [From ἔξω, "without," and θήκη, a "case."] The name given by Purkinje to the coat of the anther.

Ex-ot'ic. [**Exot'icus;** from ἔξω, "without."] Foreign; belonging to what is without, or beyond the limits of, our own country.

Ex-pan-sĭ-bil'ĭ-tỹ. [**Expansibil'itas, a'***tis;* from *ex,* "out," and *pan'do, pan'sum,* to "spread."] The capability of being expanded or dilated.

Ex-pan'sion. [**Expan'sio, o'***nis;* from the same.] The increase of bulk, or of surface, of which natural bodies are susceptible.

Ex-pec'to-rant. [**Expec'torans;** from *expec'toro, expectora'tum,* to "discharge from the breast" (from *ex,* "out," "from," and *pec'tus,* the "breast").] Facilitating or promoting the ejection of mucus, or other fluids, from the lungs and trachea.

Ex-pec-to-rā'tion. [**Expectora'tio, o'***nis;* from the same.] The [illegible] of ejecting from the lungs, or trachea, by spitting; also, the substance ejected.

Ex-pel'lent. [**Expel'lens;** from *expel'lo,* to "drive out."] Driving out.

Ex-pĭ-rā'tion. [**Expira'tio, o'***nis;* from *expi'ro, expira'tum,* to "breathe forth."] The act of breathing out, or expelling air from the lungs.

Ex-plo-rā'tion. [**Explora'tio, o'***nis;* from *explo'ro, explora'tum,* to "search diligently."] The investigation of the *physical signs* attending disease, as distinguished from what are commonly termed the *symptoms;* consisting of auscultation, inspection, mensuration, palpation, and percussion.

Ex-pressed' Oils. Oils obtained from bodies by pressure. See EXPRESSION.

Ex-pres'sion. [**Expres'sio, o'***nis;* from *ex,* "out," and *pre'mo, pres'sum,* to "press."] The process of forcing out the juices and oils of plants by means of a press. Also, the manifestation of the feelings, by the countenance, attitude, or gesture.

Ex-pul'sion. [**Expul'sio, o'***nis;* from *ex,* "out," and *pel'lo, pul'sum,* to "drive," to "force."] The act of voiding the bowels or bladder. The delivery of the placenta; also, the extrusion of an immature fœtus.

Ex-pul'sive. [**Expel'lens;** from the same.] (Fr. *Expulsif,* ĕx'pül'sēf'.) Applied to the pains in the second stage of childbirth, by which the child is expelled. Applied in Surgery to a bandage so adjusted as to expel pus or other fluid.

Ex-san'guine, Ex-san-guin'e-ous. [**Exsanguin'eus;** from *ex,* priv., and *san'guis,* "blood."] Deprived of blood: anæmial; anæmic.

Ex-san-guin'ĭ-tỹ. [**Exsanguin'itas, a'***tis;* from the same.] The state of being without blood: anæmia.

Ex-sert'ed. [**Exser'tus;** from *ex'sero, exser'tum,* to "thrust out."] Protruding beyond, as the stamens out of the corolla.

Ex-sic-cā'tion. [**Exsicca'tio, o'***nis;* from *exsic'co, exsicca'tum,* to "dry up."] The process of drying moist bodies by applying heat, or atmospheric air, or absorbing the moisture by soft spongy substances.

Ex-stip'u-late. [**Exstipula'tus;** from *ex,* priv., and *stip'ula,* a "stipule."] Without stipules.

Ex'stro-phỹ. [**Exstro'phia,** or **Ec'strophe;** from ἐκ, "out," and στρέφω, to "turn" or "twist."] Applied to a congenital malformation, in which, from deficiency in the abdominal wall, the bladder appears to be turned inside out, having the internal surface of the posterior *paries* situated outwardly on the lower part of the body.

Exsudation. See EXUDATION.

Extenseur. See EXTENSOR.

Ex-ten'sion. [**Exten'sio, o'***nis;* from *ex,* "out," and *ten'do, ten'sum,* to "stretch."] The pulling of a fractured limb in a direction from the trunk, to obviate retraction of the lower fragments; also, similar treatment in dislocations.

Ex-ten'sor, o'r*is.** [From the same.] (Fr. *Extenseur,* ĕx'tōnᵍ'sur'.) An extender. Applied to several muscles.

Exten'sor Bre'vis Dig-ĭ-to'rum Pe'dis.* ("Short Extensor of the Toes.") A muscle situated on the back of the foot, having for its office to extend the first four toes.

Exten'sor Com-mu'nis Digito'rum Pe'dis.* ("Common Extensor of the Toes.") A muscle situated on the anterior part of the leg, and attached to the phalanges of the last four toes, which it extends.

Exten'sor Digito'rum Commu'nis.* ("Common Extensor of the Fingers.") A muscle of the forearm, the tendons of which are inserted into the phalanges of all the fingers, which it extends.

Exten'sor Pro'prĭ-us Pol'lĭ-cis Pe'dis.* ("Extensor Proper of the *Thumb of the Foot,* or *Great Toe.*") A muscle on the anterior part of the leg: its office is to extend the toe.

Ex-tir-pā'tion. [**Extirpa'tio, o'**nis; from *extir'po, extirpa'tum,* to "root out."] The complete removal or eradication of a part, by the knife or caustic.

Ex'tra.* A Latin preposition signifying "without," "on the outside," "beyond," "over and above."

Ex'tract. [**Extrac'tum;** from *ex,* "out," and *tra'ho, trac'tum,* to "draw."] (Fr. *Extrait,* ĕx'tRå'.) Literally, "that which is drawn out or extracted" from any thing. The soluble parts of vegetable substances, dissolved in spirit, or water, and reduced to the consistence of a syrup or paste by evaporation. Also, the product of an aqueous decoction.

Ex-trac'tạ,* the plural of EXTRACTUM, which see.

Ex-trac'tion. [**Extrac'tio, o'**nis; from the same.] The drawing of a tooth, or taking foreign substances out of the body, or a tumor out of its cavity, etc.

Ex-trac'tĭve. [**Extracti'vus;** from the same.] (Fr. *Extractif,* ĕx'tRåk'tĕf'.) Applied to a peculiar modification of vegetable matter forming one constituent part of common extracts.

EXTRAC'TIVE PRIN'CIPLES. The designation of a variety of compounds, most of which crystallize, and have a bitter taste, but cannot be referred to any particular series.

☞ For the names and preparation of the officinal extracts, see the U.S. Pharmacopœia, pp. 142–180.

Ex-trac'tum,* plural **Ex-trac'tạ.** [From the same.] (Fr. *Extrait,* ĕx'tRå'.) An extract; a preparation obtained by the evaporation of a vegetable solution, or a native vegetable juice. Its basis is termed *extractive,* or extractive principle.

Extrac'tum Can'nạ-bis.* ("Extract of Hemp.") The Pharmacopœial name (U.S. Ph.) for the alcoholic extract of the dried tops of the *Cannabis sativa* (variety *Indica*).

Extrac'tum Glȳç-ȳr-rhi'zæ.* ("Extract of Liquorice.") The Pharmacopœial name (U.S. Ph.) for the extract of the root of *Glycyrrhiza glabra.* This extract is the "liquorice" of the shops.

Ex-trạ-fo-lĭ-ā'ceous. [**Extrafolia'ceus;** from *ex'tra,* "without," and *fo'lium,* a "leaf."] External to the leaf. Applied to *stipulæ* below the footstalk.

Extrait, ĕx'tRå'. A French term for EXTRACT, which see.

Ex'trạ-U'ter-ĭne. [From *ex'tra,* "on the outside," and *u'terus.*] Applied to those cases of pregnancy in which the fœtus is contained in some organ outside of the uterus.

Ex-trav-ạ-sā'tion. [**Extravasa'tio, o'**nis; from *ex'tra,* "without," and *vas,* a "vessel."] The effusion of a fluid (or its state when effused) out of its proper vessel or receptacle.

Ex-trem'ĭ-tȳ. [**Extrem'itas, a'**tis; from *extre'mum,* the "outermost part" or "end" of any thing.] Any of the four limbs of animals.

Ex-tro-ver'sion. [From *extror'sum,* "outwards." and *ver'to, ver'sum,* to "turn."] That kind of malformation in which a part is turned inside outwards. The same as EXSTROPHY.

Ex-u'ber-ēs.* [From *ex,* priv,, and *u'ber,* "pap" or "udder."] Applied to weaned infants, as opposed to *Sububeres,* or those being suckled.

Ex-u-dā'tion. [**Exuda'tio, o'**nis; from *exu'do, exuda'tum,* to "sweat out" (contracted from *ex,* "out," and *su'do,* to "sweat").] A sweating; the passing out of any liquid through the walls (or membranes) of the vessel containing it. Also applied to the oozing of the *Liquor sanguinis* through the vascular walls.

Ex'u-dā-tĭve. [**Exudati'vus;** from the same.] Belonging to exudation; promoting exudation.

Ex-ul-cer-ā'tion. [**Exulcera'tio, o'**nis; from *exul'cero, exulcera'tum,* to "make sore."] A soreness; the early state, or commencement, of ulceration.

Ex-u'vĭ-æ,* gen. **Ex-u-vĭ-a'rum,** found only in the plural. [From *ex'uo,* to "strip," "spoil," or "put off."] The shells, etc., found in particular strata. In Zoology, applied to the slough, or cast skins of animals whose nature it is to throw them off at certain seasons.

Ex-u'vĭ-ạl. [**Exuvia'lis.**] Belonging to *exuviæ.*

Eȳe. [Lat. **Oc'ulus;** Gr. ὀφθαλμός; Fr. *Œil,* uy' or ul; Ger. *Auge,* ŏw'gẹh.] The organ of vision. The eyes occupy two cavities, called orbits, situated in the lower anterior part of the cranium; they communicate with the brain by means of the optic nerves. The organ consists of a ball or globe containing within itself the iris, lens, the aqueous and vitreous humors, the retina, etc. This ball moves freely in a socket, and is readily turned at will in every direction by six muscles especially appropriated to this purpose. It is covered anteriorly by a delicate mucous membrane, termed the *conjuncti'va,* and is prŏtected from external injury by the eyelashes and eyelids. At the very front part of the ball, is situated a transparent, horny membrane, termed the *cornea.* The various parts of the eye will be more particularly noticed, each in its alphabetical place.

Eye of Ty'phon. The mystic name given by the Egyptians to the *Squill,* or sea-onion.

Eyebrow. See SUPERCILIUM.

Eyelash. See CILIUM.

Eyelid. See PALPEBRA.

Eye'-Teeth. The upper *Cuspidati,* or canine teeth, the fangs of which reach almost to the orbits of the eye.

F.

F., or **Ft.** = *Fi'at,** or *Fi'ant.** "Let there be made."

Fa'ba Por-ci'na.* The fruit of *Hyoscy'amus ni'ger.*

Fa'ba Pur-ga'trix.* The bean of *Ricinus communis.*

Fa'ba Sanc'ti Ig-na'tĭ-i.* ("Bean of St. Ignatius.") See IGNATIA.

Fa'ba Su-il'la.* The fruit of *Hyoscyamus niger.*

Fabaceæ. See LEGUMINOSÆ.

Fa-bā'ceous. [**Faba'ceus;** from *fa'ba,* a "bean."] Having beans; of the nature of beans.

Face. [**Fa'cies.**] The anterior and lower part of the head. The various surfaces, or planes, by which a crystal is bounded.

Face A'gue. A form of neuralgia, which occurs in the nerves of the face.

Face Grip'pée, fåss grĕp'på'. The "pinched or contracted face;" a peculiar expression of features forming one of the symptoms in peritonitis.

Faç'ets, or **Fă'cets.** [From the French *Facette,* a "small surface."] The small circumscribed surfaces of a bone. Applied in Zoology to the different bases into which the surface of the compound eyes of the *Arachnidæ, Crustacea,* and *Insecta* is divided. Also applied in Mineralogy to the planes or faces of a crystal.

Fā'cial. [**Facia'lis;** from *fa'cies.*] Belonging to the face.

Facial Angle. See ANGLE, FACIAL.

Fa'cial Nerve. [**Ner'vus Facia'lis.**] The *Portio dura* of the seventh pair.

Fa'cial Vein. A vein which commences at the summit of the forehead; it crosses the face obliquely, and joins the internal jugular. See ANGULAR.

Facies. See FACE.

Fa'cies (fa'she-ēz) **Hip-po-crat'ĭ-ca.*** The peculiar expression of the features immediately before death, so called because first described by *Hippocrates.*

Fa'cies Ru'bra.* The red face; another name for the *Gutta rosacea.* See ACNE.

Fac-tĭ'tious. [**Factĭ'tius;** from *fa'cio, fac'tum,* to "make."] Made by art; artificial.

Fac'ul-tў. [**Facul'tas;** from *face're,* to "do," to "make."] The power or ability by which an action is performed. Also employed to denote collectively the medical professors, or those of any other department, in a university. The phrase "medical faculty" is also used in a more general sense, to signify those skilled in the science of medicine.

Fæ'cēs.* [The plural of *fæx, fæ'cis,* "sediment."] Dregs, or sediment. The alvine excretions or excrements.

Fæcula. See FECULA.

Fæculent. See FECULENT.

Fa'gin. [**Fagi'na.**] A narcotic substance obtained from the nuts of the *Fagus sylvatica.*

Fahrenheit's Thermometer. See THERMOMETER.

Faiblesse. See DEBILITY.

Faim. See FAMES.

Faint'ing. See DELIQUIUM ANIMI, and SYNCOPE.

Faisceau, få'sō'. The French term for FASCICULUS, which see.

Faix, få. The French term for FŒTUS, which see.

Făl'çĭ-form. [**Falcifor'mis;** from *falx,* a "scythe" or "sickle."] Resembling a scythe in shape.

Fal'ciform Proç'ess. [**Proces'sus**

Falcifor'mis.] A process of the *dura mater*, separating the hemispheres of the brain, and ending in the *tentorium*.

Falling. See PROCIDENTIA, and PROLAPSUS.

Falling Sickness. See EPILEPSY.

Fal-lo'pi-an. [**Fallopia'nus.**] Applied to certain tubes or canals, and a ligament, first pointed out by the celebrated anatomist Fallopius.

Fallo'pian Lig'a-ment. The round ligament of the uterus.

Fallo'pian Tubes. Two canals enclosed in the peritonæum, and extending from the sides of the *Fundus uteri* to the ovaries. See UTERUS.

Fallopius, Aqueduct of. See AQUEDUCT OF FALLOPIUS.

Fâlse. [**Fal'sus;** from *fal'lo, fal'sum*, to "deceive."] (Fr. *Faux*, fō, or *Fausse*, fōss.) A term often applied in medicine to an unnatural or diseased condition of certain parts, as *False Joint, False Membrane*.

False Aneurism. See ANEURISM.

False Conception. See CONCEPTION, FALSE.

False Joint. See ARTIFICIAL JOINT.

False Mem'brane. This is always the result of inflammation, as that produced in pleurisy, in peritonitis, in croup, etc.

False Pas'sage. A passage formed by the laceration or ulceration of the mucous membrane of the urethra, from forcible introduction of instruments in a wrong direction.

False Ribs. [**Cos'tæ Spu'riæ.**] The five inferior ribs, which (except the last two, or floating ribs) are joined anteriorly to each other and to the cartilage of the last *true* rib.

False Vision. See PSEUDOBLEPSIA.

False Wa'ters. (Fr. *Fausses Eaux*, fōss ō.) A term applied by the French to a serous fluid which accumulates between the chorion and the amnion, and is discharged at certain periods of pregnancy. This must not be confounded with the *liquor amnii*, which they term simply the "waters" *(eaux)*.

Fălx Cĕr-e-bel'li.* ("Scythe of the Cerebellum." Fr. *Faux du Cervelet*, fō dü sĕʀv'lȧ'.) A triangular portion of the *dura mater*, separating the two lobes of the *cerebellum*.

Falx Cĕr'e-bri.* ("Scythe of the Cerebrum." Fr. *Faux du Cerveau*, fō dü sĕʀ'vō'.) The same as FALCIFORM PROCESS, which see.

Falx Major. See FALCIFORM PROCESS.

Falx Minor. See FALX CEREBELLI.

Fa'mēs.* (Fr. *Faim*, fănᵍ.) A Latin term signifying "hunger." Hence the terms *cura famis*, abstinence from food; and *fames canina*, voracious or canine appetite. See BULIMIA.

Fam'i-lȳ. [**Fami'lia.**] A number of genera having some organic resemblances.

Fang. [Ger. *Fan'gen*, to "take" or "seize" as prey, to "bite."] Applied to the sharp-pointed, perforated tooth in the superior maxillary bone of venomous serpents, through which a poisonous fluid flows into the wound made by it. Also, the root of a tooth.

Farcimen. See FARCY.

Far-cim-i-na'lis.* [From *farci'men*, "sausage-meat."] The same as ALLANTOID, which see.

Farc'tus.* [From *far'cio, farc'tum*, to "stuff."] Stuffed, filled, crammed.

Far'cȳ, or **Far-ci'men***(called, also, **Equi'nia*** and **Glan'ders**). [From *far'cio*, to "stuff."] A disease in which numerous small tumors suppurate and form ulcers. It occurs in the horse, ass, and mule; and is often communicated by contagion to men attending on those animals. In its aggravated form it is generally fatal.

Fa-ri'na.* [From *far*, all kinds of corn.] Wheat flour. The Pharmacopœial name for the flour from the seeds of *Triticum vulgare*.

Făr-i-nā'ceous. [**Farina'ceus.**] Belonging to or containing farina; of the nature of farina.

Far-Sightedness. See PRESBYOPIA.

Fascia,* fash'e-a. [From *fas'cis*, a "bundle."] Originally, a "swathe," "bandage," or "roller." The tendinous expansion of muscles; an aponeurosis.

Fas'cia Crib-ri-for'mis.* ("Sieve-like Fascia.") A web of cellular substance stretched from the lower edge of Poupart's ligament over the inguinal glands; so called because it is pierced with numerous openings for the transmission of the lymphatic vessels.

Fas'cia Il-i'a-ca.* ("Iliac Fascia.") A strong fascia which covers the inner surface of the iliac and psoas muscles.

Fas'cia In-fun-dib'u-li-for'mis.* ("Funnel-shaped Fascia.") A portion of cellular membrane which passes down on the spermatic cord, where it penetrates the *Fascia transversalis*.

Fas'cia La'ta.* ("Broad Fascia.")

A broad tendinous expansion continued from the tendons of the *Glutei* and neighboring muscles, and maintaining in their proper position the various muscles of the thigh.

FASCIA LATA is also the name of a muscle at the upper and exterior part of the thigh. See TENSOR VAGINÆ FEMORIS.

Fas'cia Pro'pri-a.* The proper cellular envelope of a hernial sac.

Fas'cia Spi-ra'lis.* ("Spiral Roller.") A name for the common roller which is wound spirally round a limb.

Fas'cia Su-per-fiç-i-a'lis.* ("Superficial Fascia.") A very thin layer of cellular membrane, which covers the abdominal muscles immediately under the skin.

Fas'cia Tor'ti-lis.* A name for the tourniquet.

Fas'cia Trans-ver-sa'lis.* The cellular membrane lining the inner surface of the *Transversalis abdominis* muscle.

Fascial, fash'al. [**Fascia'lis.**] Belonging to a *fascia*.

Fasciate, fash'e-at, or **Fasciated,** fash'e-āt-ed. [**Fascia'tus;** from *fas'cia*.] Flattened like a little band.

Fasciation, fash-e-ā'shŭn, or **Fasciatio,*** fash-e-a'she-o. [From *fas'cia*, a "bandage."] The binding up of a diseased or wounded part; also, a bandage.

Fascicle. See FASCICULUS.

Fas-çic'u-lar. [**Fascicula'ris;** from *fascic'ulus*, a "little bundle."] Bundled together; clustered. Applied to roots.

Fas-çic'u-late. [**Fascicula'tus;** from *fascic'ulus*, a "little bundle."] Bundled together; clustered.

Fas-çic'u-lus,* plural **Fas-çic'u-li.** [Diminutive of *fas'cis*, a "bundle."] (Fr. *Faisceau*, få'sō'.) Applied to a little bundle of muscular or nervous fibres, etc. A fascicle or compact cyme, as in the Sweet William. Also, a handful of leaves, roots, etc.

Fas-ci'o-la He-pat'i-ca.* [From *fasci'ola*, a "little strip of cloth."] Another name for the DISTOMA, which see.

Fas-ti'di-um Ci'bi.* ("Loathing of Food.") See ANOREXIA.

Fas-tig'i-ate. [**Fastigia'tus;** from *fasti'gium*, the "top."] Applied to umbelliferous flowers which rise together to the same height, forming a flat top.

Fat. (Fr. *Graisse*, grĕss or gråss.) See ADEPS, AXUNGIA, and SEVUM.

Fa-tu'i-ty. [**Fatu'itas, a'tis;** from *fat'uus*, "silly."] Weakness of understanding, or idiocy. See AMENTIA.

Fau'cēs,* gen. **Faucium,** fau'she-ŭm. [The plural of *Faux*.] The cavity at the back of the mouth from which the pharynx and larynx proceed.

Fault. [From the French *Faute*, an "error" or "defect."] A complete fracture of the mass of strata along a vertical or inclined plane, parallel to which the beds on one side are uplifted, and on the other depressed; a *slip*.

Fau'na.* [From *Fau'nus*, a sylvan deity of the ancient Romans.] The entire assemblage of animals, especially Mammalia, which nature has assigned to a particular country.

Faux,* gen. **Fau'cis.** The gorge or mouth. (See FAUCES.) Applied, by analogy, to the opening of the tube of a monopetalous corol.

Faux, fō, feminine **Fausse,** fōss. The French for FALSE, which see. *Faux* is also the French term for *Falx*. See next article.

Faux du Cerveau, fō dü sĕʀ'vō'. The French term for *Falx Cerebri*. See FALCIFORM PROCESS.

Faux du Cervelet, fō dü sĕʀv'lå'. The French term for FALX CEREBELLI, which see.

Fa-vose'. [**Favo'sus;** from *fa'vus*, a "honeycomb."] Belonging to, or like, a honeycomb.

Fa'vus.* A honeycomb. Applied to a kind of pustule. See PORRIGO.

Fay'nard's Pow'der. A celebrated powder for stopping hæmorrhage, said to have been nothing more than the charcoal of beech-wood, finely-powdered.

Feather-Veined. See PINNATELY-VEINED.

Fe'brēs,* the plural of **Fe'bris.** Fevers. An order of the class *Pyrexiæ* of Cullen's Nosology.

Fe-bric'u-la.* [Diminutive of *fe'bris*, a "fever."] A slight fever.

Feb'ri-fuge. [**Febrif'ugus;** from *fe'bris*, a "fever," and *fu'go*, to "drive away."] Having the property of moderating or abating the violence of fevers.

Feb'rile. [**Febri'lis;** from *fe'bris*, a "fever."] Belonging to fever; feverish.

Fe'bris.* [From *fer'veo*, to "be hot."] A fever. See FEVER.

Feb'ure's Lo'tion. A once celebrated remedy for cancer, consisting of ten grains of the white oxide of arsenic dissolved in a pint of distilled water, to which are added one ounce of the *Extractum conii*, three ounces of the *Liquor plumbi subacetatis*, and a drachm of laudanum.

Feces. See FÆCES.

Fécond, fā'kōnᵍ'. The French term for FECUND, which see.

Fec'u-la. [**Fæc'ula,** the diminutive of *fæx, fæ'cis*, "dregs."] Originally, the grounds or sediment of any liquor; any substance derived by spontaneous subsidence from a liquid. The term was afterwards applied to starch, which was thus deposited by agitating the flour of wheat in water; and, lastly, it denoted a peculiar vegetable principle, which, like starch, is insoluble in cold, but completely soluble in boiling water, with which it forms a gelatinous solution.

Fec'u-lent. [**Fæculen'tus;** from *fæ'ces*, "dregs."] Having dregs or fæces; of the nature of dregs or fæces.

Fe'cund. [Lat. **Fœcun'dus;** Fr. *Fécond*, fā'kōnᵍ'.] Fruitful; prolific.

Fe-cun-dā'tion. [**Fœcunda'tio, o'nis;** from *fœcun'do, fœcunda'tum*, to "make fruitful."] In Botany, the action of the pollen on the ovule, which thereby becomes impregnated. In Physiology, the act of impregnating, or the state of being impregnated.

Fe-cun'di-tȳ. [**Fœcun'ditas, a'tis;** from *fœcun'dus*, "fruitful."] The power of reproducing; fruitfulness.

Feeling. See TOUCH.

Feet, Distortion of. See TALIPES.

Fel,* gen. **Fel'lis.** (Fr. *Fiel*, fe-ĕl'.) Gall, or bile; a secretion found in the *cystis fellea*, or gall-bladder. See BILE.

Fel Bo-vi'num,* or **Fel Tau'ri.*** Gall, or bile, of the ox. See BILE.

Fel-lif'lu-a Pas'sio* (pash'e-o). Gall-flux disease; an ancient name for cholera.

Fel-lif'lu-us.* [From *fel*, "bile," and *flu'o*, to "flow."] Flowing with, or discharging, bile. See preceding article.

Fel'lin-ate. [**Fel'linas, a'tis.**] A combination of fellinic acid with a base.

Fel-lin'ic. [**Fellin'icus;** from *fel*, "gall," or "bile."] Belonging to bile, or gall.

Fellin'ic Aç'id. A peculiar substance obtained by digesting bilin with dilute hydrochloric acid.

Fe'lo de se.* [Low Latin *fe'lo*, a "felon," *de*, "with respect to," and *se*, "himself."] Literally, "one guilty of felony with respect to himself." A term in Medical Jurisprudence for one who commits suicide.

Fel'on. The name of malignant whitlow, in which the effusion is beneath the periosteum.

Feminine. See FŒMINEUS.

Fem-o-ræ'us.* Another name for the *cruræus* muscle, an extensor of the leg.

Fem'o-ral. [**Femora'lis;** from *fe'mur*, the "thigh."] Belonging to the thigh: crural.

Fem'o-ro-çēle.* [From *fe'mur*, the "thigh," and κήλη, a "tumor."] The disorder termed *Hernia cruralis*.

Fe'mur,* gen. **Fem'o-ris.** The thigh. Also, the long cylindrical bone of the thigh, or *Os femoris*. (Fr. *Os de la Cuisse*, ō dęh lā kwēss.) The second articulation of the feet of the *Arachnides, Crustacea*, and *Insecta*.

Fe-nes'tra.* [From φαίνω, to "make to appear."] A window. Applied to two *foramina* of the tympanum of the ear.

Fe-nes'tral. [**Fenestra'lis;** from *fenes'tra*.] Belonging to windows; like windows.

Fe-nes'trate. [**Fenestra'tus;** from *fenes'tra*.] Pierced with holes, or with openings like windows.

Fen'nel, Sweet. The *Anethum fœniculum*.

Fen'u-Greek, or **Fen'u-grĕc.** The *Trigonel'la Fœ'num*, a plant forming, it is said, an article of food in Egypt. It grows also in the south of France. Used chiefly in veterinary medicine.

Fer (Fr.), fêr. See IRON.

Fer-men-tā'tion. [**Fermenta'tio, o'nis;** from *fermen'to, fermenta'tum*, to "leaven."] The spontaneous changes which aqueous combinations of animal or vegetable matter undergo when exposed to the air at an ordinary temperature.

Fer-men'tum.* Ferment. The substance which excites fermentation. The Pharmacopœial name (U.S. Ph.) for "yeast." See preceding article.

Fermen'tum Cerevi'sia* (sĕr-e-vish'e-a). The scum or froth of beer during fermentation; barm; yeast. This substance has been placed on the primary list of the U.S. Pharmacopœia for 1860.

Fern, Male. See ASPIDIUM FILIX MAS.

Fe-ro'ni-a El-e-phan'tum.* [From *Fero'nia*, the goddess of groves.] An Indian tree of the order *Aurantiaceæ:* it yields a gum resembling gum Arabic.

Fer'ri,* genitive of FERRUM, which see.

Fer'ri Fer-ro-çy-an'ĭ-dum.* ("Ferrocyanide of Iron.") The Pharmacopœial name (U.S. Ph., 1860) for Prussian blue.

Fer'ri Fi'lum.* The Pharmacopœial name (Ed. Ph.) for iron wire; the *Ferrum in fila tractum* of the London Pharmacopœia.

Fer'ri, Ra-men'ta.* ("Raspings of Iron.") A name for iron filings.

Fer'ri Sul-phu-re'tum.* ("Sulphuret of Iron.") The Pharmacopœial name (U.S. Ph.) for the protosulphuret of iron, prepared by melting together sublimed sulphur and iron in small pieces.

Fer-rif'er-ous. [**Ferrif'erus;** from *fer'rum,* "iron," and *fe'ro,* to "bear."] Containing iron in some form, usually in the state of oxide or carbonate.

Fer'ro-. (From *fer'rum,* "iron.") A prefix in compound names, denoting connection with iron.

Fer'ro-çy-an'ic Aç'id. A compound of cyanogen, metallic iron, and hydrogen; also called *ferruretted chyazic acid.* It contains the elements of hydrocyanic acid, but differs from it totally in its properties. Its salts, once termed triple prussiates, are now called *ferro-cyanates.*

Fer-ru'ġin-ous, or **Fer-ru-ġin'e-ous.** [**Ferrugin'eus,** or **Ferrugino'sus;** from *ferru'go,* the "rust of iron."] Full of iron-rust; containing iron-rust; of a yellowish-brown color.

Ferrum. See Iron.

Fer'tile. [**Fer'tilis;** from *fe'ro,* to "bring forth."] Fruitful. Applied to flowers having a pistil, or producing seeds capable of vegetation.

Fertilization. See Fecundation.

Fer'u-la.* [From *fe'rio,* to "strike."] A Linnæan genus of the class *Pentandria,* natural order *Apiaceæ* (or *Umbelliferæ*).

Fer'ula As-sa-fœt'i-da.* The plant which yields *assafœtida.*

Fer'vor. [From *fer'veo,* to "boil."] A violent and scorching heat. *Ardor* denotes an excessive heat; *Calor,* a moderate or natural heat.

Fessier, fĕs'se'à'. The French term for Gluteal or Glutæus, which see.

Fĕs'ter-ing. A word applied to a sore, signifying the discharge either of pus or of a morbid watery fluid.

Fes-tooned' Rings. A popular designation of the fibrous zones or tendinous circles which surround the orifices of the heart.

Fe'tal. [**Fœta'lis.**] Belonging to the fœtus.

Feticide. See Fœticide.

Fet'id. [**Fœ'tidus;** from *fœ'teo,* to "become putrid."] Having a bad smell.

Fe'tor. [**Fœ'tor, o'ris;** from *fœ'teo,* to "stink."] A bad smell, or stink.

Fe'ver. [Lat. **Fe'bris;** Fr. *Fièvre,* fe-ĕvR' or fe-âvR'.] A condition characterized by accelerated pulse, increased heat of surface, loss of appetite, thirst, languor, debility, unwillingness to move, and general disturbance of all the functions. See Febris, and Pyrexia.

Fever, Slight. See Febricula.

Fe'ver-ish. [Lat. **Feb'riens;** Fr. *Fiévreux,* fe-à'vRuh'.] A term applied to the state of one laboring under fever; also to that which causes fever.

Fi'ber.* The Latin term for the "beaver."

Fi'bre. [**Fi'bra;** from *fi'ber,* "extreme;" because originally applied to the thread-like radicles at the extremity of a root.] The minute threads or filaments which occur in the structure of parts in animals and vegetables.

Fi'bre, An'i-mal. [**Fi'bra Anima'lis.**] The filaments which compose the muscular fasciculi, the cellular membrane, etc.

Fi'bre, Wood'y. [**Fi'bra Lig'nea.**] The filaments of which any woody substance is composed.

Fibreux, fè'bRuh'. The French term for Fibrous, which see.

Fi'bril. [**Fibril'la;** the diminutive of *fi'bra,* a "fibre."] Applied in the plural to the extremely slender filaments seen by the microscope, and by the collection of a number of which in a sheath, or *sarcolemma,* a muscular fibre (of animal life) is formed.

Fib-ril-la'tus.* [From *fibril'la,* a "little fibre."] Disposed in very delicate filaments.

Fi'brin, or **Fi'brine.** [**Fibri'na;** from *fi'bra,* a "fibre."] A peculiar whitish, solid, insipid, and inodorous compound substance found in animal and vegetable matter; coagulable lymph.

Fib-rin-og'e-nous. [From *fibri'na,* "fibrin," and γεννάω, to "produce."] Producing fibrin. Applied by Virchow to a substance which exists in lymph and is converted into fibrin by exposure to air.

Fi'bro-. [From *fi'bra,* a "fibre."] A prefix denoting a fibrous condition.

Fi'bro-Car'ti-laġe. Membraniform cartilage. The substance, intermediate between proper cartilage and ligament, constituting the base of the ear, determining the form of that part; and composing the rings of the trachea, the epiglottis, etc. By the older anatomists it was termed *ligamentous cartilage,* or *cartilaginiform ligament.* Fibro-cartilages are sometimes formed as the result of a morbid process in different organs.

Fi'bro-Plas'tic. [**Fi'bro-Plas'ti-cus;** from *fi'bro-*, and πλάσσω, to "form."] Forming fibres. Applied to an organized tissue, from the corpuscles exuded on sores.

Fi'brous. [**Fibro'sus;** from *fi'bra*, a "fibre."] (Fr. *Fibreux*, fè'bruh'.) Having fibres, or composed of fibres.

Fib'u-la.* Literally, a "clasp." The long bone extending from the knee to the ankle, on the outer side of the leg.

Fib'u-lar. [From *fib'ula*.] Belonging to the fibula.

Ficatio,* fi-ka'she-o, or **Fi'cus.*** [From *fi'cus*, a "fig."] A fig-like tubercle about the anus or pudenda.

Fi'coid. [**Ficoi'des;** from *fi'cus*, a "fig," and εἶδος, a "form."] Resembling a fig.

Ficoideæ,* fi-ko-i'de-ē. A natural order of plants. See MESEMBRYACEÆ.

Fi'cus.* A Linnæan genus of the class *Polygamia*, natural order *Urticaceæ*. Also, the Pharmacopœial name ‖ for the dried fruit of *Ficus carica*, or fig.

FICUS* is also the name of a fleshy substance, or *condyloma*, resembling a fig. See FICATIO.

Fi'cus Car'i-ca.* The fig-tree; also called *F. commu'nis*, *F. sati'va*, and *F. vulga'ris*.

Fi'cus E-las'ti-ca.* The tree which affords caoutchouc, or Indian rubber.

Fid'gets. [**Tituba'tio.**] A term denoting general restlessness, with a desire of changing one's position.

Fi-diç-i-na'lēs.* [From *fid'icen*, a "harper."] A designation of the lumbricales (muscles) of the hand, from their usefulness in playing upon musical instruments.

Fièvre, fe-àvr' or fe-ĕvr'. The French term for FEVER, which see.

Fièvre Algide. See ALGIDA FEBRIS.

Fièvre Hectique. See HECTIC FEVER.

Fièvre Jaune. See YELLOW FEVER.

Fiévreux. See FEVERISH.

Fifth Pair of Nerves. See TRIGEMINI.

Fig. See FICUS.

Fil'a-ment. [**Filamen'tum;** from *fi'lum*, a "thread."] A small, delicate, thread-like substance; a fibre. The thread-like part of a stamen.

Fi-la'ri-a.* [From *fi'lum*, a "thread."] A thread-like parasitic worm, which infests the cornea of the eye of the horse.

Fila'ria Med-i-nen'sis.* The systematic name of the Guinea-worm.

Filicales. See FILICES.

Filices,* fil'e-sēz, the plural of **Fi'lix.** Ferns. A natural order of cryptogamous plants, which abound in temperate and tropical regions, remarkable for their beautiful plumy foliage.

Fil'i-coid. [**Filicoi'des;** from *Fi'lix*, and εἶδος, a "form."] Fern-like.

Fil-i-col'o-ġy. [From *Fi'lix*, a "fern," and λόγος, a "discourse."] That branch of Botany which treats of ferns.

Fil'i-form. [**Filifor'mis;** from *fi'lum*, a "thread."] Having the appearance of thread.

Fi'lix,* gen. **Fil'i-cis.** The Latin word for "fern." Applied in the plural to a Linnæan order of *Cryptogamia*. (See FILICES.) Also, the Pharmacopœial name (Br. Ph.) of the rhizoma of *Aspidium filix mas*.

Fi'lix Mas.* Male Fern. The Pharmacopœial name (U.S. Ph.) for the rhizoma of ASPIDIUM FILIX MAS, which see.

Film. The popular name for opacity of the cornea.

Fil'ter. [**Fil'trum.**] An apparatus of various construction, for the purposes of filtration.

Fil'trate. [From *fil'trum*, a "filter."] Any liquid strained or filtered.

Fil-trā'tion. [**Filtra'tio, o'nis;** from *fil'trum*, a "filter."] The process by which a fluid is gradually separated from the particles or impurities that may be floating or suspended in it; straining.

Fil'trum.* Literally, a "filter." Sometimes applied to the superficial groove across the upper lip from the partition of the nose to the tip of the lip.

Fim'bri-a.* [From *fi'brum*, an "extremity."] A border, or fringe. Applied in the plural (*fim'briæ*) to the extremities of the Fallopian tubes.

Fim'bri-ate, or **Fim'bri-āt-ed.** [**Fimbria'tus;** from *fim'bria*, a "fringe."] Having a fringe, or border.

Fin'ger [**Dig'itus Ma'nus**], in anatomical language denotes one of the five extremities of the hand; in popular parlance, one of the four besides the thumb.

Fingered. See DIGITATE.

Fins. [**Pin'næ.**] Membranous organs in fishes, somewhat analogous to hands and feet.

Fire Damp. A name given by miners to the explosive gas, consisting chiefly of light carburetted hydrogen, found in mines.

First In-ten'tion. Union by the first intention means adhesive inflammation without suppuration, as when the lips of a wound made by a sharp knife are brought into immediate contact, and quickly healed without much inflammation.

Fish-Glue. See ICHTHYOCOLLA.

Fish-Skin. See ICHTHYOSIS.

Fis'sĭle. [**Fis'silis;** from *fin'do, fis'sum*, to "cleave."] Cleavable; easily cleft or cloven.

Fis-sip'ar-ous. [**Fissip'arus;** from *fin'do, fis'sum*, to "cleave," and *pa'rio*, to "produce."] Producing offspring by portions being separated from the parent individual. See next article.

Fissip'arous Çen-e-rā'tion. That generation which occurs either by spontaneous division of the body of the parent into two or more parts, each part, when separated, becoming a distinct individual, as in the monad, vorticella, etc., or by artificial division, as in the hydra, planaria, etc. The propagation of plants by slips furnishes another example of this kind of reproduction.

Fis-sĭ-pā'tion. [**Fissipa'tio, o'***nis*.] A faulty term for FISSIPAROUS GENERATION, which see.

Fis-sĭ-ros'tris.* [From *fin'do, fis'sum*, to "cleave," and *ros'trum*, a "beak."] Applied in the plural (*Fissiros'tres*) to a family of birds having a broad beak with an extended commissure: fissiros'trate.

Fis-su'ra Gla-se'rĭ-i.* ("Glaser's Fissure.") A fissure situated in the deepest part of the glenoid fossa.

Fissu'ra Lon-ḡĭ-tu-dĭ-na'lis.* ("Longitudinal Fissure.") A deep fissure observed in the median line on the upper surface of the brain, occupied by the falx cerebri of the dura mater.

Fissu'ra Sȳl'vĭ-i* ("Fissure of Sylvius"), called also **Fissu'ra Mag'na Syl'vii*** ("Great Fissure of Sylvius"). A fissure which separates the anterior and middle lobes of the cerebrum. It lodges the middle cerebral artery.

Fissu'ra Um-bil-ĭ-ca'lis.* ("Umbilical Fissure.") The groove of the umbilical vein, situated between the large and small lobes, at the upper and fore part of the liver. This groove in the fœtus contains the umbilical vein.

Fis'sure. [**Fissu'ra;** from *fin'do, fis'sum*, to "cleave."] Any deep extended depression.

Fis'sure of the Spleen. The groove which divides the inner surface of the spleen. It is filled by vessels and fat.

Fis'sus.* [From *fin'do, fis'sum*, to "cleave."] Divided; cleft; cloven.

Fist. Armat. = *Fis'tula arma'ta.** "A clyster pipe and bag fit for use."

Fis'tu-la.* [Originally, a "pipe."] A sinuous ulcer, having an external opening often leading to a larger cavity, and slow to heal. A fistula is termed *blind* when it has but one opening, and *complete* if it has two, communicating with an internal cavity, and with the surface.

Fis'tula in A'no.* ("Fistula in the Anus.") A fistula in the cellular substance about the anus or rectum.

Fis'tu-lous. [**Fistulo'sus;** from *fis'tula*.] Of the nature of *fistula*. Also applied to plants having many tubes.

Fixed Air. See CARBONIC ACID.

Fixed Bod'ies. [**Cor'pora Fix'a.**] Substances which do not evaporate by heat, especially those which cannot be fused or volatilized: as carbon, silicon, etc.

Fix'ĭ-tȳ. [**Fix'itas, a'***tis*.] A property by which bodies withstand the action of heat. See preceding article.

Fl. = *Flu'idus.** "Fluid."

Fla-bel'lĭ-form. [**Flabellifor'mis;** from *flabel'lum*, a "fan."] Fanlike.

Flacourtiaceæ,* flå-koor-te-a'she-ē. [From *Flacour'tia*, one of the genera.] A natural order of exogenous trees and shrubs, natives of the hottest parts of the East and West Indies.

Flag, Sweet-Scented. See ACORUS CALAMUS.

Fla-ḡel'lĭ-form. [**Flagellifor'mis;** from *flagel'lum*, a "little whip."] Resembling a little whip. A botanical term denoting "whiplike."

Fla-ḡel'lum.* [Diminutive of *flag'rum*, a "whip."] Applied in Botany to a runner which is long and slender, like a whip.

Flake-White. The subnitrate of bismuth.

Flame. [**Flam'ma.**] The combustion of any substance yielding an inflammable gas.

Flank. (Fr. *Flanc*, flŏnᴳ, the "side.") That part of the body between the false ribs and the *Ossa innominata*.

Flash. A preparation used for coloring brandy and rum, and giving them a fictitious strength; it consists of an extract of cayenne pepper, or capsicum with burnt sugar.

Flat'u-lence, or **Flat'u-len-cȳ.** [**Flatulen'tia;** from *fla'tus*, "wind."] A collection of gas or wind in the stomach and bowels, from fermentation or chemical decomposition of the articles of food taken into the stomach.

Flat'u-lent. [**Flatulen'tus;** from

the same.] Having flatulence, or causing flatulence.

Fla'tus.* [From *flo, fla'tum,* to "blow."] Wind, or gas, in the stomach and bowels: flatulency.

Flax. The *Li'num usitatis'simum.*

Flax, Purg'ing. The *Linum catharticum.*

Flēam. [**Flam'ma,** or **Flam'mula.**] An instrument for lancing the gums and for bleeding horses.

Fléchisseur. See FLEXOR.

Flesh. [Lat. **Ca'ro, Car'nis;** Fr. *Chair,* shêR.] The muscles, and generally the soft parts, of an animal. Sometimes applied to the fruit, leaves, etc. of plants, when of a thick consistence, somewhat like flesh.

Flesh, Proud. See PROUD FLESH.

Fleshy. See CARNEUS, and CARNOSUS.

Flex'ĭle. [**Flex'ilis;** from *flec'to, flex'um,* to "bend."] Flexible; easily bent.

Flex'ion. [**Flex'io, o'**nis; from the same.] The state of being bent.

Flex'or, o'ris.* [From the same.] (Fr. *Fléchisseur,* flȧ'shė'SUR'.) Literally, a "bender;" applied to muscles.

Flex'or Car'pi Ra-dĭ-a'lis.* ("Radial Flexor of the Wrist.") See PALMARIS MAGNUS.

Flex'or Lon'gus Dĭg-ĭ-to'rum Pe'dis.* ("Long Flexor of the Fingers of the Foot.") It arises from the posterior surface of the tibia, and is inserted into the phalanges of the last four toes. It bends the toes, and extends the foot upon the leg.

Flex'or Lon'gus Pol'lĭ-cis.* ("Long Flexor of the Thumb.") A muscle which arises from the anterior part of the radius and interosseous ligament, and is inserted into the second phalanx of the thumb. It bends the thumb and hand.

Flex'or Lon'gus Pol'licis Pe'dis.* ("Long Flexor of the *Thumb of the Foot,* or *Great Toe.*") It arises from the posterior part of the fibula, and is inserted into the second phalanx of the great toe. It bends the toe.

Flex'u-ous, or **Flex'u-ose.** [**Flexuo'sus;** from the same.] Having many bendings, or turnings; zigzag.

Flint. [**Si'lex.**] A mineral consisting of silicious earth, nearly pure.

Flint, Liq'uor of, or **Liq'uor Sil'ĭ-cum.*** A name formerly given to the solution of silicated alkali.

Floating. See NATANS.

Float'ing Ribs. [**Cos'tæ Fluctuan'tes.**] The last two false ribs, whose anterior extremities are not connected with the rest, or with each other.

Floc'çi,* the plural of *floc'cus,* a "lock or little particle of wool, cotton," etc.

Floc'çi Vol-ĭ-tan'tēs.* The imaginary objects floating before the eyes, in cases of depraved sight. See MUSCÆ VOLITANTES.

Floccilatio,* flok-se-la'she-o. See FLOCCILLATION.

Floc-çil-lā'tion. [**Floccilla'tio, o'**nis; from *floc'cus,* a "lock of wool," the "nap of clothes."] The picking of the bedclothes,—a symptom betokening extreme danger. See CARPHOLOGY.

Floc'cu-lus,* otherwise called **Lo'bus Ner'vi Pneū-mo-gas'trĭ-ci.*** ("Lobe of the Pneumogastric Nerve.") A term applied to the pneumogastric lobule of the cerebellum; its form is that of a small foliated or lamellated tuft.

Flood'ing. [**Hæmorrha'gia Ute-ri'na.**] The popular term for uterine hæmorrhage; more particularly in connection with parturition.

Flo'ra.* [From *flos, flo'ris,* a "flower."] Originally, the Goddess of Flowers. The Flora of any country (or district) is the entire assemblage of plants which nature has allotted to it. Also, a systematic description of those plants.

Flo'ral. [**Flora'lis;** from *flos,* a "flower."] Belonging to flowers.

Floral Leaf. See BRACTEA.

Flor'en-tine Or'ris. The *Iris Florentina.*

Flo'rēs.* (The plural of FLOS, which see.) "Flowers." A term formerly used to denote such bodies as assume a pulverulent form by sublimation or crystallization.

FLO'RES ANTIMO'NII.* ("Flowers of Antimony.") They consist of small, elongated, and very brilliant crystals of the sesquioxide of antimony.

FLO'RES BISMU'THI.* ("Flowers of Bismuth.") A yellowish oxide of bismuth.

FLO'RES SUL'PHURIS.* ("Flowers of Sulphur.") Sublimed sulphur.

FLO'RES ZIN'CI.* ("Flowers of Zinc.") Oxide of zinc, or philosophical wool.

Flo-rĕs'çence. [**Florescen'tia;** from *flores'co,* to "flower," to "flourish."] The act of flowering, in plants; also, the season of flowering.

Floret. See FLOSCULUS.

Florideæ. See CERAMIACEÆ.

Flo-rif'er-ous. [**Florif'erus;** from *flos*, a "flower," and *fe'ro*, to "bear."] Bearing flowers.

Flos,* gen. **Flo'ris.** A "flower." That part of a plant which comprises the organs of reproduction, the essential parts of which are stamens and pistils. These in a complete flower are surrounded by two envelopes, of which the inferior or exterior is called the calyx, or cup; the superior or interior is termed the corolla. See COROLLA, and CALYX.

Flos Æ-ru'gi-nis.* ("Flower of Verdigris.") *Cupri acetas*, or acetate of copper, sometimes called *distilled* or *crystallized verdigris*.

Flos'cu-lous. [**Flosculo'sus;** from *flos'culus*.] Having many florets: flos'culose.

Flos'cu-lus.* [Diminutive of *flos*, a "flower."] A little flower; a floret.

Flour. See FARINA, and POLLEN.

Flower. See FLOS.

Flowers. See FLORES.

Flowers of Antimony, Sulphur, etc. See FLORES.

Flu'āte. [**Flu'as, a'tis.**] A combination of fluoric acid with a base.

Fluc-tu-ā'tion. [**Fluctua'tio, o'nis;** from *fluc'tuo*, *fluctua'tum*, to "rise in waves."] Applied to the undulation of a fluid within the body, ascertained by the proper application of the fingers, or the hand, or by *succussion*.

Flu'id. [**Flu'idus;** from *flu'o*, to "flow."] Having particles easily separable, yielding to the least pressure, and moving over each other in every direction.

Flu'id of Co-tun'ni-us. It has been also called *A'qua Labyrin'thi* ("Water of the Labyrinth"), and by Breschet, the *perilymph*. A thin gelatinous fluid, found in the bony cavities of the labyrinth of the ear: so called from the name of the anatomist who first distinctly described it.

Flu-id'i-ty. [**Fluid'itas, a'tis.**] The quality of being fluid.

Flu'i-drachm. [**Fluidrach'ma;** from *flu'idus*, "fluid," and *drach'ma*, a "drachm."] Sixty minims: a fluid drachm.

Flu-id-un'cia* (-un'she-a). [From *flu'idus*, and *un'cia*, an "ounce."] Eight fluidrachms: a fluid ounce.

Fluke. An intestinal worm. See DISTOMA.

Flu-o-bo'rāte. [**Fluobo'ras, a'tis.**] A combination of fluoboric acid with a base.

Flu-o-bo'ric. [**Fluobo'ricus;** from *fluo'rium*, "fluorin," and *bo'rium*, "boron."] Composed of fluorin and boron. Applied to an acid.

Flu'or, o'ris.* [From *flu'o*, to "flow."] A flowing, or flux. Also, fluorin, a simple body, the existence of which is predicated on mere analogy. The term is sometimes applied to a diseased condition of the mucous secretion of the vagina. See LEUCORRHŒA.

Flu'or Al'bus.* ("White Flux.") See LEUCORRHŒA.

Flu'or Spar. (So called from its assisting the fusion of earthy minerals in metallurgic operations.) Derbyshire spar; properly, fluoride of calcium.

Flu-or-a'tus.* Having or containing fluorine: flu'orated. Hydrofluoric acid has been called *fluorated hydrogen*.

Flu-or'ic. [**Fluor'icus.**] Belonging to fluorin.

Fluor'ic Aç'id. An acid obtained by treating fluor spar with sulphuric acid. Owing to its destructive properties, it has been termed *phthore* (from φθόριος, "destructive").

Flu'o-ride. A combination of fluorin with a base.

Flu'or-in, or **Flu'or-ine.** [**Fluo'rium.**] The supposed primary principle of hydrofluoric acid, found chiefly in fluor spar. See FLUOR.

Flu-or'u-ret. [**Fluorure'tum;** from *fluo'rium*.] A combination of fluorin with a simple body.

Flu'vi-al, Flu'vi-a-tile. [**Fluviat'ilis;** from *flu'vius*, a "river."] Belonging to a river.

Flux. [**Flux'us;** from *flu'o*, *flux'um*, to "flow."] Any excessive discharge from the bowels or other organs. Applied in Chemistry to any substance used to promote the fusion of metals. See FLUX, CHEMICAL.

Flux, Black. See BLACK FLUX.

Flux, Chem'i-cal. A substance or mixture much employed to assist the fusion of minerals. Alkaline fluxes are generally used, which render the earthy mixtures fusible by converting them into glass.

Flux'ion. [**Flux'io, o'nis;** from *flu'o*, *flux'um*, to "flow."] The change of metals or other bodies from solid to fluid by the agency of heat; fusion.

Flux'us Cap-il-lo'rum.* ("Flowing or Passing Away of the Hair.") A term applied by Celsus to alopecia, or the falling off of the hair.

Fly Pow'der. (Fr. *Poudre à Mouches*, pood'r â moosh'.) A black powder formed by the exposure of metallic arsenic to a moist atmosphere till it becomes partly oxidized.

Flying Blisters. See BLISTERS, FLYING.

Fo'cus,* plural **Fo'çi.** Literally, a "hearth" or "fireplace." Applied in Astronomy to the two points (*Fo'ci*) within the elliptical orbit of a planet round the sun. In Optics, the point of convergence of the rays of light after passing through a convex lens, or being reflected from a concave mirror.

Fœcunditas. See FECUNDITY.

Fœm-in'e-us.* [From *fœm'ina*, a "woman."] Belonging to a female; feminine.

Fœ-nic'u-lum.* Fennel. The Pharmacopœial name ‖ for the fruit of *Fœniculum vulgare, dulce,* or *officinale;* the *Anethum fœniculum.* Fennel-seed is a grateful aromatic, and is much used as a carminative, and especially to correct the action of other medicines, as senna, rhubarb, etc.

Fœnic'ulum Dul'ce,* **Fœnic'u-lum Ger-man'i-cum.*** The *Anethum fœniculum,* or sweet fennel.

Fœticide, fē'tĭ-sīd. [**Fœtici'dium;** from *fœ'tus,* and *cæ'do,* to "kill."] The murder of the fœtus *in utero;* criminal abortion.

Fœ'tus,* or **Fe'tus.** (Fr. *Faix,* få.) The child *in utero* from the fifth month of pregnancy till birth.

Foie (Fr.), fwå. See LIVER.

Folia. See FOLIUM.

Fo'lia Cĕr-e-bel'li.* [From *fo'lium,* any sort of leaf.] An assemblage of gray laminæ observed on the surface of the cerebellum.

Fo-li-ā'ceous. [**Folia'ceus;** from *fo'lium,* a "leaf."] Full of leaves; leafy.

Fo'li-ate. [**Folia'tus;** from the same.] Clothed with leaves; leafy.

Fo-li-ā'tion. [**Folia'tio, o'nis;** from the same.] The putting forth of leaves; arrangement of leaves in the bud. Also, the act of beating a metal into thin leaves.

Folie, fo'lē'. The French term for INSANITY, which see.

Fo-lif'er-ous. [**Folif'erus,** or **Folif'erus;** from *fo'lium,* a "leaf," and *fe'ro,* to "bear."] Bearing or producing leaves.

Fo'li-ole. [**Foli'olum.**] Diminutive of *Fo'lium.* A little leaf, or leaflet.

Fo'li-um,* plural **Fo'li-a.** [From φύλλον, a "leaf."] The leaf of a plant. A thin plate of metal.

Fol'li-cle. [**Follic'ulus;** diminutive of *fol'lis,* a "bag."] A little bag. Applied in Anatomy to a very small secretory cavity. In Botany it denotes a simple pod opening by the inner suture, differing from the legume, which opens by both sutures.

Fol-lic'u-late. [**Follicula'tus;** from *follic'ulus,* a "follicle."] Having follicles.

Fol-lic'u-lose, or **Fol-lic'u-lous.** [**Folliculo'sus;** from *follic'ulus,* a "follicle."] Having numerous follicles.

Folliculus. See FOLLICLE.

Fol-lic'u-lus A'er-is.* ("Little Bag of Air.") The space at the broad end of an egg.

Fo-men-tā'tion. [**Fomenta'tio, o'nis;** from *fo'veo,* to "keep warm."] The application of any warm, soft, medicinal substance to some part of the body, by which the vessels are relaxed, and their morbid action sometimes removed.

Fo'mēs,* gen. **Fom'i-tis.** [From the same.] Any porous substance capable of absorbing contagious effluvia, as woollen clothing, etc. See FOMITES.

Fom'i-tēs,* the plural of **Fo'mes.** Applied to goods, clothing, or other materials imbued with contagion.

Fonction, fôɴɢ'se-ôɴɢ'. The French term for FUNCTION, which see.

Fongosité, fôɴɢ'go'zē'tå'. The French term for FUNGOSITY, which see.

Fongueux, fôɴɢ'guh'. The French term for FUNGOUS, which see.

Fongus, fôɴɢ'güss'. The French term for FUNGUS, which see.

Fons Pul-sa'til-is.* ("Pulsating Fountain.") The anterior fontanel, because for years after birth arterial pulsation may be there perceived. See FONTANEL.

Fon'ta-nel. [**Fontanel'la;** diminutive of *fons,* a "fountain:" so named because the pulsating of the artery was imagined to resemble the bubbling of a fountain.] (Fr. *Fontanelle,* fôɴɢ'tå'nĕll'.) The quadrangular space between the frontal and two parietal bones in very young children. A smaller one, triangular, sometimes exists between the occipital and parietal bones.

Fon-tic'u-lus.* [Diminutive of *fons,* a "fountain."] An issue, or artificial ulcer. See ISSUE.

Food. See ALIMENT, ALITURA, and PABULUM.

Foot. See PES.

Foot-Bath. See PEDILUVIUM.

Foot-Jaws. The extremities of the last three pairs of feet in most *Crustacea.*

Foot-Stalk. See PEDICEL, PEDUNCLE, PETIOLE.

Fo-ra'men,* gen. **Fo-ram'ĭ-nis,** nominative plural **Fo-ram'ĭ-na.** [From *fo'ro,* to "bore a hole."] A hole, or opening.

Fora'men Çæ'cum.* ("Blind Hole.") The hole at the root of the spine of the frontal bone; so called from its not perforating the bone or leading to any cavity. Also the designation of a little sulcus of the brain, situated between the *Corpora pyramidalia* and the *Pons Varolii.*

Fora'men Cæ'cum (of Morgag'-ni, mor-gân'yè). A deep mucous follicle, situated at the meeting of the *papillæ circumvallatæ* upon the middle of the root of the tongue.

Fora'men In-cĭ-si'vum.* The opening immediately behind the incisor teeth.

Fora'men Mag'num Oc-cip'ĭ-tis.* ("Great Opening of the Occiput.") The great opening at the under and fore part of the occipital bone, through which the spinal marrow passes, with its vessels and membranes.

Fora'men of Mon-ro', Fora'men Com-mu'ne An-te'rĭ-us.* An opening under the arch of the fornix of the cerebrum, by which the lateral ventricles communicate with each other, with the third ventricle, and with the infundibulum.

Fora'men of Wins'low. An aperture situated behind the capsule of Glisson, first described by Winslow, and forming a communication between the large sac of the omentum and the cavity of the abdomen.

Fora'men O-va'le.* ("Oval Opening.") An opening situated in the partition which separates the right and left auricles in the fœtus. It is also called the FORAMEN OF BOTAL. The same term is applied to an oval aperture communicating between the tympanum and the vestibule of the ear.

Fora'men Pneumat'icum* (num ăt'ĭ-kŭm). ("Pneumatic Foramen.") A large aperture near one end of the long air-bones of birds, communicating with the interior.

Fora'men Ro-tun'dum.* ("Round Opening.") The round, or, more correctly, triangular aperture of the internal ear. This, and the *Foramen ovale,* are respectively synonymous with *Fenestra ovalis* and *Fenestra rotunda.*

Fora'men Su'pra-Or-bit-a'rĭ-um.* ("Supra-Orbital Opening.") The supra-orbital hole or notch, situated on the ridge over which the eyebrow is placed. It gives passage to the superciliary artery.

Fora'men Ve-sa'lĭ-i.* ("Foramen of Vesalius.") An indistinct hole, situated between the *foramen rotundum* and *foramen ovale* of the sphenoid bone: it was particularly pointed out by Vesalius.

Fo-ram'ĭ-na.* The plural of FORAMEN, which see.

Fo-ram'ĭ-nāt-ed. [Foramina'tus; from *fora'men,* a "hole."] Pierced with small holes.

Fo-ram-ĭn-if'er-ous. [Foraminif'erus; from *fora'men,* a "hole," and *fe'ro,* to "bear."] Bearing or having *foramina.*

For'ceps,* gen. **For'çĭ-pis.** [As if *Fer'riceps;* from *fer'rum,* "iron," and *ca'pio,* to "take."] Originally, a "pair of tongs or pincers." Applied in Obstetrics to an instrument consisting of a pair of curved blades, for the purpose of grasping the head of the fœtus and bringing it through the passages, in certain cases of difficult labor. Also, to various surgical instruments, of diverse construction, for seizing hold of objects, etc. Applied in Zoology to the claws of certain *Crustaceæ.*

Forces of Medicines. See DYNAMICS.

Fore'-Arm. [Antibra'chium.] The *cubitus,* that portion of the arm between the elbow and wrist. In Ornithology, the second part of the anterior extremity which supports the wing.

Forehead. See FRONS, and SINCIPUT.

For'eign Bod'ȳ. Any substance which is left in a wound and keeps up irritation, preventing its cure, as a bullet, a piece of broken glass, a splinter, nail, etc.

Fo-ren'sic Med'ĭ-cine. Such parts of medicine as are connected with judicial inquiries. See MEDICAL JURISPRUDENCE.

Fore-Skin. See PREPUCE.

Forgetfulness. See AMNESIA.

Forked. See FURCATE.

For'māte, For'mĭ-āte. [For'mas, or **For'mias, a'tis.]** A combination of formic acid with a base.

For'mic. [Formi'cus; from *formi'ca,* the "ant."] Applied to an acid obtained by distillation of ants and water.

For-mi'ca.* Literally, an "ant." A term applied by the Arabians to *Herpes*, from its creeping progress.

Formi'ca Ru'fa.* The ant, emmet, or pismire, which contains an acid juice and oil supposed to possess aphrodisiac virtues.

For-mi-că'tion. [**Formica'tio, o'nis**, a tingling like the stinging of ants; from *formi'ca*, an "ant."] (Fr. *Fourmillement*, fooR'mēl'mŏNᵍ'.) A sense of pricking or tingling on the surface of the body.

For-miç'ic. The same as FORMIC.

For'mu-la.* [Diminutive of *for'ma*, a "form."] A short form of prescription in practice, in place of the more full instruction in the Pharmacopœias.

For'myle, Per-chlo'ride of. The fluid substance Chloroform.

For'ni-cate. [**Fornica'tus**; from *for'nix*, a "vault," *for'nicor*, to "be arched."] Arched; vaulted.

For-niç'i-form. [**Fornicifor'mis**; from *for'nix*, a "vault."] Resembling an arch, or vault; vaulted.

For'nix,* gen. **For'ni-cis.** An arch or vault. A white, fibrous, triangular substance of the brain beneath the *Corpus callosum* and *Septum lucidum;* so called because it has a somewhat arched appearance: also termed *Corpus psaloides*.

Fos'sa.* [From *fo'dio, fos'sum*, to "dig."] Originally, a "ditch" or "fosse." A depression, or sinus. Also, the *Pudendum muliebre*.

Fos'sa Hy-a-lo-i'de-a.* [See HYALOID.] The cup-like excavation of the vitreous humor, in which the crystalline lens is imbedded.

Fos'sa In-nom-i-na'ta.* ("Unnamed Fossa.") The space between the helix and the anthelix of the ear.

Fos'sa Lach-ry-ma'lis.* ("Lachrymal Fossa.") A depression in the frontal bone for the reception of the lachrymal gland.

Fos'sa Na-vic-u-la'ris.* ("Navicular or Boat-Shaped Fossa.") The superficial depression which separates the two roots of the anthelix; also called *Sca'pha*, or "little boat." Applied also to the dilatation towards the extremity of the spongy portion of the urethra. Also, the name of a small cavity immediately within the fourchette.

Fos'sa O-va'lis.* ("Oval Fossa.") The oval depression presented by the septum of the right auricle of the heart.

Fos'sa Pi-tu-i-ta'ri-a.* ("Pituitary Fossa.") The *sella turcica*, or cavity in the sphenoid bone, for receiving the pituitary body.

Fos'sa Sca-pho-i'dēs.* A term synonymous with FOSSA NAVICULARIS.

Fos'sa Syl'vi-i.* ("Fossa of Sylvius.") A designation of the fifth ventricle of the brain.

Fos'sil. [**Fos'silis**; from *fo'dio, fos'sum*, to "dig."] That which is dug out of the earth. Applied to organic remains, animal and vegetable, found in the strata of the earth.

Fos-sil-if'er-ous. [**Fossilif'erus**; from *fos'silis*, and *fe'ro*, to "bear."] Bearing, or containing, fossil specimens.

Fos-sil-i-ză'tion. [**Fossiliza'tio, o'nis**; from *fos'silis*, "fossil."] The process of converting into a fossil.

Fotus. See FOMENTATION.

Fou, foo. The French term for INSANE, which see.

Fourchette (Fr.), fooR'shĕtt'. [Lat. **Fur'cula.**] Literally, a "fork." The posterior commissure of the *Labia majora pudendi*. In Comparative Anatomy, the prominent portion in the centre of the plantar surface of the horse's foot, shaped like the letter V, called in common language the "frog of the foot." Applied also to the breast-bone (merry-thought) of birds.

Fourmillement, fooR'mēl'mŏNᵍ'. The French term for FORMICATION, which see.

Fousel Oil. See FUSEL OIL.

Fo've-ate. [**Fovea'tus**; from *fo'vea*, a "pit," a "depression."] Having a depression or depressions; pitted.

Fo-ve'o-late, Fo-ve-o-lā'ri-ous. [**Foveola'tus, Foveola'rius**; from *fove'ola*, diminutive of *fo'vea*, a "pit."] Having little unequal pits or depressions.

Fo-vil'la.* [Perhaps from *fo'veo*, to "foster;" because it fosters or keeps alive the vital principle in the plant.] The fecundating liquor contained in the grains of pollen.

Fowler's Solution. See LIQUOR ARSENICALIS.

Fox'-Glove. The *Digitalis purpurea*.

Frac-tu'ra.* [From *fran'go, frac'tum*, to "break."] Fracture. A genus of the order *Dialyses*, class *Locales*, of Cullen's Nosology. In Surgery, the solution of continuity of a bone, generally by external force, but occasionally by the powerful action of muscles.

Fracture. See FRACTURA.

Frac'ture, Com'min-ūt-ed. A fracture in which the bone is broken or crushed into several pieces.

Fracture, Compound. See COMPOUND FRACTURE.

Frac'ture, Sim'ple. A fracture in which the bone only is divided, without any external wound.

Fræ'na,* the plural of FRÆNUM, which see.

Fræ'na Ep-ĭ-glot'tĭ-dis.* ("Curbs of the Epiglottis.") Three folds of mucous membrane which unite the epiglottis to the os hyoïdes and the tongue.

Fræ'na of the Valvule of Bauhin. The name given by Morgagni to the rugæ or lines observed at the extremities of the lips of the valvule of Bauhin, or ileo-colic valve.

Fræn'u-lum.* [Diminutive of *fræ'num*, a "bridle."] A "little bridle." Sometimes used for *Frænum*.

Fræ'num,* plural **Fræ'na.** (Fr. *Frein*, fRăNG.) Literally, a "bridle," or "curb." A part which performs the office of a check or curb.

Fræ'num Lab-ĭ-o'rum.* The fourchette, or lower commissure of the *labia majora pudendi*.

Fræ'num Lin'guæ.* ("Bridle of the Tongue.") A fold formed at the under surface of the tongue by the mucous membrane lining the mouth. Infants are said to be *tongue-tied* when the frænum is very short, or continued too far forward towards the tip of the tongue.

Fræ'num of the Un'der Lip. [**Fræ'num La'bii Inferio'ris.**] A fold of the mucous membrane of the mouth, formed opposite to the symphysis of the chin.

Fræ'num Præpu'tii* (pre-pu'she-i). A triangular fold, connecting the prepuce with the under part of the glans penis.

Fra-gil'ĭ-tas Os'sĭ-um.* A morbid "brittleness of the bones." See MOLLITIES OSSIUM.

Frag'ment. [**Fragmen'tum**; from *fran'go*, to "break."] A piece of a thing broken. A splinter or detached portion of a fractured bone.

Frambœsia,* fram-bē'she-a. (Fr. *Framboise*, a "raspberry.") The yaws. A genus of the order *Impetigenes*, class *Cachexiæ*, of Cullen's Nosology.

Francoaceæ,* fran-ko-a'she-ē. [From *Fran'coa*, one of the genera.] A natural order of exogenous herbaceous plants, found in Chili.

Fran-gĭ-pan'. An extract of milk, for preparing artificial milk, made by evaporating skimmed milk to dryness, mixed with almonds and sugar.

Frankeniaceæ,* fran-ke-ne-a'she-ē. [From *Franke'nia*, one of the genera.] A small natural order of exogenous plants, found in Europe, Africa, and Australia.

Frankincense. See OLIBANUM, and THUS.

Frank'in-cense, Com'mon. The *Abietis resina*.

Fra-se'ra.* American Columbo. The Pharmacopœial name (U.S. Ph.) for the root of *Frasera Walteri*.

Frax'ĭ-nine. [**Fraxini'na.**] A crystallizable bitter principle obtained from the *Fraxinus excelsior*, a species of ash.

Frax'ĭ-nus.* (Fr. *Frêne*, fRĕn or fRån.) A Linnæan genus of the class *Polygamia*, natural order *Oleaceæ*. The ash-tree.

Fraxinus Ornus. See ORNUS.

Frax'inus Ro-tun-dĭ-fo'lĭ-a.* A tree from which *manna* is said to be obtained.

Freckle. See ÆSTATES, EPHELIS, and LENTIGO.

Freez'ing Mix'ture. A mixture by which artificial cold is produced.

Freez'ing Point. The point at which water freezes, being 32° above zero in Fahrenheit's thermometer; in Reaumur's and the Centigrade, it is taken as zero.

Frein, fRăNG. The French term for FRÆNUM, which see.

Frem'ĭ-tus.* [From *fre'mo, frem'itum*, to "roar," to "fret," to "murmur."] An irregular, rapid, oscillating commotion of the muscular system.

French Ber'ries. The fruit of several species of *Rhamnus* (or Buckthorn), called by the French *Graines d'Avignon* (grĕn or grån då'vèn'yòNG'): they yield a yellow color.

French Pol'ish. Gum lac dissolved in spirits of wine.

French Red, or **Rouge** (roozh). Genuine carmine, mixed with fine sifted starch powder, according to the shade required.

French White. The common designation of finely pulverized talc.

Frêne. See FRAXINUS.

Fri-a-bil'ĭ-tȳ. [**Friabil'itas, a'tis**; from *fri'o*, to "crumble."] The quality of being easily reducible into small pieces.

Fri'ar's Bâl-sam. Another name for the *Tinctu'ra Benzo'ini Compos'ita,* formerly called *Bal'samum Traumat'icum.*

Fric'tion. [From *fri'co, fric'tum,* to "rub."] A therapeutical agent of great power, by means of which the circulation is stimulated, and medicinal applications enter the pores of the skin.

Fries'land Green. Otherwise called **Bruns'wick Green.** An ammoniaco-muriate of copper.

Frig-ĭ-da'rĭ-um.* [From *frig'idus,* "cold."] Another name for the cold bath. See BATH.

Frig'id Zone. The space between each Polar circle and the Pole.

Frig-o-rif'ic. [**Frigorif'icus;** from *fri'gus,* "cold," and *fa'cio,* to "make" or "cause."] Having power to make cold.

Fri'gus,* gen. **Frig'o-ris.** [From *fri'geo,* to "be cold."] Cold; trembling with cold. This term differs from *Algor,* which implies suffering or starving with cold.

Fringe. See FIMBRIA.

Fringed. See FIMBRIATE, LACINIATUS, CILIATE.

Frit, or **Fritt.** The mass produced by the materials of glass, on calcination.

Froissement, Bruit de, brwē dęh fRwåss'mōNG'. ("Sound of Rubbing.") A French term applied to certain sounds of the lungs or heart.

Frond. [From *frons, fron'dis,* a "leaf," or "green branch."] A term applied to the leaves of ferns and other cryptogamic plants, from their partaking at once of the nature of a leaf and a branch.

Fron-dĕs'çence. [**Frondescen'tia;** from *frons, fron'dis,* a "leaf."] The development of the leaves, or fronds of plants.

Fron-dif'er-ous. [**Frondif'erus;** from *frons, fron'dis,* a "leaf," and *fe'ro,* "to bear."] Bearing fronds.

Frons,* gen. **Frondis.** See FROND.

Frons,* gen. **Fron'tis.** [Perhaps from φροντίζω, to "study."] The forehead; that part of the head between the eyebrows and commencement of the hairy scalp.

Fron'tal. [**Fronta'lis;** from *frons,* the "forehead."] Belonging to the forehead.

Frost'-Bite. A state of numbness or torpefaction of a part of the body, caused by intense cold, which, unless relieved by proper remedies, is followed by the death of the part. In such cases it is very important that heat should not be applied suddenly. If a finger be frozen, the best remedy is to place it in water reduced almost to the freezing-point, by which means the frost is extracted very slowly.

Frottement (Fr.), fRŏtt'mŏNG'. A term signifying "rubbing." See FROISSEMENT.

Frozen Sulphuric Acid. See GLACIAL SULPHURIC ACID.

Fruc-tif'er-ous. [**Fruc'tifer;** from *fruc'tus,* "fruit," and *fe'ro,* to "bear."] Bearing fruit.

Fruc-tĭ-fĭ-cā'tion. [**Fructifica'tio, o'nis;** from *fructif'ico, fructifica'tum,* to "make fruitful," to "bear fruit."] That part of a plant, embracing the organs appropriated to generation, and comprehending both flowers and fruit, terminating the old plant and beginning the new.

Fru-ġiv'or-ous. [**Frugiv'orus;** from *frux, fru'gis,* "fruit," or "corn," and *vo'ro,* to "devour."] Eating or living on grains or seeds.

Fruit. [From *fru'or, fruc'tus,* to "enjoy."] In Botany, the matured ovary, with all its contents and appendages.

Fruit-Stalk. See PEDUNCLE.

Fru-men-tā'ceous. [**Frumenta'ceus;** from *frumen'tum,* "wheat."] Applied to all plants that resemble wheat or corn.

Fru-men'tum.* All kinds of corn or grain for making bread, especially wheat.

Frust. = *Frustilla'tim.** "In small pieces."

Frus'tum.* That part of a pyramid or cone which remains when any part next the vertex is cut off by a plane parallel to the base.

Fru-tĕs'çence. [From *fruc'tus,* "fruit."] The ripe or mature state of a fruit.

Fru'tex,* gen. **Fru'tĭ-cis.** A shrub; a plant whose branches are perennial and proceed directly from the surface of the earth, without any supporting trunk.

Fru-tĭ-cose'. [**Frutico'sus;** from *fru'tex,* a "shrub."] Full of shrubs; like a shrub: shrubby.

Ft. = *Fi'at,** or *Fi'ant.** "Let there be made."

Fucaceæ,* fu-ka'she-ē. [From *Fu'cus,* a kind of sea-weed.] Sea-weeds. A natural order of cryptogamous plants.

Fu-civ'or-ous. [**Fuciv'orus;** from *fu'cus,* a "sea-weed," and *vo'ro,* to "devour."] Living on sea-weed.

Fu'cus.* [From φῦκος, "sea-wrack."] A Linnæan genus of the class *Cryptogamia*, natural order *Fucaceæ*.

Fu'cus Ve-sic-u-lo'sus.* The systematic name of bladder-fucus, sea-oak, or sea-wrack.

Ful'crum,* plural **Ful'cra.** A "stay," or "prop." In the plural, the various appendages of a plant, as tendrils, prickles, stipules. In Natural Philosophy, applied to a fixed point on which a lever rests.

Ful-gu-rā'tion. [**Fulgura'tio, o'***nis;* from *ful'gur*, "brightness," "lightning."] The electrical phenomenon of flashes of light in the atmosphere unaccompanied by thunder.

Fu-lig'in-ous. [**Fuligino'sus;** from *fuli'go*, "soot."] Full of soot; sooty; smoky.

Fu-li'go,* gen. **Fu-lig'i-nis.** The Latin term for "soot."

Fuli'go Lig'ni.* ("Soot of Wood.") Wood-soot is the condensed smoke of burning wood. Made into an ointment, it has been found an efficacious remedy in some cutaneous affections, such as tetter, *psora, porrigo favosa*, etc.

Ful'ler's Earth. A variety of clay, containing about twenty-five per cent. of alumina, and so named from its being used by fullers to remove the grease from cloth before the soap is applied.

Ful'mi-nāte. [**Ful'minas, a'***tis.*] A combination of fulminic acid with a base.

Ful'mi-nāt-ing Gold. [**Au'rum Ful'minans.**] The aurate of ammonia, or ammoniuret of the peroxide of gold. It is produced by precipitating a solution of gold by ammonia.

Ful'minating Mer'cu-ry. A powder obtained by treating the nitrate of mercury with alcohol. It is employed in the manufacture of percussion-caps.

Ful'minating Sil'ver. [**Argen'tum Ful'minans.**] An argentate of ammonia, prepared by leaving oxide of silver for ten or twelve hours in contact with a strong solution of ammonia. It is in the form of a black powder which is extremely explosive.

Ful-mi-nā'tion. [**Fulmina'tio, o'***nis;* from *ful'men*, "thunder," *ful'mino, fulmina'tum*, to "thunder."] A quick explosion, with noise; as of fulminating powder, or the combustion of inflammable gas with oxygen: detonation.

Ful-min'ic. [**Fulmin'icus.**] Applied to an acid obtained from the fulminate of silver.

Fu-ma'ri-a Of-fiç-i-na'lis.* Fumitory. (Fr. *Fumeterre*, füm'têr'.) A plant common in Europe, and cultivated in the United States. An infusion of the dried leaves has been recommended in leprous affections.

Fumariaceæ,* fu-ma-re-a'she-ē. [From *Fuma'ria*, one of the genera.] A natural order of exogenous herbaceous plants, found in many or all temperate climates. It includes the *Coryd'alis* and some others which are cultivated for their beauty.

Fu-mi-gā'tion. [**Fumiga'tio, o'***nis;* from *fu'migo, fumiga'tum*, to "perfume a place."] The employment of certain fumes for the purpose of counteracting contagious effluvia.

Func'tion. [**Func'tio, o'***nis;* from *fun'gor, func'tus*, to "fulfil an office."] (Fr. *Fonction*, fònk'se-òng'.) A power, or faculty, by the exercise of which the vital phenomena are produced.

Func'tion-al Dis-ease'. A disease in which the function or secretion of an organ is vitiated, but its structure is but little if at all changed.

Func'tions, Vi'tal. Functions immediately necessary to life; viz., those of the brain, the heart, the lungs, etc.; whence these have been called the tripod of life.

Fund'a-ment. [**Fundamen'tum;** from *fun'dus*, the "bottom of a thing."] The anus.

Fun'gāte. [**Fun'gas, a'***tis.*] A combination of fungic acid with a base.

Fun'gi,* the plural of **Fun'gus,** a "mushroom." A large natural order of cryptogamous plants, of a very low organization. They grow on dead and decaying organic bodies, and infest living plants. They are of great importance to man, either for their useful or mischievous qualities.

Blight, mildew, and rust are caused by the ravages of microscopic fungi. The common mushroom and truffle are used as food. Many other fungi are dangerous poisons. The fungus called ergot is a valuable medicine for its specific action on the uterus. See PRIMALIA.

Fun-gic'o-lus.* [From *fun'gus*, a "mushroom," and *co'lo*, to "inhabit."] Living on or in mushrooms. Applied in the plural neuter (*Fungic'ola*) to a family of coleopterous insects.

Fun'gi-form. [**Fungifor'mis;** from *fun'gus*, a "mushroom."] Resembling a mushroom.

Fun'gin. [**Fungi'na;** from *fun'gus*,

a "mushroom."] The residual fleshy substance of *fungi*, after being subjected to the action of alcohol and water.

Fun'goid. [**Fungoi'des;** from *fun'gus*, a "mushroom," and εἶδος, a "form."] Resembling a mushroom, or the disease termed *fungus*.

Fun'gous. [**Fungo'sus;** from *fun'gus*, a "mushroom."] (Fr. *Fongueux.*) Having fungi, or the disease termed *fungus;* resembling *fungus*.

Fun'gus.* [Gr. σπόγγος, or σφόγγος; Fr. *Fongus*, fôNᴳ'güss'.] One of a natural order of plants. (See FUNGI.) Also, a redundant growth of flesh on an ulcer; proud flesh; any large, soft, spongy excrescence arising from diseased structure.

Fungus Cerebri. See HERNIA CEREBRI, and ENCEPHALOCELE.

Fun'gus Hæm-a-to'dĕs.* [From αἱματώδης, "bloody."] "Bleeding Fungus;" otherwise called Soft Cancer, Medullary Sarcoma, Spongoïd Inflammation, etc. It is a cancerous affection of a very malignant character, spreading rapidly, and almost invariably fatal.

Fu-nic'u-lus.* [Diminutive of *fu'nis*, a "rope."] A botanical term applied to the small filament, or podosperm, connecting the imperfect seed to the receptacle. Also, the navel-string.

Fu'nis.* [From σχοῖνος, a "rope plaited from the bulrush"?] Literally, a "rope." Generally applied to the *Funis umbilicalis*, or navel-string.

Fu'nis Um-bil-i-ca'lis.* (Fr. *Cordon ombilicale*, koR'dôNᴳ' ôM'bè'lè'kâl'.) The umbilical cord; the means of communication between the fœtus and the placenta. Its length is almost two feet. It consists of the umbilical arteries and vein, with the enveloping membranes, etc.

Funnel-Shaped. See INFUNDIBULIFORMIS.

Fur'cate. [**Furca'tus;** from *fur'ca*, a "fork."] Divided into two parts; forked: dichotomous.

Furcula. See FOURCHETTE.

Fur'fur, ur*is*.* [From *far*, "corn."] Bran, the husk or skin of wheat. The diseased condition of the head called dandriff, or scurf, a species of *Pityriasis*.

Fur'fur Trit'i-ci.* ("Bran of Wheat.") A material employed to make bread for dyspeptics.

Fur-fur-ā'ceous. [**Furfura'ceus;** from *fur'fur*, "bran," or "dandriff."] Resembling bran or dandriff.

Fur-fur-a'tio* (fŭr-fŭr-a'she-o), **o'***nis*. [From *fur'fur*, "dandriff."] The state of having *Pityriasis*, or a scaliness of the skin.

Fur'nace. [**Fur'nus.**] A fireplace employed for pharmaceutical operations. Furnaces are termed *evaporatory* when employed to reduce substances into vapor by heat; *reverberatory*, when so constructed as to prevent the flame from rising; *forge furnaces*, when the current of air is determined by bellows.

Furoncle, or **Froncle.** See FURUNCULUS.

Fu'ror U-te-ri'nus.* Another term for *Nymphomania*, or *Hysteromania*.

Furrowed. See SULCATED.

Fu-run'cu-lus.* (Fr. *Furoncle*, fü'-rôNkl'.) A boil, or inflammatory tumor; a blain.

Fu'sel Oil. [**Al'cohol Amyl'icum.**] An oily, poisonous liquid, of a highly disagreeable smell and nauseous taste, produced in the manufacture of potato spirit, and of ardent spirit obtained from the various kinds of grain. It is valuable in Pharmacy as the artificial source of valerianic acid.

Fu'si.* The plural of FUSUS, which see.

Fu-ṡĭ-bil'ĭ-tȳ. [**Fusibil'itas, a***tis*.] The capability of being fused.

Fu'ṡĭ-ble. [**Fu'silis;** from *fun'do, fu'sum*, to "pour," to "melt."] Capable of being made fluid by the application of heat.

Fu'ṡĭ-form. [**Fusifor'mis;** from *fu'sus*, a "spindle."] Resembling a spindle; tapering.

Fu'ṡion. [**Fu'sio, o'***nis;* from *fun'do, fu'sum*, to "pour," to "melt."] The act of melting, or state of being melted, by heat.

Fu'sion, A'que-ous. The liquefaction of salts which contain water of crystallization, on exposure to increased temperature.

Fu'sion, Dry. The liquefaction produced by heat after the water has been expelled.

Fu'sion, Ig'ne-ous. The melting of anhydrous salts by heat without undergoing any decomposition.

Fus'tic. A yellow dye-wood, consisting of two kinds: *Old fustic*, the product of the *Morus Tinctoria*, or Dyer's Mulberry, an American tree; and *Young fustic*, the *Rhus Cotinus*, or Venice Sumach, a shrub growing in Italy and the south of Europe.

Fu'sus,* plural **Fu'si.** Literally, a "spindle." Applied in the plural to the *papillæ* through which, in the *Arachnides*, the delicate threads pass.

G.

G, or Γ, denoted, among Greek physicians, *Uncia,* or an ounce.

Gad'o-lin-īte. The name of a mineral, so called from the Swedish chemist Gadolin, who discovered it in the earth called *yttria.*

Gad'u-in. [**Gadui'na;** from *Ga'dus mor'rhua,* the "cod-fish."] A peculiar substance found in cod-liver oil.

Ga'dus.* A genus of fishes of the order *Jugulares.*

Ga'dus Mor'rhu-a.* The cod-fish, abounding in the northern seas, from the liver of which cod-fish oil is obtained.

Ga-lac'ta-gogue. [**Galactago'gus;** from γάλα, γάλακτος, "milk," and ἄγω, to "lead or bring away."] Causing the flow of milk.

Ga-lac'tĭ-a.* [From γάλα, γάλακτος, "milk."] A genus in Good's Nosology, embracing defective, excessive, or morbid secretions of the milk: mislactation.

Ga-lac'tic. The same as LACTIC, which see.

Ga-lac'tin. [**Galacti'na**; from γάλα, γάλακτος, "milk."] The coagulating principle of milk.

Ga-lac-tir-rhœ'a.* [From γάλα, "milk," and ῥέω, to "flow."] An excessive flow of milk.

Ga-lac'to-çēle.* [From γάλα, "milk," and κήλη, a "tumor."] A tumor or swelling containing a milky fluid.

Gal-ac-tom'e-ter. [**Galactom'etrum;** from γάλα, "milk," and μέτρον, a "measure."] An instrument for measuring or ascertaining the quality of milk.

Gal-ac-toph'a-gous. [**Galactoph'agus;** from γάλα, "milk," and φάγω, to "eat."] Living on milk. See LACTIVOROUS.

Gal-ac-toph'o-rous. [**Galactoph'orus;** from γάλα, "milk," and φέρω, to "bear."] Milk-bearing; lactiferous.

Ga-lac-to-poi-et'ic. [**Galactopoiet'icus;** from γάλα, "milk," and ποιέω, to "make."] Milk-making, or milk-producing.

Ga-lac-to-po'sĭ-a.* [From γάλα, "milk," and πίνω, to "drink."] Milk diet.

Gal'ba-num.* The Pharmacopœial name ‖ for a resinous substance obtained from an undetermined plant. It is expectorant and antispasmodic, somewhat resembling ammoniac in its action.

Gal'bu-lus.* A kind of cone, differing from the strobile only in being round and having the heads of the carpels much enlarged. The fruit of the juniper is a galbulus.

Gale, gål. The French term for "itch." See PSORA.

Ga'le-a.* Literally, a "helmet." In Botany, the superior arched lip of ringent and personate corollas. A form of headache extending all over the head. In Surgery, a bandage for the head, somewhat like a helmet. Also, a large vaulted membrane, movable, and covering the jaws of orthopterous and some other insects.

Ga'le-ate. [**Galea'tus;** from *ga'lea,* a "helmet."] Formed like a helmet; helmeted.

Ga-le'ga Vir-ġin-ĭ-a'na.* A plant growing native in the United States, said to be diaphoretic and powerfully anthelmintic.

Ga-le'na.* [From γάλειν, to "shine" or "glister."] Lead-glance, the native sulphuret of lead. See MOLYBDÆNUM.

Ga-len'ic. [**Galen'icus.**] After the manner of Galen, whose practice of medicine was remarkable for multiplying herbs and roots in the same composition.

Ga'len's Ban'dage. A term sometimes applied to the four-tailed bandage, or single split cloth.

Galeux, gå'luh'. The French term for PSORIC, which see.

Galiaceæ,* ga-le-a'she-ē, or **Stellatæ,*** stel-la'tē (because the leaves are placed round the stem in the form of a star). A natural order of exogenous herbaceous plants, found in cold and temperate climates. It includes *Galium* and *Rubia tinctoria,* which produces madder.

Gal-ĭ-pe'a Cus-pa'rĭ-a.* The tree which, according to the London Pharmacopœia, produces the Angustura bark.

Galipe'a Of-fiç-ĭ-na'lis.* The tree which, according to the United States and Edinburgh Pharmacopœias, produces Angustura or Cusparia bark.

Gal'ĭ-pot. An earthen pot, painted and glazed, wherein ointments, etc., are kept. Also, a resin obtained from the several species of *Pinus.*

Gall. The bile, or secretion of the liver. See BILE.

Gall-Blad'der. [Lat. **Vesi'ca Fel'lis;** Fr. *Vésicule du Fiel*, và'zè'kül' dü fe-ĕl'.] A membranous reservoir containing the bile, situated on the lower surface of the right lobe of the liver.

Gall-Ducts. See CYSTIC DUCTS.

Gall-Nut. See GALLA.

Gall-Sick'ness. The remittent fever (otherwise called **Wal'cheren Fe'ver**) produced by marsh *miasmata* in the Netherlands; so named because accompanied with a vomiting of bile.

Gall'-Stone. A *calculus* formed in the gall-bladder.

Găl'la,* plural **Gal'læ.** The Pharmacopœial name ‖ for the nutgall, or galls, found on the branches of the *Quercus infectoria*. They are excrescences caused by the sting of an insect belonging for the most part to the genus *Cynips;* though the Chinese gall is said to be produced by an *Aphis*.

Galls are powerfully astringent. Although sometimes prescribed in chronic diarrhœa and similar complaints, they are chiefly used in external applications, such as lotions, gargles, ointments, etc.

Gal'læ,* the plural of GALLA, which see.

Găl'lāte. [**Gal'las, a'**tis.] A combination of gallic acid with a base.

Găl'lic. [**Gal'licus;** from *Gal'lia*, "Gaul."] Belonging to the French. See GALLICUS MORBUS.

Găl'lic. [**Gal'licus;** from *gal'la*, a "gall-nut."] Belonging to galls. Applied to an acid found in astringent vegetable substances, but very abundantly in the gall-nut.

Gal-lic'o-læ.* [From *gal'la*, a "gall," and *co'lo*, to "inhabit."] Literally, "inhabiters of the gall-nut." A tribe of hymenopterous insects, or *Diplolepariæ*, which produce those excrescences on plants called *galls*. Latreille comprehends all the insects of this tribe in one genus, viz.: *Cynips*. See GALLA.

Găl'lĭ-cus Mor'bus.* ("French Disease.") Another name for SYPHILIS, which see.

Găl-lĭ-nā'ceous. [**Gallina'ceus;** from *gal'lus*, a "cock," or *galli'na*, a "hen."] Resembling the domestic hen. See GALLINÆ.

Gallinadæ. See GALLINÆ.

Găl-lī'næ*(the plural of *galli'na*, a "hen"), or **Gallina'ceous Birds.** A family of birds so named from their affinity to the domestic hen.

Gallinaginis Caput. See CAPUT GALLINAGINIS.

Găl-lĭ-na'go, *inis.** [Probably from *gal'lus*, a "cock."] The Latin name for the wood-cock.

Găl-van'ic. [**Galvan'icus.**] Pertaining to galvanism.

Galvan'ic Bat'te-rȳ or **Trough.** An apparatus for accumulating galvanism, consisting of plates of zinc and copper alternately fastened together, and cemented into a wooden or earthenware trough, so as to form a number of cells; the trough is then filled with diluted acid.

Galvan'ic Mox'a. A term applied by Fabré Palaprat to the employment of voltaic electricity as a therapeutical agent for producing the cauterizing effects of the moxa.

Găl'van-ism. [**Galvanis'mus;** from Professor *Galvani*, of Bologna, who first observed the manifestations of this fluid or principle.] A form of electricity usually developed or produced by the mutual action of various metals and chemical agents upon each other. The additional discoveries of Volta led to the term Voltaism, or Voltaic Electricity, and its effect on the muscles of animals newly killed, suggested the term Animal Electricity.

Gal-van-om'e-ter. [**Galvanom'etrum;** from *galvanism*, and *μέτρον*, a "measure."] An instrument for ascertaining the nature and degree of excitement produced by galvanic action.

Gal-van'o-scope. [**Galvanos'copus;** from *galvanism*, and *σκοπέω*, to "observe."] An instrument capable of exhibiting electric phenomena. The term has been applied by M. Hall to a frog properly prepared and placed under certain conditions for experiment.

Gambir, or **Gambier,** găm-beer'. The Malay name of an astringent extract procured from the *Nau'clea Gambir* (or *Unca'ria Gambir*). The substance called square catechu, and *terra japonica*, is the produce of this plant. See CATECHU.

Gamboge. See GAMBOGIA.

Gam-boge', A-mer'ĭ-can. A secretion similar to gamboge, yielded by several species of *Vismia*.

Gam-bo'gĭ-a.* The Pharmacopœial name (U.S. and Dub. Ph.) for gamboge, or camboge; the concrete juice of an undetermined tree. Gamboge is a powerful hydragogue cathartic, and as such is often given in dropsy. It is also recommended as a remedy for the tape-worm. In large doses its action is extremely violent, and has sometimes proved fatal. See CAMBOGIA.

Gam-o-pet'al-ous. [**Gamopet'alus**; from γάμος, "marriage," or "union," and πέταλοι, a "petal."] Having petals joined together by the borders.

Gam-o-sep'al-ous. [**Gamosep'alus**; from γάμος, "marriage," or "union," and *sep'alum*, a "sepal."] Having sepals joined together by their borders.

Gang'li-form. [**Ganglifor'mis**; from *gang'lion*.] Of the nature, likeness, or appearance of a ganglion.

Gan'gli-on. [Lat. **Gan'glion**; Gr. γαγγλίον, a "knot."] An enlargement in the course of a nerve, resembling a knot. Also, a collection of vesicular neurine which serves as a centre of nervous power to certain fibres connected with it. Applied in Surgery to an encysted tumor occurring on a tendon or aponeurosis, sometimes on the knee, or on the back of the hand or foot. Also, a genus of the order *Tumores*, class *Locales*, of Cullen's Nosology.

Gan'glion Im'par.* A small ganglion on the coccyx.

Ganglion of Gasser. See GASSERIAN GANGLION.

Ganglion of Meckel. See MECKEL, GANGLION OF.

Gan-gli-on'ic. [**Ganglion'icus**; from *gan'glion*.] Pertaining to a ganglion, or to ganglions; consisting of ganglions.

GANGLION'IC SYS'TEM, or GANGLION'IC NERV'OUS SYS'TEM. A name applied to the Trisplanchnic (or Great Sympathetic) nerve, with its system of ganglia, constituting, according to Bichat, the nervous system of organic life. See ORGANIC.

Gan-gli-on'i-ca.* [From γαγγλίον, a "nerve-knot."] A class of medicinal agents which affect the sensibility or muscular motion of parts supplied by the ganglionic or sympathetic system of nerves.

Gangræna. See GANGRENE.

Gan-græ'na O'ris.* ("Gangrene of the Mouth.") A name for *Stomacace*, *Cancrum Oris*, or canker of the mouth.

Gan'grēne. [Lat. **Gangræ'na**; Gr. γάγγραινα, from γραίνω, or γράω, to "gnaw," to "consume."] (Fr. *Gangrène*, gōNᵍ'grĕn' or gōNᵍ'grÂn'.) The state of incipient mortification. It is sometimes termed *hot mortification*. See next article.

Gan'grene, Hot. [**Gangræ'na Cal'ida.**] A name applied by some writers to that form of mortification which is preceded or accompanied by inflammation, in other words, to gangrene proper; while they term that which is unattended by inflammation *cold gangrene*.

Gan'grene, Hu'mid. [**Gangræ'na Hu'mida.**] A term applied to that form of the disease in which the affected part contains more or less of decomposed or other fluids. In *dry gangrene* (*Gangræ'na Sic'ca*), these fluids are not present, or only in very small quantity. The latter form, being frequently found to affect old people, has been sometimes called *Gangræna Senilis*.

Gaping. See PANDICULATIO.

Găr'an-cine. [From *Garance*, gå'rŏNss', the French name of "madder."] The coloring matter of madder, mixed with the carbonized residue resulting from the action of the oil of vitriol on the woody fibre and other constituents of madder. It is a brownish or puce-colored powder used in dyeing.

Gar-cin'i-a.* [Named after Dr. *Garcin*.] A Linnæan genus of the class *Dodecandria*, natural order *Guttiferæ*.

Garcin'ia Cam-bo'gi-a,* or **Garcin'ia Cam-bo-gi-oi'dēs.*** A plant considered to afford the best gamboge. See CAMBOGIA, and GAMBOGIA.

Gar'diner's Al-i-men'ta-ry Prep-a-rā'tion. A nutritious article, consisting of very finely-ground rice meal.

Garg. = *Gargaris'ma*.* A "gargle."

Gar-ga-ris'ma, atis,* **Gar-ga-ris'mum,*** **Gar-ga-ris'mus.*** [From γαργαρίζω, to "wash the throat."] A wash for the throat: a gar'gle.

Gargle. See GARGARISMA.

Gar'lic. The common English name of the plant *Al'lium sati'vum*. Its bulbous root or roots constitute what are termed the cloves of garlic.

Gar'rot. (Fr. a "stick," a "kind of lever.") A cylindrical piece of wood, or ivory, for tightening circular bandages.

Garryaceæ,* gar-re-a'she-ē. [From *Garrya*, one of the genera.] A small natural order of exogenous shrubs, found in North America.

Ga'rum.* A sauce or pickle made by the Romans, from the γάρος, a small fish. It resembled the modern anchovy sauce in nature and use.

Gas, gass. [From the Anglo-Saxon *gast*, "breath," "wind," "spirit."] An aeriform, elastic fluid.

Gaseous, gaz'e-ŭs. [**Gaseo'sus.**] Belonging to gas; of the nature of gas.

Gaseous Pulse. See PULSE.

Gas'i-form. [**Gasifor'mis.**] Having the form or nature of gas.

Gas-om'e-ter. [**Gasom'etrum;** from *gas*, and μέτρον, a "measure."] A measurer of gas. Usually applied, however, to a reservoir for containing gas.

Gas-se'rĭ-an Gan'glĭ-on. The semilunar ganglion. A ganglion of the fifth pair of nerves, first discovered by Gasser.

Gas'ter (Gr. γαστήρ). The Greek name for the stomach.

Gas-ter-an-gem-phrax'is.* [From γαστήρ, the "stomach," ἄγγος, a "vessel," and ἔμφραξις, an "obstruction."] Congestion of the blood-vessels of the stomach.

Gas-ter'ic. The same as GASTRIC, which see.

Gasteropoda, or **Gasteropods.** See next article.

Gas-ter-op'o-dus.* [From γαστήρ, the "belly," or "stomach," and πούς, a "foot."] Gasterop'odous. Applied in the plural neuter (*Gasterop'oda*) to a class of Mollusks which crawl by means of a fleshy disk on their belly. The common snail belongs to this class.

Gas-ter-os'to-mus.* [From γαστήρ, the "stomach," and στόμα, a "mouth."] Gasteros'tomous. Having a mouth in the belly, or stomach. Applied to a species of *Tænia*, or tape-worm.

Gas-træ'mĭ-a.* [From γαστήρ, the "stomach," and αἷμα, "blood."] Congestion of the veins of the stomach, and, so, nearly synonymous with *Gasterangemphraxis*.

Gas-trăl'gĭ-a.* [From γαστήρ, the "stomach," and ἄλγος, "pain."] Pain in the stomach: gastral'gy.

Gas-trel-co'sis.* [From γαστήρ, the "stomach," and ἑλκόω, to "ulcerate."] Ulceration of the stomach.

Gas-tren-çeph-a-lo'ma, *atis.** [From γαστήρ, the "stomach," and *encephalo'ma*, a "tumor of brain-like substance."] A brain-like fungus of the stomach.

Gas-tren-çeph-a-lo'sis.* The formation and progress of *gastrencephaloma*.

Gas-tren'chy̆-ta.* [From γαστήρ, the "stomach," and ἐγχέω, to "pour in."] A stomach-syringe, or stomach-pump.

Gas'tric. [**Gas'tricus;** from γαστήρ, the "stomach."] Belonging to the stomach.

Gas'tric Fe'ver. A name given by some to *bilious* fever, which was thought to depend on gastric derangement. It is the *Meningo-gastric* of Pinel.

Gas'tric Juice. [**Suc'cus Gas'tricus.**] The juice secreted in the stomach, by the action of which on the food, digestion is carried on.

Gas'trĭ-çiṡm. [**Gastricis'mus;** from γαστήρ, the "stomach."] A term for gastric affections in general; but usually applied to the theory that all diseases are caused by the accumulation of impurities in the stomach and bowels, suggesting their removal by vomiting and purging.

Gas-tric'o-la.* [From γαστήρ, the "stomach," and *co'lo*, to "inhabit."] Literally, an "inhabitant of the stomach." Applied to those *Œstridæ* (the common bott, for example) the larvæ of which are found in the intestines of various animals.

Gas-tril'o-quus.* [From γαστήρ, the "stomach," and *lo'quor*, to "speak."] The same as VENTRILOQUOUS, which see.

Gas-tri'tis, *idis.** [From γαστήρ, the "stomach."] Inflammation of the stomach. A genus of the order *Phlegmasiæ*, class *Pyrexiæ*, of Cullen's Nosology.

Gas'tro-çēle.* [From γαστήρ, the "stomach," and κήλη, a "tumor."] Hernia in which a portion of the stomach is protruded: *Hernia ventriculi*.

Gas-tro-cho'lĭ-a.* [From γαστήρ, the "stomach," and χολή, "bile."] Bilious disease of the stomach.

Gas-tro-cho-lo'sis.* [From the same.] Gastric bilious fever.

Gas-troc-ne'mĭ-us.* [From γαστήρ, the "stomach," or "belly," and κνήμη, the "leg."] (Fr. *Gastrocnémien*, gås'trok'-nå'me-ăNº'.) Literally, "belonging to the belly (or calf) of the leg." The name of a muscle constituting the chief part of the calf of the leg.

Gas-tro-col'ĭ-ca.* [From γαστήρ, the "stomach," and *col'ica*, the "belly-ache."] Severe colic-like pain in the stomach. Sometimes applied to neuralgia of the stomach.

Gas-tro'dēṡ.* [From γαστήρ, the "stomach."] A term used in Comparative Anatomy and Botany, and applied to that which has many swellings like the belly, or conjoined with a belly.

Gas-tro-dy̆n'ĭ-a.* [From γαστήρ, the "stomach," and ὀδύνη, "pain."] Spasmodic pain in the stomach.

Gas-tro-en-ter-i'tis.* [From γαστήρ, the "stomach," and ἔντερον, an "intestine."] Inflammation of the gastro-intestinal mucous membrane.

Gas-tro-ep-ĭ-plo'ic. [From γαστήρ, the "stomach," and ἐπίπλοον, the "omentum."] Belonging to the stomach and omentum, as applied to a branch of the hepatic artery, lymphatic glands of the abdomen, etc.

Gas'troid. [**Gastroi'des;** from *γαστήρ*, the "stomach," and *εἶδος*, a "form."] Resembling the belly, or stomach.

Gas-trol'ĭ-thus.* [From *γαστήρ*, the "stomach," and *λίθος*, a "stone."] A calculus in the stomach: a gas'trolith.

Gas-trol'o-ġy̆. [**Gastrolo'gia;** from *γαστήρ*, the "stomach," and *λόγος*, a "discourse."] A dissertation on the stomach, its structure, function, etc. Also, the science of the stomach.

Gastromalacia,* gas-tro-ma-la'-she-ạ. [From *γαστήρ*, the "stomach," and *μαλακός*, "soft."] Softening of the stomach; a disease occurring in infants, and usually preceded by hydrocephalus, acute exanthematous disease, or some disease of the respiratory organs.

Gas-tron'o-sos,* or **Gas-tron'o-sus.*** [From *γαστήρ*, the "stomach," and *νόσος*, a "disease."] Disorder of the stomach.

Gas-tro-path'ic. [**Gastropath'i-cus.**] Belonging to gastropathy.

Gas-trop'ạ-thy̆. [**Gastropathi'a;** from *γαστήρ*, the "stomach," and *πάθος*, "affection," or "disease."] Disease of the stomach.

Gas'tro-pe'rĭ-o-dy̆n'ĭ-ạ.* [From *γαστήρ*, the "stomach," *περίοδος*, a "period," and *ὀδύνη*, "pain."] A disease said to be peculiar to India, attended with severe neuralgic pains, returning at intervals. So distressing are the paroxysms, that they are supposed to be produced by the terrible weapon of Siva, the deity of destruction.

Gastropodus. See GASTEROPODUS.

Gas-tror'rhạ-ġy̆. [**Gastrorrha'-gia;** from *γαστήρ*, the "stomach," and *ῥήγνυμι*, to "break" or "burst," to "break through."] Escape of the contents of the stomach through a lesion of its several coats; also, the oozing of blood from its internal surface.

Gas-tror'rhạ-phy̆. [**Gastror'rha-phe,** or **Gastrorrha'phia;** from *γαστήρ*, the "stomach," or "belly," and *ῥαφή*, a "suture."] The sewing of wounds which penetrate through the belly.

Gas-tror-rhœ'ạ.* [From *γαστήρ*, the "stomach," or "belly," and *ῥέω*, to "flow."] Undue increase of the secretion of the mucous glands of the stomach; also, a flux from the belly.

Gas-tros'co-py̆. [**Gastrosco'pia;** from *γαστήρ*, the "belly," and *σκοπέω*, to "examine."] Examination of the abdomen.

Gas-tro'sis.* [From *γαστήρ*, the "stomach."] A name given by Alibert to a family including all diseases of the stomach.

Gas-tro-splen'ic O-men'tạ. A term applied to the laminæ of the peritonæum which are comprised between the spleen and the stomach.

Gas-tros'to-my̆. [**Gastrosto'mia;** from *γαστήρ*, the "stomach," and *στόμα*, an "orifice."] The operation of forming an artificial opening into the stomach.

Gas-tro-tom'ic. [**Gastrotom'i-cus.**] Belonging to gastrotomy.

Gas-trot'o-my̆. [**Gastroto'mia;** from *γαστήρ*, the "stomach," or "belly," and *τέμνω*, to "cut."] The operation of cutting open the abdomen, as in the Cæsarean section; also, cutting through the stomach itself.

Gas-try̆-păl'ġĭ-ạ.* [From *γαστήρ*, the "stomach," *ὑπο*, "under," "in a slight degree," and *ἄλγος*, "pain."] Slight or gentle pains in the stomach.

Gas-try̆'per-pa-thi'ạ.* [From *γαστήρ*, the "stomach," *ὑπέρ*, "above," "excessive," and *πάθος*, "disease."] Severe affection of the stomach.

Gas-try̆-po-pa-thi'ạ.* [From *γαστήρ*, the "stomach," *ὑπο*, "under," and *πάθος*, "disease."] Slight affection of the stomach.

Gâteau Fébrile, gâ'to' fâ'brêl'. The French term for AGUE CAKE, which see.

Gath'er-ing. The same as ABSCESS, and SUPPURATION.

Gaul-the'rĭ-ạ.* The Pharmacopœial name (U.S. Ph.) for the leaves of *Gaul-the'ria procum'bens.*

Gaul-thĕr'ic Aç'id. The heavy oil of partridge-berry, or *Gaultheria procumbens,* formerly a constituent of the commercial *oil of wintergreen.* It combines with bases, and forms salts called gaultherates. The light oil of partridge-berry is called *gaultherylene.*

Gayacine. See GUAIACIN.

Gaz. See GAS.

Gaziform. See GASIFORM.

Gazometer. See GASOMETER.

Ġe'ĭne (or **Ġe'ic**) **Aç'id.** [From *γέα*, "earth," *γήϊνος*, "earthy."] A name given by Berzelius to *humus,* or vegetable mould, the result of the decomposition of vegetable substances.

Ġel-ạ-tiġ'en-ous. [From *gelat'ina,* "gelatine," and *γεννάω*, to "produce."] Yielding gelatine, or forming the gelatinous structures of the body.

Ġel'ạ-tĭne. [**Gelat'ina;** from *ge'lo,*

gela'tum, to "congeal," to "harden."] Jelly. A substance obtained from bone, cartilage, sinew, ligament, skin, cellular tissue, and serous membrane, by long-continued boiling in water. The glue and isinglass of commerce are forms of gelatine.

Gel'atine Cap'sules. Capsules prepared from a concentrated solution of gelatine, and filled with medicines. When swallowed, the capsules dissolve in the gastro-intestinal juices, and the nauseous taste of the medicine is avoided.

Gelatine, Sugar of. See GLYCICOLL.

Gel-a-tin'ĭ-form. [**Gelatinifor'mis.**] Resembling gelatine.

Ge-lat-ĭ-no'sus.* [From *gelat'ina*, "gelatine."] Gelat'inous. Like gelatine, or full of gelatine. Applied in the plural masculine (*Gelatino'si*) to an order of *Polypi*.

Ge-lat'ĭ-nous. [**Gelatino'sus.**] Like gelatine; composed of gelatine.

Gelat'inous Tis'sues. Tissues which yield to boiling water a substance which, on cooling, forms a jelly, or may be called gelatine. They are chiefly found in the cellular membrane, the membranes in general, the tendons, ligaments, bones, cartilages, etc.

Gelatio (je-la'she-o), **o'***nis*.* [From *ge'lo*, *gela'tum*, to "freeze."] Literally, a "freezing." Sometimes applied to the rigid state of the body in catalepsy.

Gel. Quâv. = *Gelat'inâ quâ'vis*.* "In any kind of jelly."

Gel-se'mĭ-um.* Yellow jasmine. The Pharmacopœial name for the root of *Gelse'mium semper'vi'rens*. This plant has been placed in the secondary list of the U.S. Pharmacopœia for 1860.

Gemelli. See GEMELLUS.

Ge-mel-lĭ-flo'rus.* [From *gemel'lus*, "double," or "twin," and *flos*, a "flower."] Having flowers disposed two and two: gemelliflo'rate.

Ge-mel'lus,* plural **Ge-mel'li.** [Diminutive of *gem'inus*, "double."] Applied to the *Gastrocnemius externus* muscle, because it has a double origin.

Gemini. See GEMINUS.

Gem'iniflo'rus.* See GEMELLIFLORUS.

Gem'ĭ-nus,* plural **Gem'ĭ-ni.** "Double," or "twin." Applied to certain parts of plants when in pairs. Applied also to the *gemelli* muscles, and to leaves, etc.

Gem'ma.* A bud which contains the rudiments of a plant in a latent state till the season favors its evolution. Also, a precious stone; a gem.

Gem-mā'ceous. [**Gemma'ceus;** from *gem'ma*, a "bud."] Belonging to buds; having buds.

Gem-mā'tion. [**Gemma'tio, o'***nis*; from *gem'ma*, a "bud."] The state or process of budding; the arrangement of leaves or petals in a bud.

Gem-mif'er-ous. [**Gemmif'erus;** from *gem'ma*, a "bud," or "gem," and *fe'ro*, to "bear."] Bearing buds, or containing gems.

Gem-mĭ-fĭ-cā'tion. [**Gemmifica'tio, o'***nis*; from *gem'ma*, a "bud," and *fa'cio*, to "make."] The manner in which the bud or gem is developed. Also, synonymous with RAMIFICATION.

Gem-mĭ-flo'rus.* [From *gem'ma*, a "bud," and *flos*, a "flower."] Having flowers like buds: gemmiflo'rate.

Gem-mĭ-for'mis.* [From *gem'ma*, a "bud."] Bud- or gem-like: gem'miform.

Gem-mip'a-rous. [**Gemmip'arus;** from *gem'ma*, a "bud," and *pa'rio*, to "bring forth."] Applied to the multiplication of the species by *buds*, or *gemmules*, arising from germs, as exemplified in the vegetable kingdom and in many of the Infusoria.

Gem-mu-lā'tion. [**Gemmula'tio, o'***nis*; from *gem'mula*, a "little bud."] A kind of reproduction consisting in simple growth and development without the agency of sexes. See GEMMIPAROUS.

Gem'mule. [**Gem'mula;** diminutive of *gem'ma*, a "bud."] The rudiment of the stem, afterwards becoming stem and branches; a plumule.

Ge'na,* plural **Ge'næ.** [From γένυς, the "cheek-bone."] (Fr. *Joue*, zhoo.) The cheek, or cheeks, forming the lateral walls of the mouth. They are composed chiefly of muscular tissue, lined internally with a mucous membrane.

Gencives, zhŏN°'sēv'. The French term for the "gums." See GINGIVA.

Gen-e-an'thro-pȳ. [From γενεά, "birth," and ἄνθρωπος, a "man."] The same as ANTHROPOGENY.

Gen'e-ra,* plural of GENUS, which see.

Gen'er-al Prac-tĭ'tion-er. A term applied to those practitioners in England and Wales who do not profess to advise as *pure* physicians, or to act as *pure* surgeons, but perform in their daily vocation the duties of both, with those of the obstetrician in addition.

Gen-er-ā'tion. [**Genera'tio, o'***nis*;

from *gen'ero, genera'tum,* to "beget."] The act of reproducing; reproduction.

Generation, Fissiparous. See FISSIPAROUS GENERATION.

Genera'tion, Or'gans of. In woman, the external are the *Mons veneris, labia, perinæum, clitoris,* and *nymphæ;* the internal, the *vagina, uterus, ovaria,* and *Fallopian tubes;* in man, the *penis, testes, vesiculæ seminales, vasa deferentia,* and *prostate gland.*

Ge-nĕr'ic. [**Gener'icus.**] Belonging to the same genus.

Ge-ne'sĭ-al. [**Genesia'lis;** from γένεσις, "origin," "generation."] Belonging to generation.

Gen-es'ic-us.* Belonging to *genesis.*

Gen'e-sis.* [From γένω, to "be born."] Birth, origin, or generation.

Genêt des Teinturiers. See GENISTA TINCTORIA.

Ge-net'ĭ-ca.* [See GENETICUS.] The name of a class in Dr. Good's Nosology, comprising diseases connected with the sexual function.

Gen-et'ĭ-cus.* [From γένεσις, "generation," or γεννάω, to "beget."] Belonging to the procreative function: genet'ic.

Ge-ne'va.* [From *Gene'va,* where first made.] (Fr. *Genièvre,* zheh-ne-ĕvʀ' or zh'ne-àvʀ'.) Gin, distilled from malt or rye, and afterwards subjected to the same process with juniper-berries. A spurious kind, from turpentine and cardamom-seeds, with very few, if any, juniper-berries, is largely consumed in the English metropolis, etc., as *British gin.*

Gen-ic'u-late. [**Genicula'tus;** from *genic'ulum.*] Bent like a little joint, or like the knee.

Ge-nic'u-lum.* [Diminutive of *ge'nu,* the "knee."] A small knot or joint; a little knee.

Ge'nĭ-o-. [From γένειον, the "chin."] A prefix denoting attachment to, or connection with, the chin.

Ge-nis'ta Tinc-to'rĭ-a.* ("Dyers' Broom.") (Fr. *Genêt des Teinturiers,* zh'nà dà tăɴᵍ'tü're-à'.) A shrub cultivated in Europe and the United States, and sometimes used in medicine.

Gen'ĭ-tal. [**Genita'lis;** from *gig'no, gen'itum,* to "beget."] Belonging to generation.

Gen'ĭ-tals. [**Genita'lia,** plural neuter of **Genita'lis;** from the same.] The organs or parts contributing to generation in the male or female. See GENERATION, ORGANS OF.

Gen'ĭ-to-. [From *genita'lia.*] A prefix denoting connection with the genital organs.

Gen'ĭ-to-Cru'ral. The name of a nerve proceeding from the first lumbar, and dividing into an *internal branch,* which accompanies the spermatic cord; and an *external,* which is distributed into filaments at the crural arch.

Genneticus. See GENETICUS.

Genou. See GENU.

Gentian. See GENTIANA LUTEA.

Gentiana,* jen-she-a'na. [From *Gen'tius,* a king of Illyria.] The Pharmacopœial name ‖ of the root of *Gentiana lutea.* Gentian is an excellent bitter tonic, and is particularly adapted to cases of simple debility of the digestive organs.

Gentia'na Cat-es-bæ'i.* Blue gentian. The Pharmacopœial name (U.S. Ph.) for the root of *Gentiana Catesbæi.*

Gentia'na Lu'te-a,* Gentia'na Ru'bra.* The gentian-plant; felwort.

Gentia'na Ra'dix.* ("Gentian Root.") See GENTIANA LUTEA.

Gentianaceæ,* jen-she-an-a'she-ē. [From *Gentia'na,* one of the genera.] A natural order of exogenous herbaceous plants, found in nearly all parts of the world. Their characteristic property is intense bitterness, which resides in the root, stem, leaf, etc., and renders them tonic, stomachic, and febrifugal. The gentian-root is an example. Some species are prized for their beauty.

Gen-tĭ-an-ā'ceous. [**Gentiana'ceus.**] Resembling the *Gentian* plant. See GENTIANACEÆ.

Gen-tĭ-a'næ Lu'te-æ Ra'dix.* ("Root of Gentiana Lutea.") See GENTIANA.

Gentianin, jen'she-a-nin. [**Gentiani'na.**] The bitter principle of the plant *Gentiana lutea.*

Gentianius, or **Gentianus.** See GENTIANACEOUS.

Ge'nu,* plural **Gen'u-a.** (Fr. *Genou,* zheh-noo'.) The knee; the articulation of the leg with the thigh.

Gen'u-a,* the plural of **Ge'nu,** the "knee."

Gen'ua Văl'ga.* [From *val'gus,* "crooked," or "bowed."] ("Bowed or Crooked Knees.") The deformity vulgarly called *knock-knees.*

Ge'nus,* gen. **Gen'e-ris.*** [From γένος, a "family."] A group or assemblage of species subordinate to a class or order.

Ge-o-cen'tric. [**Geocen'tricus;** from γῆ, or γέα, the "earth," and κεντρικός, "centric."] Having the earth for the centre. Applied to the place in which any heavenly body, as seen from the earth, appears.

Ge'ode. [**Geo'des;** from γῆ, or γέα, the "earth."] Belonging to earth; earthy. Applied in Mineralogy to a stone containing a cavity usually lined within with crystals, but sometimes containing loose earth or a nodule of stone. The term *Geode* is also applied to the cavity itself.

Ge-od'e-sy̆. [**Geodæ'sia;** from γῆ, or γέα, the "earth," and δαίω, to "divide."] That science by which the extent and figure of the earth (or of a portion of its surface) are ascertained.

Ge-of-fræ'a.* [Named after Dr. *Geoffroy.*] A Linnæan genus of the class *Diadelphia,* natural order *Leguminosæ,* or *Fabaceæ.*

Geoffræ'a In-er'mis.* The systematic name of the cabbage-tree.

Ge-o-gen'ĭ-cus.* Belonging to geogony: geogen'ic.

Geogeny. See GEOGONY.

Ge-og-nos'tic. [**Geognos'ticus.**] Belonging to geognosy.

Ge-og'no-sy̆. [**Geogno'sia;** from γῆ, or γέα, the "earth," and γνῶσις, "knowledge."] The knowledge or science of the structure of the globe. It may be regarded as essentially the same as GEOLOGY, which see.

Ge-og'o-ny̆, or **Ge-og'e-ny̆.** [**Geoge'nia;** from γῆ, or γέα, the "earth," and γένω, to "be born."] The doctrine of the formation of the earth.

Ge-og'ra-phy̆. [**Geogra'phia;** from γῆ, or γέα, the "earth," and γράφω, to "write."] A description of the known world, its mountains, seas, rivers, parts, limits, situation, and all other remarkable things belonging to it.

Ge-ol'o-gy̆. [**Geolo'gia;** from γῆ, or γέα, the "earth," and λόγος, a "discourse."] That branch of science which treats of the structure or formation of the earth, including the rocks, strata, etc., of which it is composed. It is distinguished from Mineralogy by treating of mineral substances in the aggregate, while Mineralogy is chiefly confined to the consideration of particular species.

Ge-o-met'ric, Ge-o-met'rĭ-cal. [**Geomet'ricus.**] Belonging to geometry.

Ge-om'e-try̆. [**Geome'tria;** from γῆ, or γέα, the "earth," and μετρέω, to "measure."] Originally, the art of measuring the earth, or any distance or dimensions on it. Now applied to the science of quantity and extension, irrespective of matter.

Ge-on'o-my̆. [**Geono'mia;** from γῆ, or γέα, the "earth," and νόμος, a "law."] That branch of general Physics which treats of the laws regulating the changes that have taken place, or are now taking place, in the structure of the earth, or in the atmosphere.

Ge-oph'ĭ-lus.* [From γῆ, or γέα, the "earth," and φιλέω, to "love."] Earth-loving. Applied as a specific name to plants that grow on the earth, to distinguish them from others of the same genus or order growing on trees, etc. Also applied in the plural neuter (*Geoph'ila*) to a division of *Gasteropoda* that live upon the land.

Geor'gĭ-a Bark. The bark of the *Pinckneya pubens,* an American plant, used as a substitute for *Cinchona.*

Ge-ra'nĭ-a,* plural of **Ge-ra'nĭ-um,** forming the Jussieuan name of a natural order of plants. See GERANIACEÆ.

Geraniaceæ,* je-ra-ne-a'she-ē, or **Ge-ra'nĭ-a.*** A natural order of exogenous plants, including the *Geranium.* An astringent principle and an aromatic or resinous flavor characterize this order.

Ge-ra'nĭ-um.* Cranesbill. The Pharmacopœial name (U.S. Ph.) for the rhizoma of *Gera'nium macula'tum.*

Ge-rat'ĭ-cus.* [From γῆρας, "old age."] Belonging to old age. Applied (in the plural, *Gerat'ici*) to an order of diseases.

Germ. [**Ger'men, Ger'minis.**] The first principle of any thing that has life, whether animal or vegetable. Applied in Botany to the *corculum* or embryo of a germinating seed, lying between the cotyledons, and constituting the exact point from which the life and organization of the future plant are to spring.

Ger'man Sil'ver (called by the Chinese **Packfong**). The white alloy of nickel, formed by fusing together one hundred parts of copper, sixty of zinc, and forty of nickel.

Ger'man Tin'der. (Fr. *Amadou,* å'må'doo'.) A substance prepared from the *Polyp'orus fomenta'rius* and *ignia'rius,* by cutting the fungi into slices, beating, and soaking them in a solution of nitre.

Ger'men,* gen. **Ger'mĭ-nis.** The rudiment of the young fruit and seed of vegetables at the base of the pistil; also the same as GERM, which see.

Germinal Membrane. See BLASTODERM.

Ger-mĭ-nā'tion. [**Germina'tio,**

o'*nis;* from *ger'mino, germina'tum,* to "bud."] The act of sprouting.

Ger-min'a-tive. [**Germinati'vus;** from the same.] Having power to bud, or develop.

Gĕr-o-co'mĭ-a.* [From γέρας, "old age," and κομέω, to "care for."] That department of hygiene which treats of the regimen and medical attention proper for old age.

Gérofle. The same as GIROFLE.

Ger-on-tox'on.* [From γέρων, γέροντος, an "old man," and τόξον, a "bow."] The same as ARCUS SENILIS, which see.

Gesneraceæ,*jes-ner-a'she-ē. [From *Gesne'ra,* one of the genera.] A natural order of exogenous plants (shrubs or herbs), found in India, Europe, etc.

Ges-tā'tion. [**Gesta'tio, o**'*nis;* from *ges'to, gesta'tum,* to "carry often," to "carry about" (from *ge'ro, ges'tum,* to "carry").] The condition of a pregnant female; pregnancy; gravidity, or uterine gestation. Also, applied to a species of exercise without bodily exertion; as swinging, riding in a carriage, or sailing.

Ge'um.* A Linnæan genus of the class *Icosandria,* natural order *Rosaceæ.* Also, the Pharmacopœial name (U.S. Ph.) for the root of *Ge'um riva'le* (Water Avens).

Ge'um Ur-ba'num.* The herb avens, or bennet.

G. G. G. = *Gum'mi Gut'tæ Gam'biæ.** "Gamboge."

Gib-bĭ-for'mis.* [From *gib'bus,* a "hump on the back."] Resembling a hump: gib'biform.

Gib-bos'ĭ-tў. [**Gibbos'itas, a**'*tis;* from *gib'bus,* "crooked," or "bossed."] The state of being irregularly swelled or bunched; crookedness.

Gib'bous. [**Gib'bus;** from ὕβος, the "hump on a camel's back."] Convex; bunched out.

Giddiness. See VERTIGO.

Gil-le'nĭ-a.* The Pharmacopœial name (U.S. Ph.) for the root of *Gille'nia trifolia'ta,* and of *Gille'nia stipula'cea.*

Gilliesiaceæ,* jil-le-se-a'she-ē. [From *Gillie'sia,* one of the genera.] A small natural order of endogenous and bulbous plants, found in Chili.

Gil-lĭ-flow'er, or **Gil'lў-Flow'er.** The *Dian'thus caryophyl'lus.*

Gills. [From *gu'la,* the "throat." Lat. **Bran'chiæ.**] The organs of respiration in fishes. See BRANCHIÆ.

Gimbernat's (jim-bęr-nats'; Sp. pron. Hĕm-bĕr-nât') **Lig'a-ment.** The broad, thin, triangular insertion of Poupart's ligament.

Gin. See GENEVA.

Gin'ger. The root of *Zingiber officinale.*

Gin-gī'va.* [Derived, according to some, from *gig'no,* to "beget," because they seem to produce the teeth.] (Fr. *Gencive,* zhŏnᴳ'sĕv'.) The gum; the highly vascular, fleshy substance covering the *alveoli,* and necks of the teeth.

Gin-gĭ-vi'tis, idis.* [From *gingi'va,* the "gum."] Inflammation of the gum.

Gin'glў-moid. [**Ginglymoi'des;** from γιγγλυμός, a "hinge," and εἶδος, a "form."] Resembling a hinge; hinge-like.

Gin'glў-mus.* [Gr. γιγγλυμός.] A species of diarthrosis. A hinge-like articulation, in which the bones move upon each other in two directions only, viz.: forwards and backwards. Examples occur in the elbow, the wrist, the knee, the ankle, the lower jaw, etc.

Gin'seng. [A Chinese word, signifying, it is said, the "power of man;" so called because it is supposed to increase virility.] The Chinese name of the root of the *Pa'nax quinquefo'lium.* See PANAX.

Girofle, zhē'rofl'. A French term for the "clove." See EUGENIA.

Giz'zard. [**Ventric'ulus Callo'sus.**] The proper stomach of birds.

Gla-bel'la.* [Diminutive of *gla'bra,* the feminine of *gla'ber,* "smooth."] The small space between the eyebrows, and immediately above a line from one to the other; also called INTERCILIUM.

Gla-bel'lar. [**Glabella'ris.**] Belonging to the *glabella.* The same as ANTINIAL.

Gla'brous. [**Gla'ber;** from γλαφυρός, "fair."] Without hairs or pubescence; smooth.

Glace, glâss. The French term for "ice." See GLACIES.

Glacial, glā'she-al. [**Glacia'lis;** from *gla'cies,* "ice."] Pertaining to ice; like ice; icy. The term is often applied to acids existing in a crystalline form like ice.

Gla'cial A-cet'ic Aç'id. The strongest acetic acid which can be procured. It exists in a *crystallized* state under 50° of Fahrenheit, and contains 79 per cent. of real acid. See ACETUM.

Gla'cial Phos-phor'ic Aç'id. [**Aç'idum Phosphor'icum Glacia'le.**] A colorless, glass-like substance, sometimes used as a tonic and refrigerant. It has been placed on the primary list of the Materia Medica in the U.S. Pharmacopœia for 1860.

Glacies,* gla'she-ēz. [From *gelas'co,* to "freeze."] The Latin term for "ice," or congealed water.

Glad'i-ate. [**Gladia'tus;** from *gla'dius,* a "sword."] Sword-like; ensiform.

Gla'dĭ-us Pis-to-rĭ-en'sis.* (A "Pistorian Sword-Knife.") A bistoury: so called because the town of *Pistori* was once famous for their manufacture. See BISTOURY.

Glăire, or **Glăir.** The white of egg.

Glair'in, or **Glair'ĭne.** [**Glairi'na.**] A peculiar vegetable or animal substance, somewhat resembling dried albumen (or glaire), produced at the sulphureous spring of Aix, in Savoy.

Glance. A name given to certain minerals which have a metallic or pseudometallic lustre, as glance coal, etc.

Gland. [**Glans, Glan'dis;** from *glans,* an "acorn."] An organ consisting of blood-vessels, absorbents, and nerves, for secreting or separating some particular fluid from the blood. Also, the bulbous extremity of the *penis* and *clitoris.* In Botany, applied to a secretory vessel.

Gland, Pain of. See ADENALGIA.

Glanders. See FARCY.

Glan'dĭ-form. [**Glandifor'mis.**] Formed or shaped like a gland. The same as ADENIFORM, and ADENOID.

Glan'dŭ-la.* [Diminutive of *glans.*] A little gland: a glan'dule.

Glandula Prostata Muliebris. See CORPUS GLANDULOSUM.

Glan'du-læ Ag-gre-ga'tæ,* or **Glan'dulæ Con-gre-ga'tæ.*** ("Aggregated or Clustered Glandules.") See PEYER'S GLANDS.

Glan'dulæ An-tĭ-pros-tat'ĭ-çæ.* The antiprostatic glandules or glands.

Glandulæ Brunneri. See BRUNNER'S GLANDS.

Glandulæ Cowperi. See GLANDULÆ ANTIPROSTATICÆ.

Glandulæ Meibomii. See MEIBOMIAN GLANDS.

Glandulæ Myrtiformes. See CARUNCULÆ MYRTIFORMES.

Glandulæ Nabothi, Glandulæ Nabothianæ. See NABOTH'S GLANDS.

Glandulæ Odoriferæ. See TYSONI GLANDULÆ.

Glandulæ Pacchioniæ. See PACCHIONIÆ, GLANDULÆ.

Glandulæ Solitariæ. See BRUNNER'S GLANDS.

Glandulæ Tysoni. See TYSONI GLANDULÆ.

Glan'du-lar. [**Glandula'rius,** from *glan'dula.*] Pertaining to, or like, a gland, in appearance, function, or structure.

Glan'du-lous. [**Glandulo'sus;** from *glan'dula.*] Having little elevations like glands.

Glans. See GLAND.

Glans Clĭ-tor'ĭ-dis.* A term applied to the extremity of the clitoris.

Glans Pe'nis.* The nut-like head of the *Mem'brum viri'le.*

Glaserian Fissure, or **Fissure of Glaserius.** See FISSURA GLASERII.

Glass. See CYATHUS.

Glass, Sol'u-ble, is formed by combining potash or soda with silicic acid or silica, without any third ingredient. It presents the usual vitreous aspect, but is easily dissolved in water. It is employed as a kind of paint for paper, cloth, wood, etc., to prevent or retard their inflammation on the contact of an ignited body.

Glau'ber's Salts. [**Sal Glau'beris.**] The sulphate of soda.

Glau-co'ma, atis.* [From γλαυκός, "blue green," also "light gray."] Dimness or defect of vision from opacity of the vitreous humor.

Glau-co-mat'ĭ-cus.* Pertaining to glaucoma.

Glau-com'a-tous, or **Glau-com'a-tose.** [**Glaucomato'des, Glaucomato'sus;** from *glauco'ma.*] Having glaucoma, or like glaucoma: green.

Glau-co'sis.* Another name for GLAUCOMA, which see.

Glau'cous. [**Glau'cus;** from γλαυκός, a "blue green," or "light gray."] Light gray. Applied to leaves or fruits covered with a whitish bloom which is easily rubbed off, as the cabbage-leaf or the plum.

Gleet. [Anglo-Saxon *Glidan,* to "glide," to "flow down gently."] A thin matter issuing out of ulcers, but generally applied to a result of gonorrhœal disease.

Gle'noid. [**Glenoi'des;** from γλήνη, a "cavity," and εἶδος, a "form."] Resembling a pit or cavity.

Gleucose. See GLUCOSE.

Gli'a-din. [**Gliadi'na;** from γλία, "glue."] One of the constituents of vegetable gluten.

Glis'son, Cap'sule of. [**Cap'sula Glisso'nii.**] A thin, strong sheath of peritonæum surrounding the vessels of the liver, and entering the transverse fissure, throughout the entire organ.

Glo'bate. [**Globa'tus;** from *glo'bus*, a "ball."] Shaped like a ball.

Glo'bose. [**Globo'sus;** from *glo'bus*, a "ball."] Round like a ball; globular.

Glob'u-lar. [**Globula'ris;** from *glo'bus*, a "globe."] Like a globe.

Glob'ule. [**Glob'ulus;** diminutive of *glo'bus*, a "globe."] Applied to such particles of matter as are of a globular or spherical figure, like the globules of the blood, or of milk.

Glob'u-lin, or **Glob'u-line.** [**Globuli'na;** from *glob'ulus*, a "globule."] The colorless substance which remains after the red coloring matter has been removed from the globules of the blood.

Glob'u-lism. [From *glob'ulus*, a "little globe," or "pill."] A name for *Homœopathy*.

Glo'bus Hys-tĕr'ĭ-cus.* ("Hysterical Ball.") A sensation as if a ball were ascending in the throat, caused by a portion of air arising in the *œsophagus*, and prevented from escaping by spasm.

Glo'bus Ma'jor.* The head of the *epididymis*.

Glo'bus Mi'nor.* The lower enlargement of the *epididymis*.

Glo-chid'ĭ-ate, Glo'chin-ate. [**Glochidia'tus, Glochina'tus;** from γλωχίς, the "point of a dart."] A botanical term signifying "barbed," bent back at the point, like the barb of a fish-hook.

Glom'er-ate. [**Glomera'tus;** from *glom'ero, glomera'tum*, to "wind on a ball" (from *glo'mus*, a "clue," or "ball").] Crowded together; congregated. Applied to glands formed of a clue, as it were, of sanguineous vessels having an excretory duct but no cavity.

Glom'e-rule. [**Glomeru'lus;** diminutive of *glo'mus*, a "clue of thread."] A botanical term signifying a small tuft or *capitulum*, mostly in the axilla of the peduncle.

Glos'sa.* [Gr. γλῶσσα.] The tongue; the chief organ of taste. See Tongue.

Glos'sa-gra.* [From γλῶσσα, the "tongue," and ἄγρα, a "seizure."] Violent pain in the tongue; nearly the same as *glossalgia*.

Glos-săl'ġĭ-a.* [From γλῶσσα, the "tongue," and ἄλγος, "pain."] Pain in the tongue. See Glossagra.

Glos-săl'ġĭ-cus.* Belonging to *glossalgia:* glossal'gic.

Glos-san'thrax, *acis*.* [From γλῶσσα, the "tongue," and ἄνθραξ, a "burning coal."] Carbuncle of the tongue, of rare occurrence in human beings, but not unfrequent in some domestic animals.

Glos-sep-ĭ-glot'tĭ-cus.* [From γλῶσσα, the "tongue," and *epiglot'tis*.] Belonging to the tongue and epiglottis. Applied to a ligament: glossepiglot'tic.

Glos-sit'ĭ-cus.* Belonging to *glossitis:* glossit'ic.

Glos-si'tis, *idis*.* [From γλῶσσα, the "tongue."] Inflammation of the tongue.

Glos-so-cat'o-chus.* [From γλῶσσα, the "tongue," and κατέχω, to "hold down."] An instrument for depressing the tongue.

Glos'so-çēle.* [From γλῶσσα, the "tongue," and κήλη, a "tumor."] Extrusion, or a hypertrophied condition of the tongue, causing it to be partially projected.

Glos-soc'o-mum.* [From γλῶσσα, the "tongue," and κομέω, to "guard."] Formerly, a case for the tongue of a hautboy; but, metaphorically, a kind of long box or case for containing a fractured leg.

Glos-sog'ra-phy̆. [**Glossogra'phia;** from γλῶσσα, the "tongue," and γράφω, to "write."] A description of the tongue.

Glos-so-hy̆'al. [**Glossohya'lis;** from γλῶσσα, the "tongue," and *hyoi'des*, "hyoid."] Applied by Geoffroy St. Hilaire to the posterior *cornua* of the hyoid bone, and by Owen to the *Os linguale* in birds and fishes.

Glos-so-i'dēs.* [From γλῶσσα, the "tongue," and εἶδος, a "form."] Resembling the tongue: glos'soid.

Glos-sol'o-ġy̆. [**Glossolo'gia;** from γλῶσσα, the "tongue," and λόγος, a "discourse."] A treatise on the powers and functions of the tongue; the science of the tongue. Also used nearly synonymously with Terminology.

Glos-sol'y̆-sis.* [From γλῶσσα, the "tongue," and λύσις, a "solution."] Paralysis of the tongue. See Glossoplegia.

Glossomantia,* glos-so-man'she-a. [From γλῶσσα, the "tongue," and μαντεία, a "divination."] Prognosis from the state of the tongue. See Glossoscopia.

Glosso-Pharyngeal. See Glosso-Pharyngeus.

Glos'so-Phăr-y̆n-ġe'al Nerves. Another name for the eighth pair.

Glos'so-Phăr-y̆n-ġe'us.* [From γλῶσσα, the "tongue," and φάρυγξ, the "pharynx."] Belonging to the tongue and pharynx. A synonym of the *constrictor superior* of the pharynx, from its origin in the root of the tongue, and its insertion into the pharynx.

Glos-so-ple'gi-a.* [From γλῶσσα, the "tongue," and πληγή, a "stroke."] Paralysis of the tongue: glos'soplegy.

Glos-sop-to'sis.* [From γλῶσσα, the "tongue," and πτῶσις, a "falling."] A falling or lengthening of the tongue.

Glos-sor-rha'gi-a.* [From γλῶσσα, the "tongue," and ῥήγνυμι, to "burst forth."] An incomplete term, intended to mean hæmorrhage from the tongue.

Glos-sor-rha'phi-a.* [From γλῶσσα, the "tongue," and ῥαφή, a "suture."] The suture, or sewing up of a wound, of the tongue.

Glos-sos-co'pi-a.* [From γλῶσσα, the "tongue," and σκοπέω, to "examine."] Examination of the tongue, as a principal means of diagnosis: glossos'copy.

Glos-so-staph-y̆-li'nus.* [From γλῶσσα, the "tongue," and σταφυλή, the "uvula."] A designation of the *constrictor isthmi faucium*, from its origin in the tongue and its insertion into the uvula.

Glos-sos-te-re'sis.* [From γλῶσσα, the "tongue," and στερέω, to "deprive."] Excision or extirpation of the tongue.

Glos-sot'o-my̆. [**Glossoto'mia;** from γλῶσσα, the "tongue," and τέμνω, to "cut."] Dissection of the tongue.

Glos-sy'per-tro'phi-a.* [From γλῶσσα, the "tongue," and *hypertro'phia*, "hypertrophy."] Hypertrophy of the tongue: glossyper'trophy.

Glot-ti-do-spas'mus.* [From *glot'tis*, and *spas'mus*, a "spasm."] Spasm of the glottis.

Glot'tis, idis.* [Gr. γλωττίς, the small chink or aperture of a pipe.] The aperture of the larynx.

Glot-ti'tis.* Inflammation of the glottis.

Glu-çi'na,* or **Glu'çine.** [From γλυκύς, "sweet."] One of the primitive earths.

Glu-çin'i-ŭm,* or **Glu-çi'num.*** The metallic base of *glucina*.

Glu'cose. [From γλυκύς, "sweet."] A kind of sugar obtained from grapes; also from starch and sulphuric acid.

Glue. [Lat. **Glu'ten,** or **Glu'ti-num;** Gr. γλία, "paste," or "glue."] A jelly obtained by boiling the parings of hides and other offal.

Glu-co-su'ri-a.* [From *glucose*, and οὖρον, "urine."] Applied to the urine in *diabetes mellitus*.

Glu-mā'ceous. [**Gluma'ceus;** from *glu'ma*, a "glume."] Having glumes; like a glume.

Glume. [**Glu'ma;** from *glu'bo*, to "pull off bark."] The husk of corn; chaff; a species of calyx peculiar to corn and grasses.

Glumous. See GLUMACEOUS.

Glu-tæ'us.* [From γλουτός, the "buttock."] (Fr. *Fessier*, fĕs'se-à'.) The name of three muscles forming the greater part of the fleshy mass beneath the ischia. They are termed the *Glutæus maximus*, the *Glutæus medius*, and the *Glutæus minimus*. Belonging to the buttock: glute'al.

Glu'ten,* gen. **Glu'ti-nis.** Glue. Usually applied to vegetable gluten, or the residue after the farina of wheat has been deprived of its starch; paste.

Glu'ten, An'i-mal. The same as GELATINE, which see.

Gluten, Vegetable. See GLUTEN.

Glu'tin, or **Glu'tĭne.** [**Gluti'na;** from *glu'ten*, "glue."] A distinct form of gelatine obtained from common glue, of which it forms the chief ingredient.

Glutineux. See GLUTINOUS.

Glu'tin-ous. [Lat. **Glutino'sus;** Fr. *Glutineux*, glü'tè'nuh'.] Having the properties of gluten; gluey; adhesive.

Glutinum. See GLUE.

Glu-ti'tis, idis.* [From γλουτός, the "buttock."] Inflammation of the buttocks, or of the *glutæi* muscles.

Gly̆ç'er-id, or **Gly̆ç'er-ide.** A compound of glycerin with a fatty acid.

Gly̆ç'er-in, or **Gly̆ç'er-ine.** [**Gly̆ç-eri'na;** from γλυκύς, "sweet."] A yellowish, transparent, syrup-like fluid, without smell, and of a sweet taste, obtained from the residue in making litharge plaster, and from the refuse in the manufacture of soap, etc. It is alterative and demulcent.

Gly̆ç-er-i'na.* The Pharmacopœial name (U.S. Ph.) for GLYCERIN, which see.

Gly̆ç'i-coll. [**Glycicol'la;** from γλυκύς, "sweet," and κόλλα, "glue."] Sugar of gelatine, obtained by boiling gluten in an excess of caustic alkali.

Glycocholic. See TAUROCHOLIC.

Gly̆c'o-gen. [From *glu'cose*, and γεννάω, to "produce."] Literally, "producing glucose." A peculiar substance in the tissue of the liver, which may be changed into glucose.

Gly̆ç'y̆r-rhi'za.* [From γλυκύς, "sweet," and ῥίζα, a "root."] The Pharmacopœial name ‖ for the root of *Glycyrrhiza glabra;* the *Glycyrrhizæ Radix* of the Edinburgh and Dublin Pharmacopœias.

Glycyrrhi'za Gla'bra.* The liquorice-plant.

Glȳ-çȳr'rhī-zin. [**Glycyrrhizi'na.**] The saccharine juice of the *Glycyrrhiza*, or liquorice-plant.

Glȳ-phog'ra-phȳ. [**Glyphogra'phia**; from γλυφή, a "carving" or "graving," and γράφω, to "paint."] A new kind of engraved drawing, by which prints are produced in colors from the printing-press.

Glyster. See CLYSTER, and ENEMA.

Gna-thăl'ğĭ-a* (na-thăl'je-a). [From γνάθος, the "jaw," or "cheek," and ἄλγος, "pain."] Pain of the jaw or cheek.

Gna-thit'ĭ-cus.* Belonging to *gnathitis*.

Gna-thi'tis, *idis*.* [From γνάθος, the "jaw," or "cheek."] Internal inflammation of the cheek or *maxilla*.

Gnath-o-neū-răl'ğĭ-a.* [From γνάθος, the "jaw," or "cheek," νεῦρον, a "nerve," and ἄλγος, "pain."] Pain of a nerve of the cheek, or *maxilla*; maxillary neuralgia.

Gnath-o-plas'tic. [**Gnathoplas'ticus.**] Belonging to gnathoplasty.

Gnath'o-plas-tȳ. [**Gnathoplas'tia**; from γνάθος, the "jaw," or "cheek," and πλάσσω, to "form."] Operation for repairing any deficiency of the cheek by appropriating a sufficient portion of the sound parts contiguous.

Gnetaceæ,* ne-ta'she-ē. A natural order of plants (Gymnogens), found in the temperate parts of Europe, Asia, and South America. It includes *Gne'tum*, and one other genus.

Gōad'bȳ's So-lu'tion. A preparation for preserving animal substances, made with bay-salt, corrosive sublimate or arsenious acid, and water.

God'frey's Cor'dĭ-al. A quack medicine, composed of an infusion of sassafras, coriander, caraway, and aniseseeds, treacle, and laudanum.

Goître. (French, probably derived from *guttur*, the "throat.") A Swiss term for BRONCHOCELE, which see.

Gold. [Lat. **Au'rum**; Fr. *Or*, OR.] A yellow metal, of great malleability and ductility. It is found generally native, either massive, or disseminated in threads through a rock, or in grains among the sands of rivers. Gold is remarkable for resisting, under all circumstances, the action of the air and of the ordinary acids. It is, however, dissolved by chlorine and by nitro-muriatic acid, forming a chloride of gold. The specific gravity of gold is 19.3, it being, next to platinum, the heaviest of all metals.

Gold-Leaf E-lec-trom'e-ter. An instrument for detecting the presence of electricity by the divergence of two slips of gold-leaf.

Gomme, gomm. The French term for GUM, which see.

Gom-pho'sis.* [From γομφόω, to "drive in a nail."] A variety of *Synarthrosis*, in which one bone is fixed in another like a nail in wood, as the teeth in their sockets.

Gon-a-cra'tĭ-a.* [From γονή, "semen," and ἀκρατής, "impotent," or "incontinent."] *Gonorrhœa*, in its proper signification, being the same as *Spermatorrhœa*, arising from debility induced by excess.

Gon'a-gra.* [From γόνυ, the "knee," and ἄγρα, a "seizure."] Gout in the knee, or knee-joint.

Gon-ar-thri'tis, *idis*.* [From γόνυ, the "knee," and ἄρθρον, a "joint."] Inflammation of the knee-joint; also, of the knee.

Gon-ar-throc'a-cē.* [From γόνυ, the "knee," ἄρθρον, a "joint," and κάκη, "evil," or "disease."] A cancerous or ulcerated condition of the knee-joint.

Gon-e-çȳs'tis.* [From γονή, "semen," and κύστις, a "bladder."] Applied in the plural (*Gonecys'tides*) to the seminal vesicles.

Gon-e-poi-e'sis.* [From γονή, "semen," and ποιέω, to "make."] The secretion of the semen.

Gon-e-poi-et'ic. [**Gonepoiet'icus.**] Belonging to *gonepoiesis*.

Gonflement, gôNfl'mŏNᵍ'. The French term for "swelling." See TUMEFACTION.

Gong Met'al. An alloy of eighty parts of copper and twenty of tin.

Gon'gȳle. [Lat. **Gon'gylus**; Gr. γογγύλος, "round."] A round, hard body prolonged from the wood into the bark of the plant, and detached by the progress of age.

Gon'gȳ-lus.* [Gr. γογγύλος, "round."] Round; globular: gon'gylous.

Go-nĭ-om'e-ter. [**Goniom'etrum**; from γωνία, an "angle," and μέτρον, a "measure."] An instrument for measuring the angles of crystals.

Go-noc'a-cē.* [From γόνυ, the "knee," and κάκη, an "evil."] White swelling of the knee.

Gon'o-çēle.* [From γονή, "semen," and κήλη, a "tumor."] Effusion of semen out of the ruptured seminal vesicles, into the cellular texture; also, a swelling of the testicle and spermatic cord, from supposed retention of the semen.

Go'noid. [**Gonoi'des;** from γονή, "semen," and εἶδος, a "form."] Resembling the semen.

Gon'o-phore. [**Gonoph'orus;** from γόνος, "seed," "offspring," and φέρω, to "bear."] In Botany, a prolongation of the receptacle which proceeds from the bottom of the calyx, and sustains the stamens and pistil.

Gon-o-phy̆-se'ma, a*tis.** [From γόνυ, the "knee," and φύσημα, an "inflation."] The same as GONOCACE, GONYOCELE, GONYONCUS, which see.

Gonopoesis. See GONEPOIESIS.

Gon'or-rho-bleph'ar-rhœ'a.* [From γονόῤῥοια, a "flow of semen," βλέφαρον, the "eyelid," and ῥέω, to "flow."] Gonorrhœal inflammation, and discharge of purulent matter from the eye and eyelids. See OPHTHALMIA.

Gonorrhœa,* gon-or-rē'a. [From γονή, "semen," and ῥέω, to "flow."] Involuntary discharge of semen without copulation. The same as SPERMATORRHŒA. Applied, however (erroneously, if we regard the etymology), to a discharge of purulent infectious matter from the urethra of males, the vagina, labia, nymphæ, clitoris, frequently the mouth and neck of the uterus, and sometimes the urethra, of females. A genus of the order *Apocenoses*, class *Locales*, of Cullen's Nosology.

Gonorrhœ'a Bal'a-ni.* [From *bal'anus*, the "glans penis."] A purulent discharge from the surface of the entire *glans penis*, which is then in a highly inflamed and raw state.

Gonorrhœa Dormientium. See SPERMATORRHŒA DORMIENTIUM.

Gon-or-rhœ'al. [**Gonorrho'icus.**] Belonging to *gonorrhœa.*

Gon'or-rho-pros'ta-ti'tis, i*dis.** Inflammation of the prostate gland produced by *gonorrhœa.*

Go-nos'che-o-çēle.* [From γονή, "semen," ὄσχεον, the "scrotum," and κήλη, a "tumor."] Swelling of the testicle, or epididymis, from accumulation of the semen: spermatocele.

Gon-os-per'mous. [**Gonosper'mus;** from γωνία, an "angle," and σπέρμα, a "seed."] Having angular seeds.

Gon-os-tro'ma, a*tis.** [From γόνος, "offspring," and στρῶμα, a "stratum," or "bed."] A gon'ostrome. The germinal layer or bed in the ovule of *Mammalia;* the *Stratum proligerum* of Baer.

Go'ny̆-ăl'gĭ-a.* [From γόνυ, the "knee," and ἄλγος, "pain."] Pain in the knee.

Go'ny̆-o-cam'psis.* [From γόνυ, the "knee," and κάμψις, a "curvature."] Curvature of the knees.

Go'ny̆-o-çēle.* [From γόνυ, the "knee," and κήλη, a "tumor."] White swelling, or what has been called hernia of the knee.

Go'ny̆-on'cus.* [From γόνυ, the "knee," and ὄγκος, a "tumor."] Swelling, or tumor, of the knee. See GONYOCELE.

Gon-y̆-ty'le.* [From γόνυ, the "knee," and τύλη, a "callus."] Callus, or a hard thick skin, of the knee.

Goodeniaceæ,* goo-de-ne-a'she-ē. A natural order of exogenous plants, mostly herbaceous, found in Australia.

Goose-Skin. See CUTIS ANSERINA.

Gor'dĭ-us,* called also **Se'ta E-qui'na,*** or "horse-hair." The horse-hair worm of the old writers. It is supposed to occasion *Intestinal disease*, occurring among the peasantry of Lapland from drinking water containing this worm; and *Cuticular disease* when it is lodged under the skin, constituting the *morbus pilaris* of Horst, and the *malis à crinonibus* of Sauvages.

Gordius Medinensis. See GUINEA-WORM.

Gor'get. An instrument for the operation of lithotomy, formed like a knife, with a beak which fits the groove in the staff.

Gos-sy̆p'ĭ-i Ra'dix.* ("Root of Gossypium.") The Pharmacopœial name (U.S. Ph.) for the root of the *Gossypium herbaceum* and other species of *Gossypium.*

Gos-sy̆p'ĭ-um.* [**Gossip'ion.**] A Linnæan genus of cotton-producing plants, class *Monadelphia*, natural order *Malvaceæ.* Also, the Pharmacopœial name (U.S. Ph.) for cotton, a filamentous substance separated from the seed of *Gossypium herbaceum*, and of other species of *Gossypium.*

Gossyp'ium Herba'ceum* (her-ba'she-ŭm). The systematic name of the cotton-plant.

Goulard's (goo'lardz') **Ce'rate.** The *Ceratum plumbi subacetatis.* It received its name from Goulard (Fr. pron. goo'lar'), a Frenchman, by whom it was introduced to the notice of the public. Its refrigerant properties often render it a most useful and grateful application to blistered surfaces indisposed to heal; also, to burns, excoriations, and cutaneous eruptions, especially if attended with much heat or irritation of the surface.

Gou'lard's' Ex'tract. The *Liquor plumbi subacetatis.*

Gōurd. [**Cucur'bita.**] The fruit of the *Cucurbita pepo;* also, the plant itself.

Gourd, Bit'ter. The *Cucumis colocynthis,* plant and fruit.

Gout. [From the Latin *gut'ta;* Fr. *Goutte,* goott, a "drop;" so named from the idea that the disease was produced by a morbid fluid gradually distilling into the part.] *Arthri'tis,* characterized by pain in the joints, chiefly of the great toe, or of the feet and hands; also termed PODAGRA, which see.

Gout'-Stone. The *Cal'culus arthrit'icus,* or *podag'ricus.* A stony concretion deposited in the affected part in gout.

Goutte. See GOUT.

Gr. = *Gra'num,** or *Gra'na.** A "grain," or "grains."

Grāā'fĭ-an Fol'lĭ-cles [**Follic'uli Graafia'ni**], or **Graa'fian Ves'ĭ-cles** [**Vesic'ulæ Graafia'næ**]. Applied to small spherical bodies found in the stroma of the ovary. They consist of two coats or layers. The interior, immediately enclosing the *ovum,* is termed the *ovisac.*

Graç'ĭ-lis.* ("Slender.") Applied to a slender muscle of the thigh, and to a process of the *malleus,* an ossicle of the ear.

Grad'u-āt-ed Com'press. A compress formed of a number of circular pieces of cotton cloth, progressively decreasing in size, the whole forming a sort of pyramid, the apex of which can be applied on the precise point wished, in cases of wounded arteries, etc.

Grain. [Lat. **Gra'num;** Fr. *Graine,* grĕn or grȧn.] Literally, "a grain or seed of wheat, barley," etc. In Pharmacy, the twentieth part of a scruple, or sixtieth of a drachm.

Graines d'Avignon. See FRENCH BERRIES.

Grains of Paradise. See AMOMUM GRANA PARADISI.

Graisse, grĕss or grȧss. The French term for "fat." See ADEPS.

Gral'læ,* gen. **Gral-la'rum,** used only in the plural. (Literally, "stilts.") Another term for GRALLATORES.

Gral-la-to'rēs.* [The plural of *gralla'tor,* "one who goes on stilts."] The name of an order of waders, or wading birds, having long legs and bills, by which they wade and catch their prey in the water. Also termed *Grallæ, Grallatoriæ, Grallidæ.*

Gral-la-to'rĭ-us.* [From *gral'læ,* "stilts."] Belonging to stilts or crutches. Sometimes applied in the plural feminine (*Grallato'riæ*) to an order of birds. See GRALLATORES.

Gra'men Ca-ni'num.* The *Triticum repens,* couch-grass, or dog's-grass.

Gram'ĭ-na,* the plural of *gra'men,* "grass," forming the Jussieuan name of a natural order of plants. See GRAMINACEÆ.

Graminaceæ,* gram-ĭ-na'she-ē. [From *gra'men,* "grass."] An important natural order of endogenous plants, very widely distributed. It includes the grasses, wheat, maize, and various other kinds of cultivated cereals, the sugar-cane, and the bamboo. Their habits are gregarious or social. Some tropical species assume the form of trees, and attain the height of fifty feet. Sugar is a general product of this order, and silex is found in the cuticle of many species.

Gram-ĭ-nā'ceous, Gra-min'e-ous. [**Gramina'ceus, Gramin'eus;** from *gra'men,* "grass."] Belonging to grass; grass-like.

Gram-ĭ-nic'o-lus.* [From *gra'men,* "grass," and *co'lo,* to "inhabit."] Growing among grass; as, *Agaricus graminicola,* etc.

Gram-ĭ-nĭ-fo'lĭ-ous. [**Graminifo'lius;** from *gra'men,* "grass," and *fo'lium,* a "leaf."] Having leaves like those of grass.

Gram'ĭ-nĭ-form. [**Graminifor'mis;** from *gra'men,* "grass."] Resembling grass.

Gram-ĭ-niv'o-rous. [**Graminiv'orus;** from *gra'men,* "grass," and *vo'ro,* to "devour."] Feeding upon grass.

Gram-ĭ-nol'o-ġȳ. [**Graminolo'gia;** from *gra'men,* "grass," and λόγος, a "discourse."] A treatise on the grasses; the science of grasses.

Gram'ma, *atis.** [From γράμμα, a "letter," a "note" or "point" in music; and, hence, a scruple, the smallest of Roman weights.] A scruple; the twenty-fourth part of an ounce. See SCRUPULUS.

Gram'mē.* [From γραμμή, a "letter," or "line."] Another name for the iris, because it has the appearance of minute lines drawn upon it. See IRIS.

Gramme, grăm. A French weight, equal to 15.434 grains troy.

Gra'na, the plural of GRANUM, which see.

Grana Paradisi. See AMOMUM GRANA PARADISI.

Gra'na Se-ca'lis De-ġen-er-a'ti.* ("Seeds of Degenerate [or Diseased] Rye.") See ERGOT.

Gra'na Tig'lĭ-i.* The seeds of the *Croton tiglium.*

Granadia. See next article.

Gran'a-din, or **Gran'a-dine.** [**Grana'dia.**] A white, crystalline, volatile, and exceedingly sweet substance, neither alkaline nor acid, obtained from the root of the pomegranate, *Pu'nica grana'tum;* and now decided to be mannite.

Gra-na'ti Fruc'tûs Cor'tex.* ("Rind of the Pomegranate Fruit.") The Pharmacopœial name (U.S. Ph.) for the rind of the fruit of the *Pu'nica grana'tum.*

Grana'ti Ra-di'cis Cor'tex.* ("Bark of Pomegranate Root.") The Pharmacopœial name (U.S. Ph.) for the bark of the root of the *Pu'nica grana'tum.*

Gran-dĭ-den-ta'tus.* [From *gran'dis,* "large," and *dens,* a "tooth."] Having large teeth, or indentations: granditen'tate.

Gran-dĭ-flo'rus.* [From *gran'dis,* "large," and *flos,* a "flower."] Having large flowers: grandiflo'rate.

Gran-dĭ-fo'lĭ-us.* [From *gran'dis,* "large," and *fo'lium,* a "leaf."] Having large leaves: grandifo'liate.

Gran'dĭ-nēs,* the plural of *gran'do,* a "hailstone." A term applied by Wesser to tubercles as they become enlarged.

Gran-dĭ-no'sus.* [From *gran'do, gran'dinus,* "hail."] Literally, "full of hail;" also, "resembling a hailstone." Applied to the *Os cuboides,* from its irregular form.

Gran'do,* gen. **Gran'dĭ-nis.** ("Hail, or Hailstone.") A small, hard tumor on the eyelid, supposed to resemble a hailstone. See CHALAZA.

Gra-nif'er-ous. [**Gran'ifer;** from *gra'num,* a "grain," and *fe'ro,* to "bear."] Bearing or producing grain.

Gran'ite. [**Grani'tes;** from *gra'num,* a "grain."] A kind of primitive rock, consisting essentially of quartz, felspar, and mica.

Gran-it'ic. [**Granit'icus.**] Belonging to granite.

Gra-niv'o-rous. [**Graniv'orus;** from *gra'num,* a "grain," and *vo'ro,* to "devour."] Eating grain.

Gran'u-lar. [**Granula'ris;** from *gran'ulum,* a "little grain."] (Fr. *Granuleux,* gRå'nü'luh'.) In the form of grains; of the nature or appearance of granulations.

Gran'u-lāt-ed. [**Granula'tus;** from the same.] Having grains, or granular.

Gran-u-lā'tion. [**Granula'tio, o'nis;** from the same.] The division of metallic substances into small particles, or grains, to facilitate their combination with other substances. Also, the process by which little grain-like, fleshy bodies form on ulcers and suppurating wounds, filling up the cavities, and bringing nearer together and uniting their sides.

Gran'ule. [**Gran'ulum;** the diminutive of *gra'num,* a "grain."] A little grain.

Granuleux. See GRANULAR.

Gran'u-lĭ-cau'lis.* [From *gran'ulum,* a "little grain," and *cau'lis,* a "stem."] Having stem and branches covered with little tubercles.

Gran-u-lif'er-ous. [**Granu'lifer;** from *gran'ulum,* a "little grain," and *fe'ro,* to "bear."] Bearing granules; as the shell of the *Mitra granulifera.*

Gran'u-lĭ-form. [**Granulifor'mis;** from *gran'ulum,* a "little grain."] Resembling little grains.

Gran-u-los'ĭ-tȳ. [**Granulos'itas, a'tis;** from the same.] A mass of small tubercles, like granules.

Gran'u-lous. [**Granulo'sus;** from the same.] Having granules; full of granules.

Gra'num,* plural **Gra'na.** A grain; a small seed of any kind. The sixtieth part of a drachm, or twentieth of a scruple.

Grape-Sugar. See GLUCOSE.

Graph-ĭ-o-i'dēs.* [From γραφίς, a "style," or "writing-instrument," and εἶδος, a "form."] Resembling a style; styloid. Applied to the styloid process of the temporal bone.

Graph'ite. [From γράφω, to "write," and λίθος, a "stone;" from its use in making pencils.] Plumbago, or black lead.

Grass Oil of Na'mur. A volatile oil, procured, according to Boyle, from the *Andropogon Calamus aromaticus.* It is sometimes incorrectly called *oil of spikenard.*

Gratiola (grash'e-o-la) **Of-fiç-ĭ-na'lis.*** The systematic name of the hedge-hyssop.

Gra-ve'do, dinis.* [From *gra'vis,* "heavy."] Literally, "heaviness." A term for *coryza;* so called, probably, from the sense of weight or oppression experienced in a severe catarrh.

Grav'el. [Lat. **Lithi'asis;** Fr. *Gravelle,* grå'vĕll'; from the French *gravier,* grå've'å', "gravel" or "coarse sand."] A popular term applied either to calculous matter formed in the kidneys, passing off in the urine, or to small distinct *calculi* or concretions. It is distinguished from *stone in the bladder* by being of smaller size. See CALCULUS.

Gravelle. See GRAVEL.

Grave'-Wax. Adipocere.

Grav'id U'ter-us. [**U'terus Grav'idus.**] The womb in the impregnated state, or during gestation.

Gra-vid'ĭ-tȳ. [**Gravid'itas, a'**_tis_; from _grav'idus,_ "pregnant."] The condition of a woman who is pregnant; gestation; pregnancy.

Grav-ĭ-gra'di-us.* [From _gra'vis,_ "heavy," and _gra'dior,_ to "march."] Walking with a heavy tread. Applied in the plural neuter (_Gravigra'dia_) to an order of Mammals, as the elephant, etc.

Grav-im'e-ter. [**Gravim'etrum;** from _gra'vis,_ "heavy," and μέτρον, a "measure."] An instrument for ascertaining the specific gravity of bodies.

Grav-ĭ-tā'tion. [**Gravita'tio, o'**_nis;_ from _grav'itas,_ "weight."] That power or tendency by which all material bodies are drawn towards each other, or by which a stone or other body on the surface of the earth is drawn towards the centre.

Grav'ĭ-tȳ. [**Grav'itas, a'**_tis;_ from _gra'vis,_ "heavy."] The cause or power by which bodies naturally tend towards the centre of the earth; weight.

Gravity, Centre of. See CENTRE OF GRAVITY.

Grav'ity, Spe-cif'ic. The comparative density (or gravity) of one body considered in relation to another assumed as the standard. In measuring the specific gravity of liquids or solids, water is usually taken as the standard of comparison, being reckoned as a unit; in measuring gases, common air or hydrogen is assumed as the standard.

Great Sympathetic Nerve. See TRISPLANCHNIC NERVE.

Gre'ci-an Wa'ter. A solution of nitrate of silver disguised, for dyeing the hair black; the hair thus dyed soon becomes purple on exposure to the light.

Green Milk. See COLOSTRUM.

Green Sickness. See CHLOROSIS.

Green Vit'ri-ol. The sulphate of iron.

Green Wa'ters. Popularly, the _Lochia,_ when of a dark, dirty, greenish aspect.

Grenadia. See GRANADIN.

Grey Lo'tion. The _Lotio nigra._

Grif'fith's Mix'ture, otherwise called **Mis-tu'ra Fer'ri Com-pos'ĭ-ta*** ("Compound Mixture of Iron"). It is composed chiefly of myrrh, carbonate of potash, sulphate of iron, and spirit of lavender. It is used as a tonic in dyspepsia, chlorosis, and similar affections.

Grippe, grĭp or grĕp. The French name for INFLUENZA, which see.

Groats, grawts. The decorticated grains of the common oat.

Gro'cer's Itch. The _ecze'ma impetigino'des_ of some writers. See ACARUS SACCHARI.

Groin. See INGUEN.

Grooved. See SULCATED.

Grossesse, gro'sĕss'. The French term for PREGNANCY, which see.

Grossulaceæ,* gros-u-la'she-ē, or **Gros-su-la-ri-a'ce-æ.*** [From _gros'sula,_ a "gooseberry," _grossula'ria,_ a "gooseberry-bush."] A natural order of exogenous shrubs, found in the temperate parts of Europe, Asia, and America. It includes the currant and gooseberry.

Gros'su-line. [From _gros'sula,_ a "gooseberry."] The name given by Guibourt to a peculiar principle procured from gooseberries and other acid fruits, forming the basis of jelly.

Grot'to del Ca'ne (kå'nå). ("Dog's Grotto.") A grotto near Naples, in which carbonic acid gas rises about eighteen inches above the surface of the ground, so that it affects dogs and other small animals.

Growth. [Lat. **Incremen'tum;** Fr. _Croissance,_ krwå'sŏnss'.] Increase or augmentation of the body in all its parts, without reference to the peculiar structure, or function, and, so, distinct from, though nearly connected with, _Development._

Grub. The larva of insects; also, a sort of maggot, hatched from the egg of the beetle (_Scarabæ'us_).

Gru'mous. [**Grumo'sus;** from _gru'mus,_ a "clot."] Thickened; clotted; curdled.

Gru'mus.* A clot of milk, or of blood; a curd.

Gru'tum,* or **Gru'tum Mil'ĭ-um.*** A small white tubercle of the skin, resembling a millet-seed.

Grȳl'lus Ver-ru-cĭv'o-rus.* [From _verru'ca,_ a "wart," and _vo'ro,_ to "eat."] The wart-eating grasshopper of Sweden, which is caught for the purpose, as it is said, of biting off the excrescence, when it also discharges a corrosive liquor on the wound.

Gtt. = _Gut'ta,*_ a "drop," or _Gut'tæ,*_ "drops."

Guaiac, gwī'ak or gwā'ak. The same as GUAIACI RESINA, which see.

Guaiacanæ,* gwī-ạ-ka'nē. The Jussieuan name of a natural order of plants. See EBENACEÆ.

Guai'aci (gwī'ạ-si) **Lig'num.*** ("Wood of Guaiacum.") The Pharmacopœial name ‖ for the wood of the *Guai'acum officina'le*, popularly called *Lig'num Vi'tæ* ("Wood of Life"), in allusion to its great medicinal virtues. It is a stimulant diaphoretic, and is principally used in cases of secondary syphilis and other diseases dependent on a vitiated condition of the system.

Guai'aci Re-si'nạ.* ("Resin of Guaiacum.") Guaiac. The Pharmacopœial name ‖ for the concrete juice of the *Guai'acum officina'le*. It is alterative and stimulant, and is much used as a remedy in rheumatism.

Guaiacin, or **Guaiacine,** gwī'ạ-sin. A resinoid principle found in guaiac. It differs from most other resins, by being converted by nitric acid into oxalic acid, instead of artificial tannin.

Guaiacum,* gwī'ạ-kŭm or gwā'ạ-kŭm. (Sp. *Guaiaco*, gwå-yå'ko.) The guaiac-tree; a Linnæan genus of the class *Decandria*, natural order *Rutaceæ*. Also, the Pharmacopœial name (Lond. and Ed. Ph.) for the resin obtained from the *Guai'acum officina'le*.

Guai'acum Lig'num.* The Pharmacopœial name (Lond. and Ed. Ph.) for the wood of *Guaiacum officinale*.

Guai'acum Of-fiç-ĭ-na'le.* The tree which yields *Guaiacum*.

Guano, gwå'no. (Said to be derived from the Peruvian *Huanu*, hwå'-noo, "dung.") A species of manure recently discovered and much employed, on account of its great strength as a fertilizer. It is the excrement of sea-fowl, usually deposited on small islands and cliffs near the coast. In some places it is found in such enormous beds as could only be produced by the accumulation of thousands of years.

Gu-ber-nac'u-lum.* [From *guber'-no, guberna'tum*, to "guide," to "govern."] Something which guides or directs. See next article.

Gubernac'ulum Tes'tis.* A fibro-vascular cord between the testicle and scrotum in the fœtus. So named because it is supposed to guide the testicle in its descent from the abdomen.

Guin'ea (ğin'e) **Grains.** Another name for Malaguetta pepper. See AMOMUM GRANA PARADISI.

Guinea Pepper. See CAPSICUM ANNUUM.

Guin'ea Worm, otherwise called **Ma'lis Fi-la'rĭ-æ*** (which is equivalent to "skein worm," so called because it is wound off like a skein of thread). A worm found chiefly in the East and West Indies. It is said to be frequently twelve feet long, and about the thickness of a horse-hair; it burrows under the cuticle, and "may be felt under the skin, and traced by the fingers like the string of a violin. . . . It should be drawn out with great caution, by means of a piece of silk tied round its head; for if, by being too much strained, the animal break, the part remaining under the skin will grow with double vigor, and often occasion a fatal inflammation."—(GOOD.)

Guin'ea-hen Weed. The vulgar name of the *Peteve'ria Allia'cea*, an extremely acrid plant, used in Jamaica as a sialagogue.

Gul, gŏŏl. A Persian word signifying a "rose."

Gul Attar. See ATTAR OF ROSES.

Gu'lạ.* The *œsophagus*, or gullet; popularly, the throat.

Gum. = *Gum'mi.** "Gum."

Gum. [Lat. **Gum'mi;** Fr. *Gomme*, gomm.] The mucilage of vegetables.

Gum Arabic. See GUMMI ACACIÆ.

Gum Boil. [**Paru'lis.**] Inflammation, abscess, or boil of the gums.

Gum E-las'tic. A term for *Caoutchouc*.

Gum Ju'nĭ-per. A concrete resin which exudes in white tears from the *Junip'erus commu'nis*. It has been called *sandarach*, and, hence, confounded with the σανδαράχη of Aristotle, which was a sulphuret of arsenic. Reduced to powder it is called *pounce*, which prevents ink from sinking into paper from which the exterior coating of size has been scraped away.

Gum of the Teeth. See GINGIVA.

Gum, Rank Red. The common name for the *Stroph'ulus confer'tus*.

Gum Rash. Red gum. A genus of cutaneous diseases. See STROPHULUS.

Gum, Red. The common name for *Stroph'ulus intertinc'tus*.

Gum Res'in. [**Gum'mi-Resi'na.**] The concrete juice of certain plants, consisting of resin, essential oil, gum, and extractive vegetable matter; as aloes, ammoniac, assafœtida, euphorbium, scammony, &c.

Gum, White. The common name for *Stroph'ulus al'bidus*. See STROPHULUS.

Gum'mạ.* A soft tumor, so named

from the resemblance of its contents to gum.

Gum'mi Aca'ciæ*(a-ka'she-ē). The Pharmacopœial name (Ed. Ph.) of gum Arabic, obtained from the *Acacia vera*, and other species of *Acacia*.

Gummi Rubrum Gambiense. See KINO.

Gum'mi Scor-pĭ-o'nis,* Gum'mi Sen'e-gạ,* Gum'mi Sen-e-gal-en'-sē,* Gum'mi The-ba'ĭ-cum.* Names for gum Arabic.

Gun-Cot'ton. An explosive substance, prepared by steeping cotton freed from all impurities in a mixture of sulphuric and nitric acids, and then washing it carefully and drying it. It is principally used for the manufacture of COLLODION, which see.

Gun'jah. The dried plant *Cannabis Indica*.

Gun'pow-der. A mixture of five parts of nitre, one of sulphur, and one of charcoal, finely powdered and very accurately blended. The grains are smoothed by friction, and are then said to be glazed.

Gus'tạ-to-rỹ, Gus'tạ-tĭve. [**Gustato'rius, Gustati'vus**; from *gus'to, gusta'tum*, to "taste."] Belonging to the sense of taste.

Gus'tatory Nerve. The lingual branch of the deep portion of the inferior maxillary, or third branch of the fifth pair of nerves.

Gus'tus.* [From γεύομαι, to "taste."] The sense of taste.

Gutt. = *Gut'tæ.** "Drops."

Gutt. quibusd. = *Gut'tis quibus'-dam.** "With a few drops."

Gut'tạ.* [Fr. *Goutte*, goot, a "drop."] A minim, or the sixtieth part of a fluidrachm.

Gut'ta A-nod'ỹ-nạ.* ("Anodyne Drop.") A solution of acetate of morphia.

Gutta Nigra. See BLACK DROP.

Gut'ta O-pa'cạ.* ("Opake Drop.") The disease called cataract, as distinguished from GUTTA SERENA, which see.

Gut'ta Per'chạ.* A name applied to the concrete juice of the *Isonandra gutta*. This substance has been placed on the primary list of the Materia Medica of the U.S. Pharmacopœia for 1860.

Gutta Rosacea, or **Gutta Rosea.** See ACNE ROSACEA.

Gut'ta Se-re'nạ.* ("Drop Serene.") A name for *amaurosis*, in which the disease being in the retina, and not in the lens or humors of the eye, this organ appears clear and natural.

Guttat. = *Gutta'tim.** "By drops."

Gut-ta'tim.* [From *gut'ta*, a "drop."] In prescriptions, "drop by drop."

Gut'tĭ-fer.* Resin-producing. See GUTTIFEROUS.

Gut-tif'er-æ.* [See GUTTIFEROUS.] The Jussieuan name of a natural order of plants. See CLUSIACEÆ.

Guttiferal. See next article.

Gut'tĭ-fer-a'lēs,* or **Gut-tif'er-als.** Applied by Lindley to an alliance or division of plants (or trees) comprising those which produce resin. (See GUTTIFEROUS.) The Guttiferal alliance comprises, among others, the important natural orders *Clusiaceæ* and *Dipteraceæ*.

Gut-tif'ĕr-ous. [**Gut'tifer,** or **Guttif'erus**; from *gut'ta*, a "drop," and *fe'ro*, to "bear."] Literally "drop-bearing," that is, "resin-producing." Applied to a natural division of plants.

Gut'tur, ur*is*.* The throat; also, the larynx or trachea. See GULA.

Ģỹm-nan'thus.* [From γυμνός, "naked," and ἄνθος, a "flower."] Having naked flowers: gymnan'thous.

Gymnasium,* jim-nā'zhe-ŭm. [Gr. γυμνάσιον; from γυμνός, "naked."] The place where the ancient *Athletæ* and others exercised themselves; so named because, previously to the exercises, they stripped themselves naked.

Ģỹm-nas'tic. [Lat. **Gymnas'ticus**; Gr. γυμναστικός; see preceding article.] Belonging to gymnastics. See next article.

Ģỹm-nas'tics. [**Gymnas'tica,** or **Gymnas'tice.**] The science or system by which the health is promoted and the strength of the body developed by the regular practice of active exercises.

Ģỹm-no-blas'tus.* [From γυμνός, "naked," and βλαστός, a "germ."] Having a naked germ. Applied to flowers.

Ģỹm-no-car'pous. [**Gymnocar'-pus**; from γυμνός, "naked," and καρπός, "fruit," or "seed."] Having naked seed.

Ģỹm'no-ġens. [**Gymnog'enæ**; from γυμνός, "naked," and γένω, to "be born," to "grow."] A division or class of exogenous plants, which have no ovary, style, or stigma, but are so constructed that the pollen falls immediately upon the naked ovules, without the introduction of any intermediate apparatus. The *Coniferæ* may be cited as an example of this class of plants.

Gymnospermes, jim'no-sperms.

[See GYMNOSPERMIUS.] Applied in the same manner as GYMNOGENS, which see.

Gym-no-sper'mi-a.* The name of a Linnæan order. See GYMNOSPERMIUS.

Gym-no-sper'mi-us.* [From γυμνός, "naked," and σπέρμα, a "seed."] Gymnosper'mious, or gymnosper'mous. Having naked seeds. Applied to a Linnæan order of the class *Didynamia.*

Gym-nos'to-mus.* [From γυμνός, "naked," and στόμα, a "mouth."] Gymnos'tomous. Applied in the plural masculine (*Gymnos'tomi*) to a division of Mosses, in which the orifice of the urn is naked.

Gyn-an'dri-a.* The name of a Linnæan class. See GYNANDRIOUS.

Gyn-an'dri-ous, or **Gyn-an'drous.** [**Gynan'drius;** from γυνή, a "woman," or "female," and ἀνήρ, ἀνδρός, a "man," or "male."] Having the male and female portions of the flower united. Applied to a Linnæan class, the stamens of which grow upon the pistil.

Gyn'a-phore. [**Gynaph'ora;** from γυνή, a "woman," or "female," and φορέω, to "bear."] Literally, "that which bears the female" portion of the plant; a prolongation of the receptacle, to which the pistil is often attached; a thecaphore.

Gyn-a-tre'si-a.* [From γυνή, a "woman," or "female," α, negative, and τίτρημι, to "perforate."] A term for the obliteration or imperforation of the vagina.

Gyn-e-co-log'i-cal. [**Gynæcolog'icus.**] Belonging to gynecology.

Gyn-e-col'o-gy. [**Gynæcolo'gia;** from γυνή, γυναικός, a "woman," and λόγος, a "discourse."] A treatise on woman, and the peculiarities of her constitution as compared with man; the science which treats of the female constitution.

Gy-ni'a-cus.* [From γυνή, a "woman."] Pertaining to women. Applied in the plural (*Gyni'aci*) to an order of diseases.

Gy-nob'a-sis.* [From γυνή, a "woman," or "female," and βάσις, a "base."] The base of a style or pistil.

Gynophorum. See GYNAPHORE.

Gyp'sum.* [Gr. γύψος.] The sulphate of lime, or *plaster of Paris.*

Gy'rans.* [From *gy'ro, gyra'tum,* to "turn about."] Turning about; rotating itself: gy'rant. Applied to certain plants.

Gy'rate. [**Gyra'tus;** from *gy'ro,* to "turn about."] Literally, "turned about." The same as CIRCINATE.

Gy-ra'tion. [**Gyra'tio, o'nis;** from *gy'ro, gyra'tum,* to "turn about."] The sensation of dizziness.

Gyr-en-ceph'a-lus.* [From γυριόω, to "wind," and ἐγκέφαλον, the "brain."] Applied by Owen to a sub-class of Mammals, having the brain convoluted, but in less degree than in man: gyrenceph'alous.

Gy'ri.* [The plural of *gy'rus,* a "circuit."] The spiral cavities of the internal ear. Also, the convolutions of the brain.

Gy-rose', or **Gy'rous.** [**Gyro'sus;** from γυρός, a "circle."] Having circles, or full of circles.

H.

H. = *Ho'ra.** "Hour." Hence **H. S.** = *Ho'râ som'ni,** "at the hour of sleep," in other words, "at bedtime."

Hab'it. [**Hab'itus;** from *ha'beo, hab'itum,* to "have," to "have oneself," or to "be."] Temperament, or diathesis. Also, a power of doing any thing acquired by frequent repetition of the same action. See DIATHESIS, and HEXIS.

Hab'i-tat.* [From *hab'ito,* to "inhabit," or "dwell."] Literally, "it dwells." Applied to a place where a plant best grows, or an animal is generally found.

Hab-ro-ma'ni-a.* [From ἁβρός, "light," or "gay," and μανία, "madness."] Insanity or delirium in which the patient is cheerful or merry. Compare AMENOMANIA.

Hæ'ma,* gen. **Hæm'a-tos.** [Gr. αἷμα.] Another term for "blood."

Hæm-a-çel-i-no'sis.* [From αἷμα, "blood," κῆλις, a "spot," and νοσός, a "disease."] Blood-spot disease, the name given by Royer to *purpura.*

Hæmacyanina. See HÆMATOCYANINA.

Hæm-a-dyn-a-mom'e-ter. [**Hæmadynamom'etrum;** from αἷμα, "blood," δύναμις, "power," and μέτρον, a "measure."] An instrument for ascertaining the force of the circulation of the blood.

Hæm'a-gogue. [**Hæmago'gus;** from αἷμα, "blood," and ἄγω, to "carry away," to "expel."] Applied to medicines favoring the access of the catamenia, or the hemorrhoidal discharge.

Hæ'mạl, or **He'mạl.** [**Hæma'lis;** from *αἷμα*, "blood."] Relating to blood, or the blood-vessels.

Hæ'mal Arch. A name applied to the arch formed by the sternum and ribs with the vertebræ, because it protects or encloses the most important portion of the vascular system.

Hæ'mal Ax'is. A name applied by Owen to the central organ and large trunks of the vascular system.

Hæ'mal Spine. Another name for the sternum. Used by Owen for the homologue of the sternum and ensiform cartilage, or (in the abdomen) for the *linea alba.*

Hæm-ạ-leū-çi'nạ.* [From *αἷμα*, "blood," and λευκός, "white."] The buffy coat, or fibrin, of the blood: hæmaleu'cin.

Hæm-ạ-lo'pĭ-ạ.* [From *αἷμα*, "blood," and *ὤψ, ὠπός*, the "eye."] A disease of the eye, in which every object appears of a blood color: hæm'alopy.

Hæ-man'thus.* [From *αἷμα*, "blood," and *ἄνθος*, a "flower."] The Blood Flower, a plant of the natural order *Amaryllidaceæ.* The Hottentots are said to dip their arrow-heads in the juice of its bulbs, on account of its poisonous properties.

Hæ-maph'e-in, or hem-ạ-fe'in. [**Hæmaphæi'na;** from *αἷμα*, "blood," and *φαιός*, "of a fawn color."] The substance which gives the pale amber color to urine.

Hæm-ạ-poph'ÿ-sis.* [From *αἷμα*, "blood," and *apoph'ysis.*] Applied by Owen, in Comparative Anatomy, to the laminæ of a vertebra, which form an irregular canal, lodging the *hæmal axis;* also, the homologue of the cartilage of a rib, or its sternal portion, named in reference to the *hæmal arch.*

Hæ-mas-the-no'sis.* [From *αἷμα*, "blood," and *ἀσθένεια*, "debility."] Poverty, or deterioration, of the blood.

Hæm-ạ-tan-ạ-go'gē.* [From *αἷμα*, "blood," and *ἀναγωγή*, a "raising" or "bringing up."] A raising, or vomiting, of blood. See HÆMATEMESIS.

Hæm-ạ-tan-ġĭ-on'o-sos,* or **Hæm-ạ-tan-ġĭ-on'o-sus.*** [From *αἷμα*, "blood," *ἀγγεῖον*, a "vessel," and *νόσος*, a "disease."] Disease of the blood-vessels.

Hæm-ạ-tan-ġĭ-o'sis.* The same as HÆMATANGIONOSOS.

Hæm'ạ-tạ-po'rĭ-ạ.* [From *αἷμα*, "blood," and *ἀπορία*, "defect."] The same as ANÆMIA.

Hæm-ạ-tạ-por'ĭ-cus.* Belonging to *hæmataporia:* hæmatapor'ic.

Hæm-ạ-tap-or-rho'sis.* [From *αἷμα*, "blood," *ἀπό*, "from," and *ὀῤῥός*, "serum."] The separation of serum from the blood, as in the profuse discharges of *Cholera.*

Hæm'ạ-tạ-pos'tạ-sis.* [From *αἷμα*, "blood," and *ἀπόστασις*, a "departure."] *Metastasis*, or transposition of the blood to another part.

Hæm'ạ-tạ-pos-tat'ĭ-cus.* Belonging to *hæmatapostasis:* hæmatapostat'ic.

Hæm'ạ-te-læ'um.* [From *αἷμα*, "blood," and *ἔλαιον*, "oil."] A concrete oil existing in the blood.

Hæm-ạ-tem'e-sis.* [From *αἷμα*, "blood," and *ἐμέω*, to "vomit."] Vomiting of blood. See HÆMATANAGOGE.

Hæm-ạ-te-met'ĭ-cus.* Belonging to *hæmatemesis:* hæmatemet'ic.

Hæm-ạ-tep-ạ-go'gē.* [From *αἷμα*, "blood," and *ἐπαγωγή*, an "attack," or "invasion."] Congestion of blood in a part.

Hæm-ạ-ther'mus.* [From *αἷμα*, "blood," and *θέρμη*, "heat."] Having warm blood: hæmather'mous.

Hæm'ạt-hĭ-dro'sis.* [From *αἷμα*, "blood," and *ἵδρωσις*, a "sweating."] An oozing of blood-colored perspiration.

Hæmathorax. See HÆMATOTHORAX.

Hæm-ạ-tĭ'ạ-sis.* [From *αἷμα*, "blood."] The same as HÆMATONOSUS.

Hæ-mat'ĭ-cạ.* [From *hæmat'icus*, "relating to the blood, or system of blood-vessels."] A name applied by Dr. Good to a class of his Nosology, comprising diseases of the sanguineous function. *Hæmatica* is also used to denote medicines which are supposed to modify in some way the condition of the blood. See HÆMATINICA.

Hæ-mat'ĭ-cus.* [From *αἷμα*, "blood."] Hæmat'ic. Relating to the blood.

Hæm'ạ-tin, or **Hæm'ạ-tīne.** [**Hæmati'na;** from *αἷμα*, "blood."] The coloring matter of the blood; sometimes, though improperly, termed *globulin.* Also applied to the coloring matter of logwood, from its resemblance to blood.

Hæm-ạ-tin'ĭ-cạ.* [The plural neuter of *hæmatin'icus*, "belonging to hæmatine."] A class of the *Hæmatica* which augment the amount of *hæmatin* in the blood. They consist chiefly, if not exclusively, of iron and its compounds.

Hæm-a-tis'che-sis.* [From αἷμα, "blood," and ἴσχω, another form of ἔχω, to "hold," to "restrain."] Stoppage of discharges of blood.

Hæm-a-tisth'mus.* [From αἷμα, "blood," and ἰσθμός, the "fauces."] Hæmorrhage from the fauces.

Hæm'a-tīte, or **Hem'a-tīte.** [**Hæmati'tes;** from αἷμα, "blood."] The blood-stone; a species of iron ore.

Hæm-a-ti'tis, *idis.** [From αἷμα, "blood."] Inflammation of the blood.

Hæm'a-to-car'pus.* [From αἷμα, "blood," and καρπός, "fruit."] Having fruit spotted with red: hæmatocar'pous.

Hæm'a-to-çēle.* [From αἷμα, "blood," and κήλη, a "tumor."] Enlargement of the scrotum, from blood being within one or other of its tunics.

Hæm'a-to-çeph'a-lus.* [From αἷμα, "blood," and κεφαλή, the "head."] A monster-fœtus, in which effusion of blood into the cerebral hemispheres has produced a marked deformity.

Hæm'a-to-che'zĭ-a.* [From αἷμα, "blood," and χέζω, to "evacuate the bowels."] A bloody stool.

Hæm'a-to-çœ'lĭ-a.* [From αἷμα, "blood," and κοιλία, the "belly."] Effusion or escape of blood into the peritonæal cavity.

Hæm'a-to-col'pus.* [From αἷμα, "blood," and κόλπος, a "sinus," sometimes the "vagina."] Effusion of blood into the vagina. Also, a collection of blood, or of menstrual secretion, there.

Hæm'a-to-Crys'tal-line. [From αἷμα, "blood," and κρύσταλλον, "crystal."] A crystalline body found in the remains of extravasations of blood. In man the crystals are very small and rectangular. They are remarkable from their becoming larger and smaller under the influence of external agencies, without change of form. They become bright red under the influence of oxygen, dark red under that of carbonic acid.

Hæm'a-to-çy'a-ni'na.* [From αἷμα, "blood," and κύανος, "blue."] The blue coloring matter of the blood: hæmatocy'anin.

Hæm'a-to-çys'tis.* [From αἷμα, "blood," and κύστις, a "bladder."] A cyst containing blood. Also, effusion of blood into the urinary bladder. Also, encysted *hæmatoma:* a hæm'atocyst.

Hæm-a-to'dēs.* [From αἷμα, "blood."] Full of blood: hæm'atose.

Hæmatodynamometer. See HÆMADYNAMOMETER.

Hæm-a-to-glob-u-li'na.* The same as GLOBULIN.

Hæm-a-tog'ra-phy̆. [**Hæmatogra'phia;** from αἷμα, "blood," and γράφω, to "write."] A description of the blood, its nature and quality.

Hæm'a-toid. [**Hæmatoi'des;** from αἷμα, "blood," and εἶδος, a "form."] Resembling blood.

Hæm-a-toi'din. [**Hæmatoidi'na;** from *hæmati'na,* "hæmatin."] A crystalline body produced spontaneously from hæmatin during the drying of blood.

Hæm-a-tol'o-gy̆. [**Hæmatolo'gia;** from αἷμα, "blood," and λόγος, a "discourse."] The history of the nature and constitution of the blood; the science of the blood.

Hæm'a-to-ly̆t'ĭ-ca.* [From αἷμα, "blood," and λύω, to "dissolve," to "weaken."] A term applied by some writers to a class of remedies which impoverish the blood. See SPANÆMIA, and SPANÆMICA.

Hæm-a-to'ma, *atis.** [From αἱματόω, to "turn into blood."] A bloody tumor: a hæm'atome.

Hæm-a-to-ma-to'sus.* Having *hæmatoma:* hæmatom'atous.

Hæm'a-to-met-ach'y̆-sis.* [From αἷμα, "blood," μετά, "beyond," and χύσις, an "effusion."] Transfusion of blood.

Hæm-a-tom'e-ter. [**Hæmatom'etrum;** from αἷμα, "blood," and μέτρον, a "measure."] An instrument for measuring the force of blood.

Hæm'a-to-me'tra.* [From αἷμα, "blood," and μήτρα, the "womb."] A filling of the womb with blood.

Hæm'a-to-me'trĭ-a.* [From αἷμα, "blood," and μετρέω, to "measure."] The measuring of the force of the blood in its course: hæmatom'etry.

Hæm-a-tom'pha-lo-çēle.* [From αἷμα, "blood," ὀμφαλός, the "navel," and κήλη, a "tumor."] Tumor at the navel, turgid with blood.

Hæm-a-tom'y̆-çēs, *e'tis.** [From αἷμα, "blood," and μύκης, a "fungus."] *Fungus hæmatodes,* or bloody fungus. See FUNGUS HÆMATODES.

Hæm-a-ton'o-sos,* or **Hæm-a-ton'o-sus.*** [From αἷμα, "blood," and νόσος, "disease."] Disease of the blood.

Hæm'a-to-pĕr'ĭ-car'dĭ-um.* [From αἷμα, "blood," and *pericar'dium.*] Effusion of blood into the *pericardium.*

Hæm'a-to-phy̆l'lus.* [From αἷμα, "blood," and φύλλον, a "leaf."] Having leaves tinged with a blood color: hæmatophyl'lous.

Hæm'a-to-plas'ma, atis.* [From *αἷμα*, "blood," and *πλάσμα*, a "formation."] The plastic principle of the blood.

Hæm'a-to-poi-e'sis.* [From *αἷμα*, "blood," and *ποίησις*, a "making."] Assimilation of the chyle to blood. The same as HÆMATOSIS.

Hæm'a-to-poi-et'i-cus.* Belonging to *hæmatopoiesis:* hæmatopoiet'ic.

Hæm-a-top-ty'si-a,* **Hæm-a-top'ty-sis.*** The same as HÆMOPTYSIS.

Hæm-a-tor'rha-chis.* [From *αἷμα*, "blood," and *ῥάχις*, the "spine."] Effusion of blood into the spine, or into the theca of the spinal marrow.

Hæm'a-tor-rhœ'a.* [From *αἷμα*, "blood," and *ῥέω*, to "flow."] A passive flowing of blood; hæmorrhage.

Hæmatosine. See HÆMATIN.

Hæm-a-to'sis.* [From *αἱματόω*, to "make bloody."] A flow, or flux, of blood; a hæmorrhage.

Hæm'a-to-spil'i-a.* [From *αἷμα*, "blood," and *σπῖλος*, a "spot."] A name for *Purpura hæmorrhagica.*

Hæm'a-to-spon-go'sis.* The formation or growth of *hæmatospongus.*

Hæm'a-to-spon'gus.* [From *αἷμα*, "blood," and *σπόγγος*, a "sponge."] *Fungus hæmatodes,* or bloody fungus. See FUNGUS HÆMATODES.

Hæm'a-to-sym'pho-re'sis,* or **Hæm'a-to-syn'a-go'gē.*** [From *αἷμα*, "blood," and *συμφόρησις*, or *συναγωγή*, an "assembling together," a "collection."] Congestion of blood. See HÆMATEPAGOGE.

Hæmatothorax. See HÆMOTHORAX.

Hæm-a-to-tox'ic, Hæm-a-tox'ic. [**Hæmatotox'icus, Hæmatox'icus;** from *αἷμα*, "blood," and *τοξικός*, "poison."] Belonging to a vitiated state of the blood.

Hæm-a-tox-i'na,* or **Hæm-a-tox-y-li'na.*** The coloring matter of logwood.

Hæm-a-tox'y-lon.* [From *αἷμα*, "blood," and *ξύλον*, "wood."] Logwood. A Linnæan genus of the class *Decandria,* natural order *Leguminosæ.* Also, the Pharmacopœial name (Ed. and U.S. Ph.) of the wood of *Hæmatoxylon Campechianum,* otherwise called the *Hæmatoxyli lignum* ("Wood of Hæmatoxylon"). See HÆMATOXYLUM.

Hæmatox'ylon Cam-pe-chi-a'num.* The logwood-tree.

Hæm-a-tox'y-lum.* The Pharmacopœial name (Lond. Ph.) of logwood.

Hæm-a-to-zo'on.* [From *αἷμα*, "blood," and *ζῶον*, an "animal."] An animalcule discovered in the blood.

Hæm-a-tu-re'sis,* or **Hæm-a-tu'ri-a.*** [From *αἷμα*, "blood," and *οὖρον*, the "urine."] A disease in which blood is discharged with urine.

Hæm-a-tu'ri-cus.* Belonging to *hæmaturia:* hæmatu'ric.

Hæmidrosis. See HÆMATHIDROSIS.

Hæ'min, or **Hæ'mine.** [**Hæmi'na;** from *αἷμα*, "blood."] A crystalline substance obtained from dried blood by the action of dry salt and glacial acetic acid at a boiling temperature. It occurs in flat rhombic plates, which are remarkable for their insensibility to reagents, not being affected by strong mineral acids.

Hæmodoraceæ,* hem-o-do-ra'she-ē. [From *Hæmodo'rum,* one of the genera.] A natural order of endogenous herbaceous plants, found in New Holland, and some other parts of the world.

Hæmometer. See HÆMATOMETER.

Hæmopathia. See HÆMATONOSUS.

Hæm-oph-thal'mus.* [From *αἷμα*, "blood," and *ὀφθαλμός*, the "eye."] Effusion of blood into the chambers of the eye.

Hæm-o-proc'tos,* or **Hæm-o-proc'tus.*** [From *αἷμα*, "blood," and *πρωκτός*, the "anus."] Discharge of blood from the bowels.

Hæm-op'ti-cus.* Belonging to *hæmoptœ* or *hæmoptysis:* hæmop'tic.

Hæmoptoicus. See HÆMOPTICUS.

Hæ-mop'ty-sis,* or **Hæ-mop'to-e.*** [From *αἷμα*, "blood," and *πτύω*, to "spit."] (Fr. *Hémoptysie,* à'mop'tè'zè'.) A spitting of blood; hæmorrhage from the lungs. A genus of the order *Hæmorrhagiæ,* class *Pyrexiæ,* of Cullen's Nosology.

Hæmorrhage. See HÆMORRHAGIA.

Hæm-or-rha'gi-a.* [From *αἷμα*, "blood," and *ῥήγνυμι*, to "burst."] (Fr. *Hémorrhagie,* à'mo'rà'zhè'.) Hæm'orrhage, or hæm'orrhagy. A bursting forth of blood, from whatever cause. In the plural, an order of the class *Pyrexiæ* of Cullen's Nosology.

Hæm-or-rhag'i-cus.* Belonging to hæmorrhage: hæmorrhag'ic.

Hæm-or-rhin'i-a.* [From *αἷμα*, "blood," and *ῥίν*, the "nose."] The same as EPISTAXIS.

Hæm-or-rhœ'a.* The same as HÆMATORRHŒA, which see.

Hæmorrhœ'a Pe-te-chi-a'lis.* (See PETECHIÆ.) A term which has been applied to a chronic form of *purpura.*

Hæm-or-rho'ĭ-cus.* Belonging to *hæmorrhœa:* hæmorrho'ic.

Hæm'or-rhoid. [**Hæmor'rhois,** *ides;* from αἷμα, "blood," and ῥέω, to "flow."] Literally, a "hæmorrhage," and originally used in this sense in general, but now restricted to the piles. These are termed *open,* when they discharge blood; and *blind,* when there is no discharge. A genus of the order *Hæmorrhagiæ,* class *Pyrexiæ,* of Cullen's Nosology.

Hæm-or-rhoi'dal. [**Hæmorrhoida'lis;** from *hæmorrhŏi'des,* "piles."] Belonging to hæmorrhoides, or piles.

Hæm-or-rho-i'de-us.* The same as HÆMORRHOIDAL.

Hæm-o-spa'sĭ-a.* [From αἷμα, "blood," and σπάω, to "draw to."] The forming of a vacuum over a considerable surface of the body, being an extension of the principle of dry cupping. See HÆMOSPASTIC SYSTEM.

Hæm-o-spas'tic. [From the same.] Drawing or attracting the blood.

Hæmospas'tic Sys'tem. A new system of medicine, introduced by Dr. Junod, of Paris. He employs a pneumatic apparatus of peculiar construction, in which the arm or leg is so placed as to attract the blood to the extremities, without diminishing the mass of this liquid.

Hæm-os-ta'sĭ-a,* **Hæ-mos'ta-sis.*** [From αἷμα, "blood," and στάσις, a "standing."] A stoppage, or stagnation, of the blood; also applied to any operation for stopping blood.

Hæm-os-tat'ic. [**Hæmostat'icus.**] Belonging to *hæmostasia,* or *hæmostasis.* Also applied to means employed for staunching or arresting hæmorrhage; styptic.

Hæm-os-tat'ĭ-ca.* [From αἷμα, "blood," and στατική, the "science of weights."] The powers or motions of the blood, and the laws by which these are regulated in the vessels of the body: hæmostat'ics.

Hæm-o-tex'ĭ-a,* **Hæm-o-tex'is.*** [From αἷμα, "blood," and τῆξις, a "liquefaction."] Dissolution or liquefaction of the blood.

Hæm-o-tho'rax, a'*cis,** or **Hæm'a-to-tho'rax.*** [From αἷμα, "blood," and θώραξ, the "chest."] The escape of blood into the thorax, through a wound or otherwise.

Hæmotoxicus. See HÆMATOTOXICUS.

Hæm-ot'ro-phy̆. [From αἷμα, "blood," and τροφή, "nourishment."] An excess of sanguineous nutriment, as distinguished from hypertrophy and hyperæmia.

Hair. [Lat. **Capil'lus,** and **Pi'lus;** Gr. θρίξ; Fr. *Poil,* pwăl.] A substance like horn, growing from the skin of animals, in nearly cylindrical filaments.

Hair-Dyes. [**Tinctu'ræ Capillo'rum.**] The basis of most of the powders, pastes, and liquids sold under this name, is either lead or silver. To these are sometimes added litharge, slaked lime, and starch.

Hair, Morbid. See TRICHOSIS.

Hairy. See HIRSUTE.

Hai'ry̆ Scalp. That part of the integument of the head which is covered with hairs.

Halberd-Shaped. See HASTATE.

Haleine. See HALITUS.

Haligraphia. See HALOGRAPHIA.

Hal'ĭ-hoo'. [A corruption of *Holy hood.*] A Scotch term for the *caul,* which was formerly carefully preserved by the superstitious, on account of the many virtues attributed to it.

Hal'ĭ-tus.* [From *ha'lo, hala'tum,* to "breathe," or "breathe out," to "exhale."] (Fr. *Haleine,* ă'lĕn' or ă'lăn'.) Vapor, or breath.

Hal'itus of the Blood. The vapor which arises from the blood when newly drawn from the body.

Hal-lu-cĭ-nā'tion. [**Hallucina'tio, o'***nis;* from *hallu'cinor, hallucina'tus,* to "mistake."] Mental error, or foolish imagination.

Hal'lus,* **Hal'lux,*** and **Hal'lex.*** Names for the great toe.

Ha'lo, o'*nis.** [From ἅλως, a "circle."] The circle which surrounds the sun, moon, or stars, when their rays are refracted in their passage through a mist. The *areola,* or brownish circle, around the female nipple. Also, the red margin, or *areola,* around pustules.

Hal'o-ġen, or **Hal'o-ġene.** [From ἅλς, "salt," and γεννάω, to "produce."] A term employed by Berzelius to denote bodies which form salts with metals, as chlorine, bromine, iodine, fluorine, and cyanogen.

Ha-log'ra-phy̆. [**Halogra'phia;** from ἅλς, "salt," and γράφω, to "write."] A description of salts.

Hā'loid. [**Haloi'des;** from ἅλς, "salt," and εἶδος, a "form."] Applied to salts compounded of the metals with chlorine, iodine, bromine, because similar in nature or composition to common salt.

Ha-lol'o-ġy̆. [**Halolo'gia;** from

ἅλς, "salt," and λόγος, a "discourse."] A treatise on the salts.

Ha-lom'e-ter. [**Halom'etrum;** from ἅλς, "salt," and μέτρον, a "measure."] An instrument for measuring the form, angles, etc., of salts.

Ha-loph'i-lous. [**Haloph'ilus;** from ἅλς, "salt," and φίλεω, to "love."] Delighting in a soil impregnated with salt. Applied to plants.

Hal'o-phȳtes. [**Haloph'yta,** plural of *haloph'yton;* from ἅλς, "salt," and φύτον, a "plant."] A class of plants which inhabit salt marshes, and by combustion yield barilla, as *Salsola, Salicornia,* and *Chenopodium.*

Halophyton, or **Halophytum.** See HALOPHYTE.

Haloragaceæ,* ha-lor-a-ga'she-ē. [From *Halor'agis,* one of the genera.] A natural order of exogenous plants, found in damp places, ditches, etc.

Hăl'ter,* gen. **Hăl-te'ris.** [From ἁλτήρ, an instrument anciently used in gymnastic exercise.] Applied in the nominative plural (*Halte'res*) to two small movable bodies which are situated or hang above the wings in the *Diptera.*

Hal'ur-ġȳ. [**Halur'gia;** from ἅλς, "salt," and ἔργον, a "work."] The process of forming, extracting, or producing salts.

Hamamelidaceæ,* ham-a-mel-e-da'she-ē. [From *Hamame'lis,* one of the genera.] A natural order of exogenous trees and shrubs, found in Asia, North America, and Africa. It includes the Witch-Hazel.

Hā'mate. [**Hama'tus;** from *ha'mus,* a "hook."] A botanical term signifying having a hook, or hooked.

Ham'i-form. [**Hamifor'mis;** from *ha'mus,* a "hook."] Resembling a hook.

Hā'mose. [**Hamo'sus;** from *ha'mus,* a "hook."] Having a hooked appearance.

Ham'string, Out'er. The *Biceps flexor cruris* muscle.

Ham'u-lose, or **Ham'u-lous.** [**Hamulo'sus;** from *ham'ulus,* a "little hook."] Having little hooks.

Ham'u-lus.* [Diminutive of *ha'mus,* a "hook."] A little hook. Applied to the hook-like portion of the pterygoid process of the sphenoid bone, or any similar object.

Hanche, hŏNsh. The French term for "hip." See COXA.

Hand. [Lat. **Ma'nus;** Fr. *Main,* măNº.] The organ of prehension in man, extending from the wrist to the extremities of the fingers. It consists of three parts, the WRIST (or *Carpus*), the METACARPUS, and the FINGERS, which will be noticed under their respective heads. In Ornithology, it denotes the third portion of the anterior extremity which supports the wing, having one finger, and vestiges of two others.

Handful. See MANIPULUS, PUGILLUS.

Hang'ing. [**Suspen'sio, o'nis.**] Suspension by the neck, causing *Asphyxia suffocationis.*

Hap-lo-car'di-ac. [From ἅπλοος, "without fold," "simple," or "single," and καρδία, a "heart."] Having a single heart. Applied to fishes, etc., as distinguished from Mammals, which have a double heart, and are hence termed diplocardiac.

Hap-tot'i-ca.* [From ἅπτομαι, to "touch."] The doctrine (or science) of the phenomena of touch, or sensation.

Har'der-i Glan'du-la.* ("Gland of Harder.") A gland in ruminant and pachydermatous quadrupeds, and in birds, near the inner angle of the eye.

Hare'-Lip. [Lat. **La'bium Lepori'num;** Fr. *Bec de Lièvre,* bĕk dẹh le-ĕvr'.] A congenital cleft, or division, of one or both lips, most frequently the upper. It is sometimes double.

Hargne, harñ. A French term for HERNIA, which see.

Har'ma-lane. A beautiful coloring substance obtained from the seed of the hermal-plant (*Peganum harmala*), which grows wild in the salt steppes of the Crimea.

Har'mo-nȳ. [**Harmo'nia;** from ἁρμόζω, to "adapt."] A variety of *Synarthrosis,* denoting a simple joining together, as the nasal and other bones of the face.

Har. pil. sum. iij. = *Ha'rum pilula'rum suman'tur tres.** "Let three of these pills be taken."

Harts'horn. The horn of certain kinds of the hart, or stag. The substance *Cornu Cervi.* The popular name for *Liquor Ammoniæ,* or *Ammoniæ Aqua.*

Har'vest Bug. The *Ac'arus Autumna'lis.* A variety of the tick insect which infests the skin in the autumn, producing intolerable itching, succeeded by glossy wheals. It is also called the *wheal-worm.*

Hashish, or **Haschisch,** hå-sheesh'. A preparation of *Cannabis Indica,* or hemp, used as an intoxicating drug by the

Arabs, and generally throughout Syria. It is made by boiling the leaves and flowers of the plant with water and fresh butter. See BHANG.

Has'tate. [**Hasta'tus;** from *has'ta*, a "spear."] Like a spear, or halberd.

Has-ti-fo'li-ous. [**Hastifo'lius;** from *has'ta*, a "spear," and *fo'lium*, a "leaf."] Having hastate leaves.

Has-ti-for'mis.* [From *has'ta*, a "spear."] Resembling a spear: hastate.

Haunch. [Lat. **Clu'nis;** Fr. *Hanche*, hŏnsh.] The region formed by the lateral parts of the pelvis and the hip joint; the hip.

Haust. = *Haus'tus.** "A draught."

Haus'tus.* [From *hau'rio, haus'tum*, to "drink greedily."] A liquid preparation forming one dose, generally about two ounces in quantity; a draught.

Haut Mal, hō mål. A French term for epilepsy in its full development, that is, accompanied with convulsions. See EPILEPSY.

Ha-ve'ri Glan'du-læ.* ("Glands of Haver.") See next article.

Haversian (ha-ver'she-an) **Glands.** The name of the fatty bodies which are found in connection with most of the joints, and in general lying behind the synovial fringes. Havers supposed them to be the agents of the synovial secretion, and called them *glandulæ mucilaginosæ*. Weitbrecht called them *adipo-glandulosæ*.

Haver'sian Tubes, or **Ca-nāls'.** A term given, from the name of their discoverer, to a very complicated apparatus of minute canals, found in the substance of bone, and containing medullary matter. The central canal, as well as the separate cells, may be regarded as enlargements of them.

Hb. = *Her'ba.** "The plant."

H. d. or **decub.** = *Ho'râ decu'bitûs.** "At going to bed."

Hĕad. [Lat. **Ca'put;** Gr. κεφαλή; Fr. *Tête*, tĕt or tāt.] In higher animals, that portion which contains the brain, with the chief organs of sense, as sight, hearing, etc., as well as the mouth and organs of mastication. In lower animals, it contains the mouth, or opening to the stomach, and the principal organs of sense when these exist. The human head is distinguished into *cranium* and face. The term "head" is often applied to the upper end of a long bone, the origin of a muscle, the beginning of a part, or to any round protuberance which can be supposed to resemble a head.

Head'ache. [**Cephalal'gia.**] Pain in the head, differently denominated according to the part affected, or its cause. See BHANG

Hĕad'ing. A preparation of equal parts of alum and green vitriol, used in brewing.

Hĕalth. [**San'itas.**] The proper disposition and condition of the several parts of the body for performing their functions without impediment or sensation of weariness.

Hĕal'thȳ Pus. That discharged from abscesses, the result of phlegmonous inflammation; or from wounds and ulcers in the healing state; laudable pus.

Hear'ing. [**Audi'tus.**] That sense by which sounds are distinguished, the organ of which is the ear.

Hearing, Morbid. See PARACUSIS.

Heart. [Lat. **Cor, Cor'dis;** Gr. καρδία; Fr. *Cœur*, kur.] A hollow muscular viscus situated between the lungs, but more under the left one, and enclosed in the *pericardium;* from which proceeds the circulation of the blood. In man and in other Mammals, it is double, that is, it consists of two parts, the right ventricle and auricle for the pulmonic circulation, and the left ventricle and auricle for the general or systemic circulation.

Heart'-Burn. The popular name for *Cardialgia.*

Heart'-Shaped. The same as CORDATE.

Heat. In a general sense, the same as CALORIC. Heat in a mild form is necessary to the life of plants and animals. In the latter, the needful temperature is in part furnished by the respiratory apparatus. Heat is also one of the most important agents the chemist or pharmacist can command, for effecting both chemical union and decomposition, according to the manner in which it is applied, or the character of the substance submitted to its action.

Heat, Ab'so-lūte. The whole quantity of caloric existing in a body; absolute caloric.

Heat, Animal. See CALOR ANIMALIS.

Heat, Latent. See CALORIC, LATENT.

Heat, Prick'lȳ. Common term for the *Lichen tropicus.*

Heat, Sensible. See CALORIC, FREE.

Heat-Spots. See ÆSTATES.

Heavy Spar. See BARYTA.

Hebd. = *Hebdom'ada.** "A week."

He'be.* [Gr. ἥβη, "down," or "incipient beard;" hence, "youth."] Youth;

or the goddess of Youth, fabled by the ancients to have been cup-bearer to Jupiter.

He-be-an'thus.* [From ἥβη, "youth," "down," and ἄνθος, a "flower."] Having tomentose corols: hebean'thous.

Heb-e-car'pus.* [From ἥβη, "youth," "down," and καρπός, "fruit."] Having pubescent fruits: hebecar'pous.

He-bec'la-dus.* [From ἥβη, "youth," "down," and κλάδος, a "branch."] Having pubescent branches: hebec'ladous.

He-beg'ȳ-nus.* [From ἥβη, "youth," "down," and γυνή, a "woman," or "female."] Having pubescent ovaries: hebeg'ynous.

Heb-e-pet'a-lus.* [From ἥβη, "youth," "down," and πέταλον, a "petal."] Having pubescent petals: hebepet'alous.

He-bet'ĭ-cus.* [From ἥβη, "youth," or "puberty."] Belonging to puberty; youthful: hebet'ic.

Heb'e-tude. [Hebetu'do, dinis.] Dulness, or insensibility.

Heb-ra-den'dron Cam-bo-gĭ-o-ī'dēs.* A guttiferous plant, which yields a kind of gamboge not distinguishable from that of Siam. See GAMBOGE.

Hec-a-to-phȳl'lus.* [From ἑκατόν, a "hundred," and φύλλον, a "leaf."] Having leaves composed of a hundred (or a great number of) folioles: hecatophyl'lous.

Hec'tic. [Hec'ticus; from ἕξις, "habit."] (Fr. *Hectique*, ĕk'tēk', or *Étique*, ā'tēk'.) Belonging to habit or state of body, as distinguished from diseases which are the result of miasma or contagion.

Hec'tic Fe'ver. [Lat. **Fe'bris Hec'tica;** Fr. *Fièvre Hectique*, fe-āvʀ' ĕk'tēk'.] A slow, insidious fever, idiopathic or symptomatic; the latter arising in consequence of some incurable local disease.

Hec-tĭ-co-pȳr'e-tos,* or **Hec-tĭ-cop'ȳ-ra.*** [From ἕξις, "habit," and πῦρ, or πυρετός, a "fever."] Hectic fever.

Hec'to-grămme. [Hectogram'ma, atis; from ἑκατόν, a "hundred," and *gramme*.] 100 grammes; equal to 3 oz. 8 dr. 2.152 gr. avoirdupois.

Hectolitre, ĕk'to'lētr'. [From ἑκατόν, a "hundred," and *li'tre*.] 100 litres; equal to 3.5377 English cubic feet, or 22 Imperial gallons, or 2¾ Imperial bushels.

Hectometre, hĕk-to-mē'ter or ĕk'to'-mêtʀ'. [From ἑκατόν, a "hundred," and *mètre*.] 100 metres; or 109 yards, 1 foot, 1 inch.

He-de-o'ma.* American Pennyroyal. The Pharmacopœial name (U.S. Ph.) for the herb of the *Hedeoma pulegioides*. Pennyroyal is a stimulant aromatic and emmenagogue.

Hedeo'ma Pu-le-gĭ-o-ī'dēs.* The systematic name of the plant Pennyroyal. See preceding article.

Hed'e-ra He'lix.* (Fr. *Lierre*, le-ĕr'.) The systematic name of the ivy.

Hed-e-rā'ceous. [Hedera'ceus; from *Hed'era*, the "ivy."] Resembling the *Hedera*, or ivy.

Hedge-Hys'sop. Common name for *Gratiola officinalis*.

Hel-coc'a-çē.* [From ἕλκος, an "ulcer," and κάκη, "corruption."] Malignant ulcer.

Hel-co'dēs.* [From ἕλκος, an "ulcer."] Having ulcers, or full of ulcers.

Hel-çœ-de'ma, atis.* [From ἕλκος, an "ulcer," and οἴδημα, a "tumor."] Œdematous ulceration.

Hel'coid. [Helcoi'des; from ἕλκος, an "ulcer," and εἶδος, a "form."] Resembling an ulcer.

Hel-col'o-gȳ. [Helcolo'gia; from ἕλκος, an "ulcer," and λόγος, a "discourse."] A history of ulcers.

Hel-co-me'nĭ-a.* [From ἕλκος, an "ulcer," and μήν, a "month."] *Metastasis* of the catamenia to an ulcer; a sort of vicarious menstruation.

Hel-coph-thăl'mĭ-a.* [From ἕλκος, an "ulcer," and ὀφθαλμός, the "eye."] Ulcerous ophthalmia.

Hel-co'sis.* [From ἕλκος, an "ulcer."] The progress of ulceration.

Hel'e-nin, or **Hel'e-nīne.** Elecampane Camphor. A volatile, crystalline solid, obtained from the *In'ula hele'nium*.

Hel-ĭ-an'the-mum.* Frostwort. The Pharmacopœial name (U.S. Ph.) for the herb of the *Helianthemum Canadense*.

Hel-ĭ-co'dēs.* [From ἕλιξ, a "coil," or any thing spiral.] Full of windings: hel'icose.

Hel'ĭ-coid. [Helicoi'des; from ἕλιξ, a "coil," and εἶδος, a "form."] Resembling that which is spiral.

He-lic'u-lus.* [Diminutive of *he'lix*, or ἕλιξ, a "coil."] Applied in the plural (*Helic'uli*) to the spiral vessels of plants: a hel'icule.

He-lĭ-o-çen'tric. [Heliocen'tricus; from ἥλιος, the "sun," and κεντρικός, "centric."] Having the sun for the centre, or point of observation.

He-lĭ-o-ī'dēs.* [From ἥλιος, the

"sun," and εἶδος, a "form."] Resembling the sun: he'lioid.

He-li-om'e-ter. [**Heliom'etrum;** from ἥλιος, the "sun," and μέτρον, a "measure."] An instrument for measuring the apparent diameter of the sun.

He'li-o-scope. [**Heliosco'pium;** from ἥλιος, the "sun," and σκοπέω, to "observe."] An instrument for observing the sun.

He'li-o-stat.* [From ἥλιος, the "sun," and ἵστημι, to "stand," to "cause to stand still."] An instrument by which the sunbeam can be steadily directed to one spot during the whole of its diurnal period.

He-li-o-tro'pi-ous. [**Heliotro'pius;** from ἥλιος, the "sun," and τρέπω, to "turn."] Applied to plants, the flowers of which turn constantly towards the sun.

He'li-o-tro-pis'mus.* [From ἥλιος, the "sun," and τρέπω, to "turn."] That faculty by which certain plants constantly turn their flowers to the sun: heliot'ropism.

He'lix, i*cis*.* [Gr. ἕλιξ; from εἰλέω, to "wind about."] Literally, a "coil," or any thing spiral. The outer border of the *Pinna*, or external ear. Also, the snail, a genus of *Mollusca*, order *Pulmonea*.

Hel-le-bo-ra'ceous. [**Hellebora'ceus.**] Having an arrangement of parts as in *Helleborus*.

Hel'le-bore. [Gr. ἐλλέβορος.] A plant. See HELLEBORUS.

Hellebore, American. See VERATRUM VIRIDE.

Hel-le-bo're-us.* Belonging to *hellebore*.

Hel-leb'o-rin, or **Hel-leb'o-rine.** An acrid oil, said to contain the acrid principle of the *Helleborus niger*, black hellebore, or Christmas rose.

Hel-leb'o-rus.* [From ἑλεῖν, to "destroy," and βορά, "fodder"?] Black Hellebore. A Linnæan genus of the class *Polyandria*, natural order *Ranunculaceæ*. Also, the Pharmacopœial name for the rhizoma of *Helleb'orus officina'lis*, or *H. niger;* the *Hellebori Nigri Radix* ("Root of Black Hellebore") of the Dublin Pharmacopœia. Hellebore is a drastic hydragogue cathartic; it also possesses emmenagogue properties.

Helleb'orus Al'bus.* The Pharmacopœial name (Dub. Ph.) of white hellebore root. See VERATRUM ALBUM.

Helleb'orus Fœt'i-dus.* ("Fœtid Hellebore.") Bear's-Foot. The leaves have been extolled as a remedy for the *Ascaris lumbricoides*. Little used.

Helleb'orus Ni'ger,* Helleb'o-rus Of-fic-i-na'lis.* Systematic names of black hellebore, or *Melampodium*.

Helleb'orus O-ri-en-ta'lis.* ("Oriental Hellebore.") The root was formerly extolled in mania, epilepsy, and dropsy. It is still used in the Levant.

Hel-min'tha-gogue. [**Helminthago'gus;** from ἕλμινς, ἕλμινθος, a "worm," and ἄγω, to "carry or drive away."] The same as ANTHELMINTIC.

Hel-min'thes.* [From ἕλμινς, ἕλμινθος, a "worm."] A class or division in Zoology, including the various kinds of worms.

Hel-min-thi'a-sis,* or **Hel-min'thi-a.*** [From ἕλμινς, ἕλμινθος, a "worm."] The breeding of worms, or *larvæ*, in any part of the body.

Hel-min'thic. [**Helmin'thicus;** from ἕλμινς, ἕλμινθος, a "worm."] Belonging to worms.

Hel-min-tho'des.* [From ἕλμινς, a "worm."] Having worms, or full of worms.

Hel-min'thoid. [**Helminthoi'des;** from ἕλμινς, a "worm," and εἶδος, a "form."] Resembling a worm.

Hel-min-thol'o-gy. [**Helmintholo'gia;** from ἕλμινς, a "worm," and λόγος, a "discourse."] A treatise on worms,—particularly intestinal worms; that branch of medicine which treats of intestinal worms.

Hel-min-thoph'thi-sis.* [From ἕλμινς, a "worm," and φθίσις, a "wasting away."] *Tabes verminosa*, or wasting from the presence of intestinal worms.

Hel-min-thop'y-ra.* [From ἕλμινς, a "worm," and πῦρ, or πυρετός, a "fever."] Worm-fever.

He-lo'bi-us.* [From ἕλος, a "marsh," a "pool," and βίος, "life."] Living on moisture; aquatic.

He-lo'des.* [From ἕλος, a "marsh," a "pool."] Full of moisture. Applied to a fever with profuse sweating; also, to marsh fever.

He-lop'y-ra.* [From ἕλος, a "marsh," and πυρετός, a "fever."] Marsh or swamp fever.

He'los.* [Gr. ἧλος; Lat. **Cla'vus,** a "nail."] A name given to the tumor formed by prolapsus, or *procidentia iridis*, supposed to resemble a nail.

Helwingiaceæ,* hel-win-je-a'-she-ē. A natural order of exogenous shrubs, which appears to be composed of a single genus, *Helwin'gia,* found in Japan.

Hemacyanin, or **Hematocyanin.** See HÆMATOCYANINA.

Hemal. See HÆMAL.

Hémaproctie, à'mâ'prok'tè'. [From αἷμα, "blood," and πρωκτός, the "anus."] The French term for PILES, which see.

Hematic. See HÆMATIC.

Hematite. See HÆMATITE.

Hem-e-ra-lo'pi-a.* [From ἡμέρα, a "day," and ὤψ, the "eye."] A defect of vision, by which objects are seen only in broad daylight: day-sight; night-blindness.

Hem-e-ra-pho'ni-a.* [From ἡμέρα, a "day," α, priv., and φωνή, the "voice."] Loss of voice during the day.

Hem-e-rod'ro-mus.* [From ἡμέρα, a "day," and δρόμος, a "course."] Applied to a fever which runs its course in a day. The same as EPHEMERUS.

Hem-e-rot-y̆-phlo'sis.* [From ἡμέρα, a "day," and τύφλωσις, "blindness."] Day-blindness, or *Nyctalopia.*

Hem-ĭ-car'pus.* [From ἥμισυς, the "half," and καρπός, "fruit."] Each portion of a fruit which naturally separates itself into halves.

Hem-ĭ-çeph'a-lus.* [From ἥμισυς, "half," and κέφαλή, a "head."] A monster-fœtus with half a head.

Hem-ĭ-cra'nĭ-a.* [From ἥμισυς, "half," and κρανίον, the "head."] (Fr. *Migraine,* mè'grĕn' or mè'grån'.) A severe pain, generally hysterical, nervous, or bilious, affecting one half or side of the head; a megrim.

Hem-ĭ-cran'ĭ-cus.* Belonging to *hemicrania.*

Hem-ĭ-des'mus In'dĭ-cus.* An asclepiadaceous plant, the root of which is used in India under the name of *Country Sarsaparilla.* It has been called Indian or Scented Sarsaparilla, or the root of *Smilax aspera.*

Hem-ĭ-he'dral, or **Hem-ĭ-ed'ric.** [From ἥμισυς, a "half," and ἕδρα, a "base."] Having half faces, or facets.

Hem-ĭ-o-păl'gĭ-a.* [From ἥμισυς, a "half," ὤψ, the "eye," and ἄλγος, "pain."] Hemicranic pain of the eye.

Hem-ĭ-op'sy̆. [**Hemiop'sia, Hemio'pia;** from ἥμισυς, a "half," ὄπτομαι, to "see," or ὤψ, the "eye."] Defect of vision, under which only the half of objects is seen.

Hem-ĭ-ple'gĭ-a,* Hem-ĭ-plex'ĭ-a.* [From ἥμισυς, a "half," and πλήσσω, to "strike."] Paralysis, affecting one half or side of the body; *paralysis hemiplegica.*

Hem-ĭ-pleg'ic. [**Hemipleg'icus.**] Belonging to *hemiplegia.*

Hemiplexicus. See HEMIPLEGIA.

He-mip'ter-a.* [See HEMIPTERUS.] Insects which have one half of their wings thick and coriaceous, and the other half membranous, as the bug, tick, etc.

Hem-ip'ter-o-lo'gĭ-a.* [From ἥμισυς, a "half," πτέρον, a "wing," and λόγος, a "discourse."] A treatise on the *Hemiptera.*

Hem-ip'ter-ous. [**Hemip'terus;** from ἥμισυς, a "half," and πτέρον, a "wing."] Half-winged. Applied to an order of insects. See HEMIPTERA.

Hem'ĭ-sphere. [From ἥμισυς, a "half," and σφαῖρα, a "sphere."] The half of a sphere. Applied in Anatomy to the two portions which constitute the upper portion of the cerebrum. They are separated by the *falx cerebri.*

He-mit'ro-pous. [**Hemit'ropus;** from ἥμισυς, a "half," and τρέπω, to "turn."] Applied to a crystal formed of two parts or halves regularly united, but as if the superior had undergone a revolution upon the inferior.

Hem'lock. The *Conium maculatum.*

Hem'lock Pitch. The *Pix Canadensis.*

Hémoptysie, à'mop'tè'zè'. The French term for HÆMOPTYSIS, which see.

Hemorrhage. See HÆMORRHAGE.

Hémorrhagie, à'mo'râ'zhè'. The French term for HÆMORRHAGIA, which see.

Hémorrhoïdes, à'mo'ro'èd'. A French term for PILES, which see.

Hemp. See CANNABIS.

Hemp'-Seed Cal'cu-lus. The name of some varieties of the mulberry calculus, which are remarkably smooth and pale-colored, resembling hemp-seed.

Hen'bane. [**Hyoscy'amus.**] A powerful narcotic plant, said to be poisonous to the domestic fowl. See HYOSCYAMUS.

Hen'bane, Black. The *Hyoscyamus niger.*

Hen-Blind'ness. [**Nyctalo'pia.**] So termed because hens are said to be subject to it.

Hen-dec'a-gon. [**Hendecago'num;** from ἕνδεκα, "eleven," and γωνία, an "angle."] A figure having eleven equal angles and sides.

Henne, hĕn'nĕh. A substance procured in Egypt from the *Lawso'nia Iner'mis,* with which the women stain their fingers and feet. Also used for dyeing skins of a reddish yellow.

He'par,* gen. **Hep'a-tis.** [From ἧπαρ, ἥπατος, the "liver."] The liver, or organ which secretes the bile. (See LIVER.) The term *hepar*, or "liver," was formerly applied to the combinations of sulphur with alkalies, from their *liver-like* appearance.

He'par An-ti-mo'ni-i.* ("Liver of Antimony.") An oxy-sulphuret of antimony.

He'par Cal'cis,* called also **Cal'cis Sul-phu-re'tum.*** A crude bisulphuret of calcium, recommended as an external application to *Crusta lactea*.

He'par Sul'phur-is.* ("Liver of Sulphur.") The old Pharmaceutical name of a liver-brown sulphuret of potash.

Hep-a-tăl'gi-a.* [From ἧπαρ, the "liver," and ἄλγος, "pain."] Pain affecting the liver. See HEPATODYNIA.

Hep-a-taux'e.* [From ἧπαρ, the "liver," and αὔξη, "increase."] Enlargement of the liver.

Hep-a-tem-phrax'is.* [From ἧπαρ, the "liver," and ἔμφραξις, "obstruction."] Obstruction of the liver.

Hep-at-hæm-or-rha'gi-a.* [From ἧπαρ, the "liver," and αἱμοῤῥαγία, an "eruption of blood."] Hæmorrhage from the liver.

Hep-at-hel-co'sis.* [From ἧπαρ, the "liver," and ἕλκωσις, "ulceration."] Ulceration of the liver.

He-pat'ic. [**Hepat'icus;** from ἧπαρ, ἥπατος, the "liver."] Belonging to the liver. Applied to vessels, ducts, etc.

Hepat'ic Air. Another name for sulphuretted hydrogen gas; so called, it would seem, because commonly produced by the action of muriatic acid on the *Hepar Antimonii*.

Hepat'ic Flux. Bilious Flux. The name given in the East to a variety of dysentery, in which there is a frequent flow of bilious fluid from the bowels.

He-pat'i-ca.* [From *hepat'icus*, "belonging to the liver."] Liverwort. A genus of plants belonging to the Linnæan class *Polyandria*, natural order *Ranunculaceæ*, so named on account of its supposed medicinal virtues in hepatic affections. Also, the Pharmacopœial name (U.S. Ph.) for the leaves of the *Hepat'ica America'na*.

He-pat'i-cæ.* A natural order of flowerless plants, related to Mosses, found in damp, shady places.

He-pat'i-co-col'i-cus.* [From *hepat'icus*, "hepatic," and *col'icus*, "of the colon."] Belonging to the liver and colon.

He-pat'i-co-re-na'lis.* [From *hepat'icus*, "hepatic," and *rena'lis*, "of the kidney."] Belonging to the liver and kidney.

Hepaticus. See HEPATIC.

Hep-a-tir-rhœ'a.* [From ἧπαρ, the "liver," and ῥέω, to "flow."] A purging, with bilious evacuations. See HEPATORRHŒA.

Hépatite. See HEPATITIS.

Hep-a-tit'i-cus.* Belonging to *hepatitis*.

Hep-a-ti'tis, i'dis.* [From ἧπαρ, the "liver;" Fr. *Hépatite*, à'pâ'tèt'.] Inflammation of the liver. A genus of the order *Phlegmasiæ*, class *Pyrexiæ*, of Cullen's Nosology.

Hep-a-ti-zā'tion. [**Hepatiza'tio, o'nis;** from ἧπαρ, the "liver."] A change of structure in the lungs, or other texture, into a liver-like substance.

Hep'a-to-çēle.* [From ἧπαρ, the "liver," and κήλη, a "tumor."] Hernia, in which a part of the liver protrudes through the abdominal parietes.

Hep-a-to-dȳn'i-a.* [From ἧπαρ, the "liver," and ὀδύνη, "pain."] Chronic pain in the liver. Nearly the same as *hepatalgia*.

Hep-a-to-gas'tric. [From ἧπαρ, the "liver," and γαστήρ, the "stomach."] A term applied to the smaller omentum, which passes from the liver to the stomach.

Hep-a-tog'ra-phy̆. [**Hepatogra'phia;** from ἧπαρ, the "liver," and γράφω, to "write."] A description of the liver, its attachments, functions, etc.

Hep-a-tol'i-thus.* [From ἧπαρ, the "liver," and λίθος, a "stone."] *Calculus* or concretion in the liver.

Hep-a-tol'o-gy̆. [**Hepatolo'gia;** from ἧπαρ, the "liver," and λόγος, a "discourse."] A treatise on the liver; the science which treats of the anatomy, functions, and diseases of the liver.

Hep-a-ton'cus.* [From ἧπαρ, the "liver," and ὄγκος, a "swelling."] Chronic *hepatitis*, or swelling of the liver.

Hep-a-to-phleg'mon, or **Hep-a-to-phleg'mo-ne.*** [From ἧπαρ, the "liver," and φλεγμονή, "inflammation."] The same as HEPATITIS.

Hep-a-toph'thi-sis,* or **Hep-a-toph'tho-e.*** [From ἧπαρ, the "liver," and φθίσις, "consumption," or φθόη, a "wasting."] Consumption, decay, or wasting, of the liver.

Hep-a-toph-tho'i-cus.* Of, or belonging to, *hepatophthöe*.

Hep-a-to-phy'ma.* [From ἧπαρ, the "liver," and φῦμα, a "suppurating tumor."] A suppuration of the liver.

Hep-a-tor-rha'gi-a.* [From ἧπαρ, the "liver," and ῥήγνυμι, to "burst forth."] A discharge (of blood) from the liver.

Hep-a-tor-rhex'is.* [From ἧπαρ, the "liver," and ῥῆξις, a "rupture."] Rupture of the liver.

Hep-a-tor-rhœ'a.* [From ἧπαρ, the "liver," and ῥέω, to "flow."] A flow of blood from the liver.

Hep-a-to-to'mi-a,* or **Hep-a-tot'o-mў.** [From ἧπαρ, the "liver," and τέμνω, to "cut."] Dissection of the liver, or cutting into the liver.

Hep'ta-gon. [**Heptago'num;** from ἑπτά, "seven," and γωνία, an "angle."] A plane figure having seven equal angles and sides.

Hep-ta-gўn'ĭ-ous. [**Heptagyn'ius;** from ἑπτά, "seven," and γυνή, a "woman," or "female."] Having seven pistils.

Hep-tan'dri-a.* [From ἑπτά, "seven," and ἀνήρ, ἀνδρός, a "man," or "male."] The seventh Linnæan class of plants, including those which have seven stamens in each flower.

Hep-tan'dri-ous, or **Hep-tan'drous.** [**Heptan'drius;** from the same.] Having seven stamens.

Hep-ta-pet'a-lous. [**Heptapet'alus;** from ἑπτά, "seven," and πέταλον, a "petal."] Having seven petals.

Hep-ta-phўl'lous. [**Heptaphyl'lus;** from ἑπτά, "seven," and φύλλον, a "leaf."] Having seven leaves.

Hep-ta-pleū'rus.* [From ἑπτά, "seven," and πλευρόν, a "rib."] Having seven ribs.

Hep-ta-sep'a-lus.* [From ἑπτά, "seven," and *sep'alum*, a "sepal."] Having seven sepals: heptasep'alous.

Hep-ta-sper'mous. [**Hepta-sper'mus;** from ἑπτά, "seven," and σπέρμα, a "seed."] Having seven seeds.

Her-ba.* (Fr. *Herbe*, ĕRb.) An herb. A plant with a soft and succulent stalk, which dies to the root every year. A plant of which the stem does not become woody and persistent.

Her-bā'ceous. [**Herba'ceus.**] Having soft stalks, and perishing to the root each year; of the nature of an herb.

Her-ba'ri-um.* [From *her'ba*, an "herb," and *-arium*, a Latin termination denoting a repository, or the place where any thing is kept. See OVARIUM.] (Fr. *Herbier*, ĕr'be'à'.) A collection of dried specimens of plants: a *Hortus siccus.*

Herbe. See HERBA.

Herbier. See HERBARIUM.

Her-biv'o-rous. [**Herbiv'orus;** from *her'ba*, an "herb," and *vo'ro*, to "devour."] Feeding on herbs.

Héréditaire. See HEREDITARY.

He-red'ĭ-ta-rў. [**Hæredita'rius;** from *hæ'res*, *hære'dis*, an "heir."] (Fr. *Héréditaire*, à'rà'dè'têR'.) Derived by inheritance; transmitted from parent to offspring.

Her-maph'ro-dīte. [**Hermaphrodi'tus;** Hermaphroditus was fabled to be the son of *Her'mes* (or Mercury) and *Aphrodi'te* (or Venus), and to have united both sexes in one person.] One in whom either the male organs of generation are too slightly, or the female too highly, developed, in either case approaching in size and resemblance those of the opposite sex. Applied in Botany to a flower which contains stamens and pistils within the same calyx and petals.

Her-maph-ro-dit'ic. [**Hermaphrodit'icus.**] Belonging to a hermaphrodite.

Her-met'ic, or **Her-met'ĭ-cal.** [**Hermet'icus;** from Ἑρμῆς, Mercury, who is said to have invented chemistry.] Belonging to chemistry.

Hermet'ic Seal. The closing of the end of a glass vessel or tube, while in a state of fusion.

Her-mo-dac'tў-lus.* The ancient name of a plant supposed to be colchicum.

Her'ni-a.* [From ἔρνος, a "branch, or something given off."] (Fr. *Hargne*, haRñ, or *Hernie*, ĕR'nè'.) In popular language, a "rupture;" a tumor formed by the protrusion of any of the viscera of the abdomen beyond its parietes; also, displacement of any part from its normal cavity. A genus of the order *Ectopiæ*, class *Locales*, of Cullen's Nosology.

HER'NIA CER'EBRI.* ("Hernia of the Brain.") Protrusion of the substance of the brain through the fontanels, or through an opening made by a fracture, a trephine, etc.

HER'NIA CONGEN'ITAL. [*Her'nia Congen'ita.*] Hernia existing at birth.

HER'NIA CRURA'LIS.* ("Crural Hernia.") Femoral hernia, or a protrusion under Poupart's ligament. The passage through which the hernia descends is variously called the crural, or femoral, ring, and crural canal.

HER'NIA HUMORA'LIS.* ("Humoral Hernia.") Acute inflammation of the testicle, or swelled testicle. See ORCHITIS.

HER'NIA, IN'GUINAL. [*Her'nia Inguina'lis.*] Bubonocele, or hernia at the groin. It is termed *incomplete*, or *oblique*, when it does not protrude through the abdominal ring, and *complete*, or *direct*, when it passes out at that opening.

HER'NIA, UMBIL'ICAL. [*Her'nia Umbilica'lis.*] Omphalocele, or exomphalos. Hernia of the bowels at the umbilicus.

HER'NIA VARICO'SA.* ("Varicose Hernia.") Another name for *Circocele.*

Herniaire. See HERNIAL.

Her'ni-al. (Fr. *Herniaire*, ĕr'nè'ĕR', *Hernié*, ĕR'nè'à', or *Hernieux*, ĕR'nè'uh'.) Belonging to hernia.

Hernie. See HERNIA.

Hernie Ombilicale. See HERNIA, UMBILICAL.

Hernié. See HERNIAL.

Hernieux. See HERNIAL.

Her-ni-ot'o-my̆. [**Hernioto'mia;** from *her'nia*, and τέμνω, to "cut."] The operation for strangulated hernia.

He-ro'ic. [**Hero'icus;** from ἥρως, a "hero."] Applied to certain remedies from their potency or severity.

Her'pēs, e'tis.* [From ἕρπω, to "creep."] *Serpigo*, or Tetter; a skin-disease in which little itchy vesicles increase, spread, and cluster together, terminating in furfuraceous scales. A genus of the order *Dialyses*, class *Locales*, of Cullen's Nosology.

Her'pes Cir-ci-na'tus.* Ringworm; also called *Herpes Serpigo.*

Her'pes Ex'e-dens.* ("Corroding Herpes.") A species of herpes in which there is a rapid spreading of the disease.

Her'pes Lab-i-a'lis.* ("Herpes of the Lip.") A form of herpes attacking the lips: it is occasionally diffused on the velum and palate.

Her'pes Ser-pi'go.* *Herpes circinatus*, or ringworm.

Her'pes Zos'ter.* [See ZOSTER.] Herpes spreading across the waist, or thorax, like a sash or sword-belt, commonly called *shingles.*

Her-pet'ic. [**Herpet'icus.**] Belonging to *herpes*, or tetter.

Her-pet-i-for'mis.* [From *her'pes*, "tetter," or "cutaneous eruption."] Having the appearance of *herpes.*

Her-pe-tog'ra-phy̆. [**Herpetogra'phia;** from *her'pes*, "tetter," and γράφω, to "describe."] A description of *herpes.*

Her-pe-tol'o-ġy̆. [**Herpetolo'gia;** from ἑρπετός, "reptile," and λόγος, a "discourse."] The study or science of reptiles, their habits, nature, etc. Also, a dissertation on herpetic diseases. See HERPETIC.

Hes-pĕr'i-din. [From *hesperid'ium*, the "orange."] A peculiar crystallizable substance obtained from unripe oranges.

Hestern. = *Hester'nus.** "Of yesterday."

Het'er-a-can'thus.* [From ἕτερος, "other," "different," and ἄκανθα, a "thorn."] Having different spines, or spinous stipules, one of which is straight, the other hooked.

Het'er-a-del'phi-a.* [From ἕτερος, "other," "different," and ἀδελφός, a "brother."] A term applied to the union of the body of two fœtuses. In these cases, one fœtus generally attains its perfect growth; the other remains undeveloped or acephalous, maintaining a parasitic life upon its brother.

Het'er-a-de'ni-a,* or **Het'er-o-de'ni-a.*** [From ἕτερος, "different," and ἀδήν, a "gland."] A heterologous formation of glandular substance.

Het-er-an'drus.* [From ἕτερος, "different," and ἀνήρ, ἀνδρός, a "man," or "male."] Having stamens or anthers of different form.

Het-er-an'thus.* [From ἕτερος, "different," and ἄνθος, a "flower."] Having different flowers.

Het'er-o-car'pous. [**Heterocar'pus;** from ἕτερος, "different," and καρπός, "fruit."] Bearing different fruits.

Het'er-o-çeph'a-lus.* [From ἕτερος, "different," and κεφαλή, the "head."] A monster-fœtus with two unequal heads.

Het-er-o-chro'ni-a.* [From ἕτερος, "different," and χρόνος, "time."] A deviation from the normal condition of a part, consisting in the development of some mass or tissue at a time when, according to the laws of health, it ought not to have been developed.

Het'er-o-clite. [**Heteroc'litus;** from ἕτερος, "different," and κλίνω, to "incline."] Literally, "anomalous," or "irregular." Applied to plants which have the sexes separated.

Het'er-o-ga'mi-us,* **Het-er-og'a-mus.*** [From ἕτερος, "different," and γάμος, a "marriage."] Having flowers, monœcious, diœcious, or polygamous.

Heterogangliata. See ZOOLOGY.

Het'er-o-ġe'ne-ous. [**Heteroge'neus;** from ἕτερος, "different," and γένος, a "kind."] Of different or opposite kinds.

Het'er-o-la'li-a.* [From ἕτερος, "different," and λαλία, "speech."] A defect in speech. See HETEROPHONIA.

Het-er-ol'o-bus.* [From ἕτερος, "different," and λόβος, a "lobe."] Applied to plants, or parts of plants, having unequal lobes.

Het-er-ol'o-gous. [**Heterol'ogus;** from ἕτερος, "different," and λόγος, a "discourse," "proportion," or "relation."] Applied to certain formations, consisting of the presence of a solid or fluid substance different from any of the solids or fluids which enter into the healthy composition of the body.

Het-er-om'e-rus.* [From ἕτερος, "different," and μέρος, a "part," or "portion."] Having, or consisting of, different portions. See ISOMEROUS.

Het-er-o-me'tri-a.* [From ἕτερος, "different," and μέτρον, a "measure."] A variation from the normal condition of a part with respect to the "measure" or quantity of material which it contains.

Het'er-o-mor'phous. [**Heteromor'phus;** from ἕτερος, "different," and μορφή, "form."] Differing in form, shape, or external appearance. See ISOMORPHOUS.

Het'er-o-ne'mus.* [From ἕτερος, "different," and νῆμα, a "thread," or "fillet."] Having unequal filaments.

Het-er-op'a-thy. [**Heteropathi'a;** from ἕτερος, "different," and πάθος, "affection."] That mode of treating diseases by which a morbid condition is removed, by inducing a different or opposite condition to supplant it; such, for example, as resorting to cold water or refrigerating medicines to get rid of fever. The opposite of *Homœopathy*, and, so, the same as *Allopathy.*

Het'er-o-pet'a-lus.* [From ἕτερος, "different," and πέταλον, a "petal."] Having dissimilar or unequal petals.

Het'er-o-pho'ni-a.* [From ἕτερος, "different," and φωνή, the "voice."] An abnormal state of the voice.

Het'er-o-pla'si-a.* [From ἕτερος, "different," and πλάσις, "formation," or "structure."] The increase of a part by the addition of structural elements different from those of its normal condition.

Het-er-op'o-dus.* [From ἕτερος, "different," and πούς, a "foot."] Having feet different (from the other orders). Applied in the plural neuter (*Heterop'oda*) to an order of *Mollusca Gasteropoda.*

Het-er-op'te-rus.* [From ἕτερος, "different," and πτερόν, a "wing."] Applied in the plural neuter (*Heterop'tera*) to a section of *Hemiptera*, in which the *elytra* are membranous only at the extremity.

Het'er-o-rhyn'chus,* **Het-er-o-ros'tris.*** [From ἕτερος, "different," and ῥύγχος, a "beak," *ros'trum*, a "beak."] Having different beaks.

Het'er-o-ste'mo-nus.* [From ἕτερος, "different," and στήμων, a "stamen."] Having dissimilar stamens.

Het-er-ot'ro-pous. [**Heterot'ropus;** from ἕτερος, "different," and τρόπος, "manner."] Applied to the embryo of a plant when it lies across the *hilum.*

Het'er-o-typ'i-a.* [From ἕτερος, "different," and τύπος, a "type."] A variation from the normal condition, by the production of a mass in a part differing in type from the remaining structure of the part.

Heu-che'ra.* Alum-root. The Pharmacopœial name (U.S. Ph.) for the root of *Heuchera Americana.*

Hex'a-gon. [**Hexago'num;** from ἕξ, "six," and γωνία, an "angle."] A plane figure having six equal angles and sides.

Hex-ag'o-nal. [**Hexag'onus.**] Belonging to a hexagon.

Hex-ag'yn-ous, or **Hex-a-gyn'i-ous.** [**Hexagyn'ius;** from ἕξ, "six," and γυνή, a "woman," or "female."] Having six pistils. Applied to a Linnæan order.

Hex-a-he'dral. [**Hexahe'drus.**] Belonging to a hexahedron.

Hex-a-he'dron. [**Hexahe'drum;** from ἕξ, "six," and ἕδρα, a "base."] A regular solid figure bounded by six equal sides; a cube.

Hex-an'dri-a.* [From ἕξ, "six," and ἀνήρ, ἀνδρός, a "man," or "male."] The sixth class of the Linnæan system of plants, including those which have six equal stamens in each flower.

Hex-an'drous, or **Hex-an'dri-ous.** [**Hexan'drius.**] Having six equal stamens. See HEXANDRIA.

Hex-an'gu-lar. [**Hexangula'ris;** from ἕξ, "six," and *an'gulus*, an "angle."] Having six angles.

Hex-a-pet'a-lous. [**Hexapet'alus;** from ἕξ, "six," and πέταλον, a "petal."] Having six petals.

Hex-a-phyl'lous. [**Hexaphyl'lus;** from ἕξ, "six," and φύλλον, a "leaf."] Having six leaves.

Hex-ap'o-dus.* [From ἕξ, "six," and πούς, a "foot."] Having six feet. Applied particularly to insects.

Hex-ap'te-rous. [**Hexap'terus;** from ἕξ, "six," and πτέρον, a "wing."] Provided with six wings.

Hex-a-sep'a-lus.* [From ἕξ, "six,"

and *sep'alum*, a "sepal."] Composed of six sepals.

Hex-a-sper'mus.* [From ἕξ, "six," and σπέρμα, a "seed."] Having six seeds.

Hex-a-ste'mo-nus.* [From ἕξ, "six," and στήμων, a "stamen."] Having six stamens. See HEXANDROUS.

Hex'is.* [Gr. ἕξις; from ἔχω, to "have," to "have one's self," or to "be."] The same as *habit* of body. See DIATHESIS.

Hi-a'tus Fal-lo'pi-i.* [From *hi'o, hia'tum*, to "gape."] An opening in the tympanum, named from Fallopius.

Hibernaculum. See HYBERNACULUM.

Hibiscus Moschatus. See ABELMOSCHUS.

Hiccough, Hiccup. See SINGULTUS.

Hid'den Seiz'ure. A term used by M. Hall for such a paroxysm in convulsive diseases, as may have been unobserved, because occurring in the night, or away from the patient's home and friends, or limited to the deeply-seated muscles.

Hi-dro'a.* [From ἱδρώς, "sweat."] The term given by Sauvages and Vogel to *eczema*, or heat eruption.

Hi-dro'dēs.* [From ἱδρώς, "sweat."] Full of sweat; sweaty.

Hi-dron'o-sus.* [From ἱδρώς, "sweat," and νόσος, a "disease."] See ANGLICUS SUDOR.

Hi-drop-e-de'sis.* [From ἱδρώς, "sweat," and πήδησις, a "spring."] Excessive sweating.

Hidropyretus. See HYDRONOSUS.

Hid-ror-rhœ'a.* [From ἱδρώς, "sweat," and ῥέω, to "flow."] Profuse sweating.

Hi-dro'sis.* [From ἱδρώς, ἱδρῶτος, "sweat."] The condition of sweating.

Hi-drot'ic. [**Hidrot'icus**; from the same.] Causing sweat; sudorific; diaphoretic.

Hi-drot-o-pœ'ia,* Hi-drot-o-poi-e'sis.* [From ἱδρώς, "sweat," and ποιέω, to "make."] Excretion of the sweat.

Hi-er-an'o-sos.* [From ἱερός, "holy," and νόσος, "disease."] *Mor'bus Sa'cer.* An ancient term for "epilepsy."

Hi'er-a Pi'cra.* [From ἱερός, "holy," and πικρός, "bitter."] A name applied to *Pulvis Aloes cum Canellâ.*

High-mo-ri-a'num An'trum.* A cavity in the superior maxillary bone, described by Highmore; otherwise called the *Antrum maxillæ*, or *A. maxillare.*

Hi-lif'er-us.* [From *hi'lum*, and *fe'ro*, to "bear."] Having *hila.*

Hilon. See HILUM.

Hi'lum,* plural **Hi'la.** Sometimes improperly written **Hi'lus.** (Fr. *Hilon*, ē'lôNᴳ'.) The point of attachment of a seed to its seed-vessel, or receptacle by which it obtains its nourishment; the umbilicus of the seed.

Hi'lus Li-e-na'lis.* [From *li'en*, the "spleen."] The concave part of the spleen.

Hip. See COXA.

Hip-Bath. See SEMICUPIUM.

Hip-Ber'ries. The ripe fruit of the *Rosa canina.*

Hip-Joint Disease. See COXALGIA.

Hip'-Tree. The *Rosa canina.*

Hip-po-cam'pus.* [From ἱππόκαμπος, a small marine animal with a head closely resembling that of a horse.] The small animal named the sea-horse.

Hippocam'pus Ma'jor,* called also **Cor'nu Am-mo'nis.*** A large white curved body in the *inferior cornu* of the lateral ventricles of the brain.

Hippocam'pus Mi'nor.* A small eminence of white substance in the *posterior cornu* of the lateral ventricles of the brain.

Hippocastanaceæ,* hip-po-kas-ta-na'she-ē, or **Hippocastaneæ,*** hip-po-kas-ta'ne-ē. [From *Hippocas'tanum*, the specific name of the "horse-chestnut."] A name given by some botanists to a natural order of plants. See SAPINDACEÆ.

Hip'po-co-ry'za.* [From ἵππος, the "horse," and κορύζα, "inflammation of the mucous membrane of the nostrils."] Applied to coryza in horses, such as occurs in farcy or glanders; likewise to the same affection in cattle, etc. It is also termed *Hippomyxa.* See FARCY.

Hippocrateaceæ,* hip-po-kra-te-a'-she-ē. [From *Hippocra'tea*, one of the genera.] A natural order of exogenous shrubs, mostly natives of South America.

Hip-poc'ra-tēs' Sleeve. [**Man'ica Hippoc'ratis.**] A name given to a conical-shaped strainer of linen or flannel.

Hip-po-crat'ic. [**Hippocrat'icus.**] Belonging to Hippocrates.

Hippocratic Countenance. See FACIES HIPPOCRATICA.

Hippocraticeæ,* hip-po-kra-tish'-e-ē. The Jussieuan name of a natural order of plants. See HIPPOCRATEACEÆ.

Hip'po-lith. [**Hippol'ithus**; from ἵππος, a "horse," and λίθος, a "stone."]

The *Bezoar equinum;* a concretion in the gall-bladder, or intestines, of the horse.

Hip-pol'o-ġy̆. [Hippolo'gia; from ἵππος, a "horse," and λόγος, a "discourse."] A term for a dissertation on the horse; the science which treats of the horse.

Hip-po-my̆x'ạ.* [From ἵππος, a "horse," and μύξα, "mucus."] The same as HIPPOCORYZA, which see.

Hip'po-no-sol'o-ġy̆. [Hipponosolo'gia.] The same as HIPPOPATHOLOGY, which see.

Hip'po-path-o-loġ'ĭ-cạl. [Hippopatholoġ'icus.] Belonging to hippopathology.

Hip'po-pạ-thol'o-ġy̆. [Hippopatholo'gia; from ἵππος, a "horse," πάθος, "disease," and λόγος, a "discourse."] That branch of general medicine which treats of the diseases of the horse.

Hip-pos-te-ol'o-ġy̆. [Hipposteolo'gia; from ἵππος, a "horse," and ὀστεολογία, a "treatise upon bones."] A treatise on the bones of the horse; that branch of Comparative Anatomy which treats of the skeleton of the horse.

Hip-pot'o-my̆. [Hippoto'mia; from ἵππος, a "horse," and τέμνω, to "cut."] The anatomy, or dissection, of the horse.

Hip-pu'rāte. [Hippu'ras, a'*tis.*] A combination of hippuric acid with a base.

Hip-pu'ric. [Hippu'ricus; from ἵππος, a "horse," and οὖρον, "urine."] Applied to an acid found plentifully in the urine of the horse and cow, and in that of the *Graminivora* generally.

Hip'pus.* [Gr. ἵππος, a "horse," also, an "affection of the eyelids."] A disease of the eyelid, in which there is a constant tendency to wink; so called, it is said, because the lid goes up and down, like a man on horseback.

Hip'pus Pu-pil'læ.* ("Hippus of the Pupil.") A tremulous condition of the iris, attended with alternate contractions and dilatations of the pupil.

Hir'cāte. [Hir'cas, a'*tis.*] A combination of hircic acid with a base.

Hir'cic, or **Hir-cin'ic. [Hircin'icus.]** Applied to an acid obtained from the fat of the goat.

Hir'cin, or **Hir'cine. [Hirci'na;** from *hir'cus*, the "male goat."] A peculiar substance found in the fat of the goat, and on which its strong odor depends. It yields by saponification the *hircic*, or *hircinic*, acid.

Hir-çis'mus.* [From *hir'cus*, a "male goat."] The strong odor, peculiar to the human axilla, which resembles that of the male goat.

Hir'sute. [Hirsu'tus.] Hairy; rough; shaggy.

Hirsuties,* hir-su'she-ēz. [From *hirsu'tus*, "hairy."] A disease in which hair grows in morbid excess or on a part where it is unnatural.

Hir-ti-flo'rus.* [From *hir'tus*, "hairy," and *flos*, a "flower."] Having hairy flowers.

Hir'tus.* [Contraction of *hirsu'tus*, "hairy," or "shaggy."] Rough-haired; hairy.

Hirud. = *Hiru'do,** or *hiru'dines.** A "leech, or leeches."

Hĭ-ru-dĭ-for'mis.* [From *hiru'do*, a "horse-leech."] Resembling the leech. Applied by Latreille, in the neuter plural (*Hirudifor'mia*), to an order of animals.

Hĭ-ru'do, d*inis.** [From *hau'rio*, to "drink up"?] A genus of worms, or worm-like animals, belonging to the class *Anellata* (or *Anellides*). The Pharmacopœial name (Brit. Ph.) of the *Sanguisuga medicinalis* (Fr. *Sangsue*, sŏnᵍ'sü'), the *Hirudo medicinalis*.

Hiru'do Me-diç-ĭ-na'lis.* The European leech, an animal much employed for local depletion. It will draw nearly a half an ounce of blood. The American leech, or *Hiru'do deco'ra*, does not make so deep an incision as the European, and draws less blood.

His'pid. [His'pidus.] Having bristles; bristly.

His-pid-u-la'tus.* [From *hispid'ulus*, the diminutive of *his'pidus*, "rough," "bristly."] In a slight degree rough.

His-pĭd-u-lo'sus.* [From the same.] Having stiff hairs.

His-to-dĭ-al'y̆-sis.* [From ἱστός, a "web," or "tissue," and διάλυσις, a "dissolution."] A resolution of organic texture.

His-to-dĭ-ạ-ly̆t'ĭ-cus.* Belonging to *histodialysis*.

His-to-ġe-net'ic. [Histogenet'icus.] Belonging to histogeny: promoting the formation of organic textures.

His-toġ'e-ny̆. [Histogen'esis; from ἱστός, a "web," or "tissue," and γένω, to "be born."] The origin or formation of organic tissue.

His-to-graph'ĭ-cus.* Belonging to histography.

His-tog'ra-phy̆. [**Histogra'phia;** from ἱστός, a "web," or "tissue," and γράφω, to "write."] A description of the organic tissues.

His-to-log'ĭ-cal. [**Histolog'icus.**] Belonging to histology.

His-tol'o-ğy̆. [**Histolo'gia;** from ἱστός, a "web," or "tissue," and λόγος, a "discourse."] The science or doctrine of the minute structure and composition of the different textures of organized bodies.

His-ton'o-my̆. [**Histono'mia;** from ἱστός, a "web," or "tissue," and νόμος, a "law."] History of the laws which regulate the formation and arrangement of organic tissues.

His-tot'o-my̆. [**Histoto'mia;** from ἱστός, a "web," or "tissue," and τέμνω, to "cut."] Dissection of organic tissues.

His-trĭ-on'ic. [From *his'trio,* a "play-actor."] A term applied by German writers to affections of the muscles of expression, inducing spasms and paralysis.

Hive Syr'up. A syrup prepared as a remedy for croup. See SYRUPUS SCILLÆ COMPOSITUS.

Hives, hīvz. A popular name for the croup. It is also applied to different species of rash.

Hoarseness. See RAUCEDO.

Hoary. See GLAUCUS, and INCANOUS.

Hoff'mann's An'o-dyne Liq'uor. [**Hoffman'ni Liq'uor Anod'ynus.**] See SPIRITUS ÆTHERIS COMPOSITUS.

Hog's Lard. See ADEPS SUILLUS, and AXUNGIA PORCINA.

Hol-o-car'pus.* [From ὅλος, "whole," or "entire," and καρπός, "fruit."] Having entire fruit-capsules.

Hol-o-pet'a-lus.* [From ὅλος, "whole," or "entire," and πέταλον, a "petal."] Having entire petals.

Homaliaceæ,* ho-ma-le-a'she-ē. [From *Homa'lium,* one of the genera.] A natural order of exogenous trees and shrubs, all of which are tropical.

Hom'berg's Phos'pho-rus. Muriate of lime, which, on being reduced by heat to a vitreous mass, Homberg found to emit a phosphoric light, when struck by a hard body.

Hom-berg's Py̆-roph'o-rus. A mixture of alum and brown sugar, which takes fire on exposure to the air.

Home-Sickness. See NOSTALGIA.

Hom'ĭ-cide. [**Homici'dium;** from *ho'mo,* "man," and *cæ'do,* to "kill."] The killing of a man, woman, or child by accident, in distinction from that done in malice, with set purpose; manslaughter, chance-medley, etc.

Ho'mo-. [From ὁμός, "equal," "same."] A prefix denoting equality, or sameness.

Ho-mœ-o-mor'phus.* [From ὅμοιος, "like," and μορφή, "form."] Having a similar form.

Ho-mœ-o-path'ic. [**Homœopath'icus.**] Belonging to homœopathy.

Homœopathie. See HOMŒOPATHY.

Ho-mœ-op'a-thy̆. [**Homœopathi'a;** from ὅμοιος, "like," and πάθος, "disease."] (Fr. *Homœopathie,* o'mā'o'pâ'tē'.) A doctrine propounded by Hahnemann, professing to cure diseases by the action of infinitesimal doses of medicines, of a quality to excite in the healthy a disease similar to that which is to be cured.

Ho-mœ-o'sis.* [From ὅμοιος, "like."] Assimilation.

Homogangliata. See ZOOLOGY.

Ho-mo-ğe-ne'ĭ-ty̆. [**Homogene'itas, a'tis.**] Homogeneousness.

Ho-mo-ğe'ne-ous. [**Homoge'neus;** from ὁμός, "equal," "same," and γένος, a "kind."] Of the same kind or quality throughout.

Ho-mol'o-gous. [**Homol'ogus;** from ὁμός, "equal," "same," and λόγος, a "discourse," also, "relation," "analogy," "ratio," or "proportion."] Applied to things of the same essential nature, however different in form or name, in different animal bodies. See HOMOLOGY.

Homologue, hom'o-log. [**Homol'ogum;** from the same.] A term applied to a part of an animal which corresponds to another part in a different animal, or to a different portion of the same animal. See next article.

Ho-mol'o-ğy̆ [**Homolo'gia;** from the same], or **Ho-mol'o-ğies, Doc'trine of.** That branch of anatomical science which investigates the correspondence of parts and of plan in the construction of animals.

1. *Special Homology* relates to the correspondence of parts in different animals. Thus, the wing of a bird is the homologue of the arm in a man, or of the fore-leg of a horse.

2. *Serial Homology* relates to the correspondence of parts in the same animal. Thus, the wing of a bird is the homologue, in one segment of its body,

of the leg of the bird in another segment.

3. *General Homology* relates to correspondencies of parts viewed with reference to the ideal archetype of the vertebrate skeleton. Thus, the arm is the *diverging appendage* of its segment; the supra-occipital bone is the *neural spine;* the ex-occipital bone, or condyloid part of the occipital bone, in the human subject, is the *neurapophysis.*

Hom-o-mor'phous. [Homomor'phus; from ὁμός, "equal," "same," and μορφή, "form."] Having the same form. See HETEROMORPHUS.

Ho-mon'ȳ-mous [from ὁμός, "same," and ὄνομα, a "name"], and **Ho-mo-ty'pal** [see HOMOTYPE]. These terms denote, in Anatomy, a correlation of parts: the frontal bone is the *homonym* or *homotype* of the super-occipital bone, the humerus of the femur, etc. It is the aim of *serial homology* to determine homonymous or homotypal relations. See HOMOLOGY.

Hom-o-pet'a-lus.* [From ὁμός, "equal," "same," and πέταλον, a "petal."] Applied to flowers in which the petals are alike.

Hom-o-phȳl'lus.* [From ὁμός, "equal," "same," and φύλλον, a "leaf."] Having leaves or leaflets all alike.

Ho-mop'ter-ous. [Homop'terus; from ὁμός, "equal," "same," and πτερόν, a "wing."] A term applied to a section of hemipterous insects, having *elytra* of the same consistence throughout, and almost similar to the wings.

Ho-mot'ro-pous, or **Ho-mot'ro-pal. [Homot'ropus;** from ὁμός, "equal," "same," and τρέπω, to "turn."] Applied to the embryo when it has the same direction as the seed.

Hom'o-type. [Homot'ypus; from ὁμός, "equal," "same," and τύπος, "form," or "nature."] A term employed by Owen for a repeated part in the segments of the same skeleton.

Hon'ey. [Mel, Mel'lis.] A sweet substance collected from the nectaries of flowers by the *A'pis Mellif'ica,* or Honey-Bee.

Hon'ey-Dew. A sweetish substance secreted and deposited upon the leaves of plants by the *Aphides,* a genus of small insects popularly called plant-lice.

Hoop'er's Pills. A nostrum which has been extensively used as a purgative and emmenagogue. See PILULÆ ALOES ET MYRRHÆ.

Hooping-Cough. See PERTUSSIS.

Hop. The *Humulus lupulus;* also, the *bracteæ,* or floral leaves, of the same. See HUMULUS.

Hôpital, ō'pē'tȁl'. The French term for HOSPITAL, which see.

Hoquet, ho'kȁ'. The French term for "hiccup." See SINGULTUS.

Hor-de-ā'ceous. [Hordea'ceus; from *hor'deum,* "barley."] Of the nature of barley; resembling barley.

Hor'de-i Dis'ti-chi Sem'ĭ-na.* ("Seeds of the Hordeum Distichon.") See HORDEUM.

Hor'de-i Sem'ĭ-na.* ("Seeds of Barley.") Pearl Barley; the grains of the *Hordeum Distichon,* or common barley, deprived of the husk or skin. See HORDEUM.

Hor'de-ĭ-for'mis.* [From *hor'deum,* "barley."] Formed like barley.

Hor'de-in. [Hordei'na; from *hor'deum,* "barley."] A peculiar substance found in barley, allied to starch, but constituting a distinct substance.

Hor-de'o-lum.* [Diminutive of *hor'deum,* "barley."] A small, highly-inflammatory tumor on the edge of the eyelid: popularly, a stye.

Hor'de-um.* Barley. A Linnæan genus of the class *Triandria,* natural order *Graminaceæ.* Also, the Pharmacopœial name ‖ of the seeds of *Hor'deum dis'tichon,* or barley.

Hor'deum Dis'ti-chon.* The French barley-plant.

Hor'deum Vul-ga're.* The Scotch, or common, barley-plant.

Hore'hound. The *Marrubium vulgare.*

Hore'hound Tea. Prepared by infusing an ounce of the *Marrubium vulgare,* or white horehound, in a pint of boiling water.

Hor. interm. = *Ho'ris interme'diis.** "At the intermediate hours" between what has been ordered at stated times.

Ho-rī'zon. [From ὁρίζων, the present participle of ὁρίζω, to "bound."] The great circle dividing the heavens from the earth, and forming the boundary to our sight.

Hor-ĭ-zon'tal. [Horizonta'lis.] Parallel with the horizon: on a level.

Horn'blende. A mineral of dark-green or black color, abounding in oxide of iron and entering into the composition of several of the trap rocks.

Horn Pock. A name given by some writers to a form of Variola, in which the pimples are imperfectly suppurating, ichorous, or horny, and semi-transparent.

Hor'ri-dus.* [From *hor'ror*, a "shivering or quaking from fear or cold."] Shivering with cold. Applied to a fever, etc.

Hor-ri-pi-lā'tion. [**Horripila'tio, o'***nis*; from *hor'reo*, to "have one's hair stand on end," to "shiver," or "tremble," and *pi'lus*, the "hair."] A sensation of creeping, or as if each hair were stiff and erect, in different parts of the body. It is often a symptom of the approach of fever.

Hor'ror, o'*ris*.* [From *hor'reo*, to "shake from cold."] A shivering, or cold fit.

Horse-Ches'nut. The fruit of the *Æs'culus Hippocas'tanum.*

Horse-Mint. The common name of the *Monar'da puncta'ta.*

Horse-Rad'ish. The common name of the *Cochlea'ria armora'cia.*

Hor-tic'o-lus.* [From *hor'tus*, a "garden," and *co'lo*, to "inhabit."] Growing in a garden.

Hor'tus Sic'cus.* (Literally, a "dry garden.") A *herbarium*, or collection of dried plants.

Hor. un. spatio = *Ho'ræ uni'us spa'tio.** "At the end of an hour."

Hos'pi-tal. [**Hospita'lium**; from *hos'pes*, a "host;" also, a "guest."] (Fr. *Hôpital*, ō'pȧ'tȧl'.) Originally, a place for exercising hospitality towards strangers, or the sick and poor. A charitable establishment for the relief of the sick, and for their lodgment and maintenance during treatment; an infirmary.

Hos'pital Fe'ver. [**Fe'bris Nosocomia'lis.**] A fever peculiar to the inmates of a hospital, from their condition and circumstances.

Hos'pital Gan'grēne. [**Gangræ'na Nosocomia'lis.**] A severe and peculiar species of humid gangrene, combined with phagedenic ulceration of a highly infectious nature.

Houblon, hoo'blôɴᴳ'. The French term for the "hop." See Humulus.

Hour-Glass Con-trac'tion. An irregular and transverse contraction of the uterus, in which it assumes the form of an hour-glass.

H. S., or **Hor. som.** = *Ho'râ som'ni.** "Just before going to sleep."

Huile, wēl. The French term for "oil." See Oleum, and Oil.

Hum'bold-tite. A mineral consisting of oxalate of lime, and forming the basis of a urinary calculus.

Hu-mec'tant. [**Humec'tans**; from *humec'to, humecta'tum*, to "make moist."] Rendering moist; moistening. The same as Diluent.

Hu-mec-tā'tion. [**Humecta'tio, o'***nis*; from the same.] The act or process of making moist.

Hu'me-ral. [**Humera'lis**; from *hu'merus*, the "arm," or "shoulder."] Belonging to the *humerus*; brachial.

Hu'me-rus,* gen. **Hu'me-ri.** [From ὦμος, the "shoulder."] (Fr. *Épaule*, ā'pōl'.) Originally, the "shoulder." In Anatomy, the *brachium*, or arm proper, from the shoulder to the elbow; also, the long bone, or *Os humeri* itself. In Ornithology, the first portion of the superior extremity supporting the wing.

Hume's Test. A test for arsenious acid, consisting of the ammonio-nitrate of silver. If solutions of these substances be mixed, a yellow arsenite of silver is precipitated, and nitrate of ammonia remains in solution.

Humeur Aqueuse, ü'mᴜʀ' ȧ'kᴜᴢ'. The French term for Aqueous Humor, which see.

Hu'mic. [**Hu'micus**; from *hu'mus*, the "ground."] Pertaining to the ground, or earth. The same as Geic. Applied to an acid found in earth.

Hu'mi-fuse. [**Humifu'sus**; from *hu'mus*, the "ground," and *fu'sus*, "spread," or "lying along."] A botanical term which signifies "running along the surface of the ground."

Hu'mi-lis.* [From *hu'mus*, the "ground."] Mean; humble; dwarfish. Applied to plants which grow close to the ground.

Humiriaceæ,* hu-me-re-a'she-ē. A natural order of exogenous trees and shrubs, which are found in the tropical parts of America. It includes the *Humir'ium*, which produces Balsam of Umiri, resembling copaiva in properties.

Hu'mor. [**Hu'mor, o'***ris*.] Moisture, or sap. Any fluid of the body other than the blood.

Humor, Aqueous. See Aqueous Humor.

Humor, Vitreous. See Vitreous Humor.

Hu'mo-ral. [**Humora'lis**; from *hu'mor*, "moisture," or "humor."] Belonging to the humors of the body.

Hu'moral Pa-thol'o-gy̆. A system in medicine which attributed all diseases to morbid changes in the *humors*, or fluid parts of the body, without assigning any influence to the state of the solids.

Hu-mor'ic. [**Humor'icus**; from

hu'mor, "moisture," or "humor."] Applied to the sound produced by percussion on the stomach when distended with air and fluid.

Hu'mu-lin. [**Humuli'na.**] The narcotic principle of the *Hu'mulus lu'pulus.*

Hu'mu-lus.* Hops. The Pharmacopœial name (U.S. Ph.) for the strobiles of the *Hu'mulus lu'pulus.*

Hu'mulus Lu'pu-lus.* (Fr. *Houblon*, hoo'blòN'.) The systematic name of the hop, which is both a tonic and hypnotic.

Hu'mus.* Vegetable mould; woody fibre in a state of decay.

Hunger. See FAMES.

Husk. See GLUME, INVOLUCRE, and SILIQUA.

Hux'ham's (hŭx'amz) **Tinc'ture of Bark.** The same as TINCTURA CINCHONÆ COMPOSITA, which see.

Hy-a-li'nus.* [From ὕαλος, "glass."] Transparent, like glass: hy'aline.

Hy'a-li-pen'nis.* [From ὕαλος, "glass," and *pen'na*, a "wing."] The same as HYALOPTERUS.

Hyalitis, idis. See HYALOIDITIS.

Hy'a-lo-dec'crȳ-sis.* [From ὑαλώδης, "glassy," and ἔκρυσις, a "flowing out."] Escape of part of the vitreous body or humor.

Hy-a-lo'de-o-ma-la'ci-a* (-ma-la'-she-a). [From ὑαλώδης, "glassy," and μαλακία, "softness."] A softening of the vitreous body.

Hy-a-lo'de-o-mal-a-co'sis.* The progress of *hyalodeomalacia.*

Hy-a-lo'dēs.* [From ὕαλος, "glass."] Glassy.

Hȳ'a-loid. [**Hyaloi'des;** from ὕαλος, "glass," and εἶδος, a "form."] Resembling glass; transparent.

Hy'aloid Mem'brane. [**Membra'na Hyaloi'des.**] The extremely delicate membrane of the eye whose numerous cells contain the vitreous humor.

Hy-a-loi-di'tis, idis.* [From *hyaloi'des*, "hyaloid."] Inflammation of the hyaloid membrane.

Hy-a-lop'te-rus.* [From ὕαλος, "glass," and πτέρον, a "wing."] A term applied to insects having transparent wings: hyalop'terous.

Hy-a-lo-sper'mus.* [From ὕαλος, "glass," and σπέρμα, a "seed."] Having transparent seeds: hyalosper'mous.

Hy-ber-nac'u-lum.* [From *hyber'na*, "winter quarters," or a "wintering place."] An organic body which springs from the surface of a plant, in order to protect the new shoot which it encases from injury.

Hȳ-ber'nal. [**Hyber'nus;** from *hyber'no, hyberna'tum*, to "winter."] Belonging to winter.

Hȳ'ber-nāt-ing. [**Hyber'nans;** from the same.] Passing the winter.

Hȳ-ber-nā'tion. [From the same.] The state of torpor or winter-sleep peculiar to certain animals.

Hȳ'brid. [**Hyb'rida,** or **Hy'bris, idos;** from ὕβρις, "mongrel."] (Fr. *Métis*, mà'tès'.) The offspring of two different species of animals or plants. As an adjective it signifies "mongrel."

Hydarthrosis. See HYDRARTHROSIS.

Hydarthrus. See HYDRARTHRUS.

Hȳ-dat'id. [**Hyd'atis, idis;** from ὑδατίς, a "vesicle" (from ὕδωρ, "water").] A small vesicular tumor, containing a watery fluid; also, a genus of the *Entozoa*, formed of a membrane containing a water-like fluid. See AQUULA.

Hydatidodes. See HYDATIDOSUS.

Hȳ-dat-i-do-i'dēs.* [From *hyd'atis*, a "hydatid," and εἶδος, a "form."] Resembling a hydatid.

Hȳ-dat-i-do'ma, atis.* [From *hyd'atis*, a "hydatid."] A tumor containing hydatids.

Hȳ-dat-i-do'sis.* [From *hyd'atis*, a "vesicle," or "hydatid."] The formation of *hydatidoma.*

Hȳ-dat-i-do'sus.* [From *hyd'atis*, a "vesicle," or "hydatid."] Having, or full of, hydatids.

Hȳ-dat-i-for'mis.* [From *hyd'atis*, a "vesicle," or "hydatid."] Having the appearance of a hydatid: hydat'iform.

Hȳd-a-tig'e-nus.* [From ὑδατίς, a "vesicle," and γένω, to "be born."] Proceeding from a hydatid.

Hȳd-a-to-gen'e-sis.* [From ὕδωρ, "water," and γένεσις, "origin," "birth."] A term for the formation of water, or of a watery fluid, in the body.

Hȳd-a-ton'cus.* [From ὕδωρ, "water," and ὄγκος, a "tumor."] A watery swelling.

Hyderoncus. See HYDATONCUS.

Hy'de-ros,* or **Hy'de-rus.*** [From ὕδωρ, "water."] Literally, "water-flux." A name given by the Greeks to diabetes.

Hȳ'dra.* [From ὕδωρ, "water."] A polypus, destitute of brain, viscera, or lungs, found in brooks and pools in temperate countries.

Hȳ-drac'id. [**Hydrac'idum;** from ὕδωρ, "water," and *ac'idum*, an "acid."] Applied to acids containing hydrogen.

Hy'dra-de-ni'tis, *idis.** [From *hy'-draden*, a "lymphatic gland."] Inflammation of a lymphatic gland. See LYMPHADENITIS.

Hy-dræ'ma,* or **Hy-dræ'mi-a.*** [From ὕδωρ, "water," and αἷμα, "blood."] A state of the blood in which the serum is transparent, with a small quantity of coloring matter.

Hy'dra-gŏgue. [**Hydrago'gus;** from ὕδωρ, "water," and ἄγω, to "bring or drive away."] Applied to medicines which increase the secretions, and so tend to remove water from the system.

Hydrangeaceæ,* hi-dran-je-a'she-ē. [From *Hydrange'a*, one of the genera.] A natural order of exogenous shrubs, found in China, Japan, and America.

Hy-dran-ge-i'tis, *idis.** [From *hydrangi'on*, a "lymphatic vessel" (from ὕδωρ, "water," or "lymph," and ἀγγεῖον, a "vessel").] Inflammation of the lymphatic vessels.

Hy-dran-gi-o-gra'phi-a.* [From *hydrangi'on*, a "lymphatic vessel," and γράφω, to "write."] A term for a description of the lymphatic vessels, their situation, function, etc.

Hy-dran-gi-o-to'mi-a.* [From *hydrangi'on*, a "lymphatic vessel," and τέμνω, to "cut."] Dissection of the lymphatic vessels.

Hy-drar'gy̆-ri Bi-chlo'ri-dum.* The *Mercurius sublimatus corrosivus*, or corrosive sublimate. See HYDRARGYRI CHLORIDUM CORROSIVUM.

Hydrar'gyri Chlo'ri-dum.* The submuriate of mercury. See HYDRARGYRI CHLORIDUM MITE.

Hydrar'gyri Chlo'ridum Cor-ro-si'vum.* ("Corrosive Chloride of Mercury.") Corrosive sublimate. A substance occurring in colorless crystals, or crystalline masses, which are fusible by heat, sublime without residue, and are entirely soluble in water, alcohol, and ether. Except in very minute doses, corrosive sublimate, if taken internally, is a dangerous poison. It is sometimes applied externally, as a stimulant and escharotic, to indolent or malignant ulcers. Albumen forms an insoluble and comparatively harmless compound with corrosive sublimate. Hence, in cases of poisoning from this substance, the white of eggs beaten up with water affords an excellent antidote. In case eggs cannot be procured, copious draughts of milk, or wheat flour mixed with water, may be substituted. See POISONS.

Hydrar'gyri Chlo'ridum Mi'te.* ("Mild Chloride of Mercury.") The Pharmacopœial name (U.S. Ph.) for the substance popularly known as *Calomel* It occurs in the form of a white powder, which is tasteless and inodorous, wholly volatilizable by heat, and insoluble in water, alcohol, and ether. Calomel is esteemed the most valuable of all mercurial preparations. In minute doses it is an excellent alterative; in larger ones it is a purgative and anthelmintic. It possesses this great advantage, that in small doses it is not liable to be rejected by the most irritable stomach. But unhappily, like other mercurials, it acts unequally on different constitutions; so that the prudent physician will always be on his guard against salivation and other more serious results from its too free use,—more especially if he be not thoroughly acquainted with the constitutional peculiarities of his patient. Even a very moderate and cautious exhibition of this remedy has sometimes been followed by the most terrible and fatal effects.

Hydrar'gyri Çy-an'i-dum* ("Cyanide of Mercury"), otherwise called **Hydrar'gyri Çy-an-u-re'tum*** (U.S. Ph., 1850). A substance occurring in white prismatic crystals wholly soluble in water. It is an active poison, but it is sometimes given in very minute doses in syphilitic complaints.

Hydrar'gyri I-od'i-dum Ru'-brum.* ("Red Iodide of Mercury.") A red powder, which becomes yellow when heated, and red again when cold. It is wholly volatilized by heat. It is insoluble in water, but is dissolved by boiling alcohol. The red iodide of mercury is a powerful and irritant poison. It is highly recommended, in very minute doses, as a remedy in rheumatism dependent on syphilitic taint.

Hydrar'gyri Iod'idum Vir'i-de* ("Green Iodide of Mercury"), otherwise called **Hydrar'gyri Iod'idum*** (U.S. Ph., 1850). A greenish-yellow powder, which becomes red when heated. It is insoluble in water and alcohol. Its properties are similar to those of the preceding preparation, but it is less active.

Hydrar'gyri Ox'i-dum Ru'-brum.* ("Red Oxide of Mercury.") Red Precipitate. An orange-red powder, entirely soluble in muriatic acid. When heated, it gives off oxygen. As an external application it is used in the form of ointment and in powder.

Hydrar'gyri Sub-mu'rĭ-as.* ("Submuriate of Mercury.") See HYDRARGYRI CHLORIDUM MITE.

Hydrar'gyri Sul'phas Fla'va* ("Yellow Sulphate of Mercury"), otherwise called **Hydrar'gyri Sul'phas Fla'vus*** (U.S. Ph., 1850). Turpeth mineral. A lemon-yellow powder, sparingly soluble in water. It is entirely dissipated by heat. It is used as an alterative, emetic, and errhine.

Hydrar'gyri Sul-phu-re'tum Ni'grum.* ("Black Sulphuret of Mercury.") See ÆTHIOPS MINERAL.

Hydrar'gyri Sulphure'tum Ru'brum.* ("Red Sulphuret of Mercury.") Cin'nabar. A substance occurring in brilliant crystalline masses of a deep-red color and fibrous texture. It is entirely volatilized by heat.

Hydrargyri Unguentum. See UNGUENTUM HYDRARGYRI.

Hy-drar-ġȳr'ĭ-a.* [From *hydrar'gyrum*, "mercury."] An erythematous redness sometimes produced by an over-use of mercury; also applied to any morbid effects arising from its abuse as a medicine.

Hy-drar-ġȳ-ri'a-sis.* [From ὑδράργυρος, "mercury."] The effect arising from the administration of mercury; mercurialism. See HYDRARGYROSIS.

Hȳ-drar-ġȳr'ic. [**Hydrargyr'icus.**] Belonging to *hydrargyrum*, or mercury.

Hydrargyris. See HYDRARGYRIA.

Hy-drar-ġȳ-ro'sis.* The same as HYDRARGYRIASIS, which see.

Hy-drar'ġȳ-rum,* gen. **Hy-drar'ġȳ-ri.** [From ὕδωρ, "water," or "liquid," and ἄργυρος, "silver."] (Fr. *Mercure*, mĕR'küR', or *Vif Argent*, vĕf aR'zhŏNᵒ'.) Literally, "liquid silver." The Pharmacopœial name ‖ for quicksilver, or mercury. See MERCURY.

Hydrar'gyrum Am-mo-nĭ-a'tum.* ("Ammoniated Mercury.") White Precipitate. A substance occurring in white powder, or pulverulent masses, decomposed and entirely dissipated by a strong heat, insoluble in water and alcohol, but dissolved without effervescence by muriatic acid. It is used in medicine only as an external application.

Hydrar'gyrum cum Cre'tâ.* ("Mercury with Chalk.") A mixture composed of three parts of mercury and five of chalk; used as a mild mercurial alterative for children.

Hȳd-rar-thro'sis.* The morbid diathesis indicated by the occurrence of *hydrarthrus*.

Hȳ-drar'thrus.* [From ὕδωρ, "water," and ἄρθρον, a "joint."] The disease white-swelling; sometimes called *Spina Ventosa*. A genus of the order *Tumores*, class *Locales*, of Cullen's Nosology.

Hy-dras'tis.* The Pharmacopœial name (U.S. Ph.) for the root of the *Hydrastis Canadensis*.

Hȳ'drāte. [**Hy'dras, a'***tis*; from ὕδωρ, "water."] A combination of water with an oxide: a hydro-oxide.

Hȳ'drāt-ed. [**Hydra'tus;** from *hy'dras*, a "hydrate."] Applied to substances combined with water.

Hȳ-drau'lic. [**Hydraul'icus;** from ὕδωρ, "water," and αὐλικός, "belonging to a pipe."] Belonging to the conveyance of water through pipes.

Hȳ-drau'lics. [**Hydraul'ica;** from the same.] The art of constructing engines to convey or raise water through pipes; a branch of hydrodynamics. That branch of Natural Philosophy which treats of the motions of liquids, and the laws by which they are regulated.

Hy-dren-çeph-a-li'tis, i*dis*.* [From *hydrenceph'alus*.] *Hydrocephalus*, with inflammation.

Hy-dren-çe-phal'o-çēle.* [From ὕδωρ, "water," and *encephal'ocele*, "tumor of the head."] Hydrocephalic tumor, or hernia.

Hy-dren-çeph'a-lus.* [From ὕδωρ, "water," and ἐγκέφαλος, "within the head."] Water in the head. The same as *hydrocephalus*.

Hȳ-drī'o-dāte. [**Hydrio'das, a'***tis*.] A combination of hydriodic acid with a base.

Hȳ-drī-od'ic. [**Hydriod'icus;** from ὕδωρ, "water," and *iod'inum*, "iodine."] Belonging to water and iodine. Applied to an acid.

Hy-dro-a'rĭ-um.* [From ὕδωρ, "water," and ὠάριον, an "ovule," the "ovary"?] Dropsy of the ovary.

Hȳ-dro-bro'māte. [**Hydrobro'mas, a'***tis*.] A combination of hydrobromic acid with a base.

Hȳ-dro-brom'ic. [**Hydrobrom'icus.**] Belonging to a combination of hydrogen and bromine. Applied to an acid.

Hȳ-dro-car'bo-nāte. [**Hydrocarbo'nas, a'***tis*.] A combination of a carbonate with a hydrate, or of a carbonate and water.

Hȳ-dro-car'bu-ret. [**Hydrocar-**

bure'tum.] A combination of hydrogen and carbon with another body.

Hy-dro-cau'lis.* [From ὕδωρ, "water," and *cau'lis*, a "stem."] Applied to a knotty stem with sheathed leaves, which float on the water.

Hȳ'dro-çēle.* [From ὕδωρ, "water," and κήλη, a "tumor."] Dropsy of the testicle. Water, or other fluid, in the membranes of the scrotum, the coats of the testicle, or the cellular texture of the spermatic cord. A genus of the order *Intumescentiæ*, class *Cachexiæ*, of Cullen's Nosology.

Hy'dro-çe-no'sis.* [From ὕδωρ, "water," and κένωσις, an "evacuation."] An evacuation of water, as in dropsy, either by paracentesis, or hydragogue medicines.

Hydrocéphale. See HYDROCEPHALUS.

Hy'dro-çe-phal'ĭ-cus.* Belonging to *hydrocephalus*.

Hydrocephalitis. See HYDRENCEPHALITIS.

Hy'dro-çeph'a-lo-çen-te'sis.* [From *hydroceph'alus*, and κέντησις, a "puncturing."] The operation of puncturing the head in *hydrocephalus*.

Hȳ-dro-çeph'a-loid. [**Hydrocephaloi'des**; from *hydroceph'alus*, and εἶδος, a "form."] Resembling *hydrocephalus*.

Hy-dro-çeph'a-lus.* [From ὕδωρ, "water," and κεφαλή, the "head."] (Fr. *Hydrocéphale*, è'dRo'sà'fâl'.) Literally, "water in the head." Dropsy of the brain. A genus of the order *Intumescentiæ*, class *Cachexiæ*, of Cullen's Nosology.

Hydrocharidaceæ,* hi-dro-kăr-ĭ-da'she-ē. [From *Hydroch'aris*, one of the genera.] A natural order of endogenous aquatic plants, natives of fresh water, in Europe, India, and North America. It includes the *Vallisneria spiralis*.

Hydrocharides,* hi-dro-kăr'e-dēz. The Jussieuan name of a natural order of plants. See HYDROCHARIDACEÆ.

Hȳ-dro-chlo'rāte. [**Hydrochlo'ras, a'tis.**] A combination of hydrochloric acid with a base.

Hȳ-dro-chlo'ric. [**Hydrochlo'ricus.**] Belonging to hydrogen or chlorine. Applied to an acid formerly termed muriatic acid.

Hȳ-dro-chlo'rine. [**Hydrochlori'na.**] A compound of hydrogen and chlorine.

Hy-dro-chol-e-çȳs'tis, idis.* [From ὕδωρ, "water," χολή, "bile," and κύστις, a "bag."] Dropsy of the gall-bladder.

Hy-dro-chol-e-çȳs-ti'tis, idis.* [From *hydrocholecys'tis*.] Dropsy of the gall-bladder, with inflammation.

Hy-dro-çir'so-çēle.* [From ὕδωρ, "water," κιρσός, a "varix," and κήλη, a "tumor."] Hydrocele, with varicose veins, of the spermatic cord.

Hy-dro-çœ'lĭ-a.* [From ὕδωρ, "water," and κοιλία, the "belly."] The same as ASCITES, which see.

Hy-dro-cor'mus.* [From ὕδωρ, "water," and κορμός, a "trunk."] A stem or stalk that is horizontal, and floats on the water.

Hy-dro-cra'nĭ-a.* [From ὕδωρ, "water," and κρανίον, the "head."] The same as HYDROCEPHALUS, which see.

Hȳ-dro-çȳ'a-nāte. [**Hydrocy'anas, a'tis.**] A combination of hydrocyanic acid with a base.

Hȳ'dro-çȳ-an'ic. [**Hydrocyan'icus.**] Belonging to hydrogen and cyanogen. Applied to an acid also termed cyanic.

Hy-dro-çȳs'tis, idis.* [From ὕδωρ, "water," and κύστις, a "vesicle."] A hydatid or hy'drocyst.

Hy-dro-der'ma, atis.* [From ὕδωρ, "water," and δέρμα, the "skin."] The same as ANASARCA, which see.

Hy-dro'dēs.* [From ὕδωρ, "water."] Full of water: hy'drous.

Hȳ-dro-dȳ-nam'ic. [**Hydrodynam'icus**; from ὕδωρ, "water," and δύναμις, "power."] Belonging to the power of water, or other fluids.

Hȳ-dro-dȳ-nam'ics. [**Hydrodynam'ica**; from the same.] The science which applies the principles of dynamics to determine the conditions of motion or rest in fluid bodies. It is usually divided into two branches, hydrostatics and hydraulics.—(BRANDE.)

Hy-drœ-de'ma, atis.* [From ὕδωρ, "water," and οἴδημα, a "swelling."] Watery œdema.

Hydroëncephalus. See HYDRENCEPHALUS.

Hȳ-dro-flu'āte. [**Hydrof'luas, a'tis.**] A combination of hydrofluoric acid with a base.

Hȳ-dro-flu-or'ic. [**Hydrofluor'icus.**] Belonging to hydrogen and fluorine. Applied to an acid, also termed fluoric.

Hȳ'dro-ġen. [**Hydroge'nium**; from ὕδωρ, "water," and γεννάω, to "produce."] (Fr. *Hydrogène*, è'dRo'zhĕn.) The lightest ascertained substance; a gas forming one of the constituents of water; inflammable air.

Hy̆'dro-gen-āt-ed. [**Hydrogena'tus.**] Having hydrogen in combination.

Hydrogène. The French term for HYDROGEN, which see.

Hy̆-dro-ge-nif'e-rous. [**Hydrogenif'erus;** from *hydroge'nium*, "hydrogen," and *fe'ro*, to "bear."] Containing hydrogen.

Hy̆-drog'no-sy̆. [**Hydrogno'sia;** from ὕδωρ, "water," and γνῶσις, "knowledge."] A history of the waters of the terrestrial globe.

Hy̆-drog'ra-phy̆. [**Hydrogra'phia;** from ὕδωρ, "water," and γράφω, to "write."] A description of the waters distributed on the earth's surface, particularly with reference to the course and magnitude of rivers, the bearings of the coasts, the depths, currents, and other circumstances required to be known for the purposes of navigation.

Hy-dro-hæ'mĭ-a.* [From ὕδωρ, "water," and αἷμα, "blood."] Wateriness, or a poor state, of the blood: hydrohe'my.

Hy̆-dro-hæm'ic, or **Hy̆-dro-hem'ic.** [**Hydrohæm'icus.**] Belonging to *hydrohæmia*, or an impoverished condition of the blood.

Hy-dro-hy̆s'te-ra.* [From ὕδωρ, "water," and ὑστέρα, the "womb."] The same as HYDROMETRA.

Hy̆-drol'o-gy̆. [**Hydrolo'gia;** from ὕδωρ, "water," and λόγος, a "discourse."] The science which treats of water, its properties, uses, etc.

Hy-dro-ma'nĭ-a.* [From ὕδωρ, "water," and μανία, "madness."] A rage for water.

Hy̆'dro-mel. [**Hydrom'eli;** from ὕδωρ, "water," and μέλι, "honey."] Water impregnated with honey.

Hy-dro-men-in-gi'tis, i*dis*.* [From ὕδρωψ, "dropsy," and *meningi'tis*.] Dropsy complicated with inflammation of the membranes of the brain. See MENINGITIS.

Hy̆-drom'e-ter. [**Hydrom'etrum;** from ὕδωρ, "water," and μέτρον, a "measure."] An instrument for ascertaining the specific gravity of fluids. See AREOMETER.

Hy-dro-me'tra.* [From ὕδρωψ, "dropsy," and μήτρα, the "womb."] Dropsy of the *uterus*, or womb. A genus of the order *Intumescentiæ*, class *Cachexiæ*, of Cullen's Nosology.

Hy-drom'pha-lon,* or **Hy-drom'pha-lum.*** [From ὕδρωψ, "dropsy," and ὀμφαλός, the "navel."] A tumor of the umbilicus, containing water.

Hy-dron'e-phros,* or **Hy-dron'e-phrus.*** [From ὕδρωψ, "dropsy," and νεφρός, the "kidney."] Dropsy of the kidney.

Hy-dro-ne-phro'sis.* The progress of *hydronephrus*.

Hy-dron'o-sos,* or **Hy-dron'o-sus.*** [From ὕδωρ, "water," and νόσος, "disease."] Water-disease; dropsy. Incorrectly put for the *Anglicus Sudor*, or sweating sickness.

Hy̆-dro-path'ic. [**Hydropath'icus.**] Belonging to hydropathy.

Hy̆-drop'a-thy̆. [**Hydropathi'a;** from ὕδωρ, "water," and πάθος, "disease."] A system of treating diseases by the plentiful use, internal and external, of water, mostly cold or tepid.

Hy-dro-pe-de'sis.* [From ὕδωρ, "water," and πηδάω, to "spring or rush forth."] Excessive perspiration.

Hy-dro-pel-tid'e-æ.* [From *Hydropel'tis*, a name of one of the genera (from ὕδωρ, "water," and πέλτη, a "kind of small shield," because the leaves are shaped like a shield).] A synonym of a natural order of aquatic plants, called "Water-shields." See CABOMBACEÆ.

Hy-dro-pĕr-ĭ-car'dĭ-um.* [From ὕδρωψ, "dropsy," and *pericar'dium*.] Dropsy of the pericardium.

Hy-dro-pĕr-ĭ-to-næ'um.* [From ὕδρωψ, "dropsy," and *peritonæ'um*.] The same as ASCITES.

Hy̆'dro-phāne. [From ὕδωρ, "water," and φαίνομαι, to "appear."] A variety of opal which becomes transparent, when immersed in pure water.

Hy-dro-phi-mo'sis.* [From ὕδωρ, "water," and φίμωσις, a "constriction."] Phimosis with, or consequent upon, œdema of the prepuce.

Hy-dro-pho'bĭ-a.* [From ὕδωρ, "water," and φοβέω, to "fear;" because a dread or horror of water is one of its symptoms.] (Fr. *Rage*, råzh.) Madness caused by the bite of a rabid dog, or other animal. A genus of the order *Spasmi*, class *Neuroses*, of Cullen's Nosology. See LYSSA, and RABIES.

Hy̆-dro-phob'ic. [**Hydrophob'icus.**] Belonging to *hydrophobia*.

Hy̆-droph-thal'my̆. [**Hydrophthal'mia;** from ὕδρωψ, "dropsy," and ὀφθαλμός, the "eye."] Dropsy of the eye; also, anasarcous swelling of the eyelid; *Oculus Elephantinus*.

Hydrophyllaceæ,* hi-dro-fil-la'-she-ē. [From *Hydrophyl'lum*, one of the genera.] A natural order of exogenous plants, mostly natives of America.

Hy-dro-phy̆l'le-us.* [From ὕδωρ, "water," and φύλλον, a "leaf."] Applied in the plural feminine (*Hydrophyl'leæ*) to a family of plants, having for their type the *Hydrophyllum.*

Hy-dro-phy̆s'o-çēle.* [From ὕδωρ, "water," φῦσα, "flatus," and κήλη, a "tumor."] Hernia, the sac of which contains fluid and air.

Hy-dro-phy̆s-o-me'tra.* [From ὕδωρ, "water," φῦσα, "flatus," and μήτρα, the "womb."] Accumulation of serum and gas in the womb.

Hy̆'dro-phy̆te. [Hydroph'yton; from ὕδωρ, "water," and φυτόν, a "plant."] A plant which grows in water.

Hy̆-dro-phy̆-tog'ra-phy̆. [Hydrophytogra'phia; from *hydroph'yton,* a "hydrophyte," and γράφω, to "write."] A description of *Hydrophyta,* or water-plants.

Hy̆-dro-phy̆-tol'o-ġy̆. [Hydrophytolo'gia; from *hydroph'yton,* a "hydrophyte," and λόγος, a "discourse."] A treatise on water-plants.

Hy̆-drop'ic. [Lat. **Hydrop'icus;** Fr. *Hydropique,* è'dro'pèk'.] Belonging to *hydrops,* or dropsy.

Hydropisie. See HYDROPS.

Hy'dro-pneū'mo-tho'rax.* The complication of pneumo-thorax with dropsical effusion.

Hy-dro-po-i'dēs.* [From ὕδρωψ, "dropsy," and εἶδος, a "form."] Resembling dropsy.

Hy'drops,* gen. **Hy-dro'pis.** [Gr. ὕδρωψ, from ὕδωρ, "water;" Fr. *Hydropisie,* è'dro'pè'zè'.] The dropsy. An unnatural or morbid collection of serous fluid in the cellular tissue, or in any of the cavities of the body. When this fluid is diffused through the entire cellular tissue of the body, the disease is termed General Dropsy, or ANASARCA; if contained in the abdomen, it is called ASCITES; if in the head, HYDROCEPHALUS,—of which a notice will be found in their alphabetical places.

Hy'drops Ar-tic'u-li.* Dropsy of a joint; generally occurring in that of the knee, in which the synovial membrane is filled with a fluid less glairy, and thinner, than the natural *synovia.*

Hy'drops Sic'cus.* ("Dry Dropsy.") An absurd term for *tympanites.*

Hydropyretus. See HYDRONOSUS.

Hy-dror'chis.* [From ὕδωρ, "water," and ὄρχις, a "testicle."] Dropsy of the testicle.

Hy-dror-rha-chi'tis, *idis,** or **Hy-dror'rha-chis.*** [From ὕδωρ, "water," and ῥάχις, the "vertebral column."] Dropsy of the spine. A genus of the order *Intumescentiæ,* class *Cachexiæ,* of Cullen's Nosology. See RHACHIOCHYSIS.

Hy-dro-sar'ca.* [From ὕδωρ, "water," and σάρξ, "flesh."] The same as ANASARCA.

Hy-dros'ta-sis.* [From ὕδωρ, "water," and στάσις, a "standing."] The equilibrium, weight, or pressure of water, or liquid bodies.

Hy̆-dro-stat'ic. [Hydrostat'icus; from ὕδωρ, "water," and στατική, the "science of weights."] Belonging to the weight, pressure, or equilibrium of liquid bodies.

Hydrostat'ic Bed. Otherwise called a Water Bed. A kind of bed or trough, capable of holding water, and covered with water-proof cloth; or a bed-tick made of water-proof cloth and filled with water. The great advantage of such a bed is that it presses equally on every part of the lower surface of the body; and it is always ready for use without being shaken up.

Hydrostat'ic Test. The putting the lungs of a dead child in water, to ascertain, by their *floating* or *sinking,* whether it has been born alive.

Hy̆-dro-stat'ics. [Hydrostat'ica; from the same.] That science which explains the properties of the equilibrium and pressure of liquids.

Hy̆-dro-sul'phu-ret. [Hydrosulphure'tum; from ὕδωρ, "water," and *sul'phur.*] A combination of sulphuretted hydrogen with a base.

Hy-dro-sul-phu'ric Aç'id. Sulphuretted hydrogen gas.

Hy-dro-tho'rax, *a'cis.** [From ὕδωρ, "water," and θώραξ, the "chest."] (Fr. *Hydropisie de Poitrine,* è'dro'pè'zè' dęh pwå'trèn'.) Dropsy of the chest. A genus of the order *Intumescentiæ,* class *Cachexiæ,* of Cullen's Nosology.

Hydrous. See HYDRODES.

Hydrovarium. See HYDROARIUM.

Hy-dro-zo'on,* **Hy-dro-zo'um.*** [From ὕδωρ, "water," and ζῶον, an "animal."] Applied in the plural (*Hydrozo'a*) to certain animals, including the *Mollusca* and *Zoophyta,* to which water is indispensable.

Hy̆'dru-ret. [Hydrure'tum; from ὕδωρ, "water."] A combination of hydrogen with a metal, or inflammable substance.

Hy̆-dru-ret'ted. [Hydrure'tus;

from ὕδωρ, "water."] Containing hydrogen.

Hy-e-to-gra'phĭ-a.* [From ὑετός, "rain," and γράφω, to "write."] An account or description of rain, and the quantity fallen within a given period.

Hȳ-e-tom'e-ter. [**Hyetom'etrum;** from ὑετός, "rain," and μέτρον, a "measure."] An instrument for ascertaining the quantity of rain that falls in a given period.

Hy-ġe'ia,* or **Hy-ġĭ-e'ia.*** [Gr. Ὑγίεια, "health;" also, the goddess of Health; from ὑγιής, "sound," "healthy."] See HYGIENE.

Hy-ġĭ-as'tĭ-ca.* [From *hygias'ticus*, "relating to health."] The science of health, its conditions and relations.

Hy-ġĭ-as'ti-cus.* [From ὑγίεια, "health."] Relating to health.

Hy-ġĭ-eī-o-co'mĭ-um.* [From ὑγίεια, "health," and κομέω, to "take care of."] A house or residence for the convalescent.

Hȳ'ġĭ-ēne. [From ὑγίεια, "health."] That department of medicine which has for its direct object the preservation of health, or the prevention of disease.

Hȳ-ġĭ-en'ic. [Lat. **Hygien'icus;** Fr. *Hygiénique*, è'zhe-à'nèk'.] Belonging to *hygiene*.

Hȳ-ġĭ-ol'o-ġȳ, or **Hȳ-ġe-ol'o-ġȳ.** [**Hygeiolo'gia,** or **Hygieiolo'gia;** from ὑγίεια, "health," and λόγος, a "discourse."] The doctrine or consideration of health; the science of health.

Hy-gre-che'ma, atis.* [From ὑγρός, "moist," and ἠχή, a "sound."] The sound of fluid heard by means of the stethoscope, or by percussion.

Hȳ-grol'o-ġȳ. [**Hygrolo'gia;** from ὑγρός, "moist," and λόγος, a "discourse."] A treatise on fluids, or humors.

Hy-gro'ma, atis.* [From ὑγρός, "moist."] A tumor containing serum or other fluid, not pus.

Hȳ-grom'a-tous. [**Hygromato'sus.**] Having *hygroma*.

Hȳ-grom'e-ter. [**Hygrom'etrum;** from ὑγρός, "moist," and μέτρον, a "measure."] An instrument for ascertaining the degree of moisture in atmospheric air.

Hȳ-gro-met'ric. [**Hygromet'ricus.**] Belonging to hygrometry.

Hȳ-grom'e-trȳ. [**Hygromet'ria;** from ὑγρός, "moist," and μετρέω, to "measure."] The art of measuring or ascertaining the degree of moisture in atmospheric air.

Hȳ'gro-scope. [From ὑγρός, "moist," and σκοπέω, to "observe," or "examine."] An instrument for ascertaining the degree of moisture in the air, or in any substance; nearly synonymous with HYGROMETER.

Hȳ-gro-sco-piç'ĭ-tȳ. [**Hygroscopiç'itas, a'tis;** from the same.] The property by which vegetable tissues absorb or discharge moisture according to circumstances.

Hȳ-gros'co-pȳ. [**Hygrosco'pia;** from the same.] Synonymous with HYGROMETRY.

Hy-log-no'sĭ-a.* [From ὕλη, "material," or "matter," and γνῶσις, "knowledge."] A knowledge of the properties of matter.

Hȳ-lol'o-ġȳ. [**Hylolo'gia;** from ὕλη, "material," or "matter," and λόγος, a "discourse."] The doctrine or science of matter.

Hy'men,* gen. **Hy'men-is.** [From ὑμήν, a "thin membrane."] Any membrane. Usually applied to a thin membrane, of a circular, semilunar, or irregular form, extending across the vagina at its entrance.

Hy-men'ĭ-cus.* Belonging to the hymen: hymen'ic.

Hy-me-ni'tis, idis.* [From *hy'men*, a "membrane."] Inflammation of the hymen.

Hy-me'nĭ-um.* [From *hy'men*, a "membrane."] The dilated exposed membrane of gymnocarpous mushrooms in which the seed is contained.

Hy-me-nog'ra-phȳ. [**Hymenogra'phia;** from ὑμήν, a "membrane," and γράφω, to "write."] A description of the membranes of animal bodies.

Hy-me-nol'o-ġȳ. [**Hymenolo'gia;** from ὑμήν, a "membrane," and λόγος, a "discourse."] A treatise on the membranes; the science of the membranes.

Hy'me-no-ma-la'cĭ-a* (-ma-la'-she-a). [From ὑμήν, a "membrane," and μαλακός, "soft."] Morbid softening of the (serous) membranes.

Hy-me-nop'ter-ous. [**Hymenop'terus;** from ὑμήν, a "membrane," and πτερόν, a "wing."] Having membranous wings. Applied in the neuter plural (*Hymenop'tera*) to an order of insects including the bee, the wasp, and also the ant.

Hy-me-not'o-mȳ. [**Hymenoto'mia;** from ὑμήν, a "membrane," and τέμνω, to "cut."] Dissection of membranes.

Hy'o-. A prefix denoting connection with the *os hyoides*.

Hy-o-glos'sus.* [From *hy'o-*, and

γλῶσσα, the "tongue."] A large muscle of the neck, connecting the *Os hyoides* with the tongue.

Hȳ'oid. [**Hyoi'des;** from υ, a Greek letter,and εἶδος, a "form."] Resembling the Greek letter *υ*.

Hy-os-çy'a-mi Fo'lĭ-um or **Fo'lĭ-a.*** ("Henbane Leaf or Leaves.") The Pharmacopœial name (U.S. Ph.) for the leaves of the *Hyoscy'amus ni'ger.* See HYOSCYAMUS.

Hyoscy'ami Se'men.* ("Henbane Seed.") The Pharmacopœial name (U.S. Ph.) for the seed of the *Hyoscy'amus ni'ger.*

Hy-os-çy'a-min. A vegetable alkali obtained from *Hyoscyamus niger.*

Hy-os-çy'a-mus.* [From ὗς, a "sow," and κύαμος, a "bean."] (Fr. *Jusquiame,* zhüs'ke-âm'.) A Linnæan genus of the class *Pentandria,* natural order *Solanaceæ.* Also, the Pharmacopœial name (Brit. Pharm.) for the fresh and dried stalk-leaves of *Hyoscyamus niger;* the *Hyoscyami Folia et Semina* ("Leaves and Seeds of Hyoscyamus") of the Dublin Pharmacopœia. Hyoscyamus (including both leaves and seed) is a narcotic, and is much used as an anodyne and soporific. It possesses this great advantage over opium, that it has no tendency to constipate the bowels.

Hyoscy'amus Ni'ġer.* The black henbane.

Hyp-. [From ὑπό, "under."] A prefix denoting a slight degree.

Hȳp-ăl'ġĭ-a.* [From *hyp-,* and ἄλγος, "pain."] Slight pain.

Hȳp-ăl'ġĭ-cus.* Belonging to *hypalgia:* hypal'gic.

Hy'per (ὑπέρ). A Greek preposition signifying "above," "beyond," and, hence, "excessive" (*i.e.* implying excess); as, *hyper-carbonate,* a carbonate with an excess of carbonic acid, now called a *bicarbonate; hypercatharsis,* excessive catharsis or purging, etc.

Hy-per-a-cu'sis.* [From ὑπέρ, "over," "excessive," and ἄκουσις, "hearing."] Morbid exaltation of the sense of hearing.

Hy'per-ad'e-no'ma, a*tis.** [From ὑπέρ, "over," "excessive," and ἀδήν, a "gland."] An enlarged, or hypertrophied, gland.

Hy'per-ad'e-no'sis.* [From the same.] The progress, or gradual advancing, of *hyperadenoma.*

Hy-per-æ'mĭ-a.* [From ὑπέρ, "over," "excessive," and αἷμα, "blood."] (Fr. *Hypérémie,* è'pȧ'rȧ'mè'.) Excess of blood in any part.

Hy-per-æs-the'sis.* [From ὑπέρ, "over," "excessive," and *æsthe'sis,* "sensibility."] Morbid increase of sensibility.

Hy-per-æs-thet'ĭ-cus.* Belonging to *hyperæsthesis:* hyperesthet'ic.

Hy-per-a'phĭ-a.* [From ὑπέρ, "over," "excessive," and ἁφή, "touch," or "tact."] Over-tension, or excessive sensibility of touch.

Hy-per-aph'ĭ-cus.* Belonging to *hyperaphia:* hyperaph'ic.

Hy-per-as-the'nĭ-a.* [From ὑπέρ, "over," "excessive," and *asthe'nia,* "loss of strength."] Excessive debility.

Hy-per-as-then'ĭ-cus.* Belonging to *hyperasthenia.*

Hȳ-per-bo're-an. [**Hyperbo're-us;** from ὑπέρ, "above," or "beyond," and βορέας, the "north wind."] Dwelling in the far northern parts of the globe.

Hy-per-ca-thar'sis.* [From ὑπέρ, "over," or "excessive," and *cathar'sis,* "purgation."] Excessive purging.

Hy-per-ca-thar'tĭ-cus.* Belonging to *hypercatharsis:* hypercathar'tic.

Hȳ-per-cĭ-ne'sis.* Increased irritability of the muscles, producing spasm.

Hȳ-per'crĭ-sis.* A crisis of unusual severity.

Hy-per-cro'max, a'*cis.** [From ὑπέρ, "over," "on," and κρῶμαξ, a "heap of stones," also a "lump."] The small carnosity on the white of the eye.

Hy-per-çy-e'ma, a*tis,* or **Hy-per-çy-e'sis.*** [From ὑπέρ, "over," "excessive," and κύησις, "uterine gestation."] Superfœtation.

Hy-per-çy-et'ĭ-cus.* Belonging to *hypercyesis.*

Hy-per-dȳ-na'mĭ-a.* [From ὑπέρ, "over," "excessive," and *dyna'mia,* "vital force."] Excessive *dynamia,* or vital force.

Hy-per-dȳ-nam'ĭ-cus.* Belonging to *hyperdynamia:* hyperdynam'ic.

Hy-per-em'e-sis.* [From ὑπέρ, "over," "excessive," and *em'esis,* "vomiting."] Excessive vomiting.

Hȳ'per-e-met'ic. [**Hyperemet'i-cus.**] Belonging to *hyperemesis.*

Hypérémie. See HYPERÆMIA.

Hȳ-per-en'er-ġȳ. [**Hyperener'gia;** from ὑπέρ, "over," "excessive," and ἐνέργεια, "action."] Increased action or energy.

Hȳ-per-ġen'e-sis.* [From ὑπέρ, "over," "excessive," and γένω, to "be born."] A congenital excess, or redundancy of parts.

Hy̆-per-ge-net'ic. [Hypergenet'icus.] Belonging to *hypergenesis*.

Hyperhæmia. See HYPERÆMIA.

Hy-per-hi-dro'sis.* [From ἱδρώς, "sweat."] A term applied by Swediaur to morbidly profuse perspiration. It is also termed EPHIDROSIS.

Hy̆-pĕr'ĭ-ca,* the plural of **Hyper'icum,** forming the Jussieuan name of a natural order of plants. See HYPERICACEÆ.

Hypericaceæ,* hi-pĕr-e-ka'she-ē. A natural order of exogenous plants, found in nearly all parts of the world. It includes the *Hyper'icum* (St. Johnswort). Some of the species are astringent, and are used as tonics.

Hy-per-ĭ-no'sis.* [From ὑπέρ, "over," "excessive," and ἴς, ἰνός, the "fibre of flesh."] A form of diseased blood, consisting in excess of fibrin.

Hy-per-ĭ-not'ic. [Hyperinot'icus.] Belonging to *hyperinosis*.

Hy-per-ner'vĭ-a,* **Hy-per-neū'rĭ-a.*** [From ὑπέρ, "over," "excessive," and νεῦρον, a "nerve."] Excessive nervous action.

Hy-per-op'sĭ-a.* [From ὑπέρ, "over," and ὄψις, "vision."] Extremely acute vision.

Hy-per-os'mĭ-a.* [From ὑπέρ, "over," "excessive," and ὀσμή, "odor."] A keen sense of smell, or excessive odor.

Hy-per-os-phre'sis.* [From ὑπέρ, "over," "excessive," and ὄσφρησις, the "faculty of smelling."] A morbidly acute sense of smell. See HYPEROSMIA.

Hy̆-per-os-to'sis.* [From ὑπέρ, "over," or "excessive," and ὀστέον, a "bone."] Enlargement of a bone, or its membranous covering.

Hy-per-pla'sĭ-a.* [From ὑπέρ, "over," "excessive," and πλάσις, "formation," or "structure."] The increase of a part by an increase in the number of its individual structural elements. See HYPERTROPHY.

Hy̆-per-troph'ic. [Hypertroph'icus.] Belonging to hypertrophy.

Hy̆-per'tro-phy̆. [Hypertro'phia; from ὑπέρ, "over," or "excessive," and τρέφω, to "nourish."] Excessive growth, thickening, or enlargement of any organ. In a more restricted sense, it signifies the increase of a part by the increase in bulk of its individual structural elements. See HYPERPLASIA.

Hy̆-phæ'ma, a*tis*.* [From ὑπό, "under," and αἷμα, "blood."] Sugillation.

Hy̆p-ĭ-no'sis.* [From ὑπό, "under," implying deficiency, and ἴς, ἰνός, the "fibre of flesh."] A form of diseased blood, consisting in deficiency of fibrin.

Hy̆p-ĭ-not'ic. [Hypinot'icus.] Belonging to *hypinosis*.

Hy̆p-næs-the'sis.* [From ὕπνος, "sleep," and αἴσθησις, "sense," or "feeling."] Dulled sensibility; drowsiness.

Hy̆p'nĭ-cus.* [From ὕπνος, "sleep."] Belonging to sleep: hypnic. Applied in the neuter plural (*Hyp'nica*) to medicines or agents affecting sleep, either by inducing it or preventing it.

Hy̆p-no'dēs.* [From ὕπνος, "sleep."] Sleepy, or full of sleep.

Hy̆p-no'dĭ-a.* [From *hypno'des*, "sleepy."] The same as HYPNÆSTHESIS, which see.

Hy̆p-nol'o-gy̆. [Hypnolo'gia; from ὕπνος, "sleep," and λόγος, a "discourse."] The doctrine or science of sleep, its proper periods of indulgence, duration, regulation, etc.

Hy̆p-not'ic. [Hypnot'icus; from ὕπνος, "sleep."] Having power to induce sleep; somnif'erous.

Hy̆p'no-tism. [Hypnotis'mus; from ὕπνος, "sleep."] A term denoting a state of sleep; sometimes used for MESMERISM.

Hy̆p-no-ty'phus.* [From ὕπνος, "sleep," and *ty'phus*.] Typhus, with morbid drowsiness.

Hy̆'po (ὑπό). A Greek particle signifying "under," "beneath," sometimes "in," or "behind." It often implies *diminution* or *deficiency*.

Hy̆p-o-æ'ma Scor-bu'tĭ-cum.* [From ὑπό, "under," "in," or "within," and αἷμα, "blood."] A scorbutic, bloodshot appearance of the eye.

Hy̆p-o-branch'ĭ-al. [Hypobranchia'lis; from ὑπό, "under," and βράγχια, the "gills."] Applied by Owen to the homologues of the lateral lingual bones in fishes, etc.

Hypocalycius,* hĭp'o-ka-lish'e-us. [From ὑπό, "under," and *ca'lyx*.] Situated under the calyx.

Hy̆p-o-ca-thar'sis.* [From ὑπό, "under," and καθαίρω, to "purge."] A slight purging.

Hy̆p-o-chon'drĭ-a, the plural of HYPOCHONDRIUM, which see.

Hy̆p-o-chon'drĭ-ac. [Hypochondri'acus; from ὑπό, "under," and χονδρός, a "cartilage."] (Fr. *Hypocondriaque*, ē'po'kôɴᵍ'dRē'ăk'.) Belonging to the *hypochondria*, or spaces beneath the cartilages of the false ribs. Applied to one affected with *hypochondriasis.*

Hўp-o-chon-drī'ạ-çism. [**Hypochondriacis'mus;** from *hypochon'drium.*] Hypochondriac disease.

Hўp-o-chon-drī'ạ-sis.* [From *hypochon'drium,* the supposed seat of the disease.] (Fr. *Hypocondrie,* è'po'-kȯnᵍ'dRè'.) Vapors; low spirits. A genus of the order *Adynamiæ,* class *Neuroses,* of Cullen's Nosology. Hypochondriasis is almost invariably connected with dyspepsia, and is doubtless often produced by it; though some physiologists consider the seat of the disease to be in the brain.

Hўp-o-chon'drĭ-um,* plural **Hўp-o-chon'drĭ-ạ.** [From ὑπό, "under," and χονδρός, a "cartilage."] The *Regio hypochondriaca,* or space beneath the cartilages of the false ribs on either side.

Hypocondrie. See Hypochondriasis.

Hўp-o-crạ-tĕr'ĭ-form. The same as Hypocraterimorphous.

Hўp-o-crạ-tĕr-ĭ-mor'phous. [From ὑποκρατήριον, the "support of a bowl or cup," a "salver," and μορφή, "form."] Salver-shaped: applied to flowers.

Hўp-o-der'mic. [**Hypoder'micus;** from ὑπό, "under," and δέρμα, the "skin."] A term for the application of medicines under the skin; that is, to the denuded surface after the skin has been removed by a blister.

Hўp-og'ạ-lạ.* [From ὑπό, "under," "in," or "within," and γάλα, "milk."] The effusion of a milk-like fluid into the chambers of the eye.

Hўp-o-gas-trăl'ġĭ-ạ.* [From *hypogas'trium,* and ἄλγος, "pain."] Pain in the hypogastrium.

Hўp-o-gas'tric. [**Hypogas'tricus.**] Belonging to the *hypogastrium.*

Hypogas'tric Plex'us. A plexus on the sides and back part of the rectum, and lower and back part of the bladder, formed by the inferior mesenteric plexus with the sacral.

Hўp-o-gas-trĭ-o-to'mĭ-ạ.* [From *hypogas'trium,* and τέμνω, to "cut."] Dissection of the hypogastric region.

Hўp-o-gas-trī'tis, ĭdis.* [From ὑπό, "under," and *gastri'tis,* "inflammation of the stomach."] Slight inflammation of the stomach.

Hўp-o-gas'trĭ-um.* [From ὑπό, "under," and γαστήρ, the "stomach."] The abdominal space above the *pubes* and below the line of the anterior superior spinous processes of the iliac bones.

Hўp-o-gas'tro-çēle.* [From ὑπό, "under," γαστήρ, the "stomach," and κήλη, a "tumor."] Hernia in the hypogastric region.

Hўp-o-gas-tror-rha'ġĭ-ạ.* [From ὑπό, "under," "in a slight degree," and *gastrorrha'gia.*] Literally, a "slight discharge [of any kind] from the stomach," but usually applied to a slight hæmorrhage from the stomach.

Hўp-o-gas-tror-rhex'is.* [From *hypogas'trium,* and ῥῆξις, a "rupture."] Rupture of the abdomen, with laceration of the peritonæum.

Hўp-o-gas-tror-rhœ'ạ.* [From ὑπό, "under," "in a slight degree," and *gastrorrhœ'a,* a "discharge from the stomach."] A slight flow of mucus from the stomach.

Hўp-o-ġe'an. [**Hypoge'us;** from ὑπό, "under," and γῆ, or γέα, the "earth."] Applied to cotyledons which, filled with nutritious matter, remain below the ground during germination.

Hўp-o-ġe-o-car'pus.* [From ὑπό, "under," γῆ, or γέα, the "earth," and καρπός, "fruit."] Having fruit under the surface of the earth.

Hўp-o-glos'sạl. [**Hypoglos'sus;** from the same.] Situated on the under part of the tongue.

Hўp-o-glos'sĭ-um,* or **Hўp-o-glos'sis, ĭdis.*** [From ὑπό, "under," and γλῶσσα, the "tongue."] The under-surface of the tongue. See Par Nonum.

Hўp-o-glot'tis, ĭdis.* [From ὑπό, "under," and γλῶττα, the "tongue."] The inferior part of the tongue adhering to the lower jaw.

Hўp-o-ġўn'ĭ-cus.* [From ὑπό, "under," and γυνή, a "woman," or "female."] Applied to the insertion of stamens, petals, etc., when the point of attachment is under the ovary: hypogynic.

Hўp-oġ'ў-nous. [**Hypoġ'ynus;** from the same.] Growing or inserted under the pistil, and free, as the stamens, calyx, and corolla of some plants.

Hўp-o-hæ'mĭ-ạ.* [From ὑπό, "under," and αἷμα, "blood."] Deficiency or loss of blood.

Hўp-o-hæm'ic. [**Hypohæm'icus.**] Belonging to *hypohæmia.*

Hўp-o-ner'vĭ-ạ,* or **Hўp-o-neū'rĭ-ạ.*** [From ὑπό, "under," and νεῦρον, a "nerve."] Morbidly slight, or diminished, nervous power.

Hў-po-nī'trīte. [**Hyponi'tris, ĭ'tis.**] A combination of hyponitrous acid with a base.

Hўp-o-pe-ta'le-us.* [From ὑπό,

"under," and πέταλον, a "petal."] Applied in the plural feminine (*Hypopeta'leæ*) to dicotyledonous, polypetalous plants, in which the stamens are hypogynous.

Hȳ-po-phos'phīte. [**Hypophos'phis, i'tis.**] A combination of hypophosphorous acid with a base.

Hȳp-o-phȳl'lous. [**Hypophyl'lus;** from ὑπό, "under," and φύλλον, a "leaf."] Growing on the lower side of a leaf.

Hȳp-o'pȳ-um.* [From ὑπό, "under," and πύον, "pus."] An accumulation of a puriform fluid under the cornea, or in either chamber of the eye.

Hȳp-o-spa'dĭ-a.* [From ὑπό, "under," and σπάζω, to "tap," or "open"?] An unnatural perforation of the penis, the extremity of the urethra terminating on the under part of it.

Hȳp-o-spa-di'a-sis.* [From *hypospa'dia.*] The state of *hypospadia.*

Hȳp-o-sta-min'e-us.* [From *hy'po-,* "under," and *sta'men.*] Applied in the plural feminine (*Hypostamin'eæ*) to dicotyledonous, apetalous plants, in which the stamens are hypogynous.

Hȳp-os'ta-sis.* [From ὑφίστημι, to "throw down."] The subsidence of sediment in liquids, or of blood in the body after death, by gravitation of the fluids; but, more particularly, of the urine in health and disease.

Hȳp-os-the'nĭ-a.* [From ὑπό, "under," and σθένος, "strength."] A state of weakness, or a reduction of strength.

Hȳp-os-then'ic. [**Hyposthen'icus.**] Belonging to *hyposthenia.*

Hȳ-po-sul'phāte. [**Hyposul'phas, a'tis.**] A combination of hyposulphuric acid with a base.

Hȳ-po-sul'phīte. A combination of hyposulphurous acid with a base.

Hȳ-pot'e-nuse, or **Hȳ-poth'e-nuse.** [Gr. ὑποτείνουσα, the present participle feminine of ὑποτείνω, to "subtend."] That side of a right-angled triangle which subtends the right angle.

Hȳp-o-tȳm'pa-nic. [**Hypotympan'icus;** from ὑπό, "under," and *tympan'icus,* "tympanic."] Applied by Owen to the inferior subdivision of the tympanic pedicle which supports the mandible in fishes.

Hy-po-zo'ĭ-cus.* [From ὑπό, "under," and ζῶον, an "animal."] Applied to an order of rock formations, inferior to all those in which are found the traces of organic bodies.

Hȳp-sĭ-lo-i'dēs.* [From Υ, "upsilon," a Greek letter, and εἶδος, a "form."] The same as HYOIDES.

Hȳp-so-met'rĭ-cal. [**Hypsomet'ricus.**] Belonging to hypsometry.

Hȳp-som'e-trȳ. [**Hypsomet'ria;** from ὕψος, "height," and μετρέω, to "measure."] The art of measuring the relative height of a place, or of a portion of terrestrial ground.

Hȳs'so-pin. [**Hyssopi'na;** from *hysso'pus,* the "hyssop-plant."] A salifiable base, said to have been discovered in the hyssop.

Hȳs'te-ra.* [From ὑστέρα, the "womb," or "uterus."] The *uterus,* or womb; also, the vulva.

Hȳs-te-răl'ġic. [**Hysteral'gicus.**] Belonging to *hysteralgia.*

Hȳs-te-răl'ġȳ. [**Hysteral'gia;** from ὑστέρα, the "womb," and ἄλγος, "pain."] Pain in the womb, from whatever cause.

Hȳs-te-ran'drĭ-us.* [From ὑστέρα, the "womb," or "ovary," and ἀνήρ, ἀνδρός, a "man," or "male."] Having stamens and ovary. Applied in the plural neuter (*Hysteran'dria*) to a class of a modified sexual system, which comprehends plants having more than ten stamens inserted in one ovary.

Hȳs-ter-a-tre'sĭ-a.* [From ὑστέρα, the "womb," and *atre'sia,* "occlusion."] Occlusion of the womb, or an impervious condition of its opening.

Hȳs-ter-el-co'sis.* [From ὑστέρα, the "womb," and ἕλκος, an "ulcer."] Ulceration of the womb.

Hȳs-ter-em-phȳ-se'ma, a*tis.** [From ὑστέρα, the "womb," and *emphyse'ma,* a "windy swelling."] The same as *Physometra,* or the presence of air in the womb.

Hȳs-te'rĭ-a.* [From ὑστέρα, the "womb."] (Fr. *Hystérie,* ès'tà'rè'.) Hysterics, attacking in paroxysms or fits, usually preceded by dejection, anxiety, tears, difficult breathing, sickness, and palpitation of the heart. Termed, also, *Pas'sio hyster'ica* (Fr. *Passion hystérique,* pâ'se-ôɴᵒ' ès'tà'rèk'). A genus of the order *Spasmi,* class *Neuroses,* of Cullen's Nosology.

Hȳs-tĕr'ĭ-cal, Hȳs-tĕr'ic. [**Hyster'icus.**] Belonging to *hysteria.*

Hystérie. See HYSTERIA.

Hȳs-te-ri'tis, idis.** [From ὑστέρα, the "womb."] Inflammation of the womb. A genus of the order *Phlegmasiæ,* class *Pyrexiæ,* of Cullen's Nosology. See METRITIS, and UTERITIS.

Hy̆s'te-ro-car'çĭ-no'ma, *atis.** [From ὑστέρα, the "womb," and *carci-no'ma*, "cancer."] Cancer of the womb. See METROCARCINOMA.

Hy̆s'te-ro-cat'a-lep'sis.* [From ὑστέρα, the "womb," and *catalep'sis*, "catalepsy."] Cataleptic *hysteria*.

Hy̆s'te-ro-çēle.* [From ὑστέρα, the "womb," and κήλη, a "tumor."] Hernia, in which the *uterus*, or womb, is protruded.

Hy̆s-te-ro-col'ĭ-ca.* [From ὑστέρα, the "womb," and *col'ica*, "colic."] Pains in the womb, like those of colic: uterine colic.

Hy̆s-te-ro-dy̆n'ĭ-a.* [From ὑστέρα, the "womb," and ὀδύνη, "pain."] Pain of the womb. The same as HYSTERALGIA.

Hy̆s'te-rœ-de'ma, *atis.** [From ὑστέρα, the "womb," and *œde'ma*, a "swelling."] Enlargement of the substance of the womb.

Hy̆s'te-ro-lĭ-thi'a-sis.* [From ὑστέρα, the "womb," and *lithi'asis*, the "generation of calculus."] The formation of *calculus* in the womb.

Hy̆s-te-rol'ĭ-thus.* [From ὑστέρα, the "womb," and λίθος, a "stone."] Stone or *calculus* in the womb: a hysterolith.

Hy̆s-te-rol'o-ġy̆. [**Hysterolo'gia;** from ὑστέρα, the "womb," and λόγος, a "discourse."] A treatise on the womb, its functions, etc.

Hy̆s'te-ro-mal-a-co'ma, *atis.** [From ὑστέρα, the "womb," and μαλακός, "soft."] Softening of the womb.

Hy̆s'te-ro-mal-a-co'sis.* The formation or progress of *hysteromalacoma*, or softening of the womb.

Hy̆s'te-ro-ma'nĭ-a.* [From ὑστέρα, the "womb," and μανία, "madness."] Another term for *Furor uterinus*, or NYMPHOMANIA, which see.

Hy̆s-te-rom'e-ter. [**Hysterom'e-trum;** from ὑστέρα, the "womb," and μέτρον, a "measure."] An instrument or means of ascertaining the size of the *uterus*, or womb.

Hy̆s-te-roph'y̆-tal. [From ὑστέρα, the "womb," or "matrix," and φυτόν, a "plant."] Living on a matrix either of dead or living organic matter. Applied to Fungi.

Hy̆s'te-ro-phy̆te. [From the same.] A name for a fungus.

Hy̆s'te-ror-rha'ġĭ-a.* [From ὑστέρα, the "womb," and ῥήγνυμι, to "burst forth."] The same as METRORRHAGIA.

Hy̆s'te-ror-rhex'is.* [From ὑστέρα, the "womb," and ῥῆξις, a "rupture."] Rupture of the *uterus*, or womb.

Hy̆s'te-ror-rhœ'a.* [From ὑστέρα, the "womb," and ῥέω, to "flow."] The same as METRORRHŒA.

Hy̆s'te-ro-sçir'rhus.* [From ὑστέρα, the "womb," and σκιῤῥός, a "hard tumor."] Scirrhus, or incipient cancer, of the womb.

Hy̆s'te-ro-spas'mus.* [From ὑστέρα, the "womb," and σπασμός, a "convulsion."] Spasm of the *uterus*, or womb; also, hysterical spasm.

Hy̆s'te-ro-tome. [**Hysterot'o-mus;** from ὑστέρα, the "womb," and τέμνω, to "cut."] An instrument for dividing the neck of the womb.

Hy̆s-te-rot'o-my̆. [**Hysteroto'-mia;** from the same.] The *Cæsarean operation*, or cutting into the womb to extract the child, in cases where, from malformation, or other cause, natural delivery is impracticable. See CÆSAREAN OPERATION.

Hystriasis. See HYSTRICIASIS.

Hy̆s-trĭ-çi'a-sis.* [From ὕστριξ, a "hedge-hog."] A rare disease of the hairs, in which they stand erect like the spines or prickles of the hedge-hog.

I.

I-am-a-tol'o-ġy̆. [**Iamatolo'gia;** from ἴαμα, a "remedy," and λόγος, a "discourse."] That branch of therapeutics which treats of remedies.

I-at-ra-lip'tic Meth'od. [From *ia'tro-*, and ἀλείφω, to "anoint."] The application of medicines to the skin, aided by friction.

I-a-treū-so-lo'ġĭ-a.* [From ἰατρεύω, to "cure," and λόγος, a "discourse."] A term applied to general therapeutics.

I-a-tri'a.* [Gr. ἰάτρεια; from ἰατρός, a "physician."] The art of healing, or curing; also, a cure.

Iatro-. A prefix signifying connection with the healing art.

I-a-trol'o-ġy̆. [**Iatrolo'gia;** from *iatro-*, and λόγος, a "discourse."] A treatise on medicine, or on physicians; also, the science of medicine, or the healing art.

Iatropha. See JATROPHA.

Iatrophate. The same as JATROPHATE.

-Ic. A terminal syllable, generally denoting that acid compound which has most oxygen,—as nitr*ic*, sulphur*ic*, etc., which are thus distinguished from those ending in *-ous*, such as nitr*ous*, sulphur*ous*, etc., implying a smaller proportion of oxygen.

Ice. See GLACIES.

Ice Pōul'tice. A bladder containing pounded ice, to be applied to hernial tumors.

Ice'land Moss. The *Li'chen Islan'dicus*, or *Cetra'ria Islan'dica*.

Ice'land Spar. One of the purest varieties of calcareous spar, or crystallized carbonate of lime.

I'chor, o'ris.* [From ἰχώρ, "serum," or "pus."] A thin aqueous and acrid discharge from a wound, sore, or diseased surface.

Ich-or-æ'mĭ-a,* or **Ich-or-hæ'mĭ-a.*** [From ἰχώρ, "pus, or sanious fluid," and αἷμα, "blood."] A term denoting the poisoning of the blood from the absorption of sanious matter.

Ich-o-ro-i'dēs.* [From ἰχώρ, "serum," or "pus," and εἶδος, a "form."] Resembling ichor, or pus.

Ich'o-rous. [**Ichoro'sus;** from *i'chor*, "serum," or "pus."] Having ichor; of the nature of ichor.

Ich-thy̆-i'tēs.* [From ἰχθύς, a "fish," and λίθος, a "stone."] The same as ICHTHYOLITE.

Ich-thy'ĭus.* [From ἰχθύς, a "fish," and ἰός, "poison."] The same as ICHTHYOTOXICUM.

Ich-thy̆-o-col'la.* [From ἰχθύς, a "fish," and κόλλα, "glue."] Isinglass; fish-glue. The Pharmacopœial name (U.S. Ph.) for the swimming bladder of the *Acipenser Huso*.

Ich-thy̆-og'ra-phy̆. [**Ichthyogra'phia;** from ἰχθύς, a "fish," and γράφω, to "write."] A description of fishes.

Ich-thy̆-o-i'dēs.* [From ἰχθύς, a "fish," and εἶδος, a "form."] Resembling a fish; ichthyoid.

Ich'thy̆-o-līte. [**Ichthyol'ites;** from ἰχθύς, a "fish," and λίθος, a "stone."] Applied to petrified fish, or their fossil remains.

Ich-thy̆-o-log'ĭ-cal. [**Ichthyolog'icus.**] Belonging to Ichthyology.

Ich-thy̆-ol'o-gy̆. [**Ichthyolo'gia;** from ἰχθύς, a "fish," and λόγος, a "discourse."] A treatise on the nature and habits of fishes; also, the science which treats of fishes, their classification, structure, etc.

Ich-thy̆-oph'a-gous. [**Ichthyoph'agus;** from ἰχθύς, a "fish," and φάγω, to "eat."] Fish-eating; piscivorous.

Ich-thy̆-o-sau'rus.* [From ἰχθύς, a "fish," and σαῦρος, a "lizard."] A genus of extinct marine animals, which combined the characters of saurian reptiles and of fishes with some of the peculiarities of Cetaceous Mammalia.

Ich-thy̆-o'sis.* [From ἰχθύα, the "scale of a fish."] A disease in which the skin becomes thickened, hard, and rough, with a tendency to scaliness; the fish-skin disease.

Ich-thy̆-ot'o-my̆. [**Ichthyoto'mia;** from ἰχθύς, a "fish," and τέμνω, to "cut."] Dissection of fishes.

Ich'thy̆-o-tox'ĭ-cum.* [From ἰχθύς, a "fish," and τοξικόν, a "poison."] A morbid and poisonous product sometimes found in fish.

I-con-o-graph'ic. [**Iconograph'icus.**] Belonging to Iconography.

I-co-nog'ra-phy̆. [**Iconogra'phia;** from εἰκών, an "image," and γράφω, to "write."] A description by images, or figures; or a description of pictures, statues, etc.

I-co-san'drĭ-a.* [From εἴκοσι, "twenty," and ἀνήρ, a "man," or "male."] The twelfth Linnæan class of plants, including those which have twenty or more unconnected stamens inserted on the calyx.

I-co-san'drĭ-ous, or **I-co-san'drous.** [**Icosan'drius;** from the same.] Having twenty stamens or more.

I'co-sĭ-go'nus.* [From εἴκοσι, "twenty," and γωνία, an "angle."] Having twenty angles.

I'co-sĭ-he'dral. [**Icosihe'drus.**] Belonging to an icosihedron.

I'co-sĭ-he'dron, or **I'co-sa-he'dron.** [**Icosihe'drum;** from εἴκοσι, "twenty," and ἕδρα, a "base."] A solid figure bounded by twenty equilateral and equal triangles.

I'co-sĭ-tet-ra-he'dral. [**Icositetrahe'drus.**] Belonging to an icositetrahedron; twenty-four-sided.

I'co-sĭ-tet-ra-he'dron. [**Icositetrahe'drum;** from εἴκοσι, "twenty," τέτρα, "four," and ἕδρα, a "base."] A solid figure of twenty-four equal sides, or faces.

Ictère. See ICTERUS.

Ic-ter-ep-a-ti'tis, ĭdis.* [From *ic'terus*, "jaundice," and *hepati'tis*, "inflammation of the liver."] *Hepatitis* and jaundice, or icteric hepatitis.

Ic-tĕr'ic. [**Icter'icus.**] Belonging to *icterus*.

Ic-ter-o'dēs.* [From *ic'terus*, "jaundice."] Like jaundice, or having a yellow color resembling jaundice. Sometimes applied to the yellow fever.

Ic'ter-oid. [**Icteroi'des;** from *ic'terus*, "jaundice," and εἶδος, a "form."] Resembling *icterus*.

Ic-ter-oph'thi-sis.* [From *ic'terus*, "jaundice," and *phthis'is*, "consumption."] *Tabes icterica*, or *phthisis* with jaundice.

Ic'ter-us.* [Gr. ἴκτερος.] (Fr. *Ictère*, ĕk'têR', or *Jaunisse*, zhō'nĕss', *i.e.* "yellowness.") Jaundice,—characterized by yellowness of the skin and eyes. A genus of the order *Impetigines*, class *Cachexiæ*, of Cullen's Nosology.

Ic'tus So'lis.* ("Stroke of the Sun.") The same as Coup de Soleil, which see.

-Idæ. A terminal employed (in imitation of the classical patronymic) to denote a family or group exhibiting some points of likeness to the type; as *Leporidæ*, the family of the *Lepus*, or hare, etc.

-Idæus, or **-Ideus.** A terminal applied to objects belonging to, or connected with, others, which are designated by terms ending in *-oid* or *-ides;* as, *Arytænoidæus*, the muscle between or belonging to the *Arytenoid* (*Arytenoides*) cartilage, etc. The terminations *-ideus* or *-idæus* are sometimes equivalent to *-ides* or *-oid;* thus, *Ligamentum coracoideum* is the same as *Ligamentum coracoides* (the "coracoid ligament").

-Ide. A terminal affixed to oxygen, chlorine, fluorine, and iodine, when combined with each other, or with simple combustibles, or metals, in proportions not forming an acid.

I-de'al-ism. [**Idealis'mus;** from ἰδέα, an "idea," a "thought."] A system of metaphysics in which no real existence is attributed to any thing except to thought or mind.

I-den'ti-tў. [**Iden'titas,** **a'***tis;* from *i'dem*, the "same."] Absolute or essential sameness of two apparently different things, as, for example, that of the electric spark and lightning.

I-de-og'ra-phў. [**Ideogra'phia;** from ἰδέα, an "idea," and γράφω, to "write."] A description or definition of ideas.

I-de-ol'o-ġў. [**Ideolo'gia;** from ἰδέα, an "idea," and λόγος, a "discourse."] The doctrine or science of thought or of the mind; the philosophy of the origin and development of ideas.

-Ides. An affix of many words. See Oid.

Idiocy. See Idiotism, and Amentia.

Id'i-o-e-lec'tric. [From ἴδιος, "one's own," "peculiar," and *elec'tric.*] Literally, "having electricity of its [or their] own." A term applied to bodies, such as amber, resin, or glass, which, when rubbed, acquire electricity, without any communication with another electrified body.

Id-i-o-path'ic. [**Idiopath'icus.**] Relating to idiopathy; opposed to *sympathetic*, or *symptomatic*.

Id-i-op'a-thў. [**Idiopathi'a;** from ἴδιος, "one's own," "peculiar," or "private," and πάθος, "affection," or "disease."] A disease arising spontaneously, not from another; an affection the opposite of *sympathy*.

Id-i-o-sўn'cra-sў. [**Idiosyncra'sia;** from ἴδιος, "one's own," "peculiar," or "private," and σύγκρασις, a "mixing or tempering together," and, hence, "temperament," or "constitution."] The disposition or habit of body peculiar to an individual.

Id-i-o-sўn-crat'ic. [**Idiosyncrat'icus.**] Belonging to idiosyncrasy.

Id'i-ot. [**Idio'ta;** from ἰδιώτης, "private," because unfit for intercourse with the world.] One who is silly, or without understanding; a fool.

Id-i-o-ti'a.* [Gr. ἰδιωτεία.] Literally, "a state of privacy or obscurity." A state of idiotism. See Idiot.

Id-i-ot'ic. [**Idiot'icus.**] Like an idiot.

Id'i-o-tism. [**Idiotis'mus;** from ἰδιώτης, "private."] The state or condition of an idiot; idiocy.

Id'ri-a-lin. [**Idriali'na.**] A fossil, fatty substance, found in mercury-mines.

Idrosis. See Hidrosis.

If, ĕf. The French term for the "yew." See Taxus.

Ig-a-su'ri-a.* [See next article.] An alkaloid found in the different species of *Strychnos*.

Ig-a-su'ric. [**Igasu'ricus;** said to be derived from *Igasur*, the Malay name for St. Ignatius's bean.] Of or belonging to the *Faba Sancti Ignatii* (the seed of the *Strychnos Ignatia*).

Igasu'ric Aç'id. [**Igasu'ricum Aç'idum.**] An acid, somewhat resembling the malic, existing in the *Strychnos Ignatia* and *Nux vomica*.

Ignatia,* ig-na'she-a. Bean of St. Ignatius. The name applied to the seed of the *Strychnos Ignatia*. It has been placed on the primary list of the Materia Medica of the U.S. Pharmacopœia for 1860. Its medical properties are essentially the same as those of *Nux vomica*.

Ignes Fatui. See IGNIS FATUUS.

Ig'nis.* Fire; the evolution of light and heat which attends combustion.

Ig'nis Ac-tu-a'lis.* ("Actual Fire.") See ACTUAL CAUTERY.

Ig'nis Fat'u-us,* plural **Ig'nēs Fat'u-ī.** ("Vain or Foolish Fire;" so called, probably, because it makes fools of those who pursue it.) The luminous appearance of flame frequently seen in the night in marshy places, and popularly called *Jack with the lantern*, or *Will o' the Wisp*. It is produced by phosphorus evolved from decaying vegetable matter.

Ig'nis Potentia'lis,* po-ten-she-a'-lis. ("Potential Fire.") A name for the potential cautery.

Ig'nis Sa'cer.* ("Sacred Fire.") The same as ERYSIPELAS, which see.

Ig'nis Sanc'ti An-to'nī-i.* ("Saint Anthony's Fire.") A name for *erysipelas*.

Ig'nis Vo-lat'ī-cus.* Literally, "flying fire." A term for *erysipelas*.

Ig-nī'tion. [From *ig'nis*, "fire."] The state of being heated so as to resemble fire; in other words, so as to emit heat and light like a burning body.

Ileac Passion. See ILIAC PASSION.

Il-e-i'tis, i*dis*.* [From *il'eum*.] Inflammation of the *ileum* or *ilium*.

Ileo-. A prefix denoting connection with, or relation to, the *ileum* or *ilium*.

Il'eo-Cæ'cal Valve. The inferior semilunar fold of mucous membrane which secures against any matter re-entering the *ileum* from the *cæcum*.

Il'eo-Col'ic Valve. The superior semilunar fold of mucous membrane which secures the *ileum* against regurgitation from the *colon*.

Il'e-um,* or **Il'ī-um.*** [From εἰλέω, to "turn about."] The third or last portion of the small intestine, ending at the valve of the *cæcum*.

Il'e-us.* [Gr. εἰλεός.] The same as ILIAC PASSION, which see.

I'lex Aq-uī-fo'lī-um.* (Fr. *Houx*, hoo.) The systematic name of the common European holly, the leaves of which have been reputed as tonic, astringent, and antiseptic.

Il'ī-a.* [The nominative plural of *i'le*; from εἰλέω, to "involve."] The flanks, which enclose the small intestines; also, the small intestines themselves.

Il'ī-ac. [Lat. **Ili'acus**; Fr. *Iliaque*, ē'lē'āk'.] Belonging to the flanks.

Il'iac Ar'te-ries. [**Arte'riæ Ili'-acæ.**] These are termed the common iliac arteries immediately after they are given off by the aorta. They afterwards divide into the external iliac, and the internal iliac, or hypogastric, arteries.

Il'iac Fos'sa. [**Fos'sa Ili'aca.**] A broad and shallow cavity at the upper part of the inner surface of the *Os iliacum*. It is also called the *internal iliac fossa*.

Il'iac Fos'sa, Ex-ter'nal. A fossa or depression on the external surface of the *Os iliacum*.

Il'iac Pas'sion. [**Pas'sio Ili'aca**; from *il'ia*.] A disease characterized by severe griping pain, vomiting of fecal matter, and costiveness, with retraction and spasm of the abdominal muscles.

Il'iac Re'gion. The side of the abdomen, between the ribs and hips.

Iliacum Os. See OS ILIACUM.

Il-ī-a-del'phus.* [From *i'le*, the "flank," and ἀδελφός, a "brother."] Applied to monsters which are double above and united at and below the pelvis.

Iliaque. See ILIAC.

Il'ī-cin, or **Il'ī-cine.** [**Ilici'na.**] An active principle obtained from the ilex, and recommended as a febrifuge.

Il'ī-um,* plural **Il'ī-a.** The haunch-bone. The upper portion of the *os innominatum*; in the fœtus it is distinct from the other parts. See ILIA.

Illacrymatio* (il-lak-re-ma'she-o), **o'***nis*; from *illac'rymo*, *illacryma'tum*, to "weep greatly, or involuntarily."] Excessive involuntary weeping. Sometimes synonymous with EPIPHORA.

Illecebraceæ,* il-le-se-bra'she-ē. [From *Illece'brum*, one of the genera.] A natural order of exogenous plants, found in Europe and Africa.

Il-lu'sion. [**Illu'sio, o'***nis*; from *illu'do*, *illu'sum*, to "mock," or "deceive."] A deception, false appearance, or mockery; a hallucination.

Im. A Latin particle. See IN.

Im'age. [From *ima'go*, a "resemblance," "picture," or "image."] An idea; a picture of the imagination. In Optics, the spectrum or picture of an object, formed by the reflection or refraction of the rays of light from its various points. Optical images form an essential part of the process or function of vision.

I-ma'go,* gen. **I-mag'i-nis.** [From *im'itor*, to "imitate," or "copy."] Literally, an "image," "picture," or "portrait." Applied to the perfect insect, which has undergone all its metamorphoses. The origin of this appellation would seem to be, that, as a portrait is not merely the first rude outline of the artist, but the perfect elaboration of his idea; so, after the several preparatory stages of the egg, the *larva*, and the *pupa* (or *chrysalis*), the *imago* is the full and final elaboration of nature's idea respecting the insect.

Im'be-cile. [**Imbecil'lis**; from *in*, "on," and *bac'ulus*, a "staff."] Feeble; weak; but generally applied to weakness of the mental faculties.

Im-bibe'. [From *in*, "in," and *bi'bo*, *bib'itum*, to "drink."] To drink in; to absorb.

Im-bi-bi'tion. [**Imbibi'tio, o'nis**; from the same.] The act of drinking in or sucking up moisture.

Im'bri-cate. [**Imbrica'tus**; from *im'brico*, *imbrica'tum*, to "cover with tiles" (from *im'brex*, a "roof-tile").] Having an appearance of tiles successively overlapping each other.

Im'bri-cāt-ing. [**Im'bricans**; from the same.] Applied to the folioles of a compound leaf, when, during the *sleep* of the plant, they apply themselves along the petiole, which they entirely conceal, covering each other like tiles on a house-top, directed from the base to the summit.

Im'bri-că-tive. [**Imbricati'vus**; from the same.] See Imbricating.

Im-mar'gi-nate. [**Immargina'tus**; from *in*, priv., and *mar'go*, a "border."] Having no marked border.

Im-me-di-a'tus.* [From *in*, negative, or privative, and *me'dium*, "something between, or intervening."] Literally, "with nothing intervening." (Fr. *Immédiat*, ēm'mā'de-ā'.) Applied in Botany to the insertion of stamens when they are attached directly under the ovary, upon the calyx, or upon the pistil.

Im-mersed'. [**Immer'sus**; from *immer'go*, *immer'sum*, to "plunge under, or into, water."] Beneath the surface of water.

Im-mo'bil-is.* [From *in*, priv., and *mo'veo*, to "move."] Applied to anthers wholly attached to the filament: immov'able.

Im-pac'ted. [**Impac'tus**; from *impin'go*, *impac'tum*, to "drive, or dash against," to "drive in."] Used in reference to the head of the child when fixed in the pelvic cavity.

Im'par, a'ris.* [From *in*, negative, and *par*, "equal."] Odd, not even; unequal. See Ganglion Impar.

Im-par-i-ner-va'tus.* [From *im'par*, "unequal," and *ner'vus*, a "nerve."] Having unequal nervures: impariner'vate.

Im-par-i-pen'nate. [**Imparipenna'tus**; from *pen'na*, a "feather," or "quill."] The same as Imparipinnate.

Im-par-i-pin'nate. [**Imparipinna'tus**; from *im'par*, "unequal," and *pin'na*, a "feather," a "wing."] Unequally pinnate; having unequal leaves or folioles.

Im-pen-e-tra-bil'i-tў. [**Impenetrabil'itas, a'tis**; from *in*, negative, and *pen'etro*, to "pierce," to "penetrate," to "enter into."] A property of matter, by which no portion of it can occupy the same place at the same time with another.

Im-per'fect. [**Imperfec'tus**; from *in*, negative, and *perfi'cio*, *perfec'tum*, to "finish."] Incomplete. Applied to flowers which want either anthers or pistils.

Im-per-fo-li-a'tus.* [From *in*, negative, and *perfolia'tus*, "pierced through the leaves."] Having leaves that are not perfoliate.

Im-per'fo-rate. [**Imperfora'tus**; from *in*, negative, and *per'foro*, *perfora'tum*, to "bore through."] Abnormally occluded; applied to the *anus*, *vagina*, etc.

Im-pe'ri-al. A cooling beverage prepared by mixing half an ounce each of cream of tartar and fresh lemon-peel, bruised, with four ounces of white sugar, and three pints of boiling water.

Im-pe-tig'i-nous. [**Impetigino'des, Impetigino'sus**; from *impeti'go*.] Having *impetigo*.

Im-pe-ti'go,* gen. **Im-pe-tig'i-nis.** [From *im'peto*, to "invade."] (Fr. *Dartre*, dartr.) A skin-disease marked by small, irregularly circumscribed pustules, chiefly on the extremities, slightly elevated, and terminating in a laminated scab, unaccompanied by fever, and not contagious; humid or running tetter.

Im-pe-ti-o-la'ris.* [From *in*, priv., and *peti'olus*, a "petiole."] Having no petiole.

Im-plan-ta'tus.* [From *in*, "in," and *plan'to*, *planta'tum*, to "set," to "plant."] Applied to crystals attached by one of their ends to the walls of an excavation in a rock.

Im-plĭ-ca'tus.* [From *in*, "in," or "into," and *pli'co*, *plica'tum*, to "fold," or "wrap."] The same as COMPLICATED, which see.

Im-plu'vĭ-ŭm.* [From *in*, "upon," and *plu'via*, "rain."] A shower-bath.

Im-pon-der-a-bil'ĭ-tў. [**Imponderabil'itas, a'tis.**] The quality of being imponderable.

Im-pon'der-a-ble. [**Impondera'bilis**; from *in*, negative, and *pon'dero*, to "weigh."] Incapable of being weighed. Applied to light, heat, electricity, magnetism, etc.

Im-pos'thume. [Probably a corruption of *aposte'ma*.] Another term for an abscess. See ABSCESS.

Im'po-tence, Im'po-ten-cў. [**Impoten'tia**; from *in*, negative, and *pos'sum*, to "be able."] (Fr. *Impuissance*, ăɴ'pwē'sŏɴss'.) Weakness; want of power, especially of virile power. See ADYNAMIA, ANAPHRODISIA, and STERILITY.

Im'po-tent. [**Im'potens**; from the same.] Incapable of procreating or impregnating.

Im-preg-nā'tion. [**Impregna'tio, o'nis**; from the Low Latin *impreg'no*, *impregna'tum*, to "make fruitful," to "make pregnant."] The act of making, or state of being, pregnant; fecundation.

Impregnation, Diseases affecting the. See CARPOTICUS.

Im-pu'ber, eris.* [From *in*, negative, and *pu'ber*, "of ripe age."] Without hair on the *pubes*; not arrived at adult age.

Impuissance. See IMPOTENCE.

Im-pus-tu-la'tus.* [From *in*, negative, and *pustula'tus*, "having pustules."] Having no red spots: impus'tulate.

I'mus Ven'ter.* ("Lowest Belly.") The lowest part of the abdomen, between the *umbilicus* and *pudenda*.

In. A Latin particle signifying "in," "within," "into," "on," "against." It is often negative, and sometimes intensive. Before *b*, *m*, and *p*, the *n* is changed to *m*: *e.g.*, *imbibe*, instead of *inbibe*; *immobilis* for *inmobilis*, *impotent* for *inpotent*, etc.

In-æ-qual-ĭ-fo'lĭ-us.* [From *inæqua'lis*, "unequal," and *fo'lium*, a "leaf."] Having unequal leaves.

In-al-bu-mĭ-na'tus.* [From *in*, priv., and *albu'men*.] Applied to the embryo of plants not having albumen.

In-an-a-gen'e-sis.* [From ἴς, ἰνός, a "fibre," and *anagen'esis*, "regeneration."] Muscular regeneration, or reproduction of muscular fibre.

In-a-naph'ў-sis.* [From ἴς, ἰνός, a "fibre," and *anaph'ysis*, "renewed growth."] Similar to INANAGENESIS.

In-an-ĭ'tion. [**Inani'tio, o'nis**; from *ina'nio*, *inani'tum*, to "empty" (from *ina'nis*, "empty").] Emptiness of the body, its viscera, or its vessels, from want of food; starvation.

In-an-the-ra'tus.* [From *in*, priv., and *anthe'ra*, an "anther."] Applied to the filaments of stamens when they do not bear anthers.

In-an-ther-if'er-us.* [From *in*, priv., *anthe'ra*, an "anther," and *fe'ro*, to "bear."] The same as INANTHERATUS, which see.

In-ap-pen-dic-u-la'tus.* [From *in*, priv., and *appen'dix*, an "addition."] Having no *appendices*. Applied mostly to plants.

In-ap'pe-ten-cў. [**Inappeten'tia**; from *in*, negative, and *ap'peto*, to "desire."] The same as ANOREXIA. A want or loss of appetite.

In-ar-tic'u-late. [**Inarticula'tus**; from *in*, priv., and *articula'tus*, "articulated."] Having no articulation: inarticulated. Also, not having distinct utterance.

In-cal-ў-ca'tus.* [From *in*, priv., and *ca'lyx*.] Without a calyx.

In-can-dĕs'çence. [**Incandescen'tia**; from *incandes'co*, to "grow very hot."] The bright appearance presented by solids and liquids when heated to a sufficient degree.

In-can-dĕs'çent. [**Incandes'cens**; from the same.] Applied to a body heated till its surface becomes white and brilliant.

In-cā'nous. [**Inca'nus**; from *in*, intensive, and *ca'nus*, "hoary."] Hoary; covered with a white down. Applied to the stems, leaves, etc. of plants.

In-can-tā'tion. [From *incan'to*, *incanta'tum*, to "charm."] A mode of curing disease by charms, etc.

In-car'cer-āt-ed. [**Incarcera'tus**; from *in*, "in," and *car'cer*, a "prison."] Applied to the portion of bowel or other substance confined by the stricture in strangulated hernia.

Incarceration. See STRANGULATION.

In-car-nā'tion. [From *in*, "in," or "upon," and *ca'ro*, *car'nis*, "flesh."] Growth of flesh or granulations.

In-cer-nic'u-lum.* [From *incer'no*, to "sift," or "strain."] The pelvis of the kidney into which the urine is strained from the *papillæ renis*.

In'ci-dence. [**Inciden'tia**; from *in'cido*, to "fall upon."] A term for the direction in which one body strikes upon another.

In'cidence, An'gle of. The angle formed by the line in which a body or ray of light moves, and the straight line perpendicular to the plane against which the body or ray strikes.

Incidentia,* in-se-den'she-a. [From *inci'do*, to "cut in."] A name formerly given to medicines which were supposed to consist of sharp particles, as acids and salts.

In-cin-er-ā'tion. [**Incinera'tio, o'***nis;* from *incin'ero, incinera'tum*, to "burn to ashes."] The act of reducing animal or vegetable matter to ashes.

In-cīsed'. [**Inci'sus.**] Cut irregularly and sharply. Applied to leaves.

In-cis'ion. [**Inci'sio, o'***nis;* from *inci'do, inci'sum*, to "cut into," to "cut."] The cutting into the integuments or flesh with an instrument.

In-cī-si'vus.* [From the same.] Belonging to the incisor teeth.

In-cī'sor,* plural **In-cī-so'rēs.** [From the same.] The four front teeth of both jaws which have sharp, cutting edges.

In-clī-nā'tion. [**Inclina'tio, o'***nis;* from *incli'no, inclina'tum*, to "bend down," to "incline."] The state of a body or vessel placed obliquely. The angle made by two planes or two lines, or by a plane and a line; or the angle which they would make if they were extended until they met.

In-com-pat'ī-ble. [From *in*, negative, and *compa'tior*, to "suffer together."] Literally, "that cannot be suffered (or allowed) together." Applied to substances which act chemically on each other, and therefore cannot with propriety be prescribed together.

In-com-plete'. [From *in*, negative, and *com'pleo, comple'tum*, to "fulfil," to "finish."] A term applied to a flower which wants some one or more kinds of organs.

In-com-pres-sī-bil'ī-tў. [**Incompressibil'itas, a'***tis;* from *in*, negative, and *com'primo, compres'sum*, to "press together."] Incapability of being compressed.

In-con'tī-nence. [**Incontinen'tia**; from *in*, negative, and *conti'neo*, to "contain."] Inability to retain the natural evacuations.

In-cor-po-rā'tion. [**Incorpora'tio, o'***nis;* from *in*, "into," and *cor'pus*, a "body."] The mixing of particles of different bodies together so that they appear to be formed into one body, or into a uniform substance.

Incrassantia,* in-kras-san'she-a. [The neuter plural of *incras'sans*, the present participle of *incras'so, incrassa'tum*, to "make thick."] Applied to medicines supposed to have the power of thickening the humors or the blood when too thin.

In-crus-tā'tion. [**Incrusta'tio, o'***nis;* from *incrus'to, incrusta'tum*, to "rough-cast," to "incrust."] The act or process of forming a crust. A crust or deposit of stony molecules on bodies plunged or habitually bathed in water charged with calcareous salts.

In-cu-bā'tion. [**Incuba'tio, o'***nis;* from *in'cubo, incuba'tum*, to "lie upon," to "sit on," as eggs.] The act or process by which most birds hatch their eggs. Also applied to the period between the implanting of a disease, or subjection to its causes, and its development.

In'cu-bus.* [From *in'cubo*, to "lie or sit upon."] (Fr. *Cauchemar*, kōsh'-mar'.) The night-mare. See EPHIALTES.

In'cubus Vigilan'tium* (vij-e-lan'she-ŭm). See DAY-MARE.

In-cum'bent. [From *incum'bo*, to "lie or lean upon."] Leaning or lying upon. Applied to anthers which lie on the inner side of the filaments, etc.

In-cur'vate. [**Incurva'tus, Incur'vus**; from *incur'vo, incurva'tum*, to "bend," to "curve."] Bent, or bowed, inwards; incurved.

In-cur-vā'tion. [**Incurva'tio, o'***nis;* from the same.] A bowing or bending. Applied to the back, etc.

In'cus,* gen. **In-cu'dis.** (Fr. *Enclume*, ŏNᴳ'klüm'.) Literally, an "anvil." The largest of the ossicles of the internal ear; so named from its fancied resemblance to a smith's anvil.

Ind. = *In di'es.** "From day to day," or "daily."

In-def'ī-nite. [From *in*, negative, and *defi'nio, defini'tum*, to "limit," to "define."] Either uncertain in number or too many to be readily counted. Applied to petals, stamens, etc.

In-de-his'çent. [**Indehis'cens**; from *in*, negative, and *dehis'co*, to "gape open."] Applied to a pericarp that does not open spontaneously, when ripe.

In'dex,* gen. **In'dī-cis.** [From *in'dico*, to "point out," to "show."] Applied to the fore-finger, because it is used for pointing.

In'dĭ-an Ar'row-Root. The root of the *Maranta arundinacea.*

In'dian Corn. The *Zea Mays,* or maize-plant.

In'dian Hemp. The *Cannabis Indica.*

In'dian Pink. The *Spigelia marilandica.*

In'dian Rub'ber. A name for caoutchouc.

In'dian To-bac'co. The *Lobelia inflata.*

In-dĭ-a'na Ra'dix.* A name for Ipecacuanha.

In-dĭ-cā'tion. [**Indica'tio, o'***nis;* from *in'dico, indica'tum,* to "point out."] That which indicates or points out what ought to be done by the practitioner.

In-dĭ-ca'tor, o'*ris.** [From the same.] A muscle of the fore-finger. Also termed *Extensor Indicis.* See INDEX.

In'dĭ-cus Mor'bus.* ("Indian Disease.") A name for the venereal disease; so called because it was believed to have been first brought to Europe from the West Indies (or the neighboring coast of America) by the Spaniards.

In-dĭg'en-ous. [**Indig'enus;** from *in'du,* for *in,* "in," and *ge'no,* an ancient form of *gig'no,* to "beget," to "produce."] Native to a country; originally produced in a country or place.

In-dĭ-ġes'tion. [**Indiges'tio, o'***nis;* from *in,* negative, and *dig'ero, diges'tum,* to "set in order," to "digest."] The disease *Dyspepsia.*

In-dĭg-ĭ-tā'tion. [**Indigita'tio, o'***nis;* from *in,* "into," and *dig'itus,* a "finger."] The passing or thrusting of one part of the intestines into another; the part which enters being compared to a finger. See INTUSSUSCEPTION.

In-dig-na-bun'dus.* [From *indig'nor,* to "be indignant."] Literally, "angry." A name given to the *rectus externus* (a muscle of the eye), from the expression of anger or scorn which the action of this muscle imparts.

In'dĭ-go. [A corruption of *In'dico,* the Portuguese and Spanish for "Indian;" Latin *In'dicum;* so called because it was originally procured exclusively from India.] A blue coloring matter extracted from the *Indigofera tinctoria,* the anil, or indigo-plant.

In-dĭ-gof'er-a An'il.* Another name for the *Indigofera tinctoria.*

Indigof'era Tinc-to'rĭ-a.* The plant which yields indigo. It belongs to the natural order *Leguminosæ.*

In-dĭ-gof'er-us.* [From *in'digo,* and *fe'ro,* to "bear."] Bearing, or producing, indigo. Applied to plants.

In'dĭ-go-tāte. [**Indig'otas, a'***tis.*] A combination of indigotic acid with a base.

In-dig'o-tin. [**Indigoti'na.**] The coloring principle of indigo.

In'do-lēs.* The natural disposition or character.

In-duc'tion. [**Induc'tio, o'***nis;* from *indu'co, induc'tum,* to "lead into."] The act or process of inferring or establishing a general proposition from several particular ones; also, the proposition thus established.

In-duc'tĭve. [From the same.] Capable of leading to; inferring, or persuading by induction.

In-du-men'tum.* [From *in'duo,* to "put on," to "cover."] Any hairiness or downy covering of plants.

In-du'plĭ-cate. [From *in,* "in," or "inwards," and *du'plico, duplica'tum,* to "double."] A term applied to valvate æstivation, in which the margins of the leaves are inflexed.

In'du-rate. [**Indura'tus;** from *indu'ro, indura'tum,* to "harden."] Made hard; hardened.

In-du-rā'tion. [**Indura'tio, o'***nis;* from the same.] (Fr. *Endurcissement,* ŏNᴳ'dür'sêss'mŏNᴳ'.) The state or process of hardening: the hardening of any part from the effect of disease.

In-du-sĭ-a'tus.* Having an *indusium.*

In-du'sĭ-um.* [From *in'duo, indu'tum,* to "put on," to "cover."] The proper covering of the fruit-dots of ferns; any peculiar membranous covering. Applied to the *amnion,* because it covers the fœtus.

In-du'vĭ-al. [**Induvia'lis;** from the same.] Applied to a calyx when it is persistent, and covers the fruit, as that of the *Physalis alkekengi.*

In-du'vĭ-ate. [**Induvia'tus;** from the same.] Applied to fruit that is covered by *induvia.*

In-du'vĭ-um,* plural **In-du'vĭ-a.** [From *in'duo,* to "cover."] Applied to the whole perianth, or every accessory part of the flower which persists and covers the fruit, after maturity of the ovary.

In-em'brȳ-o-nate. [**Inembryona'tus;** from *in,* negative, and *em'bryo.*] Having no embryo, germ, or *corculum.*

In-e-quĭ-lat'er-al. [**Inæquilat'erus;** from *in,* negative, or priv., *æ'quus,* "equal," and *la'tus,* a "side."] Having unequal sides, as the leaves of certain plants.

In-er'mis.* [From *in*, priv., and *ar'ma*, "arms."] Without spines, or prickles; unarmed.

Inertia,* in-er'she-ạ. [From *in'ers*, "slothful."] This term is used to denote the principle or law of the material world that all bodies are absolutely passive or indifferent to a state of rest or motion, and would continue forever at rest, or persevere in the same uniform and rectilinear motion, unless disturbed by the action of some extrinsic force.—(BRANDE.)

Inf. = *Infu'sum*,* an "infusion;" also, *Infun'de*,* "pour in."

In'fạn-cỹ. [Lat. **Infan'tia;** see INFANT; Fr. *Enfance*, ŏɴɢ'fŏɴss'.] Early childhood, usually reckoned from birth to the seventh year. See ÆTAS.

In'fạnt. [Lat. **In'fans;** from *in*, negative, and *fans*, "speaking;" Fr. *Enfant*, ŏɴɢ'fŏɴɢ'.] Originally, a child so young as to be unable to speak; now applied somewhat indefinitely to any young child. See INFANCY.

In-fan'ti-cide. [**Infantici'da;** from *in'fans*, a "child," or "infant," and *cæ'do*, to "kill."] One who kills, murders, or destroys an infant.

Infan'ticide. [**Infanticid'ium;** from the same.] Child-murder, distinguished into that which is perpetrated by omission, and that by commission.

In-farc'tion. [**Infarc'tio, o'***nis;* from *infar'cio*, *infarc'tum*, to "fill in."] A sense of oppression, fulness, or stuffing of the chest.

In-fec'tion. [**Infec'tio, o'***nis;* from *infi'cio*, *infec'tum*, to "infect."] The communication of a disease by personal contact with the sick, or by means of *effluvia* arising from the body of the sick; contagion.

Infecundity. See STERILITY.

In-fe'ri-or. A term applied to the ovary when the calyx is attached to it, or to the calyx when it is free.

Infe'rior Lon-gi-tu'di-nal Si'nus. A vein of the *dura mater*, running along the lower margin of the *falx cerebri*.

In'fe-ro-bran-chi-a'tus.* [From *in'ferus*, "beneath," and *bran'chiæ*, "gills."] Applied in the plural neuter (*Inferobranchia'ta*) to an order of *Mollusca Gasteropoda*, having the *branchiæ* on both sides of the body under the border of the mantle.

In-fil'trāt-ed. [**Infiltra'tus;** from *in*, "into," and *fil'trum*, a "strainer."] Strained through; filtered. Applied to an organ or part in the state of filtration.

In-fil-trā'tion. [**Infiltra'tio, o'***nis*, from the same.] A straining of fluid substances into the *areolæ* or cellular tissue of a structure.

In-fin-i-tes'i-mal. [**Infinites'imus;** from *in*, negative, and *fi'nis*, a "boundary."] Infinitely small.

Infirmary. See HOSPITAL.

In-flamed'. [**Inflamma'tus;** from *inflam'mo*, *inflamma'tum*, to "set on fire," to "inflame."] (Fr. *Enflammé*, ŏɴɢ'flâm'mà'.) In a state of inflammation.

In-flam'mạ-ble. [**Inflamma'bilis;** from the same.] Applied to gases or substances that are easily set on fire.

Inflammable Air. See HYDROGEN.

In-flam-mā'tion. [**Inflamma'tio, o'***nis;* from the same.] A state of disease characterized by redness, pain, heat, and swelling, attended or not with fever; termed, also, *Phlogosis*. It is often expressed by the terminal *-itis* added to the name of the organ or part affected; as, *bronchitis*, inflammation of the bronchia; *tonsillitis*, inflammation of the tonsils. See PHLEGMASIA, and PHLOGOSIS.

In-flam'mạ-to-rỹ. [**Inflammato'rius;** from the same.] Belonging to inflammation; phlogistic.

Inflam'matory Crust. The *buffy coat* of the blood.

Inflam'matory Fe'ver. The state of fever called *synocha*.

Inflatio. See EMPHYSEMA.

In-flexed'. [**Inflex'us;** from *in*, "in," or "inwards," and *flec'to*, *flex'um*, to "bend."] Abruptly bent or curved inwards.

In-flo-rĕs'çence. [**Inflorescen'tia;** from *inflores'co*, to "blossom."] A mode of flowering; the arrangement of flowers on the stem or branch; the particular manner of flowering.

In-flu-en'zạ. An Italian word signifying "influence;" because the disease seems to reside in, or be dependent upon, some atmospheric influence. (Fr. *Grippe*, gʀĕp or gʀipp.) An epidemic disease characterized by the suddenness of its attack, general depression, great heaviness over the eyes, and by a peculiarly distressing fever.

In-frạ-max-il-la'ris.* [From *in'fra*, "beneath," and *maxil'la*, the "jaw."] Situated under the jaw: inframax'illary.

In-fra-or'bĭ-tar, or **In-fra-or'bĭ-ta-rȳ.** [**Infraorbita'rius,** or **Infra-orbita'ris;** from *in'fra,* "beneath," "below," and *or'bita,* the "orbit."] Situated beneath the orbit of the eye.

In-fra-scap'u-lar. [**Infrascapu-la'ris;** from *in'fra,* "beneath," "below," and *scap'ula,* the "shoulder-blade."] Below the shoulder-blade.

In-fra-spi'nate. [**Infraspina'tus;** from *in'fra,* "beneath," "below," and *spi'na,* a "spine."] Below a spinous process.

In-fun-dib'u-lar, or **In-fun-dib'-u-lĭ-form.** [**Infundibulifor'mis;** from *infundib'ulum,* a "funnel."] Shaped like a funnel.

In-fun-dib'u-lum,* plural **In-fun-dib'u-la.** [From *infun'do, infu'sum,* to "pour in."] (Fr. *Entonnoir,* ŏɴɢ'ton'-nwåʀ'.) A funnel. Applied in the plural to three small tubes in the kidney, of a funnel-like shape; also to the canal leading from the third ventricle of the brain to the pituitary gland.

In-fu'sa,* the plural of INFUSUM, which see.

In-fu'sion. [**Infu'sio, o'nis,** or **Infu'sum;** from *in,* "in," or "upon," and *fun'do, fu'sum,* to "pour."] Literally, a "pouring in or upon." The act of steeping some substance in cold or hot water, for the purpose of obtaining a solution of its soluble principle; also, the name of such solution. See INFUSUM.

Infusoria. See next article.

In-fu-so'rĭ-us.* [From the same.] Belonging to infusions: infu'sory. Applied in the plural neuter (*Infuso'ria*) to a class of *Radiata,* so extremely minute as to be invisible to the naked eye; found in infusions of various substances, and in stagnant water. See ANIMALCULE.

In-fu'sum.* [From the same.] An aqueous solution of vegetable substances, obtained without the aid of ebullition.

Infu'sum An-gus-tu'ræ.* ("Infusion of Angustura.") Take of Angustura, in moderately coarse powder, half a troyounce; water, a sufficient quantity. Moisten the powder with two fluidrachms of water, pack it firmly in a conical percolator, and gradually pour water upon it, until the filtered liquid measures a pint. This infusion may also be prepared by macerating the Angustura in a pint of boiling water, for two hours, in a covered vessel, and straining.

Infu'sum An-them'ĭ-dis.* ("Infusion of Chamomile.") Take of chamomile, half a troyounce; boiling water, a pint. Macerate for ten minutes in a covered vessel, and strain.

Infu'sum Ca-lum'bæ,* or **Infu'-sum Co-lom'bæ*** (U.S. Ph., 1850). ("Infusion of Columbo.") Prepared in the same manner as the INFUSUM ANGUSTURÆ, only substituting Columbo for Angustura.

Infu'sum Cap'sĭ-çi.* ("Infusion of Capsicum.") Take of capsicum, in coarse powder, half a troyounce; boiling water, a pint. Macerate for two hours in a covered vessel, and strain.

Infu'sum Căr-ȳ-o-phȳl'lĭ.* ("Infusion of Cloves.") Take of cloves, bruised, one hundred and twenty grains; boiling water, a pint. Macerate for two hours in a covered vessel, and strain.

In-fu'sum Cin-cho'næ Fla'væ.* ("Infusion of Yellow Cinchona.") Take of yellow cinchona, in moderately fine powder, a troyounce; aromatic sulphuric acid, a fluidrachm; water, a sufficient quantity. Mix the acid with a pint of water; then moisten the powder with half a fluidounce of the mixture, and, having packed it firmly in a conical glass percolator, gradually pour upon it the remainder of the mixture, and afterwards water, until the filtered liquid measures a pint.

Infu'sum Cincho'næ Ru'bræ,* or **Infu'sum Cincho'næ Com-pos'ĭ-tum*** (U.S. Ph., 1850). ("Infusion of Red Cinchona," or "Compound Infusion of Cinchona.") Prepared exactly as the preceding, only substituting the red for the yellow cinchona.

Infu'sum Dĭg-ĭ-ta'lis.* ("Infusion of Digitalis.") Take of digitalis, in coarse powder, sixty grains; tincture of cinnamon, a fluidounce; boiling water, half a pint. Macerate the digitalis with the water for two hours in a covered vessel, and strain; then add the tincture of cinnamon, and mix.

In-fu'sum Eu-pa-to'rĭ-i.* ("Infusion of Thoroughwort.") Take of thoroughwort, a troyounce; boiling water, a pint. Macerate for two hours in a covered vessel, and strain.

In-fu'sum Gentia'næ (jen-she-a'-nē) **Com-pos'ĭ-tum.*** ("Compound Infusion of Gentian.") Take of gentian, in moderately coarse powder, half a troyounce; bitter orange peel, in moderately coarse powder, coriander, in moderately coarse powder, each sixty grains; alcohol, two fluidounces; water, a sufficient quantity. Mix the alcohol with fourteen fluidounces of water, and, having moistened the mixed powders with three fluidrachms of the menstruum, pack them firmly in a conical percolator, and gradually pour upon them, first the remainder of the menstruum, and afterwards water, until the filtered liquid measures a pint.

Infu'sum Ju-nip'e-ri.* ("Infusion of Juniper.") Take of juniper, bruised, a troyounce; boiling water, a pint. Macerate for an hour in a covered vessel, and strain.

Infu'sum Pi'cis Liq'ui-dæ.* ("Infusion of *Liquid Pitch* or *Tar*.") Tar-water. Take of tar, a pint; water, four pints. Mix them, and shake the mixture frequently during twenty-four hours; then pour off the infusion, and filter through paper.

Infu'sum Pru'ni Vir-ġin-ĭ-a'næ.* ("Infusion of Wild Cherry Bark.") Take of wild cherry bark, in moderately coarse powder, half a troyounce; water, a sufficient quantity. Moisten the powder with six fluidrachms of water, let it stand for an hour, pack it gently in a conical glass percolator, and gradually pour water upon it, until the filtered liquid measures a pint.

Infu'sum Quas'siæ* (kwŏsh'e-ē). ("Infusion of Quassia.") Take of quassia, rasped, one hundred and twenty grains; water, a pint. Macerate for twelve hours in a covered vessel, and strain.

Infu'sum Sen'næ.* ("Infusion of Senna.") Take of senna, a troyounce; coriander, bruised, sixty grains; boiling water, a pint. Macerate for an hour in a covered vessel, and strain.

Infu'sum Ser-pen-ta'rĭ-æ.* ("Infusion of Serpentaria, or Snake-root.") Prepared in the same manner as the INFUSUM ANGUSTURÆ, only substituting Serpentaria for Angustura.

Infu'sum Spi-ġe'lĭ-æ.* ("Infusion of Spigelia.") Take of spigelia, half a troyounce; boiling water, a pint. Macerate for two hours in a covered vessel, and strain.

Infu'sum Ta-rax'a-çi.* ("Infusion of Dandelion.") Take of dandelion, bruised, two troyounces; boiling water, a pint. Macerate for two hours in a covered vessel, and strain.

Infu'sum Va-le-rĭ-a'næ.* ("Infusion of Valerian.") Prepared in the same manner as the INFUSUM ANGUSTURÆ.

Infu'sum Zin-ġib'e-ris.* ("Infusion of Ginger.") Take of ginger, bruised, half a troyounce; boiling water, a pint. Macerate for two hours in a covered vessel, and strain.

In-ġes'tus.* [From *in'gero, inges'tum*, to "carry in."] Applied in the plural neuter (*Inges'ta*) to the aliments taken into the body by the mouth.

In-glu'vĭ-ēs.* [Perhaps from *in*, "in," and *gu'la*, the "throat."] The craw, or crop, of birds.

In-gras'sĭ-as, Wings of. Two portions of the symmetrical halves of the sphenoid bone, termed the large and small wings.

In-grav-ĭ-dā'tion. [**Ingravida'tio, o'***nis*; from *in*, intensive, and *grav'ido, gravida'tum*, to "impregnate."] Impregnation; being with young.

In-gre'dĭ-ent. [**Ingre'diens;** from *ingre'dior*, to "enter in."] Any substance which enters into the composition of a compound body.

In'guen,* gen. **In'guĭ-nis.** The lower and lateral part of the abdomen, just above the thigh; the groin.

In'guĭ-nal. [**Inguina'lis;** from *in'guen*.] Belonging to the groin.

Inguinal Canal, Inguinal Ring. See SPERMATIC CANAL.

Inguinal Hernia. See BUBONOCELE.

In'guinal Lig'a-ment. The same as POUPART'S LIGAMENT, which see.

Ingulatio (in-gu-la'she-o), **o'***nis*.* [From *in*, "into," and *gu'la*, the "throat."] The introducing or putting any thing into the throat: ingula'tion.

In-hab'ĭ-tive-ness. [From *inhab'ito*, to "dwell in."] A term used by phrenologists to indicate the propensity, observed to be much stronger in some men and some animals than in others, to remain in the place in which they have long resided; or to be attached to their home simply because they have become accustomed to it.

In-ha-lā'tion. [**Inhala'tio, o'***nis*; from *inha'lo, inhala'tum*, to "breathe in."] Originally, a drawing of the air into the lungs. Usually applied to the inspiring of medicated or poisonous fumes with the breath.

In-hā'ler. [From the same.] A name applied to an apparatus constructed for the convenient inhalation of medicinal vapors; sometimes resorted to in pulmonary affections.

In'ĭ-ad. Applied the same as INIAL, used adverbially.

In'i-al. [From ἰνίον, the "occiput."] Belonging to the occiput; looking to the occiput. A term used by Dr. Barclay in reference to the aspects of the head.

In-i'tis, idis.* [From ἴς, ἰνός, "fibre."] Inflammation of muscular fibre or substance. Applied by Feuerstein to rheumatism.

Inj. enem. = *Injicia'tur en'ema.** "Let a clyster be given."

Inject. = *Injec'tio.** "An injection."

In-jec'tion. [**Injec'tio, o'***nis;* from *inji'cio, injec'tum,* to "throw into."] Any medicated liquor thrown into a natural or preternatural cavity by means of a syringe, or an injection-bag; when intended for the rectum, it is termed an *enema,* or clyster. In Anatomy, the term injection is applied to the filling of the vessels of any part of the body with some bright or highly colored substance, in order to exhibit their form or number to better advantage. Thus, a mercurial injection is often used for the minute vessels or capillaries, as, from its perfect fluidity, it readily penetrates the smallest passages, while its metallic brilliancy enables the minutest vascular ramifications to be clearly seen. But a resinous compound—colored red or blue, according as the design is to represent the arteries or veins—is, perhaps, most generally used.

In-Knees. A vulgar name for the deformity termed *Genua valga.*

In-nāte'. [From *in,* "in," or "on," and *nas'cor, na'tus,* to "be born."] Literally, "inborn," or "produced upon." Applied to anthers which are attached by their base to the apex of the filament.

In-ner-vā'tion. [**Innerva'tio, o'***nis;* from *in,* "into," or "to," and *ner'vus,* a "nerve," or "strength."] That vital process by which nervous energy is communicated to any part.

In-ner'vis.* [From *in,* priv., and *ner'vus,* a "nerve."] Applied to cotyledons and leaves when the nervures, enveloped by the parenchyma, are not seen externally, and seem not to exist.

Innominata Artery. See Arteria Innominata.

In-nom-ĭ-na'tus.* [From *in,* priv., and *no'men,* a "name."] Having no name; unnamed.

In-nu-trĭ'tion. [**Innutri'tio, o'***nis;* from *in,* priv., and *nu'trio, nutri'tum,* to "nourish."] Want of nourishment.

In-o-car'pus.* [From ἴς, ἰνός, a "fibre," and καρπός, "fruit."] Having fibrous fruit.

In-o-chon-drī'tis, idis.* [From ἴς, ἰνός, a "fibre," and χόνδρος, a "cartilage."] Inflammation of tendons and cartilages.

In-oc-u-lā'tion. [**Inocula'tio, o'***nis;* from *inoc'ulo, inocula'tum,* to "ingraft."] The insertion of *virus* into any part of the body in order to communicate a disease.

In-o-ġen'e-sis.* [From ἴς, ἰνός, a "fibre," and γένω, to "be born."] The production of fibre.

In-o'ma, atis.* [From ἴς, ἰνός, a "fibre."] A fibrous tumor.

Inonction. A French term for Inunction, which see.

In-o-pol'ȳ-pus.* [From ἴς, ἰνός, a "fibre," and *pol'ypus.*] A fibrous polypus.

In-or-gan'ic. [**Inorgan'icus;** from *in,* priv., and *or'ganum,* an "organ."] Destitute of organs. Applied to minerals as distinguished from animals and vegetables.

In-os'cu-lāt-ing. [From *in,* "into," and *os'culum,* a "little mouth."] Opening into each other; anastomosing, as the tubes of some plants. See Inosculation.

In-os-cu-lā'tion. [**Inoscula'tio, o'***nis;* from the same.] The junction or interunion of different branches of arteries, or veins, or extremities of arteries with the origins of veins.

In. pulm. = *In pulmen'to.** "In gruel."

Inquest. See Inquisitio.

In'quest, Cor'o-ner's. An inquisition appointed by a coroner in a case of sudden death, by summoning a jury to make inquiry upon examination of the body, respecting the cause of death, etc.

In-quĭ-sĭ'tion. [**Inquisi'tio, o'***nis;* from *inqui'ro, inquisi'tum,* to "search into," to "inquire."] An inquiry or inquest of jurors, in causes civil and criminal, on proof made of the fact on either side, as in cases of the lunacy of criminals, etc.

In-sal-ĭ-fī'a-ble. [**Insalifiab'ilis;** from *in,* priv., and *salifiab'ilis,* "capable of being formed into a salt."] Applied to oxides which are not acids, nor capable of neutralizing them.

In-sal-ĭ-vā'tion. [**Insaliva'tio, o'***nis;* from *in,* "by," and *saliva'tio,* a "filling with saliva."] The process of mixing the saliva with the food in the act of mastication.

In-sāne'. [**Insa'nus;** from *in,* negative, and *sa'nus,* "sane," or "sound."]

(Fr. *Fou*, foo.) Mad; wanting intellect; deranged in mind.

In-săn'ĭ-tў. [**Insa'nia, Insan'itas,** a'*tis*; from the same.] (Fr. *Folie*, fo'lè'.) Deranged intellect; madness or lunacy.

Insatiable Appetite. See BULIMIA.

In'sect. [See INSECTUS.] A name applied to any small animal having the body deeply incised, or, so to speak, divided between the head and the belly; as the common fly, the bee, the ant, the locust, etc.

In-sec'ta,* the plural of **In-sec'tum,** an "insect."

In-sec-tif'er-us.* [From *insec'tum*, an "insect," and *fe'ro*, to "bear."] Applied to amber (*Succinum*) when it contains insects imbedded in its substance.

In-sec-tiv'or-ous. [**Insectiv'orus**; from *insec'ta*, "insects," and *vo'ro*, to "devour."] Insect-devouring. Applied in the plural neuter (*Insectiv'ora*) to a family of *Mammalia*.

In-sec-tol'o-ġў. [**Insectolo'gia**; from *insec'tum*, an "insect," and λόγος, a "discourse."] A treatise upon insects. The same as ENTOMOLOGY.

In-sec'tum.* [I.e. *an'imal* **insec'tum**; *an'imal*, a "living creature," and *insec'tus*, "cut in," "incised."] Literally, an "incised animal." A small animal of a particular description. See INSECT.

In-sec'tus.* [From *in'seco*, *insec'tum*, to "cut into."] Insec'ted. Applied in the plural neuter (*Insec'ta*) to a class of *Articulata*. See INSECTUM.

In-ser'tion. [**Inser'tio,** o'*nis*; from *in'sero*, *inser'tum*, to "implant," or "insert," to "set in."] The attachment of muscle to a bone; also, the entrance of a nerve into a muscle or organ. Also, the place or the mode of junction of leaves with the stem, etc.

In-ses-so'rēs.* [From *insi'deo*, *inses'sum*, to "sit upon," to "perch."] "Perchers." A name applied somewhat loosely to various orders or divisions of birds. C. Bonaparte includes under this term the *Pas'seres scanso'res* and *Accip'itres*.

In'sĭ-dens, en'*tis*.* [From *insi'deo*, to "sit upon."] Sitting upon; resting, or floating on, the surface. Applied formerly to matters supernatant on the urine.

In Si'tu* (ablative of *si'tus*, "situation"). In its natural position or situation.

In-so-lā'tion. [**Insola'tio,** o'*nis*; from *inso'lo*, *insola'tum*, to "dry in the sun," to "expose to the sun."] Exposure to the sun to promote the action of one substance upon another; blanching; bleaching. Exposure to the sun as a cause of disease.

Insoluble, or **Insolubility.** See SOLUBILITY.

In-som'nĭ-a.* [From *in*, priv., and *som'nus*, "sleep."] Want of sleep; wakefulness. See AGRYPNIA, PERVIGILIUM.

In-spec'tion. [**Inspec'tio,** o'*nis*; from *inspi'cio*, *inspec'tum*, to "observe," or "examine," to "behold."] Examination by the eye. See EXPLORATIO.

In-spĭ-rā'tion. [**Inspira'tio,** o'*nis*; from *in*, "in," and *spi'ro*, *spira'tum*, to "breathe."] The act of drawing in the breath.

Inspissantia,* in-spis-san'she-a. [From *in*, intensive, and *spis'so*, *spissa'tum*, to "thicken."] Agents which augment the density of the plasma, or colorless portion of the blood.

In'spis-sāt-ed. [**Inspissa'tus**; from the same.] Made thick by evaporation of the thinner parts. Applied to vegetable juices.

In'stinct. [**Instinc'tus**; from *insting'uo*, *instinc'tum*, to "move," or "excite."] That power by which animals are moved, independently of instruction or experience, to perform such acts as are necessary for the preservation of the individual or the race.

In'stru-ment. [**Instrumen'tum**; from *in'struo*, to "provide with," or "furnish."] Any mechanical appliance, tool, or agent used in manipulations or operations.

In-suf-flā'tion. [**Insuffla'tio,** o'*nis*; from *in*, "into," and *suf'flo*, *suffla'tum*, to "blow."] The act of blowing into any cavity, or hollow part, by mechanical means, or otherwise.

In'su-lāt-ed. [**Insula'tus**; from *in'sula*, an "island."] Surrounded by non-conductors. Also, in Entomology, applied to discoid *areolæ* of the wing which are without connection with others. See INSULATION.

In-su-lā'tion. [**Insula'tio,** o'*nis*; from the same.] The state of being insulated, detached, or separated from surrounding bodies (as an island is detached or separated from the main land). Applied in electrical experiments to the state of a body surrounded by non-conductors.

In'te-grant. [**In'tegrans**; from

in'tegro, to "make whole," to "complete" or "perfect;" hence, to constitute an essential part of any thing.] Applied to the atoms of simple bodies. Applied, also, to the smaller particles into which a mineral may be divided without its nature undergoing alteration.

In-teg-rĭ-fo'lĭ-us.* [From *in'teger*, "entire," and *fo'lium*, a "leaf."] Having entire leaves.

In-teg'u-ments. [From *in'tego*, to "cover."] (Fr. *Tégument*, tå'gü'mŏng'.) The cuticle, *rete mucosum*, *cutis*, and adipose tissue, together forming the covering of every part of the body except the nails, therefore termed *common integuments*. The covering of seeds, etc. See TEGUMENT.

Intellect, Diseases affecting the. See PHRENICA.

In-tense'. [**Inten'sus;** from *inten'do*, *inten'sum*, to "stretch," or "put to the utmost stretch," as the string of a harp or bow.] Literally, "kept on the stretch," or "put to the utmost stretch:" thus, we say, "intense application." Hence, the term signifies carried or raised to the highest degree. Applied to heat, cold, pain, etc.

In-ter-ar-tic'u-lar. [**Interarticula'ris;** from *in'ter*, "between," and *artic'ulus*, a "joint."] Situated between the joints.

In-ter-cal'a-rȳ. [**Intercala'ris, Intercala'rius;** from *in'ter*, "between," and *Cal* (from the Sanscrit *Kâlă*, "time"), an ancient root, signifying a "time," or a "portion of time"?] Applied to a day inserted in the calendar every fourth year, called leap-year. Applied also to any time between the paroxysms of periodical diseases.

In-ter-cel'lu-lar. [**Intercellula'ris;** from *in'ter*, "between," and *cel'lula*, a "little cell."] Between the cellules of animal or vegetable tissue.

In-ter-cil'ĭ-um.* [Probably a contraction of *intersupercil'ium*, "between the eyebrows."] The space between the eyebrows; the *glabella*.

In-ter-cla-vic'u-lar. [**Interclavicula'ris;** from *in'ter*, "between," and *clavic'ula*, the "collar-bone."] Between the clavicles.

In-ter-cos'tal. [**Intercosta'lis;** from *in'ter*, "between," and *cos'ta*, a "rib."] Between the ribs.

In-ter-cur'rent. [**Intercur'rens, en'tis;** from *in'ter*, "between," and *cur'ro*, to "run."] Occurring, or running, between. Applied to diseases which occur sporadically during the prevalence of epidemic or endemic diseases.

In-ter'cus, utis.* [From *in'ter*, "between," and *cu'tis*, the "skin."] Between the skin and flesh. Applied to dropsy of the cellular tissue.

In-ter-cu-ta'ne-us.* [From the same.] The same as SUBCUTANEUS.

In-ter-fo-lĭ-ā'ceous. [**Interfolia'ceus;** from *in'ter*, "between," and *fo'lium*, a "leaf."] Applied to flowers growing alternately between each couple of opposing leaves.

In-ter-lob'u-lar. [**Interlobula'ris;** from *in'ter*, "between," and *lob'ulus*, a "little lobe."] Between lobes, or lobules.

In-ter-max'il-la-rȳ. [**Intermaxilla'ris;** from *in'ter*, "between," and *maxil'la*, a "jaw."] Applied to a small osseous piece between the maxillary bones.

In-ter-mis'sion. [**Intermis'sio, o'nis;** from *intermit'to*, to "leave off for a time," to "discontinue."] A temporary cessation. Applied to fevers, etc.

In-ter-mit'tent. [**Intermit'tens, en'tis;** from the same.] Applied to a disease which disappears and returns again and again at regular or uncertain periods.

Intermit'tent Fe'ver. (Lat. **Fe'bris Intermit'tens;** Fr. *Fièvre intermittente*, fe-ĕvR' ăNG'tĕR'mĕt'tŏNT'.) A generic term applied to all fevers in which the paroxysm intermits and returns,—usually at nearly regular intervals. Dr. Good employs *An'etus* (from *ανίημι*, to "send or let back," to "unstring" as a bow; hence, to "relax," to "intermit") as the systematic name of this genus, which includes three principal species, viz.: (1) *Quotid'ian* (*quotidia'nus*), the paroxysms of which return every day; (2) *Ter'tian* (*tertia'nus*), in which the disease returns every third day, that is, on alternate days; (3) *Quar'tan* (*quarta'nus*), in which it returns every fourth day, thus leaving two days between the paroxysms. A more particular notice of these different forms of intermittent will be found under their alphabetical heads. To the above species may be added a fourth, termed *Erratic* (*errat'icus*), in which the fever occurs at irregular intervals.

In'ter-node. [**Interno'dium**, or **Interno'dius;** from *in'ter*, "between," and *no'dus*, a "joint."] Applied to the phalanges of the hand, being between the joints formed by their united extremities. In Botany, the space between two joints, or nodes, of a stem.

In-ter-oc'u-lar. [**Interocula'ris;** from *in'ter*, "between," and *oc'ulus*, the "eye."] Between the eyes.

In-ter-o-per'cu-lar. [**Interopercula'ris.**] Belonging to the *interoperculum*.

In-ter-o-per'cu-lum.* [From *in'ter*, "between," and *oper'culum*, a "lid."] A bony formation which, with the *operculum* and *suboperculum*, between which it lies, composes a sort of lid for the great opening of the gills of fishes.

In-ter-os'se-ous. [**Interos'seus;** from *in'ter*, "between," and *os*, a "bone."] (Fr. *Interosseux*, ăNᵍ'têR'o'suh'.) Situated between bones.

Interosseux. See Interosseous.

In-ter-pa-ri'e-tal. [**Interparieta'lis;** from *in'ter*, "between," and *parieta'lis*, "relating to a wall."] Applied to a cranial bone between the parietal, frontal, and superior occipital bones in the *Mammifera*.

In-ter-pet'i-o-lar. [From *in'ter*, "between," and *peti'olus* or *pet'iolus*, a "petiole."] A term applied to stipules which are between two opposite leaves.

In-ter-pleū-rī-cos-ta'lis.* [From *in'ter*, "between," and *cos'ta*, a "rib."] Applied to the internal intercostal muscles.

In-ter-pos-ĭ-ti'vus.* [From *in'ter*, "between," and *po'no*, *pos'itum*, to "place."] That which is situated between.

In-ter-rup-te-Pin-na'tus.* [From *interrup'tus*, "interrupted," and *pinna'tus*, "pinnate."] Interruptedly-pinnate. Having small pinnate leaflets, intermixed with larger ones.

In-ter-scap'u-lar. [**Interscapula'ris;** from *in'ter*, "between," and *scap'ula*, the "shoulder-blade."] Between the shoulder-blades.

In-ter-sec'tion. [**Intersec'tio, o'nis;** from *in'ter*, "between," or "across"? and *sec'tio*, a "cutting."] A "cutting across," or crossing, of two lines or objects. See Chiasma.

In-ter-spī'nal. [**Interspina'lis;** from *in'ter*, "between," and *spi'na*, a "spine."] Between spines or spinous processes.

In'ter-stice. [**Intersti'tium;** from *in'ter*, "between," and *sto*, to "stand."] The slight separation between organs, or parts of organs; the minute interval which separates the molecules of bodies.

Interstitial, in-ter-stish'al. [**Interstitia'lis;** from the same.] Situated between; pertaining to interstices.

Intersti'tial Absorp'tion, also termed Inter'nal Absorp'tion. The absorption, in cases of abscess, of textures between the cyst and the skin, by which the cyst gradually approaches the surface. Also applied to the process by which the effete materials of the various organs and tissue are removed.

In-ter-trans'verse, or **In-ter-trans-ver'sal.** [**Intertransversa'lis;** from *in'ter*, "between," and *transver'sus*, "across."] Between the transverse processes of the *vertebræ*.

In-ter-tri'go, g'inis.* [From *in'ter*, "between," and *te'ro*, *tri'tum*, to "rub," or "wear."] An excoriation, or galling, of the skin about the *anus*, *axilla*, or other part of the body, with inflammation and moisture.

In-ter-val'var, or **In'ter-valved.** [**Intervalva'ris,** or **Interval'vis;** from *in'ter*, "between," and *val'va*, a "valve."] Between valves.

In-ter-ver'te-bral. [**Intervertebra'lis;** from *in'ter*, "between," and *ver'tebra*.] Between the *vertebræ*.

In-tes'tĭ-nal. [**Intestina'lis;** from *intesti'num*, an "intestine."] (Fr. *Entérique*, ŏNᵍ'tà'rēk'.) Belonging to the intestines.

In-tes'tĭne, or **Intes'tines.** [**Intesti'num,** plural **Intesti'na;** from *in'tus*, "within."] The long membranous tube continuing from the stomach to the anus, in the cavity of the abdomen; th bowels, or entrails.

In-to-nā'tion. [**Intona'tio, o'nis;** from *in'tono*, *intona'tum*, to "thunder."] The same as Borborygmus.

In-tor'tion, or **In-tor'sion.** [**Intor'tio** or **Intor'sio, o'nis;** from *intor'queo*, *intor'tum* or *intor'sum*, to "twist," to "twine."] The phenomenon presented by certain plants twining their flexible stalks around others for support.

In-tox-ĭ-cā'tion. [**Intoxica'tio, o'nis;** from *in*, "into," and *tox'icum*, a "poison."] Literally, the "infusing of poison into" the system. Applied to the effects of alcoholic liquors or narcotic substances used in excess; ebriety. See Temulentia.

In-tra-fo-li-ā'ceous. [**Intrafolia'ceus;** from *in'tra*, "within," and *fo'lium*, a "leaf."] Situated within the leaf, or between the leaf and stem, as certain stipules.

In-tra-mar'gĭ-nal. [**Intramargina'lis;** from *in'tra*, "within," and *mar'go*, a "border."] Situated within the margin.

In-tra-ver'te-brāt-ed. [**Intra-vertebra'tus;** from *in'tra*, "within," and *vertebra'tus*, "vertebrated," or "having vertebræ."] Applied to animals having their osseous system within the body. The same as *vertebrated* in its ordinary acceptation.

In-tri-ca-tu'ra.* [From *intri'co, intrica'tum*, to "entangle."] An entangling or matting of the hair. See PLICA. Also, the same as CHIASMA.

In-tro-flexed'. [From *in'tro*, "inwards," and *flec'to, flex'um*, to "bend."] Bent strongly inwards.

In-tro'ĭ-tus.* [From *in'tro*, "inwards," and *e'o, i'tum*, to "go."] Entrance. Hence the term introitus (or *apertura*) *pelvis* superior is applied to the upper or abdominal strait of the pelvis.

In-trorse'. [**Intror'sus.**] Turned inwards, towards the axis or pistil, as some anthers.

Introsusception. See INTUSSUSCEPTION, and INVAGINATION.

In-tu-mĕs'çence. [**Intumescen'tia;** from *intumes'co*, to "swell."] A swelling; an increase in volume of the tissue of any part or organ. Applied in the plural (*Intumescen'tiæ*) to an order of the class *Cachexiæ* of Cullen's Nosology.

In-tus-sus-çep'tion. [**Intussuscep'tio, o'nis;** from *in'tus*, "within," and *suscip'io, suscep'tum*, to "receive."] The taking of nourishment into the interior as a principal part of the process of nutrition of plants and animals. Also, a condition in which a portion of intestine has passed, for some length, within another portion (as a small tube might slide into a larger one), thereby obstructing the passage of their contents, and causing serious disease; indigitation; invagination.

In'u-la.* [Corruption of *Hele'nium*.] A Linnæan genus of the class *Syngenesiæ*, natural order *Asteraceæ* of Lindley (or *Compositæ* of Jussieu). Also, the Pharmacopœial name (U.S. and Lond. Ph.) for the root of *Inula helenium*.

In'ula He-le'nĭ-um.* The plant elecampane.

In'u-lin, or **In'u-līne.** [**Inuli'na.**] A vegetable product discovered in the *Inula helenium*, or elecampane.

In-unc'tion. [**Inunc'tio, o'nis;** from *in*, "into," "upon," and *un'guo, unc'tum*, to "anoint."] (Fr. *Onction*, ôɴk'se-ôɴᵍ', or *Inonction*, è'nôɴk'se-ôɴᵍ'.) The act of rubbing in ointment, or simply of anointing.

In-un'dāt-ed. [**Inunda'tus;** from *inun'do, inunda'tum*, to "overflow."] Applied to plants which, in certain seasons, live under water.

In-us'tion. [**Inus'tio, o'nis;** from *in*, "in," and *u'ro, us'tum*, to "burn."] A term applied to the burning operation of the cautery.

In-vag-ĭ-nā'tion. [**Invagina'tio, o'nis;** from *invagi'no, invagina'tum*, to "sheathe."] Another term for INTUSSUSCEPTION. Also, an operation for hernia, in which, after reduction, the skin is thrust by the finger of the operator into the canal, so as to form a *cul de sac* open externally, retained by means of sutures, etc., till inflammation and adhesion ensue, with the view of obliterating the canal.

In'va-lid. [**Inval'idus;** from *in*, negative, and *val'idus*, "strong."] Applied to those affected by sickness.

In-vā'sion. [**Inva'sio, o'nis;** from *inva'do, inva'sum*, to "invade," to "seize."] The first development of the phenomena of a disease; access.

In-ver-mĭ-nā'tion. [From *in*, "within," and *ver'mino, vermina'tum*, to "have worms."] The diseased condition caused by the presence of *Entozo'a*, or worms in the intestinal canal.

In-ver'te-brāte. [**Invertebra'tus;** from *in*, negative, and *vertebra'tus*, "vertebrated."] Having no *vertebræ*. Applied to animals in the plural neuter (*Invertebra'ta*), in contradistinction to the *Vertebrata*.

In-vol'u-cel. [**Involucel'lum;** diminutive of *involu'crum*.] A secondary or partial involucre.

In-vo-lu'cral. [**Involucra'lis;** from *involu'crum*, an "involucre."] Belonging to an involucre.

In-vo-lu'crāt-ed. [**Involucra'tus;** from the same.] Having involucres.

In'vo-lu-cre. [**Involu'crum;** from *invol'vo, involu'tum*, to "wrap up."] A membrane covering any part. A set of bracts surrounding a flower-cluster, or a whorl of bracts situated at the base of an umbel or a capitulum. Sometimes it forms a kind of outer calyx to each flower, as in the Mallow.

In-vo-lu'crĭ-form. [**Involucrifor'mis;** from the same.] Resembling an involucre.

In'vo-lūt-ed. [**Involu'tus;** from *in*, "inward," and *vol'vo, volu'tum*, to "roll."] Rolled inwards.

In-vo-lu-tĭ-fo'lĭ-ous. [**Involutifo'lius;** from *involu'tus*, "folded in," and *fo'lium*, a "leaf."] Having leaves folded inward from summit to base.

I'o-dāte. [**I'odas, a'**tis.] A combination of iodic acid with a base.

I'o-dāt-ed. [**Ioda'tus;** from *io'dium*, "iodine."] Containing iodine.

Iode. See IODINIUM.

I-o'dēs.* [From ἰός, "verdigris," "poison."] Full of verdigris.

I-od'ic. [**Iod'icus;** from *io'dium*, "iodine."] Belonging to iodine. Applied to an acid, also termed *oxyodic*.

I-od'ĭ-ca.* [The neuter plural of *iod'icus*: see IODIC.] A class of pharmaceutical remedies, consisting of preparations of iodine.

I'o-dide. [**Iod'idum;** from *io'dium*, "iodine."] A combination of iodine with a simple body.

Iodina. See IODINIUM.

Iodine. See IODINIUM.

I-o-din'ĭ-um;* also written **I-o'-dĭ-um,* I-od'ĭ-na,*** and **I-od'ĭ-num.*** [From ἰώδης, "violet-colored."] (Fr. *Iode*, ē'od'.) Iodine. The Pharmacopœial name of a simple body obtained from certain sea-weeds, and from sponge. Iodine operates as a general excitant of the vital actions, especially of the absorbent and glandular systems. It is much employed as a remedy in scrofula, in nearly all the forms of this disease. In over-doses, it is an irritant poison. A serious objection to its extensive employment as a medicine, arises from its operating very unequally on different persons. A dose which would act very moderately in a large majority of cases, will sometimes produce, in certain constitutions, the most distressing symptoms, such as extreme restlessness, nausea, palpitations, vomiting and purging, violent cramps, etc., attended with permanently injurious effects on the system. The physician should, therefore, unless he is thoroughly acquainted with the idiosyncrasy of his patient, commence the use of this remedy with great caution; after observing its effects, he may gradually increase the dose, if it should seem advisable to do so.

I'o-dism. [**Iodis'mus;** from *io'dium*, "iodine."] That derangement of the system produced by the continued administration of iodine.

Iodium. See IODINIUM.

I-od'o-form. [From *io'dium*, "iodine," and *for'myle*.] A body analogous to formic acid when the oxygen is replaced by iodine.

I-o-dog-no'sis.* [From *io'dium*, "iodine," and γινώσκω, to "know."] A knowledge of the properties of iodine.

I-o-dom'e-the.* [From *io'dium*, "iodine," and μέθη, "drunkenness."] The nervous state induced by too free use of iodine. See IODISM.

I-o-doph'thĭ-sis.* [From *io'dium*, "iodine," and *phthis'is*, a "wasting."] *Tabes*, or wasting, caused by the abuse, or excessive use, of iodine. See IODISM.

I'o-dous. [**Iodo'sus;** from *io'dium*, "iodine."] Belonging to iodine. Applied to an acid.

I-od'u-ret. [**Iodure'tum;** from *iodin'ium*, "iodine."] A combination of iodine with a simple body.

I-on'thus.* [From ἴονθος, "down."] The down, or soft hair, which precedes the beard. Also, a pimple on the face, resembling, or identical with, *Acne*.

I-op'ter-us.* [From ἴον, a "violet," and πτερόν, a "wing."] Having wings of a violet color: iop'terous.

Ip-e-cac-u-an'ha.* (This word is used in South America to signify *vomiting root*.) A name given to several and very different species of plants. The Pharmacopœial name ‖ of the root of *Cephaëlis Ipecacuanha*, otherwise called the *Ipecacuanhæ Radix* ("Root of Ipecacuanha"). Ipecacuanha, in small doses, is a diaphoretic and expectorant, in large doses it is an emetic. A moderate dose sometimes acts on the bowels.

I-po-mæ'a.* [From ἴψ, a "worm," and ὅμοιος, "like."] A Linnæan genus of the class *Pentandria*, natural order *Convolvulaceæ*.

Ipomæ'a Ja-la'pa,* **Ipomæ'a Pur'ga.*** Names for the jalap-plant.

I-ral'gĭ-a.* [From *i'ris*, and ἄλγος, "pain."] Pain of the iris: iral'gy.

Ir-ĭ-an-kis'trĭ-um,* Ir-ĭ-an-kis'-tron.* [From *i'ris*, and ἄγκιστρον, a "fish-hook."] An instrument, hook-shaped, used in the operation for artificial pupil by separation.

Iridaceæ,* ir-e-da'she-ē, or **Ir'ĭ-dēs.*** A natural order of endogenous herbaceous plants, including the *Iris*, *Crocus*, and *Gladiolus*, which are prized for their beauty. Saffron is procured from the *Crocus Sativa*.

Ir-ĭ-dæ'mĭ-a.* [From *i'ris*, *ir'idis*, the "iris," and αἷμα, "blood."] Hæmorrhage from the iris.

Iridalgia. See IRALGIA.

Ir-ĭ-da'tio, o'*nis*.* [From *i'ris*, *ir'idis*, the "rainbow."] The property of producing the appearance of the colors of the rainbow: irida'tion.

Ir-i-daux-e'sis.* [From *i'ris*, and αὔξησις, "increase."] Thickening or growth of the iris, from exudation into its substance.

Ir-i-dec'to-mus.* [From *i'ris*, and ἐκτέμνω, to "cut out."] An instrument or kind of knife used for the operation of iridectomy: an iridec'tome.

Ir-i-dec'to-mȳ. [**Iridecto'mia;** from the same.] The operation of removing or cutting out a portion of the iris. See Corectomia.

Ir-i-dec-tro'pi-um.* [From *i'ris*, and *ectro'pium*, "eversion."] Eversion of a portion of the iris: iridec'tropy.

Ir-i-den-tro'pi-um.* [From *i'ris*, and *entro'pium*, "inversion."] Inversion of a portion of the iris.

Ir-i-de-re'mi-a.* [From *i'ris*, and ἐρημία, "destitution," "deficiency."] Defect, or imperfect condition, of the iris.

Irides,* ĭr'e-dēz, the plural of **I'ris,** forming the Jussieuan name of a natural order of plants. See Iridaceæ.

Ir-i-dĕs'çent. [From *i'ris*, the "rainbow."] Applied to minerals exhibiting the colors of the rainbow.

I-rid'i-um.* [From *i'ris*, the "rainbow."] A metal named in allusion to the variety of colors exhibited by its solutions. It is extremely hard, and the most infusible of all known metals. Specific gravity, about 18.6. It was discovered in 1803, associated with the ore of platinum.

Ir'i-do-çēle.* [From *i'ris*, and κήλη, a "tumor."] Hernia, in which a portion of the iris is protruded.

Ir'i-do-çi-ne'sis.* [From *i'ris*, and κίνησις, "motion."] The movement of the iris, its contraction and expansion.

Ir'i-do-di-al'ȳ-sis.* [From *i'ris*, and διάλυσις, a "separation."] The operation for artificial pupil by separation. See Coredialysis.

Ir'i-do-do-ne'sis.* [From *i'ris*, and δόνησις, an "agitation."] Trembling or agitation of the iris.

Iridomalacia,* ĭr'e-do-ma-la'she-a. [From *i'ris*, and μαλακία, "softness."] Softening of the iris.

Ir-i-don'cus.* [From *i'ris*, and ὄγκος, a "tumor."] Tumor or swelling of the iris; a tumid iris.

I-rid-o-pla'ni-a.* [From *i'ris*, and πλανάω, to "wander."] The same as Iridodonesis, which see.

Ir-i-dot'o-mȳ. [**Iridoto'mia;** from *i'ris*, and τέμνω, to "cut."] The operation for artificial pupil by incision. See Corectomia.

Ir-i-dot'ro-mus.* [From *i'ris*, and τρόμος, a "trembling."] The same as Iridodonesis, which see.

I'ris,* gen. **Ir'i-dis.** Originally, a "rainbow." A delicate circular membrane of the eye, floating in the aqueous humor, suspended vertically behind the *cornea*, and perforated to form the pupil. It received its name from the variety of its colors. Also, the name of a plant.

I'ris Flor-en-ti'na.* ("Florentine Orris.") The Pharmacopœial name (U.S. Ph.) for the rhizoma of the *Iris Florentina*.

I'ris Ver-sic'o-lor.* Blue Flag. The Pharmacopœial name (U.S. Ph.) for the rhizoma of the *Iris versicolor*.

Ir-i-sā'tion. [**Irisa'tio, o'nis;** from *i'ris*, the "rainbow."] The effect of decomposition of light by the prism, and observed in many bodies, shells, and insects, caused by the particular arrangement of the molecules on their surface, by fissures, etc.

I'rish Moss. The *Chondrus crispus*.

I-rit'i-cus.* Belonging to *iritis*: irit'ic.

I-ri'tis.* Inflammation of the iris.

I'ron. [Lat. **Fer'rum;** Gr. σίδηρος; Fr. *Fer*, fêr; Ger. *Eisen*, ī'zen.] The strongest, most common, and most useful of the metals. Some of its compounds afford medicines of great value. Combined with a small quantity of carbon, thus forming steel, it possesses great hardness. Iron has the rare property of capability of being welded. Specific gravity, about 7.7.

Iron Filings. See Ferri Ramenta.

Iron Wire. See Ferri Filum.

Ir-rā-di-ā'tion. [**Irradia'tio, o'nis;** from *irra'dio, irradia'tum*, to "shine upon."] The phenomenon of the apparent enlargement of a body strongly illuminated, as a fixed star, the image of which is never a point, but a disk having a sensible diameter.

Ir-re-du'ci-ble. [From *in*, negative, and *redu'co, reduc'tum*, to "reduce."] (Fr. *Irréductible*, è'rà'dük'tèbl'.) A term applied to fractures, luxations, hernia, etc., when they cannot be reduced.

Irréductible. See Irreducible.

Ir-ri-gā'tion. [From *ir'rigo, irriga'tum*, to "water."] The continual application of a lotion, by dropping water on an affected part.

Ir-ri-ta-bil'i-tȳ. [**Irritabil'itas, a'tis;** from *irri'to, irrita'tum*, to "provoke," to "excite."] A property peculiar to muscular substance, by which it contracts on the application of a stimulus.

Ir-ri-tā'tion. [From the same.] The excessive action of any stimulus, causing a morbid increase in the circulation or sensibility.

Ir'rĭ-tā-tive Fe'ver. That violent derangement of the system excited by great irritation, as from wounds, ulcers, etc.

Is-a-del'phus.* [From ἴσος, "equal," and ἀδελφός, a "brother."] Having diadelphous stamens forming two equal packets: isadel'phous.

Is-an-the'rus.* [From ἴσος, "equal," and *anthe'ra*, an "anther."] Having anthers equal or alike: isanthe'rous.

I-san'thus.* [From ἴσος, "equal," and ἄνθος, a "flower."] Having the teguments of all their flowers alike: isan'thous.

I-sa'tis Tinc-to'rĭ-a.* Woad. A plant from which an inferior kind of indigo is procured.

Is-chĭ-ad'ic. The same as ISCHIATIC, which see.

Ischiadocele. See ISCHIOCELE.

Is-chi'a-gra.* [From ἰσχίον, the "haunch," and ἄγρα, a "seizure."] Gout in the haunch. Also, *Sciatica.*

Is-chĭ-ăl'gĭ-a.* [From ἰσχίον, the "hip," and ἄλγος, "pain."] Is'chialgy. Pain in the *ischium.*

Is'chĭ-as, adis.* [From ἰσχίον, the "hip."] Gout, or a rheumatic affection, of the hip-joint.

Is-chĭ-at'ic. [**Ischiat'icus.**] Belonging to the *ischium.*

Is-chĭ-a-ti'tis.* Inflammation of the ischiatic nerve.

Ischiatocele. See ISCHIOCELE.

Is-chĭ-dro'sis.* [From ἴσχω, to "suppress," and ἱδρώς, "sweat."] Deficiency, or suppression, of sweat, or of transpiration.

Is-chĭ-drot'ĭ-cus.* Belonging to *ischidrosis.*

Is'chĭ-o-. [From ἰσχίον, the "hip."] A prefix denoting connection with the *ischium*, or with the hip-joint.

Is'chĭ-o-çēle.* [From ἰσχίον, the "hip," and κήλη, a "tumor."] Hernia at the ischiadic foramen.

Ischion. See ISCHIUM.

Is'chĭ-o-neū-răl'gĭ-a.* [From *is'chium*, the "hip," and *neural'gia*, "pain of a nerve."] Ischiatic neuralgy; *sciatica.*

Is-chĭ-oph'thĭ-sis.* [From *is'chium*, the "hip," and φθίσις, a "wasting."] Literally, "consumption, or wasting, of the hip-joint." Hip-joint disease. See COXARUM MORBUS.

Is'chĭ-um.* [From ἴσχις, the "loin."] (Fr. *Os de l'assiette*, ō d'lå'se'ētt'.) The posterior and inferior bone of the pelvis, distinct and separate in the fœtus or infant; or the corresponding part of the *Os innomina'tum* in the adult.

Is-chu'rĭ-a.* [From ἴσχω, to "suppress," and οὖρον, "urine."] Retention or stoppage of the urine. A genus of the order *Epischeses*, class *Locales*, of Cullen's Nosology.

Is-chu-rĭ-oph-thăl'mĭ-a.* [From *ischu'ria*, and *ophthal'mia*, "inflammation of the eyes."] Ophthalmy from suppression of the urine.

I'ṡin-glass. [Probably a corruption of *Hausenblase*, how'zẹn-blå'zẹh, or how'zẹn-blås; from *hause*, a "sturgeon," and *blase*, a "bladder."] Fish-glue, prepared chiefly from the air-bladder of the sturgeon. See ICHTHYOCOLLA.

I-soch'ro-nous, or **I-soch'ro-nal.** [**Isoch'ronus**; from ἴσος, "equal," and χρόνος, "time."] Enduring an equal space of time, or performed in equal times, as the vibrations of a pendulum

I-soch'ro-us.* [From ἴσος, "equal," and χρόα, "color of the skin."] Of uniform color: isoch'röous.

Is-o-cli'nal, Is-o-clin'ĭ-cal. [**Isoclin'icus**; from ἴσος, "equal," and κλίνω, to "incline."] Of equal inclination.

I-sod'ro-mus.* [From ἴσος, "equal," and δρόμος, a "course."] Similar to ISOCHRONUS, which see.

Is-o-dȳ-nam'ic. [**Isodyn'amus**; from ἴσος, "equal," and δύναμις, "power."] Having equal powers: isodyn'amous.

Is-o-gon'ic. [**Isogon'icus**; from ἴσος, "equal," and γωνία, an "angle."] Having equal angles.

Is'o-lāt-ed. [From the Italian *isola*, ē'so-lå, an "island."] The same as INSULATED, which see.

Is-o-mĕr'ic. [From ἴσος, and μέρος, a "part."] Composed of the same elements in the same proportions, but chemically and physically different.

I-som'er-iṡm. [**Isomeris'mus**; from the same.] The state of compounds that are isomeric. Identity in respect to the quality and quantity of the constituents, with essential difference of chemical properties.

Isomerus. See ISOMERIC.

Is-o-mor'phiṡm. [**Isomorphis'mus.**] The state or arrangement of bodies that are isomorphous.

Is-o-mor'phous. [**Isomor'phus**;

from ἴσος, "equal," and μορφή, "form."] Of the same form. Applied to substances which resemble each other in their crystalline forms, but differ in their component parts.

Is-o-path′ĭ-cus.* Belonging to Isopathy: isopath′ic.

I-sop′a-thy̆. [**Isopathi′a;** from ἴσος, "equal," "exactly like," or "the same," and πάθος, an "affection," or "disease."] A branch of Homœopathy which recommends the administration of virus as a remedy, in the same disease by which it is produced. Thus, it is said that small-pox may be cured by minute doses of variolous matter, etc. The difference between Isopathy and Homœopathy, as the latter is commonly understood, is indicated by the etymology of the terms. The one (Homœopathy) aims to cure disease by inducing a condition of the system *similar* to that produced by the disease. The other (Isopathy) would combat disease by employing *the same* (that is, the disease itself) as a weapon.

Is-o-pet′a-lous. [**Isopet′alus;** from ἴσος, "equal," and πέταλον, a "petal."] Having equal petals.

I-sop′o-dous. [**Isop′odus;** from ἴσος, "equal," and πούς, a "foot."] Equal-footed.

I-sos′çe-lēs.* [From ἴσος, "equal," and σκέλος, a "leg."] Having equal legs, or sides.

Is-o-ste′mo-nous. [**Isoste′monis;** from ἴσος, "equal," and στήμων, a "stamen."] Having stamens equal to the number of petals.

Is-o-ther′mal, or **Is-o-ther′mous.** [**Isother′mus;** from ἴσος, "equal," and θέρμη, "heat."] Of the same degree of heat; of the same temperature. In Physical Geography, *isothermal lines* are those passing on the surface of the earth through those points at which the mean annual temperature is the same. *Isothermal zones* are spaces on opposite sides of the equator, having the same mean temperature, and bounded by corresponding isothermal lines.

Is′sue. [Lat. **Fontic′ulus;** Fr. *Fonticule*, fôɴᵍ′tè′kül′.] A small ulcer or sore produced by art, and kept open by inserting a pea or other small body, with a view to relieve irritation or morbid action in a neighboring part. See REVULSION.

Isth′mĭ-cus.* [From *isth′mus*, a "neck," or "narrow passage."] Belonging to the *isthmus faucium*, or to a neck of land.

Isth-mi′tis, idis.* [From *isth′mus fau′cium.*] Inflammation of the *isthmus faucium.*

Isthmodes. See ISTHMOIDES.

Isth-mo-dy̆n′ĭ-a.* [From *isth′mus* fau′cium, and ὀδύνη, "pain."] Pain in the fauces.

Isth-mo-i′dēs.* [From *isth′mus* fau′cium, and εἶδος, a "form."] Resembling the *isthmus faucium:* isth′moid.

Isth-mo-pa-thi′a.* [From *isth′mus* fau′cium, and πάθος, "disease."] Disease of the fauces.

Isth-mo-ple′gĭ-a.* [From *isth′mus* fau′cium, and πληγή, a "stroke."] Paralysis of the *isthmus faucium.*

Isth-mop′y̆-ra.* [From *isth′mus* fau′cium, and πῦρ, "fire."] Inflammation of the fauces.

Isth′mus.* [Gr. ἰσθμός, a "neck."] A term denoting a neck, or narrow passage; as, *isthmus faucium*, literally, "the narrow passage of the fauces."

Itch. See SCABIES, PSORA, and PSORIASIS.

-Ite. A terminal denoting a salt from a combination of an acid, the name of which ends in *-ous*.

I′ter.* A passage of communication between two or more parts.

I′TER AD INFUNDIB′ULUM.* ("Passage to the Infundibulum.") The passage of communication between the third ventricle of the brain and the infundibulum. It is also termed *fora′men commu′ne ante′rius.*

I′TER A PALA′TO AD AU′REM.* ("Passage from the Palate to the Ear.") The Eustachian tube.

I′TER A TER′TIO AD QUAR′TUM VENTRIC′ULUM.* ("Passage from the Third to the Fourth Ventricle.") See AQUEDUCT OF SYLVIUS.

Ith-y̆-phy̆l′lus.* [From ἰθύς, "straight," and φύλλον, a "leaf."] Having straight leaves.

-Itis. A terminal, denoting inflammation of any organ or part indicated by the word to which it is added. Thus, *gastri′tis* [from γαστήρ, the "stomach"] signifies "inflammation of the stomach:" *spleni′tis* [from σπλήν, the "spleen"], inflammation of the spleen, etc.

Iulaceous. See JULACEOUS.

Ivoire. See IVORY.

I′vo-ry̆. (Fr. *Ivoire*, è′vwȧʀ′.) The bone-like matter of the tusks of the elephant and some other animals.

Ivory Black. See CARBON, ANIMAL.

Ivresse. See TEMULENTIA.

Ivy. See HEDERA.

J.

Jacobi Membrana. See MEMBRANA JACOBI.

Jac-tĭ-tā'tion. [**Jactita'tio, o**'*nis;* from *jac'tito, jactita'tum,* to "toss often."] The constant tossing from one position to another, the effect of restlessness in acute diseases.

Jaf'na Moss. A species of moss found in Ceylon, yielding a semi-opaque jelly, nutritious for invalids; also called Ceylon moss.

Ja-la'pa.* [From *Jala'pa,* or *Xala'pa,* its native place.] Jalap. The Pharmacopœial name ‖ of the root of *Exogonium purga,* otherwise called the *Ipomæ'a Jala'pa.* Jalap is an active cathartic, producing copious watery discharges. It is usually given in connection with other medicines which assist or qualify its operation. Combined with the bitartrate of potash, it is much employed as a remedy in dropsy, in the hip-disease, and in other scrofulous affections of the joints.

Jala'pa Al'ba.* ("White Jalap.") A name for the *Convolvulus mechoacana,* or mechoacan.

Jal'a-pin, or **Jal'a-pine.** [**Jalapi'na.**] The active principle of jalap.

Jamaica Bark. See BARK, CARIBEAN.

Ja-mai'ca Pep'per. Dried berries of *Myrtus pimenta.*

Jamaica Spirit. [**Spir'itus Jamaicen'sis.**] A name for rum.

James's Pow'der. [**Pul'vis Jaco'bi;** from *Dr. James,* its inventor.] A febrifuge preparation for which the *Pulvis antimonialis* is substituted.

Jan'ĭ-pha Man'ĭ-hot,* or **Jat'ropha Man'ihot.*** A plant from which tapioca and Cassava bread are obtained.

Ja-pan' Earth. The substance termed *catechu.*

Jarret, zhâ'râ'. The French term for POPLES, which see.

Jasmin. See JASMINUM.

Jasminaceæ,* jas-mĭ-na'she-ē. A natural order of exogenous shrubs, growing abundantly in tropical India. It includes the Jasmine (*Jas'minum*), which yields a fragrant oil.

Jas-min'e-æ.* The Jussieuan name of a natural order of plants. See JASMINACEÆ.

Jas'mĭ-num Of-fiç-ĭ-na'le.* (Fr. *Jasmin,* zhâs'mănᵍ'.) A plant of the Linnæan class *Diandria,* natural order *Jasminaceæ.* The flowers yield an essential oil used as an external application in paralysis and rheumatism.

Jas'per. [**Jas'pis.**] A silicious mineral, prized for its variegated colors. It is used in jewelry.

Jat'ro-pha.* A Linnæan genus of the class *Monœcia,* natural order *Euphorbiaceæ.*

Jat'ropha Cur'cas.* A plant which grows in South America, the West Indies, and Western Africa. The oil obtained from the seeds is similar in its medicinal properties to croton oil, but is less powerful.

Jatropha Manihot. See JANIPHA MANIHOT.

Jat'ro-phāte. [**Jat'rophas, a**'*tis.*] A combination of jatrophic acid with a base.

Jaun'dice. [From the French *jaunisse,* zhō'nĕss', "yellowness," or the "yellows;" so named from its color.] See ICTERUS.

Jaunisse, zhō'nĕss'. A French term for "jaundice." See ICTERUS.

Jaw. See MAXILLA.

Jecur. See LIVER.

Je-ju'num.* [From *jeju'nus,* "fasting," "jejune," "empty."] The second portion of the small intestine; so named because it is usually found empty, or nearly so, in the dead body.

Jel'ly̆. The common name for gelatine.

Je-ru'sa-lem Ar'tĭ-choke. The *Helianthus Tuberosus,* a species of sunflower, the root of which resembles the artichoke in taste. The term *Jerusalem* as applied to artichoke is a curious corruption of the Italian term *gira-sole* (jee'râ so'lâ), that is, *turn-sun* in English and *heliotrope* (ἡλιοτρόπιον) in Greek.—(HOBLYN.)

Jes'u-it's Bark. A name for *Cinchona,* because introduced into Europe by a Jesuit.

Jet. A black, bituminous substance, used for ornaments, vessels, etc.

Jeunesse, zhuh'nĕss'. The French term for "youth," or ADOLESCENCE, which see.

Joint. See ARTICULUS.

Joint, Contraction of, Joint, Stiffened. See ANKYLOSIS.

Joue, zhoo. The French word for "cheek." See GENA.

Ju'gạ,* the plural of JUGUM, which see.

Jugale Os. See OS MALÆ.

Ju-ga'lēs,* plural of **Juga'lis.** A name of the superficial temporal, or zygomatic, nerves, given off from the facial.

Ju-ga'lis.* Belonging to the *Os jugale*, or cheek-bone.

Juglandaceæ,* jug-lan-da'she-ē. A small natural order of exogenous trees, natives of the temperate parts of North America and Asia. It includes the Walnut (*Juglans*), and Hickory (*Carya*). A valuable oil is obtained from some species of *Juglans.* The bark is purgative.

Jug'lans.* Butternut. The Pharmacopœial name (U.S. Ph.) for the inner bark of the root of *Juglans cinerea.* It is a mild cathartic, resembling rhubarb in its operation.

Ju'gu-lạr. [**Jugula'ris;** from *ju'gulum*, the "throat."] Belonging to the throat.

Ju'gular Veins. The large veins which run from the head down the sides of the neck, and are termed, according to their situation, *internal* or *external.*

Ju'gu-lum.* [From *ju'gum*, a "yoke."] The throat, or fore-part of the neck.

Ju'gum,* plural **Ju'gạ.** A Latin word, signifying originally a "yoke;" also, a "ridge," or "hill." Applied in Botany to the ridges, or ribs, on the fruit of umbelliferous plants.

Ju'jube. [**Juju'ba.**] The fruit of the *Rham'nus Ziz'yphus*, a native of the south of Europe, from which a pectoral lozenge is prepared.

Jul. = *Jule'pus.** "A julep."

Ju-lā'ceous. [From *ju'lus*, a "catkin."] Resembling a catkin.

Ju'lep. [Lat. **Jula'pium,** or **Jule'pus;** Arab. *Juleb*, a "sweet potion."] A liquid medicine of an agreeable taste.

Ju'lus.* A Latin term signifying "catkin."

Ju-men-to'sus.* [From *jumen'tum*, a "beast of burden."] Applied to the urine, when of a strong rank odor.

Juncaceæ,* jun-ka'she-ē. A natural order of endogenous glumaceous plants, found chiefly in the colder parts of the world. It includes the common Rush (*Juncus*).

Jun-cā'ceous. [**Junca'ceus;** from *jun'cus*, a "rush."] Resembling the *Juncus*, or rush.

Juncaginaceæ,* jun-kaj-e-na'she-ē. [From *Junca'go*, one of the genera.] A natural order of endogenous aquatic plants, found in most parts of the world.

Jun'ce-us.* The same as JUNCACEOUS.

Jun'ci,* the plural of *Juncus*, a "rush," forming the Jussieuan name of a natural order of plants. See JUNCACEÆ.

Jun-ci-for'mis.* [From *jun'cus*, a "rush."] Formed like a rush.

Jungermanniaceæ,* jung-ẹr-man-ne-a'she-ē. [From *Jungerman'nia*, one of the genera.] A natural order of cryptogamic moss-like plants, found in damp, shady places.

Ju'ni-per. The *Juniperus communis.*

Ju-nip'e-ri Ca-cu'mĭ-nạ.* ("Tops of Juniper.") The Pharmacopœial name (Ed. Ph.) for the tops of the *Juniperus communis.*

Ju-nip'e-rus.* A Linnæan genus of the class *Diœcia*, natural order *Coniferæ.* The Pharmacopœial name (U.S. and Lond. Ph.) for the fruit of *Juniperus communis.*

Junip'erus Com-mu'nis.* (Fr. *Genévrier*, zhẹh-nå'vRE-å'.) The juniper-tree.

Junip'erus Sa-bi'nạ.* (Fr. *Sabine*, så'bėn'.) The common savin-tree.

Junip'erus Vir-ġin-ĭ-a'nạ.* Red Cedar. The Pharmacopœial name (U.S. Ph.) for the tops of the *Juniperus Virginiana.*

Ju'pi-ter.* An ancient name for tin.

Ju-ras'sic. [**Juras'sicus;** from *Ju'ra.*] A term applied to a particular group of öolitic rocks found in Mount Jura, and to the corresponding strata of other regions.

Jurisprudence, Medical. See MEDICAL JURISPRUDENCE.

Jus,* gen. **Ju'ris.** Broth or soup.

Jusquiame, zhüs'ke-åm'. The French term for HYOSCYAMUS, which see.

Jussieuan, jŭs-sū'ạn. Belonging to Jussieu: applied to a system of arranging plants according to their resemblance to each other; or what is termed the Natural Method.

Juvantia,*ju-van'she-ạ. [Plural neuter of *ju'vans*, present participle of *ju'vo*, to "help."] Helping, or aiding; applied to medicines or applications which assuage pain, nervous distress, etc.

Ju-ven'tus,* gen. **Ju-ven-tu'tis.** [From *ju'venis*, "young;" Fr. *Jeunesse*, zhuh'nĕss'.] Youth. (See ADOLESCENCE.) Applied by some writers to the third stage of life, between about the twenty-fifth and thirty-fifth years.

K.

Kajeput. See CAJUPUTI OLEUM.

Ka'li.* [From the Arabic.] The vegetable alkali; potash.

Ka'li Pu'rum.* ("Pure Potash.") The *Potassa fusa.*

Ka-liġ'e-nous. [**Kaliġ'enus;** from *ka'li,* an "alkali," "potash," and γεννάω, to "generate."] Applied to metals which form alkalies with oxygen.

Ka'lĭ-um.* [From *ka'li,* "potash."] A synonymous term for potassium, the base of potash.

Kā'o-lin,* or **Kā'o-līne.** (Chinese, *Kao-ling,* kå'o-ling'.) China clay; a fine, pure clay, procured by levigation from the felspar of mouldering granite, and employed in the manufacture of porcelain.

Kas'su'. A black astringent extract prepared from the seeds of the *Areca catechu.*

Keel. See CARINA.

Kéloïde, kà'lo'ėd'. [From κήλη, a "tumor," and εἶδος, a "form."] The French name for a disease resembling Cancer, or Scirrhus, also termed *Cancroide,* and *Scirrhoide.*

Kelotomia. See CELOTOMY.

Kelp. The crude soda obtained from the ashes of sea-weed in Holland, and on the northern coast of France. It is used in the manufacture of glass and of soap.

Kĕr-a-ti'a-sis.* [From κέρας, a "horn."] A horn-like excrescence on the temple or forehead.

Kĕr-a-to-de-i'tis.* [From κερατώδης, the "cornea."] The same as CORNEITIS.

Kĕr'a-tome. [**Kerato'ma,** *atis;* from κέρας, a "horn."] A horn-like tumor, or swelling.

Ke-rat'o-nȳx'is,* or **Ce-rat'o-nȳx'is.*** [From κέρας, a "horn," or the "cornea," and νύσσω, to "puncture."] An operation by which the crystalline is depressed by a needle passed through the cornea.

Ke-rat'o-plas'tic. [**Keratoplas'ticus.**] Belonging to keratoplasty.

Ker-at'o-plas'tȳ. [**Keratoplas'tia;** from κέρας, a "horn," or the "cornea," and πλάσσω, to "form."] An operation by which the *cornea* of an animal has been excised and reapplied, or a new one from another animal put in its place. Also written *Ceratoplasty,* or *Ceratoplastica.*

Keratotome. See CERATOTOME.

Ke-rec'to-mȳ. [**Kerecto'mia;** from κέρας, a "horn," or the "cornea," and ἐκτέμνω, to "cut off."] The operation of excising the outward layers of the cornea, by which a clear aperture in the middle of a generally opaque *cornea* may be obtained.

Ker'mēs An'ĭ-mal, or **Ker'mes Ber'rȳ.** [**Coc'cus Il'icis.**] A name applied to insects found upon the *Quercus coccifera,* which grows in Southern Europe and in the Levant. They are in the form of round, reddish grains, about the size of peas, found adhering to the branches. They were formerly used for dyeing scarlet. Kermes is a Latin form of a word found in several Asiatic languages, and signifying a little worm or insect.

Ker'mes Min'e-ral. The precipitated sulphuret of antimony, named from its resemblance in color to the kermes insect.

Kibe. See CHILBLAIN.

Kid'ney. [**Ren, Re'nis.**] The kidneys are two glandular bodies situated in the lumbar region, consisting of an external or cortical, and an internal or tubular, substance. Their office is to secrete the urine, and thus to carry off the superfluous fluid matter from the system.

Kid'ney-Shaped'. [**Renifor'mis.**] A term applied to a roundish or broadly cordate leaf, concave at the base.

Kiestein, or **Kiestin.** See KYESTEIN.

Kil'o-gram, or **Kil'o-gramme.** [From χίλιοι, a "thousand," and *gramme.*] A French weight of a thousand grammes, equal to 2.68 (or about $2\frac{2}{3}$) lbs. troy, or $2\frac{1}{5}$ lbs. avoirdupois.

Kilolitre, kė'lo-lėtr', or kil'o-lė't'r. [From χίλιοι, a "thousand," and *litre.*] A French measure of a thousand litres, equal to 35.3171 English cubic feet.

Kilometre, kil'o'mē'ter (French pron. kė'lo'mêtr'). [From χίλιοι, a "thousand," and *mètre.*] A French measure of a thousand metres, or 4 furlongs, 213 yards, 1 foot, and 10.2 inches.

Ki'na-Ki'na.* A name for *Cinchona.*

Ki'nāte. [**Ki'nas,** *a'tis.*] A combination of kinic acid with a base.

Kin-e-sip'a-thȳ. [**Kinesipathi'a;** from κινέω, to "move," and πάθος, an "affection," or "disease."] A system of athletic exercises and feats of muscular strength, adopted as a means of curing disease.

King's E'vil. A name given to *scrofula*, from the belief that it might be cured by the touch of royalty.

Kī'nic, or kin'ik. [**Kin'icus.**] (Called, also, **Cinchon'ic** and **Quin'ic.**) Applied to an acid obtained from *Cinchona*.

Kinkina. See KINA-KINA.

Kī'no.* The Pharmacopœial name ‖ for the inspissated juice of the *Pterocar'pus marsu'pium* (or of the *Pterocar'pus erina'ceus*, according to the Edinburgh Pharmacopœia for 1830).

Kirsch Wasser, kēērsh vås'sẹr. ("Cherry Water.") The German name of a liquor distilled from cherries, stones and all. It is sometimes called "the brandy of Switzerland."

Klep-to-ma'nĭ-ạ.* [From κλέπτω, to "steal," and μανία, "madness."] A supposed species of moral insanity, actuating the subjects of it to pilfer and steal.

Knee. See GENU.

Knee-Jointed. See GENICULATE.

Knee-Pan. The *patella*.

Knit'ted. [**Connex'us.**] That stage in the union of fractured bones in which a certain degree of firmness is attained.

Knock-Knees. See GENUA VALGA.

Knotted. See ARTICULATUS.

Korectomia. See CORECTOMIA.

Kousso,* **Koosso,*** or **Cusso,*** koos'so. The flowers of the *Braye'ra anthelmin'tica*, long used in Abyssinia, and more recently in Europe, as a remedy against *Tænia*, or tapeworm.

Kra-me'rĭ-ạ.* Rhatany. The Pharmacopœial name ‖ for the root of the *Krameria triandra*.

Krame'ria Tri-an'drạ.* The systematic name of a plant used as an astringent, diuretic, and detergent. It belongs to the natural order *Polygalaceæ*.

Kreasote. See CREASOTE.

Kreatin. See CREATIN.

Kreatinin. See CREATININ.

Kȳ-ĕs'te-in, or **Kȳ-ĕs'te-ïne** (frequently pronounced kī'ĕs-tīn), written also **Cyestein** and **Kiestein.** [From κύω or κυέω, to "be pregnant," and ἐσθής, a "garment," or "covering," and, hence, used for "pellicle."] An albuminoid substance discovered floating as a pellicle on the urine of pregnant women; not confined, however, to utero-gestation, but connected with the lacteal secretion. Taken in connection with other symptoms, it is considered a valuable aid in the diagnosis of pregnancy.

Kystotome. See CYSTOTOME.

L.

Labdanum, or **Ladanum.** See CISTUS CRETICUS.

La-bel'lum.* [Diminutive of *la'bium*, a "lip."] The lip or lower petal of ringent, personate, or orchideous flowers.

La'bĭ-ạ,* gen. **La-bĭ-o'rum.** The plural of LABIUM, which see.

La'bia Pu-den'di.* The thick orifice of the vulva, or parts external to the *nymphæ*.

Lā'bĭ-ạl. [**Labia'lis.**] Belonging to the *labium*.

Labialis (Muscle). See ORBICULARIS ORIS.

La-bĭ-a'tæ,* or **Lamiaceæ,*** la-me-a'she-ē. A natural order of exogenous plants, mostly herbaceous, which abound in temperate regions. It includes Peppermint (*Mentha*), Lavender (*Lavandula*), and Sage (*Salvia*). Their aromatic qualities render many species valuable as carminative medicines.

Lā'bĭ-ate. [**Labia'tus;** from *la'bium*, a "lip."] Having two lips, as the snapdragon flower.

La-bĭ-at-ĭ-flo'rus.* [From *la'bium*, a "lip," and *flos*, a "flower."] Having labiate flowers.

Lab-ĭ-dom'e-ter. [**Labidom'etrum;** from λαβίς, a "forceps," and μέτρον, a "measure."] An instrument for ascertaining the dimensions of the child's head in the pelvis, etc.

La'bĭ-um,* plural **La'bĭ-ạ.** [From λαβεῖν (from λαμβάνω), to "receive;" because they receive the food.] (Fr. *Lèvre*, lĕvR or låvR.) The lip; but often applied to other parts from their resemblance to a lip.

La'bium Lep-o-ri'num.* The malformation called hare-lip.

Lā'bor.* [From *labo'ro, labora'tum*, to "work," to "labor," to "be in distress."] The process of parturition, or childbirth. See PARTURITION.

La'bor, Com'plĭ-cāt-ed. That which is attended with some dangerous or troublesome accident or disease, connected in particular instances with the process of parturition.

Labor, Morbid. See PARODYNIA.

Lab'o-ra-to-ry̆. [**Laborato'rium;** from *labo'ro, labora'tum,* to "work," to "labor."] (Fr. *Laboratoire,* lå'bo'rå'-twåʀ'.) The place in which chemical operations are performed.

La'brum.* [From *la'vo,* to "wash;" a "bathing-tub," the "brim of a vessel."] The lip, especially the upper lip.

Lab'y̆-rinth. [**Labyrin'thus;** from λαβύρινθος, a "place having many windings."] That portion of the internal ear comprising the *cochlea, vestibulum,* and semicircular canals.

Lab-y̆-rin'thĭ-form. [**Labyrinthifor'mis;** from *labyrin'thus,* a "labyrinth."] Formed like a labyrinth.

Lab-y̆-rinth'o-don.* [From λαβύρινθος, a "labyrinth," and ὀδούς, a "tooth."] A genus of extinct, gigantic reptiles, characterized by remarkable complexity in the structure of the teeth.

Lac,* gen. **Lac'tis.** [From γάλα, γάλακτος, "milk;" also, the "sap" or "juice" of a plant.] The Latin word for "milk." Also, the common name for a substance deposited by an insect on the branches of several kinds of trees in the East Indies.

Lac'ca,* or **Gum Lac.** A resinous substance formed by an insect on several species of East Indian trees. It yields a fine red dye, and is used to make sealing-wax. When melted, it is called *Shell-lac.*

Laç'er,* neuter **Laç'er-um.** [From λακίς, a "rent," or "cleft."] Torn; rent: laç'erated.

Laç-e-rā'tion. [**Lacera'tio, o'nis;** from *laç'ero, lacera'tum,* to "tear."] The act of tearing or rending.

La-cer'tĭ-dæ.* [From *lacer'ta,* a "lizard."] A group of Saurians forming the second family in the Cuvierian system.

La-cer'tĭ-form. [**Lacertifor'mis;** from *lacer'ta,* a "lizard."] Formed like a lizard.

La-çer-tin'ĭ-dæ.* [From *lacer'ta,* a "lizard."] A family of Saurian reptiles.

La-cer-to-ĭ'dēs.* [From *lacer'ta,* a "lizard."] Resembling the lizard: lacer'toid.

Laç'er-um Fo-ra'men,* plural **Laç'er-a Fo-ram'ĭ-na.** ("Torn Opening.") The name applied to two irregular openings, appearing as if they were torn, between the occipital and temporal bones.

Lach'ry̆-ma,* or **Lac'ry̆-ma.*** [Gr. δάκρυμα; from δακρύω, to "weep."] (Fr. *Larme,* laʀm.) The limpid secretion of the lachrymal gland. See TEAR.

Lach'ry̆-mal. [**Lachryma'lis,** or **Lacryma'lis;** from *lach'ryma,* a "tear."] Belonging to the tears.

Lachrymal Bone. [**Os Lachrymale.**] See UNGUIS OS.

Lachrymal Caruncle. See CARUNCULA LACHRYMALIS.

Lachrymal Duct. See DUCTUS AD NASUM.

Lach'rymal Gland. [**Glan'dula Lachryma'lis.**] The glomerate gland, situated above the external angle of the orbit, which secretes the tears.

La-cin'ĭ-ate. [**Lacinia'tus;** from *lacin'ia,* a "fringe," or "rag."] Fringed; jagged; slashed. Applied to flowers.

La-cin-ĭ-flo'rus.* [From *lacin'ia,* a "fringe," or "rag," and *flos,* a "flower."] Having fringed petals: laciniflo'rous.

La-cin-ĭ-fo-lĭ-a'tus.* [From *lacin'ia,* a "fringe," or "rag," and *fo'lium,* a "leaf."] Having laciniated or fringed leaves.

La-cin'ĭ-form. [**Lacinifor'mis;** from *lacin'ia,* a "fringe," or "rag."] Formed like a fringe.

La-cin-u-la'tus.* [From *lacin'ula,* a "little fringe."] Having irregular divisions.

La-cin-u-lo'sus.* [From *lacin'ula,* a "little fringe."] Having, or full of, little fringes.

Lacis, lå'sè'. The French term for PLEXUS, which see.

Lac'mus. Synonymous with LITMUS.

La-con'ĭ-cum.* [From *Lacon'icus,* "belonging to Laconia," or Lacedæmon.] A name applied to a vapor bath, from its having been much used by the ancient Lacedæmonians.

Lacryma. See LACHRYMA.

Lact-ăl-bu'men. [From *lac,* "milk," and *albu'men.*] Literally, the "albumen of milk." Another name for CASEIN.

Lac'tāte. [**Lac'tas, a'tis.**] A combination of lactic acid with a base.

Lac-tā'tion. [**Lacta'tio, o'nis;** from *lac'to, lacta'tum,* to "suckle."] The act or the period of giving suck.

Lac'te-al. [**Lac'teus;** from *lac, lac'tis,* "milk."] (Fr. *Lacté,* låk'tà'.) Belonging to milk. Applied to certain vessels, because they absorb and convey a fluid (chyle) of a milky appearance.

Lac'te-als. [**Va'sa Chylif'era,** or **Va'sa Lac'tea.**] The chyliferous vessels. See LACTEAL.

Lac'te-in. [**Lactei'na;** from the same.] A substance obtained by the evaporation of milk, concentrating its essential qualities; solidified milk.

Lac'te-ous. [**Lac'teus;** from *lac, lac'tis,* "milk."] Milk-white.

Lac-tĕs'çence. [**Lactescen'tia;** from *lactes'co,* to "become like milk," to "have milk."] The quality of any liquid that is thick, white, and resembles milk.

Lac-tĕs'çent. [**Lactes'cens;** from the same.] Resembling milk, or yielding a milky juice, as some plants.

Lac'tic. [**Lac'ticus;** from *lac, lac'tis,* "milk."] (Fr. *Lactique,* lăk'tēk', or *Laiteux,* lā'tuh'.) Applied to an acid obtained from milk; also termed *Galactic.*

Lac'tic Aç'id. [**Aç'idum Lac'ticum.**] A syrupy, nearly transparent, liquid, of a pale wine color, having a slight, bland odor, and a very sour taste. Its specific gravity is 1.212. It is found in a number of animal secretions, and exists abundantly in the juice of flesh. It is usually obtained by decomposing the lactate of iron by alcohol. Lactic acid has been assigned a place on the primary list of the U.S. Pharmacopœia for 1860. Lactic acid has been used with advantage in some forms of dyspepsia.

Lac-tif'er-ous. [**Lactif'erus;** from *lac, lac'tis,* "milk," and *fe'ro,* to "bear."] Producing or conveying milk.

Lactif'erous Ducts. The milk-conveying ducts of the mammillary glands.

Lac-tĭ-flo'rus.* [From *lac,* "milk," and *flos,* a "flower."] Having flowers white like milk: lactiflo'rous.

Lac-tif'u-gus.* [From *lac,* "milk," and *fu'go,* to "drive away."] Lactifuge. Preventing, or checking, the secretion of milk.

Lac'tin, or **Lac'tīne.** [From *lac,* "milk."] Sugar of milk.

Lac'tis,* the genitive of Lac, which see.

Lac-tiv'or-ous. [**Lactiv'orus;** from *lac,* "milk," and *vo'ro,* to "devour."] Milk-devouring, or living on milk.

Lac'to-çēle.* [From *lac,* "milk," and κήλη, a "tumor."] A collection of a milk-like fluid; also termed *Galactocele.*

Lactometrum. See Galactometer.

Lac'to-scope. [**Lactos'copus;** from *lac,* "milk," and σκοπέω, to "examine."] An instrument for ascertaining the quantity and value of milk.

Lac-tu'cą.* [From *lac,* "milk;" named on account of its milky juice.] (Fr. *Laitue,* lā'tü'.) A Linnæan genus of the class *Syngenesia,* natural order *Compositæ,* or *Chicoraceæ.* Also, the Pharmacopœial name (Lond. Ph., 1851) for *Lactuca sativa.*

Lactu'ca Sa-ti'vą.* Garden lettuce.

Lactu'ca Vī-ro'są.* The strong-scented lettuce (termed also Opium-lettuce) from which *lactucarium* is obtained.

Lac-tu-ca'rĭ-um.* [From *lactu'ca,* "lettuce."] The Pharmacopœial name for the inspissated juice of *Lactuca sativa* and *Lactuca virosa.*

Lą-cu'ną,* plural **Lą-cu'næ.** [From *la'cus,* a "lake," or "ditch."] Literally, a "ditch," "hole," or "chasm." Applied in Anatomy to the excretory ducts of mucous glands. Applied in Botany to punctures on stems, leaves, etc.

Lacu'na Mag'ną.* ("Large Lacuna.") A small opening, or hollow larger than the rest, situated near the *Fossa navicularis* of the male *urethra.*

Lą-cu'næ,* the plural of Lacuna.

Lą-cu'nar. Having, or resembling, *lacunæ.* Also, a "roof." See next article.

Lacu'nar Or'bĭ-tæ.* ("Roof of the Orbit.") The roof of the orbit of the eye.

Lac-u-nose'. [**Lacuno'sus;** from *lacu'na,* a "gap," or "cavity."] Having *lacunæ;* full of depressions, or cavities.

Lą-cus'trīne. [**Lacus'tris;** from *la'cus,* a "lake."] Belonging to a lake.

Læsio. See Lesion.

Lævigatio. See Levigation.

La-ġen'ĭ-form. [**Lagenifor'mis;** from *lage'na,* a "bottle."] Having the form of a Florence flask.

Lag-ne'sis.* [From λάγνης, "lustful."] Lust. The name of a genus in Good's Nosology.

La-goon'. [**Lagu'na;** from *la'cus,* a "lake."] A shallow channel, or creek, mostly on the margin of the sea.

Lag-oph-thăl'mĭ-ą.* [From λαγώς, a "hare," and ὀφθαλμός, the "eye."] A disease in which, from a defect in the upper eyelid, there is imperfect power of closing the eye: so named, it is said, because this is the natural condition of the eye of the hare when asleep.

Lag-oph-thăl'mĭ-cus.* Belonging to *lagophthalmia.*

La-gop'o-dous. [**Lagop'odus;** from λαγώς, a "hare," and πούς, a "foot."] Applied to certain birds, having the feet covered with soft hair or down.

La-go'pus, p'*odis.** [From the same.] Hare-footed. Applied to the grouse genus; also to the fox, and other animals.

La-gos'to-ma.* [From λαγώς, a "hare," and στόμα, a "mouth."] Another name for hare-lip.

Lait, là. The French for MILK, which see.

Laiteux. See LACTIC.

Lake. A term applied to certain insoluble compounds,—pigments composed of aluminous earth and vegetable or animal coloring matter, as carmine lake, madder lake. It appears to have been originally applied to *red* pigments only: it is perhaps a corruption of *lac*, a reddish resinous substance. See LAC.

Lal-lā'tion. [**Lalla'tio, o'***nis.*] A term for the faulty pronunciation in which *l* is rendered unduly liquid, or substituted for an *r*.

Lamb-da-cis'mus.* [From *lamb'da*, the name of the Greek λ, or *l*.] The same as LALLATION, which see.

Lamb'doid, or **Lamb-doi'dal.** [From *lamb'da*, and εἶδος, a "form."] The same as LAMBDOIDES.

Lamb-do-i'dēs.* [From Λ, and εἶδος, a "form."] Resembling the Greek *l*, or *lambda*.

Lambdoi'des Os.* The *Os hyoides*, so called from its resembling the Greek letter Λ.

Lam'el-lar, or **Lam'el-late.** [**Lamella'ris;** from *lamel'la*, a "thin plate."] Composed of flat plates; having lamellæ.

La-mel-lĭ-bran'chĭ-ate. [**Lamellibranchia'tus,** or **Lamellibran'-chius;** from *lamel'la*, a "thin plate," and βράγχια, "gills."] Having the gills disposed symmetrically in large semicircular plates.

La-mel-lĭ-cor'nis.* [From *lamel'la*, a "thin plate," and *cor'nu*, a "horn."] Applied to insects having lamellar horns (or *antennæ*): lamellicornate.

Lam-el-lif'er-ous. [**Lamellif'er-us;** from *lamel'la*, a "thin plate," and *fe'ro*, to "bear."] Bearing or having lamellæ. Applied to certain plants.

La-mel'lĭ-form. [**Lamellifor'mis;** from *lamel'la*, a "thin plate."] Formed of, or like, small plates.

Lam-el-lig'er-us.* [From *lamel'-la*, a "thin plate," and *ge'ro*, to "carry."] The same as LAMELLIFEROUS: lamellig'-erous.

La-mel'lĭ-pēs, e*dis.** [From *lamel'la*, a "thin plate," and *pes*, a "foot."] Having flattened and lamelliform feet. Applied to a section of *Conchifera*.

Lam-el-lĭ-ros'trēs,* or **La-mel-lĭ-ros'trals.** [From *lamel'la*, a "thin plate," and *ros'trum*, a "beak."] The name of a tribe of swimming birds, the fourth in the system of Cuvier, comprising those in which the margins of the beaks are furnished with numerous lamellæ or dental plates, arranged in a regular series, as in the swan, goose, and duck.

Lam'ĭ-na,* plural **Lam'ĭ-næ.** Any thin plate or layer of bone, membrane, or other substance. The border of a polypetalous corolla; the blade of a leaf or petal.

Lam'ĭ-nāt-ed. [**Lamina'tus.**] Applied to parts that consist of thin layers, or laminæ, lying closely upon each other.

Lam'ĭ-nĭ-form. [**Laminifor'mis;** from *lam'ina*, a "thin plate."] Flattened in the form of a thin plate.

Lamp'black. A species of charcoal, of which the finest sort is produced by collecting the smoke from a lamp.

Lam-po-car'pus.* [From λάμπω, to "shine," and καρπός, "fruit."] Having shining fruit: lampocarpous.

Lam-pro-pho'nĭ-a.* [From λαμπρός, "bright," "clear," and φωνή, the "voice."] A clear and sonorous state of the voice.

Lam-pro-phȳl'le-us.* [From λαμπρός, "bright," "clear," and φύλλον, a "leaf."] Applied to plants having smooth and bright leaves.

Lam'pro-pus.* [From λαμπρός, "bright," "clear," and πούς, a "foot."] Having the *stipes*, or foot, of a bright appearance.

Lam'pȳ-ris, i*dis.** [From λάμπω, to "shine," and πῦρ, "fire."] The glow-worm.

Lam'pyris Noc-tĭ-lu'ca.* The systematic name of the glow-worm.

La'na.* Wool. Applied to a kind of pubescence which covers the surfaces of plants.

La'na Phil-o-soph'ĭ-ca.* ("Philosophical Wool.") Flowers of zinc, or the snowy flakes of the white oxide of zinc, which arise and float in the air from the combustion of that metal.

Lā'nate. [**Lana'tus;** from *la'na*, "wool."] Woolly; having a pubescence like wool.

Lan-ce'o-la.* [Diminutive of *lan'-cea*, a "lance."] A little lance; a lancet, and, so, the same as LANCET, which see.

Lan'ce-o-late. [**Lanceola'tus;** from *lance'ola*, a "little lance."] Having the form of a little lance, or spear.

Lan'cet. [Lat. **Lancet'ta;** Fr. *Lancette*, lŏNᵍ'sĕt'.] A two-edged instrument for bleeding, or other purposes.

Lan-ci-fo'li-ous. [**Lancifo'lius;** from *lan'cea*, a "lance," and *fo'lium*, a "leaf."] Having lanceolated leaves, or divisions of leaves.

Lan'ci-form. [**Lancifor'mis;** from *lan'cea*, a "lance."] Having the form of a lance, or head of a lance; applied to teeth, etc.

Lan'ci-nāt-ing. [**Lan'cinans, an'***tis;* from *lan'cino*, to "thrust through," or "rend."] Piercing, as with a lance; lacerating.

Langue, lŏNḡ. The French word for Tongue, which see.

Lan'guor, o'r*is*.* A listless unwillingness to use exertion, with faintness.

La-nif'er-ous. [**Lanif'erus;** from *la'na*, "wool," and *fe'ro*, to "bear."] Bearing or producing wool.

Lan-ĭ-flo'rus.* [From *la'na*, "wool," and *flos*, a "flower."] Having woolly flowers: laniflo'rous.

La-nig'er-ous. [**Lan'iger,** or **Lanig'erus;** from *la'na*, "wool," and *ge'ro*, to "carry."] The same as Laniferous.

La'nĭ-pēs, p'e*dis*.* [From *la'na*, "wool," and *pes*, a "foot."] Having hairy petioles, or feet.

La-nose'. [From *la'na*, "wool."] The same as Lanate, which see.

Lantanium. See Lanthanum.

Lantanum. See Lanthanum.

Lan'tha-num,* Lan'ta-num,* or **Lan-ta'nĭ-um.*** [From λανθάνω, to "be concealed."] A newly discovered metal, so named from its properties being concealed by those of cerium, with which it is found united.

La-nu'gĭ-nous. [**Lanugino'sus;** from *lanu'go*, "down," or "soft hair."] Having soft hairs or down.

La-nu'go,* gen. **La-nu'gĭ-nis.** [From *la'na*, "wool."] Soft hairs, wool, or down.

Lan-u-lo'sus.* [From *la'na*, "wool."] Having wool; full of wool.

Lap-a-rom-no-did'y̆-mus.* [From λαπάρα, the "flank," or "loins," μόνος, "single," and δίδυμος, "double."] Applied in the plural (*Laparomnodid'ymi*) to twins born adhering together by the loins.

Lap-a-ro-sco'pĭ-a.* [From λαπάρα, the "flank," or "loins," and σκοπέω, to "examine."] The examination of the loins, or side, by means of the stethoscope, pleximeter, etc.

Lap-a-ro-to'mĭ-a.* [From λαπάρα, the "flank," or "loins," and τέμνω, to "cut."] Cutting into the abdomen in the region of the loins.

Lap-a-rot'o-mus.* [From the same.] A name of the instrument for performing laparotomy: a lap'arotome.

Lap'a-rȳs'te-ro-to'mĭ-a.* [From λαπάρα, the "flank," or "loins," ὑστέρα, the "womb," and τέμνω, to "cut."] Cutting into the womb through the flank or abdomen.

Lap'a-thum.* [From λαπάζω, to "empty;" because it is an aperient, or purgative.] The dock. See Rumex.

Lap-ĭ-ci'dus.* [From *la'pis*, a "stone," and *cæ'do*, to "cut," or "dig."] Digging into stone; imbedded in rocks, etc. Applied to animals and shells so found, as if they had dug their retreat there.

La-pid'e-ous. [**Lapid'eus;** from *la'pis*, a "stone."] Stony; belonging to stone.

Lap'ĭ-dēs,* the plural of Lapis, which see.

Lapides Cancrorum. See Cancrorum Lapilli.

Lap-ĭ-dĕs'çent. [**Lapides'cens, en'***tis;* from *la'pis*, a "stone," and *-esco*, a Latin termination signifying to "grow."] Resembling a stone in hardness.

La-pid-ĭ-fĭ-cā'tion. [**Lapidifica'tio, o'***nis;* from *la'pis*, a "stone," and *fa'cio*, to "make."] Conversion into stone.

La-pil'li,* the plural of Lapillus, which see.

La-pil-lĭ-for'mis.* [From *lapil'lus*, a "little stone."] Having the appearance of small stones: lapilliform.

Lap-il-lo'sus.* [From the same.] Having *lapilli*.

La-pil'lus,* plural **La-pil'li.** [Diminutive of *la'pis*, a "stone."] A little stone. See Cancrorum Lapilli.

La'pis,* gen. **Lap'ĭ-dis.** [Gr. λᾶας, a "stone."] A Latin word signifying a "stone." The alchemists called by this term every fixed thing which does not evaporate, and, hence, even human blood was termed *La'pis anima'lis*.

Lapis Calaminaris. See Calamina.

La'pis Cal-ca'rĭ-us.* The native carbonate of lime, or limestone.

La'pis Dĭ-vi'nus.* A substance

composed of sulphate of copper, nitrate of potash, alum, and camphor, used as a collyrium, and named "divine," on account of its supposed virtues.

Lapis Infernalis. See POTASSA FUSA.

Lapis Philosophorum. See PHILOSOPHER'S STONE.

Lap'pa.* Burdock. The Pharmacopœial name (U.S. Ph.) for the root of the *Lappa minor* (or *Arc'tium lappa*).

Lappaceus,* lap-pa'she-ŭs. [From *lap'pa*, the "clitbur."] Curved at the extremity like the *bracteæ* of the burdock.

Laq'ue-us Gut'tur-is.* Literally, "noose of the throat." A name applied to a malignant inflammation of the tonsils.

Larch-Tree. The *Pinus Larix.*

Lardacé. See LARDACEOUS.

Lar-dā'ceous. [**Larda'ceus**; from *lar'dum*, "lard."] (Fr. *Lardacé*, lar'då'-så'.) Resembling lard, or the fat of bacon.

Larda'ceous De-ġen-e-rā'tion, otherwise called **Wax'y Degenera'tion.** A term applied to certain organic alterations in the tissues, whereby these assume a translucent, wax-like appearance. One form of substance resulting from this change (found as a deposit between the proper elements of the tissues) has the remarkable property of becoming blue, like vegetable starch, by the simple action of iodine; whence Virchow applies to these altered structures the term *amyloid* (i.e. "starch-like") *degeneration.* The tissues themselves participate in this peculiar change, and usually exhibit a blue or violet color, if the application of iodine be followed by a cautious addition of sulphuric acid.

Lar'de-us.* [From *lar'dum*, the "fat of bacon," or "lard."] Belonging to lard.

Lar'dum.* The fat of bacon. See ADEPS SUILLUS.

La'rix Eū-ro-pæ'a.* A name of the larch-tree, from which Venice turpentine is procured. See PINUS LARIX.

Larme, larm. See LACHRYMA.

Larmoiement, lar'mwå'mŏnᴳ'. [From *larme*, a "tear."] A French term for EPIPHORA, which see.

Lar'va,* plural **Lar'væ.** A Latin word, signifying, originally, a "mask," or "spectre." A grub, or larve. Applied in Entomology to the first condition of the metamorphosis of insects hatched from the egg. So called because, in this condition, their real character seems to be masked.

Lar'val. [**Larva'lis**; from *lar'va* a "mask," a "spectre."] Belonging to a mask, or to *larvæ*. Applied to diseases in which the skin of the face is disfigured, as if covered by a mask.

Lar-vic'o-lus.* [From *lar'va*, a "mask," a "spectre," and *co'lo*, to "inhabit."] Applied to certain small insects existing in *larvæ*.

Lar'vi-form. [**Larvifor'mis.**] Formed like *larvæ*.

Lar-vip'a-rous. [**Larvip'arus**; from *lar'væ*, and *pa'rio*, to "bring forth."] Producing *larvæ* in the place of eggs.

Larynge. See LARYNGEAL.

Lăr-ўn-ġe'al. [**Larynge'us**; from λάρυγξ, the "larynx."] (Fr. *Larynge*, lå'rănᴳ'zhå', or *Laryngien*, lå'rănᴳ'zhe-ănᴳ'.) Belonging to the larynx.

Laryngien. See LARYNGEAL.

Lăr-ўn-ġis'mus.* [From λαρυγγίζω, to "vociferate."] Spasm of the muscles closing the larynx.

Lăr-ўn-ġī'tis, idis.* [From λάρυγξ, the "larynx."] Inflammation of the larynx.

La-rўn-go-gra'phi-a.* [From λάρυγξ, the "larynx," and γράφω, to "write."] A description of the larynx.

Lăr-ўn-gol'o-ġў. [**Laryngolo'gia**; from λάρυγξ, the "larynx," and λόγος, a "discourse."] A treatise on the larynx; the science of the larynx.

Lăr-ўn-goph'o-nў, or **Lăr-ўn-goph'o-nism.** [**Laryngopho'nia,** or **Laryngophonis'mus**; from λάρυγξ, the "larynx," and φωνή, the "voice."] The sound of the voice, heard by means of the stethoscope, within the larynx.

Lăr-ўn-goph-this'ĭ-cus.* Belonging to *laryngophthisis.*

Lăr-ўn-goph'thi-sis.* [From λάρυγξ, the "larynx," and φθίσις, a "wasting."] A disease of the larynx, connected with pulmonary consumption: laryngeal phthisis.

La-rўn-gor-rhœ'a.* [From λάρυγξ, the "larynx," and ῥέω, to "flow."] A pituitous or serous flow from the larynx.

La-rўn-go-spas'mus.* [From λάρυγξ, the "larynx," and σπασμός, a "spasm."] The same as LARYNGISMUS, which see.

La-rўn-go-ste-no'sis.* [From λάρυγξ, the "larynx," and στένωσις, a "contraction."] Contraction of the larynx.

Lăr-ўn-got'o-mus.* [From λάρυγξ, the "larynx," and τέμνω, to "cut."] An instrument for performing laryngotomy: a laryn'gotome.

Lăr-ўn-got'o-mў. [**Laryngoto'mia;** from the same.] The operation of cutting into the larynx.

Lăr'ўnx,* gen. **La-rўn'gis.** [Gr. λάρυγξ.] The upper part of the *trachea*, or windpipe; in a general sense, the organ of the voice.

La-sĭ-an'thus.* [From λάσιος, "hairy," and ἄνθος, a "flower."] Having hairy or rough flowers.

La-sĭ-o-car'pus.* [From λάσιος, "hairy," and καρπός, "fruit."] Having hairy fruit.

La-sĭ-o-pe-ta'le-us.* [From λάσιος, "hairy," and πέταλον, a "petal."] Having hairy petals.

La-sĭ-op'ter-us.* [From λάσιος, "rough," or "hairy," and πτερόν, a "wing."] Having hairy wings, as the *Vespertil'io lasiop'terus*, a species of bat.

La-si'o-pus.* [From λάσιος, "hairy," and πούς, a "foot."] Having the *stipes* hairy.

La-sĭ-o-sper'mus.* [From λάσιος, "hairy," and σπέρμα, a "seed."] Having hairy fruit or seed.

La-sĭ-os'ta-chўs.* [From λάσιος, "hairy," and στάχυς, an "ear of corn."] Having flowers in rough, hairy ears.

La'sĭ-pēs, p'edis.* The same as LASIOPUS.

La-sĭ-u'rus.* [From λάσιος, "hairy," and οὐρά, a "tail."] Having hairy peduncles, or tails.

Las'sĭ-tude. [**Lassitu'do, dinis;** from *las'sus*, "weary," "tired."] Literally, "weariness," or "fatigue;" but usually denoting a sensation of exhaustion and weakness, independent of fatigue.

Lat. dol. = *Lat'eri dolen'ti.** "To the side affected."

Lā'tent. [**La'tens;** from *la'teo*, to "lie hid."] Lurking; concealed; lying hid.

La'tent Pe'rĭ-od. That space of time during which certain diseases lurk in the system, before their presence is manifested by symptoms.

Lat'er-al. [**Latera'lis;** from *la'tus, lat'eris*, the "side."] Belonging to the side; on the side, as distinguished from *medial* or *central*.

Lat'eral Op-e-rā'tion. [**Opera'tio Latera'lis.**] One of the operations of lithotomy; being performed on the left side of the perinæum.

Lat'eral Si'nus-es. Two veins of the *dura mater;* the right and left lateral sinuses, running along the crucial spine of the occipital bone.

Lat-e-rĭ-flo'rus.* [From *la'tus*, the "side," and *flos*, a "flower."] Having lateral flowers.

Lat-e-rĭ-fo'lĭ-ous. [**Laterifo'lius;** from *la'tus*, the "side," and *fo'lium*, a "leaf."] Growing at the side of a leaf.

Lat-e-rig'ra-dus.* [From *la'tus*, the "side," and *gra'dior*, to "go," to "step."] Going or moving sideways.

Lat-e-rĭ-ner'vus.* [From *la'tus*, the "side," and *ner'vus*, a "nerve."] Applied to leaves in which the nervures diverge from the middle.

Lat-e-rĭ'tious. [**Lateri'tius;** from *la'ter*, a "brick."] Applied to a sediment like brick-dust in the urine.

La'tex,* gen. **Lat'ĭ-cis.** A Latin term for "liquor" or "juice" in general. Applied to the proper juice, or vital fluid, of plants.

Lat-ĭ-cif'er-ous. [**Laticif'erus;** from *la'tex, lat'icis*, a "liquor," or "juice," and *fe'ro*, to "bear."] Producing or containing elaborated sap, or special juices of plants, as the *laticiferous tissue*.

Lat-ĭ-flo'rus.* [From *la'tus*, "broad," and *flos*, a "flower."] Having broad flowers: latiflo'rous.

Lat-ĭ-fo'lĭ-ous. [**Latifo'lius;** from *la'tus*, "broad," and *fo'lium*, a "leaf."] Having broad leaves.

La-tis'sĭ-mus.* [The superlative degree of *la'tus*, "broad."] The "broadest;" applied to the *Platysma myodes*, which is called the *Latissimus colli* (The "Broadest [Muscle] of the Neck"), and to the *Aniscalptor* of Cowper, more frequently called the *Latissimus dorsi* (The "Broadest [Muscle] of the Back").

Lat'ĭ-tude. [**Latitu'do;** from *la'tus*, "broad."] Literally, "breadth." The distance of a heavenly body from the ecliptic, or of a place from the equator.

Latticed. See CANCELLATUS.

Laudable Pus. See HEALTHY PUS.

Lau'da-num.* [From *lau'do*, to "praise."] The *Tinctu'ra o'pii.*

Lauraceæ,* lau-ra'she-ē. A natural order of exogenous trees, found in the cooler parts of the tropics, and some temperate countries. It comprises the Cinnamon, *Lau'rus* (including the Bay-tree, or true laurel), and Sassafras. The species are generally tonic, stimulant, and aromatic. Camphor is an abundant product of this order.

Lau-rā'ceous. [**Laura'ceus.**] Resembling the *Laurus.*

Lau'rel. The genus *Laurus.*

Lau'rel, Al-ex-an'dri-an. The *Prunus laurocerasus.*

Laurier. See LAURUS.

Lau'ro-Cĕr'a-sus.* The Pharmacopœial name (Br. Ph.) for the *Prunus laurocerasus.*

Lau'rus.* (Fr. *Laurier,* lō're-å'.) A Linnæan genus of the class *Enneandria,* natural order *Lauraceæ.* The Pharmacopœial name (Lond. Ph., 1851) for the fruit of *Laurus nobilis.*

Lau'rus Cam'pho-ra.* The Linnæan name of the camphor-tree. See CAMPHORA OFFICINARUM.

Lau'rus Cas'sia* (kash'e-a). The systematic name of the *Cassia lignea* (or wild cinnamon) tree, the bark of which, according to some authorities, is called *Cassia lignea,* and the leaves *Folia malabathri.*

Lau'rus Cin-na-mo'mum.* The name (Dub. Ph.) of the cinnamon-tree.

Lau'rus Cu-li-la'wan.* The systematic name of a species, the bark of which is called *Cortex culilawan,* and closely resembles cinnamon.

Lau'rus Nob'i-lis.* The bay-laurel, or sweet-bay.

Lau'rus Sas'sa-fras.* The sassafras-tree.

La'va. [From the German *Lau'fen,* to "run," to "flow"?] A generic term for all mineral substances melted by volcanic fire, and cast forth in the form of burning streams.

Lav-a-men'tum.* [From *la'vo,* to "wash."] A clyster, or injection.

Lavande. See LAVANDULA.

La-van'du-la.* [From *la'vo,* to "wash;" because it was much used in lotions.] (Fr. *Lavande,* lå'vŏnd'.) Lavender. A Linnæan genus of the class *Didynamia,* natural order *Labiatæ.* The Pharmacopœial name (U.S. and Ed. Ph.) for the flowers of *Lavandula spica,* or *Lavandula vera;* the *Lavandulæ Spicæ Flores* ("Flowers of Lavandula Spica") of the Dublin Pharmacopœia.

Lavan'dula Spi'ca.* The common lavender-plant.

Lavandula Ve'ra.* The same as LAVANDULA SPICA.

Lavender. See LAVANDULA.

Lavendula. See LAVANDULA.

Lav-i-pe'di-um.* A bath for the feet.

Law-so'ni-a In-er'mis.* The systematic name of the plant from which the henné of Egypt is obtained.

Lax-ā'tion. [**Laxa'tio, o'nis;** from *lax'o, laxa'tum,* to "loosen."] A loosening, or purgation.

Lax'a-tive. [**Laxati'vus;** from the same.] Slightly purgative.

Lax-a'tor, o'ris.* [From the same.] A relaxer. Applied to muscles.

Laxa'tor Tўm'pa-ni.* A muscle of the tympanum attached to the handle of the malleus.

Lax-i-cos-ta'tus.* [From *lax'us,* "loose," "free," and *cos'ta,* a "rib."] Furnished with solitary or distinct ribs.

Lax-i-flo'rus.* [From *lax'us,* "loose," or "free," and *flos,* a "flower."] Having distinct flowers: laxiflo'rous.

Lax-i-fo'li-us.* [From *lax'us,* "loose," or "free," and *fo'lium,* a "leaf."] Having distinct leaves: laxifo'lious.

Lax'us.* Literally, "loose;" hence, spread out; diffused. Applied to a condition of animal fibre.

Laz-a-ret'to. (Italian.) A hospital for persons afflicted with contagious diseases. A building set apart for the performance of quarantine.

Lb. or **Lib.** = *Li'bra.** A "pound."

Lead. [Lat. **Plum'bum;** Gr. μόλυβδος; Fr. *Plomb,* plŏn°.] A soft, flexible, inelastic metal, of a bluish-gray color. It is ductile and malleable, but possesses very little tenacity. It has a bright metallic lustre when freshly cut, but quickly tarnishes on exposure to air. Its specific gravity is 11.38. It fuses at about 600°. The most important ore of lead is the sulphuret, the galena of the mineralogists. For the compounds of lead, see PLUMBUM, PLUMBI. etc.

Lead, Sugar of. See PLUMBI ACETAS.

Leaf. [**Fo'lium, Frons.**] An organ performing in plants the functions of respiration and assimilation. It consists of the *lamina* and petiole, and is the type of the other organs. See TYPE.

Leaf-Stalk. See PETIOLE.

Leaflet. See FOLIOLE.

Leafy. See FOLIACEOUS.

Leanness. See EMACIATION.

Leather-Like, or **Leathery.** See CORIACEUS.

Lec'tus.* A bed or couch.

Lecythidaceæ,* le-sith-e-da'she-ē. [From *Lec'ythis,* one of the genera.] A natural order of exogenous trees, found in South America. The well-known Brazil-nut is a product of this order.

Ledoyen's (leh-dwå'yŏnz') **Dis-in-fec'ting Flu'id.** A solution of nitrate of lead in water.

Leech. See HIRUDO MEDICINALIS.

Leg'ume. [**Legu'men, Legu'-**

minis; from *le'go*, to "gather up."] (Fr. *Légume*, lā'güm'.) A pericarp of two oblong valves in which the seeds are ranged along one suture only.

Le-gu-mi-na'ris.* [From *legu'men*, a "legume."] Applied to the dehiscence of pericarps by a marginal suture: legu'minar.

Le-gu'mĭ-nĭ-for'mis.* [From *legu'men*, a "legume."] Having the form of a legume: leguminiform.

Le-gu-mĭ-no'sæ,* or **Fabaceæ,*** fa-ba'she-ē. A large and important natural order of exogenous plants, found in all parts of the world. It includes a variety of useful and beautiful species, some of which, as clover and lucern, are cultivated for cattle; others, as peas and beans, form part of the food of man. Indigo, liquorice, gum-Arabic, and senna are products of this order. The properties of many species are tonic, purgative, or narcotic.

Le-gu'mĭ-nous. [Legumino'sus; from *legu'men*, a "legume."] Having legumes.

Leim'ma.* [Gr. λεῖμμα; from λείπω, to "leave."] The residue, or what is left of a thing.

Leī-o-car'pus.* [From λεῖος, "smooth," and καρπός, "fruit."] Having smooth fruit, as the *Heylandia leiocarpa*, and *Panicum leiocarpum*.

Leī-o-çeph'a-lus.* [From λεῖος, "smooth," and κεφαλή, the "head."] Having a smooth head, or hat. Applied to a species of mushroom.

Leī-o-phȳl'lus.* [From λεῖος, "smooth," and φύλλον, a "leaf."] Having smooth leaves: smooth leaved.

Leī-o-pi'lus.* [From λεῖος, "smooth," and πῖλος, a "hat."] Having a smooth or glabrous hat. Used in the same manner as LEIOCEPHALUS.

Leī'o-pus, p'odis.* [From λεῖος, "smooth," and πούς, a "foot."] Having a smooth *stipes*, as the *Helotium leiopus*.

Leī-o-sper'mus.* [From λεῖος, "smooth," and σπέρμα, a "seed."] Having smooth seed, as the *Galium leiospermum*.

Leī-o-sta'chȳ-us.* [From λεῖος, "smooth," and σταχύς, an "ear of corn."] Having smooth ears; the glumes which compose them being smooth and glabrous, as the *Trista'chya leiosta'chya*.

Leī-po-thȳm'ĭ-a.* [From λείπω, to "relinquish," to "fail," and θυμός, the "mind."] The sensation of sinking, or fainting; *Deliquium animi:* syncope.

Lem'ma,* gen. **Lem'ma-tis.** [Gr. λέμμα; from λέπω, to "decorticate."] The *cortex*, or bark; the coat, or covering of plants.

Lem'ma.* [Gr. λῆμμα; from λαμβάνω, to "receive," or "take."] Something assumed or taken for granted as the basis of an argument; also, the demonstration of some premise, in order to render what follows more easy.

Lemnaceæ,* lem-na'she-ē, or **Pistiaceæ,*** pis-te-a'she-ē. A natural order of endogenous plants, often found in ditches. It includes the *Lemna* (Duckweed).

Lem'on. [Li'mon, o'nis.] The fruit of the *Citrus medica*.

Lem-on-āde'. A beverage composed of lemon-juice diluted with water and sweetened.

Lem'on Scur'vȳ-Grass. The *Cochlea'ria officina'lis*, regarded as a powerful antiscorbutic.

Lem'ons, Aç'id of. Citric acid.

Lem'ons, Salt of. Oxalic acid, with a small portion of potash.

Lenientia,* le-ne-en'she-a. [From *le'nio*, to "allay."] Medicines which allay irritation.

Len'ĭ-tĭve. [Leniti'vus; from the same.] Assuaging, gently palliating.

Len'itive E-lec'tu-a-rȳ. The *Confectio sennæ composita*.

Lens,* gen. **Len'tis.** [A "lentil;" because it is usually convex like a lentil.] A piece of glass, or transparent substance, formed so as, by its refraction, to converge or scatter the rays of light. See EYE.

Lentibulariaceæ,* len-tib-u-la-re-a'she-ē. [From *Lentibula'ria*, one of the genera.] A natural order of exogenous herbaceous plants, found in marshes and streams in all parts of the world.

Len-tĭ-cel'la,* plural **Len-tĭ-cel'læ.** [From *lens*, a "lentil."] Applied to ruddy oval points upon the bark of the branches of trees. Also, the same as LENTICULA, which see.

Len-tĭ-cel-la'tus.* Having *lenticellæ*.

Len-tic'u-la.* [Diminutive of *lens*, a "lentil."] A smaller kind of lentil. Also, an instrument for removing irregularities of bone from the edge of the perforation made in the cranium with the trephine.

Len-tic'u-lar. [Lenticula'ris; from *lens*, a "lentil."] Lens-shaped; double-convex.

Lentic'ular Gan'glĭ-on. A small reddish body near the back part of the orbit of the eye, between the optic nerve and the external *rectus* muscle; also termed *Ophthalmic ganglion.*

Lentic'ular Pa-pil'læ. The papillæ situated at the posterior part of the tongue.

Len-tif'er-us.* [From *lens*, a "lentil," and *fe'ro*, to "bear."] Applied to flowers having receptacles in the form of lentils.

Len'ti-form. [**Lentifor'mis**; from *lens*, a "lentil."] Formed like a lens.

Len-tig'er-us.* [From *lens*, a "lentil," and *ge'ro*, to "carry."] The same as LENTIFERUS: lentigerous.

Len-tig'i-nose. Freckled or dusty-dotted, as the parts of some plants.

Len-ti'go, ġ'inis.* [From *lens*, a "lentil."] A cutaneous affection chiefly of the face, in which there are spots of the color and size of the lentil seed.

Len'til. The genus *Ervum:* the seed of *Ervum.*

Len'tor, o'ris.* [From *len'tus*, "slow," "tough," "viscid."] Viscidity, or gluey consistence, of any fluid.

Le-on-ti'a-sis.* [From λέων, a "lion"?] A name applied to the disease known as the *Elephantiasis Græcorum*, and other forms of leprosy.

Le-on'to-don, on'tis.* [From λέων, the "lion," and ὀδούς, a "tooth;" named from the tooth-like sections of the leaves.] A Linnæan genus of the class *Syngenesia*, natural order *Compositæ.*

Leon'todon Ta-rax'a-cum.* The plant *Dandelion;* also called *Dens Leonis.*

Le-o-nu'rus.* [From λέων, a "lion," and οὐρά, a "tail."] Like the tail of a lion: leonu'rous.

Lĕop'ard's Bane. The common name for the plant *Arnica montana.*

Lep'al. A sterile transformed stamen.

Lep-i-dan'the-us.* [From λεπίς, λεπίδος, a "scale," or "husk," and ἄνθος, a "flower."] Having flowers like scales; squamiflorous.

Lep-i-do-den'dron.* [From λεπίς, a "scale," and δένδρον, a "tree."] A genus of fossil trees found in coal-beds. They are sometimes several feet in diameter, and are covered with regular rhomboidal projections, like scales, arranged in spiral rows, extending around the tree from base to summit.

Lep-i-do'dēs.* [From λεπίς, a "scale."] Resembling scales; scaly.

Lep'i-doid. [**Lepidoi'des**; from λεπίς, a "scale," and εἶδος, a "form."] Resembling a scale.

Lep-i-do-phyl'lous. [**Lepidophyl'lus**; from λεπίς, a "scale," and φύλλον, a "leaf."] Having leaves in the form of scales.

Lep-i-do-plas'tus.* [From λεπίς, a "scale," and πλάσσω, to "form."] Forming scales.

Lepidoptera. See LEPIDOPTERUS.

Lep-i-dop'ter-us.* [From λεπίς, a "scale," and πτερόν, a "wing."] Lepidop'terous; having wings sprinkled, or partially covered, with scales. Applied in the plural neuter (*Lepidop'tera*) to an order of insects having four wings so covered. It includes the butterfly, and what are popularly called "millers."

Lep-i-do'sis.* [From λεπίς, a "scale."] A name for ICHTHYOSIS, which see.

Lep'i-dote. [**Lepido'tus**; from λεπίς, a "scale."] Furnished with scales; scaly, or scurfy.

Lep-o-ri'num La'bi-um,* Lepori'num Ros'trum.* The defect called hare-lip.

Lep'ra.* [Gr. λέπρα, "leprosy."] (Fr. *Lèpre*, lĕpr or lȧpr.) Leprosy. A disease of the skin distinguished by circular scaly patches. A genus of the order *Impetigenes*, class *Cachexiæ*, of Cullen's Nosology.

Lep'ra Ar'a-bum.* An epithet of *Elephantiasis Græcorum*, or tubercular *Elephantiasis.*

Lèpre. See LEPRA.

Lépreux. See LEPROUS.

Lep-ri'a-sis.* [From λεπρός, "rough."] The specific name for leprosy, or *Lepidosis lepriasis.*

Lep'ri-cus.* Belonging to *lepra:* lep'ric.

Lep-roph-thăl'mi-a.* [From λέπρα, the "leprosy," and ὀφθαλμός, the "eye."] Leprous ophthalmia.

Lep-roph-thăl'mus.* [From the same.] The eye affected by lepropthalmy; also, the patient laboring under that affection.

Lep-ro-sa'ri-um.* A hospital for the treatment of leprosy; a leper-house, or *Domus leprosarius.*

Lep-ro-sa'ri-us.* [From λέπρα, "leprosy."] Belonging to *lepra.*

Lep-ro'sis.* [From λέπρα, "leprosy."] The progress of leprosy.

Leprosy. See LEPRA.

Lep'rous. [**Lepro'sus**; from *lep'ra.*] (Fr. *Lépreux*, lȧ'pruh'.) Belonging to *lepra;* scaly.

Lep-ta-can'thus.* [From λεπτός, "slender," and ἄκανθα, a "spine."] Having slender spines.

Lep-tan'dra.* A name applied to the root of the *Veronica Virginica.* It has been placed on the primary list of the Materia Medica in the U.S. Pharmacopœia for 1860. The active principle of the plant, called *Leptan'drin*, is regarded as an excellent cholagogue cathartic, and is extensively used as a substitute for mercury.

Lep-tan'drin. [**Leptandri'na.**] See preceding article.

Lep-to-cau'lis.* [From λεπτός, "slender," and καύλος, a "stem."] Having a slender stem.

Lep-to-çeph'a-lus.* [From λεπτός, "slender," and κεφαλή, a "head."] Having a small head. Applied to plants or flowers.

Lep-toch'ro-a,* or **Lep-toch'ros.*** [From λεπτός, "fine," or "slender," and χρόα, the "skin."] A fine, thin, soft, or delicate membrane.

Lep'to-don, on'tis.* [From λεπτός, "fine," or "slender," and ὀδούς, a "tooth."] Having very small teeth.

Lep-to-pet'a-lus.* [From λεπτός, "slender," and πέταλον, a "petal."] Having strait or narrow petals.

Lep-to-phўl'lus.* [From λεπτός, "slender," and φύλλον, a "leaf."] Having slender leaves.

Lep-top'o-dus.* [From λεπτός, "slender," and πούς, a "foot."] Having a slender *stipes*, or foot.

Lep-to-rhi'zus.* [From λεπτός, "slender," and ῥίζα, a "root."] Having slender roots.

Lep-to-sep'a-lus.* [From λεπτός, "slender," and *sep'alum*, a "sepal."] Having narrow, linear sepals.

Lep-to-sper'me-us.* Applied in the plural feminine (*Leptosper'meæ*) to a tribe of *Myrtaceæ*, having the *Leptospermum* for their type: leptosper'meous.

Lep-to-sper'mus.* [From λεπτός, "slender," and σπέρμα, a "seed."] Having very small seeds: leptosper'mous.

Lep-to-sta'chў-us.* [From λεπτός, "slender," and στάχυς, an "ear of corn."] Having slender ears.

Lep-to-sty'lus.* [From λεπτός, "slender," and στύλος, a "style."] Having a filiform style.

Lep-to-trich'ĭ-a.* [From λεπτός, "slender," or "fine," and θρίξ, "hair."] Fineness, or thinness, of the hair.

Le'sion. [**Læ'sio, o'**nis; from *læ'do, læ'sum*, to "hurt."] Literally, an "injury." A vitiated or depressed condition of any organ or part. Applied in Surgery to a hurt, wound, or injury of a part.

Le'sion of Nu-trĭ'tion. A term for those pathological alterations which originate in the capillary system, consisting in any excess or deficiency of the particles of blood in the process of assimilation and absorption, etc.

Le'thal. [**Letha'lis**; from *le'thum*, "death."] Belonging to death; mortal; fatal.

Le-thal'ĭ-tў. [**Lethal'itas, a'**tis; from *letha'lis*, "deadly."] The quality of being deadly, or fatal; mortality.

Le-thar'gic. [**Lethar'gicus.**] Belonging to a state of lethargy.

Leth'ar-gў. [**Lethar'gus**; from λήθη, "forgetfulness."] A state of marked drowsiness, or sleep, which cannot be driven off.

Lettuce. See LACTUCA.

Lettuce Opium. See LACTUCARIUM.

Lettuce, Opium- or **Strong-scented.** See LACTUCA VIROSA.

Leucæmia. See LEUCHÆMIA.

Leū-çæ-thĭ-o'pĭ-a.* [From λευκός, "white," and αἰθίοψ, an "Ethiopian," or "negro."] The same as ALBINISM, which see.

Leū-çæ'thĭ-ops, opis.* [From the same.] See ALBINO.

Leū-can'thous. [**Leucan'thus**; from λευκός, "white," and ἄνθος, a "flower."] White-flowered.

Leūc-hæ'mĭ-a,* or **Leū-kæ'mĭ-a.*** [From λευκός, "white," and αἷμα, the "blood."] Literally, "white blood." Applied by Virchow to a morbid condition of the blood, in which there is a continual increase in the colorless corpuscles, so that in some cases the number of the colorless globules is almost equal to that of the red ones. See LEUCOCYTOSIS.

Leū'çin. [**Leuci'na**; from λευκός, "white."] A white, pulverulent substance obtained from beef-fibre, etc.

Leū-çi'tis, idis.* [From λευκός, "white."] The same as SCLEROTITIS, which see.

Leū-co-car'pus.* [From λευκός, "white," and καρπός, "fruit."] Having white fruit: leucocar'pous.

Leū-co-çeph'a-lus.* [From λευκός, "white," and κεφαλή, the "head."] Having white flowers joined together in capitules.

Leū-co-çў-thæ'mĭ-a.* [From λευκός, "white," κύτος, a "cell," and αἷμα, "blood."] Sometimes applied, like *leuchæmia*, to a state of the blood in which there is a superabundance of colorless corpuscles; more properly, fatty blood in which there is a milky, opalescent appearance; white-cell blood.

Leū-co-çў-to'sis.* [From λευκός,

"white," and κύτος, a "cell."] A term applied by Virchow to a morbid condition, in which there is an increase in the colorless corpuscles of the blood, dependent (as he supposes) on an affection of the lymphatic glands. He considers *leukæmia* to be a "sort of permanent progressive *leucocytosis;*" and the latter, a "transitory process connected with fluctuating conditions in certain organs."

Leū-co-den'dron,* Leū-co-den'drum.* [From λευκός, "white," and δένδρον, a "tree."] The specific name of the *Melaleuca leucodendron.*

Leū'col. [From λευκός, "white," and *o'leum,* "oil."] A basic substance found in the naphtha of coal gas.

Leū-co-lo'mus.* [From λευκός, "white," and λῶμα, a "frame."] Bordered with white.

Leū-co'mạ, a'tis.* [From λευκός, "white."] A milky opacity of the *cornea,* the effect of an ulcer or wound, with loss of substance; the *pin* and *web.* See Albugo.

Leū-com-ạ-to'dēs.* Having *leucoma:* leucom'atous.

Leū-co-mạ-to-i'dēs.* [From *leuco'ma,* and εἶδος, a "form."] Resembling *leucoma:* leucom'atoid.

Leū-com'mạ, a*tis.** [From λευκός, "white," and ὄμμα, "appearance."] A white opacity of the cornea.

Leū-co-no'tus.* [From λευκός, "white," and νῶτος, the "back."] White on the under-surface. Applied to leaves.

Leū-co-pạ-thi'ạ.* [From λευκός, "white," and πάθος, "disease."] A disease affecting negroes, by which they become white, and termed Albinos.

Leū-co-path'ĭ-cus.* Belonging to *leucopathia.*

Leū-co-phleg'mạ-sȳ. [**Leucophlegma'sia;** from λευκός, "white," and φλέγμα, "phlegm."] A dropsical tendency, denoted by a pale, tumid, and flabby condition of body.

Leū-co-phleg-mat'ic. [**Leucophlegmat'icus.**] Belonging to leucophlegmasy.

Leū-co-phleg-mạ-to'dēs.* [From *leucophlegma'sia.*] Having leucophlegmasy.

Leū-co-phleg-mạ-to-i'dēs.* [From *leucophlegma'sia,* and εἶδος, a "form."] Resembling leucophlegmasy.

Leū-co-phȳl-la'tus,* Leū-co-phȳl'lus.* [From λευκός, "white," and φύλλον, a "leaf."] Having white leaves.

Leū-cop'ĭ-per, er*is.** [From λευκός, "white," and πέπερι, "pepper."] The *Piper album,* or white pepper. See Piper.

Leū-co-po'dĭ-us,* Leū-cop'o-dus.* [From λευκός, "white," and πούς, a "foot."] Having a white *stipes,* or white petioles.

Leū-cop'ter-us.* [From λευκός, "white," and πτερόν, a "wing."] Having white wings: leucop'terous.

Leū-co'pus, p'*odis.** The same as Leucopodius, which see.

Leū-cor-rhœ'ạ.* [From λευκός, "white," and ῥέω, to "flow."] (Fr. *Leucorrhée,* lŭh'ko'rā'.) A whitish mucous secretion of the vagina, arising from debility, or from inflammatory action; the whites; also termed *Catarrhus vaginæ,* and *Fluor albus.*

Leū-cor-rho'ĭ-cus.* Belonging to *leucorrhœa;* leucorrho'ic.

Leū-co'sis.* The formation or progress of *leucoma.*

Leū-co-sper'mus.* [From λευκός, "white," and σπέρμα, a "seed."] Having white fruit or seed: leucosper'mous.

Leū-cos'to-mus.* [From λευκός, "white," and στόμα, a "mouth."] Having a white peristome, or white mouth.

Leū-cot'ĭ-cus.* Belonging to *leucoma.*

Leukæmia. See Leuchæmia.

Levain, lęh-văng'. The French term for Ferment, which see.

Le-va'tor, o'r*is.** [From *le'vo, leva'tum,* to "raise," to "lift up."] An elevator, or lifter up. Applied to muscles.

Le'ver. [From *le'vo,* to "lift up."] A mechanical power, consisting of a rod or bar resting upon a certain determinate point, termed its *fulcrum,* which, if the object be to gain *power,* should always be nearer to the resistance to be overcome than to the force applied; but when the object is to gain *time,* the fulcrum should be nearer to the force than to the resistance. See Vectis.

Lev-ĭ-cos'tate. [**Lævicosta'tus;** from *læ'vis,* "smooth," and *cos'ta,* a "rib."] Having smooth ribs.

Lev-ĭ-fo'lĭ-ous. [**Lævifo'lius;** from *læ'vis,* "smooth," and *fo'lium,* a "leaf."] Having smooth leaves.

Lev'ĭ-gate. [**Læviga'tus;** from *læv'igo, læviga'tum,* to "smooth."] Smoothly polished.

Lev-ĭ-gā'tion. [**Læviga'tio, o'*nis;*** from the same.] The process of rubbing down any hard substance to an impalpable powder, so that no roughness or grittiness is perceptible.

Lev'ĭ-pede. [**Læ'vipes, p'*edis;***

from *læ'vis*, "smooth," and *pes*, a "foot."] Having smooth feet.

Lèvre, lĕvr or lâvr. The French term for "lip." See Labium, and Lip.

Lexipharmic. See Alexipharmic.

Ley. See Lye.

Leyden (lī'dẹn) **Bat'te-rȳ.** A number of *Leyden jars*, connected externally by being placed on tinfoil, or other good conductor, and internally by a metallic rod or wire communicating with the internal coating of each jar.

Ley'den Jar. A glass jar or bottle, coated to within a short distance from the top with tinfoil, within and without, and having a rod with a ball at the top passing through the cork to the interior coating. It is used for accumulating electricity in larger quantity than in the prime conductor.

Lī-as'ic, or **Lī-as'sic. [Lias'sicus.]** Applied to a group of strata, of which the rock which forms the type has been named *Lias* by English geologists.

Li'ber.* The interior fibrous bark of exogenous plants. It serves to convey downwards the secretions elaborated in the bark and leaves.

Lĭ-bi'do, d'inis.* [From *li'beo*, to "please," or "like."] Venereal desire.

Li'brạ.* [From λίτρα, a "silver coin," or a "pound."] A pound-weight.

Lich'en. [Lat. **Li'chen, e'nis**; Gr. λειχήν.] A Linnæan genus of the class *Cryptogamia*. Also, a disease consisting in extensive eruption of *papulæ*, usually terminating in scurf.

Li'chen Ce-tra'ri-ạ.* Iceland moss, or liverwort, now called *Cetraria Islandica*.

Li'chen Is-lan'dĭ-cạ.* The same as Lichen Cetraria.

Li'chen Roc-çel'lạ.* The herb from which *Litmus*, or *Lacmus*, is obtained; the *Roccella tinctoria*.

Li'chen Sax-at'ĭ-lis.* The *Mus'cus cra'nii huma'ni*, a plant sometimes growing on the human skull.

Lich'e-nāte. [Liche'nas, a'tis.] A combination of lichenic acid with a salifiable base.

Li-che'nēs,* the plural of Lichen, which see.

Lĭ-chen'ic. [Lichen'icus.] Belonging to lichens; applied to an acid discovered in the *Cetraria Islandica*.

Lich-e-nic'o-lus.* [From *li'chen*, and *co'lo*, to "inhabit."] That which grows upon lichens.

Li-chen-ĭ-for'mis.* [From *li'chen*.] Having the appearance of lichen: licheniform.

Lich'e-nin. [Licheni'na.] A substance obtained from the *Lichen Islandica*.

Lich-e-no-graph'ic. [Licheno-graph'icus.] Belonging to lichenography.

Lich-e-nog'rạ-phȳ. [Licheno-gra'phia; from *li'chen*, and γράφω, to "write."] A description of lichens.

Li-chen-o-i'dēs.* [From *li'chen*, and εἶδος, a "form."] Resembling a lichen: lich'enoid.

Lich-e-nol'o-ġȳ. [Lichenolo'-gia; from *li'chen*, and λόγος, a "discourse."] The part of Botany devoted to lichens.

Lich'en-ous. [Licheno'sus; from *li'chen*.] Pertaining to lichens; resembling a lichen.

Lid. See Operculum.

Lieberkü'hnii (lee-ber-ku'ne-i) **Glan'du-læ.*** ("Glands of Lieberkühn.") See Lieberkühn's Glands.

Lieberkühn's (lee'bẹr-künz') **Glands,** or **Fol'lĭ-cles. [Glan'dulæ** or **Cryp'tæ Lieberkuhnia'næ.]** The minute tubular glands of the small intestine, first described by Lieberkühn.

Li'en,* gen. **Li-e'nis.** The organ or viscus of the abdominal cavity called the spleen.

Lienomalacia,* le-en-o-mạ-la'she-ạ. [From *li'en*, the "spleen," and μαλακία, a "softening."] Morbid softening of the spleen.

Lī'en-ter-ȳ. [Liente'ria; from λεῖος, "smooth," and ἔντερον, an "intestine."] A species of *diarrhœa*, in which the food passes rapidly through the bowels undigested.

Life. [Lat. **Vi'ta**; Gr. βίος and ζωή; Fr. *Vie*, vè.] That mysterious principle existing in organized beings, whereby they are endowed with certain powers or functions peculiar to themselves, and not possessed by any form of inorganic matter. As soon as life has ceased in any animal (or plant), the matter of which this is composed, being no longer protected by the vital forces, is thenceforth subject to those laws of affinity which regulate the composition of inorganic bodies, and that combination of elements which was the result of life, gives place to new combinations, formed in obedience to the laws of chemistry. Bichat defined life to be the "aggregate of those functions which resist death."

Lig'ạ-ment. [Ligamen'tum;

from *li'go, liga'tum,* to "bind."] A peculiar, elastic, membranous substance, connecting the ends of movable bones.

Lig-a-men'ta,* the plural of *Ligamentum.* See LIGAMENT.

Ligamen'ta Sub-fla'va* ("Yellowish Ligaments"), otherwise called **Yel'low Lig'aments.** The ligaments occupying the intervals between the *vertebræ,* which thus complete the back part of the spinal canal. They are composed of dense, yellow, elastic fibres.

Lig-a-men'tous. [**Ligamento'sus;** from *ligamen'tum,* a "ligament."] Of the nature of a ligament; belonging to a ligament.

Lig'a-ments, Vag'i-nal. [**Ligamen'ta Vagina'lia.**] A term for the sheath-like ligaments of the flexor tendons of the fingers.

Ligamentum Coracoideum. See CORACOID LIGAMENT.

Li-gā'tion. [**Liga'tio, o'nis;** from *li'go, liga'tum,* to "bind."] The act of tying, or of applying a ligature, as to an artery, etc.

Lig'a-ture. [**Ligatu'ra;** from the same.] A thread of silk, flax, or other suitable material, for tying arteries, or other parts.

Light. [Lat. **Lux;** Gr. φῶς; Fr. *Lumière,* lü'me-ėR'.] The agent of vision. It is distinguished into two kinds, viz.: natural light, proceeding from the sun and stars, and artificial light, proceeding from terrestrial bodies which burn or which are strongly heated. The phenomena of light may be referred to the following heads:—

1. *Radiation,* the emission of light, or of caloric, in all directions, in the form of *radii,* or rays. A collection of such rays, passing nearly in the same direction, is termed a *pencil.* The radiant point is the point from which diverging rays proceed; the *focus,* the point to which converging rays are collected.

2. *Reflection,* the rebound of a ray of light, or of caloric, from a polished surface: the angle of incidence being equal to the angle of reflection.

3. *Refraction,* the *break* of the natural course of a ray of light as it passes into a transparent substance, as glass, or water; this is termed *ordinary refraction.* If a ray fall upon the surface of Iceland spar, or certain other substances, it will be split into two portions, making an angle with each other, and each pursuing its own separate course; this is called *double refraction,*—one of these rays following the same rule as if the substance were glass or water, the other undergoing *extraordinary refraction.*

Ligne, lėñ. The French term for "line." See LINEA.

Ligne Blanche, lėñ blŏNsh. The French term for LINEA ALBA, which see.

Lig'ne-ous. [**Lig'neus;** from *lig'num,* "wood."] (Fr. *Ligneux,* lėn'yuh'.) Of the nature of wood; resembling wood; woody.

Lig-nif'er-ous. [**Lignif'erus;** from *lig'num,* "wood," and *fe'ro,* to "bear."] Bearing wood.

Lig'nĭ-form. [**Lignifor'mis;** from *lig'num,* "wood."] Resembling wood.

Lig'nin, or **Lig'nĭne.** [**Ligni'na;** from the same.] The woody fibre constituting the fibrous structure of vegetable substances, the most abundant principle in plants.

Lig'nous. [**Ligno'sus;** from the same.] Wooden, or like wood; woody.

Lig'num.* A Latin word signifying "wood," used in medicine chiefly in such phrases as *Lignum Quassiæ, Lignum Vitæ,* etc. See WOOD.

Lig'num Cam-pe-chi-a'num.* ("Campeachy Wood.") See HÆMATOXYLON.

Lig'num Col-u-bri'num.* ("Snake Wood.") Another name for the ARISTOLOCHIA SERPENTARIA.

Lig'num In'dĭ-cum.* ("Indian Wood.") The wood of the *Hæmatoxylon Campechianum.*

Lignum Quassiæ. See QUASSIA.

Lig'num Vi'tæ.* ("Wood of Life.") The wood of *Guaiacum officinale.* See GUAIACI LIGNUM.

Lig'u-la.* [As if *lin'gula,* diminutive of *lin'gua,* a "tongue."] A little tongue. The tongue of the *Crustacea, Arachnides,* and *Insecta.*

Lig'u-late. [**Ligula'tus;** from *lig'ula,* a "little tongue," also, a "strap."] Strap-shaped.

Lig'ule. [**Lig'ula,** a "little tongue," or "strap."] A strap-shaped corolla.

Lig-u-lif'er-us.* [From *lig'ula,* a "little tongue," and *fe'ro,* to "bear."] Bearing ligules.

Lig-u-lĭ-flo'rus.* [From *lig'ula,* a "little tongue," and *flos,* a "flower."] Having ligulated corollas.

Lig-u-lĭ-fo'lĭ-us.* [From *lig'ula,* a "little tongue," and *fo'lium,* a "leaf."] Having linear leaves.

Lig'u-lĭ-form. [**Ligulifor'mis;** from *lig'ula,* a "little tongue."] Like a ligulated corolla.

Lil'ĭ-a,* the plural of **Lil'ĭ-um,** forming the Jussieuan name of a natural order of plants. See LILIACEÆ.

Liliaceæ,* lil-e-a'she-ē. [From *Lil'ium,* one of the genera.] A large natural order of endogenous plants, natives of many tropical and temperate regions. It includes the lily, tulip, hyacinth, asparagus, onion, and other plants prized for beauty or utility. Among the products of this order are aloes, squills, and New Zealand flax. Several species are used as purgatives or emetics.

Lil-ĭ-ā'ceous. [**Lilia'ceus;** from *lil'ium,* a "lily."] Resembling the lily, or *Liliaceæ.*

Lil-ĭ-ĭ-flo'rus.* [From *lil'ium,* a "lily," and *flos,* a "flower."] Having flowers resembling the lily.

Lil-ĭ-ĭ-for'mis.* [From *lil'ium,* a "lily."] Having the form of a lily.

Lil'ĭ-um.* The lily. A Linnæan genus of the class *Hexandria,* natural order *Liliaceæ.*

Lim. = *Limo'nes.** "Lemons."

Limaçon, lè'mâ'sòNᵍ'. The French term for COCHLEA, which see.

Lim-a-tu'ra.* [From *li'ma,* a "file."] The filings of a metal.

Limatu'ra Fer'ri.* ("Filings of Iron," or "Iron Filings.") A preparation used as a mild chalybeate.

Limb. [From *lim'bus,* a "border"?] One of the extremities of an animal, as a leg, or arm. Applied in Botany to the blade or lamina of a petal, a sepal, etc.; the expanded part of a corolla, or calyx.

Lim'bate. [From the same.] Bordered.

Lim-bif'er-us.* [From *lim'bus,* a "border," and *fe'ro,* to "bear."] Having a border, or margin.

Lime. [Lat. **Calx, Cal'cis;** Fr. *Chaux,* shō.] Oxide of calcium; one of the primitive earths, abundant in nature, but always united to an acid, most frequently the carbonic.

Lime. [**Li'mon, o'nis.**] The fruit of the *Citrus limetta,* or *Citrus limonum.*

Lime, Chlo'ride of. A compound of chlorine and lime, much used as a disinfecting agent. For this purpose, one pound may be dissolved in, or mixed with, six gallons of water.

Lime'stone. [**La'pis Calca'reus.**] Carbonate of lime; one of the most abundant and most important of stratified rocks.

Lime-Water. See LIQUOR CALCIS

Lim'ĭ-cus.* [From λιμός, "hunger."] Belonging to hunger.

Lim-ĭ-for'mis.* [From *li'ma,* a "file."] Having the appearance of a file.

Lim-no-me-phi'tis, idis.* [From λίμνη, a "stagnant pool," or "marsh," and *mephi'tis,* a "stink;" a "strong, heavy smell."] Marsh-miasm, or the effluvia arising from vegetable matter in a putrescent state, as in moist or marshy ground.

Lim-no-pol'ў-pus.* [From λίμνη, a "stagnant pool," or "marsh," and πολύπους, a "polypus."] Applied in the plural masculine (*Limnopol'ypi*) to a family of the *Pol'ypi brachios'toma.*

Li'mon,* gen. **Li-mo'nis.** The Pharmacopœial name for the fruit of the *Ci'trus limo'num;* and of the *Ci'trus med'ica.*

Li-mo'nēs,* gen. **Li-mo'num,** the plural of LIMON, which see.

Li-mo'nis Cor'tex.* ("Rind of Lemon," or "Lemon-Peel.") The Pharmacopœial name ‖ for the rind of the fruit of the *Citrus limonum.*

Limo'nis Suc'cus.* ("Lemon-juice.") The name applied to the juice of the fruit of the *Citrus limonum.* It has been placed on the primary list of the Materia Medica of the U.S. Pharmacopœia for 1860.

Li-mo'num Cor'tex.* ("Rind of Lemons.") The Pharmacopœial name (Lond. and Ed. Ph.) for the fresh and dry exterior rind of the fruit of the *Citrus limonum.*

Li-moph'thĭ-sis.* [From λιμός, "hunger," "famine," and φθίσις, a "wasting."] *Tabes,* or wasting, from privation of food.

Lim-op-so'ra.* [From λιμός, "famine," and ψώρα, "scabies."] A kind of *scabies* which attacks man and the lower animals from long privation of food.

Li-mo'sis.* [From λιμός, "famine."] Morbid appetite. A genus of diseases characterized by depraved, excessive, or defective appetite.

Lim-o-thĕr-a-pi'a.* [From λιμός, "hunger," and θεραπεία, the "system of healing."] The treatment of disease by abstinence.

Li'mous, or **Li-mose'.** [**Limo'sus;** from *li'mus,* "mud," "clay," "slime."] Applied to plants growing in muddy soils. Sometimes applied to soil or strata composed of mud, argillaceous marl, or sand, either separate or combined.

Linaceæ,* li-na'she-ē. [From *Li'num,* one of the genera.] A small natural order of exogenous plants, natives of

Europe, Africa, etc. It includes *Linum* (flax). The chief characters of this order are the tenacity of the fibres and the mucilage of the seeds.

Lin-a-go'gus.* [From λίνον, a "flaxen thread," and ἄγω, to "lead."] An instrument used in the operation for vesico-vaginal fistula.

Linamentum. See LINT.

Linc'tus.* [From *lin'go, linc'tum*, to "lick," or "lap."] A *looch* (or *lohoch*), or electuary; any medicine licked off the spoon because of its adhesive consistence.

Line. See LINEA.

Lin'e-a,* plural **Lin'e-æ.** [From *li'num*, a "thread."] A line, or thread; the twelfth part of an inch. In Geometry, that which has length without breadth.

Lin'ea Al'ba.* ("White Line.") (Fr. *Ligne Blanche*, lēñ blōnsh.) The central tendinous line extending from the ensiform cartilage to the pubes.

Lin'ea As'per-a.* ("Rough Line.") A rough prominence observed along the posterior surface of the femur.

Lin'ea In-nom-i-na'ta.* Literally, the "unnamed line." An elevated line forming a part of the brim of the pelvis.

Lin'e-æ Al-bi-can'tēs.* ("Whitish Lines.") Applied to certain shining reddish and whitish lines on the abdomen, extending from the groins and pubes to the navel, sometimes occurring in women during the first three or four days after delivery.

Lin'eæ Sem-i-lu-na'rēs.* ("Semilunar Lines.") The lines which bound the exterior margin of the *recti* muscles of the abdomen.

Lin'eæ Trans-ver'sæ.* ("Transverse Lines.") The lines which cross the *recti* muscles; also applied to some fibres which run across the raphe of the *corpus callosum*.

Lin'e-ar. [**Linea'ris;** from *lin'ea*, a "line."] (Fr. *Linéaire*, lè'nà'èr'.) Disposed in lines; pertaining to, or in the form of, a line. In Botany, narrow, and much longer than broad, with parallel margins, as a leaf of grass.

Lin-e-ar-i-fo'li-us.* [From *linea'ris*, "linear," and *fo'lium*, a "leaf."] Having linear leaves.

Lin'e-ate. [**Linea'tus;** from *lin'ea*, a "line."] Marked with lines; streaked.

Lin-e-at-i-fo'li-us.* [From *linea'tus*, "linear," and *fo'lium*, a "leaf."] Having leaves of which the nervures run parallel from base to apex.

Li-ne'o-la.* [Diminutive of *lin'ea*, a "line."] Applied to certain small white lines sometimes seen on the female breast.

Lin'e-o-late. [**Lineola'tus;** from *line'ola*, a "little line."] Marked with fine or obscure lines.

Lin'gual. [**Lingua'lis;** from *lin'gua*, a "tongue."] Belonging to the tongue.

Lin-gui-fo'li-us.* [From *lin'gua*, a "tongue," and *fo'lium*, a "leaf."] Having linguiform leaves.

Lin'gui-form. [**Linguifor'mis;** from *lin'gua*, a "tongue."] Formed like a tongue.

Lin'gu-la.* [Diminutive of *lin'gua*, a "tongue."] A little tongue; a latchet.

Lin'gu-late. [**Lingula'tus;** from *lin'gula*, a "little tongue."] Having a little tongue; tongue-shaped.

Li'ni,* the genitive of LINUM, which see.

Li'ni Fa-ri'na.* ("Meal of Flaxseed," or "Flaxseed Meal.") The Pharmacopœial name (Br. Ph.) for meal of the seeds of *Linum usitatissimum*, deprived of their fixed oil by expression: lintseed meal. It has been placed on the primary list of the Materia Medica of the U.S. Pharmacopœia for 1860.

Li'ni Se'men.* ("Seed of Flax.") The Pharmacopœial name (Brit. Ph.) for flaxseed, lintseed, or linseed.

Li'ni Sem'i-na.* ("Seeds of Flax.") The Pharmacopœial name (Br. Ph.) for the seeds of *Linum usitatissimum*.

Liniment. See LINIMENTUM.

Lin-i-men'ta,* the plural of LINIMENTUM, which see.

Lin-i-men'tum,* plural **Lin-i-men'ta.** [From *li'no*, to "anoint."] A thin ointment: a lin'iment.

Linimen'tum Am-mo'ni-æ.* ("Liniment of Ammonia.") Take of water of ammonia, a fluidounce; olive oil, two troyounces. Mix them.

Linimen'tum Căl'cis.* ("Liniment of Lime," or "Lime Liniment.") Take of solution of lime, eight fluidounces; flaxseed oil, seven troyounces. Mix them.

Linimen'tum Cam'pho-ræ.* ("Liniment of Camphor.") Take of camphor, three troyounces; olive oil, twelve troyounces. Dissolve the camphor in the oil.

Linimen'tum Can-thăr'i-dis.* ("Liniment of Cantharides.") Take of cantharides, in fine powder, a troyounce; oil of turpentine, half a pint. Digest the cantharides with the oil for three hours in a close vessel, by means of a water-bath, and strain.

Linimen'tum Chlo-ro-for'mi.* ("Liniment of Chloroform.") Take of purified chloroform, three troyounces; olive oil, four troyounces. Mix them.

Linimen'tum Sa-po'nis.* ("Liniment of Soap," or "Soap Liniment.") *Tinctura Saponis Camphorata*, Pharm., 1850. Take of soap, in shavings, four troyounces; camphor, two troyounces; oil of rosemary, half a fluidounce; water, four fluidounces; alcohol, two pints. Mix the alcohol and water, digest the soap with the mixture by means of a water-bath until it is dissolved; then filter, and, having added the camphor and oil, mix the whole thoroughly together.

Linimen'tum Tĕr-e-bin'thĭ-næ.* ("Liniment of Turpentine.") Take of resin cerate, twelve troyounces; oil of turpentine, half a pint. Add the oil to the cerate previously melted, and mix them.

Lin-næ'an. Belonging to Linnæus, the naturalist. In Botany, the Linnæan, or sexual, system, is founded on the number of stamens which determines the primary divisions, or Classes; the subdivisions, or Orders, generally depend on the number of pistils. The term is applied in a more general sense to a system of arranging the productions of the animal, vegetable, and mineral kingdoms laid down by Linnæus.

Lin-o-sper'mum.* [From λίνον, "flax," and σπέρμα, "seed."] Linseed, or lintseed, afforded by the *Linum usitatissimum*. See LINI SEMEN.

Linseed. See LINTSEED.

Lint. [**Lin'teum;** from *li'num*, "flax."] (Fr. *Charpie*, shar'pè'.) A soft material made by scraping old linen cloth, and used as a dressing in all cases of wounds, ulcers, etc.

Lin-te-ĭ-for'mis.* [From *lin'teum*, "lint."] Having the appearance or texture of lint: lin'teiform.

Lint'seed. The seeds of *Linum usitatissimum*. See LINI SEMEN, or LINI SEMINA.

Li'num,* gen. **Li'ni.** [From λίνον, "flax."] A Linnæan genus of the class *Pentandria*, natural order *Linaceæ*. Also, the Pharmacopœial name (U.S. Ph.) for the seed of the *Li'num usitatis'simum.*

Li'num Ca-thar'tĭ-cum.* The Pharmacopœial name (Ed. Ph.) of the purging flax.

Lip. (Fr. *Lèvre*, lĕvr or låvr.) See LABIUM, and LABRUM.

Lip'a-ro-çēle.* [From λιπαρός, "fat," and κήλη, a "tumor."] A fatty tumor in the *scrotum.*

Lip-a-ro'dēs.* [From λιπαρός, "fat," or "obese."] Full of fat; obese.

Lip-a-ro-dȳsp-nœ'a.* [From λιπαρός, "fat," and δύσπνοια, "difficult breathing."] *Dyspnœa* caused by obesity.

Lip-a-ro-i'dēs.* [From λιπαρός, "fat," or "obese," and εἶδος, a "form."] Resembling fat.

Lip-a-rom'pha-lus.* [From λιπαρός, "fat," and ὀμφαλός, the "navel."] A fatty tumor at the *umbilicus.*

Lip-a-ro-scir'rhus.* [From λιπαρός, "fat," and σκίῤῥος, "incipient cancer."] A fatty, scirrhous tumor.

Lipocele. See LIPAROCELE.

Lĭ-po'ma,* plural **Lĭ-pom'a-ta.** [From λίπος, "fat."] A species of fatty tumor.

Lĭ-pom-a-to'dēs.* [From *lipo'ma*, a "fatty tumor."] Resembling *lipoma;* conjoined with *lipoma.*

Lĭ-pom-a-to-i'dēs.* [From *lipo'ma*, a "fatty tumor," and εἶδος, a "form."] Resembling *lipoma:* lipom'atoid.

Lipomphalus. See LIPAROMPHALUS.

Lip-o-scir'rhus.* [From λίπος, "fat," and σκίῤῥος, "incipient cancer."] The same as LIPAROSCIRRHUS, which see.

Lĭ-po'sis.* [From λίπος, "fat."] The progressive accumulation of fat.

Lip-o-sphȳx'ĭ-a.* [From λείπω, to "fail," and σφύξις, the "pulse."] Absence, or cessation, of the pulse.

Lipothymia. See LEIPOTHYMIA.

Lip'pĭ-tude. [**Lippitu'do, dinis;** from *lip'pus*, "blear-eyed."] A raw, tumid state of the margin of the eyelids, from which a puriform humor exudes.

Liq. = *Li'quor.** See LIQUOR.

Liquatio (le-qua'she-o), **o'***nis.** [From *li'quo, liqua'tum*, to "melt."] Strictly, the same as FUSION; also, LIQUEFACTION.

Liq-ue-fā'cients. [From *liquefa'cio*, to "melt."] Agents which augment the secretions, arrest the solidifying, and promote the liquefying processes of the animal economy.

Liq-ue-fac'tion. [**Liquefac'tio, o'***nis;* from *liquefa'cio, liquefac'tum*, to "make liquid."] The conversion of a solid into a liquid.

Liqueur (Fr.), lè'kur'. A spirituous liquor composed of water, alcohol, sugar, and some aromatic infusion extracted from fruits, seeds, etc.

Liq'uid. [**Liq'uidum;** from *liq'uidus*, "liquid," "moist."] Any substance, not aeriform, which is fluid, like water.

Liq-uid-am'bar.* [From *liq'uidus*, "liquid," and *am'ber;* so called because the tree yields on incision a fluid, amber-like substance.] A genus of plants, several species of which afford a fragrant resin, called storax.

Liquiritia,* lik-we-rish'e-ạ. Liquorice. See GLYCYRRHIZA.

Li'quor,* gen. **Li-quo'ris,** nominative plural **Li-quo'rēs.** [From *li'queo*, to "become liquid." (Fr. *Liqueur*, lè'-KUR'.) A term applied to many liquids, particularly those composed chiefly of water, or of alcohol. As a Pharmacopœial term it signifies "solution."

Liquor Aluminis Compositus. See BATES'S ALUM-WATER.

Li'quor Am-mo'nĭ-æ.* ("Liquor of Ammonia.") A solution of ammoniacal gas in water; otherwise called *Aqua Ammoniæ* ("Water of Ammonia").

Liquor Ammoniæ Acetatis. See MINDERERI SPIRITUS.

Li'quor Am'nĭ-i.* ("Liquor of the Amnion.") The watery fluid in which the fœtus is suspended. See AMNION.

Li'quor Ar-sen-ĭ-ca'lis.* ("Arsenical Liquor.") A Pharmacopœial preparation, also called *Fowler's Solution*, and *Tasteless Ague Drop*, consisting of arseniate of potash dissolved in water, and flavored and colored by spirit of lavender. This has been recommended as a remedy in intermittents, and has been found very useful in *lepra* and other inveterate cutaneous affections.

Li'quor Căl'cis,* otherwise called **A'qua Cal'cis.*** ("Water of Lime," or "Lime-Water.") A saturated solution of lime in water. It may be prepared by pouring upon some freshly slacked lime a quantity of pure water. In a few hours, the solution will become clear by the settling of such particles of lime as are not dissolved by the water. The solution, with the undissolved lime, should be kept in a well-stopped bottle; pour off the clear liquid as it is wanted for use. The U.S. Pharmacopœia directs the preparation to be made in the proportion of four ounces of lime to eight pints of water. But if the lime be in excess, no disadvantage can result; the superfluous portion will, in that case, simply remain undissolved.

Lime-water is antacid, tonic, and astringent. Mixed with an equal quantity of milk, which completely covers its offensive taste, it often proves an excellent remedy for nausea and vomiting dependent on irritability of the stomach. It may be employed with great advantage in dyspepsia accompanied with acidity of the stomach, as well as in some forms of diarrhœa, and in calculous affections attended with a superabundant secretion of uric acid. Externally, it is often used as a wash in *porrigo* and similar affections, and as an application to foul ulcers.

Liquor Morgagni. See MORGAGNI, LIQUOR.

Li'quor Po-tas'sæ Ar-se-ni'tis.* ("Liquor of the Arsenite of Potash.") The Pharmacopœial name (Lond. and Dub. Ph.) for the LIQUOR ARSENICALIS, which see.

Li'quor San'guĭ-nis.* ("Liquor of the Blood.") The colorless fluid which holds the globules of the blood in suspension during life.

Li'quor Sil'ĭ-cum.* ("Liquor of Flints.") See GLASS, SOLUBLE.

Li-quo'rēs,* the plural of LIQUOR, which see.

Liquorice, lik'or-ĭss. [**Liquiri'tia.**] See GLYCYRRHIZA.

Lir-ĭ-o-den'dron.* [From λείριον, a "lily," a "tulip" (?) and δένδρον, a "tree."] A Linnæan genus of the class *Polyandria*, natural order *Magnoliaceæ.* Also, the Pharmacopœial name (U.S. Ph.) for the bark of *Lirioden'dron tulipif'era.*

Lisp'ing. A species of *psellismus*, or defective enunciation, commonly called speaking through the teeth, and produced by an abnormal length of tongue, or by affectation.

Lith'ạ-gogue. [**Lithago'gus;** from λίθος, a "stone," and ἄγω, to "carry off," to "expel."] Having power to expel calculi from the bladder or kidneys.

Lith'arge. [**Lithar'gyrum, Lithar'gyrus;** from λίθος, a "stone," and ἄργυρος, "silver;" so named from its being obtained from an ore (or stone) containing lead and silver.] An oxide of lead imperfectly vitrified.

Lith'āte. [**Li'thas,** *atis.*] A combination of lithic acid with a base. See URATE.

Lith-ec'tạ-sy̆. [**Lithecta'sia;** from λίθος, a "stone," and ἐκτείνω, to "extend."] The operation of removing calculi of moderate size through the urethra, by first extending or dilating it.

Lith'ĭ-ạ.* [From λίθος, a "stone."] The protoxide of lithium, an alkali discovered in 1818.

Lith'ia.* [From the same.] The

name of a genus in Dr. Good's Nosology, comprising the different species of urinary calculus. See LITHIASIS.

Lith'ĭ-æ Car-bo'nas.* ("Carbonate of Lithia.") A white powder sparingly soluble in water, and having a feeble alkaline reaction. It has been placed on the primary list of the Materia Medica of the U.S. Pharmacopœia for 1860. It is recommended as a remedy in calculous diseases.

Lĭ-thi'ạ-sis.* [From the same.] The formation of stone, or urinary calculus. Also, a disease of the eyelids, in which small hard tumors grow upon their margins.

Lith'ic. [**Lith'icus;** from the same.] Applied to an acid obtained from calculi and urine. See URIC.

Lith'ĭ-cạ.* [From the same.] Medicines which counteract the predisposition to the formation of calculous concretions in the urinary organs.

Lith'ĭ-um.* The metallic base of lithia.

Lith-o-çe-no'sis.* [From λίθος, a "stone," and κένωσις, an "evacuation."] The removal or extraction of the fragments of a calculus broken in the operation of lithotrity.

Lith-o-çe-not'ĭ-cus.* Belonging to *lithocenosis*.

Lith'o-clast, or **Lith'o-claste.** [From λίθος, a "stone," and κλαστάω, to "break."] An instrument introduced through the urethra for the purpose of reducing calculi to small fragments in the bladder.

Lith-o-dec-ta'sĭ-ạ.* [From λίθος, a "stone," ὁδός, a "passage," or "way," and ἔκτασις, an "extension."] The same as LITHECTASY, which see.

Lĭ-tho'dēs.* [From λίθος, a "stone."] Full of calculi; of the nature of calculi.

Lith-o-dĭ-a'lĭ-ạ,* or **Lith-o-dĭ-al'ȳ-sis.*** [From λίθος, a "stone," and διαλύω, to "dissolve."] A dissolving of stone or calculus in the bladder.

Lith-o-dȳsp-nœ'ạ.* [From λίθος, a "stone," and δύσπνοια, "difficult breathing."] Calculous *dyspnœa*, or difficult breathing caused by calcareous concretions in the lungs or other air-passages.

Lithœcius,* lith-e'she-us. [From λίθος, a "stone," and οἶκος, a "habitation."] Growing upon stones.

Lith-o-fel-lĭ'nus.* [From λίθος, a "stone," and *fel*, the "bile."] Pertaining to a gall-stone or biliary calculus. See CHOLOLITHIC.

Lith-o-ġen'e-sȳ. [**Lithogene'sia;** from λίθος, a "stone," and γένεσις, "generation."] The science which treats of the origin and formation of minerals.

Lĭ-thog'rạ-phȳ. [**Lithogra'phia;** from λίθος, a "stone," and γράφω, to "engrave," or to "write."] Engraving on stone. The art by which impressions or prints are obtained from drawings made on calcareous stone.

Lith'oid. [**Lithoi'des;** from λίθος, a "stone," and εἶδος, a "form."] Resembling stone.

Lĭ-thol'o-ġȳ. [**Litholo'gia;** from λίθος, a "stone," and λόγος, a "discourse."] A treatise on stones; the science which treats of the nature or properties of stones, or of calculi.

Lith-o-me'trạ.* [From λίθος, a "stone," and μήτρα, the "womb."] A term for ossification of the uterus.

Lithontriptic. See LITHOTRIPTIC.

Lĭ-thoph'ĭ-lus.* [From λίθος, a "stone," and φιλέω, to "lŏve."] Growing upon rocks or stony places.

Lith'o-phȳte. [**Lithoph'yton;** from λίθος, a "stone," and φύτον, a "plant."] Certain productions having the qualities both of stone and plant, as corals; also, *Polypi* that have an interior stony axis.

Lith-o-sco'pĭ-um.* [From λίθος, a "stone," and σκοπέω, to "examine."] An instrument for ascertaining the size and form of a calculus; a lith'oscope.

Lith-o-sper'mus.* [From λίθος, a "stone," and σπέρμα, a "seed."] Having fruit hard and like stones: lithospermous.

Lĭ-thot'o-mȳ. [**Lithoto'mia;** from λίθος, a "stone," and τέμνω, to "cut."] (Fr. *Taille*, tăl.) The operation of cutting into the bladder to withdraw a stone or calculus: cystot'omy.

Lith-o-tre'sis.* [From λίθος, a "stone," and τρῆσις, a "perforation."] The same, nearly, as LITHOTRITY.

Lith'o-trip-sȳ. [**Lithotrip'sia;** from λίθος, a "stone," and τρίβω, to "wear by friction."] The operation of rubbing down calculi in the bladder by means of a lithotriptor.

Lith-o-trip'tic. [**Lithotrip'ticus;** from the same.] Applied to medicines that tend to counteract the formation of calculi.

Lith-o-trip'tor, o'ris.* [From the same.] An instrument for crushing calculi in the bladder into fragments so minute that they may pass the urethra.

Lĭ-thot'rĭ-tor, o'ris.* [From λίθος, a "stone," and *te'ro*, *tri'tum*, to "rub," to "break."] The same as LITHOTRIPTOR.

Li-thot'ri-tÿ. [From the same.] The operation of breaking a stone or calculus in pieces by means of the *lithoclaste.*

Li-thox'ÿ-lum.* [From λίθος, a "stone," and ξύλον, "wood."] Fossil, or petrified, wood.

Lith-u-re'sis.* [From λίθος, a "stone," and οὖρον, the "urine."] The passing of small calculi with the urine.

Lith-u-ror-rhœ'a.* [From λίθος, a "stone," οὖρον, the "urine," and ῥέω, to "flow."] Calculous diabetes.

Lit'mus,* or **Lac'mus.*** A test, of a bluish color, obtained from the *Croton tinctorium* and the *Lichen roccella.*

LIT'MUS PA'PER is prepared by digesting powdered litmus in water, and painting with it white paper which is free from alum.

Litra. The same as LIBRA.

Litre, lē'tẹr or lētR. A French measure, equal to 61.028 English cubic inches, or 0.22 of an imperial gallon.

Lit'to-ral. [**Littora'lis;** from *lit'tus, lit'toris,* the "shore."] Applied to plants that grow on the banks or shores of waters, chiefly of rivers and lakes. Written also LITORAL.

Liv'er. [Lat. **Je'cur,** or **He'par;** Gr. ἧπαρ; Fr. *Foie,* fwå.] The gland whose office it is to secrete the bile. It is situated on the right side of the abdominal cavity, immediately below the diaphragm, and is divided into three lobes, the right lobe, the left lobe, and the inferior or lesser lobe, also called the *Lobulus Spigelii.* The liver is the largest gland in the body.

Liver, Inflammation of the. See HEPATITIS.

Liver-Wort. See HEPATICA.

Liver-Wort, Iceland. See CETRARIA ISLANDICA.

Li'vor, o'ris.* [From *li'veo,* to "grow black and blue."] The mark of a blow; lividness.

Lix,* gen. **Li'cis.** Lye, or water impregnated with the alkali of wood-ashes.

Lix-iv'i-al. [**Lixivia'lis.**] Belonging to a lixivium.

Lix-iv'i-āt-ed. [**Lixivia'tus;** from *lixiv'ium,* "lye."] Having undergone lixiviation.

Lix-iv'i-ā'tion. [**Lixivia'tio;** from *lixiv'ium,* "lye."] The process of dissolving an alkali or a salt in water or other fluid, to form a lixivium.

Lix-iv'i-um.* [From *lix,* "lye."] A liquid impregnated with an alkali, or a salt; lye.

Lixiv'ium Sap-o-na'ri-um.* The *Liquor potassæ,* or solution of potash.

Load'stone. [**Mag'nes.**] A species of iron ore which has the peculiar properties of attracting iron and of turning towards the magnetic pole of the earth when freely suspended.

Loasaceæ,* lo-a-sa'she-ē. [From *Loasa,* one of the genera.] A natural order of exogenous herbaceous plants, natives of America.

Lo'bate. [**Loba'tus;** from *lo'bus,* a "lobe."] Lobed. Having lobes, as the lungs, liver, leaves, tumors, etc.

Lobe. [Lat. **Lo'bus;** Gr. λοβός.] Applied to parts of certain viscera, more or less distinct from the rest, and to the lower part of the external ear. In Botany, any division, or projecting part, of an organ, especially a rounded one.

Lobed. See LOBATUS.

Lo-be'li-a.* [From *Lo'bel,* a botanist.] A Linnæan genus of the class *Monadelphia,* natural order *Lobeliaceæ.* Also, the Pharmacopœial name ‖ of the herb of *Lobelia inflata.* Lobelia is emetic, and in small doses diaphoretic and expectorant.

Lobe'lia In-fla'ta.* The systematic name of the plant called Indian Tobacco.

Lobeliaceæ,* lo-be-le-a'she-ē. A natural order of exogenous plants, found in many warm and temperate regions. It includes the *Lobelia inflata,* a powerful emetic, and several poisonous plants.

Lo-be-li-ā'ceous. [**Lobelia'ceus.**] Resembling the lobelia.

Lob'e-lin. [**Lobeli'na.**] The active, volatile, organic base obtained from *Lobelia inflata,* by macerating the herb in alcohol, previously prepared with sulphuric acid and powdered caustic lime.

Lo-bi'o-lus.* [Diminutive of *lo'bus,* a "lobe."] Applied to the small segments at the edges of the *thallus* of lichens, when their form approaches that of leaves.

Lob'u-lar. [**Lobula'ris;** from *lob'ulus,* a "lobule."] Belonging to a lobule; shaped like a lobe or lobule.

Lob'u-late. [From the same.] Bearing or having small lobes. Applied to leaves.

Lob'u-li,* the plural of LOBULUS.

Lob'uli Tes'tis.* ("Lobules of the Testicle.") The lobules formed by the convolutions of the *tubuli seminiferi* of the testis.

Lob'u-lus,* plural **Lob'u-li.** [Diminutive of *lo'bus,* a "lobe."] A lob'ule.

Lob'u-lus Ac-ces-so'rĭ-us,* **Lob'-ulus A-non'y̆-mus,*** or **Lob'ulus Quad-ra'tus.*** A small lobe on the under-surface of the liver, forming the anterior point of the right lobe; otherwise that space of the great lobe between the *fossa* of the umbilical vein and gall-bladder, extending to the anterior margin.

Lob'ulus Cau-da'tus.* A tail-like process of the liver, stretching downward from the middle of the great right lobe to the *Lobulus Spigelii.*

Lob'ulus Spi-ge'lĭ-i.* ("Lobule of Spigelius.") The inferior, or smallest, lobe of the liver, first particularly described by Spigelius.

Lo'ca,* gen. **Lo-co'rum,** the plural of Locus.

Lo'cal. [**Loca'lis;** from *lo'cus,* a "place."] Belonging to a place or part; limited to a particular place. See Topical.

Lo-ca'lēs.* [Plural of *loca'lis,* "local."] Local diseases. Applied to a class of Cullen's Nosology.

Lo-cel'late. [From *locel'lus,* a "little cell."] Having secondary cells.

Loch. See Linctus.

Lo-chi'a,* or **Lo'chĭ-a,** *o'rum.** [Gr. λοχεῖα or λόχια, from λοχός, a "lying in," or "confinement," also the discharge after childbirth.] (Fr. *Suites de Couches,* swēt deh koosh.) The serous discharge from the uterus and vagina after delivery; the cleansings.

Lo-chĭ-op'y̆-ra.* [From λοχεῖος, "pertaining to childbed," and πῦρ, a "fever."] Puerperal or childbed fever.

Lo-chĭ-or-rha'gĭ-a.* [From λοχεῖα, or λόχια, the discharge after childbirth, and ῥήγνυμι, to "burst forth."] An excessive flow of the *lochia.*

Lo-chĭ-or-rhœ'a.* [From λοχεῖα, or λόχια, "childbirth," the "lochia," and ῥέω, to "flow."] A more than natural discharge of the *lochia.*

Lo-chĭ-os'che-sis.* [From λοχεῖα, "childbirth," and σχέσις, "holding," or "retention."] Retention or stoppage of the *lochia.*

Loch-o-cac-o-col'pĭ-a.* [From λοχός, "confinement," κακός, "evil," and κόλπος, a "sinus."] Puerperal putridity or disease of the vulva.

Loch-o-do-chi'um.* [From λοχός, "confinement," and δοχεῖον, a "receptacle."] A lying-in hospital.

Loch-o-me-tri'tis, idis.* [From λοχός, "confinement," and *metri'tis,* "inflammation of the womb."] Puerperal *metritis.*

Loch-o-pĕr-ĭ-to-ni'tis, *idis,** or **Loch-o-pĕr-ĭ-to-ne-i'tis.*** [From λοχός, "confinement," and *peritoni'tis.*] Inflammation of the peritonæum in childbed.

Lo-chop'y̆-ra.* [From λοχός, "confinement," and πῦρ, a "fever."] Puerperal fever.

Loch-o-ty'phus.* [From λοχός, "confinement," and τῦφος, "stupor."] Contagious puerperal fever; puerperal typhus.

Lo'çi,* gen. **Lo-co'rum,** the plural of Locus, which see.

Lock Hos'pĭ-tal. A general name, in Great Britain, for a hospital for the treatment of venereal diseases.

Locked Jaw. See Tetanus.

Lo-co-mo'tion. [**Locomo'tio,** *o'nis;* from *lo'cus,* a "place," and *mo'veo, mo'tum,* to "move."] The act or power of moving from place to place.

Loc'u-la-ment. [**Loculamen'-tum;** from *loc'ulus,* a "cell," "box," or "case."] A cell of an ovary.

Loc-u-lam-en-to'sus.* [From *loculamen'tum.*] Having loculaments, or cells.

Loc'u-lar. [**Locula'ris;** from *loc'-ulus,* a "box," or "case."] Divided into cells or cavities; pertaining to a cell.

Loc-u-la'tus.* [From the same.] Having loculi: loculate.

Loc'u-li,* the plural of Loculus.

Loc-u-lĭ-cī'dal. [**Loculici'dus;** from *loc'ulus,* a "cell," or "box," and *cæ'do,* to "cut," to "cut through."] Opening or breaking directly into the back of a cell.

Loc'u-lus,* plural **Loc'u-li.** [Diminutive of *lo'cus,* a "place."] A locule: a name for a cell of the ovary (or anther) of a plant; also applied to any small cavity.

Lo'cus,* gen. **Lo'çi,** plural **Lo'ci** and **Lo'ca.** A place; a topic.

Lo'cus Ni'ger.* ("Black Place.") A quantity of dark-colored matter in the centre of the *Crura cerebri,* or limbs of the brain.

Lo-cus'ta.* A spikelet or flower-cluster of grasses.

Lœmia. See Loimia.

Lœmology. See Loimology.

Log'wood. The wood of the *Hæmatox'ylon Campechia'num.*

Lo'hoch. The same as Looch. See Eclegma.

Loi'mĭ-a.* [From λοιμός, the "plague."] The plague, or other epidemic disease.

Loi'mic. [**Loi'micus;** from the same.] Belonging to the plague, or to epidemic disease.

Loi-mo'dēs.* [From the same.] Like the plague; pestilential.

Loi-mog'ra-phy̆. [**Loimogra'-phia;** from λοιμός, the "plague," and γράφω, to "write."] A description, or history, of the plague.

Loi-mo-i'dēs.* [From λοιμός, the "plague," and εἶδος, a "form."] Resembling the *pestis*, or plague: loi'moid.

Loi-mol'o-ġy̆. [**Loimolo'gia;** from λοιμός, the "plague," and λόγος, a "discourse."] A treatise on the plague; the science of the plague or pestilential diseases.

Loi-moph-thăl'mĭ-a.* [From λοιμός, the "plague," and *ophthal'mia.*] Contagious ophthalmia.

Loi-mop'y̆-ra.* [From λοιμός, the "plague," and πῦρ, a "fever."] Pestilential fever.

Loins. See Lumbi.

Lom-a-to-car'pus.* [From λῶμα, a "fringe," or "border," and καρπός, "fruit."] Having flattened fruit with a thick border.

Lom-a-to-phy̆l'lus.* [From λῶμα, a "fringe," or "border," and φύλλον, a "leaf."] Having the borders of the leaf different from the rest: lomatophyl'lous.

Lombes, lòmb. The French term for "loins." See Lumbi.

Lo'ment. [**Lomen'tum.**] A jointed legume or pod, resembling a legume divided transversely into two or more joints.

Lo-men-tā'ceous. [**Lomenta'-ceus.**] Bearing or resembling a loment.

Lon-cho-phy̆l'lus.* [From λόγχη, a "lance," and φύλλον, a "leaf."] Having very long leaves, linear and slightly lanceolated.

Lon-ġev'ĭ-ty̆. [From *lon'gus*, "long," and *æ'vum*, "age."] The prolongation of life to an advanced period.

Lon-ġĭ-brac-te-a'tus.* [From *lon'gus*, "long," and *brac'tea*, a "floral leaf."] Having long bracts.

Lon-ġĭ-car'pus.* [From *lon'gus*, "long," and καρπός, "fruit."] Having very long fruit.

Lon-ġĭ-cau-da'tus,* or **Lon-ġĭ-cau'dus.*** [From *lon'gus*, "long," and *cau'da*, a "tail."] Having a long tail.

Lon-ġĭ-cau'lis.* [From *lon'gus*, "long," and *cau'lis*, a "stem."] Having a long stem.

Lon-ġĭ-col'lis.* [From *lon'gus*, "long," and *col'lum*, a "neck."] Applied to mosses that have urns in the form of a very elongated pear.

Long'ing. The peculiar, and often capricious, desires of females during pregnancy.

Lon-ġĭ-pen'nēs,* or **Lon-ġĭ-pen'-nates.** [From *lon'gus*, "long," and *pen'na*, a "wing."] A family of swimming birds, comprising those in which the wings reach as far as, or beyond, the tail; as the tropic bird, the albatross, etc. They are all denizens of the high seas, and, from their powers of flight, are met with in various latitudes.

Lon-ġis'sĭ-mus.* [Superlative degree of *lon'gus*, "long."] The longest. Applied as a name to certain muscles.

Longis'simus Dorsi.* ("The Longest [Muscle] of the Back.") It arises from the posterior surface of the sacrum, and is attached to the transverse processes of all the lumbar and dorsal vertebræ; it serves to keep the body in an erect posture.

Longis'simus Oc'uli.* ("The Longest [Muscle] of the Eye.") Another name for the *obliquus superior*.

Lon'ġĭ-tude. [**Longitu'do,** *dinis;* from *lon'gus*, "long."] Originally, "length." The longitude of a heavenly body is its distance from the vernal equinox, reckoned on the ecliptic. The longitude of a place on the earth is the number of degrees, minutes, etc., measured on a parallel of latitude between the place and some conventional fixed meridian, as Greenwich, Paris, Washington, etc., from which the measurements are made east and west to the 180th degree.

Lon-ġĭ-tu'dĭ-nal. [**Longitudina'lis;** from *longitu'do*, "length," or "longitude."] Belonging to longitude, or length.

Longitu'dinal Si'nus. A triangular canal within the skull, along the upper margin of the *Falx cerebri*.

Longitu'dinal Si'nus, In-fe'rĭ-or. A vein running along the lower margin of the *Falx cerebri*.

Lon-go-phy̆l'lus.* [From *lon'gus*, "long," and φύλλον, a "leaf."] Having very long leaves.

Longsightedness. See Presbyopia.

Lon'gus.* A Latin word signifying "long." See next article.

Lon'gus Col'li.* ("The Long [Muscle] of the Neck:" Fr. *Long du Cou*, lòNº dü koo.) A long muscle at the back of the œsophagus: it supports and bends the neck.

Looch, lōk. A French term for Eclegma, which see.

Lo'ra.* [From *lo'rum*, a "leathern thong."] Applied to the caulescent and aphyllous part of filamentous lichens and *Confervæ*.

Loranthaceæ,* lo-ran-tha'she-ē. [From *Loran'thus*, one of the genera.] A natural order of exogenous parasitical plants, mostly found in the equinoctial regions of Asia and America. It includes the Mistletoe of the Oak (*Viscum album*), well known in connection with the Druidical religion.

Lor-do'ma, a*tis*.* [From λορδόω, to "bend forwards or inwards."] A projection or protuberance forwards, the product or effect of *lordosis*.

Lor-do'sis.* [From the same.] An incurvation forwards; recurvation.

Lo-ri'ca.* Literally, a "coat of mail." A kind of lute with which vessels are coated before they are put on the fire.

Lor'ĭ-cate. [**Lorica'tus;** from *lori'ca*, a "coat of mail."] Having a coat of mail; mailed. Applied to certain plants and insects.

Lor-ĭ-cā'tion. [**Lorica'tio, o'***nis*; from the same.] Application of a lute of clay, or other substance, to vessels exposed to the fire.

Lor-ĭ-fo'lĭ-us.* [From *lo'rum*, a "leathern thong," and *fo'lium*, a "leaf."] Having long leaves, like thongs.

Lor'u-lum.* [Diminutive of *lo'rum*, a "leathern thong."] Applied to the *thallus* of filamentous or ramose lichens.

Lot. = *Lo'tio*.* "A lotion."

Lo'tion. [**Lo'tio, o'***nis*; from *la'vo*, *lava'tum* or *lo'tum*, to "wash."] A medicated fluid used as an external application to a wound, bruise, sore, or swelling.

Lo'vi's Beads. Specific Gravity Beads. Hollow globes of glass, each of which is a small hydrometer, sinking or rising, according as the liquid in which they are placed is lighter or heavier than the standard. They are useful in making test-acids.

Low Spir'its. See ALUSIA, and HYPOCHONDRIASIS.

Lo-we'ri Tu-ber'cu-lum.* ("Tubercle of Lower.") A thickening of the lining membrane on the posterior wall of the right auricle of the heart.

Lox'a Bark. The *Cinchona pallida*, or pale Peruvian bark.

Lox-an-the'rus.* [From λοξός, "oblique," and ἀνθηρός, an "anther."] Having oblique anthers.

Lox-ar'thron,* **Lox-ar'thrum,*** **Lox-ar'thrus.*** [From λοξός, "oblique," and ἄρθρον, a "joint."] The abnormal direction of a joint, caused neither by spasm nor luxation, as in the varieties of *Talipes*, or club-foot.

Lox'ĭ-a.* [From λοξός, "oblique."] Wry-neck, a distortion of the head towards one side.

Lox-o-çȳ-e'sis.* [From λοξός, "oblique," and κύησις, "pregnancy."] An oblique position of the gravid uterus.

Lox-oph-thăl'mos,* or **Lox-oph-thăl'mus.*** [From λοξός, "oblique," and ὀφθαλμός, an "eye."] Having oblique or squinting eyes.

Lox-ot'o-me,* **Lox-o-to'mĭ-a.*** [From λοξός, "oblique," and τέμνω, to "cut."] An oblique section or cutting; applied to a peculiar method of amputation: loxot'omy.

Lu'brĭ-cāt-ing. [**Lu'bricans;** from *lu'brico*, *lubrica'tum*, to "make slippery."] Literally, "making slippery," or making smooth. Applied to medicines which by their lubricating effects soothe irritation in the throat, fauces, etc. Also an epithet of the synovial fluid.

Lu-briç'ĭ-tȳ. [**Lubriç'itas, a'***tis*; from the same.] The quality of slipperiness, or of lubricating.

Lu'cid In'ter-val. An interval between the paroxysms of insanity, during which the mind is clear, and the patient capable of judging like other men.

Lu-cif'u-gus.* [From *lux*, *lu'cis*, "light," and *fu'gio*, to "fly."] Shunning the light: lucif'ugous.

Lu-cĭ-noc'tis.* [From *lux*, "light," and *nox*, "night."] Applied to plants to which night seems like day, inasmuch as they open their leaves by night and shut them during the day.

Lu'ēs.* [From λύω, to "melt away."] A plague, or pestilence.

Lu'es Ve-ne're-a.* ("Venereal Plague.") The true venereal disease. See SYPHILIS.

Lu'gol's' So-lu'tions. Preparations of iodine and iodide of potassium of various strengths, employed as caustics, rubefacients, and stimulants.

Lum-ba'go, ğ'*inis*.* [From *lum'bus*, the "loins."] A rheumatic affection of the muscles about the loins.

Lumbalis. See LUMBAR.

Lum'bar. [**Lumba'ris;** from *lum'bus*, the "loins."] Belonging to the loins.

Lum'bar Ab'scess. An abscess occurring in the lumbar region; called also *Psoas* abscess.

Lum'bi,* gen. **Lum-bo'rum.** [The plural of **Lum'bus.**] (Fr. *Lombes*, lōmb.) The loins, forming the posterior wall of the abdomen, between the base of the chest and the pelvis, and comprising portions of the *longissimus dorsi*, the *latissimus dorsi*, the *quadratus lumborum*, and several other muscles.

Lum'bri-cal. [**Lumbrica'lis**, plural **Lumbrica'les;** from *lumbri'cus*, the "earth-worm."] Resembling the earth-worm.

Lum-bri-ca'lēs.* The name of four muscles of the hand and foot, so called from their resemblance to the earth-worm.

Lumbricodes. See LUMBRICOIDES.

Lum-bri-co-i'dēs.* [From *lumbri'cus*, the "earth-worm," also the long round worm found in the intestines, and εἶδος, a "form."] Resembling the *lumbricus*; lumbricoid.

Lum-bri'cus.* The common earth-worm; also, the long round worm found in the intestines of man.

Lumbri'cus Ter-res'tris.* The earth-worm.

Lumbus. See LUMBI.

Lu'mi-nous. [**Lumino'sus;** from *lu'men, lu'minis*, "light."] Emitting light; shining; full of light.

Lu'na.* (Fr. *Lune*, lün.) The moon; also the alchemical name of silver.

Lu'na-cy. [From *lu'na*, the "moon;" from its supposed influence.] Insanity, but specially that in which there are lucid intervals. See INSANITY.

Lu'nar. [**Luna'ris;** from *lu'na*, the "moon," also the "goddess Diana."] Pertaining to the moon, and, hence, to silver (of which the moon was the alchemical symbol). Applied to a bone of the *carpus*, from its shape.

Lu'nar Caus'tic. The nitrate of silver (*Nitras argenti*): one of the most convenient and useful of all caustic applications. It also forms the principal ingredient of indelible ink.

Lu-nar-i-fo'li-us.* [From *luna'ris*, "lunar," and *fo'lium*, a "leaf."] Having orbicular leaves.

Lu'nate. [**Luna'tus;** from *lu'na*, the "moon."] Crescent-shaped, or having the form of a half-moon.

Lu'na-tic. [**Lunat'icus;** from *lu'na*, the "moon."] Pertaining to, or affected with, lunacy.

Lunes, lün. [The plural of *lune*, "moon," or "month."] A French term for the MENSES, which see.

Lungs. [Lat. **Pul'mo, mo'***nis*; Fr. *Poumons*, poo'môNG'.] The organs of respiration, occupying the thorax, or chest.

Lu'nu-lar, or **Lu'nu-late.** [**Lunula'ris**, or **Lunula'tus;** from *lu'nula*, a "lunule."] Belonging to a little half-moon, or crescent.

Lu'nule. [**Lu'nula;** diminutive of *lu'na*, the "moon."] The crescentic white mark near the root of the nails of certain fingers.

Lu'pi-a.* [From λυπέω, to "molest"?] A malignant, corroding, and fatal ulcer. (See LUPUS.) Sometimes applied to a soft, spongy, fungous tumor in the knee and elbow joints; also, to a species of wen. A genus of the order *Tumores*, class *Locales*, of Cullen's Nosology.

Lu-pi-no'sus.* [From *lupi'nus*, the "lupin."] Having lupins: lupinose. Applied to a disease of the skin, the *Porrigo lupinosa*.

Lu'pu-lin, or **Lu'pu-line.** [**Lupuli'na.**] A fine, yellow powder, obtained from the hop, or floral leaves of *Humulus lupulus*, being the peculiar principle on which its virtues depend.

Lu-pu-li'na.* Lupulin. The Pharmacopœial name (U.S. Ph.) for the yellow powder attached to the strobiles of the *Humulus lupulus*.

Lu'pu-lus.* The Pharmacopœial name (Br. Ph.) of hops, or the strobiles of *Humulus lupulus*.

Lu'pus.* (A "Wolf;" so named from its destructiveness.) A corroding disease like cancer; also, the disease *Noli me tangere*, and other slow tubercular affections, especially about the face.

Lu'pus Ex'e-dens.* ("Corroding Lupus.") The same as NOLI ME TANGERE.

Lus'ci-tas, a'*tis.** [From *lus'cus*, "blind of one eye."] An affection in which an eye is turned to one or other side, as in *strabismus*, the other being unaffected.

Lu'sus Na-tu'ræ.* Literally, a "sport or freak of nature." Another term for a monstrosity, or MONSTER, which see.

Lute. [From *lu'tum*, "clay;" Fr. *Lut*, lüt.] A composition for closing the junctures of vessels, to prevent the escape of gas or vapor in distillation.

Lux-ā'tion. [**Luxa'tio, o'***nis*; from *lux'o, luxa'tum*, to "dislocate."] A dislocation of a bone. A genus of the order *Ectopiæ*, class *Locales*, of Cullen's Nosology.

Ly-can'thro-py. [**Lycanthro'pia;** from λύκος, a "wolf," and ἄνθρωπος, a "man."] A species of insanity in which the patient believes himself to be a wolf.

Ly-co-ma'ni-a.* [From λύκος, a

"wolf," and μανία, "madness."] The same as LYCANTHROPY, which see.

Lycopodiaceæ,* li-ko-po'de-a'she-ē. A natural order of cryptogamic, moss-like plants, which abound in humid places in the tropics. It includes the *Lycopodium*, a violent cathartic.

Ly-co-po'dĭ-um.* The name applied to the sporules of the *Lycopodium clavatum*, and of other species of *Lycopodium*. It has been placed on the primary list of the Materia Medica of the U.S. Pharmacopœia for 1860.

Lўc'o-pus.* Bugle-weed. The Pharmacopœial name (U.S. Ph.) for the herb of the *Lycopus Virginicus*.

Ly-co-rex'ĭ-ạ.* [From λύκος, a "wolf," and ὄρεξις, "hunger."] The same as BULIMIA, which see.

Lye. [**Lix, Li'cis.**] A solution of the alkali of ashes in water.

Lўmph. [**Lym'pha;** from Νύμφη, a goddess presiding over fountains.] Primarily, "water." Applied to the colorless, transparent liquid in the lymphatic vessels.

Lўm'phạ-den, en*is.** [From *lym'pha*, "lymph," and ἀδήν, a "gland."] A lymphatic gland.

Lўm-phạ-de-ni'tis, i*dis.** [From *lym'phaden.*] Inflammation of a lymphatic gland.

Lўm-phan-ġe-i'tis,* or **Lўm-phan-ġĭ-i'tis, i***dis.** [From *lymphangi'on*, or *lymphange'on*, a "lymphatic vessel."] Inflammation of a lymphatic vessel.

Lўm-phan-ġe'on.* The same as LYMPHANGION, which see.

Lўm-phan-ġĭ-o-gra'phĭ-ạ.* [From *lymphangi'on*, a "lymphatic vessel," and γράφω, to "write."] A description of the lymphatic vessels.

Lўm-phan-ġĭ-o-lo'ġĭ-ạ.* [From *lymphangi'on*, a "lymphatic vessel," and λόγος, a "discourse."] A treatise on the lymphatic vessels.

Lўm-phan-ġĭ'on,* or **Lўm-phan-ġĭ'um.*** [From *lym'pha*, "water," or "lymph," and ἀγγεῖον, a "vessel."] A term for a lymphatic vessel.

Lўm-phan-ġĭ-o-to'mĭ-ạ.* [From *lymphangi'on*, a "lymphatic vessel," and τέμνω, to "cut."] Dissection of the lymphatic vessels.

Lўm-phat'ic. [**Lymphat'icus;** from *lym'pha*, "water," or "lymph."] Applied to vessels conveying lymph, forming with the lacteal vessels the absorbent system of the animal economy. Applied in Botany to analogous vessels containing sap or watery juices, slightly elaborated.

Lymphat'ic Glands (or **Gan'glĭ-ons**). The glands of the absorbent or lymphatic system. Also called CONGLOBATE GLANDS.

Lymphat'ic Sўs'tem. [**Syste'ma Lymphat'icum.**] A collective term, comprising the lymphatic glands, or ganglions, and the lymphatic vessels.

Lymphat'ics, or **Lymphat'ic Ves'-sels.** [**Lymphangi'a,** or **Va'sa Lymphat'ica.**] See LYMPHATIC.

Lўm-phen-te-ri'tis, i*dis.** [From *lym'pha*, "lymph," and *enteri'tis.*] Serous *enteritis*.

Lўm-pheū-rўs'mạ, a*tis.** [From *lym'pha*, "lymph," and εὐρύνω, to "dilate."] A morbid dilatation of the lymphatic vessels.

Lўm-pho'sis.* [From *lym'pha*, "lymph."] A term for the formation or elaboration of lymph.

Lymphotomia. See LYMPHANGIOTOMIA.

Lўp-o-thўm'ĭ-ạ.* [From λύπη, "sadness," and θυμός, the "mind."] Mental grief, or affliction.

Ly'rạ.* [Gr. λύρα, a "lyre."] An appearance on the inferior surface of the *Fornix cerebri*, like the strings of a harp; also termed *Corpus psalloides*. See PSALLOIDES.

Ly'rate. [**Lyra'tus;** from *ly'ra*, a "lyre."] Formed like a lyre.

Lўr-ĭ-for'mis.* [From *ly'ra*, a "lyre."] Formed like a lyre, as the leaves of the *Arabis lyriforma*.

Lўs-ĭ-ma'chĭ-æ,* the plural of *Lysimach'ia*, forming the Jussieuan name of a natural order of plants. See PRIMULACEÆ.

Lўs'sạ.* [Gr. λύσσα, "rage," or "madness."] A term for *rabies;* rage, or madness. Usually applied to HYDROPHOBIA, which see.

Lўs'sĭ-cus.* Belonging to *hydrophobia:* hydrophobic.

Lўs'sin. [**Lyssi'na;** from *lys'sa*, "madness."] A term for the zymotic principle of *hydrophobia*.

Lўs-so-i'dēs.* [From *lys'sa*, "madness," and εἶδος, a "form."] Resembling *rabies*, rage, or madness.

Lythraceæ,* lith-ra'she-ē. A natural order of exogenous plants, mostly herbaceous, found in Europe, America, etc. It includes *Ly'thrum Salica'ria*, which yields an astringent medicine.

Lўt'tạ.* [From λυττάω, to "rage."] A genus of insects.

Lyt'ta Ves-ĭ-cạ-to'rĭ-ạ.* The blistering fly. See CANTHARIS.

M.

M. = *Manip'ulus*,* a "handful;" or, at the end of a formula, *Mis'ce*,* "mix;" also, *Mensu'râ*,* "by measure;" and *Min'imum*,* a "minim."

Mac. = *Ma'cera*.* "Macerate."

Mace. A thin, flat, membranous substance which envelops the nutmeg. See Macis, and Nutmeg.

Maç-e-rā'tion. [**Macera'tio, o**'*nis*; from *ma'cero, macera'tum*, to "make soft by steeping."] The process of steeping or infusing a substance in water, with or without heat, to extract its virtues.

Macies,* ma'she-ēz. Wasting, atrophy, or emaciation.

Ma'cis.* Mace. The Pharmacopœial name (U.S. Ph.) for the aril of the fruit of the *Myris'tica fra'grans*.

Mac-ran'thus.* [From μακρός, "long," or "great," and ἄνθος, a "flower."] Having large flowers.

Mac-ro-bī-o'sis,* or **Mac-ro-bī-o'-tēs, e**'*tis*.* [From μακρός, "long," or "great," and βίος, "life."] Long life; longevity.

Mac-ro-bī-ot'ic. [**Macrobiot'icus.**] Belonging to *macrobiosis*.

Mac-ro-bī-ot'ĭ-ca.* [From the same.] The art or system of instructions for attaining long life.

Mac-ro-car'pus.* [From μακρός, "long," or "great," and καρπός, "fruit."] Having large fruit: macrocar'pous.

Mac-ro-çe-pha'lĭ-a.* [From μακρός, "long," or "great," and κεφαλή, the "head."] A genus of organic deviations characterized by excessive size of the head.

Mac-ro-çeph'a-lous. [**Macroceph'alus**; from the same.] Having a large head.

Mac'ro-cosm. [**Macrocos'mus**; from μακρός, "long," or "great," and κόσμος, a "world."] The greater world, as distinguished from *Microcosm*, the smaller, or man.

Mac-ro-cos'mĭ-cus.* Belonging to the *macrocosm*.

Mac-ro-me'lĭ-a.* [From μακρός, "long," or "great," and μέλος, a "member."] A class of monsters characterized by excessive development of some member.

Mac-ro-phȳl'lous. [**Macrophyl'-lus**; from μακρός, "long," or "great," and φύλλον, a "leaf."] Having large leaves.

Mac-rop'ĭ-per, er'*is*.* [From μακρός, "long," or "great," and πέπερι, "pepper."] The *Piper longum*.

Ma-crop'ter-us.* [From μακρός, "long," or "great," and πτερόν, a "wing."] Applied to seeds having wings of unusual length.

Mac-ros-çe'lĭ-a.* [From μακρός, "long," or "great," and σκέλος, a "leg."] A genus of organic deviations characterized by excessive development of the legs.

Mac-ro'sĭ-a,* or **Mac-ro'sis.*** [From μακρός, "long," or "great."] Increase of bulk, or length; augmentation; elongation.

Macrosomatia,* mak-ro-so-ma'-she-a. [From μακρός, "long," or "great," and σῶμα, a "body."] Applied to monsters characterized by the greatness of the entire body.

Mac-ro-sta'chȳ-us.* [From μακρός, "long," or "great," and στάχυς, an "ear of corn."] Having flowers disposed in long and thick spikes, or ears.

Mac-ro-sty'lus.* [From μακρός, "long," or "great," and στῦλος, a "style."] Having a very long style, as the *Cnicus macrostylus*.

Mac'u-la,* plural **Mac'u-læ.** Literally, a "spot," or "stain." Applied to a dark spot on the sun's surface, or to a permanent spot or stain on some part of the skin, unconnected with disorder of the constitution.

Mac'ula Matri'cis.* ("Spot of, or from, the Mother.") See Nævus Maternus.

Mac'u-læ,* the plural of Macula, which see.

Mac'u-lar. [**Macula'ris.**] Belonging to *maculæ*; resembling *maculæ*.

Mac'u-lāte. [**Macula'tus.**] Having *maculæ*.

Mac-u-lĭ-for'mis.* [From *mac'ula*, a "spot."] Having spots, or stains.

Mac-u-lose', or **Mac'u-lous.** [**Macu-lo'sus**; from *mac'ula*, a "spot."] Full of spots; spotted.

Madar. See Mudar.

Mad-a-ro'sis.* [From μαδαρός, "bald."] Loss of hair, particularly of the eyebrows or eyelashes.

Mad'der. The *Rubia tinctorum*.

Mad-e-fac'tion. [**Madefac'tio, o**'*nis*; from *madefa'cio, madefac'tum*, to "make wet."] The act of wetting.

Madjoun, må-joon'; written also

Madjound. An intoxicating preparation composed of powdered hemp and honey, and used by the Turks and Algerines.

Madness. See INSANITY, LUNACY, and MANIA.

Madness, Canine. See HYDROPHOBIA.

Mad're-pore. [Fr. *madré*, "speckled," or "spotted," and *pore*, a "pore."] A genus of corals, or zoophytes, having stems shaped like trees.

Maġ-el-lan'ic Clouds. [Named from *Magel'lan*, a strait not very far from the south pole.] Two whitish spots in the heavens, near the south pole, composed of nebulæ, or clusters of fixed stars.

Ma-gen'ta. A beautiful crimson dye obtained from aniline.

Maġ'is-ter-ȳ. [From *magis'ter*, a "master."] A term formerly applied to almost all precipitates supposed to be subtle and masterly preparations.

Ma-ġis'tral. [**Magistra'lis;** from *magis'ter*, a "master."] Applied to medicines prescribed for the occasion, by a competent person, in distinction from such as are officinal, or kept prepared in the shops. As the latter are prepared according to a certain formula, an intelligent apprentice is generally equal to the task; but the knowledge of a master is needed to give directions for an original preparation.

Mag'ma, a*tis*.* [Gr. μάγμα, "any kneaded mass."] Dregs; sediment; a squeezed mass of a certain consistence.

Mag'nēs,* gen. **Mag-ne'tis.** The same as MAGNET, which see.

Mag'nes Ar-sen-ĭ-ca'lis.* A corrosive preparation of equal parts of sulphur, white arsenic, and common antimony, mixed by fusion.

Magnesia,* mag-ne'zhe-a. [From *Magne'sia*, a district of Lydia, where the earth was originally obtained.] One of the primitive alkaline earths; an oxide of magnesium.

Magne'sia Us'ta.* ("Burnt Magnesia.") Calcined magnesia.

Magne'siæ (mag-ne'zhe-ē) **Car-bo'nas.*** ("Carbonate of Magnesia.") A white substance, occurring in powder or pulverulent masses, wholly dissolved by dilute sulphuric acid.

Magne'siæ Sul'phas.* ("Sulphate of Magnesia.") A substance occurring in colorless crystals, which slowly effloresce on exposure to the air, and are very soluble in water. The sulphate of magnesia, popularly known as Epsom salts, is one of the most valuable of all the saline cathartics. It is especially adapted to cases where it is desirable to combine a refrigerant with a mild and safe purgative.

Mag-ne'śian. [**Magnesia'nus;** from *magne'sia*.] Belonging to magnesia; containing magnesia. Applied to a group of rocks.

Magnesium,* mag-ne'zhe-um. The metallic base of magnesia.

Mag'net. [Lat. **Mag'nes, ne'***tis*; Gr. μάγνης; Fr. *Aimant*, à'mōnᵒ', or *Pierre d'Aimant*, pe-ēr'dà'mōnᵒ'.] Loadstone; a native oxide of iron which attracts iron. (See LOADSTONE.) More usually applied, however, to a bar of steel or iron to which the magnetic property has been imparted.

Mag-net'ic. [**Magnet'icus.**] Belonging to the magnet.

Mag'net-iśm. [**Magnetis'mus;** from μάγνης, a "magnet."] The property of attraction, or repulsion, possessed by the loadstone. The science which investigates the phenomena presented by natural and artificial magnets, and the laws by which they are connected.

Magnetism, Animal. See MESMERISM.

Mag-net-ol'o-ġȳ. [**Magnetolo'gia;** from μάγνης, a "magnet," and λόγος, a "discourse."] A treatise on the magnet and magnetism; the science of magnetism.

Mag-net-om'e-ter. [**Magnetom'etrum;** from μάγνης, a "magnet," and μέτρον, a "measure."] An apparatus for ascertaining the force with which the magnet attracts iron in different places.

Mag-no'lĭ-a.* (Fr. *Magnolier*, måg'-no'le-à'.) A Linnæan genus of the class *Polyandria*, natural order *Magnoliaceæ*; also, the Pharmacopœial name (U.S. Ph.) for the bark of *Magno'lia glau'ca*, *Magno'lia acumina'ta*, and *Magno'lia tripet'ala*. This bark is a mild aromatic tonic, and has been employed with success as a remedy in intermittent fevers.

Magnoliaceæ,* mag-no-le-a'she-ē, or **Mag-no'lĭ-æ.*** A natural order of exogenous trees and shrubs, natives of the tropical and temperate parts of America and Asia. It includes the Magnolia, the Tulip-tree, and other trees of great beauty. Many species are valuable as tonics.

Mag-no-lĭ-ā'ceous. [**Magnolia'ceus.**] Resembling the Magnolia.

Mag-no'lĭ-æ,* the plural of MAGNOLIA, forming the Jussieuan name of a natural order of plants. See MAGNOLIACEÆ.

Ma-hog'a-ny̆. The wood of the *Swiete'nia Mahag'oni*, or Mahogany-tree, the bark of which is used as a substitute for Peruvian bark, though it is inferior.

Main, mănᵍ. The French term for HAND, which see.

Maize. A common name for the *Zea mays*, or Indian-corn plant.

Ma-jor-a'na.* The plant marjoram; also spelled *Marjorana*. See ORIGANUM VULGARE.

Majora'na Sy̆-ri'a-ca.* A name for the *Teu'crium ma'rum*, or Syrian herb mastich.

Ma'la.* [Contraction of *maxil'la*, the "jaw"?] The prominent part of the cheek, or cheek-ball.

Malacia,* ma-la'she-a. [From μαλακός, "effeminate."] Literally, "softness," "luxury," or "effeminacy." Depraved or fanciful appetite, as in *chlorosis*, pregnancy, etc. So called, it would seem, because effeminate or luxurious habits often create capricious desires.

Mal-a-col'o-gy̆. [From μαλάκια, the Aristotelian name of Mollusca, and λόγος, a "discourse."] The science which treats of the *Mollusca*, which Cuvier divided into six classes, *Cephalop'oda, Pterop'oda, Gasterop'oda, Aceph'ala, Brachiop'oda*, and *Cirrop'oda*. A notice of these will be found under their respective heads. See MOLLUSCA.

Mal-a-co'ma, atis.* [From μαλακόω, to "soften."] A softening of a part, as of the brain, kidneys, bones, etc.

Mal-a-co-phy̆l'lus.* [From μαλακός, "soft," and φύλλον, a "leaf."] Having leaves soft to the touch.

Mal-a-co'sis.* [From μαλακόω, to "soften."] The progress of *malacoma*.

Mal-a-cos'te-on.* [From μαλακός, "soft," and ὀστέον, a "bone."] Softness of the bones.

Mal-a-co-zo-o-lo'ġĭ-a.* [From μαλακός, "soft," ζῶον, an "animal," and λόγος, a "discourse."] A treatise on *Mollusca*.

Mal-a-co-zo'on.* [From μαλακός, "soft," and ζῶον, an "animal."] The same as MOLLUSCUM.

Mal-ac-tin'ĭ-a.* [From μαλακός, "soft," and ἀκτίν, a "ray," "radius."] The same as *Acalepha*. See ACALEPHUS.

Maladie, mâ'lâ'dè'. The French term for DISEASE, which see.

Maladie du Pays, mâ'lâ'dè' dü pà'è'. A common French term for NOSTALGIA.

Ma-lag'ma, atis.* [From μαλάσσω, to "soften."] See CATAPLASMA.

Malaise (Fr.), mâ'lĕz', or mâ'lâz'. [From *mal*, "ill," and *aise*, "ease."] Discomfort or uneasiness.

Ma-lam'bo Bark, or **Matias Bark.** The bark of a tree found in Colombia, and used as a substitute for cinchona.

Ma'lar. [**Mala'ris;** from *ma'la*, the "cheek."] Belonging to the cheek-bone.

Ma-la'rĭ-a.* [From the Italian *ma'la*, "bad," and *a'ria*, "air."] A term for marsh *miasmata*, or infectious effluvia from decayed animal or vegetable matter.

Ma-lā'rĭ-al, or **Ma-lā'rĭ-ous.** Belonging to, or caused by, malaria.

Mal'āte. [**Ma'las, a'tis.**] A combination of malic acid with a base.

Male Fern. See ASPIDIUM FILIX MAS.

Malesherbiaceæ,* măl-zĕr-be-a'-she-ē. [From *Malesherbia*, one of the genera.] A small natural order of exogenous plants, found in Chili and Peru.

Mal-for-mā'tion. A deviation from the natural or proper form of an organ.

Mal'ic. [**Mal'icus;** from *ma'lum*, an "apple."] Belonging to an apple. Applied to an acid obtained from the juice of apples, and other fruits.

Mal'ice Pre-pense'. [Fr. *malice*, "ill will," *pre*, "before," and *penser*, to "think."] Premeditated ill will; in legal phrase, "malice *aforethought*."

Mal-ĭ-for'mis.* [From *ma'lum*, an "apple."] Having the form of an apple.

Ma-lig'nant. [**Malig'nus;** from *ma'lus*, "evil."] (Fr. *Malin*, mâ'lănᵍ'.) Applied to diseases that endanger life, more especially to such as are characterized by their violence or *atrocity*, so to speak (as *cancer*, the *plague*, etc.), and by their rapid progress to a fatal termination.

Malin. See MALIGNANT.

Ma-lin'ger-er. [From the French *Malingre*, "sickly."] One who simulates or feigns disease, to avoid labor or punishment.

Ma'lis.* [Gr. μάλις, a "cutaneous disease."] A Greek term, according to Dr. Good, for cutaneous vermination, or the skin being infested with animalcules.

Ma'lis Fi-la'rĭ-æ.* ("Skein-Worm.") See GUINEA-WORM.

Mal-le-a-bil'ĭ-ty̆. [**Malleabil'itas, a'tis;** from *mal'leus*, a "hammer," or "mallet."] The property possessed by certain metals of being beaten into form without cracking.

Mal-le-ā'tion. [**Mallea'tio, o'nis;**

from *mal'leus*, a "hammer," or "mallet."] A species of *Chorea*, in which the hands convulsively act in striking on the knees, as if with a hammer.

Mal-le'o-lar. [From *malle'olus*, a "little hammer."] A term applied to two branches of the posterior tibial artery.

Mal-le'o-lus.* [Diminutive of *mal'leus*, a "hammer."] Applied to the projections of bone on the *tibia* and *fibula*, forming the inner and outer ankles.

Mal'le-us.* ("A Hammer.") One of the small bones of the internal ear; named from its resemblance to a hammer.

Mal-lo-coc'cus.* [From μαλλός, a "fleece," and κόκκος, a "berry."] Having hairy fruit.

Mal'lōw. The *Malva sylvestris*.

Malpighiaceæ,* mal-pe-ḡe-a'she-ē. [From *Malpi'ghia*, one of the genera.] A natural order of exogenous trees and shrubs, nearly all of which are tropical. Many of them have beautiful flowers.

Malpi'ghian (măl-pee'ḡe-ạn) **Bod'ies.** [**Cor'pora Malpi'ghi.**] Applied to small bodies or corpuscles found in the kidney: also to certain white corpuscles found in the spleen, similar in structure to the follicles of the lymphatic glands.

Malpi'ghii (măl-pee'ḡe-ē) **Re'te.*** The *Rete muco'sum* of the negro, first pointed out by Malpighi.

Mâlt. Barley which has been prepared for the manufacture of beer by incipient germination.

Ma'lus Med'ĭ-cạ.* The same as CITRUS MEDICA, which see.

Măl'vạ.* [From μαλάχη, "softness."] A Linnæan genus of the class *Monadelphia*, natural order *Malvaceæ*. The Pharmacopœial name (Lond. and Ed. Ph.) of the *Malva sylvestris*.

Mal'va Sўl-ves'tris.* The common mallow-plant.

Malvaceæ,* măl-va'she-ē. A natural order of exogenous plants, which abound in tropical and temperate regions. It includes the *Malva* (Mallow), *Hibiscus*, and *Gossypium*, the true cotton-plant. The uniform character of the order is to abound in mucilage, which is used as a demulcent or emollient.

Mamelle. See MAMMA.

Mamelon, mảm'lỏnᵍ'. See NIPPLE.

Mam'mạ,* plural **Mam'mæ.** [From μάμμα, the "instinctive cry of an infant."] (Fr. *Mamelle*, mả'měll'.) The breast; an organ forming, in the human female, a globular projection on each side of the thorax; being the seat of the lactiferous (or milk-producing) glands. Applied also to the corresponding part of all animals that suckle their young.

Mammaire. See MAMMARY.

Mam'mạl. [**Mamma'lis;** from *mam'ma*, a "breast."] Having breasts, or teats. Applied to a class of animals. See MAMMALIA.

Mam-ma'lĭ-ạ,* or **Mam'mals.** [The plural neuter of *mamma'lis*, "having breasts, or teats." See MAMMA.] The most highly organized class of the animal kingdom, constituting the first or highest section of Cuvier's grand division *Vertebrata*. They possess mammary glands, and suckle their young. A great majority of them are four-footed and are covered with hair. The Cetaceans instead of four feet have corresponding or analogous fins. One of the principal anatomical characteristics of the Mammalia is the condition of the lungs, which are suspended freely in a thoracic cavity and separated from the abdomen by a perfect diaphragm.

Mam-măl'o-ġў. [**Mammalo'gia.**] A treatise on Mammalia; the science which treats of mammiferous animals.

Mam'mạ-rў. [**Mamma'rius;** from *mam'ma*, a "breast."] (Fr. *Mammaire*, mảm'mêʀ'.) Belonging to the *mamma*, or female breast.

Mam'mary Gland. The organ which secretes the milk; a gland placed beneath the adipose layer of the mamma.

Mam-ma'tus.* Having *mammæ*, or breasts: mammate.

Mam-mif'er-us.* [From *mam'ma*, the "breast," and *fe'ro*, to "bear."] Having breasts, or teats. Applied in the plural neuter (*Mammif'era*) to a class of animals, the same as MAMMALIA.

Mam'mĭ-form. [**Mammifor'mis;** from *mam'ma*, the "breast."] Having the form of the breast.

Mam-mil'lạ,* plural **Mam-mil'læ.** [Diminutive of *mam'ma*, the "breast."] A little breast; a nipple. Also applied to the male breast. See NIPPLE.

Mam'mil-lạ-rў. [**Mammilla'ris;** from *mammil'la*, a "nipple."] Belonging to the nipple, or resembling a nipple or small breast.

Mam'mil-late. [**Mammilla'tus.**] Having *mammil'læ*, or nipples. In Botany, bearing little prominences on the surface.

Mam-mil-lā'tion. [**Mammilla'tio, o'nis;** from *mammil'la*, a "nipple."] Applied to the appearances of little prominences like granulations on a mucous surface, as of the stomach sometimes in *phthisis*, etc.

Mam-mil-lif'er-us.* [From *mammil'la*, a "nipple," and *fe'ro*, to "bear."] Bearing *mammillæ*, or something resembling them.

Mam-mil-li-for'mis.* [From *mammil'la*, a "nipple."] Having the form of *mammillæ:* mammilliform.

Mam-mil-lo'sus.* [From *mammil'la*, a "nipple."] Having *mammillæ*, or prominent tubercles.

Mam'mose. [**Mammo'sus;** from *mam'ma*, the "breast."] Having breasts, or prominences like breasts.

Mam'moth. A word of Tartar origin, applied in Siberia to burrowing animals. It is usually applied to an extinct species of elephant, the *El'ephas primige'nius*. An entire animal of this species has been found in Siberia, with the soft parts preserved in the ice.

Mam'mu-la.* [Diminutive of *mam'ma*, the "breast."] Applied to the swollen conceptacles on the *thallus* of certain lichens.

Man. = *Manip'ulus.** "A handful."

Man. [**Ho'mo, Hom'inis.**] In general, a human being, classed with mammiferous animals, and constituting the sole genus of the order *Bimana* of the *Mammalia*. Man (Latin, *Vir*), in a restricted sense, denotes the male of the human species.

Ma-na'tus.* [From *ma'nus*, a "hand;" so called in allusion to its hand-like fins.] A genus of herbivorous Cetaceans, including the species usually called the sea-cow.

Man-chi-neel', or **Man-chi-nēal'.** The *Hippom'ane Mancinel'la*, a poisonous tree of South America. With its juice the aborigines poison their arrows.

Man'di-ble. [**Mandib'ula,** or **Mandib'ulum;** from *man'do*, to "chew."] Applied in the plural to the anterior or superior pair of jaws in certain insects; also to the jaws of birds.

Man'dible. [**Mandib'ula;** from the same.] A name for the lower jaw (*maxilla inferior*).

Man-dib'u-lar. [**Mandibula'ris;** from *mandib'ula*, a "mandible."] Belonging to a mandible, or the lower jaw.

Man-dib-u-la'ta,* or **Man-dib'u-lates.** [From *mandib'ula*, a "jaw."] A grand section of insects, including all those which preserve their organs of mastication in their last or perfect stage of metamorphosis.

Man-dib'u-li-form. [**Mandibuli-for'mis;** from *mandib'ula*, a "mandible."] Applied to the jaws of insects when hard and horny.

Mandioc. See JATROPHA MANIHOT.

Man-drag'o-ra.* The narcotic plant *Atropa Mandragora*, or mandrake.

Mandrake. See MANDRAGORA.

Man-du-cā'tion. [**Manduca'tio, o'nis;** from *mandu'co*, *manduca'tum*, to "chew."] The same as MASTICATION, which see.

Man'ga-nāte. [**Man'ganas, a'tis.**] A combination of manganic acid and a base.

Man'ga-nese. [**Mangane'sium.**] A peculiar metallic substance, which is gray, hard, brittle, and very difficult of fusion. In its metallic form it has not been applied to any use. The specific gravity is about 8.

Man-ga-ne'sic. [**Manganes'icus;** from *mangane'sium*.] Applied to an acid obtained from manganese.

Mangane'sii (man-ga-ne'she-i) **Ox'i-dum Ni'grum.*** ("Black Oxide of Manganese.") The name applied to the native impure deutoxide of manganese in powder. This substance has been placed on the primary list of the Materia Medica in the U.S. Pharmacopœia for 1860. Black oxide of manganese is regarded as a tonic and alterative; it has been employed in syphilis and various cutaneous diseases. When slowly introduced into the system, as happens to those engaged in grinding this mineral, it acts (like lead or mercury) as a cumulative poison, often producing paraplegia.

Mangane'sii Sul'phas.* ("Sulphate of Manganese.") This substance occurs in colorless, or pale rose-colored, transparent crystals. It has been placed on the primary list of the Materia Medica in the U.S. Pharmacopœia for 1860. It acts as a cholagogue purgative, and also as an alterative.

Manganium. See MANGANESE.

Man'ga-nous. [**Mangano'sus;** from *mangane'sium*.] Applied to an oxide of manganese.

Man'go. (Called by the Hindoos *âm*.) The fruit of the *Mangif'era In'dica*, a large fruit-tree, inhabiting the tropical parts of Asia, throughout all which it is cultivated nearly as extensively as the apple and pear are in Europe. The fruit is somewhat like a nectarine, but longer. It contains a large stone covered with coarse fibres, which are surrounded with succulent flesh, or rather a thick, pulpy juice.

Ma'nĭ ạ.* [Gr. μανία; from μαίνομαι, to "rage."] Delirium unaccompanied by fever; madness. A genus of the order *Vesaniæ,* class *Neuroses,* of Cullen's Nosology. See INSANITY.

Ma'nia a Po'tu.* ("Madness from Drinking.") Insanity resulting from excessive indulgence in drinking. See DELIRIUM TREMENS.

Mạ-nī'ạ-cạl. [**Maniaca'lis.**] Affected with mania; resembling mania.

Man'ĭ-cate. [**Manica'tus;** from *man'ica,* a "glove," or "sleeve."] Gloved; covered with a woolly coat which may be stripped off whole, as some plants.

Manie sans Délire, må'nē' sŏNᵍ dā'-lēR'. ("Madness, without Delirium.") See MORAL INSANITY.

Mạ-nip-u-lā'tion. [From *manip'ulus,* a "handful."] The mode of handling utensils, materials, etc., in experimental philosophy; the performance of experiments.

Mạ-nip'u-lus.* [From *ma'num im'pleat,* "what fills the hand."] A handful.

Man'nạ.* A substance supposed to resemble the manna of the Holy Scriptures, obtained from several species of ash-tree. The Pharmacopœial name ‖ for "the concrete juice, in flakes, of the *Frax'inus or'nus,* and *Frax'inus rotundifo'lia.*"

Man-nif'er-us.* [From *man'na,* and *fe'ro,* to "bear."] Bearing or affording manna.

Man'nīte. [**Man'nis, i'tis.**] A white substance, chiefly obtained from manna, and on which its laxative virtues depend; sugar of manna.

Man. pr. = *Ma'ne pri'mo.** "Very early in the morning."

Man'tle. [**Pal'lium.**] A development of the skin which covers the body or a portion of the body of nearly all *Mollusca.*

Ma-nu'brĭ-um.* [From *ma'nus,* the "hand," and *ha'beo,* to "hold."] Literally, a "hilt," or "handle." Applied in Anatomy to the uppermost part of the *sternum.*

Manu'brium Ma'nus.* An epithet applied to the *radius.*

Man-u-lu'vĭ-um.* [From *ma'nus,* a "hand," and *la'vo,* to "wash."] A hand-bath.

Ma'nus.* (Fr. *Main,* măNᵍ.) The hand. See HAND.

Manustupratio. See MASTURBATION.

Mạ-ran'tạ.* Arrow-root. The Pharmacopœial name (Lond. and Ed. Ph.) for the *fecula* of the tubers of the *Maranta arundinacea,* and *Maranta Indica.*

Maran'ta Arundina'cea* (a-run-dĭ-na'she-ạ). The arrow-root plant.

Maran'ta Gạ-lan'gạ.* A plant believed to yield *galangal,* a pungent aromatic root formerly used as a substitute for ginger. This root is brought from China and the East Indies.

Maran'ta In'dĭ-cạ.* A species of *Maranta,* from which arrow-root is obtained.

Marantaceæ,* măr-an-ta'she-ē. A natural order of endogenous plants, found in the tropical parts of Africa and America. It includes the *Maran'ta,* from which arrow-root is procured.

Măr-an-tā'ceous. [**Maranta'ceus.**] Resembling *Maran'ta.*

Măr-as-mo'dēš.* [From *maras'mus,* a "withering," or "wasting away."] Resembling, or having, *marasmus.*

Mạ-ras-mo-i'dēš.* [From *maras'mus,* a "withering," or "wasting away," and εἶδος, a "form."] Resembling *marasmus:* maras'moid.

Măr-as-mop'ȳ-rạ.* [From *maras'mus,* a "withering," or "wasting away," and πῦρ, a "fever."] Hectic fever.

Mạ-ras'mus.* [From μαραίνω, to "wither."] Literally, a "withering," or "wasting away." Consumption of the whole body.

Mar'ble. (Fr. *Marbre,* maRbR.) A species of limestone, or hard carbonate of lime, capable of a high polish. See MARMOR.

Mar-cēs'çent. [**Marces'cens;** from *mar'ceo,* to "wither."] Withering; gradually withering, without falling off.

Marcgraviaceæ,* mark-gra-ve-a'-she-ē. [From *Marcgra'via,* one of the genera.] A small natural order of exogenous trees and shrubs, found in equinoctial America.

Marchantiaceæ,* mar-shan-te-a'-she-ē. [From *Marchan'tia,* one of the genera.] A name given by Lindley to a natural order of plants. See HEPATICÆ.

Mar'cor,* plural **Mar-co'rēš.** [From *mar'ceo,* to "wither."] Leanness or wasting of the body. Applied in the plural to diseases characterized by emaciation of the body, constituting an order of the class *Cachexiæ* of Cullen's Nosology. See MARASMUS.

Mar'gạ.* Marl, a fertilizing substance found in nature, consisting of a mixture of calcareous and argillaceous earths.

The calcareous portion often consists of the fragments or *débris* of small shells.

Mar'ga-rāte. [**Mar'garas, a'***tis.*] A combination of margaric acid with a base.

Mar-găr'ic. [**Margar'icus;** from *margari'na.*] Applied to an acid obtained from margarin.

Mar'ga-rin, or **Mar'ga-rīne.** [**Margari'na;** from μάργαρον, a "pearl."] A simple fat, a constituent of the radical termed *margaryl;* named from its pearly appearance.

Mar'ga-rȳl. [From *margari'na,* "margarin," and ὕλη, "material."] A radical, of which stearin and margarin are constituents.

Mar'ġi-nal. [**Margina'lis;** from *mar'go, mar'ginis,* a "border."] Placed upon, or belonging to, the margin.

Mar'ġin-ate. [**Margina'tus;** from *mar'gino, margina'tum,* to "make borders."] Having a border, edge, or margin.

Marine (ma-reen') **Aç'id.** Muriatic or hydrochloric acid, formerly termed the spirit of salt.

Marine' Salt. Chloride of sodium; common salt: formerly called muriate of soda.

Măr'ĭ-time. [**Marit'imus;** from *ma're,* the "sea."] Belonging to the sea, or bordering on the sea.

Mar'jo-ram, Com'mon. The *Orig'anum vulga're.*

Mar'joram, Sweet. The *Orig'anum majora'na.*

Mar'joram, Wild. The *Orig'anum vulga're.*

Marl. See MARGA.

Mar-măr'ȳ-ga,* or **Mar-măr'ȳ-ġe,*** plural **Mar-măr'ȳ-ġæ.** [From μαρμαίρω, to "shine."] In the plural, the appearance of sparks or coruscations before the eyes.

Mar-măr-ȳ-go'dēs.* [From *marmar'ygæ.*] Having, or resembling, *marmarygæ.*

Mar'mor, or*is.** [From μαρμαίρω, to "shine."] (Fr. *Marbre,* marbr.) Marble. The Pharmacopœial name for the crystalline, or white granular, carbonate of lime. See MARBLE.

Mar'mo-rate. [From *mar'mor,* "marble."] Marbled; applied to some vegetable products.

Mar'rōw. [Lat. **Medul'la;** Gr. μυελός; Fr. *Moëlle,* mo'ĕll'.] The fatty oleaginous substance in the cavities of long cylindrical bones.

Marrow, Spinal. See MEDULLA SPINALIS.

Mar-ru'bĭ-um.* Horehound. A Linnæan genus of the class *Didynamia,* natural order *Labiatæ.* Also, the Pharmacopœial name (U.S. Ph.) for the herb of *Marru'bium vulga're.*

Marru'bium Al'bum.* ("White Horehound.") Another name for the *Marrubium vulgare.*

Marru'bium Vul-ga're.* ("Common Horehound.") The systematic name of the common or white horehound, also called *Marrubium album.*

Mars,* gen. **Mar'tis.** [The name of the god of war, also used for "war" itself.] One of the planets. Also, the alchemical name of iron, given on account of its importance in war; hence the salts of iron were called Martial Salts.

Marseilles (mar-sālz') **Vin'e-gar.** *Thieves' Vinegar.* A solution of essential oils and camphor in vinegar. The reputation of this prophylactic in contagious fevers is said to have arisen from the confession of four thieves, who, during the plague at Marseilles, plundered the dead bodies with perfect security, being preserved from contagion by this aromatic vinegar, which has, hence, been called *Le Vinaigre des Quatre Voleurs,* lẹh vẽ'nĕgr' dȧ kȃtr vo'lur' ("the Vinegar of the Four Thieves").

Marsh Mal'lōw. The *Althæa officinalis.*

Marsh's Test. A test for arsenious acid, consisting in the action upon the acid of nascent hydrogen, obtained by dissolving zinc in dilute sulphuric acid; the arsenious acid is deoxidyzed, with evolution of arseniuretted hydrogen gas.

Marsileaceæ,* mar-sil-e-a'she-ē. [From *Marsil'ea,* one of the genera.] A natural order of cryptogamic plants, resembling mosses, found in ditches or wet places.

Mar-su'pĭ-al. [**Marsupia'lis;** from *marsu'pium,* a "pouch."] Pouched, or resembling a pouch.

Mar-su-pĭ-a'lĭ-a,* or **Mar-su'pĭ-als.** [From the same.] An order of mammiferous quadrupeds, of which the females have a portion of the abdominal integument folded inwards, forming either a depression containing the *mammæ,* or a pouch serving also as a temporary abode for the young. It includes the kangaroo, opossum, and wombat.

Mar-su'pĭ-ĭ-flo'rus.* [From *marsu'-*

pium, a "pouch," and *flos*, a "flower."] Having pouch-like flowers.

Mar-su'pi-um.* [From μάρσυπος, a "little sack."] A pouch. Applied to the large cavity of the peritonæum; also, to the scrotum. In Zoology, the pouch or receptacle near the *mammæ* of the opossum, kangaroo, etc.

Marteau, maʀ'tō'. The French term for MALLEUS, which see.

Martial. See MARS.

Ma'rum Sȳ-ri'a-cum,* or **Teu'-cri-um Ma'rum.*** An aromatic plant of the natural order *Labiatæ*, formerly used as a tonic, antispasmodic, or errhine.

Mas,* gen. **Ma'ris.** The male of any kind of animal.

Mas-cu-lĭ-flo'rus.* [From *mas'culus*, "male," and *flos*, a "flower."] Having male flowers: masculiflo'rous.

Mas'cu-line. [**Mas'culus**; from *mas*, a "male."] Male, or belonging to the male sex; resembling a man or male.

Masked. [From the French *masquer*, to "disguise."] See PERSONATE.

Mas'sa.* [From μάσσω, to "knead."] Any compound from which pills are to be made.

Mas'sa de Hy-drar'gȳ-ro,* or **Mas'-sa ex Hydrar'gyro*** ("Mass [prepared] from Mercury.") See BLUE MASS.

Mas-se'ter, e'ris.* [Gr. μασσητήρ; from μασσάομαι, to "chew."] A short, thick muscle of the lower jaw, on each side of the face.

Mas-se-tĕr'ic. [**Masseter'icus.**] Belonging to the *masseter* muscle.

Mas'sĭ-cot. Yellow oxide of lead.

Mas'ta-den, enis.* [From μαστός, the "breast," and ἀδήν, a "gland."] The mammary gland, or female breast.

Mas-ta-de-ni'tis, idis.* [From *mas'taden*, the "mammary gland."] Inflammation of the mammary gland.

Mas-tăl'ġĭ-a.* [From μαστός, the "breast," and ἄλγος, "pain."] Pain of the mammary gland, or breast.

Mas-taux'e.* [From μαστός, the "breast," and αὔξη, "increase."] Swollen or enlarged female breast.

Mast-hel-co'sis.* [From μαστός, the "breast," and ἕλκωσις, "ulceration."] Ulceration of the *mamma*, or female breast.

Mas'tic, or **Mas'tich.** [Gr. μαστίχη.] A resinous substance obtained from the *Pistacia lentiscus*. It is a stimulant and tonic, but it is rarely given internally, except in combination. (See MASTICHE.) Dissolved in alcohol or oil of turpentine, it is used as a varnish.

Mas-tĭ-cā'tion. [**Mastica'tio, o'nis**; from *mas'tico*, *mastica'tum*, to "chew."] The act or process of chewing; also, the taking, chewing, and insalivation of the food.

Mas'tĭ-ca-to-rȳ. [**Masticato'rius**; from the same.] Relating to mastication. Also, a medicine to be masticated, or chewed.

Mas'tich Tree. The *Pista'cia lentis'cus*.

Mas'tĭ-che,* gen. **Mas'tĭ-chēs.** [Gr. μαστίχη; from μαστιχάω, to "chew."] Mastic. The name applied to the concrete juice of the *Pista'cia lentis'cus*. It has been placed on the primary list of the Materia Medica of the U.S. Pharmacopœia for 1860. It forms one of the ingredients of the *Pilulæ Aloës et Mastiches*. See MASTIC.

Mas'tĭ-cin, or **Mas'tĭ-cine.** A peculiar principle obtained by the action of alcohol upon mastic.

Mastick. See MASTIC.

Mas'tĭ-cot. The same as MASSICOT.

Mas'tĭ-cus.* [From μαστός, the "breast."] Mastic. Belonging to the *mammæ*.

Mas-ti'tis, idis.* [From the same.] Phlegmonous inflammation of the female breast.

Mas-to-car-çĭ-no'ma, atis.* [From μαστός, the "breast," and *carcino'ma*.] *Carcinoma*, or incipient cancer of the breast.

Mas-to'dēs.* [From μαστός, the "breast."] Having large breasts.

Mas'to-don.* [From μαστός, the "breast," "teat," or "nipple," (?) and ὀδούς, a "tooth."] A genus of extinct, gigantic quadrupeds, allied to the elephant; so called from the conical projections upon the surfaces of the molar teeth.

Mas-to-dyn'ĭ-a.* [From μαστός, the "breast," and ὀδύνη, "pain."] Pain occurring in the *mamma*, or female breast.

Mas'toid. [**Mastoi'des**; from μαστός, the "breast," and εἶδος, a "form."] Resembling the breast or nipple.

Mas'toid Proç'ess. [**Proces'sus Mastoi'deus.**] A prominence of the temporal bone, resembling a nipple or teat.

Mas-toi'de-al. [**Mastoi'deus**; from *mastoi'des* proces'sus.] Belonging to the mastoid process of the temporal bone.

Mas-to-i-de-ăl'ġĭ-a.* [From *mastoi'des* proces'sus, and ἄλγος, "pain."] Pain in the mastoid process.

Mas-to-i-de-o-çen-te'sis.* [From the *mas'toid* proç'ess, and κέντησις, a "puncturing."] Perforation of the mastoid process.

Mas-tol'o-ġy̆. [**Mastolo'gia;** from μαστός, the "breast," and λόγος, a "discourse."] The natural history of Mammalia; also, that branch of Anatomy which treats of the female breast.

Mas-to-me'nĭ-ạ.* [From μαστός, the "breast," and μῆνες, the "menses."] Metastasis of the menstrual flow to the *mammæ*, or breasts.

Mas-ton'cus.* [From μαστός, the "breast," and ὄγκός, a "tumor."] A tumor of the *mamma*, mammary gland itself, or nipple.

Mas-to-pạ-rec'tạ-mạ, *atis*.* [From μαστός, the "breast," and παρέκταμα, "immoderate extension."] Excessive distension of the breasts.

Mas-to-pạ-thi'ạ.* [From μαστός, the "breast," and πάθος, "affection," or "disease."] Pain in the female breast: mastop'athy.

Mas-to-path'ĭ-cus.* Belonging to *mastopathia*.

Mas-to-pim-e-lon'cus,* or **Mas-to-pĭ-on'cus.*** [From μαστός, the "breast," πιμελή, "fat," and ὄγκός, a "tumor."] A fatty swelling or tumor in the breast.

Mas-tor-rha'ġĭ-ạ.* [From μαστός, the "breast," and ῥήγνυμι, to "break forth."] Sudden hæmorrhage from the breast.

Mas-to-scir'rhus.* [From μαστός, the "breast," and σκίῤῥος, a "hard tumor."] Scirrhus of the breast.

Mas-tur-bā'tion. [**Masturba'tio, o'nis**, a contraction of *ma'nu-stupra'tio* ("defilement by the hand"); from *ma'nus*, the "hand," and *stu'pro, stupra'tum*, to "ravish," to "defile."] Self-pollution, or the secret vice.

Maté, mȧ-tȧ'. See PARAGUAY TEA.

Ma'ter A-ce'ti.* ("Mother of Vinegar.") A mould plant, belonging to the genus *Mycoder'ma*, which is developed in vinegar.

Ma-te'rĭ-ạ Med'ĭ-cạ.* ("Medical Material," or "Medical Substances." Fr. *Matière Médicale*, mȧ'te'ȇr' mȧ'dè'kȃl'.) A collective term, comprising all medicines, or all substances, natural or artificial, which are used in the cure of diseases. These substances may be divided into two great classes. 1. *Natural*, or those which are found ready prepared by nature: as *cinchona bark, nutmeg, opium*, etc. 2. *Artificial*, or those which have been produced or modified by chemical agency: as *quinia, morphia, calomel, lunar caustic*, etc. Medicines may be again divided into—1. Those which owe their effects to some peculiar specific property or principle which acts upon the vital irritability of the different organs or parts of the body: as *tartar emetic*, which has a specific action directed chiefly to the stomach; *calomel*, whose action is principally directed to the liver and salivary glands; and *alcohol*, which exerts a special influence on the brain and nervous system, etc. 2. Those which owe their effects to merely mechanical properties, as emollient poultices, lubricating substances used for allaying cough, etc. To this last division may be referred bran bread, bran mush, etc., which owe their aperient effects to the mechanical irritation of the alimentary canal, arising from the rough particles contained in the food.

Matias. See MALAMBO.

Matico,* mȧ-tee'ko. The South American name of the *Artan'the elonga'ta*, a shrub growing wild in the interior of Peru. Also, the Pharmacopœial name for the leaves of the *Artanthe elongata*. They have been assigned a place on the primary list of the Materia Medica in the U.S. Pharmacopœia for 1860. Matico is an aromatic stimulant and tonic, with a tendency like cubebs to act on the urinary passages. Hence it has been employed in gonorrhœa and other affections of the mucous membrane of the urethra, vagina, etc. It has also been highly recommended as a styptic in *hæmatemesis, hæmaturia*, etc.

Matière Médicale. See MATERIA MEDICA.

Mat'rass. A vessel of glass, metal, or earthen-ware, used in the processes of digestion, distillation, etc. Its shape is usually ovoid or globular.

Mat-rĭ-ca'rĭ-ạ.* German Chamomile. The Pharmacopœial name (U.S. Ph.) for the flowers of *Matricaria chamomilla*.

Matrice, mȧ'trėss'. The French term for UTERUS, which see.

Ma'trix, ĭ'cis.* [From μήτηρ, a "mother."] The uterus, or womb; sometimes used almost synonymously with "mother."

Ma'trix of Teeth. The formative organ of a mammalian tooth, consisting of a pulp and a capsule; the former is converted into *dentine*, the latter into cement.

Matter. See PUS.

Ma-tu'rans.* [From *matu'ro, matura'tum*, to "ripen."] Literally, "ripening." Having power to ripen, or mature. Applied in the plural neuter (*Maturantia*, mat-u-ran'she-a) to substances which promote the suppuration of tumors.

Mat-u-rā'tion. [**Matura'tio, o'**nis; from the same.] The process succeeding to inflammation, by which pus or matter is formed in an abscess.

Ma-tu'rĭ-tў̆. [From *matu'rus*, "ripe."] A term used in reference to fruits and seeds which have reached their full development.

Maw'-Worm. The *As'caris vermicula'ris*, or thread-worm; the *Oxyu'ris* of Rudolphi.

Max-il'la.* The upper or lower jaw. See MAXILLARY.

Maxillaire. See MAXILLARY.

Max'il-la-rў̆. [**Maxilla'ris;** from *maxil'la*, a "jaw."] (Fr. *Maxillaire*, måk'sèl'lêR'.) Belonging to the *maxilla*. Applied by Owen especially to the *maxilla superior*.

Maxillary Sinus. See HIGHMORIANUM ANTRUM.

Max'ĭ-mum.* [From *max'imus*, the superlative degree of *mag'nus*, "great."] A term denoting the greatest possible quantity or effect. It is opposed to *minimum*, or the least possible; and to *medium*, or the mean between these extremes.

Mayaceæ,* ma-ya'she-ē. [From *Maya'ca*, one of the genera.] A small natural order of endogenous herbaceous plants, found in marshes in America.

May'hem. [Old Fr. *Mehaigner*, to "hurt."] In English law, "the violently depriving another of the use of such of his members as may render him the less able, in fighting, either to defend himself, or annoy his adversary;" maim, hurt, or wound.

Mays. See ZEA MAYS.

May'weed. The common name of the *Anthemis cotula*, a plant growing abundantly both in Europe and the United States. Its medical properties are essentially the same as those of chamomile.

Ma-zol'o-ġў̆. That branch of Natural History which treats of mammiferous animals. The same as Mammalogy. See MAMMALIA.

Mēad. [Anglo-Saxon, *Médu;* Sanscrit, *Mĕdhu.*] The name of a fermented liquor produced from water sweetened with honey.

Mĕad'ow Crow'foot. The RANUNCULUS ACRIS, which see.

Mead'ow Saf'fron. The COLCHICUM AUTUMNALE, which see.

Mēa'ṡles. (Fr. *Rougeole*, roo'zhol'.) The disease RUBEOLA, which see.

Me-a'tus.* [From *me'o*, *mea'tum*, to "go," "pass," "move."] A passage. An opening leading to a canal, duct, or cavity.

Mea'tus U-rĭ-na'rĭ-us.* ("Urinary Passage, or Opening.") The orifice of the urethra.

Me-chan'ĭ-cal. [**Mechan'icus.**] Belonging to Mechanics, or to a machine. Applied to medicines which owe their effect to mere mechanical properties. See MATERIA MEDICA.

Me-chan'ics. [Lat. **Mechan'ica,** or **Mechan'ice;** Gr. μηχανική, from μηχανή, a "machine."] The science which treats of forces and powers, and their action on bodies either directly or by the intervention of machinery. Theoretical Mechanics is divided into two parts, Statics and Dynamics.

Meck'el's Gan'glĭ-on. The spheno-palatine ganglion, discovered by Meckel.

Mec'o-nāte. [**Meco'nas, a'**tis.] A combination of meconic acid with a base.

Me-con'ic. [**Mecon'icus;** from μήκων, the "poppy."] Belonging to the poppy. Applied to an acid which forms one of the constituents of opium.

Me-con'ĭ-ca.* [The plural neuter of *mecon'icus*. See MECONIC.] Opiates.

Mec'o-nin, or **Mec'o-nine.** [**Meco'nia;** from μήκων, a "poppy."] A white substance found in opium.

Me-co-nĭ-o-ī'dēṡ.* [From *meco'nium*, and εἶδος, a "form."] Resembling *meconium:* meco'nioid.

Me-co-nĭ-o-lo'ġĭ-a.* [From *meco'nium*, and λόγος, a "discourse."] A treatise on *meconium*, its nature and properties.

Me-co-nĭ-or-rhœ'a.* [From *meco'nium*, and ῥέω, to "flow."] A morbidly increased discharge of *meconium*.

Me-co'nĭ-um.* [Gr. μήκων; from resemblance to the inspissated juice of the poppy.] The dark-green excrementitious substance found in the large intestine of the fœtus.

Mec-o-nol'o-ġў̆. [**Meconolo'gia;** from μήκων, the "poppy," and λόγος, a "discourse."] A treatise on the poppy, or on opium.

Médecin, måd'săNG'. The French word for PHYSICIAN, which see.

Médecine. See MEDICINE.

Me'dĭ-a,* the plural of MEDIUM.

Me'dĭ-an. [**Media'nus;** from *me'*

dius, the "middle."] In the middle; between others · medial, or mesial.

Me'dian Ba-sil'ic Vein. A branch of the basilic vein.

Me'dian Çe-phal'ic Vein. A branch of the cephalic vein.

Me'dian Line. [**Lin'ea Media'na.**] A vertical line supposed to divide the body of an animal into two equal parts, the one right and the other left. See MESIAL.

Me'dian Nerve. The second branch of the brachial plexus, descending the inner part of the arm along the biceps muscle.

Me-di-a-sti'num.* [From *me'diostans*, "standing in the middle."] The *septum*, or duplicature of the *pleura*, which divides the cavity of the thorax into two parts; the *Septum thoracis*.

Med'i-ca, Ma'lus.* ("Apple-Tree of Media.") The LIMONUM CITRUS, which see.

Med'i-cal. [**Med'icus;** from *me'deor*, *mede'ri*, or *med'ico*, *medica'tum*, to "cure," "heal," or "treat with medicine."] Belonging to medicine, or the healing art; also, pertaining to medicines.

Med'ical Ju-ris-pru'dence. That science which applies the principles of medicine to the elucidation of doubtful questions in courts of justice; also termed Legal, or Forensic, Medicine.

Medicamen. See MEDICAMENT.

Med'i-ca-ment. [**Medicamen'tum,** plural **Medicamen'ta;** from *med'ico*, to "heal."] A medicine.

Med-i-ca-men'ta,* the plural of *Medicamen'tum*. See MEDICAMENT.

Medicamen'ta Ar-ca'na.* ("Secret Medicines.") Patent medicines.

Med'i-cāt-ed. [**Medica'tus;** from *med'ico*, *medica'tum*, to "heal."] Having the qualities of a medicine.

Med-i-ca'trix, i'cis.* [From the same.] Healing, or curing. Always joined with a feminine noun: as, *vis medicatrix* ("healing power").

Med-i-ci'na Di-æ-tet'i-ca.* ("Dietetic Medicine.") That department of medicine which especially regards the regulation of diet.

Medici'na Di-a-sos'ti-ca.* ("Preserving Medicine.") That branch of medicine which treats of the preservation of health.

Medici'na Gym-nas'ti-ca.* ("Gymnastic Medicine.") That branch of medicine which resorts to exercise, with a view of preserving or restoring health.

Medici'na Pro-phy-lac'ti-ca.* ("Prophylactic, or Preventive, Medicine.") That branch of medicine which treats of the means proper for the preservation of the health. See PROPHYLACTIC.

Me-diç'i-nal. [**Medicina'lis;** from *medici'na*, "medicine."] Belonging to medicine.

Mediç'inal Hours. Those in which it is considered that medicines may be taken with most advantage; being in the morning (fasting), an hour before dinner, four hours after it, and at bedtime.

Med'i-çine. [**Medici'na;** from *med'ico*, to "heal."] (Fr. *Médecine*, màd'-sèn'.) The science of medicine. Also, any substance employed for its medicinal effects.

Med'i-cus.* [From *me'deor*, to "cure," or "heal."] A healer of diseases; a physician.

Medioc. = *Medio'cris*,* or *Medio'cre*.* "Middle-sized."

Me-di-o-ju-ras'si-cus.* [From *me'dius*, the "middle," and *juras'sicus*, "belonging to Jura."] Applied to a group of strata comprehending the intermediary oolitic: mediojuras'sic.

Med-i-tul'li-um.* The *diplöe;* also, the medullary juice in the spongy tissue of the short bones, and extremities of the long bones.

Me'di-um,* plural **Me'di-a.** [From *me'dius*, the "middle."] The space or substance through which a moving body passes. The middle place or degree.

Me-dul'la.* [From *me'dius*, the "middle"?] The marrow. The pith or pulp of vegetables.

Medul'la Ob-lon-ga'ta.* (Fr. *Mésocéphale*, mà'zo'sà'fàl', or *Moelle allongée*, mo'ěll' ål'lôNº'zhà'.) The "oblong marrow;" so called from its shape. A name given to that portion of the brain which lies within the *cranium* on the basilar process of the occipital bone.

Medul'la Spi-na'lis.* The spinal marrow, or spinal cord.

Med'ul-la-ry. [**Medulla'ris;** from *medul'la*, "marrow."] Belonging to marrow, or to pith.

Med'ullary Rays. The radiating lines presented by a cross-section of the stem of an exogenous tree or other plant.

Med'ullary Sar-co'ma. A name for *Fungus hæmatodes*.

Me-dul'lin, or **Me-dul'line.** [**Medulli'na;** from *medul'la*, "marrow."] A term applied to the pith of plants, particularly that of the *Helianthus*, or sunflower.

Me-dul-li'tis, ĭdis.* [From *medul'la*, "marrow."] The same as MYELITIS.

Med-ul-lo'sus.* [From *medul'la*, "marrow."] Resembling marrow, or full of marrow, or pith.

Me-du'sa.* [From Μέδουσα, the name of a fabulous monster.] A genus of marine animals belonging to the class *Acalephæ*, having a body like a mass of jelly, which is phosphorescent at night. It excites irritation, and often inflammation, in any part of the human body with which it may come in contact.

Meer'schaum. (German pronunciation, mār'shŏwm.) "Sea-Foam," or "Sea-Froth." A silicate of magnesia; a greasy, soapy substance, found in Asia Minor, also in Cornwall and other places in Europe. When first dug up it is soft, has a greasy feel, and lathers like soap; and on this account it is used by the Tartars in washing their linen.—(DANA.) Tobacco-pipes are made of it in Turkey and Germany.

Meg-a-ceph'a-lus.* [From μέγας, "great," and κεφαλή, the "head."] Applied to plants that have flowers united into large heads. Also applied to animals remarkable for their large heads.

Meg-a-lan'thus.* [From μέγας, or μεγάλος, "great," and ἄνθος, a "flower."] Having large or ample flowers.

Meg-a-lo-car'pus.* [From μέγας, or μεγάλος, "great," and καρπός, "fruit."] Having large fruit: megalocar'pous.

Meg-a-lo-sau'rus.* [From μέγας, or μεγάλος, "great," and σαῦρος, a "lizard."] The name applied by Dr. Buckland to an extinct genus of gigantic Saurians, found by him in oolitic slate near Oxford. Some of them measure from forty to fifty feet in length. They partake of the structure of the crocodile and monitor.

Meg-a-lo-sper'mus.* [From μέγας, or μεγάλος, "great," and σπέρμα, a "seed."] Having large seeds.

Meg-a-lo-sple'ni-a.* [From μέγας, or μεγάλος, "great," and σπλήν, the "spleen."] Enlargement, or tumefaction, of the spleen.

Megalotherium. See MEGATHERIUM.

Meganthus. See MEGALANTHUS.

Meg-a-the'ri-um.* [From μέγας, "great," and θηρίον, a "beast."] The name given by Cuvier to a genus of extinct edentate quadrupeds, including one of the most remarkable of terrestrial mammalia. It is the type of the *Megatheridæ*, or Megatherioids of Owen.

Me'grim. [Lat. **Migræ'na**; Fr. *Migraine*, mè'grĕn' or mé'grån'.] A kind of headache, affecting one side near the eye or temple. See HEMICRANIA.

Meī-bo'mĭ-an Glands. Small glands between the *conjunctiva* and tarsal cartilages, discovered by Meibomius.

Meī-o-ste'mo-nous. [From μεῖον, "less," and στήμων, a "stamen."] Having fewer stamens than pistils.

Mel,* gen. **Mel'lis.** [Gr. μέλι.] The Pharmacopœial name‖ of the saccharine secretion of the *A'pis mellif'ica*, obtained from flowers: honey.

Mel A-e're-um,* Mel Ros'çĭ-dum.* ("Aërial Honey," "Honey-Dew.") Two names for the substance otherwise called *Aeromeli* ("Air Honey"), or manna. See HONEY-DEW.

Mel Dep-u-ra'tum,* or **Mel Despu-ma'tum.*** Clarified honey.

Mel Ro'sæ.* ("Honey of Rose," or "Rose Honey.") A preparation made with honey and rose-leaves. It is astringent and detergent.

Me-læ'na.* [From μέλας, μέλᾶνος, "black."] (Fr. *Méléna*, må'lå'nå', or *Mélène*, må'lĕn' or må'lån'.) A vomiting of a concrete, blackish blood, mixed with acid, or phlegm; the black vomit. A form of *melæna* (called by Good *Melæna cholæ'a*, "Bilious *Melæna*") in which the skin is of a very dark color, has received the name of *Melasicterus*, or black jaundice.

Melæ'na Cho-læ'a.* A name for *Icterus niger* (*Melasic'terus*), or black jaundice. See MELÆNA.

Me-læn'ĭ-cus.* Belonging to *melæna*.

Mel-a-leū'ca.* [From μέλας, "black," and λευκός, "white."] A Linnæan genus of the class *Polyadelphia*, natural order *Myrtaceæ*.

Melaleu'ca Caj-u-pu'ti,* or **Melaleu'ca Leu-ca-den'dron.*** The plant (U.S. Ph.) from which cajeput oil is obtained.

Melaleu'ca Mi'nor.* Another name for the *Melaleuca Cajeputi*.

Mel-am-po'dĭ-um.* [From *Melam'pus*, who first used it.] Another name for the HELLEBORUS NIGER, which see.

Mel-a-næ'mĭ-a.* [From μέλας, μέλᾶνος, "black," and αἷμα, "blood."] A suffocative state, by which all the blood in the body appears very dark or black. Also applied to a condition, usually resulting from chronic disease, in which the blood contains a black pigment matter floating in it.

Me-lan-an-the'rus.* [From μέλας,

"black," and ἀνθηρός, an "anther."] Having black anthers.

Mel-an-chol'ic. [**Melanchol'icus.**] Belonging to melancholy.

Mel'an-chol-ȳ. [**Melancho'lia;** from μέλας, μέλᾰνος, "black," and χολή, "bile;" because supposed by the ancients to proceed from black bile.] A disease characterized by gloomy thoughtfulness, ill-grounded fears, and general depression of mind. A genus of the order *Vesaniæ*, class *Neuroses*, of Cullen's Nosology. See ATRABILIS.

Mélané. See MELANIC.

Mel-a-neph-ĭ-dro'sis.* [From μέλας, μέλᾰνος, "black," and *ephidro'sis*, "morbid perspiration."] Black *ephidrosis*, or the *Sudor Anglicus niger*, or black English sweating fever.

Me-lan'ic. (Fr. *Mélané*, mà'lå'nà'.) Pertaining to *melanoma* or *melanosis*.

Mel-a-nis'mus.* [From μέλας, "black."] Black jaundice. See MELASICTERUS, and MELÆNA.

Mel-a-no-car-çĭ-no'ma, *atis.** [From μέλας, "black," and *carcino'ma*, "cancer."] Black cancer. The same as MELANOMA, which see.

Mel-a-no-car'pus.* [From μέλας, μέλᾰνος, "black," and καρπός, "fruit."] Having black fruit.

Mel-a-nœ-de'ma, *atis.** [From μέλας, μέλᾰνος, "black," and *œde'ma*, a "swelling."] Black *œdema*, or *melanosis*, of the lungs.

Mel-a-no'ma, *atis.** [From μελανόω, to "grow black."] (Fr. *Dégénérescence Noir*, dà'zhà'nà'rĕs'sŏnss' nwår.) A disease in which there are dark soot-colored tubercles under the integuments and in the viscera: black cancer.

Mel-a-noph-thăl'mus.* [From μέλας, "black," and ὀφθαλμός, the "eye."] *Melanoma* of the eye.

Mel-a-no-phy'ma, *atis.** [From μέλας, "black," and φῦμα, a "tuber."] A term applied to the *Seca'le cornu'tum*.

Mel-a-nop'ĭ-per, *eris.** [From μέλας, "black," and πέπερι, "pepper."] The *Piper nigrum*, or black pepper.

Mel-a-nor-rha'ġĭ-a.* [From μέλας, "black," and ῥήγνυμι, to "break forth."] The same as MELÆNA, which see.

Mel-a-no-scir'rhus.* [From μέλας, "black," and σκίῤῥος, a "tumor."] The same as MELANOMA, which see.

Mel-a-no'sis.* [From μέλας, "black."] The progress of *melanoma*.

Mel-a-no-sper'mus.* [From μέλας, "black," and σπέρμα, "seed."] Having black seed or fruit.

Mel-a-nos'to-mus.* The same as MELASTOMUS, which see.

Mel'a-no-sȳph-ĭ-lol'e-pis, *idis.** [From μέλας, "black," *syph'ilis*, and λεπίς, a "scale."] A term for a black syphilitic scaly eruption.

Mel-a-no-than'a-tos,* or **Mel-a-no-than'a-tus.*** [From μέλας, "black," and θάνατος, "death."] An epidemic disease of the middle ages. See BLACK DEATH.

Mel-a-not'ic. [**Melanot'icus.**] Belonging to *melanosis*.

Melanourin. See MELANURIN.

Melanthaceæ,* mel-an-tha'she-ē. [From *Melan'thium*, one of the genera.] A natural order of endogenous plants, found in nearly all parts of the world. Few orders of plants are more universally poisonous than this, whose qualities are indicated by *Colchicum* and *Veratrum* (White Hellebore).

Mel-an-the'rus.* [From μέλας, "black," and ἀνθηρός, an "anther."] Having black, or blackish, anthers.

Mel-a-nu'rin. [**Melanuri'na:** from μέλας, "black," and οὖρον, the "urine."] A new substance, in the form of a black pigment, found sometimes in urine.

Mel-a-sic'ter-us.* [From μέλας, "black," and ἴκτερος, the "jaundice."] Black jaundice. See MELÆNA.

Me-las'ma.* [From μέλας, "black."] A black *ecchymosis*, occurring chiefly in old people.

Melastomaceæ,* me-las-to-ma'-she-ē, or **Me-las'to-mæ.*** [From *Melas'toma*, one of the genera.] A large natural order of exogenous plants, natives of the tropical and temperate parts of America. It includes some species whose fruit is eatable.

Me-las'to-mæ.* The Jussieuan name of a natural order of plants. See MELASTOMACEÆ.

Me-las'to-mus.* [From μέλας, "black," and στόμα, a "mouth."] Having a black mouth.

Méléna, or **Mélène.** See MELÆNA.

Mélèze, mà'lĕz' or mà'làz'. The French name for "larch." See PINUS LARIX.

Me'li.* [Gr. μέλι, "honey."] See MEL.

Meliaceæ,* me-le-a'she-ē. [From *Me'lia*, one of the genera.] A natural order of exogenous trees and shrubs, natives of tropical Asia and America. Bitter astringent and tonic qualities belong to the species of this order. Some of them are purgatives and emetics.

Me'lĭ-æ,* the plural of *Melia*, forming the Jussieuan name of a natural order of plants. See MELIACEÆ.

Mel-i-çe'ra,* **Mel-i-çe'ri-a,*** **Mel-i-çe'ris,** *idis.** [From μέλι, "honey," and κηρός, "wax."] An encysted tumor, the contents of which are of the consistence and appearance of honey.

Mel-i-ce'rous. [**Melice'rus.**] Belonging to *melicera.*

Mel-i-phyl'lum.* [From μέλι, "honey," and φύλλον, a "leaf."] A name for the *Melis'sa officina'lis.*

Me-lis'sa.* [Gr. μέλισσα, a "bee."] A Linnæan genus of plants of the class *Didynamia,* natural order *Labiatæ.* Also, the Pharmacopœial name (Ed. and U.S. Ph.) for *Melissa officinalis;* (Dub. Ph.) the *Melissæ officinalis folia,* or balm-leaves.

Melis'sa Cit'ri-na.* A name for *Melissa officinalis.*

Melis'sa Of-fiç-i-na'lis.* The herb balm.

Mel-i-tæ'mi-a,* or **Mel-i-thæ'mi-a.*** [From μέλι, "honey," and αἷμα, "blood."] The presence of sugar in the blood.

Me-lit'a-gra.* [Etymology uncertain.] (Fr. *Mélitagre,* mà'lè'tâgR'.) A name for *Impetigo.* Also, pain of the limbs, arthritic or rheumatic (?)

Mel-i-tu'ri-a.* [From μέλι, "honey," and οὖρον, the "urine."] The same as *Diabetes Mellitus.* See DIABETES.

Mel-la'go,* gen. **Mel-lag'i-nis.** [From *mel,* "honey."] Any medicine having the consistence of honey.

Mel-lif'er-ous. [**Mellif'erus;** from *mel,* "honey," and *fe'ro,* to "bear."] Producing honey.

Mel-lif'i-cus.* [From *mel,* "honey," and *fa'cio,* to "make."] Making honey; mellif'ic. In the feminine singular it forms the specific name of the common honey-bee (*A'pis mellif'ica*).

Mel-li'tum,* plural **Mel-li'ta.** [From *melli'tus.*] A preparation of honey.

Mel-li'tus.* [From *mel,* "honey."] Mixed with honey: mellitous.

Mel'lon. A new radical substance obtained from the precipitate formed by the action of chlorine on a solution of sulpho-cyanide of potassium.

Mel'o-e.* [From μηλέα, an "apple-tree."] A genus of coleopterous insects.

Meloe Vesicatorius. See CANTHARIS; see also note on page 680.

Me-lon'cus.* [From μῆλον, an "apple," also, the "cheek," and ὄγκος, a "tumor."] A tumor of the cheek.

Mel-o-trid'y-mus.* [From μέλος, a "limb," and τρίδυμος, "threefold."] A monster-fœtus with threefold limbs.

Mem'bra,* gen. **Mem-bro'rum.** The plural of MEMBRUM, which see.

Mem-bra'na,* plural **Mem-bra'næ.** The Latin term for MEMBRANE, which see.

Membrana Conjunctiva. See CONJUNCTIVA.

Membra'na Cor-ti-ca'lis.* ("Cortical Membrane.") The external transparent coat of the ovum of mammalia before the formation of the embryo.

Membrana Decidua. See TUNICA DECIDUA UTERI.

Membra'na Den-ta'ta.* ("Dentate, or Serrated, Membrane.") A process between the *tunica arachnoidea* and the *pia mater.* It sends off a number of slender tooth-like processes, from which it derives its name.

Membra'na Çer-min-a-ti'va.* (The "Germinal Membrane.") A term sometimes applied to the earliest development of the germ in fishes and the Amphibia.

Mem-bra'na Ja-co'bi,* or **Tu'ni-ca Jaco'bi.*** ("Jacob's Membrane, or Tunic.") [Named from Dr. *Jacob,* of Dublin, its describer.] An extremely delicate serous membrane interposed between the retina and the choroid coat.

Membra'na Nic'ti-tans.* ("Nictitating Membrane.") A thin membrane forming a kind of third eyelid, found in certain birds, at the inner corner of the eye. It can be extended over the eye so as to protect it without obstructing the vision.

Membrana Ruyschiana. See RUYSCHIANA MEMBRANA.

Membrana Schneideriana. See SCHNEIDERIAN MEMBRANE.

Membra'na Se-rot'i-na.* (The "Late, or Later, Membrane.") [See SEROTINUS.] That portion of the *Membrana decidua reflexa,* which is formed later than the rest.

Mem-bra-na'ceous. [**Membrana'ceus;** from *membra'na,* a "membrane."] Of the nature of membrane.

Mem-bra'næ,* gen. **Mem-bra-na'rum,** the plural of **Membra'na.** See MEMBRANE.

Mem'brane. [**Membra'na.**] A skin-like tissue composed of interwoven fibres, used to cover some part of the body, and sometimes forming a secreting surface. The simple membranes are divided into three kinds, *mucous, serous,* and *fibrous.* 1. *Mucous membranes* investing or lining cavities and canals which communicate with the external air; as the mouth, the nose, etc. 2. *Serous mem-*

branes lining cavities which have no external communication, such as the cavity of the pleura and the cavity containing the intestines. They have a smooth, glossy surface, from which exudes a transparent *serous* fluid that gives to them their name. When this fluid is secreted in excess, dropsy of those parts is the result. 3. *Fibrous membranes* of various forms constitute capsules, sheaths, aponeuroses, etc.

Mem-bran-ĭ-fo'lĭ-us.* [From *membra'na*, a "membrane," and *fo'lium*, a "leaf."] Having foliaceous membranous expansions.

Mem-bran'ĭ-form. [**Membranifor'mis;** from *membra'na*, a "membrane."] Formed like membrane.

Mem-bran-o-i'dēś.* [From *membra'na*, a "membrane," and εἶδος, a "form."] Resembling membrane.

Mem-bra-nol'o-ġy̆. [**Membranolo'gia;** from *membra'na*, a "membrane," and λόγος, a "discourse."] The science of the membranes, their nature, quality, and use.

Mem'bra-nous. [**Membrano'sus;** from *membra'na*, a "membrane."] Composed of membrane; resembling membrane.

Mem-bran'u-la,* or **Mem-bran'u-lum.*** [Diminutive of *membra'na*, a "membrane."] A little membrane: a mem'branule.

Membre. See Membrum.

Mem'brum,* plural **Mem'bra.** (Fr. *Membre*, mŏmbr.) A member, or limb.

Mem'brum Vĭ-ri'le.* The male organ of generation. See Penis.

Memory, Loss of. See Amnesia.

Me-nin'ġe-al. [**Menin'geus;** from μῆνιγξ, a "membrane."] (Fr. *Meningé*, mà'năng'zhà'.) Belonging to the membranes of the brain.

Me-nin'ġēś,* the plural of Meninx, which see.

Me-nin-ġĭ-i'tis, idis.* [From *menin'gion.*] Inflammation of the *meningium.*

Me-nin'ġĭ-on,* or **Me-nin'ġĭ-um.*** [Diminutive of μῆνιγξ, a "membrane."] The arachnoid membrane.

Men-in-ġi'tis, idis.* [From μῆνιγξ, a "membrane."] Inflammation of the membranes of the brain.

Men-in-go'sis.* [From μῆνιγξ, a "membrane."] A variety of *Syndesmosis*, consisting in the union of osseous pieces by membrane, as in the cranial bones of the fœtus.

Men-in-gu'rĭ-a.* [From μῆνιγξ, a "membrane," and οὖρον, the "urine." The passing of urine containing membranous shreds.

Me'ninx,* plural **Me-nin'ġēś.** [From μῆνιγξ, a "membrane."] A membrane of the brain. Used by Chaussier specially for the *dura mater.*

Me-nis'coid. [**Meniscoi'des,** or **Meniscoi'deus;** from μηνίσκος, a "crescent," and εἶδος, a "form," or "resemblance."] Resembling a crescent; also, shaped like a concavo-convex lens.

Me-nis'cus.* [Gr. μηνίσκος, a "crescent."] Applied to a crescent-shaped cartilage between the joints; also, to a lens convex on one side and concave on the other.

Menispermaceæ,* men-is-per-ma'she-ē, or **Men-i-sper'me-æ.*** A natural order of exogenous shrubs, found in tropical Asia and America. It includes *Menisper'mum*, and *Cocculus Indicus.* Active narcotic and bitter qualities prevail among the species of this order, the former in excess rendering them poisonous, the latter causing them to be valuable tonics.

Men-ĭ-sper-mā'ceous. [**Menisperma'ceus.**] Resembling the *Menispermum.* Applied to an order of plants. See Menispermaceæ.

Men-ĭ-sper'māte. [**Menisper'mas, a'tis.**] A combination of menispermic acid with a base.

Men-ĭ-sper'me-æ.* [The feminine plural of *Menisper'meus.* The same as Menispermaceus.] The Jussieuan name of a natural order of plants. See Menispermaceæ.

Men-ĭ-sper'mic. [**Menisper'micus.**] Belonging to the *Menispermum cocculus.* Applied to an acid.

Men-ĭ-sper'mum.* [From μήνη, the "moon," and σπέρμα, a "seed;" so named because the seeds of some of the species are shaped like a half-moon.] "Moon-Seed." A Linnæan genus of the class *Diœcia*, natural order *Menispermaceæ.*

Menisper'mum Coc'cu-lus.* The moon-seed plant, the berries of which are called *Cocculus Indicus.*

Menisper'mum Pal-ma'tum.* The *Cocculus palmatus.*

Men-o-branch'ĭ-æ, a'rum.* [From μένω, to "remain," and βράγχια, the "gills of a fish."] The abiding or permanent respiratory apparatus of amphibious animals. See Menopomatia.

Men-o-lip'sis.* [From μῆνες, the "menses," and λεῖψις, a "failing."] A term for the failing, cessation, or retention of the *catamenia.*

Men-o-pau'sis.* [From μῆνες, the "menses," and παῦσις, a "cessation."] A cessation of the menses.

Men-o-pla'nĭ-ạ.* [From μῆνες, the "menses," and πλάνη, a "deviation."] A discharge of blood, at the catamenial period, from some other part of the body than the womb; an aberration of the menstrual flow.

Menopomatia,* men-o-po-ma'she-ạ. [From μένω, to "remain," and πωμάτιον, a "lid."] The *operculum*, or lid of the respiratory apparatus of amphibious animals.

Men-or-rha'ġĭ-ạ.* [From μῆνες, the "menses," and ῥήγνυμι, to "burst forth."] Immoderate flowing of the *catamenia*, or menses, or of blood from the uterus; men'orrhagy. A genus of the order *Hæmorrhagiæ*, class *Pyrexiæ*, of Cullen's Nosology.

Menorrha'gia Al'bạ.* ("White Menorrhagy.") The same as LEUCORRHŒA, which see.

Menorrha'gia Lo-chĭ-a'lis.* An excessive flow of the *lochia*.

Men-or-rhaġ'ic. [**Menorrhaġ'i-cus;** from *menorrha'gia*.] Belonging to *menorrhagia*.

Men-os-ta'sĭ-ạ,* or **Me-nos'tạ-sis.*** [From μῆνες, the "menses," and στάσις, a "standing."] Suppression of the *catamenia*.

Men-ox-e'nĭ-ạ.* [From μῆνες, the "menses," and ξένος, "strange."] Irregular menstruation.

Mens,* gen. **Men'tis.** [From μένος, "courage," "strength," or "power."] The Latin term for MIND, which see.

Men'ses,* gen. **Mensium,** men'she-ŭm. [The plural of *men'sis*, a "month."] (Fr. *Lunes*, lün.) The periodical monthly discharge from the uterus; the *catame'nia*.

Menses, Immoderate Flow of. See MENORRHAGIA.

Menses, Obstruction of. See AMENORRHŒA.

Menses, Retention of. See CHLOROSIS, EMANSIO MENSIUM, MENOLIPSIS.

Menses, Suppression of. See AMENORRHŒA, MENOSTASIA.

Mensium,* men'she-ŭm, the genitive of MENSES, which see.

Men'stru-ạ,* the plural of MENSTRUUM, which see.

Men'stru-ạl. [**Menstrua'lis;** from *men'ses*.] (Fr. *Menstruel*, mŏNᵍ'strü'ĕl'.) Belonging to the *catamenia*.

Men-stru-ā'tion. [**Menstrua'tio, o'nis;** from the same.] The monthly periods of the discharge of a red fluid from the uterus; the function of menstruating.

Menstruation, Difficult. See DYSMENORRHŒA.

Menstruel. See MENSTRUAL.

Men'stru-um.* [Said to be derived from *men'sis*, a "month," because formerly the menstruum was continued in action for a month.] A liquid used to dissolve, or extract the virtues of, ingredients by infusion, decoction, etc.; a solvent. The plural (*menstrua*) is used for the MENSES.

Men-su-rā'tion. [**Mensura'tio, o'nis;** from *mensu'ro*, *mensura'tum*, to "measure."] The act or process of measuring the thorax, abdomen, etc.

Men'tạ.* A name for the *Membrum virile;* also called *Mentula*.

Men'tạ-grạ.* [From *men'tum*, the "chin," and ἄγρα, a "seizure."] A herpetic eruption about the chin, forming a tenacious crust like that on a scald head; the same as SYCOSIS.

Men'tạl. [**Menta'lis;** from *mens, men'tis*, the "mind."] Pertaining to the mind.

Men'tạl. [**Menta'lis;** from *men'tum*, the "chin."] An anatomical term, signifying belonging to the chin.

Men'thạ.* [From *Min'the*, a daughter of Cocytus, fabled to have been changed into the herb.] A Linnæan genus of the class *Didynamia*, natural order *Labiatæ*.

Men'tha Pip-e-ri'tạ.* (Fr. *Menthe poivrée*, mŏNt pwå'vRå'.) Peppermint. The Pharmacopœial name for the peppermint herb.

Men'tha Pu-le'ġĭ-um.* (Fr. *Pouliot*, poo'le-o'.) The plant pennyroyal; used as carminative, emmenagogue, and stomachic.

Men'tha Sạ-ti'vạ,* Men'tha Spica'tạ,* Men'tha Vir'ĭ-dis,* Men'tha Vul-ga'ris.* (Fr. *Menthe verte*, mŏNt vêRt, or *Menthe sauvage*, mŏNt sō'våzh'.) Various names for spearmint. *Mentha viridis* is adopted in the Pharmacopœias.

Menthe. See MENTHA.

Men-ti'go, ġ'inis.* [From *men'tum*, the "chin."] The same as MENTAGRA.

Men'tu-lạ.* [Diminutive of *men'ta*.] The *membrum virile*, or penis; the same as MENTA. Formerly applied to the *clitoris*.

Men'tum.* The chin. Applied to the lower and solid part of the proper *labium*.

Me-nȳ-an'thēs.* [From μηνύω, to

"reveal," to "show," and ἄνθος, a "flower;" because its flowers reveal the marshy or swampy character of the ground on which they grow.—(WITTSTEIN.)] A Linnæan genus of the class *Pentandria*, natural order *Gentianaceæ*. Also, the Pharmacopœial name for the leaves of *Menyan'thes trifolia'ta*; the *Menyan'this trifolia'tæ fo'lia* (of the Dub. Ph.).

Menyan'thes Tri-fo-li-a'ta.* The trefoil, bog-bean, or buck-bean.

Me-nȳ-an'thin. [**Menyanthi'na.**] A starch-like substance obtained from the *Menyanthes trifoliata*.

Me-phit'ic. [**Mephit'icus**; from *mephi'tis*, a "stench."] Having a foul, heavy, poisonous smell or vapor.

Me-phi'tis.* (Latin word for a foul or sulphurous smell.) A foul, noxious, or poisonous exhalation.

Mer-cap'tan.* [From *Mercu'rius*, "Mercury," and *cap'to*, to "seize," or "seize upon."] A liquid of an ethereal character, named from its energetic action on peroxide of mercury. It is alcohol in which the oxygen is replaced by sulphur.

Mercure, mĕʀ'kür'. The French term for MERCURY, which see.

Mer-cu'rĭ-al. [**Mercuria'lis**; from *Mercu'rius*, "Mercury."] Consisting of or belonging to mercury, or quicksilver; also, sprightly, spirited.

Mercurial Balsam. A term for CITRINE OINTMENT, which see.

Mercurial Ointment. See UNGUENTUM HYDRARGYRI.

Mercu'rial Tre'mor. A disorder affecting those employed in trades or occupations which expose them to mercurial vapors, consisting in convulsive agitation of the voluntary muscles when in exercise. Popularly, the *Trembles*.

Mer-cu'rĭ-cus.* [From *Mercu'rius*, "Mercury."] Belonging to mercury.

Mer-cu'rĭ-us.* (The heathen god "Mercury." The name of a planet.) Applied in Chemistry to the metal quicksilver. See HYDRARGYRUM, and MERCURY.

Mercu'rius Cor-ro-si'vus.* ("Corrosive Mercury.") A name for corrosive sublimate. See HYDRARGYRI CHLORIDUM CORROSIVUM.

Mercu'rius Corrosi'vus Ru'ber.* ("Red Corrosive Mercury.") See HYDRARGYRI OXIDUM RUBRUM.

Mercu'rius Dul'cis Sub-lĭ-ma'tus.* ("Sublimated Sweet Mercury.") A name for calomel. See HYDRARGYRI CHLORIDUM MITE.

Mercu'rius Præ-cip-ĭ-ta'tus Al'bus.* ("White Precipitated Mercury.") A name for calomel.

Mercu'rius Præcipita'tus Ru'ber.* ("Red Precipitated Mercury.") See HYDRARGYRI OXIDUM RUBRUM.

Mer'cu-rȳ. [From *Mercu'rius*, the Latin name of the god Hermes; applied to quicksilver on account of its mobility and volatility; Fr. *Mercure*, mĕʀ'küʀ'.] *Hydrargyrum*. A metal which is always fluid above a temperature of about 40° below zero. Its specific gravity is 13.5. It is the only metal which is liquid at common temperatures. It boils at 660° of Fahrenheit, and its vapor condenses on cool surfaces in minute brilliant globules. For the compounds of mercury, see HYDRARGYRUM, HYDRARGYRI, etc.

Mĕr'ĭ-carp. [**Mericar'pium**; from μερίς, a "portion," and καρπός, "fruit."] Half a cremocarp; applied to each of the two portions of fruit of the *Umbelliferæ*.

Mer-ĭ-dĭ-al'ȳ-sis.* [From μέρος, a "part," and *dial'ysis*, a "dissolving."] A partial or incomplete solution of a substance.

Me-rid'ĭ-an. [**Meridia'num**; from *me'dius*, "middle," and *di'es*, a "day;" the *d* being changed to *r* for the sake of euphony. See MERIDIES.] Literally, "belonging to mid-day, or noon." In Astronomy, a great circle of the sphere, passing through the earth's axis and the zenith of the spectator. In Geography, a meridian is a great circle (or rather ellipse) passing through the poles of the earth, and crossing the equator at right angles. A particular meridian (sometimes one and sometimes another, according to the usage of different nations) is fixed upon, from which to reckon longitude.

Me-rid'ĭ-ēs.* [See MERIDIAN.] A Latin word signifying "mid-day," or "noon;" also, the "south."

Me-rid'ĭ-o-nal. [**Meridiona'lis**; from *merid'ies*, "noon," the "south."] That which is situated on a line to the south in respect to the place spoken of; southern.

Mĕr-ĭ-dro'sis.* [From μερίς, a "portion," and ἱδρώς, "sweat."] Perspiration occurring in a particular part.

Mer-is-mat'ic. [From μερίς, a "part."] In Botany, signifies dividing into parts.—(GRAY.)

Mĕr'ĭ-thall. [**Merithal'lus**; from μερίς, a "part," and θαλλός, a "branch."] A name for an internode of plants.

Mĕr'o-çēle.* [From μηρός, the "thigh," and κήλη, a "tumor."] Femoral hernia.

Mĕr-o-çel'ĭ-cus.* Belonging to *merocele.*

Me-ro'pĭ-a.* [From μέρος, a "part," and ὤψ, "vision."] Partial dulness or obscuration of sight.

Me-rop'ĭ-cus.* Belonging to *meropia.*

Me'rus.* Pure; unmixed. Applied to wine.

Mesembryaceæ,* me-sem-bre-a'-she-ē. A natural order of exogenous, succulent plants, mostly found at the Cape of Good Hope. It includes the *Mesembryan'themum* ("Ice-Plant").

Me-sen-çe-phal'ic. [**Mesencephal'icus;** from μέσος, the "middle," and ἐγκέφαλον, the "brain."] Situated over the middle portion of the contents of the head.

Mes-en-çeph'a-lum.* [From the same.] The middle or centre of the brain.

Mésentère. See MESENTERY.

Mes-en-ter-em-phrax'is.* [From μεσεντέριον, the "mesentery," and ἔμφραξις, a "stoppage."] Obstruction of the mesentery.

Mes-en-tĕr'ic. [**Mesenter'icus.**] Belonging to the mesentery.

Mes-en-te-rit'ĭ-cus.* Belonging to *mesenteritis.*

Me-sen-te-ri'tis, i*dis,** or **Me-sen-te-rĭ-i'tis, i***dis.** [From *mesente'rium,* the "mesentery."] Inflammation of the mesentery.

Me-sen-te-roph'thĭ-sis.* [From μεσεντέριον, the "mesentery," and φθίσις, a "wasting."] *Ta'bes mesenter'ica,* or a wasting of the mesenteric glands.

Mes'en-tĕr-ÿ. [**Mesente'rium;** from μέσος, the "middle," and ἔντερον, the "intestine."] (Fr. *Mésentère,* mà'zoɴᵒ'-têʀ'.) The largest process of the peritonæum, to which the *jejunum* and *ileum* intestines are attached.

Mes'ĭ-al. [From μέσος, the "middle."] Synonymous with MEDIAN.

Mes'ial Line, otherwise called **Me'-dĭ-an Line.** An imaginary line dividing the body perpendicularly into two symmetrical portions. See MEDIAN.

Mes'mer-ism. A theory or system invented or revived by F. A. Mesmer, about the year 1776, referring all phenomena of life to a magnetic fluid universally diffused; which fluid is influenced, it is alleged, by external agents, especially by certain individuals peculiarly, or pre-eminently, endowed with magnetic power.

Mes'mer-o-Phre-nol'o-ġÿ. The application of Mesmerism to Phrenology. It is alleged by the believers in Animal Magnetism, that, if mesmeric manipulations be directed to any phrenological organ, the particular faculty, or propensity, proper to that organ, will be called into active exercise.

Mes-o-branch'ĭ-us.* [From μέσος, the "middle," and βράγχια, the "gills."] Applied in the plural neuter (*Mesobran'-chia*) to an order of the *Anellata,* comprehending those of which the *branchiæ* occupy the middle of the body, or extend from this point almost to the posterior extremity: mesobranchious.

Mes-o-çæ'cum.* [From μέσος, the "middle," and *cæ'cum.*] A process of the peritonæum to which the cæcum is attached.

Mes'o-carp. [**Mesocar'pum,** or **Mesocar'pus;** from μέσος, the "middle," and καρπός, "fruit."] The middle layer of a fruit or pericarp.

Mes-o-çeph'a-lon.* [From μέσος, the "middle," and κεφαλή, the "head."] See PONS VAROLII.

Mes-o-co'lon.* [From μέσος, the "middle," and κῶλον, the "colon intestine."] A process of the peritonæum to which the colon is attached.

Mes-o-der'mum.* [From μέσος, the "middle," and δέρμα, the "skin."] The *Rete Malpighii.*

Me-sod'me.* [From μέσος, the "middle," and δόμος, a "house."] The *mediastinum.*

Mes-od-mi'tis, i*dis.** [From *mesod'me.*] Inflammation of the *mediastinum.*

Mes-o-gas'tric. [**Mesogas'tricus;** from μέσος, the "middle," and γαστήρ, the "belly."] Belonging to the middle of the stomach, or belly.

Mes-o-gas'trĭ-um.* [From the same.] The umbilical region, or middle portion of the abdomen.

Me-sol'o-bus.* [From μέσος, "middle," or "between," and λοβός, a "lobe;" because situated between the lobes (hemispheres) of the brain.] The *Corpus callosum.*

Mes-o-me'trĭ-um.* [From μέσος, the "middle," and μήτρα, the "womb."] A cellular vascular membrane, between the body of the uterus and adjacent parts.

Mes-o-phlœ'um.* [From μέσος, the "middle," and φλοιός, "bark."] That portion of the bark of plants which is between the *epiphlœum*, or outer bark, and the *liber*, or inner bark.

Mes-o-phyl'lum.* [From μέσος, the "middle," and φύλλον, a "leaf."] The parenchyma of a leaf between the skin of the two surfaces.

Me-soph'y-tum.* [From μέσος, the "middle," and φύτον, a "plant."] The *vital knot* in plants; that is to say, the line of demarcation between the ascending and descending axis.

Mes-o-rec'tum.* [From μέσος, the "middle," and *rec'tum.*] A process of the peritonæum, to which the rectum is attached.

Me-sos'ce-lo-çēle.* [From *mesos'celum*, the "perinæum," and κήλη, a "tumor."] Hernia of the perinæum.

Me-sos'çe-lo-phy'ma, atis.* [From *mesos'celum*, the "perinæum," and φῦμα, a "swelling."] Perinæal abscess.

Me-sos'çe-lum,* or **Me-sos'çe-lus.*** [From μέσος, "middle," or "between," and σκέλος, the "leg."] The perinæum.

Mes-o-tho'rax.* [From μέσος, the "middle," and θώραξ, the "chest."] That part of the chest in insects which gives origin to the second pair of legs.

Me-sot'i-ca.* [From μέσος, the "middle," or "between;" referring to the substance or matter deposited between the portions of the cellular tissue.] The name of an order in Dr. Good's Nosology, comprising diseases affecting the parenchyma. See PARENCHYMA.

Mes'o-tœ-chi'tis, idis.* [From *mesotœ'chium.*] Mediastinal *pleuritis*, or inflammation of the *mediastinum.*

Mes-o-tœ'chi-um.* [From μέσος, the "middle," and τοῖχος, a "wall."] The same as MEDIASTINUM.

Mes-o-tym'pa-nic. [**Mesotympan'icus;** from μέσος, the "middle," and *tympan'icus*, "tympanic."] Applied by Owen to the middle subdivision of the tympanic pedicle which supports the mandible in fishes.

Me-sox'a-lāte. [**Mesox'alas, a'tis.**] A combination of mesoxalic acid with a base.

Mes-ox-al'ic Aç'id. [**Mesoxal'icum Aç'idum.**] A new substance formed on heating to the boiling point a concentrated solution of alloxanate of barytes.

Me'ta (μετά). A Greek preposition signifying "with," "among," "between," "after;" sometimes "over," "beyond." When joined with other words, it often denotes *change*, and sometimes *perversion.*

Me-tab'a-sis.* [From μεταβαίνω, to "pass from one place or state to another."] A change of disease, or of treatment; or from one thing to another, either in the symptoms of a malady, or in the indications for its cure.

Me-tab'o-la,* or **Me-tab'o-le.*** [From μεταβάλλω, to "change."] A change, or mutation; a change of place. Also, the same as METABASIS.

Met-a-bol'ic. [**Metabol'icus;** from μεταβολή, "change."] Capable of changing, or being changed. Applied in Physiology to phenomena which result from chemical changes either in the cell itself, or in the surrounding *cystoblastema.*

Met-a-car'pal. [**Metacarpa'lis.**] Belonging to the *metacarpus.*

Met-a-car'pus.* [From μετά, "after," and καρπός, the "wrist."] (Fr. *Métacarpe*, må'tå'karp'.) The group of five cylindrical bones situated between the *carpus* and fingers.

Me-taç-e-ton'ic [from μετά, denoting "change," and *aç'etone?*] **Aç'id.** One of the products obtained when sugar is heated with hydrate of potash. It is similar to acetic acid.

Me-tach'y-sis.* [From μετά, "beyond," and χύσις, an "effusion."] The process of transfusion.

Met-a-çy-e'sis.* [From μετά, "after," "beyond," and κύησις, "uterine gestation."] Extra-uterine gestation.

Met-a-gen'e-sis.* [From μετά, implying "change," and γένεσις, "generation."] A term indicating a series of changes in organic development according to the law of *parthenogenesis.* Thus, the Acalephe passes through the infusorial and the polype stages, and propagates by germination, as well as by spontaneous division, before it acquires sexual organs. This differs from metamorphosis, in which the individual changes its form.

Met'al. [**Metal'lum;** from μέταλλον, a "mine," or "metal."] A substance regarded as simple or elementary, and distinguished by a peculiar lustre, resulting from its opacity and reflective power in regard to light. The metals are considered as electro-positive bodies.

Me-tal'lic. [**Metal'licus;** from the same.] Relating to metal; consisting of metal.

Met-al-li-zā'tion. [**Metalliza'tio, o'nis;** from the same.] A conversion into metal.

Me-tal-lo-dyn'i-a.* [From *met'al*, and ὀδύνη, "pain."] Pain, or illness, induced by working among metals, as the lead colic, and mercurialization.

Met-al-log'ra-phy. [**Metallogra'phia;** from μέταλλον, a "mine," or "metal," and γράφω, to "write."] A description of metals.

Met'al-loid. [**Metalloi'des;** from μέταλλον, a "mine," or "metal," and εἶδος, a "form."] Resembling metal.

Met'al-lur-gy. [**Metallur'gia;** from μέταλλον, a "mine," or "metal," and ἔργον, a "work."] The art of separating metals from their ores.

Met-a-mĕr'ic. [**Metamer'icus;** from μετά, implying "change," and μέρος, a "part."] Applied to compounds where the elements are the same as in other combinations, but arranged differently.

Met-a-mor'phi-cus.* Pertaining to change. See DEVELOPMENTAL.

Met-a-mor-phop'si-a.* [From μεταμορφόω, to "transform," and ὄψις, "vision."] (Fr. *Berlue*, bĕr'lü'.) Vision in which objects are changed or distorted.

Met-a-mor'pho-sis. [Lat. **Metamorpho'sis;** Gr. μεταμόρφωσις, from μεταμορφόω, to "transform."] The change of form which insects and some other animals undergo in passing from one stage of existence to another. The several forms which insects assume are called *larva*, *pupa* or *chrysalis*, and *imago*, which last is their perfect state. In Botany, the transformation of one organ into another homologous one.

Met-a-phys'ics. [**Metaphys'ica,** or **Metaphys'ice;** from μετά, "after," and φυσικά, the "science of physics;" because the study of mind naturally comes after, as it is more difficult than, the science of external nature.] The science which treats of the nature and laws of the mind. "A word employed in popular usage to denote all those inquiries which are conversant about objects other than merely physical and sensible."—(BRANDE).

Me-tas'ta-sis,* plural **Me-tas'ta-sēs.** [From μεθίστημι, to "transpose."] The translation, or shifting, of a disease from one part of the body to another, or to some internal organ.

Met-a-stat'ic. [**Metastat'icus.**] Belonging to *metastasis*.

Met-a-tar'sal. [**Metatarsa'lis.**] Belonging to the *metatarsus*.

Met-a-tar'sus.* [From μετά, "after," or "below," and ταρσός, the "tarsus."] (Fr. *Métatarse*, mā'tā'tars'.) The group of five cylindrical bones of the foot, between the *tarsus* and the toes. Applied in Ornithology to a single bone ending in three pulley-like productions representing the *tarsus* and *metatarsus* together.

Met-a-tho'rax, a'cis.* [From μετά, "after," or "below," and θώραξ, the "chest."] The third, or posterior, segment of the thorax of insects.

Met-a-tro'phi-a.* [From μετά, implying "change, or perversion," and τροφή, "nourishment."] Morbid nutrition.

Met-a-zo'ic. [**Metazo'icus;** from μετά, "after," or "below," and ζωή, "life."] Applied to the *strata* of the more ancient rocks which contain the *débris* of organized bodies, so that one is compelled to regard them as posterior to the appearance of vegetables and animals on the surface of the globe.

Me'te-or. [**Meteo'rum;** from μετέωρος, "aerial," "elevated," "pertaining to the sky."] A body suspended, or in motion, in the atmosphere, there becoming the agent of some phenomenon; also, the phenomena which arise in the atmosphere.

Me-te-or'ic. [**Meteor'icus.**] Belonging to a meteor, or to the sky. Applied to stones which fall from the heavens in certain circumstances, and to waters which accrue from condensation of the vapors suspended in the atmosphere.

Me'te-or-ism. [**Meteoris'mus;** from μετεωρίζω, to "raise up."] The secretion of gas or air in the abdomen.

Me'te-or-o-lite. [**Meteorol'ites;** from μετέωρος, "on high," "aerial," "pertaining to the sky," and λίθος, a "stone."] Certain stones which fall from the heavens after the appearance of meteors; an aërolite.

Me-te-o-rol'o-gy. [**Meteorolo'gia;** from μετέωρος, "aerial," "elevated," "pertaining to the sky," and λόγος, a "discourse."] The science of meteors, or the science which explains the various phenomena of the atmosphere, and treats of the changes of the weather. In its extended signification it comprises Climatology, and one division of Physical Geography.

Me-thæm'a-ta.* [From μετά, "after," "among," or "between," and αἷμα, "blood."] A term applied to the *intermediate* (or capillary) system of blood-vessels. See CAPILLARY.

Me-thod'ic Med'i-cine. [**Medici'na Method'ica.**] Medicine as practised by the sect called *Medici methodici* (Methodists), by exact rules, in opposition to empirical practice.

Meth-o-gas-tro'sis.* [From μέθη,

"drunkenness," and *gastro'sis*, "disease of the stomach."] Disease of the stomach, arising from indulgence in stimulating drinks.

Meth-o-ma'ni-a.* [From μέθη, "drunkenness," and μανία, "madness."] *Mania a potu*, or insanity resulting from drunkenness.

Meth'yl. [**Methy'le.**] A term applied to a newly discovered radical of pyroxylic spirit.

Meth-y-le'num.* [From *methy'le.*] A certain hypothetical base, supposed to be the radical base of a series of organic compounds.

Meth'y-sis.* [Gr. μέθυσις.] Drunkenness, or intoxication.

Me-thys'ti-ca.* [From the same.] Substances employed for the purposes of exhilaration and inebriation.

Métis, mà'tès'. The French term for Hybrid, which see.

Met-o-pan-tral'gi-a.* [From *metopan'trum*, the "frontal sinus," and ἄλγος, "pain."] Pain in the frontal sinuses.

Met-o-pan-tri'tis, idis.* [From *metopan'trum*, the "frontal sinus."] Inflammation in the frontal sinuses.

Met-o-pan'tron,* or **Met-o-pan'trum.*** [From μέτωπον, the "forehead," and ἄντρον, a "cave."] The frontal sinus.

Me-to'pon,* or **Me-to'pum.*** [From μετά, "beyond," and ὤψ, the "face."] The front, or forehead.

Me'tra.* [Gr. μήτρα.] The uterus, or womb.

Me-træ'mi-a.* [From μήτρα, the "womb," and αἷμα, "blood."] Turgescence, or swelling of blood, in the womb.

Me-træm-or-rha'gi-a.* [From μήτρα, the "womb," and αἱμοῤῥαγία, an "eruption of blood."] Hæmorrhage from the uterus.

Me-tral'gi-a.* [From μήτρα, the "womb," and ἄλγος, "pain."] Pain in the uterus. See Hysteralgia.

Me-tral'gi-cus.* Belonging to *metralgia:* metral'gic.

Met-ra-næ'mi-a.* [From μήτρα, the "womb," and *anæ'mia*, "deficiency of blood."] Want of blood in the uterus.

Met-ra-nas'tro-phe.* [From μήτρα, the "womb," and ἀναστροφή, an "inversion."] Inversion of the uterus.

Met-ra-tre'si-a.* [From μήτρα, the "womb," and *atre'sia*, "imperforation."] Imperforation of the uterus. See Hysteratresia.

Me-traux'e.* [From μήτρα, the "womb," and αὔξη, "increase."] Hypertrophy of the uterus.

Mètre, mē'tr (French pronunciation mêtr). [From μέτρον, a "measure."] A French measure, equal to 39.371 (or about 39⅓) inches,—in other words, about an English yard and one-tenth.

Met-rec-to'pi-a.* [From μήτρα, the "womb," and ἔκτοπος, "out of place."] Displacement, or deviation from the normal position, of the womb.

Met-rec-top'i-cus.* Belonging to *metrectopia:* metrectop'ic.

Met-rel-co'sis.* [From μήτρα, the "womb," and ἕλκος, an "ulcer."] Ulceration of the uterus.

Met-re-lo'sis.* [From μήτρα, the "womb," and εἰλέω, to "roll round."] The same as Metranastrophe, which see.

Met-rem-phrax'is.* [From μήτρα, the "womb," and ἐμφράσσω, to "obstruct."] Congestion, or an overloaded condition of the blood-vessels and substance, of the uterus, or womb.

Met-rem-phy-se'ma, atis.* [From μήτρα, the "womb," and ἐμφύσημα, a "windy swelling."] See Physometra.

Me-tren'chy-tes.* [From μήτρα, the "womb," and ἐγχύω, to "pour in."] An instrument, or a syringe, for injecting medicated liquors into the uterus.

Metria. See Puerperal Fever.

Me-trit'i-cus.* Belonging to *metritis*.

Me-tri'tis, idis.* [From μήτρα, the "womb."] Inflammation of the womb. See Hysteritis, and Uteritis.

Me-troc'a-ce.* [From μήτρα, the "womb," and κάκη, "vice," or "evil."] Decay of the uterus, or womb.

Met'ro-car'ci-no'ma, atis.* [From μήτρα, the "womb," and καρκίνωμα, "cancer."] *Carcinoma*, or cancer, of the womb.

Met-ro-dyn'i-a.* [From μήτρα, the "womb," and ὀδύνη, "pain."] Pain in the uterus.

Met-ro-mal-a-co'ma, atis.* [From μήτρα, the "womb," and μαλακός, "soft."] Softening of the womb.

Met-ro-mal-a-co'sis.* [From the same.] The progress or formation of *metromalacoma*.

Met-ro-ma'ni-a.* [From μήτρα, the "womb," and μανία, "madness."] The same as Nymphomania, which see.

Me-trom'e-ter. [**Metrom'etrum;** from μήτρα, the "womb," and μέτρον, a "measure."] The same as Hysterometer, which see.

Met-ro-neu'ri-a.* [From μήτρα, the "womb," and νεῦρον, a "nerve."] A nervous affection of the womb.

Met-ro-pa-thi'a.* [From μήτρα, the

"womb," and πάθος, "disease."] An affection of the womb.

Met-ro-pĕr-ĭ-to-ni'tis, i*dis.** [From μήτρα, the "womb," and *peritoni'tis.*] Inflammation of the uterus and peritonæum.

Met-ro-phle-bi'tis, i*dis.** [From μήτρα, the "womb," and *phlebi'tis.*] Inflammation of the veins of the womb.

Me-troph'thĭ-sis.* [From μήτρα, the "womb," and φθίσις, "wasting."] *Tabes,* or wasting, of the uterus.

Met-ro-ple-tho'ra.* [From μήτρα, the "womb," and πληθώρα, "fulness."] A plethoric or congested state of the uterus.

Met-ro-pol'ȳ-pus.* [From μήτρα, the "womb," and *pol'ypus.*] *Polypus* of the womb.

Met-ro-pȳ-oph'thĭ-sis.* [From μήτρα, the "womb," πύον, "pus," and φθίσις, "consumption."] Purulent *tabes* of the uterus.

Met-ror-rhag'ĭ-cus.* Belonging to metrorrhagy.

Met-ror'rha-ġȳ. [Metrorrha'gia; from μήτρα, the "womb," and ῥήγνυμι, to "break forth."] Excessive discharge (usually hæmorrhage) from the womb.

Met-ror-rhex'is.* [From μήτρα, the "womb," and ῥῆξις, a "rupture."] Rupture of the uterus.

Met-ror-rhœ'a.* [From μήτρα, the "womb," and ῥέω, to "flow."] A discharge from the uterus, as of blood, mucus, etc.

Met-ror'rho-is, i*dis.** [From the same.] Hæmorrhoidal affection of the womb.

Met-ro-scir'rhus.* [From μήτρα, the "womb," and σκίῤῥος, a "hard tumor."] Scirrhus of the uterus.

Met'ro-scope. [Metrosco'pium; from μήτρα, the "womb," and σκοπέω, to "examine."] An instrument for examining the uterus.

Met-ro-sco'pĭ-a.* [From the same.] Investigation of the uterus: metros'copy.

Met-ro-ste-re'sis.* [From μήτρα, the "womb," and στέρησις, "privation."] Extirpation, or removal, of the uterus.

Met'ro-tome. [Metrot'omus; from μήτρα, the "womb," and τέμνω, to "cut."] The same as Hysteratome, which see.

Met-ro-to'mĭ-a.* [From the same.] Metrot'omy. The same as Hysterotomy.

Met-ro-tom'ĭ-cus.* Of, or belonging to, *metrotomia.*

Met-ry-pĕr-æs-the'sis.* [From μήτρα, the "womb," and *hyperæsthe'sis,* "excessive sensibility."] Too great sensibility or irritability of the womb.

Met-ry-per-tro'phĭ-a.* [From μήτρα, the "womb," and *hypertro'phia,* "hypertrophy."] Hypertrophy of the womb.

Meurtrissure, mur'trė̀'sür'. The French term for Contusion, which see.

Mez-e-re'um,* or **Me-ze're-on.*** Pharmacopœial names ‖ of the root-bark of *Daph'ne mezere'um,* or mezereon. Used as a diaphoretic, diuretic, and alterative, and sometimes externally as an epispastic.

Mī'asm. [Mias'ma, a*tis;* from μιαίνω, to "pollute," to "corrupt."] Floating and impalpable morbific *effluvia,* the product of decay or putrefaction of animal and vegetable substances.

Mi-as'ma-ta,* the plural of *Miasma.* See Miasm.

Mī-as-mat'ic. [Miasmat'icus.] Belonging to miasm.

Mī'ca.* [From *mi'co,* to "glister."] A mineral of a laminated and glittering appearance. It is one of the constituents of granite.

Mi'ca.* [From μικκός, Doric for μικρός, "little."] A term for a crumb, or small portion broken off from any thing.

Mī-cā'ceous. [Mica'ceus; from *mi'ca.*] Belonging to, or resembling, mica.

Micatio (mi-ka'she-o), **o***'nis.** [From *mi'co, mica'tum,* to "glitter," to "flash."] Rapid winking of the eyelids.

Mic. pan. = *Mi'ca pa'nis.** "Crumb of bread."

Mic-ran-a-to'mĭ-a.* [From μικρός, "small," and *anato'mia,* "anatomy."] Microscopic anatomy.

Mic-ran-a-tom'ĭ-cus.* Belonging to *micranatomia.*

Mic-ris-tol'o-ġȳ. [Micristolo'gia; from μικρός, "small," and *histolo'gia,* "histology."] The science which treats of the minutest organic fibres.

Mic-ro-car'pus.* [From μικρός, "small," and καρπός, "fruit."] Having small fruit. Also applied to mosses that have small urns.

Mic-ro-çeph'a-lus.* [From μικρός, "small," and κεφαλή, the "head."] Having flowers disposed in small heads. In Zoology, having a small head.

Mic-ro-che'mĭ-a.* [From μικρός, "small," and *che'mia,* "chemistry."] Minute chemical investigation, respecting, for example, the constitution of the atmosphere, organic, vegetable, and animal juices, etc.: microchem'istry.

Mic-ro-chem'ĭ-cus.* Belonging to *microchemia:* microchem'ical.

Mī'cro-cosm. [Microcos'mus;

from μικρός, "little," "minute," and κόσμος, a "world."] Literally, a "little world." A term applied to man, as presenting in his mind, or organization, an epitome or similitude of the great world, or *Macrocosm.*

Mī-cro-cos'mic. [**Microcos'micus.**] Belonging to a microcosm.

Microcos'mic Salt. A triple salt of soda, ammonia, and phosphoric acid, obtained from urine: so named because found in the human body.

Mī-cro-cos-mog'ra-phy̆. [**Microcosmogra'phia;** from *mi'crocosm,* and γράφω, to "write."] A description of the microcosm, or human body.

Mī-cro-cos-mol'o-ġy̆. [**Microcosmolo'gia;** from *mi'crocosm,* and λόγος, a "discourse."] A treatise on the human body.

Mic'ro-don, on'*tis.** [From μικρός, "small," and ὀδούς, a "tooth."] Having short or small teeth.

Mic-ro-glos'sĭ-a.* [From μικρός, "small," and γλῶσσα, the "tongue."] Congenital smallness of the tongue.

Mic-ro-graph'ic. [**Microgaph'icus.**] Belonging to micrography.

Mī-crog'ra-phy̆. [**Microgra'phia;** from μικρός, "minute," and γράφω, to "write."] An account of microscopic investigations.

Mī-crol'o-ġy̆. [**Microlo'gia;** from μικρός, "minute," and λόγος, a "discourse."] The doctrine or science of minute objects, as microscopical animals and plants.

Mī-crom'e-ter. [**Microm'etrum;** from μικρός, "minute," and μέτρον, a "measure."] An instrument for ascertaining the dimensions of very minute objects under the microscope.

Mī-cro-met'ric. Belonging to the micrometer.

Mic-ro-pet'a-lus.* [From μικρός, "small," and πέταλον, a "petal."] Having short or small petals.

Mic-roph-thăl'mĭ-a.* [From μικρός, "little," and ὀφθαλμός, the "eye."] A morbid shrinking or wasting of the eyeballs.

Mī-cro-phy̆l'lous. [**Microphyl'lus;** from μικρός, "little," and φύλλον, a "leaf."] Having small leaves.

Mī'cro-py̆le. [**Microp'yla;** from μικρός, "little," and πυλή, a "gate."] The orifice of a seed.

Mī'cro-scope. [**Microsco'pium;** from μικρός, "minute," and σκοπέω, to "examine."] An optical instrument by which minute objects, scarcely or not at all visible to the naked eye, may be distinctly seen.

Mī-cro-scop'ic, Mī-cro-scop'ic-al. [**Microscop'icus;** from the same.] Relating to a microscope; like a microscope; so minute, as can only be seen by means of a microscope.

Mic-ro-sper'mus.* [From μικρός, "minute," and σπέρμα, a "seed."] Having very small seeds or grains.

Mic-ro-sphy̆x'ĭ-a.* [From μικρός, "little," and σφύξις, the "pulse."] Smallness and weakness of pulse.

Mic-ro-sta'chy̆-us.* [From μικρος, "little," and στάχυς, an "ear," or "spike."] Having flowers disposed in small spikes.

Mic'tion. [**Mic'tio, o'***nis;* from *min'go, mic'tum,* to "pass water."] The act of passing water.

Mic-tu-rĭ'tion. [**Micturi'tio, o'***nis;* from *mictu'rio,* to "desire to make water."] A constant inclination to pass water.

Mid'rib. The middle or main rib of a leaf.

Mid'riff. [Anglo-Saxon, *mid,* "middle," and *hrif,* the "belly."] The diaphragm.

Mid'wife. (Lat. **Obstet'rix, i***cis;* Fr. *Sage Femme,* sȧzh fȧmm, or *Accoucheuse,* ȧ'koo'shuz'.) A woman who delivers women with child; a female obstetrician.

Miel, me-ĕl'. The French term for "honey." See MEL.

Migraine, mè'gʀĕn' or mè'gʀȧn'. The French term for HEMICRANIA, which see.

Mī-grā'tion. [**Migra'tio, o'***nis;* from *mi'gro, migra'tum,* to "remove from one place to another."] The passage or flight from one country to another. Applied particularly to migratory animals.

Mī'gra-to-ry̆. [**Migrato'rius;** from the same.] Passing instinctively and habitually from one region or latitude to another, on account of the change of the season, as certain kinds of birds.

Mil-ĭ-a'rĭ-a.* [From *mil'ium,* "millet."] (Fr. *Miliaire,* mè'lè'êʀ'.) Also called *Febris miliaris.* A disease attended with eruption of small red pimples; miliary fever. A genus of the order *Exanthemata,* class *Pyrexiæ,* of Cullen's Nosology.

Miliary Fever. See MILIARIA.

Mil'ĭ-ta-ry̆ Med'ĭ-cine, Mil'itary Sur'ġe-ry̆. [**Medici'na Milita'ris.**] The treatment of the diseases and wounds of soldiers; of which some of the former, and most of the latter, are peculiar to military life.

Milium. See GRUTUM, and AQUULA.

Milk. [Lat. **Lac, Lac'tis;** Gr. γάλα, γάλακτος; Fr. *Lait*, lȧ.] A fluid secreted by the mammary glands of the female of Mammalia. According to Brande, a thousand parts of skimmed milk contain 929 parts of water, 28 parts of curd, 35 parts of sugar, and 6 parts of lactic acid. Cream is composed of about 45-1000 of butter, 35-1000 of curd, and 920-1000 of whey.

Milk-Bearing. See LACTIFEROUS.

Milk-Blotch. See PORRIGO LARVALIS.

Milk, Deficiency of. See AGALACTIA.

Milk, Excessive Flow of. See GALACTIRRHŒA.

Milk Fe'ver. [**Fe'bris Lac'tea.**] A fever accompanying or preceding the secretion of milk in women soon after delivery.

Milk of Sul'phur. [**Lac Sul'phuris.**] Precipitated sulphur.

Milk-Pump. See ANTLIA LACTEA.

Milk-Scab. See PORRIGO LARVALIS.

Milk-Sick'ness. An endemic disease in the Western States, including Ohio, Indiana, Illinois, Alabama, etc., resulting, it is supposed, from the milk being poisoned by something eaten by the cow.

Milk-Teeth. The first, or temporary, teeth.

Mil'le-ped, or **Mil'li-pede.** [**Mil'lepes, edis;** from *mille*, a "thousand," and *pes*, a "foot."] A name applied to several insects having a multitude of feet.

Mil'li-gramme. [From *mille*, a "thousand," and *gramme*.] A French weight, the 1000th part of a *gramme*, equal to 0.015 of a grain avoirdupois, or one sixty-sixth of a grain troy.

Millilitre, mil'le-le't'r or mėl'lė'lėtr'. [From *mille*, a "thousand," and *litre*.] A French measure of capacity, the 1000th part of a *litre;* equal to 0.0610 of an English cubic inch.

Millimetre, mil-le-me't'r (French pronunciation, mėl'lė'mėtr'). [From *mille*, a "thousand," and *mètre*.] A French measure, the 1000th part of a *metre*, equal to 0.039, or one twenty-sixth, of an English inch.

Mi-met'ic. [**Mimet'icus;** from μίμησις, an "imitation."] Resembling or imitating others.

Mi-mog'ra-phy̆. [**Mimogra'phia;** from μιμέομαι, to "gesticulate," and γράφω, to "write."] A treatise or dissertation on gesticulation or expression by signs.

Mi-mo'sa.* The sensitive plant. A Linnæan genus of the class *Polygamia*, natural order *Leguminosæ* or *Fabaceæ*.

Mimo'sa Cat'e-chu.* The *Acacia catechu*.

Mimo'sa Ni-lot'i-ca,* **Mimo'sa Sen'e-gal.*** The *Acacia vera*.

Mimoseæ,* me-mo'she-ē. A family, or sub-order, of plants, belonging to the natural order *Leguminosæ*. It includes the *Mimosa*.

Min. = *Min'imum.** See MINIM.

Min-der-e'ri, Spir'i-tus.* [From *Min'derer*, or *Mindere'rus*, who first exhibited it.] The *Li'quor ammo'niæ aceta'tis* ("Solution of the Acetate of Ammonia"). It is a valuable diaphoretic, and is much used in fevers and inflammatory diseases.

Min'e-ral. [**Minera'lis;** from *mi'na*, a "mine."] Literally, "belonging to a mine," and originally applied especially to metallic ores. The term now denotes any inorganic substance found in or on the earth. Minerals constitute one of the three grand divisions of nature, called the mineral kingdom.

Min'eral Green. A hydrated subcarbonate of copper, used as a pigment.

Min'eral Oil. A common name for *petroleum*.

Min'eral Pitch. A species of solid bitumen.

Min'eral Tar. The *Petro'leum Barbaden'se*.

Min'eral Tur'pen-tine. A substance obtained from coal oil, and used in painting as a substitute for turpentine. It is the same as rectified *Benzine*.

Mineral Waters. See AQUÆ MINERALES.

Min-e-ral-i-zā'tion. [**Mineraliza'tio, o'nis;** from *minera'le*, a "mineral."] The state or process of a metallic substance being deprived of its usual properties by combination with some other substance.

Min-er-a-loġ'i-cal. [**Mineraloġ'icus.**] Belonging to Mineralogy.

Min-e-răl'o-ġist. [From *minera'le*, a "mineral."] One who is well skilled or versed in Mineralogy.

Min-e-răl'o-ġy̆. [**Mineralo'gia;** from *minera'le*, a "mineral," and λόγος, a "discourse."] The science which treats of the properties, composition, and relations of minerals.

Min-e-rog'ra-phy̆. [**Minerogra'-**

phia; from *minera'le*, a "mineral," and γράφω, to "write."] The same as MINERALOGY.

Min'im. [**Min'imum**; from *min'imus*, the "smallest," implying that it is the smallest liquid measure.] The sixtieth part of a fluidrachm, nearly equivalent to a drop.

Min'ĭ-um.* The red oxide of lead; red lead.

Mint. The common name for the genus *Mentha*; also, *Mentha piperita*, or peppermint.

Mĭ-nu-tĭ-flo'rus.* [From *minu'tus*, "small," and *flos*, a "flower."] Having small flowers.

Mī'o-çene. [From μείων, "less," "fewer," and καινός, "recent."] A term applied to the middle tertiaries; so called because they contain fewer recent shells than the Pliocene, or upper tertiaries.

Mirage (Fr.), mē'râzh'. An optical illusion which is produced by unequal refraction in the lower strata of the atmosphere, and which causes remote objects on the sea or land to be seen double, or to appear to be suspended in the air. When inverted images are formed, the Italians give it the name of *Fata Morgana* (fâ'tâ mor-gâ'nâ).

Mis-an'thro-pȳ. [**Misanthro'pia**; from μῖσος, "hatred," and ἄνθρωπος, "man."] Hatred of mankind, or their society.

Miscarriage. See ABORTION.

Mis-e-re're Me'ī* (*i.e.* "Have mercy on me"). A name for *Iliac passion*, because of its torments.

Mis-lac-tā'tion. [**Mislacta'tio, o'nis.**] A defective or vitiated condition of milk; the same as GALACTIA.

Mismenstruation. See PARAMENIA.

Mismicturition. See PARURIA.

Mis-oġ'ȳ-nous. [**Misoġ'ynus**; from μῖσος, "hatred," and γυνή, a "woman."] Hating women.

Mis-op-sy'chĭ-ạ.* [From μῖσος, "hatred," and ψυχή, "life."] Hatred or weariness of life; melancholy, with disgust of life.

Misossification. See PAROSTIA.

Mis-o-zo'ĭ-ạ.* [From μῖσος, "hatred," and ζωή, "life."] Hatred or disgust of life.

Mist. = *Mistu'ra.** "A mixture."

Mis'tle-toe, Mis'el-toe, or **Mis'sel-to.** [**Vis'cum Al'bum.**] A parasitical plant, growing on the branches of many kinds of trees, and well known in connection with the Druidical ceremonies. The powder of its leaves has been used as a remedy in epilepsy.

Mis-tu'rạ.* [From *mis'ceo*, *mis'tum* or *mix'tum*, to "mix," to "mingle."] (Fr. *Mixtion*, mēks'te-ōno', and *Potion*, po'-se-ōno'.) A mixture. A fluid composed of two or more ingredients.

Mistu'ra Am-mo-nĭ'ạ-cī.* ("Mixture of Ammoniac.") Take of ammoniac, one hundred and twenty grains; water, half a pint. Rub the ammoniac with the water, gradually added, until they are thoroughly mixed, and strain.

Mistu'ra A-mȳg'dạ-læ.* ("Mixture of Almond.") Take of sweet almond, half a troyounce; gum arabic, in fine powder, thirty grains; sugar, one hundred and twenty grains; distilled water, eight fluidounces. Having blanched the almond, beat it with the gum arabic and sugar in a mortar, until they are thoroughly mixed; then rub the mixture with the distilled water, gradually added, and strain.

Mistu'ra As-sạ-fœt'ĭ-dæ.* ("Mixture of Assafœtida.") Take of assafœtida, one hundred and twenty grains; water, half a pint. Rub the assafœtida with the water, gradually added, until they are thoroughly mixed.

Mistu'ra Chlo-ro-for'mi.* ("Mixture of Chloroform.") Take of purified chloroform, half a troyounce; camphor, sixty grains; the yolk of one egg; water, six fluidounces. Rub the yolk in a mortar, first by itself, then with the camphor, previously dissolved in the chloroform, and lastly with the water, gradually added, so as to make a uniform mixture.

Mistu'ra Cre'tæ.* ("Mixture of Chalk," or "Chalk-Mixture.") Take of prepared chalk, half a troyounce; sugar, gum arabic, in fine powder, each one hundred and twenty grains; cinnamon-water, water, each four fluidounces. Rub them together until they are thoroughly mixed.

Mistu'ra Dĭ-ạ-bol'ĭ-cạ.* ("Diabolical Mixture.") A nauseous mixture sometimes given, in small doses, to persons feigning disease, but so frequently repeated as to maintain the taste of its nauseous components, and thus to provoke a confession.

Mistu'ra Fer'ri Com-pos'ĭ-tạ.* ("Compound Mixture of Iron.") Take of myrrh, sugar, each sixty grains; carbonate of potassa, twenty-five grains; sulphate of iron, in coarse powder, twenty grains; spirit of lavender, half a fluidounce; rose-water, seven fluidounces and a half. Rub the myrrh, sugar, and carbonate of potassa with the rose-water gradually added, then with the spirit of lavender, and lastly with the sulphate of iron, and pour the mixture immediately into a bottle, which must be well stopped.

Mistu'ra Glȳç-ȳr-rhi'zæ Compos'ĭ-tạ.* ("Compound Mixture of Liquorice.") Brown Mixture. Take of liquorice, in fine powder, sugar, in coarse powder, gum arabic, in fine powder, each half a troyounce; camphorated tincture of opium, two fluidounces; wine of antimony, a fluidounce; spirit of nitrous ether, half a fluidounce; water, twelve fluidounces. Rub the liquorice, sugar, and gum arabic with the water, gradually added; then add the other ingredients, and mix the whole together.

Mistu'ra Po-tas'sæ Cĭ-tra'tis* ("Mixture of Citrate of Potassa"), or **Liq'uor Potas'sæ Citra'tis,*** 1850 ("Solution of Citrate of Potassa"); also called **Neu'tral Mix'ture.** Take of lemon-juice, fresh, half a pint; bicarbonate of potassa, a sufficient quantity. Add the bicarbonate gradually to the lemon-juice, until the acid is completely saturated; then strain through muslin.

Mis-tu'ræ,* the plural of MISTURA, which see.

Mith'rĭ-date. [**Mithrida'tium;** said to have been invented or used by *Mithrida'tes,* King of Pontus.] A preparation of numerous ingredients, formerly regarded as an antidote against poisons, but now little used.

Mit'ĭ-găt-ing. [**Mit'igans, an'***tis;* from *mit'igo,* to "assuage."] Allaying, or palliative. Applied to remedies which lull, assuage, or soothe pain.

Mi'trạ.* [From μίτρα, a "mitre," or "turban."] Applied to the hat of mushrooms when it is low, thick, round, and plaited. In Surgery, a fillet or bandage applied on the head.

Mi'trạl. [**Mitra'lis;** from *mi'tra,* a "turban," or "mitre."] Belonging to a mitre, or shaped like a mitre.

Mi'tral Valves. Applied to the left auriculo-ventricular valves, from their shape.

Mi-trĭ-for'mis.* [From *mi'tra,* a "turban," or "mitre."] Having the form of a mitre.

Mitt. = *Mit'te,** "send;" *Mitta'tur** or *Mittan'tur,** "let there be drawn."

Mitt. Sang. = *Mitta'tur san'guis.** "Let blood be drawn."

Mixed Fe'ver. [**Syn'ochus.**] A mixture of the symptoms of inflammatory and typhus fever, being a combination of *Synocha* and *Typhus.*

Mixtura. See MISTURA.

Mne-mon'ic. [**Mnemon'icus.**] Belonging to mnemonics.

Mnemonics, ne-mon'iks. [**Mnemon'ica,** or **Mnemon'ice;** from μνήμη, the "memory."] The art of memory, or of remembering.

Mo-bil'ĭ-tȳ. [**Mobil'itas, a'***tis;* from *mo'bilis,* "movable."] A capability of motion; ability or tendency to move with rapidity or ease; tendency to change.

Moch'lĭ-um.* [Gr. μοχλίον, diminutive of μοχλός, a *vectis,* or "lever."] A small *vectis.* An instrument used in obstetrical surgery.

Moch'lus.* [Gr. μοχλός.] The *vectis,* or lever.

Moc-Main. The produce of the *Bombax heptaphyllum,* being a white shining substance of great lightness and elasticity.

Mo-dĭ'o-lạr. [**Modiola'ris.**] Belonging to the *modiolus;* having the form of the nave of a wheel.

Mo-dĭ'o-lĭ-form. [**Modiolifor'mis;** from *modi'olus,* a "small measure."] Having the shape or form of the nave of a wheel.

Mo-dĭ'o-lus.* [Diminutive of *mo'dius,* a "measure."] Literally, a "small measure;" also, the nave of a wheel. Applied to the central pillar of the *cochlea* of the ear.

Mo'dĭ-us,* the chief Roman measure for things dry, was equal to one-third of a cubic foot, and rather more than an English peck.

Mod. præs. = *Mo'do præscrip'to.** "In the manner directed."

Moëlle, mo'ĕll'. The French term for MARROW, which see.

Mo'lạ.* A molar tooth. The *patella,* or kneepan. Also, a shapeless, fleshy mass in the uterus. See MOLE (*Moles*).

Mo'lạr. [**Mola'ris;** from *mo'la,* a "mill."] Applied to the grinder teeth.

Mo'lar Glands. Two small bodies placed between the masseter and buccinator muscles, having the orifice of their excretory duct opposite the last molar tooth.

Mo'lar Teeth. [Lat. **Mola'res Den'tes;** Fr. *Dents Molaires,* dŏnᵍ mo'-lĕR'.] The grinders, or double-teeth, situated in the back part of the jaw.

Mo-lăr-ĭ-for'mis.* [From *mola'ris,* "molar."] Resembling the molar teeth.

Mo-las'ses. The uncrystallizable

part of the juice of the sugar-cane; also called Melasses, and Treacle.

Mole. [Anglo-Saxon, *Maal*, or *Mal*, a "spot," or "mark."] A small brownish spot (Lat. *næ'vus*, or *mac'ula*) on the skin, generally presenting a few hairs. In Zoology, the genus *Talpa*.

Mole. [**Mo'les,** *i.e.* a "mass."] A name applied to a fleshy mass or tumor sometimes found in the uterus. See MOLA.

Molecula. See MOLECULE.

Mo-lec'u-lar. [**Molecula'ris;** from *molec'ula*, a "molecule."] Belonging to a molecule; consisting of molecules.

Molec'ular At-trac'tion. [**Attrac'tio Molecula'ris.**] The power supposed inherent in molecules of matter, which exerts itself at distances inappreciable, or at the point of contact, and inclines them to combine one with the other.

Mol'e-cule. [**Molec'ula;** diminutive of *mo'les*, a "mass."] A "little mass." The smallest particle of matter conceivable. Applied to that exceedingly minute body, in morbid products, in which we can discover no determinate external circle and internal centre. Also, the same as BLASTODERM, which see.

Mol'ecules, Con-stit'u-ent. Those of each element comprised in an integrant molecule of a compound.

Mol'ecules, In'te-grant. The smallest particles into which it is conceivable to divide a simple body, or a compound body without resolving it into its elements.

Mo-len-dĭ-nā'ceous. [**Molendina'ceus;** from *molendi'num*, a "mill."] Resembling a wind-mill. Applied to seeds having many wings.

Mo-li'men, lim'inis.* [From *mo'lior*, to "labor," or "struggle."] An effort; struggle, or endeavor.

Moli'men Hæm-or-rhag'ĭ-cum,* or **Moli'men Men-stru-a'le.*** The menstrual period or effort.

Mollities,* mol-lish'e-ēz. [From *mol'lis*, "soft."] Softness; tenderness.

Mollities Cerebri. See SOFTENING OF THE BRAIN.

Molli'ties Os'sium* (osh'e-um). ("Softening of the Bones.") (Fr. *Ostéomalacie*, os'tȧ'o'mȧ'lȧ'sē'.) A disease in which the bones become preternaturally flexible, either from an inordinate absorption, or an imperfect secretion of the phosphate of lime.—(MAYNE.) According to Virchow, it is produced simply by the conversion of bone into medullary tissue.

Mol-lus'ca,* or **Mol'lusks.** [From *mol'lis*, "soft."] The second of the four great primary divisions of animals, having soft bodies, and no internal skeletons, as shell-fish.

Mol-lus'cous. [**Mollus'cus;** from the same.] Relating to the Mollusca.

Mol-lus'cum.* [From the same.] A disease of the skin in which numerous atheromatous tumors occur, varying in size from a pea to a pigeon's egg. So called because the tumors resemble in consistency the bodies of molluscous animals. They possess little sensibility, without constitutional disturbance, and have apparently no natural termination.

Mollusks. See MOLLUSCA.

Mol-uc-çen'se Lig'num.* ("Molucca Wood.") The wood of the *Croton tiglium*; also called *Lignum Pavanæ*.

Mo'ly, yos.* [Gr. μῶλυ.] The specific name of a species of garlic; the *Allium moly* of Linnæus.

Molybdænum* (mol-ib-dē'num), or **Mol-ўb-dæ'na.*** [From μόλυβδος, "lead."] A brittle metal which exists in the native sulphuret of molybdæna.

Mo-lўb'dāte. [**Molyb'das,** *a'tis*.] A combination of molybdic acid with a base.

Molybdena. See MOLYBDÆNA.

Molybdenum. See MOLYBDÆNUM.

Mo-lўb'dic. [**Molyb'dicus.**] Belonging to molybdænum. Applied to an acid obtained from it.

Mo-lўb-do-col'ĭ-ca.* [From μόλυβδος, "lead," and *col'ica*, "colic."] Molybdocolic. Lead-colic, or bowel complaint the effect of lead-poison.

Mo-lўb-do-i'dēs.* [From μόλυβδος, "lead," and εἶδος, a "form."] Resembling lead: molyb'doid.

Mo-lўb-don'o-sos,* or **Mo-lўb-don'o-sus.*** [From μόλυβδος, "lead," and νόσος, "disease."] Lead-disease, or lead-colic.

Mo-lўb-do-spas'mus.* [From μόλυβδος, "lead," and *spas'mus*, a "spasm."] Cramp or spasm caused by the poisonous influence of lead.

Mo-lўb'dous. [**Molybdo'sus;** from *molybdæ'num*.] Belonging to molybdænum.

Mo-men'tum.* [From *mo'men*, a "motion," or "impulse."] The momentum of a body is the product of its weight (or mass) and its velocity. It is synonymous with the phrase *quantity of motion*.

Mo-mor'dĭ-ca.* [From *mor'deo*, preterite *momor'di*, to "bite."] A Linnæan genus of the class *Monœcia*, natural order *Cucurbitaceæ*.

Momor'dica El-a-te'rĭ-um.* The plant which produces the wild or squirting cucumber.

Mon-a-can'thus.* [From μόνος, "alone," "single," "only one," and ἄκανθα, a "spine."] Having but one spine: monacanthous.

Mon'ad. [**Mo'nas,** *adis;* from μονάς, μονάδος, a "unit."] An ultimate atom; a primary constituent of matter. Also applied to the most minute of the Infusoria.

Mon-a-del'phĭ-a.* [From μόνος, "alone," or "single," and ἀδελφός, a "brother."] The sixteenth class in the Linnæan system of plants, including those whose filaments are united in a single brotherhood,—that is, set, or column.

Mon-a-del'phous. [**Monadel'phius;** from the same.] Having a single brotherhood: monadel'phious. See MONADELPHIA.

Mo-nan'drĭ-a.* [From μόνος, "single," and ἀνήρ, a "man," or "male."] The first class in the Linnæan system of plants, including those which have only one stamen in each flower.

Mo-nan'drous. [**Monan'drius;** from the same.] Having a single stamen: monandrious.

Mo-nar'da.* Horsemint. The Pharmacopœial name (U.S. Ph.) for the herb of *Monar'da puncta'ta*.

Monesia,* mo-ne'she-a. An astringent vegetable substance, procured from the bark of a South American tree supposed to be a *Chrysophyllum*. It has been prescribed for diarrhœa, etc.

Mo-nĭ-lif'er-us,* or **Mo-nil'ĭ-fer.*** [From *moni'le*, a "necklace," and *fe'ro*, to "bear."] Bearing a necklace, or something resembling a necklace. Applied to plants.

Mo-nil'ĭ-form. [**Monilifor'mis;** from *moni'le*, a "necklace."] Formed like a necklace.

Mon-ĭ-lig'er-us.* [From *moni'le*, a "necklace," and *ge'ro*, to "carry."] Moniligerous. The same as MONILIFERUS.

Mo-nil-ĭ-o-ĭ'dēs.* [From *moni'le*, a "necklace," and εἶδος, a "form."] Resembling a necklace.

Monimiaceæ,* mo-nim-e-a'she-ē. [From *Monim'ia*, one of the genera.] A natural order of exogenous, aromatic trees and shrubs, found in South America.

Monk's'-hood. The *Aconitum napellus;* aconite, or wolf's-bane.

Mon-o-bā'sic. [**Monobas'icus;** from μόνος, "single," and *ba'sis*, a "base."] Having a single base. Applied to certain chemical substances.

Mon-o-blep'sis.* [From μόνος, "single," and βλέπω, to "behold."] A state of vision in which objects are distinct when only one eye is used.

Mon'o-carp, or **Mon-o-car'pon.*** [See MONOCARPIC.] An annual plant; a plant which bears fruit only once.

Monocarpian. See MONOCARPIC.

Mon-o-car'pic, or **Mon-o-car'pous.** [From μόνος, "single," and καρπός, "fruit."] Bearing fruit only once.

Mon-o-car'pous. [**Monocar'peus.**] See MONOCARPIC.

Mon-o-çeph'a-lous. [**Monoceph'alus;** from μόνος, "single," and κεφαλή, the "head."] Bearing a single head, as certain flowers.

Mon-o-chla-mȳd'e-ous. [**Monochlamyd'eus;** from μόνος, "single," and χλαμύς, a "short cloak."] Having a single floral envelope, *i.e.* apetalous.

Mon-o-chron'ic. [**Monochron'icus;** from μόνος, "single," and χρόνος, "time."] Existing at one and the same time. Applied to organic remains.

Mo-noc'la-dus.* [From μόνος, "single," and κλάδος, a "branch."] Bearing but one branch.

Mon-o-clī'nous. [**Monoclin'ius;** from μόνος, "single," and κλίνη, a "bed."] Applied to plants bearing flowers with both sexes: hermaphrodite.

Mon-o-cot-ȳ-le'don, on*is*.* [From μόνος, "single," and κοτυληδών, a "cotyledon."] A plant having only one cotyledon. Applied in the plural (*Monocotyle'dones*) to a class of plants, now generally called Endogens.

Mon-o-cot-ȳ-led'o-nous. [**Monocotyledo'neus,** or **Monocotyled'onus;** from *monocotyle'don*.] Having but one cotyledon. This term was employed by Jussieu to denote endogenous plants.

Mon-o-cra'nus.* [From μόνος, "single," and κράνος, a "helmet," a "covering," or perhaps from κρανίον, the "cranium."] A monster-fœtus with a single mass of brain.

Mon-oc'u-lus.* [From μόνος, "single," and *oc'ulus*, the "eye."] Also termed **Sim'plex Oc'u-lus** (*i.e.* "Single Eye"). A bandage used in *fistula lacrymalis*, and other diseases of the eye, to cover one eye.

Mon-o-did'ȳ-mus.* [From μόνος, "single," and δίδυμος, "twin."] One of twins.

Monœcia,* mo-ne'she-ạ. [From μόνος, "single," "only one," and οἰκία, a "house," or "family."] Literally, "having one house, or family;" because the male and female flowers are found on the same plant, thus forming but one family (see DIŒCIOUS). The twenty-first class in the Linnæan system of plants, comprising those which have the stamens and pistils in separate flowers on the same plant.

Mo-nœ'cious. [**Monœ'cius;** from the same.] Having one house. Applied to a class of plants. See MONŒCIA.

Mon-o-ḡȳn'ĭ-ạ.* [From μόνος, "single," "only one," and γυνή, a "woman," or "female."] The name given by Linnæus to the first order in each of the first thirteen classes of plants, comprising such as have only one pistil in each flower.

Mon-oḡ'ȳ-nous. [**Monogyn'ius;** from the same.] Having one pistil or style: monogynious.

Mo-noi'cous. The same as MONŒCIOUS, which see.

Mon-o-loc'u-lar. [**Monolocula'-ris;** from μόνος, "single," "only one," and *loc'ulus*, a "cell."] Having only one cavity or cell; one-celled. Applied to cystic tumors so constituted.

Mon-o-ma'nĭ-ạ.* [From μόνος, "single," "only one," and μανία, "madness."] A kind of insanity in which the patient is irrational on one subject only, on all others clear and correct.

Mon-o-ma'nĭ-ac. [**Monomani'a-cus;** from *monoma'nia*, "madness on one subject."] A person laboring under monomania.

Mo-nom'ȳ-us.* [From μόνος, "single," "only one," and μῦς, a "muscle."] Having but one muscle. Applied in the plural neuter (*Monom'ya*) to an order of the *Conchifera*.

Mon-o-pĕr-ĭ-an'the-us.* [From μόνος, "single," περί, "around," and ἄνθος, a "flower."] The same as MONOCHLAMYDEOUS, which see.

Mon-o-pet'ạ-lous. [**Monopeta'-leus,** or **Monopet'alus;** from μόνος, "single," and πέταλον, a "petal."] Having but one petal, or several petals more or less united; gamopetalous. The term *Monopet'alæ* is applied by some botanists to a section of angiospermous, exogenous plants.

Mon-o-phȳl'lous. [**Monophyl'-lus;** from μόνος, "single," and φύλλον, a "leaf."] Having but one leaf.

Mon-o-phȳ'o-dont.* [From μόνος, "single," φύω, to "generate," and ὀδούς, ὀδόντος, a "tooth."] A mammal which produces but one set of teeth, as the sloth.

Mon-o-po'dĭ-ạ.* [From μόνος, "single," and πούς, a "foot."] A genus of monsters having only one foot.

Mo-nop'ter-us.* [From μόνος, "single," and πτερόν, a "wing."] Having but one wing. Applied to certain seeds.

Mo-nor'chis, idis.* [From μόνος, "single," and ὄρχις, a "testicle."] Applied to one in whom a single testicle has descended into the scrotum, or who has been deprived of one by accident or by an operation.

Mon-o-sep'ạ-lous. [**Monosep'a-lus;** from μόνος, "single," and *sep'alum*, a "sepal."] A calyx, the sepals of which are united, is called monosepalous, or, more correctly, gamosepalous.—(GRAY.)

Mon-o-sper'mal, or **Mon-o-sper'-mous.** [**Monosper'mus;** from μόνος, "single," and σπέρμα, a "seed."] Having only one seed.

Mo-nos'po-rus.* [From μόνος, "single," and σπορά, a "seed."] Applied to any concepticle of a cryptogamous plant which contains but a single sporule.

Mon-o-sta'chȳ-us.* [From μόνος, "single," and στάχυς, an "ear."] Having but one spike.

Mo-nos'tĭ-chous. [From μόνος, "single," and στίχος, a "line."] A term applied to leaves disposed in one vertical rank.

Mon-o-stig'mạ-tus.* [From μόνος, "single," and στίγμα, a "stigma."] Having but one stigma: monostig'matous.

Mon-o-sty'lous. [**Monosty'lus;** from μόνος, "single," and στῦλος, a "style."] Having but one style.

Mon-o-thal'ạ-mus.* [From μόνος, "single," and θάλαμος, a "bed."] Having but one unilocular shell: monothal'-amous. Applied to an order of Mollusks.

Mo-not'o-mous. [**Monot'omus;** from μόνος, "single," and τέμνω, to "cut."] Having a single cleavage-face. Applied to minerals.

Mon-o-trem'ạ-tous. [**Monotrem'-atus;** from μόνος, "single," and τρῆμα, an "opening."] Having only one opening or vent for semen, urine, and excrements.

Mon'o-treme. [**Monotre'ma, a***tis.*] A name for a monotrematous animal. See MONOTREMATOUS.

Monotropaceæ,* mon'o-tro-pa'-she-ē. [From *Monot'ropa*, one of the genera.] A natural order of exogenous parasitical plants, natives of Europe, Asia, and North America.

Monro's Foramen. See FORAMEN OF MONRO.

Mon'ster. [**Mon'strum,** plural **Mon'stra.**] Originally, any thing prodigious or ominous. A huge, or deformed, animal; a young animal born with a redundancy or deficiency, a confusion or transposition, of parts; a *lusus naturæ.*

Mon'stra,* gen. **Mon-stro'rum,** the plural of *Monstrum.* See MONSTER.

Mons Ven'e-ris.* The eminence in the upper and anterior part of the *pubes* of women.

Mon-tic'o-lus.* [From *mons, mon'tis*, a "mountain," and *co'lo*, to "inhabit."] Living or growing on mountains.

Moorhead. See ALEMBIC.

Moraceæ,* mo-ra'she-ē. A natural order of exogenous trees and shrubs, natives of the tropical and temperate parts of Asia and America. It comprises the Mulberry (*Mo'rus*), the Fig (*Fi'cus Car'ica*), and the Banyan-tree (*Fi'cus In'dica*). Caoutchouc is an abundant product of the *Fi'cus Elas'tica.*

Mor'al In-san'ĭ-tȳ. That in which the intellectual faculties appear to have sustained but little injury, but the feelings and affections are perverted and depraved.

Mor'bi,* gen. **Mor-bo'rum,** the plural of MORBUS, which see.

Mor'bid. [**Mor'bidus;** from *mor'bus*, a "disease."] (Fr. *Morbeux*, mor'buh'.) Diseased, or pertaining to disease.

Mor'bid Tem'per-a-ture. The difference either above or below the natural temperature of the body, as ascertained by the thermometer placed in the *axilla*, or under the tongue, of a patient: the natural temperature is from 96° to 98° Fahrenheit.

Mor-bif'ic. [**Morbif'icus;** from *mor'bus*, "disease," and *fa'cio*, to "make."] Inducing, or causing, disease.

Mor-bil'li,* gen. **Mor-bil-lo'rum** (found only in the plural). [Diminutive of *mor'bus*, a "disease."] A name for *Rubeola*, or measles. See RUBEOLA.

Mor-bil'lous. [**Morbillo'sus;** from *morbil'li*, "measles."] (Fr. *Morbilleux*, mor'bēl'luh'.) Belonging to the measles: measly.

Mor'bus,* plural **Mor'bi.** The Latin term for a disease, or sickness.

Morbus Brightii. See BRIGHT'S DISEASE, and NEPHRITIS.

Mor'bus Ca-du'cus.* ("Falling Disease or Sickness.") A name for EPILEPSY, which see.

Morbus Cæruleus. See CYANOSIS.

Morbus Coxarius, or **Morbus Coxarum.** See COXALGIA.

Mor'bus Găl'lĭ-cus.* ("French Disease.") A name for SYPHILIS, which see.

Mor'bus Her-cu'le-us.* ("Herculean Disease.") A name for EPILEPSY.

Mor'bus In'dĭ-cus.* ("Indian Disease.") A name for SYPHILIS, which see.

Mor'bus In-fan-ti'lis* ("Infantile Disease"), **Mor'bus Mag'nus.*** ("Great or Mighty Disease.") Names for EPILEPSY, which see.

Mor'bus Ni'ger.* ("Black Disease.") See MELÆNA.

Mor'bus Pe-dic-u-la'ris.* ("Lousy Disease.") See PHTHIRIASIS.

Mor'bus Re'gĭ-us.* ("Royal Disease.") A name for ICTERUS, which see.

Mor'bus Sa'cer.* ("Sacred Disease.") A name given to epilepsy, because epileptics were sometimes supposed to be divinely inspired. See EPILEPSY.

Mor-dā'cious. [**Mor'dax, a***'cis;* from *mor'deo*, to "bite."] Biting; pungent.

Mor'dant. [From *mor'deo*, to "bite;" hence, "to take a firm hold."] A substance, used by dyers, which combines with the fabric to be dyed, in order to fix the coloring matter.

More dict. = *Mo're dic'to.** "In the manner directed."

Morgag'ni (mor-găn'yee) **Co-lum'næ Rec'tæ.*** ("Strait Columns of Morgagni.") The longitudinal *plicæ* of the rectum.

Morgag'ni Li'quor* ("Liquor of Morgagni"), otherwise called **Hu'mor of Morgag'ni.** A small quantity of fluid between the crystalline lens and its capsule; discovered by Morgagni.

Morgag'ni, Si'nus-es of. Three small dilatations at the beginning of the aorta, first pointed out by Morgagni.

Morgue (Fr.), morg. [From the Persian *marg*, "death."] A dead-house, or place where dead bodies that have been found are exposed, in order to be recognized.

Mo'ri-a.* [Gr. μωρία.] Foolishness; fatuity.

Mo-ri-bun'dus.* [From *mo'rior*, to "die."] Dying; ready to die.

Mo-ri-for'mis.* [From *mo'rum*, a "mulberry."] Having the form of a mulberry.

Moringaceæ,* mor-in-ga'she-ē. A natural order of exogenous trees, found in the East Indies and Arabia. It consists of a single genus, the *Morin'ga*, which has been used as a remedy in diseases of the urinary organs.

Mo-ri-o-plas'ti-cē.* [From μόριον, a "part," and πλαστικός, "forming."] The restoration of lost parts.

Mor-o-co'mi-um.* [From μωρός, "idiotic," and κομέω, to "cure."] A lunatic asylum, or house for the reception and treatment of the insane.

Mor-o-do'chi-um.* [From μωρός, "idiotic," and δέχομαι, to "admit."] The same as MOROCOMIUM, which see.

Mor'phi-a,* Mor-phi'na,* or **Mor'phine.** [From *Mor'pheus*, the god of sleep or dreams.] A vegetable alkaloid, the most important narcotic principle of opium. It is mostly given in the form of acetate, sulphate, or muriate, which are very similar in their action. Morphia is, in many cases, preferable as an anodyne to opium, because it is less apt to constipate the bowels, and to prôduce headache or other unpleasant effects. It is, moreover, less likely to be rejected by an irritable stomach than opium or laudanum.

Mor'phine, or **Mor'phin.** The same as MORPHIA, which see.

Mor-pho-graph'ic. [**Morpho-graph'icus.**] Belonging to morphography.

Mor-phog'ra-phy. [**Morphogra'phia;** from μορφή, a "form," and γράφω, to "write."] A description of the external forms of plants or animals.

Mor-pho-log'i-cal. [**Morpholog'icus.**] Relating to morphology.

Mor-phol'o-gy. [**Morpholo'gia;** from μορφή, a "form," and λόγος, a "discourse."] The science of form in the organic kingdom. Morphology, as applied to plants, is analogous to the comparative anatomy of animals.

Mor-phol'y-sis.* [From μορφή, a "form," and λύω, to "dissolve."] The destruction of form or organization.

Mor-pho-met'ri-cal. [**Morpho-met'ricus.**] Belonging to morphometry.

Mor-phom'e-try. [**Morphome'tria;** from μορφή, a "form," and μετρέω, to "measure."] The art of measuring or ascertaining the external form of objects.

Mor-pho-no'mi-a.* [From μορφή, a "form," and νόμος, a "law."] The science of the laws of formation: morphon'omy.

Mor-pho'sis.* [From μορφόω, to "form."] A morbid formation; organic disease. In Botany, the manner of development.

Morrhuæ Oleum. See OLEUM MORRHUÆ.

Mors,* gen. **Mor'tis.** [From μόρος, "fate," or "destiny."] The absolute cessation of life; death.

Mor. sol. = *Mo're sol'ito.** "In the usual way."

Mor'sus Di-ab'o-li.* ("Devil's Bite.") A ridiculous name sometimes applied to the *fimbriæ* of the Fallopian tubes.

Mor'tar. [Lat. **Morta'rium;** Fr. *Mortier*, mor'te-à'.] A vessel used in Pharmacy for pulverizing solid substances.

Mor-ti-fi-cā'tion. [**Mortifica'tio, o'nis;** from *mors, mor'tis*, "death," and *fa'cio*, to "make."] The loss of vitality in, or death of, a part.

Mo'rus Ni'gra.* The black mulberry tree.

Mo'rus Tinc-to'ri-a.* [From *tin'go, tinc'tum*, to "dye," to "stain."] The plant which yields the yellow dye called fustic.

Morve, MORV. The French term for "glanders." See EQUINIA.

Mo-sa'ic Gold. [**Au'rum Musi'vum.**] The alchemical name of the bisulphuret of tin. It is produced in flakes of a gold color, and is used as a pigment.

Mosa'ic Sil'ver. [**Argen'tum Musi'vum.**] Made of bismuth and tin melted together, with the addition of quicksilver; used as a silver color.

Mos-chif'er-us.* [From *mos'chus*, "musk," and *fe'ro*, to "bear."] Bearing, or yielding, musk.

Mos'chus.* [Arab. *Mosch.*] Musk. The Pharmacopœial name‖ of a peculiar concrete substance obtained from the *Moschus moschiferus.*

Mos'chus Moschif'erus.* The animal from which musk is obtained; the musk-deer.

Moss, Pec'to-ral. A common name for the *Li'chen pulmona'rius.*

Mosses. See MUSCI.

Moth'er-Wa'ter. The residual fluid after evaporating sea-water, or any other solution containing salts, and taking out the crystals.

Moth'er's Mark. A name applied to any of the appearances included under the term *Næ'vus mater'nus.*

Mo'tion. [**Mo'tio, o'***nis;* from *mo'veo, mo'tum,* to "move."] This term is employed in Animal Physiology to denote the following phenomena:—

1. *Voluntary Motion.* The spontaneous act of the will of the individual; a function attached to the brain.

2. *Excited Motion,* or that of the *reflex function,* as in the closure of the larynx on the contact of acrid vapors; of the pharynx on that of food, etc.; a function of the spinal marrow.

3. *Motion of Irritability,* as the action of the heart, the intestinal canal, etc.; a function of the *muscular fibre.*

4. *Ciliary Motion.* The peculiar vibrating motion of the *cilia* of animals.

Mo'tor,* plural **Mo-to'rēs.** [From the same.] A mover. Applied to muscles, etc.

Mo-to'rēs,* gen. **Mo-to'rum,** the plural of MOTOR.

Moto'res Oc-u-lo'rum.* ("Movers of the Eyes.") The third pair of nerves distributed on the muscles that move the eyeball.

Mo'to-rȳ. [From *mo'veo, mo'tum,* to "move."] Causing motion. Applied to nerves which convey the peculiar stimulus which excites motion, to the muscles.

Moun'tain Cork. The name of the elastic variety of asbestos. See ASBESTOS.

Moutarde, moo'tard'. The French name for MUSTARD, which see.

Mouth. See OS, and FAUX.

Mox'a.* [From the Japanese.] A soft woolly substance prepared from the dried young leaves of *Artemisia Chinensis* and *A. Indica,* and burned on the skin to produce an eschar, with a view to cause revulsion.

Mox-i-bu'ri-um.* [From *mox'a,* and *u'ro,* to "burn;" the *b* being added for the sake of euphony, as in the case of *combustion* (from *con* or *com* and *ustion*).] The remedial application of the *moxa.*

Mox-os-phy'ra.* [From *mox'a,* and σφῦρα, a "hammer."] An iron hammer plunged into boiling water for one or two minutes, and the face now and then applied to the skin as counter-irritant or rubefacient.

Muc. = *Mucila'go.** "Mucilage."

Mu'cāte. [**Mu'cas, a'***tis.*] A combination of mucic acid with a base.

Mu'cic. [**Mu'cicus;** from *mu'cus,* "mucus," or "gum."] Belonging to gum. Applied to an acid obtained from it.

Mu'ci-lage. [**Mucila'go, g'***inis;* from the same.] An aqueous solution of gum.

Mu-ci-lag'i-nēs,* the plural of MUCILAGO, which see.

Mu-ci-lag'i-nous. [**Mucilagino'sus;** from *mucila'go,* "mucilage."] Belonging to mucilage, or to gum; gummy.

Mu-ci-la'go,* gen. **Mu-ci-lag'i-nis,** the Latin for MUCILAGE, which see.

Mucila'go Aca'ciæ* (a-ka'she-ē.) ("Mucilage of Acacia," or of Gum Arabic.) Take of gum arabic, in pieces, four troyounces; water, half a pint. Add the water to the gum arabic, agitate occasionally until it is dissolved, and strain.

Mucila'go Sas'sa-fras* ("Mucilage of Sassafras"), or **In-fu'sum Sas'sa-fras Me-dul'læ,*** 1850 ("Infusion of Sassafras Pith"). Take of sassafras pith, one hundred and twenty grains; water, a pint. Macerate for three hours, and strain.

Mucila'go Trag-a-can'thæ.* ("Mucilage of Tragacanth.") Take of tragacanth, a troyounce; boiling water, a pint. Macerate the tragacanth with the water for twenty-four hours, occasionally stirring; then rub them together, so as to render the mixture uniform, and strain forcibly through muslin.

Mucila'go Ul'mi* ("Mucilage of Elm," that is, Mucilage of Slippery Elm Bark), or **In-fu'sum Ul'mi,*** 1850 ("Infusion of Elm [Bark]"). Take of slippery elm bark, sliced and bruised, a troyounce; boiling water, a pint. Macerate for two hours in a covered vessel, and strain.

Mu'cin. [**Muci'na;** from *mu'cus,* "mucus," or "gum."] The peculiar animal matter of mucus.

Mu-cip'a-rous. [**Mucip'arus;** from *mu'cus,* "mucus," or "gum," and *pa'rio,* to "produce."] Producing or secreting mucus.

Mu-ci'tis, i*dis.** Inflammation of a mucous membrane. Applied to the disease named *Gonorrhœa, Baptorrhœa, Blennorrhagia,* etc.

Mu-civ'o-rous. [**Muciv'orus;** from *mu'cus,* and *vo'ro,* to "devour."] Eating mucus. Applied to certain insects.

Mu'co-çēle.* [From *mu'cus,* and κήλη, a "tumor."] Literally, a tumor involving a mucous membrane or tissue. Applied to an enlargement of the lacrymal sac, occasioning *fistula lacrymalis.*

Mu'coid. [**Mucoi'des;** from *mu'cus*, "mucus," and εἶδος, a "form."] Resembling mucus.

Mu'co-Pu'ru-lent, Mu-co'so-Pu'ru-lent. [**Mu'co-** or **Muco'so-purulen'tus;** from *mu'cus, muco'sus* "mucous," and *pus*, "matter."] Of the nature of mingled mucus and pus.

Mu'cous. [**Muco'sus;** from *mu'cus*, "mucus," or "gum."] Belonging to, or resembling, mucus.

Mu'cous Fol'li-cles. [**Follic'uli Muco'si.**] The follicles or minute glands belonging to the mucous membranes. Their office is to secrete mucus.

Mucous Membranes. See MEMBRANES.

Mucous Tumor. See MYXOMA.

Mu-cro-na'ta Car-ti-la'go.* ("Pointed Cartilage.") The ensiform cartilage of the sternum.

Mu'cro-nate, or **Mu'cro-nāt-ed.** [**Mucrona'tus;** from *mu'cro*, a "short, sharp point."] Having a sharp point.

Mu-cro-nif'er-us.* [From *mu'cro*, a "sharp point," and *fe'ro*, to "carry."] Bearing straight, stiff points: mucronif'erous.

Mu-cro-ni-fo'li-us.* [From *mu'cro*, a "sharp point," and *fo'lium*, a "leaf."] Having mucronated leaves.

Mu-cro-ni-for'mis.* [From *mu'cro*, a "sharp point."] Having the form of a point: mucron'iform.

Mu-cron'u-late. [**Mucronula'tus;** from *mucron'ula*, diminutive of *mu'cro*, a "point."] Having a minute, abrupt point.

Mu-cu'na.* Cowhage. A Linnæan genus of the class *Diadelphia*, natural order *Leguminosæ*. The Pharmacopœial name for the hairs from the pod of *Mucuna pruriens*.

Mucu'na Pru'ri-ens.* ("Itching Mucuna.") The plant which yields cowhage, or cowitch, formerly called the *Dolichos pruriens*.

Mu'cus.* [Gr. μύξα; Fr. *Muqueux animal*, mü'kuh' â'nè'mâl'.] Animal mucus, one of the primary fluids of the animal body. (See PHLEGM.) Also, gum, or vegetable mucus.

Mudar, mŭh-dar', or **Ma-dar'.** A name of the *Calot'ropis Gigante'a* (otherwise called *Calot'ropis Mada'rii*), the bark, root, and juice of which are used in India as a remedy for *elephanti'asis*.

Mud'a-rin, Mud'a-rine, or **Mad'a-rin.** The active principle of the mudar. It is remarkable for its property of coagulating by heat, and becoming again fluid on exposure to cold.

Mul'ber-rȳ. The fruit of the *Morus nigra*.

Mul'berry Cal'cu-lus. A species of urinary calculus, consisting of oxalate of lime, and named from its rough and tuberculated surface, resembling that of a mulberry.

Mul'berry-Tree. The common name for different trees of the genus *Mo'rus*, but applied especially to the *Mo'rus ni'gra*.

Mu-lo-med'i-cus.* [From *mu'lus*, a "mule," and *med'icus*, a "physician."] A veterinary surgeon, or horse-doctor.

Mul-tan'gu-lar. [**Multangula'ris;** from *mul'tus*, "many," and *an'gulus*, a "corner."] Having many angles, or corners.

Mul-tan-gu-la'tus.* [From *mul'tus*, "many," and *an'gulus*, a "corner."] Many-cornered; having many corners, or angles, as the shell of the *Telli'na multangula'ta*.

Mul-ti-ax-if'er-us.* [From *mul'tus*, "many," *ax'is*, and *fe'ro*, to "bear."] Applied to an inflorescence when it presents more than three axes of vegetation.

Mul-ti-bul-bo'sus.* [From *mul'tus*, "many," and *bul'bus*, a "bulb."] Having numerous bulbs.

Mul-ti-cap'su-lar. [**Multicapsula'ris;** from *mul'tus*, "many," and *cap'sula*, a "capsule."] Having many capsules.

Mul-ti-cau'dus.* [From *mul'tus*, "many," and *cau'da*, a "tail."] Having many tails, or many prolongations in the form of tails.

Mul-ti-cau'lis.* [From *mul'tus*, "many," and *cau'lis*, a "stem."] Having numerous stems: multicau'line.

Mul-ti-coc'cus.* [From *mul'tus*, "many," and *coc'cus*, a "berry," or "capsule."] Having many berries, or many seeds.

Mul-ti-em-bry-o-na'tus.* [From *mul'tus*, "many," and *em'bryo*.] Applied to seeds which contain more than one embryo.

Mul-tif'er-ous. [**Multif'erus;** from *mul'tus*, "many," and *fe'ro*, to "bear."] Bearing flowers and fruits many times in the course of a year.

Mul'ti-fid, or **Mul-tif'i-dous.** [**Multif'idus;** from *mul'tus*, "many," and *fin'do*, to "cleave," or "divide."] Many-cleft; having many divisions. Applied to a muscle of the spine which has numerous attachments; also, to leaves.

Mul-tif'i-dus Spi'næ.* ("Many-

Cleft [Muscle] of the Spine.") See TRANSVERSALIS DORSI.

Mul-tĭ-flo'rous. [**Multiflo'rus;** from *mul'tus*, "many," and *flos*, a "flower."] Having numerous flowers.

Mul-tif'o-rus.* [From *mul'tus*, "many," and *fo'ro*, to "pierce" (from *fo'ris*, a "door," or "opening").] Pierced by numerous holes.

Mul-tĭ-ġem'mĭ-us.* [From *mul'tus*, "many," and *gem'ma*, a "bud."] Applied to a tubercle containing many buds, as those of the potato.

Mul-tij'u-gate. [**Multijuga'tus;** from *mul'tus*, "many," and *ju'gum*, a "yoke."] Having many pairs, as a pinnate leaf with ten or more leaflets.

Mul-til'o-bate. [**Multiloba'tus;** from *mul'tus*, "many," and *lo'bus*, a "lobe."] Divided into many lobes.

Mul-tĭ-loc'u-lar. [**Multilocula'ris;** from *mul'tus*, "many," and *loc'ulus*, a "cell."] Having many cells.

Mul-tĭ-ner-va'tus.* [From *mul'tus*, "many," and *ner'vus*, a "nerve."] Applied to leaves having many nerves: multiner'vate.

Mul-tĭ-o-vu-la'tus.* [From *mul'tus*, "many," and *o'vulum*, a "little egg."] Containing many ovules.

Mul-tip'a-rous. [**Multip'arus;** from *mul'tus*, "many," and *pa'rio*, to "bring forth young."] Applied to animals bringing forth several young ones at a birth.

Mul'tip-ar-tīte, or mŭl-te-par'tīt. [**Multiparti'tus;** from *mul'tus*, "many," and *parti'tus*, "divided."] Divided into many parts.

Mul'tĭ-pēs, p'edis.* [From *mul'tus*, "many," and *pes*, a "foot."] Mul'tiped, or mul'tipede. Having many feet. Applied to the *Oniscus asellus*. See MILLIPED.

Mul-tĭ-pet-a-la'tus.* [From *mul'tus*, "many," and *pet'alon*, a "petal."] Multipet'alous. Having many petals.

Mul'tĭ-ple. [**Mul'tiplex, p'licis;** from *mul'tus*, "many," and *pli'co*, to "plait."] Multiple fruits are those which result from the aggregation of several flowers (or ovaries) into one mass, as the pine-apple.

Mul-tip'lĭ-cate. [**Multiplica'tus;** from the same.] Applied to flowers which become double by the transformation of parts of the floral whorls into petals.

Mul-tiv'o-rous. [**Multiv'orus;** from *mul'tus*, "many," and *vo'ro*, to "devour."] Devouring much; voracious.

Mumisatio (mu-me-sa'she-o), **o'nis.*** [From *mu'mia*, a "mummy."] The preservation of a dead body; also called *Balsamatio*. See EMBALMING.

Mummification. See EMBALMING.

Mum'my. [**Mu'mia.**] A body which has undergone the process of embalming.

Mumps. The common name for PAROTITIS, which see.

Mun'dic. A name for iron pyrites.

Mun'go. The root of the *Ophiorrhiza mungos*, supposed to be a specific for the bite of the cobra de capello and the rattlesnake.

Muqueux Animal. The French term for MUCUS, which see.

Mu'rex.* A genus of shell-fish noted for yielding a purple dye, the celebrated Tyrian purple of the ancients.

Mu-rex'an. A name given by Liebig to the purpuric acid of Prout.

Mu-rex'ĭ-a.* A term applied by Liebig to what Prout named the purpurate of ammonia.

Mu'rĭ-āte. [**Mu'rias, a'tis.**] Applied to the chlorides and hydrochlorates, when muriatic acid was ranged among the oxacids.

Mu'riate of Am-mo'nĭ-a [**Ammo'niæ Mu'rias**], formerly called **Sal-Am-mo'nĭ-ac.** A white, fibrous salt, with a pungent saline taste, but no smell. It was formerly imported from Ammonia, Egypt, whence its name. Muriate of ammonia has a place in the United States and British Pharmacopœias. It is employed principally as a discutient.

Mu'rĭ-āt-ed. [**Muria'tus.**] Combined with chlorine.

Mu-rĭ-at'ic. [**Muriat'icus;** from *mu'ria*, "brine."] Belonging to, or derived from, sea-salt.

Muriat'ic Aç'id. [**Aç'idum Muriat'icum.**] The common name of an acid prepared from common salt by the action of sulphuric acid. Now frequently called *hydrochloric* acid. Muriatic acid is a tonic, refrigerant, and antiseptic, and is often administered with advantage in low fevers. See HYDROCHLORIC.

Mu-rĭ-at-if'er-us.* [From *mu'ria*, "brine," and *fe'ro*, to "bear."] Applied to bodies containing chlorine, or a compound of chlorine.

Mu'rĭ-cate. [**Murica'tus;** from *mu'rica*, a "sharp point"?] Rough, with short and hard points.

Mu-rĭ-cu-la'tus.* [Diminutive of *mu'rica*, a "sharp point."] Furnished with small points: muric'ulate.

Mu'ri-dæ.* [From *mus*, *mu'ris*, a "mouse."] A name applied to a family of the *Mammifera Rodentia*, having the mouse (*Mus*) for their type.

Murmur. See Respiratory Murmur.

Musaceæ,* mu-za'she-ē, or **Mu'sæ.*** An important natural order of endogenous plants, mostly tropical. It includes the *Mu'sa sapien'tum* (the plantain), the fruit of which is perhaps the most valuable article of food used in the tropics. The *Mu'sa tex'tilis* affords a fibre from which fine muslin is made in India.

Mus'ca,* plural **Mus'cæ.** A genus of the *Dip'tera Atherice'ra*, including the common house-fly.

Mus'ca His-pan-i-o'la.* The blistering fly. See Cantharis.

Mus'cæ Vol-i-tan'tēs.* ("Hovering Flies;" Fr. *Mouches volantes*, moosh' vo'lŏnt'.) An affection of the eyes, in which mote-like objects, or those resembling gnats or small insects, are seen to hover before the sight. See Metamorphopsia.

Mus'ci* [the plural of *mus'cus*, "moss"], or **Bryaceæ,*** bri-a'she-ē. Mosses. A natural order of minute, small-leaved cryptogamic plants. They usually grow in moist situations, and are more common in temperate climates than in the tropics.

Mus-cic'o-lus.* [From *mus'cus*, "moss," and *co'lo*, to "inhabit."] Inhabiting the mosses. Applied to certain minute *fungi*.

Mus-cig'e-nus.* [From *mus'cus*, "moss," and *ge'no*, an antique form of *gig'no*, to "produce."] Produced among mosses. Applied to a species of fungus.

Muscle. See Musculus.

Muscles, Diseases affecting the. See Cineticus.

Mus'coid. [**Muscoi'des;** from *mus'cus*, "moss," and εἶδος, a "form."] Resembling moss.

Mus-co-log'i-cal. [**Muscolog'icus.**] Belonging to muscology.

Mus-col'o-gy̆. [**Muscolo'gia;** from *mus'cus*, "moss," and λόγος, a "discourse."] That branch of Botany which treats of mosses.

Mus-coph'i-lus.* [From *mus'cus*, "moss," and φιλέω, to "love."] Living or growing among mosses.

Musculaire. See Muscular.

Mus'cu-lar. [**Muscula'ris;** from *mus'culus*, a "muscle."] (Fr. *Musculaire*, müs'kü'lêr'.) Relating to a muscle, or abounding in muscle.

Mus'cular Fi'bre. [**Fibril'la Muscula'ris.**] The fibres composing the body of a muscle, disposed in distinct *fasciculi*, or bundles, divisible into smaller, and these into less. There are two well-marked varieties: the striped muscular fibre occurs in the voluntary muscles, and is named from its conspicuous cross-markings; the unstriped muscular fibre is found in the alimentary canal, the uterus, and the bladder, and is destitute of such cross-markings.

Mus'cular Mo'tion. [**Mo'tio Muscula'ris.**] The motion caused by the contraction of the muscles. Muscular motions are of three kinds, voluntary, involuntary, and mixed, according to the character of the muscles by which they are performed.

Muscular Texture or **Tissue.** See Muscular Fibre.

Mus'cu-li,* gen. **Mus-cu-lo'rum,** the plural of Musculus, which see.

Mus'culi Pec-ti-na'ti.* ("Pectinated Muscles.") [From *pec'ten*, a "comb."] The name of the muscular fasciculi found within the auricles of the heart, supposed to resemble the teeth of a comb.

Mus'cu-lo-Cu-ta'ne-ous. [**Mus'culo-Cuta'neus;** from *mus'culus*, "muscle," and *cu'tis*, the "skin."] Belonging to, or connected with, the skin and adjacent muscles. Applied to several nerves in different parts of the body.

Mus'cu-lous. [**Musculo'sus;** from *mus'culus*, a "muscle."] Muscular.

Mus'cu-lus,* plural **Mus'cu-li.** [Diminutive of *mus*, a "mouse;" from its resemblance to a flayed mouse.] Muscle, the organ (or means) of motion in animals. A muscle may be defined as a distinct portion of flesh, susceptible of contraction and relaxation, by which motion and action, voluntary, involuntary, and mixed, are produced.

Mus'culus Cu-ta'ne-us.* ("Cutaneous Muscle.") The Platysma Myodes, which see.

Mus'cus.* [From μόσχος, a "young, tender shoot."] The Latin word for "moss." See Musci.

Mus'cus Cra'ni-i Hu-ma'ni.* ("Moss of the Human Skull.") See Lichen Saxatilis.

Mus'cus Is-lan'di-cus.* ("Iceland Moss.") The *Cetra'ria Islan'dica*, or *Li'chen Islan'dicus*.

Mu-se'um.* [From μοῦσα, a "muse;" because the Muses were supposed to preside over learning, art, and science.]

Originally, a place consecrated to the Muses; a study, library, etc. A collection of curious objects in nature and art, but more especially of the former. The name is said to have been first given by Ptolemy Philadelphus to that part of the royal palace at Alexandria in which was contained the famous library.

Mushroom. See AGARICUS.

Mu'sĭ-co-Ma'nĭ-a.* A species of *Melancholia*, characterized by an extreme fondness for music.

Musk. See MOSCHUS.

Mu'so-Ma'nĭ-a.* Applied to the variety of *tarantismus* in which the patients are music-mad. See MUSICO-MANIA.

Mus'sel, Ed'ĭ-ble. The MYTILUS EDULIS, which see.

Mus-sĭ-tā'tion. [**Mussita'tio, o'***nis;* from *mus'sito, mussita'tum*, to "mutter."] Muttering; a morbid symptom consisting in the movement of the lips of the sick without the production of articulate sounds.

Must. [**Mus'tum.**] Juice of the grape newly expressed; by fermentation it becomes wine.

Mus'tard. [Lat. **Sina'pis**; Fr. *Moutarde*, moo'tard'.] The seeds of *Sinapis alba* and *S. nigra* reduced to flour, and deprived of their fixed oil by expression.

Mu'ta-çism. [**Mutacis'mus**; from *mu'tus*, "mute," "dumb."] Inability to enunciate properly certain *mute* letters, especially the labial consonants *b*, *p*, and *m*; leading to their frequent repetition, or the substitution of other letters for them.

Mu-tĭ-lā'tion. [**Mutila'tio, o'***nis;* from *mu'tilo, mutila'tum*, to "maim," to "mangle."] The condition which results from the loss or excision of a member, organ, or part.

Mutisme. See MUTITAS.

Mu'tĭ-tas, a'*tis*.* [From *mu'tus*, "dumb."] (Fr. *Mutisme*, mü'tèzm'.) Dumbness; inability to articulate. A genus of the order *Dyscinesiæ*, class *Locales*, of Cullen's Nosology.

Mu'titas A-ton'ĭ-ca.* ("Atonic Dumbness.") Dumbness arising from an affection of the nerves of the tongue.

Mu'titas Or-gan'ĭ-ca.* ("Organic Dumbness.") Dumbness resulting from removal or injury of the tongue.

Mu'titas Sur-do'rum.* ("Dumbness of the Deaf.") Dumbness arising from having been born deaf, or having become so in infancy.

My-ăl'ġĭ-a.* [From μῦς, a "muscle," and ἄλγος, "pain."] Pain in the muscles.

Mȳ-ăl'ġic. [**Myal'gicus.**] Belonging to myalgia.

My-as-the-nĭ'a.* [From μῦς, a "muscle," and ἀσθένεια, "debility."] Muscular debility.

Mȳ-as-then'ic. [**Myasthen'icus.**] Belonging to *myasthenia*.

Mȳ-çe'lĭ-um.* [From μύκης, a "fungus."] The filamentous expansion from which the fructification of a fungus is developed.

Mȳ-çet-o-ġen'e-sis.* [From μύκης, μύκητος, "mushroom," and γένεσις, "generation."] The origin, or first development, of mushrooms.

Mȳ-çet-o-ĭ'dēs.* [From μύκης, a "mushroom," and εἶδος, a "form."] Resembling a mushroom.

Mȳ-çe-tol'o-ġȳ. [**Mycetolo'gia**; from μύκης, a "mushroom," and λόγος, a "discourse."] A treatise on mushrooms; the science of mushrooms.

My-co-der'ma, a*tis*.* [From μῦκος, "mucus," and δέρμα, the "skin."] The mucous membrane: my'coderm.

Mȳc-o-der'mis, i*dis*.* [From μύκης, a "mushroom," and δέρμα, the "skin."] A genus of fungous growths, forming the crusts of *favus*.

My-co-der-mi'tis, i*dis*.* [From μῦκος, "mucus," and δέρμα, the "skin."] Inflammation of a mucous membrane.

My-co-der-mo-spha'ce-lus.* [From μῦκος, "mucus," δέρμα, the "skin," and *spha'celus*.] *Sphacelus*, or gangrene of a mucous membrane.

My-co-di-ar-rhœ'a.* [From μῦκος, "mucus," and διάῤῥοια, a "flow from the bowels."] Mucous or pituitous diarrhœa.

My-co-dȳs-en-te'rĭ-a.* [From μῦκος, "mucus," and δυσεντερία, "dysentery."] Mucous or pituitous dysentery.

My-co-dȳsp-nœ'a.* [From μῦκος, "mucus," and δύσπνοια, "difficulty of breathing."] Mucous or pituitous *dyspnœa*.

My-co-gas-tri'tis, i*dis*.* [From μῦκος, "mucus," and *gastri'tis*, "inflammation of the stomach."] Mucous gastritis.

My-co-ĭ'dēs.* [From μύκης, a "fungus."] Resembling a fungus; fungoid. See SPONGOIDES.

Mȳ-col'o-ġȳ. [**Mycolo'gia**; from μύκης, a "mushroom," and λόγος, a "discourse."] A treatise on mushrooms; or the science of the fungi.

Mȳ-coph-thăl'mĭ-a.* [From μύκης, a "mushroom," and ὀφθαλμός, the "eye."] Fungous inflammation of the eye.

My-co'sis.* [From μῦκος, "mucus."] A mucous polypus.

Mȳ-co'sis.* [From μύκης, a "fungus."] A fungous fleshy tumor.

My-dri'ą-sis.* [From μύδος, "moisture"?] A preternatural dilatation of the pupil; or, according to some writers, weakness of sight resulting from an excess of watery humors.

My-e-lăl'ġĭ-ą.* [From μυελός, "marrow," and ἄλγος, "pain."] Pain in the spinal marrow.

My-e-lăl'ġĭ-cus.* Belonging to *myelalgia:* myelal'gic.

My-e-lan-ą-lo'sis.* [From μυελός, "marrow," and ἀνάλωσις, "wasting."] *Tabes dorsalis,* or wasting of the spinal marrow.

My'el-ap-o-plex'ĭ-ą.* [From μυελός, "marrow," and ἀποπληξία, "stupor," "apoplexy."] Apoplexy of the spinal marrow; hæmorrhage or discharge of blood into the spinal marrow.

My-e-la'rĭ-us.* [From μυελός, "marrow."] Having a spinal marrow. A term applied to vertebrated animals.

My'e-lą-tro'phĭ-ą.* [From μυελός, "marrow," and ἀτροφία, "wasting."] *Tabes dorsalis,* or wasting of the spinal marrow. See MYELANALOSIS.

My-e-lą-troph'ĭ-cus.* Belonging to *myelatrophia.*

My-e-laux'e.* [From μυελός, "marrow," and αὔξη, "increase."] Morbid increase of the spinal marrow.

My'e-len-çeph'ą-lus.* [From μυελός, "marrow," also "brain," and ἐγκέφαλος, "within the head."] Having a brain; belonging to the brain.

My-e-let-e-ro'sis.* [From μυελός, "marrow," and ἑτέρωσις, "alteration."] Morbid alteration of the spinal marrow.

Mȳ'e-līne. [From μυελός, "marrow."] Applied by Virchow to the medullary matter filling the space between the *axis-cylinder* and sheath of the nerve-fibres.

My-e-lī'tis.* [From μυελός, "marrow."] Inflammation of the spinal marrow.

My'e-lo-dĭ-as'tą-sis.* [From μυελός, "marrow," and διάστασις, a "separation."] Disintegration of the spinal marrow.

Mȳ'e-loid. [**Myeloi'des;** from μυελός, "marrow," or "brain," and εἶδος, a "form."] Resembling marrow.

My-e-lo'mą, a*tis.** [From μυελός, "marrow."] Medullary tumor; a tumor containing a brain-like substance.

Myelomalacia* (-la'she-ą). [From μυελός, "marrow," and μαλακία, "softness."] Softening of the spinal marrow.

My'e-lo-men-in-ġī'tis, i*dis.** [From μυελός, "marrow," and μῆνιγξ, a "membrane."] Inflammation of the *theca,* or membrane investing the spinal marrow.

My'e-lo-me'ninx.* [From the same.] The *theca,* or tough hard membrane enclosing the spinal marrow.

My-e-lom'ȳ-cą,* or **My-e-lom'ȳ-çēs, e'***tis.** [From μυελός, "marrow," and μύκης, a "fungus."] The same as MYELOMA, which see.

My'e-lon.* [From μυελός, "marrow."] A term used by Owen for the *Medul'la spina'lis.*

My-el'o-nąl. [**Myelona'lis.**] Belonging to the *myelon.*

My'e-lo-neū'rą.* [From μυελός, "marrow," and νεῦρον, a "nerve."] The name given by Rudolphi to a group of articulated animals, because their nervous (or ganglionic) system consists of a cord analogous to the spinal marrow of higher animals.

My-e-loph'thĭ-sis.* [From μυελός, "marrow," and φθίσις, a "wasting."] The same as MYELANALOSIS, which see.

My-e-lo'sis.* The formation or growth of *myeloma.*

My'e-lo-spon'gus.* [From μυελός, "marrow," and σπόγγος, a "sponge," or "fungus."] Medullary fungus. The same as MYELOMA, which see.

My-e-ner-ġī'ą.* [From μῦς, a "muscle," and ἐνέργεια, "energy."] Muscular energy.

My-e-ner'ġĭ-cus.* Belonging to *myenergia.*

My-en'tą-sis.* [From μῦς, a "muscle," and ἔντασις, a "stretching."] A stretching or extending of the muscles.

My-ī'tis, i*dis.** [From μῦς, a "muscle."] A term for inflammation of a muscle.

Mȳl'o-don, on'*tis.** [From μύλη, a "mill," or "molar tooth," and ὀδούς, a "tooth."] An extinct gigantic animal of the sloth tribe, some remains of which, including molar teeth, have been found.

Mȳl'o-dus, d*on'tis.** [From the same.] A molar tooth.

Mȳl-o-glos'sus.* [From μύλη, a "mill," or "molar tooth," and γλῶσσα, the "tongue."] Applied to some muscular fibres, arising from the lower jaw near the molar teeth, and inserted into the base of the tongue and walls of the pharynx. It is considered to be a portion of the *Constrictor pharyngis superior.*

My'lo-Hy-o-ī'de-us.* [From μύλη, a "mill," and, hence, the molar teeth, and Os *hyoi'des,* the "hyoid bone."] A triangular muscle, arising from the inside of the lower jaw, between the molar teeth and the chin, and inserted into the *Os hyoides*. It raises the *Os hyoides*, or depresses the jaw.

My'lo-Phăr-ўn-ġe'us.* One of the muscles of the pharynx, called also the *constrictor superior*.

My-o-car-di'tis.* [From μῦς, μυός, a "muscle," and καρδία, the "heart."] Inflammation of the muscles of the heart.

My-o-çeph-a-li'tis, *idis*.* [From μῦς, μυός, a "muscle," and κεφαλή, the "head."] Inflammation of the muscles of the head.

My-o-çœ-lĭ-ăl'ġĭ-a.* [From μῦς, μυός, a "muscle," κοιλία, the "belly," and ἄλγος, "pain."] Pain in the muscles of the abdomen.

My-o-çœ-lĭ-i'tis, *idis*.* [From μῦς, μυός, a "muscle," and κοιλία, "belly."] Inflammation of the abdominal muscles.

My-o'dēs.* [Gr. μυώδης; from μῦς, μυός, a "muscle."] Like muscle; of the nature of muscle. See PLATYSMA MYODES.

My-o-des-op'sĭ-a.* [From μυῖα, a "fly," εἶδος, a "form," and ὄψις, "sight."] The same as METAMORPHOPSIA.

My-o-dў-na'mĭ-a.* [From μῦς, a "muscle," and δύναμις, "power."] Muscular strength or power: myodyn'amy.

Mў-o-dў-nam-ĭ-om'e-ter. [**Myodynamiom'etrum;** from μῦς, a "muscle," δύναμις, "power," and μέτρον, a "measure."] An instrument for ascertaining the amount of muscular power.

My-o-dўn'ĭ-a.* [From μῦς, a "muscle," and ὀδύνη, "pain."] Pain in a muscle.

My-o-gas'ter.* [From μῦς, a "muscle," and γαστήρ, the "belly."] The belly or thick portion of a muscle.

Mў-o-gas'tric. [**Myogas'tricus.**] Belonging to the belly of a muscle.

Mў-o-graph'ic. [**Myograph'icus.**] Belonging to myography.

Mў-og'ra-phў. [**Myogra'phia;** from μῦς, a "muscle," and γράφω, to "write."] A description of the muscles.

My-o-i'dēs.* [From μῦς, a "muscle," and εἶδος, a "form."] Resembling muscle, or flesh: my'oid.

My-o-lem'ma, *atis*.* [From μῦς, a "muscle," and λέμμα, a "covering."] The delicate membranous envelopment of each fibril of fleshy or muscular fibre. See SARCOLEMMA.

Mў'o-line. [**Myoli'na;** from μῦς, a "muscle."] A name for the elementary substance or tissue composing the muscles.

Mў-o-loġ'ic. [**Myoloġ'icus.**] Belonging to myology.

Mў-ol'o-ġў. [**Myolo'gia;** from μῦς, a "muscle," and λόγος, a "discourse."] A treatise on the muscles, their nature, structure, and functions. That branch of Anatomy which treats of the muscles.

Myomalacia,* mi-o-ma-la'she-a. [From μῦς, a "muscle," and μαλακία, "softness."] Softening of the muscles or flesh.

My-on'o-sos,* or **My-on'o-sus.*** [From μῦς, a "muscle," and νόσος, "disease."] Disease of a muscle. See MYOPATHIA.

My-o-păl'mus.* [From μῦς, a "muscle," and παλμός, a "rapid motion."] A nervous movement or twitching of the muscles or tendons; *subsul'tus ten'dinum*.

My-o-pa-thi'a.* [From μῦς, a "muscle," and πάθος, "affection," or "disease."] Severe muscular pains in the neighborhood of the womb, and interfering with its action.

My-o-path'ĭ-cus.* Belonging to *myopathia*.

Mў-op'ic. [**Myop'icus.**] Belonging to myopy.

My-o-pol-ў-plas-ĭ-as'mus,* or **My-o-po-lўp'la-sis.*** [From μῦς, a "muscle," πολύς, "many," and πλάσις, a "formation," or "moulding."] A modelling of the numerous muscles, represented lying over each other.

Myoporaceæ,* mi-o-po-ra'she-ē. [From *Myop'orum*, one of the genera.] A natural order of exogenous plants, found in Australia, and other tropical regions. It includes the *Avicennia* (White Mangrove) of Brazil, which is used for tanning.

Mў'o-pў. [**Myo'pia;** from μύω, to "contract," to "close," and ὤψ, the "eye;" because near-sighted people partially close the eyes when looking at distant objects.] Near-sightedness.

My-or-rheū'ma, *atis*.* [From μῦς, a "muscle," and ῥεῦμα, a "flow," or "rheum."] The lancinating pains of rheumatism. See RHEUMATISM.

My-or-rhex'is.* [From μῦς, a "muscle," and ῥῆξις, a "rupture."] Laceration of one or more muscles.

My-o-sçen-o-gra'phĭ-a.* [From μῦς, a "muscle," and σκηνογραφία, the "art of scene-painting."] A pictorial representation of the muscles: myoscenog'raphy.

My-o'sis.* [From μύω, to "contract."] Contraction, or too small perforation, of the pupil of the eye.

My-o-si'tis, idis.* [From μῦς, a "muscle."] Inflammation of a muscle.

My-o-spas'mus.* [From μῦς, a "muscle," and σπασμός, a "convulsion."] Spasm or cramp of a muscle.

My-os'tĭ-cus.* [From μῦς, "muscle," and ὀστέον, "bone."] Belonging to bone and muscle. Applied to certain diseases.

Mȳ-o-te-not'o-mȳ. [**Myotenoto'mia;** from μῦς, a "muscle," τένων, a "tendon," and τέμνω, to "cut."] The division or section of tendons.

Mȳ-ot'o-mȳ. [**Myoto'mia;** from μῦς, a "muscle," and τέμνω, to "cut."] Dissection of the muscles.

Mȳr-ĭ-a-can'thus.* [From μυρίος, "numberless," and ἄκανθα, a "spine."] Having numerous spines or prickles. Applied to certain plants.

Mȳr-ĭ-an'thus.* [From μυρίος, "numberless," and ἄνθος, a "flower."] Having numerous flowers.

Mȳr-ĭ-ap'o-da,* or **Mȳr'ĭ-a-pods.** [From μυρίος, "numberless," and πούς, a "foot."] The name of a class of *Articulata.*

Mȳr-ĭ-ap'o-dus.* [From the same.] Having an indeterminate number of feet; centipede: myriapodous.

Mȳ-ri'ca Ce-rif'e-ra.* The Wax Myrtle, or Bay-berry plant, the berries of which yield a substance very similar to the *Cera flava* of the Pharmacopœias.

Myricaceæ,* mĭr-e-ka'she-ē. A natural order of exogenous plants, found in India, the temperate parts of North America, and the tropics of South America. They are aromatic trees or shrubs, including the *Myri'ca cerif'era,* from which wax is obtained, and *Compto'nia,* which is astringent and tonic.

Mȳr'ĭ-o-gramme. [From μύριοι, "ten thousand," and *gramme.*] A French weight, equal to 22 pounds, 1 ounce, and 2 drachms avoirdupois.

Myriolitre, mĭr'e-o-lētr'. [From μύριοι, "ten thousand," and *li'tre.*] A French measure, equal to 2200 gallons, 7 pints, 13 fluidounces, 4 fluidrachms, and 48 minims imperial.

Myriometre, mĭr'e-o-me't'r. (French pronunciation mē'rē'o'mētR'.) [From μύριοι, "ten thousand," and *mètre.*] A French measure of length, equal to 6 miles, 1 furlong, 156 yards, and 6 inches.

Mȳr-ĭ-o-phȳl'lous. [**Myriophyl'lus;** from μύριοι, "ten thousand," "numberless," and φύλλον, a "leaf."] Literally, "having ten thousand leaves." Having an indefinitely great number of leaves.

Mȳ-ris'tĭ-ca.* [From μυρίζω, to "anoint with ointment."] A Linnæan genus of the class *Diœcia,* natural order *Myristicaceæ.* Also, the Pharmacopœial name‖ of the kernel of the fruit of the *Myris'tica moscha'ta,* or Nutmeg, otherwise called *Myris'tica officina'lis,* or *Myris'tica fra'grans.*

Myris'tica Ar-o-mat'ĭ-ca.* One of the names for the nutmeg-tree.

Myris'tica Mos-cha'ta.* The systematic name of the tree which produces the nutmeg and mace.

Myristicaceæ,* me-ris-te-ka'she-ē. A natural order of exogenous tropical trees, most abundant in the East Indies. It includes the *Myris'tica moscha'ta,* which produces two important spices, the nutmeg and mace. The nutmeg is the kernel, or seed, and mace is the aril which envelopes the seed.

Mȳ-ris'tĭ-çæ Mos-cha'tæ Nu'cle-i.* ("Kernels of the *Myristica moschata.*") The Pharmacopœial name (Dub. Ph.) for the nutmeg.

Myristiceus,* mĭr-is-tish'e-ŭs. [From *Myris'tica,* the "nutmeg-tree."] Resembling the genus *Myristica.*

Mȳ-ris'tĭ-cin. [**Myristici'na.**] A name given to *stereoptene,* which is deposited by the oil of the *Caryophyllus aromaticus.*

Mȳ-rob'a-lan, My-ro-bal'a-nus.* [From μύρον, "ointment," and βάλανος, an "acorn," or any similar fruit.] A dried Indian fruit of the plum kind, of different species of *Terminalia.* The myrobalans are said to have laxative as well as astringent properties.

Mȳ-roph'o-rum.* [From μύρον, an "ointment," and φέρω, to "carry."] An "Ointment-Bearer." An instrument for applying ointment through the narrow internal openings.

Mȳr-o-sper'mum.* [From μύρον, an "ointment," and σπέρμα, a "seed."] A genus of the Linnæan class *Diandria,* natural order *Leguminosæ.*

Myrosper'mum Pĕr-u-if'er-um.* One of the names of the tree which yields *Balsamum Peruvianum.*

Myrosper'mum Tol-u-ta'num.* The tree which (according to the Lond., Ed., and U.S. Ph.) affords *Balsamum Tolutanum.*

Mȳ-rox'ȳ-lon.* [From μύρον, an "ointment," and ξύλον, "wood."] A

Linnæan genus of the class *Diandria*, natural order *Leguminosæ*.

Myrox'ylon Per-u-if'er-um.* Another name for the *Myrospermum Peruiferum*.

Myrrh. See MYRRHA.

Myrrh, False. See BDELLIUM.

Mўr'rha,* gen. **Mўr'rhæ.** Myrrh. The Pharmacopœial name ‖ of the gum-resin from the *Balsamoden'dron Myr'rha*.

Myrsinaceæ,* mir-se-na'she-ē. [From *Myrsi'ne*, one of the genera.] A natural order of exogenous trees and shrubs, nearly all tropical.

Myrtaceæ,* mir-ta'she-ē, or **Myr'ti.*** An important natural order of exogenous plants (trees or shrubs), natives of hot countries, within and without the tropics. It includes the *Myr'tus* (Myrtle), the Clove-tree (*Caryophyl'lus*), and Pomegranate (*Pu'nica*), which is tonic, astringent, and anthelmintic. A fragrant aromatic or pungent volatile oil abounds in this order.

Myr-tā'ceous. [**Myrta'ceus.**] Resembling the myrtle.

Myr'ti,* the plural of **Myr'tus,** forming the Jussieuan name of a natural order of plants. See MYRTACEÆ.

Myr'ti-form. [**Myrtifor'mis;** from *myr'tum*, a "myrtle-berry."] Like the myrtle leaf (or berry?). See CARUNCULÆ MYRTIFORMES.

Myr'tle. The *Myrtus communis*.

Myr'tle, Dwarf. [**Chamæmyr'tus.**] A name for the *Ruscus aculeatus*.

Myr-to-i'dēs,* [From μύρτος, the "myrtle."] Resembling the *Myrtus*.

Myr'tus,* plural **Myr'ti.** [Gr. μύρτος.] The myrtle-tree. A Linnæan genus of the class *Icosandria*, natural order *Myrtaceæ*.

Myr'tus Pi-men'ta.* The tree which produces Jamaica pepper, or allspice.

Mўs-tā'chĭ-al. [**Mystachia'lis;** from μύσταξ, the "upper lip," or the beard on it.] Belonging to the upper lip.

Mўs'tax, a'cis.* [Gr. μύσταξ.] The upper lip; also, the hair on the upper lip, or moustache.

Mўt-ĭ-lo-i'dēs.* [From *myt'ilus*, the "mussel," and εἶδος, a "form."] Resembling the *mytilus*, or mussel.

Mўt'ĭ-lus E-du'lis.* ("Edible Mussel.") A shell-fish found in vast beds in the European seas. It is often poisonous: sometimes producing, in those who eat it, all the symptoms of *Urticaria*.

Mўx-o-col'ĭ-ca.* [From μύξα, "mucus," and *col'ica*, the "colic."] A mucous or pituitous colic.

Mўx-o'ma,* plural **Mўx-o'ma-ta.** [From μύξα, "mucus."] Applied by Virchow to certain tumors which contain mucus in their intercellular substance.

My-ў-dro-çўs'tis, idis.* [From μῦς, a "muscle," and *hydrocys'tis*, a "hydatid."] A hydatid in the flesh.

N.

N. = *Noc'te.** "At night."

Na-bo'thi Glan'du-læ,* **Nabo'thi O'vu-la,*** **Nabo'thi Ve-sic'u-læ.*** ("Glands, Ovules, or Vesicles of Naboth.") Applied to small glandular bodies within the mouth of the uterus; first described by Naboth.

Nabo'thi, Men-or-rha'ğĭ-a.* ("Menorrhagy of Naboth.") A serous discharge from the vagina of pregnant women, first noticed by Naboth.

Nac're-ous. [Lat. **Na'creus;** Fr. *Nacre*, "mother of pearl."] Belonging to mother of pearl.

Nā'dir. [From the Arabic.] The point in the heavens directly under our feet, and opposite to the zenith.

Næ'vus,* plural **Næ'vi.** A natural mark or blemish.

Næ'vus Ma-ter'nus.* ("Maternal Mark.") A mark on the skin from birth, the effect, as is said, of the mother's longing for, or aversion to, particular objects, or of some accidental occurrence affecting her own person during pregnancy.

Naiadaceæ,* na-a-da'she-ē, or **Nai'a-dēs.*** [From ναϊάς, ναϊάδος, a "water-nymph."] A natural order of endogenous aquatic plants, found within and without the tropics, in salt water and fresh. It includes the *Na'jas* or *Na'ias*.

Nail. (Fr. *Ongle*, ŏngl.) An appendage consisting of a semi-transparent substance, resembling horn, attached to the dorsal extremities of the fingers and toes. The finger-nails serve not merely to protect the part which they cover, but to give greater firmness or resistance to the ends of the fingers, in their attempt to lay hold of any small object.

Nain, năɴᵍ. The French term for "dwarf." See NANUS.

Na-nis'mus.* [From νᾶνος, or νάννος, a "dwarf," or "dwarfed."] A term ap plied by Geoffroy St. Hilaire to a genus of anomalies which characterize dwarfs.

Nan-keen′ Dye. A dye made by boiling annotto and carbonate of potash in water; about an ounce of each to a pint of water.

Nan-o-çeph′a-lus.* [From νᾶνος, a "dwarf," or "dwarfed," and κεφαλή, the "head."] A dwarfish or diminutive head.

Nan-o-i′dēs.* [From νᾶνος, a "dwarf," and εἶδος, a "form."] Resembling a dwarf; dwarf-like.

Na-nom′e-lus.* [From νᾶνος, a "dwarf," and μέλος, a "limb."] A monster with dwarfish limbs.

Na′nus.* [Gr. νᾶνος; Fr. *Nain*, năn°.] Dwarf; stunted in stature, so as to be below the ordinary height and size of those of the same species.

Nape of the Neck. [**Nu′cha.**] The back part of the neck, including the projecting spinous process of the seventh cervical vertebra.

Naph′tha.* [Gr. νάφθα.] A pale-yellow, but very pure, clear, inflammable liquid of the bituminous kind.

Naph′tha Vit-ri′o-li.* A name for sulphuric ether.

Naph-thal′i-din. [**Naphthalidi′na;** from *naphthali′na.*] A new base, produced by the action of reducing agents on naphthalin.

Naph′tha-lin, or **Naph′tha-line.** [**Naphthali′na;** from *naph′tha.*] A grayish-white substance formed in the rectification of the petroleum of coal-gas works.

Nap-i-fo′li-us.* [From *na′pus*, a "turnip," and *fo′lium*, a "leaf."] Having leaves like the turnip: napifo′lious.

Nap′i-form. [From *na′pus*, a "turnip."] A term applied to one of the textures of cancer, the *bunioïd* of Bayle.

Nar-cis′si,* the plural of **Narcis′sus,** forming the Jussieuan name of a natural order of plants. They are now included in *Amaryllidaceæ.*

Nar-cis′sus.* The Linnæan name of a genus of plants, class *Hexandria*, natural order *Amaryllidaceæ.*

Nar-co′dēs.* [From νάρκη, "stupor."] Having, or causing, stupor: narcose, or narcous.

Nar-co′ma, *atis.** [From the same.] Stupor, or the state of being under the influence of narcotic medicine.

Nar-com′a-tous. [From the same.] Pertaining to *narcoma.*

Nar-co′sis.* [From the same.] The progress of *narcoma.*

Nar-co-spas′mus.* [From νάρκη, "stupor," and σπασμός, a "convulsion."] Cramp or spasm, with an appearance of stupor.

Nar-cot′ic. [**Narcot′icus.**] Belonging to *narcosis.* Applied to a medicine that induces sleep, or stupor.

Nar′co-tin, or **Nar′co-tine.** [**Narcoti′na;** from ναρκόω, to "stupify."] An active principle of opium; also called *Derosne's Salt*, from its discoverer, and Opiane. It is procured by digesting opium in sulphuric ether.

Nar′co-tism. [**Narcotis′mus;** from νάρκη, "stupor."] The influence produced by narcotic substances.

Na′rēs,* gen. **Na′ri-um,** the plural of NARIS, which see.

Na′ris,* plural **Na′rēs.** The "nostril;" a cavity of a pyramidal form in each side of the nose, or of the septum of the nostrils.

Nar′thex, *e′cis.** [Gr. νάρθηξ.] The *Ferula*, a tall umbelliferous plant, with a slight knotted pithy stalk. See next article.

Nar′thex As-sa-fœt′i-da,* or **Nar′thex Fĕr′u-la.*** The plant the root of which yields assafœtida.

Nā′sal. [**Nasa′lis;** from *na′sus*, the "nose."] Belonging to the nose; uttered through the nose.

Nasal Duct. See DUCTUS AD NASUM.

Na′sal Fos′sæ. [**Fos′sæ Nasa′les;** from *fos′sa*, a "ditch."] Two irregular compressed cavities extending backwards from the nose to the pharynx, and constituting the internal part of the nose.

Nas′çent State. [From *nas′cens*, the present participle of *nas′cor*, to "be born."] The state of gases at the moment of their elimination, before they have acquired their full volume or their repulsive power.

Na′sus,* genitive **Na′si,** accusative **Na′sum.** (Fr. *Nez*, nȧ.) The "nose," composed of the *dorsum*, or bridge, the *alæ*, or wings, the *septum*, or partition, the lobe, or tip, and the *columna*, or lower thickened portion of the septum.

Nā′tant. [**Na′tans;** from *na′to, nata′tum*, to "swim."] Floating on the surface; swimming, as leaves or flowers.

Nat-a-to′rēs.* [Plural of *nata′tor, natato′ris*, a "swimmer;" from the same.] "Swimm rs." An order of swimming birds, including those whose toes are united by a membrane; whence the order is also termed *Palmip′edes.*

Na′tēs.* [A Latin word which is

either plural or singular, but used mostly in the plural.] The buttocks.

Na'tes Cĕr'e-bri.* The two anterior of the *Tubercula quadrigemina.*

Na'trĭ-um.* A term formerly applied to sodium.

Na'tron,* or **Na'trum.*** A native carbonate of soda which is found in Egypt; in popular language, "soda." It is the nitre of the Bible.

Na'trum Vit-rĭ-o-la'tum.* ("Vitriolated Soda.") A name of Glauber's Salt.

Nat'u-ral. [**Natura'lis;** from *natu'ra,* "nature."] Belonging to nature; produced according to the ordinary laws of nature.

Nat'ural His'to-rȳ. [**Histo'ria Natura'lis.**] Literally, the "history or description of nature." The science which treats of the natural products of the earth, whether animals, vegetables, or minerals. See PHYSICS.

Nat'ural Or'ders. Groups of genera which resemble each other in the most essential features and intrinsic qualities; or groups of genera which are supposed to bear a greater resemblance to each other than to any thing else.

Nat'ural Phĭ-los'o-phȳ. [**Philoso'phia Natura'lis.**] The science which treats of the properties of natural bodies, and their actions on each other, or which treats of the phenomena and laws of the material world: physics. See PHYSICS.

Nat-u-ra'lĭ-a.* [Plural neuter of *natura'lis,* "natural."] The parts of generation; the privities.

Naturals. See RES NATURALES.

Natus Mortuus. See STILLBORN.

Nauclea Gambir. See GAMBIR.

Nausea,* nau'she-a. [From ναῦς, a "ship."] Originally, "sea-sickness." Any sickness at the stomach, similar to sea-sickness.

Nau'sea Ma-ri'na.* [From *ma're,* the "sea."] The Latin for SEA-SICKNESS.

Nau'seous. [**Nauseo'sus;** from *nau'sea.*] Producing nausea; disgusting.

Nau'tĭ-cal. [**Nau'ticus;** from ναῦς, a "ship."] Belonging to a ship. Applied to sea-sickness, termed *Morbus nauticus.*

Nau'tĭ-cus Mus'cu-lus.* ("Nautical Muscle.") The *Tibia'lis posti'cus,* because chiefly exerted in climbing as sailors do.

Nau-tĭ-lo-ī'dēs.* [From *nau'tilus,* and εἶδος, a "form."] Resembling the nautilus: nautiloid.

Nau'tĭ-lus.* [Gr. ναυτίλος, a "sailor;" from ναῦς, a "ship."] A genus of the *Testacea* (of Cuvier), of which there are several species.

Navel. See UMBILICUS.

Nā'vel-String. The *Fu'nis umbilica'lis* (otherwise called *Funic'ulus umbilica'lis*), or umbilical cord.

Na-vic'u-lar. [**Navicula'ris;** from *navic'ula,* a "little ship or boat."] Pertaining to a boat or ship; having the shape or appearance of a boat.

Na-vic-u-la're, Os.* A bone of the *carpus;* also one of the *tarsus:* named from their fancied likeness to a boat.

Navicularis. See NAVICULAR.

Nav'ĭ-form. [**Navifor'mis;** from *na'vis,* a "ship," or "boat."] Resembling a boat: navicular.

Near-Sightedness. See MYOPY.

Neb'u-la,* plural **Neb'u-læ.** [From νεφέλη, a "cloud."] Literally, a "mist," a "cloud." A faintly luminous appearance, resembling a cloud, in the starry firmament. Many of these nebulæ have been resolved into stars by the power of the telescope. Also, a small cloud-like spot on the cornea.

Neb-u-lif'er-ous. [**Nebulif'erus;** from *neb'ula,* and *fe'ro,* to "bear."] Having nebulous spots.

Neb'u-lous, or **Neb'u-lose.** [**Nebulo'sus;** from *neb'ula.*] Literally, "cloudy." Pertaining to a nebula, or resembling a nebula.

Neck. [Lat. **Col'lum,** and **Cer'vix;** Gr. τράχηλος, and αὐχήν; Fr. *Cou,* koo.] In Anatomy, the part between the head and thorax. Also, the point between the root and stem of plants.

Nec-ro-bĭ-o'sis.* [From νεκρός, "dead," and βίος, "life."] Applied by Virchow to "the spontaneous wearing out of living parts."

Nec-ro-co-mi'um.* [From νεκρός, a "dead body," and κομέω, to "take care of."] A dead-house. See MORGUE.

Nec-ro-do-chi'um.* [From νεκρός, a "dead body," and δοχή, a "reception."] The same as NECROCOMIUM.

Nec-rol'o-ġȳ. [**Necrolo'gia;** from νεκρός, a "dead body," and λόγος, a "discourse."] A treatise on the dead body. Also, a register of deaths, the causes of death, and particulars presented on *post-mortem* examination.

Ne-croph'a-gous. [**Necroph'agus;** from νεκρός, a "dead body," and φάγω, to "eat."] Devouring dead animals, or animal substances in a state of decomposition. Applied to certain insects.

Ne-crop'sȳ. [**Necrop'sia;** from

νεκρός, a "dead body," and ὄπτομαι, to "behold."] Synonymous with NECROSCOPY.

Nec-ro-scop'ic, Nec-ro-scop'ĭ-cal. [**Necroscop'icus.**] Belonging to necroscopy.

Ne-cros'co-pȳ. [**Necrosco'pia;** from νεκρός, a "dead body," and σκοπέω, to "examine."] The examination of a dead body.

Ne-cro'sis.* [From νεκρόω, to "kill."] Literally, "mortification." Death of a bone or part of a bone; analogous to the mortification of the soft parts.

Nec-ro-tom'ic. [**Necrotom'icus.**] Belonging to necrotomy.

Ne-crot'o-mȳ. [**Necroto'mia;** from νεκρός, a "dead body," and τέμνω, to "cut."] Dissection of a dead body; otherwise termed *Sectio cadaveris.*

Nec-tan'dra.* Bebeeru (or Bibiru) Bark. The Pharmacopœial name ‖ of the bark of the *Nectandra Rodiei.* It has been placed on the primary list of the Materia Medica of the U.S. Pharmacopœia for 1860.

Nec-tar-if'er-ous. [**Nectarif'erus;** from νέκταρ, the "drink of the gods," also, "honey," and *fe'ro,* to "bear."] Bearing nectar, or honey; secreting a saccharine liquor.

Nec-ta-ro-the'ca.* [From νέκταρ, "nectar," or "honey," and θήκη, a "covering."] Any part which enwraps the organ for secreting honey.

Nec'ta-rȳ. [**Necta'rium;** from νέκταρ, "nectar," or "honey," and -*a'rium,* a terminal denoting a "repository." See HERBARIUM.] That part of a flower which contains, or secretes, honey; the honey-cup.

Nec-top'o-dus.* [From νηκτής, a "swimmer," and πούς, a "foot."] Having finlike *tarsi.* Applied to certain insects.

Ne-cu'sĭ-a.* [From νέκυς, a "dead body:" so called on account of its malignant character.] A poisoned wound.

Neg'a-tive Pole. The pole connected with the copper (or least oxidizable) plate of the galvanic battery.

Negro Cachexia, or **Cachexia Africana.** See CHTHONOPHAGIA.

Nelumbiaceæ,* ne-lum-be-a'she-ē. A natural order of exogenous aquatic plants, found in stagnant or quiet waters in temperate and tropical regions. It consists, according to Lindley, of one genus, the *Nelum'bium.* The mythic Lotus which occurs on the monuments of India and Egypt, is supposed to have been the *Nelumbium speciosum.*

Nem-a-to-çe-ra'tus.* [From νῆμα, a "thread," and κέρας, a "horn."] Having filiform horns or antennæ.

Nem'a-toid. [**Nematoi'des;** from νῆμα, a "thread," and εἶδος, a "form."] Resembling a thread.

Nem-a-to-neū'rus.* [From νῆμα, a "thread," and νεῦρον, a "nerve."] Having thread-like nerves.

Ne'me-ous. [**Ne'meus;** from νῆμα, a "thread."] Filamentose; composed of threads, as some cryptogamous plants.

Nem-o-blas'tus.* [From νῆμα, a "thread," and βλαστός, a "germ."] Applied to filiform embryos, as of mosses and ferns.

Ne-moç'er-us.* The same as NEMATOCERATUS, which see.

Nem-o-glos-sa'tus.* [From νῆμα, a "thread," and γλῶσσα, the "tongue."] Having a filiform tongue.

Nem'o-rous. [**Nemoro'sus;** from *ne'mus, nem'oris,* a "grove."] Belonging to a wood, or grove: nem'orose.

Ne-og'a-la, ac'*tis.** [From νέος, "new," and γάλα, "milk."] The *Colostrum,* or first milk of the mother after childbirth.

Ne-o-ga-lac'tĭ-cus.* Belonging to the *neogala:* neogalac'tic.

Ne-o-na'tus,* plural **Ne-o-na'ti,** genitive plural **Ne-o-na-to'rum.** [From νέος, "new," and *na'tus,* "born."] (Fr. *Nouveau-né,* noo'vō' nȧ.) A word signifying "newly-born," and occurring in such phrases as *Asphyxia Neonatorum* ("Asphyxia of New-born [Children"].) See ASPHYXIA NEOPHYTORUM.

Nepenthaceæ,* nep-en-tha'she-ē. A natural order of exogenous herbaceous plants, natives of swamps in China and India. It consists of a single genus, *Nepen'the* (Pitcher-Plant), in the dilated pitcher-shaped petiole of which water is secreted.

Ne-pen'thēs.* [From νή, negative, and πένθος, "grief."] A medicine mentioned by the ancient writers as having power to banish sorrow. It is supposed by some to have been opium.

Nep'e-ta Ca-ta'rĭ-a.* The systematic name for catnep. See CATARIA.

Nep'eta Vul-ga'ris.* The same as *Nepeta Cataria.* See CATARIA.

Neph'e-la.* [From νεφέλη, a "cloud."] The same as NEBULA, which see.

Ne-phel'ĭ-cus.* Belonging to the *nephelium:* nephel'ic.

Ne-phe'lĭ-um.* [Diminutive of νεφέλη, a "cloud."] A spot on the cornea.

Neph-e-lo'dēs.* [From νεφέλη, a

"cloud."] The same as NEBULOUS, which see.

Neph-el-o-dom'e-ter. [**Nephelo-dom'etrum;** from νεφέλη, a "cloud," and ὁδόμετρον, an "instrument for measuring distances."] An instrument for ascertaining the distances of the clouds.

Neph-e-lo-i'dēs.* [From νεφέλη, a "cloud," and εἶδος, a "form."] Resembling a little cloud: neph'eloid.

Neph-e-lol'o-ġy̆. [**Nephelolo'gia;** from νεφέλη, a "cloud," and λόγος, a "discourse."] The science of the clouds.

Neph-e-lo-pho-rom'e-ter. [**Nephelophorom'etrum;** from νεφέλη, a "cloud," φέρω, to "carry," and μέτρον, a "measure."] An instrument for ascertaining the direction, order, and speed of clouds.

Ne-phræm-or-rha'ġĭ-ạ.* [From νεφρός, the "kidney," and αἱμοῤῥαγία, "hæmorrhage."] Hæmorrhage of the kidney.

Ne-phrăl'ġĭ-ạ.* [From νεφρός, the "kidney," and ἄλγος, "pain."] Pain in the kidney: nephral'gy.

Ne-phrăl'ġic. [**Nephral'gicus.**] Belonging to *nephralgia*.

Neph-rạ-nu'rĭ-ạ.* [From νεφρός, the "kidney," α, priv., and οὖρον, the "urine."] Renal *anuria*, or non-secretion of urine.

Neph-rạ-pos'tạ-sis.* [From νεφρός, the "kidney," and ἀπόστασις, "suppurative inflammation."] Renal abscess, or suppurative inflammation of the kidney.

Neph-rạ-to'nĭ-ạ.* [From νεφρός, the "kidney," α, priv., and τόνος, "tone."] Renal atony, or paralysis of the kidneys.

Ne-phraux'e.* [From νεφρός, the "kidney," and αὔξω, to "increase."] Enlargement of the kidney.

Ne-phrel'cos,* or **Ne-phrel'cus.*** [From νεφρός, the "kidney," and ἕλκος, an "ulcer."] An ulcer of the kidney.

Neph-rel-co'sis.* The progress of *nephrelcus*: renal ulceration.

Neph-rem-phrax'is.* [From νεφρός, the "kidney," and ἔμφραξις, "obstruction."] Obstruction of the vessels of the kidney.

Ne'phrĭ-ạ.* [From νεφρός, the "kidney."] Proposed as a synonyme for Bright's Disease, or granulated kidney.

Neph'rĭ-cus.* [From νεφρός, the "kidney."] See NEPHRITIC.

Ne-phrit'ic. [**Nephrit'icus.**] Belonging to the kidney.

Ne-phri'tis, *idis*.* [From νεφρός, the "kidney."] Inflammation of the kidneys. A genus of the order *Phlegmasiæ*, class *Pyrexiæ*, of Cullen's Nosology.

Nephri'tis Al-bu-mĭ-no'sạ* or **Al-bu-mĭ-nen'sis.*** ("Albuminous Nephritis.") A name for Bright's Disease of the kidney; under which term have been confounded several distinct renal diseases, all agreeing, however, in the important symptom of albuminous urine, viz.: *acute* and *chronic desquamative nephritis*, *non-desquamative nephritis*, *fatty* and *amyloid* (or waxy) *degeneration*.

Desquamative nephritis is characterized by the shedding of the epithelium of the secreting tubes, either entire or in broken particles. Their *débris* blocks up the tubes, and, when washed into the urine, forms what have been termed the "tube casts." This process may be either acute or chronic. In *non-desquamative* nephritis (according to Johnson), the cells are not shed, but become atrophied, whilst the tubules are blocked up by a simple, albuminous deposit, which forms what he terms the small hyaline casts.

Neph'ro-çēle.* [From νεφρός, the "kidney," and κήλη, a "tumor."] Hernia of the kidney.

Neph-ro-çel'ic. [**Nephrocel'icus.**] Belonging to *nephrocele*.

Ne-phrol'ĭ-thos,* or **Ne-phrol'ĭ-thus.*** [From νεφρός, the "kidney," and λίθος, a "stone."] An old term for a renal calculus, or stone in the kidney.

Neph-ro-py̆-o'sis.* [From νεφρός, the "kidney," and πύωσις, "suppuration."] Suppuration of the kidney.

Ne-phrot'o-my̆. [**Nephroto'mia;** from νεφρός, the "kidney," and τέμνω, to "cut."] The dangerous and difficult operation of cutting into the kidney to extract a calculus.

Ne'rạ. A name for TODDY, which see.

Nerf. See NERVE.

Nervate. See NERVOSE.

Ner-vā'tion. [From *ner'vus*, a "nerve."] The arrangement of nerves in leaves.

Nerve. [Lat. **Ner'vus;** Gr. νεῦρον; Fr. *Nerf*, nĕRf.] A long, medullary cord, originating from the brain or spinal marrow, by which sensation, volition, or vital influence is conveyed to and from the sensorium. It is applied in Botany to parallel and simple veins.

Nerve-ache. See NEURALGIA.

Nerves, Pairs of. See PARIA NERVORUM.

Ner'vi,* gen. **Ner-vo'rum,** the plural of *Ner'vus*. See NERVE.

Ner'vīne. [**Nervi'nus;** from *ner'vus*, a "nerve."] Belonging to the nerves.

Nervorum Paria. See PARIA NERVORUM.

Ner-vo'rum, Res-o-lu'ti-o.* ("Loosening of the Nerves.") A name for PARALYSIS.

Ner-vose'. [**Nervo'sus.**] Abounding in nerves, as some leaves.

Ner'vous. [**Nervo'sus;** from *ner'vus*, a "nerve."] Belonging to, or connected with, nerves. Applied to fevers and affections of the nervous system, and to medicines that act on the latter. See NERVOSE.

Ner'vous Flu'id. [**Flu'idum Ner'veum.**] A fluid supposed to circulate through the nerves, and to be the medium by which sensation or motion is transmitted from one portion of the nervous system to another.

Nervous Matter. See NEURINE.

Ner'vous Sys'tem. [**Syste'ma Nervo'rum.**] A collective term, comprehending all the nerves of the body. These may be divided into two great classes:—1. Those chiefly appropriated to perception, sensation, and voluntary motion, connected more immediately with the brain and spinal marrow. 2. Those destined to the organs of involuntary motion (such as the heart, stomach, etc.), called by Bichat the "organic nervous system." The latter belong to what is often termed the *ganglionic nervous system*. See TRISPLANCHNIC NERVE.

Ner'vure. [From *ner'vus*, a "nerve."] A vein of a leaf.

Ner'vus,* gen. **Ner'vi.** The Latin term for NERVE, which see.

Ner'vus Va'gus.* ("Wandering Nerve.") The pneumogastric nerve.

Net'ted. The same as RETICULATED.

Net'ted-Veined. An awkward term, signifying having reticulated veins; that is, marked with veins like a network, as *netted-veined* leaves, which are characteristic of exogenous plants.

Nettle. See URTICA.

Nettle-Rash. See URTICARIA.

Neū-ra-dȳ-na'mi-a.* [From νεῦρον, a "nerve," *a*, priv., and δύναμις, "strength."] Nervous debility.

Neū-ra-dȳ-nam'ic. [**Neuradynam'icus.**] Belonging to *neuradynamia*.

Neū'ral. [**Neura'lis;** from νεῦρον, a "nerve."] Belonging to nerves.

Neū'ral Ax'is. Used by Owen for the trunk of the nervous system lodged in the extensive canal formed by the chain of the vertebræ.

Neū'ral Spine. Used by Owen for the autogenous part in the vertebra, above the *neurapophysis*, or parts lodging the neural axis; the homologue of the spinous process of a vertebra.

Neū-răl'gi-a.* [From νεῦρον, a "nerve," and ἄλγος, "pain."] (Fr. *Névralgie*, nȧ'vRăl'zhė'.) Pain in a nerve: neural'gy.

Neū-răl'gic. [**Neural'gicus.**] Belonging to neuralgia.

Neū-ran-a-gen-ne'ma, *atis*.* [From νεῦρον, a "nerve," and ἀναγεννάω, to "regenerate."] A renewed or regenerated portion of a nerve.

Neū-ran-a-gen-ne'sis.* [From the same.] Regeneration, or renewal, of nerves.

Neū-ra-naph'ȳ-sis.* [From νεῦρον, a "nerve," and ἀναφύω, to "produce," or "grow again."] Similar to NEURANAGENNESIS, which see.

Neū-ra-po-phȳs'i-al. [**Neurapophysia'lis.**] Belonging to *neurapophysis*.

Neū-ra-poph'ȳ-sis,* plural **Neū-ra-poph'ȳ-sēs.** [From νεῦρον, a "nerve," and ἀποφύω, to "be generated from."] In Comparative Anatomy, the lateral segments forming the sides of the superior arch of the vertebra, which encloses the axis or trunk of the nervous system, and whose base is the body of the vertebra.

Neū-rar-te'ri-a.* [From νεῦρον, a "nerve," and ἀρτηρία, an "artery."] The intimate association of minute nerves with minute arteries, distributed over the whole body.

Neū-ras-the-ni'a.* [From νεῦρον, a "nerve," and ἀσθένεια, "debility."] Nervous debility.

Neū-ras-then'ic. [**Neurasthen'icus.**] Belonging to *neurasthenia*.

Neū-rec'to-me,* or **Neū-rec-to'mi-a.*** [From νεῦρον, a "nerve," and ἐκτομή, a "cutting out."] Excision of a nerve, or part of a nerve.

Neū-rec-tom'i-cus.* Belonging to neurectomy.

Neū'ri-a.* [Diminutive of νεῦρον, a "nerve."] Fine nervous tissue or membrane, as the retina.

Neū'ri-cus.* [From νεῦρον, a "nerve."] Belonging to a nerve: neu'ric.

Neū-ri-lem'ma,* or **Neū-ri-le'ma, *atis*.*** [From νεῦρον, a "nerve," and λέμμα, "bark of plants."] (Fr. *Névrilème*, nȧ'vRė'lĕm' or nȧ'vRė'lăm'.) The membranous sheath encasing each nerve or filament of a nerve: a neu'rileme.

Neū-ri-lem-mi'tis, *idis*.* [From *neurilem'ma*.] Inflammation of the *neurilemma*.

Neū'rin, or **Neū'rine.** [**Neuri'na;**

from νεῦρον, a "nerve."] (Fr. *Névrine*, nà'vRèn'.) The matter of which nerves are composed. One of the most important substances or tissues entering into the composition of organic bodies. It exhibits two forms: the *vesicular* nervous matter, which is gray or cineritious in color and granular in texture, and contains nucleated nerve-vesicles; and the *fibrous* nervous matter, which is white and tubular, though in some parts its color is gray and its fibres solid.

Neū-rĭ-or-rhab'dĭ-um.* [From νευ-ριον, a "little nerve," and ῥάβδιον, a "little rod."] In the plural, the rod-like bodies of the retina, the *corpora virgæformia retinæ*.

Neū-rit'ic. [**Neurit'icus.**] Belonging to *neuritis*.

Neū-ri'tis, idis.* [From νεῦρον, a "nerve."] (Fr. *Névrite*, nà'vRèt'.) Inflammation of a nerve.

Neuroasthenia. See NEURASTHENIA.

Neū-ro-de-ăl'ġĭ-a.* [From *neuro'des* tu'nica, a name for the "retina," and ἄλγος, "pain."] Pain, or excessive sensibility, of the retina.

Neū-ro-de-a-tro'phĭ-a.* [From *neuro'des* tu'nica, the "retina," and *atro'phia*, "want of nutrition."] Atrophy of the retina.

Neū-ro'dēs.* [From νεῦρον, a "nerve."] Abounding in nerves or nervous substance. Applied to the retina, or *tunica neurodes*.

Neū-ro-dȳ-nam'ĭ-cus.* Belonging to *neurodynamis*: neurodynam'ic.

Neū-ro-dȳn'a-mis.* [From νεῦρον, a "nerve," and δύναμις, "strength."] Nervous strength, or energy.

Neū-ro-dȳn'ĭ-a.* [From νεῦρον, a "nerve," and ὀδύνη, "pain."] (Fr. *Névrodynie*, nà'vRo'dè'nè'.) Pain of a nerve; an affection similar to *neuralgia*, but limited by some writers to chronic pain in the nerves.

Neū-ro-dȳn'ĭ-cus.* Belonging to *neurodynia*: neurodyn'ic.

Neū-roġ'e-nȳ. [**Neuroge'nia;** from νεῦρον, a "nerve," and γένεσις, "generation."] The formation or production of nerves.

Neū'ro-Glĭ'a.* [From νεῦρον, a "nerve," and γλία, "glue," or "cement."] Nerve-cement. A term applied by Virchow to the substance or cement which binds the proper nervous elements of a nerve together, and, to a certain extent, gives to the whole its form. A remarkable peculiarity of *neuro-glia* is, that in it are always found, in greater or less number, minute corpuscles (termed *cor'pora amyla'cea*), which, in their structure and chemical properties, closely resemble vegetable starch, invariably becoming blue on the addition of iodine. See LARDACEOUS DEGENERATION.

Neū-rog'ra-phȳ. [**Neurogra'phia;** from νεῦρον, a "nerve," and γράφω, to "write."] A description of the nerves.

Neurohymenitis. See NEURILEMMITIS.

Neū-ro-hȳp'no-tism. [**Neurohypnotis'mus;** from νεῦρον, a "nerve," and ὕπνος, "sleep."] A term for the state induced by mesmerism, intended to signify partial sleep of the nervous system.

Neū'roid. [**Neuroi'des;** from νεῦρον, a "nerve."] Resembling a nerve, or nervous substance.

Neurolemma. See NEURILEMMA.

Neū-ro-loġ'ĭ-cal. [**Neurolog'icus.**] Belonging to neurology.

Neū-rol'o-ġȳ. [**Neurolo'gia;** from νεῦρον, a "nerve," and λόγος, a "discourse."] (Fr. *Névrologie*, nà'vRo'lo'zhè'.) The consideration of the nature and functions of the nerves. That part of Anatomy which treats of the nerves.

Neū-ro'ma, atis.* [From νεῦρον, a "nerve."] (Fr. *Névrome*, nà'vRom'.) A knotty swelling, or tumor, in the course of a nerve: nervous tumor.

Neuromalacia,* nu-ro-ma-la'she-a. [From νεῦρον, a "nerve," and μαλακία, "softness."] Softening of the nerves.

Neū-rom'a-tous. [**Neuromato'sus.**] Having the nature of a *neuroma*, or nervous tumor.

Neū-ro-my-e-li'tis, idis.* [From νεῦρον, a "nerve," and μυελός, "marrow."] Inflammation of nervous or medullary substance.

Neū-ro-my-e-lo'dēs.* [From the same.] Having, or resembling, medullary substance.

Neū-ro-my-e-lo-i'dēs.* [From νεῦρον, a "nerve," and εἶδος, a "form."] Resembling nervous, or medullary, substance.

Neuron. See NERVE.

Neū-ron'o-sos,* or **Neū-ron'o-sus.*** [From νεῦρον, a "nerve," and νόσος, a "disease."] Nervous disease, or disease of a nerve. See NEUROPATHY.

Neū-ro-path'ic. [**Neuropath'icus.**] Belonging to neuropathy.

Neū-rop'a-thȳ. [**Neuropathi'a;** from νεῦρον, a "nerve," and πάθος, an "affection," or "disease."] Nearly the same as NEURONOSUS.

Neū-roph-this'ĭ-cus.* Belonging to *neurophthisis*.

Neū-roph'thĭ-sis.* [From νεῦρον, a "nerve," and φθίσις, a "wasting."] Nervous *tabes*, or wasting away of the nerves.

Neuroptera. See NEUROPTEROUS.

Neū-rop-ter-ol'o-ġy̆. [**Neuropterolo'gia;** from *neurop'terus,* and λόγος, a "discourse."] A treatise on the *Neuroptera;* that branch of Entomology which treats of neuropterous insects.

Neū-rop'ter-us.* [From νεῦρον, a "nerve," and πτερόν, a "wing."] Neurop'-terous, or nerve-winged. Applied in the plural neuter (*Neurop'tera*) to an order of insects in which the surface of the wings is finely reticulated. The dragon-fly may be regarded as the type of this order.

Neū-ro-sçen-o-gra'phĭ-ạ.* [From νεῦρον, a "nerve," and σκηνογραφία, the "art of scene-painting."] Pictures, or representations, of the nerves.

Neū'rose. [From νεῦρον, a "nerve."] The same as NERVOSE, which see.

Neū-ro'sis,* plural **Neū-ro'sēs.** [From the same.] (Fr. *Névrose,* nå'vRōz'.) A nervous affection or disease; in the plural, a class of Cullen's Nosology.

Neū-ros-the-ni'ạ.* [From νεῦρον, a "nerve," and σθένεια, a "contest," a "trial or exertion of strength."] Great nervous power or excitement. See NEURODYNAMIS.

Neū-ro-the'le.* [From νεῦρον, a "nerve," and θήλη, the "nipple."] A nervous *papilla.*

Neū-ro-the-le-i'tis, i*dis.** [From *neurothe'le.*] Inflammation of nervous *papillæ.*

Neū-rot'ic. [**Neurot'icus;** from νεῦρον, a "nerve."] Of or belonging to the nerves; nervous.

Neū-rot'ĭ-cạ.* [From *neurot'icus,* "pertaining to the nerves."] The name of a class in Dr. Good's Nosology, comprising diseases of the nervous function.

Neū-rot'o-my̆. [**Neuroto'mia;** from νεῦρον, a "nerve," and τέμνω, to "cut."] (Fr. *Névrotomie,* nå'vRo'to'mè'.) Dissection of the nerves. The cutting or division of a nerve.

Neū-ro-tro'mạ, a*tis.** [From νεῦρον, a "nerve," and τρώμα for τραῦμα, a "wound."] The wound of a nerve.

Neū-ro-tro'sis.* The progress of *neurotroma.*

Neū-ry'men, en*is.** [From νεῦρον, a "nerve," and ὑμήν, a "membrane."] The same as NEURILEMMA, which see.

Neū-rym-e-ni'tis, i*dis.** [From *neury'men.*] See NEURILEMMITIS.

Neū'trạl. [Lat. **Neutra'lis; Fr.** *Neutre,* NUTR; from *neu'ter,* "neither of the two."] Applied to flowers having neither stamens nor pistils, and so producing no seed. Applied in Chemistry to substances which have neither the property of an alkali nor an acid, as creatin; also to salts in which the base is perfectly saturated without excess of either acid or alkali.

Neū-trạ-li-zā'tion. [**Neutraliza'tio, o'***nis;* from *neutra'lis,* "neutral."] Applied to the complete loss of characteristic properties attending certain combinations, when one ingredient is neutralized or saturated by the other. Thus, if forty parts of sulphuric acid be added to forty-eight parts of pure caustic potash, both the acid and alkali lose their characteristic qualities, and a neutral compound is formed, which has neither alkalinity nor acidity.

Neū-trĭ-flo'rus.* [From *neu'ter,* "neutral," and *flos,* a "flower."] Having neutral flowers: neutriflo'rous.

Névralgie. See NEURALGIA.

Nevrasthenia. See NEURASTHENIA.

Névrilème. See NEURILEMMA.

Névrine. See NEURINE.

Névrite. See NEURITIS.

Névrologie. See NEUROLOGY.

Névrome. See NEUROMA.

Névrose. See NEUROSIS.

Névrotomie. See NEUROTOMY.

New Jersey Tea. See RED ROOT.

Nez (Fr.), nå. See NASUS.

Nicaragua (nik-ạr-å'gwå) **Wood,** called also **Peach Wood.** The wood of a tree which belongs to the genus *Cæsalpinia,* and grows near Lake Nicaragua. It is used as a dye.

Nic'co-lāte. [**Nic'colas, a'***tis.*] Niccolic oxide being a base or acid, this name has been given to the compounds which it produces, when it plays the second part.

Nic-col'ĭ-cus.* Belonging to *niccolum,* or nickel: niccolic.

Nick'el. A white, hard metal, generally found in the metallic state; sometimes as an oxide. It is found in all meteoric stones. Its specific gravity is about 9. It is used extensively in the preparation of German silver, of which it constitutes one-fifth part.

Nicotia. See NICOTIN.

Nicotiana,* ne-ko-she-a'nạ. [From *Nicot,* who first brought it to Europe.] Tobacco. A Linnæan genus of the class *Pentandria,* natural order *Solanaceæ.*

Nicotia'na A-mer-ĭ-ca'nạ.* A

name for the *Nicotiana tabacum,* or tobacco-plant.

Nicotia'na Tab'a-cum.* The Virginia tobacco-plant.

Nicotianin, ne-ko'she-a-nin. [**Nicotiani'na;** from *nicotia'na.*] A fatty, volatile substance, found in tobacco, to which it gives the characteristic odor.

Ni-cot'i-cus.* Belonging to nicotin.

Nic'o-tin, or **Nic'o-tine.** [**Nicoti'na;** from *nicotia'na,* "tobacco."] An acrid colorless (or nearly colorless) fluid, forming the active principle of tobacco: it is a powerful poison.

Nictitating Membrane. See MEMBRANA NICTITATANS.

Nic-ti-tā'tion. [**Nictita'tio, o'***nis;* from *nic'tito, nictita'tum,* to "wink often."] A quick and frequent closing of the eyelids; frequent winking.

Nid-i-fi-cā'tion. [**Nidifica'tio, o'***nis;* from *ni'dus,* a "nest," and *fa'cio,* to "make."] The act or process of forming a nest.

Nid'u-lant. [**Nid'ulans, an'***tis;* from *nid'ulor,* to "nestle."] Nestling. A term sometimes used in Botany.

Nid-u-lā'tion. [**Nidula'tio, o'***nis;* from the same.] The act of sitting on a nest; incubation.

Nid-u-la'tus.* [From *nid'ulus,* a "little nest."] Nestled; in a nest; nid'ulate.

Night-Blindness. See HEMERALOPIA.

Nightmare. See EPHIALTES, INCUBUS, and ONEIRODYNIA GRAVANS.

Night'shade, Dead'ly̆. The *At'ropa belladon'na.*

Night'shade, Wood'y̆. The *Sola'num dulcama'ra.*

Night-Sight. See NYCTALOPIA.

Nig-ri-cau'lis.* [From *ni'ger,* "black," and *cau'lis,* a "stem."] Having a black stem: nigricau'line.

Nig'ri-pēs, p'*edis.** [From *ni'ger,* "black," and *pes,* a "foot."] Having a black *stipes,* or foot.

Nig-ri-sper'mus.* [From *ni'ger,* "black," and σπέρμα, a "seed."] Having black seeds.

Nigrities,* ni-grish'e-ēz. [From *ni'ger,* "black."] Literally, "blackness." A black or dark color.

Nigri'ties Os'sium* (osh'e-ŭm). ("Blackness of the Bones.") A term sometimes applied to caries.

Ni'hil Al'bum.* Literally, "white nothing." A name for the flowers of the white oxide of zinc.

Ni-o'bi-um.* A new metal discovered in the Bavarian tantalite. The name was given from *Niobe,* the daughter of Tantalus, to show the affinity or analogy of the metal to *tantalium.*

Niph-a-blep'si-a.* [From νίφα, "snow," and ἀβλεψία, "blindness."] Snow-blindness. Blindness caused by the glaring reflection of sunlight upon the snow. To guard against this disease, the Esquimaux wear goggles called snow-eyes.

Niph-o-ty̆ph-lo'sis.* The progress of *niphotyphlotes.*

Niph-o-ty̆ph'lo-tēs.* [From νίφα, "snow," and τυφλός, "blind."] Blindness produced by exposure to the glare of sunlight upon the snow: the same as NIPHABLEPSIA.

Nip'ple. [Lat. **Mammil'la;** Fr. *Mamelon,* mâm'lòng'.] The small conical projection in the centre of the breast. See MAMMILLA, and PAPILLA.

Ni'sus.* [From *ni'tor, ni'sus,* to "endeavor."] An effort made by the contraction of the diaphragm and abdominal muscles, to expel any thing from the body. Also applied to the vernal generative impulse of birds, etc.

Ni'sus For-ma-ti'vus.* Literally, a "formative effort." A principle similar to gravitation, applied by Blumenbach to organized matter, by which each organ is supposed to be endowed, as soon as it acquires structure, with a *vita propria,* or vital power peculiar to itself.

Nit'id. [**Nit'idus;** from *ni'teo,* to "shine."] Smooth and shining. Applied to some plants, or leaves.

Nit-i-di-flo'rus.* [From *nit'idus,* "shining," and *flos,* a "flower."] Having brilliant flowers: nitidiflo'rous.

Nit-i-di-fo'li-us.* [From *nit'idus,* "shining," and *fo'lium,* a "leaf."] Having shining leaves: nitidifo'lious.

Ni'tras Ar-ġen'ti.* ("Nitrate of Silver.") See LUNAR CAUSTIC.

Nitras Potassæ. See POTASSÆ NITRAS.

Ni'trāte. [**Ni'tras, a'***tis.*] A combination of nitric acid with a base.

Ni'trate of Pot'ash. Nitre, or saltpetre.

Ni'trate of Sil'ver. The *Nitras argenti,* or lunar caustic.

Ni'trāt-ed. [**Nitra'tus.**] Applied to a base converted into a salt by combination with nitric acid.

Ni'tre. [Lat. **Ni'trum;** Gr. νίτρον.] The nitrate of potash, commonly called saltpetre. It is the chief ingredient of gunpowder. See POTASSÆ NITRAS.

Nī'tric. [**Ni'tricus;** from *ni'trum,* "nitre."] Belonging to nitre. Applied to an acid.

Nī'tric Aç'id [**Aç'idum Ni'tricum**], formerly called **A'qua For'tis*** ("Strong Water"). A compound of oxygen and nitrogen, which contains five equivalents of the former to one of the latter. It is a powerful solvent, dissolving all the metals ordinarily met with, except gold and platinum. See AQUA FORTIS.

Nī-trĭ-fĭ-cā'tion. [**Nitrifica'tio,** o'*nis;* from *ni'trum,* "nitre," and *fa'cio,* to "make."] The process of conversion into nitre.

Nī'trīte. [**Ni'tris,** i'*tis.*] A combination of nitrous acid with a base.

Nī-tro-ben-zin'ic Aç'id. [**Aç'idum Nitrobenzin'icus.**] The name given to a new nitrogenous acid, into which benzoic acid is transformed when acted upon by strong nitric acid: also termed *benzoi-nitric.*

Nī-tro-ben'zōle, or **Nī-tro-ben'zule,** also called **Nī-tro-ben'zīde.** [From *ni'tric, benzo'ic,* and ὕλη, "stuff," or "substance."] A peculiar substance, produced by the action of concentrated nitric acid on benzole. It is sometimes called "artificial oil of bitter almonds;" but it differs essentially from the true oil in containing no prussic acid.

Nī'tro-ġen. [**Nitroge'nium;** from νίτρον, "nitre," and γεννάω, to "generate."] An important elementary principle, forming about four-fifths of atmospheric air; azote.

Nī'tro-ġe-nized Foods. Substances containing nitrogen, and supposed to be the only substances capable of being converted into blood, and of forming organic tissues.

Nī'tro-mu-rĭ-at'ic Aç'id. [Lat. **Aç'idum Nitromuriat'icum,** or **A'qua Re'gia;** Fr. *Eau régale,* ō rà'-gål'.] A compound acid formed by the union of nitric and muriatic acids. It is the only known acid which has the power of dissolving gold.

Nī'trous. [**Nitro'sus;** from *ni'trum,* "nitre."] Belonging to nitre.

Nī'trous Aç'id. [**Aç'idum Nitro'sum.**] An acid consisting of four equivalents of oxygen combined with one equivalent of nitrogen.

Nī'trous Ox'īde. More properly, the protoxide of nitrogen, the compound known as exhilarating or laughing gas.

Nī'trum Flam'mans* [from *flam'mo,* to "flame"]. A name given to nitrate of ammonia, from its property of exploding.

Nī'trum Sat-ur-nī'num.* Another name for nitrate of lead. See PLUMBI NITRAS.

Nī'tru-ret. [**Nitrure'tum;** from *ni'trum,* "nitre."] A combination of nitrogen with a simple body.

Nī'val. [**Niva'lis;** from *nix, ni'vis,* "snow."] Applied to plants which flower during winter: also to those which grow upon mountains covered with eternal snows, and to those that grow on the snow itself.

Niv'e-ous. [From the same.] Snow-white.

N. M. *Nux Moscha'ta.** "Nutmeg."

No. = *Nu'mero.* The Italian word for "number."

Nob'ĭ-lis.* [From *nos'co,* to "know."] Well known, distinguished: hence, "noble," as used in English. Applied to many objects, by way of eminence.

Noc-tam-bu-lā'tion. [**Noctambula'tio,** o'*nis;* from *nox, noc'tis,* "night," and *am'bulo, ambula'tum,* to "walk."] Sleep-walking, or walking during sleep; *Oneirodyn'ia acti'va.*

Noc-tĭ-flo'rus.* [From *nox,* "night," and *flos,* a "flower."] Flowering at night: noctiflo'rous.

Noc-tĭ-lu'cus.* [From *nox,* "night," and *lu'ceo,* to "shine."] Applied to flowers which open at night, and close during its course.

Noc-tur'nal. [**Noctur'nus;** from *nox, noc'tis,* "night."] Belonging to the night-time. Applied to flowers which remain open during the night and close themselves in the daytime, or shed an agreeable odor at night and are inodorous in the day. Applied in Entomology to a family of the *Lepidoptera* which fly only at night, or after sunset; in Ornithology, to a family of predaceous birds which are chiefly on the wing in the twilight and when the moon shines, and forming, according to Linnæus, but one genus (*Strix*), including the owls.

Nocturnal Blindness. See HEMERALOPIA.

Noc-tur'nal E-mis'sion. The same as NOCTURNAL POLLUTION.

Nocturnal Light. See NYCTALOPIA.

Nocturnal Pollution. See SPERMATORRHŒA DORMIENTIUM.

Nod'ding. Curved so that the apex hangs down. Applied to plants.

Node. [Lat. **No'dus,** plural **No'di;** from the Hebrew *Anad,* to "knit," or "tie;" Fr. *Nœud,* nuh.] A knot, knob, or joint. The point of intersection of the orbit of a planet with the ecliptic. In Botany, the place on a stem where a leaf is attached. Also, a hard, circumscribed tumor on a bone, arising from a swelling of the periosteum.

No'di Ner-vo'rum.* ("Knots of the Nerves.") The same as *ganglions*. See GANGLION.

No-dif'er-us.* [From *no'dus*, a "knot," or "node," and *fe'ro*, to "bear."] Bearing nodes: nodiferous.

Nod-ĭ-flo'rus.* [From *no'dus*, a "knot," or "node," and *flos*, a "flower."] Having flowers with nodes or joints.

Nod'ĭ-pēs, p'edis.* [From *no'dus*, a "knot," or "node," and *pes*, a "foot."] Having feet thickset with nodosities.

No-dose'. [**Nodo'sus;** from *no'dus*, a "knot," or "node."] Having nodes; knotty; swollen in some parts, contracted at others.

No-do'sis.* [From the same.] The progress or formation of nodes; the node disease.

No-dos'ĭ-tў. [**Nodos'itas,** *a'tis;* from the same.] The state, or quality, of being nodose.

Nod'u-lar. [**Nodula'ris.**] Belonging to a nodule; having the form of a nodule.

Nod-u-la'rĭ-us.* [From *nod'ulus*, a "nodule."] Having nodules: nodula'rious.

Nod'ule. [**Nod'ulus;** diminutive of *no'dus*, a "node."] A little node.

Nod-u-lif'er-us.* [From *nod'ulus*, a "nodule," and *fe'ro*, to "bear."] Bearing nodosities: nodulif'erous.

Nod'u-lose. [**Nodulo'sus;** from *nod'ulus*, a "nodule."] Full of nodules.

No'dus,* plural **No'di.** "A knot." See NODE.

No'dus Cĕr'e-bri.* ("Knot of the Brain.") A designation of the PONS VAROLII, which see.

Nœud. See NODE.

Noix, nwå. The French for NUT, which see.

No'li me Tan'ġe-re.* ("Touch me not.") A malignant disease affecting the skin, and sometimes the cartilages, of the nose.

No'ma.* [From νέμω, to "eat away."] A corroding, ulcerous disease of the skin, frequently attacking the mouth. It is sometimes called *Cancer Aquaticus* ("Watery Cancer"), because accompanied by a flow of saliva. Also applied to an ulceration of the *pudenda* in female children.

Nombril, nôm'bRē'. See UMBILICUS.

No'men-cla-ture. [**Nomencla-tu'ra;** from *no'men*, a "name," and *ca'lo*, to "call."] The proper arrangement and application of a set of distinctive and significant words as names of particular objects in science or language.

Non Com'pos Men'tis.* ("Not Sound of Mind.") Applied to those "who lose their intellects by disease, that grow deaf, dumb, and blind, not having been born so; or such, in short, as are judged by the Court of Chancery incapable of conducting their own affairs."

Non-Com'po-tēs.* [The plural of NON COMPOS.] Not having ability or purpose; madmen.

Nooth's Ap-pa-ra'tus. An apparatus for impregnating water with carbonic acid or other gases.

Nor'mal. [From *nor'ma*, a "rule."] Regular; without any deviation from the ordinary structure or function.

Nor'thern Light. A popular name for the *Auro'ra Borea'lis.*

Nose. See NASUS.

Nose, Bleeding of the. See EPISTAXIS.

Nos-o-co-mĭ-a'lis,* or **Nos-o-co'-mĭ-al.** Belonging to a *nosocomium.*

Nos-o-co-mi'um.* [From νόσος, a "disease," and κομέω, to "take care of."] A hospital or infirmary for the sick.

Nos-o-do-chi'um.* [From νόσος, "disease," and δοχεῖον, a "receptacle."] See HOSPITAL.

Nos-o-ġe'nĭ-a,* or **Nos-o-ġen'e-sis.*** [From νόσος, "disease," and γένεσις, "generation."] The production and progress of disease.

No-sog'ra-phў. [**Nosogra'phia;** from νόσος, "disease," and γράφω, to "write."] A description of diseases, their characters, nature, and course.

Nos-o-loġ'ĭ-cal. [**Nosoloġ'icus.**] Belonging to *nosology.*

No-sol'o-ġў. [**Nosolo'gia;** from νόσος, "disease," and λόγος, a "discourse."] The doctrine or science of diseases; also, that science or system which treats of the classification of diseases.

Nos-tăl'ġĭ-a.* [From νοστέω, to "come home," or "return," and ἄλγος, "pain."] (Fr. *Maladie du Pays*, må'lå'dē' dü på-ē'.) Nos'talgy. An intense longing to return to one's native country; longing for home; home-sickness. A genus of the order *Dysorexiæ*, class *Locales*, of Cullen's Nosology.

Nos-tăl'gic. [**Nostal'gicus.**] Belonging to *nostalgia.*

Nos-to-ma'ni-a.* [From νοστέω, to "come home," or "return," and μανία, "madness."] A kind of madness, forming the highest degree of *nostalgia*.

Nostril. See NARIS.

Nos'trum.* [Neuter of *nos'ter*, "ours;" implying that it is private property, not shared by the community at large.] A significant term for any quack or patent medicine.

No-tăl'gĭ-a.* [From νῶτον, the "back," and ἄλγος, "pain."] Pain of the back.

No-tăl'gĭ-cus.* Belonging to *notalgia*: notal'gic.

Notch. (Fr. *Echancrure*, à'shŏNᵍ'krür'.) A depression or indentation on the circumference or edge of certain bones.

No-ten-çeph'a-lo-çēle.* [From νῶτον, the "back," ἐγκέφαλον, the "brain," and κήλη, a "tumor."] Protrusion of the brain (in a monster-fœtus) from a cleft in the back of the head.

No-ten-çeph'a-lus.* [From νῶτον, the "back," and ἐγκέφαλον, the "brain."] A monster-fœtus, with the brain in a hernial mass on the back.

No'to-chord. [From νῶτον, the "back," and χορδή, a "string."] A term for the spinal marrow.

No-to-my'e-los,* or **No-to-my'e-lus.*** [From νῶτον, the "back," and μυελός, "marrow."] The *Medullæ spinalis*, or spinal marrow.

No-tor-rhi'ze-us.* [From νῶτον, the "back," and ῥίζα, a "root."] Having the radicles turned up against one of the faces of the cotyledons.

Nourrice, noo'rèss'. A French term for "nurse." See NUTRIX.

Nouure, noo'ür'. The French term for "rickets." See RACHITIS.

Nouveau-né, noo'vō nà'. The French term for "newly-born." See NEONATUS.

No-vac'u-lar. [**Novacula'ris**; from *novac'ula*, a "razor."] Literally, "pertaining to a razor." Applied to a variety of schist with which hones or razor-stones are made.

No-vac'u-lite. [From *novac'ula*, a "razor," and λίθος, a "stone."] A stone of which hones are made for sharpening razors. It is of a slaty structure, and contains silex.

No-vem-cos-ta'tus.* [From *no'vem*, "nine," and *cos'ta*, a "rib."] Having nine ribs or longitudinal projections.

No-vem-lo-ba'tus.* [From *no'vem*, "nine," and *lo'bus*, a "lobe."] Divided into nine lobes.

Nu-bec'u-la.* [Diminutive of *nu'bes*, a "cloud."] The little cloud-like appearances suspended in the urine in certain disordered conditions.

Nu-bec-u-la'tus.* Presenting appearances resembling *nubeculæ*: nubeculate.

Nu-bĭg'en-ous. [**Nubĭg'enus**; from *nu'bes*, a "cloud," and *ge'no*, to "beget."] Cloud-born. Growing upon mountains at a very great height.

Nu-ca-men'tum.* [From *nux*, a "nut," and *amen'tum*, a "catkin."] Synonymous with AMENTUM.

Nu'cēs,* the plural of NUX, which see.

Nu'cha,* gen. **Nu'chæ.** The nape, or back part, of the neck.

Nu-cha'lis.* Belonging to the *nucha*.

Nu-cif'er-ous. [**Nucif'erus**; from *nux*, *nu'cis*, a "nut," and *fe'ro*, to "bear."] Bearing nuts.

Nu-cĭ-for'mis.* [From *nux*, *nu'cis*, a "nut."] Resembling a nut; nuciform.

Nu'cle-āt-ed. [**Nuclea'tus**; from *nu'cleus*, a "kernel," or "central part."] Having nuclei.

Nu'cle-i,* the plural of NUCLEUS, which see.

Nu-cle-if'er-us.* [From *nu'cleus*, a "kernel," or "central part," and *fe'ro*, to "bear."] Bearing kernels.

Nu-cle'ĭ-form. [**Nucleifor'mis**; from *nu'cleus*, a "kernel," or "central part."] Resembling a nucleus; nut-shaped.

Nu-cle'o-lus,* plural **Nu-cle'o-li.** [Diminutive of *nu'cleus*, a "kernel," or "central part."] A little nucleus: a nu'cleole.

Nu'cle-us,* plural **Nu-cle'i.** [From *nux*, a "nut."] In Astronomy, that portion of a *macula* (or spot on the sun's surface) which is much darker than the rest; also applied to a small dense portion in the centre of a comet. In Botany, the kernel of a nut, or of the stone of fruit. Also, any solid substance, or thread, suspended in crystallizing matter, to afford points of contact for the commencement of crystallization. Synonymous with CYTOBLAST. Any thing about which a substance or matter gathers, as a cherry-stone forming the centre of a calculus.

Nu-cu-la'nĭ-um.* A name for a berry containing several seeds, as a grape.

Nu'cule. [**Nu'cula**; diminutive of *nux*, a "nut."] A little nut; a small, hard, seed-like pericarp, as in the oak.

Nu-cu-lo'sus.* [From *nu'cula,* a "nucule."] Having nucules.

Nu-dĭ-branch'ĭ-ate. [**Nudibranchia'tus;** from *nu'dus,* "naked," and *branch'iæ,* the "respiratory organs" in certain animals.] Having exposed *branchiæ.*

Nu-dĭ-cau'date. [**Nudicauda'tus;** from *nu'dus,* "naked," and *cau'da,* a "tail."] Having the tail without hairs.

Nu-dĭ-cau'lis.* [From *nu'dus,* "naked," and *cau'lis,* a "stem."] Having a leafless stem.

Nu-dĭ-flo'rus.* [From *nu'dus,* "naked," and *flos,* a "flower."] Having a naked corolla: nudiflo'rous.

Nu-dĭ-fo'lĭ-us.* [From *nu'dus,* "naked," and *fo'lium,* a "leaf."] Having smooth leaves.

Nu-dĭ-pel-lif'er-us.* [From *nu'dus,* "naked," *pel'lis,* the "skin," and *fe'ro,* to "bear."] Having the skin entirely bare.

Nu'dĭ-pēs, p'edis.* [From *nu'dus,* "naked," and *pes,* a "foot."] Having naked feet: nu'dipede.

Nul-lĭ-ner'vis.* [From *nul'lus,* "none," or "no," and *ner'vus,* a "nerve."] Applied to leaves which have neither true nor false nerves.

Nul-lip'o-rus.* [From *nul'lus,* "none," or "no," and *po'rus,* a "pore."] Having no pores on their surface.

Numbness. See Torpor.

Nu-mis-ma'lis.* [From *numis'ma,* a "coin."] Like a piece of money: numis'mal. Applied to certain shells.

Nu-mis-mat'ic. [**Numismat'icus;** from *numis'ma,* a "coin."] Pertaining to a coin or medal.

Nu-mis-mat'ics. [**Numismat'ica;** from *numismat'icus,* "pertaining to a coin."] The science of coins and medals.

Num-mĭ-for'mis.* [From *num'mus,* a "medal," or "coin."] Shaped like a piece of money: num'miform.

Num'mu-lar [**Nummula'ris**], and **Num'mu-lāt-ed** [**Nummula'tus;** from *num'mulus,* a "coin"]. Pertaining to, or resembling, a coin or coins. Sometimes applied to thick, roundish *sputa.*

Nut. [Lat. **Nux;** Fr. *Noix,* nwå.] A hard, one-celled, and one-seeded indehiscent fruit, as that of the oak, hazel, chesnut, etc.

Nu'tant. [**Nu'tans;** from *nu'to, nuta'tum,* to "nod," "bend," or "waver."] Nodding; drooping. Applied to the stems of plants.

Nu-tā'tion. [**Nuta'tio, o'nis;** from the same.] A small gyratory motion of the earth's axis, in virtue of which, if it subsisted alone without the precession of the equinoxes, the pole of the equator would describe among the stars, in a period of about nineteen years, a small ellipse.—(Brande.) The property which certain flowers have of following the apparent movement of the sun.

Nu-ta'tor, o'ris.* [From the same.] Literally, a "nodder," or "that which nods." Applied to the *Sterno-cleido-mastoideus,* because nodding is performed chiefly by its exercise.

Nutgall. See Galla.

Nut'meg. The seed of the *Myristica moschata;* also called *Nux Aromatica, Moschata,* or *Myristica.*

Nu'trĭ-ment. [**Nutrimen'tum, Nutri'men, m'inis;** from *nu'trio, nutri'tum,* to "nourish."] Nourishment. See Aliment.

Nu-trĭ'tion. [**Nutri'tio, o'nis;** from the same.] The assimilation or identification of nutritive matter to or with our organs.

Nutrition, Excessive, Nutrition, Morbid. See Alogotrophy.

Nu'trix, i'cis.* [From *nu'trio,* to "nourish."] (Fr. *Nourrice,* noo'rèss'.) One who has the charge and suckling of an infant, and then termed a wet-nurse. Also, a nurse or attendant upon the sick or infirm (Fr. *Garde-malade,* gaRd må'-låd').

Nux,* gen. **Nu'cis,** plural **Nu'çēs.** A "nut." Applied by some botanists to a fruit like that of the *Lithospermum, Borago,* etc. It is also called *Achenium.*

Nux Ar-o-mat'ĭ-ca.* The nutmeg, or seed of the *Myristica moschata.*

Nux Me-tel'la.* The seed of *Strychnos nux vomica.*

Nux Mos-cha'ta,* **Nux My-ris'tĭ-ca.*** The nutmeg, or fruit of the *Myristica moschata.*

Nux Vom'ĭ-ca.* The Pharmacopœial name ‖ of the seed of *Strychnos nux vomica.* Nux vomica has been long known to the Indian and Arabian physicians. It has been employed as a remedy in dyspepsia; also, in intermittents and other fevers in which powerful tonics are indicated. Its use, however, is dangerous, except in small doses. In large quantities, it usually proves speedily fatal, death being preceded by spasms, and sometimes permanent muscular contraction.

Nyctaginaceæ,* nik-taj-e-na'she-ē, or **Nўc-tag'ĭ-nēs.*** [From *Nycta'go,* one of the genera.] A natural order of exogenous plants, found in tropical and temperate regions. It includes the *Mirab'ilis* (the Marvel of Peru). The roots of many species are purgative.

Nўc-tag'ĭ-nēs,* the plural of *Nycta'go,* forming the Jussieuan name of a natural order of plants. See NYCTAGINACEÆ.

Nўc-ta-lop'ic. [**Nyctalop'icus.**] Belonging to *nyctalopy.*

Nўc'ta-lo-pў. [**Nyctalo'pia;** from νύξ, νυκτός, "night," and ὤψ, "vision."] Defect of vision except in the evening and at night; nocturnal sight; day-blindness.

Nўc-to-pho'nĭ-a.* [From νύξ, "night," and φωνή, the "voice."] Loss of voice during the day.

Nўc'to-tў-phlo'sis.* [From νύξ, "night," and τύφλωσις, a "making blind," also "blindness."] A term for nocturnal blindness. See NYCTALOPY.

Nўm'pha,* plural **Nўm'phæ.** [From νύμφη, a "marriageable maiden."] The membranous folds descending, one on each side, from the prepuce of the clitoris; also termed *Labia minora,* in distinction from the *Labia pudendi,* or *Labia majora.* Also, a nymph, *pupa,* or chrysalis, being the second condition in the metamorphosis of insects.

Nym'phæ,* gen. **Nўm-pha'rum,** the plural of NYMPHA, which see.

Nўm-phæ'a.* [From νύμφη, a "maiden," a "water-nymph."] A genus of beautiful floating plants, of the Linnæan class *Polyandria,* natural order *Nymphæaceæ.*

Nymphæaceæ,* nim-fe-a'she-ē. A natural order of exogenous floating plants (water-lilies), found in nearly all parts of the northern hemisphere. It includes the *Nymphæ'a* and the *Victoria regia,* the flower of which is the largest known, sometimes measuring more than four feet in circumference.

Nўm-phi'tis, idis.* [From *nym'phæ.*] Inflammation of the *nymphæ.*

Nўm'phĭ-us.* Having a *nymphium:* nym'phious.

Nўm-pho-i'dēs.* [From νυμφαία, the "water-lily," and εἶδος, a "form."] Resembling the *Nymphæa,* or water-lily. Applied to a species of *Menyanthes,* etc.

Nўm-pho-ma'nĭ-a.* [From νύμφη, a "maiden," a "woman," and μανία, "madness."] Morbid or excessive sexual desire in females. It is often associated with, or becomes a form of, insanity. Also termed *Furor uterinus,* and *Hysteromania.* A genus of the order *Dysorexiæ,* class *Locales,* of Cullen's Nosology.

Nўm-phon'cus.* [From *nym'pha,* and ὄγκος, a "tumor."] A tumor, or swelling, of the *nymphæ.*

Nўm-phot'o-mў [**Nymphoto'mia;** from *nym'phæ,* and τέμνω, to "cut"], or **Nym-pha'rum Sec'tĭo.*** The operation of cutting away the *nymphæ* when diseased or greatly enlarged.

Nўs-tag'mus.* [Gr. νυσταγμός; from νυστάζω, to "be sleepy."] Habitual squinting, or a partial rotatory movement of the eyeball from side to side.

O.

O. = *Octa'rium.** "A pint."

Oak. The name of a tree. See QUERCUS.

Oak Bark. See QUERCUS ALBA.

Oak Gall. See GALL-NUT.

Oarialgia. See OVARIALGIA.

O-ar'ĭ-cus.* [From ὠάριον, a "small egg."] Belonging to the ovary.

O-ar'ĭ-o-çēle.* [From ὠάριον, a "small egg," an "ovule," also the "ovary" (?) and κήλη, a "tumor."] A tumor, or hernia, of the ovary.

O-ar-ĭ-on'cus.* [From ὠάριον, an "ovule," or "ovary," and ὄγκος, a "tumor."] A tumor of the ovary; a tumid ovary.

O-a'rĭ-um.* [From ὠάριον, a "small egg."] The same as OVARIUM; an ovary.

Oats. The seeds of *Avena sativa.*

Ob. A Latin particle signifying "against," "in the way," implying obstruction, "opposite," and hence sometimes "inversely." Before words beginning with *c, f,* or *p,* the *b* is usually changed to the corresponding consonant: hence we have *occlusion* for *obclusion, offend* for *obfend, oppose* for *obpose,* etc.

Ob-cla'vate. [**Obclava'tus;** from *ob,* "inversely," and *cla'va,* a "club."] Having the appearance of an inverted club.

Ob-con'ĭ-cal. [**Obcon'icus;** from *ob,* "inversely," and *con'icus,* "conical."] Having the appearance of a reversed cone; inversely conical, as a conical fruit whose smaller end is next to the stem.

Ob-cor'date. [**Obcorda'tus;** from

ob, "inversely," and *corda'tus,* "heart-shaped."] Heart-shaped inverted, as a cordate leaf which is broad and concave at the apex and tapers towards the base.

Ob-cor-dĭ-for'mis.* [From *ob,* "inversely," and *cor, cor'dis,* the "heart."] Having the form of a heart reversed: obcor'diform.

Ob-dor-mĭ'tion. [**Obdormi'tio, o'**nis; from *ob,* "inversely," and *dor'mio, dormi'tum,* to "sleep."] The state of being asleep; also, what is meant by sleep applied to the limbs.

O-bes'ĭ-tȳ. [**Obes'itas, a'***tis;* from *obe'sus,* "fat."] Fatness, or grossness, of the body generally.

Ob-fus-cā'tion. [**Obfusca'tio, o'***nis;* from *obfus'co, obfusca'tum,* to "make dark."] The act of darkening, or rendering obscure; the state of being obscure. Applied to the sight.

Ob-jec'tĭve. [**Objecti'vus;** from *obji'cio, objec'tum,* to "put in the way," as an object which we see or feel.] Applied to things which are the objects of the external senses in contradistinction to *subjective,* that is, belonging to, or arising from, our own minds, independently of external objects. See SUBJECTIVE.

Ob-lan'ce-o-late. Inversely lanceolate, as a lance-shaped leaf of which the base is narrower than the apex.

Oblique, ob-līk'. [**Obli'quus.**] Crooked; indirect. Applied to muscles, stems, leaves, etc. An oblique leaf is one which is divided by the midrib into unequal portions.

Ob-li'qu-us Ex-ter'nus.* ("External Oblique [Muscle].") A muscle of the abdomen, also called *descendens,* which arises from the eight lowest ribs, and is inserted into the *linea alba* and the pubes.

Obli'quus In-fe'rĭ-or.* ("Inferior Oblique.") A muscle which arises from the outer edge of the orbitar process of the upper jaw-bone, and is inserted into the *sclerotica.* It is also called *brevissimus oculi,* from being the shortest muscle of the eye. This muscle and the *obliquus superior* roll the eye, and have hence been named *circumagentes,* and, from the expression they impart, *amatorii* ("amatory").

Obli'quus In-ter'nus.* ("Internal Oblique.") A muscle situated within the *obliquus externus,* also called *ascendens,* or *minor.* It arises from the spine of the ilium, etc., and is inserted into the cartilage of the seventh rib and of all the false ribs. This muscle and the *obliquus externus* turn the trunk upon its axis.

Obli'quus Su-pe'rĭ-or.* ("Superior Oblique.") A muscle which arises from the optic foramen, passes through the ring of the cartilaginous pulley which is in the margin of the socket, and is inserted into the sclerotica. It is also called *longissimus oculi,* from being the longest muscle of the eye; and *trochlearis,* from its passing through the trochlea, or pulley.

Ob-lit'er-āt-ed. [**Oblitera'tus;** from *oblit'ero, oblitera'tum,* to "blot out," or "erase."] Altered so that the natural condition has disappeared.

Ob-lit-e-rā'tion. [**Oblitera'tio, o'***nis;* from the same.] The alteration in appearance or function of a part, by which it no longer serves its original purpose.

Ob-li'vĭ-o In'ers,* or **Ob-li'vĭ-um In'ers.*** ("Inert or Sluggish Oblivion.") A term for lethargy.

Ob-lon-ga'tus.* Prolonged; somewhat long.

Ob-lon'ġĭ-fo'lĭ-us.* [From *oblon'gus,* "oblong," and *fo'lium,* a "leaf."] Having oblong leaves or folioles.

Obomasum. See ABOMASUM.

Ob-o'vate. [**Obova'tus;** from *ob,* "inversely," and *o'vum,* an "egg."] Inversely ovate, as a leaf of which the apex is broader than the base.

Ob-o-vat-ĭ-fo'lĭ-us.* [From *ob,* "inversely," *ova'tus,* "ovate," and *fo'lium,* a "leaf."] Having obovate leaves: obovatifo'lious.

Ob-o'void. [**Obovoi'des;** from *ob,* "inversely," *o'vum,* an "egg," and εἶδος, a "form."] Resembling an egg of which the small end is turned downwards.

Ob-sid'ĭ-ạn. [**Obsidia'num.**] A volcanic substance, or species of lava, resembling green bottle-glass. It was discovered by Obsid'ius in Ethiopia.

Ob-so-lĕs'çence. [**Obsolescen'tia;** from *obsoles'co,* to "grow out of use."] The state of ceasing to grow, and undergoing no further change.

Ob'so-lete. [**Obsole'tus;** from *obso'leo, obsole'tum,* to "grow out of use, or out of fashion."] Applied in Natural History to that which is indistinct, or is imperfectly developed, as if it were fading away.

Ob-stet'ric. [**Obstet'ricus;** from *ob'stetrix,* a "midwife."] Belonging to midwifery.

Obstetrician, ob-stet-rish'ŭn. [**Ob-**

stetri'cius; from *ob'stetrix*, a "midwife."] Belonging to an *obstetrix*.

Ob-stet-ri'cius Med'ĭ-cus.* ("Obstetrical Physician.") An accoucheur, or man-midwife.

Ob-stet'rics. [**Obstet'rica, Obstetri'cium;** from *ob'stetrix*, a "midwife."] The art of assisting women in childbirth, and of treating their diseases during pregnancy and after delivery: midwif'ery.

Ob'ste-trix, icis.* [From *ob'sto*, to "stand in the way," to "stand near;" because she watches by the side of the woman in labor.] A midwife.

Ob-stĭ-pā'tion. [**Obstipa'tio, o'nis;** from *ob*, "against," and *sti'po*, *stipa'tum*, to "stuff," or "cram."] Obstinate costiveness, there being no relief by evacuation; distinguished from constipation. A genus of the order *Epischeses*, class *Locales*, of Cullen's Nosology.

Ob'stru-ent. [**Ob'struens;** from *ob'struo*, to "stop up," or "shut up."] Shutting or closing up.

Ob-su-tu-ra'lis.* [From *ob*, "inversely," and *sutu'ra*, a "suture."] An epithet given to the *placentarium*, when applied against, or opposed to, the suture; to *septa* when their border is empty.

Ob-tec'tus.* [From *ob'tego*, *obtec'tum*, to "cover."] Applied to a *chrysalis*, in which all the parts of the insect are perfectly indicated on the outside, and delineated by compartments of the horny case, as in the *Lepidoptera*.

Ob-tun'dent. [**Obtun'dens;** from *obtun'do*, to "make blunt."] Having power to dull, or overcome, irritation.

Ob-tu-ra'tor, o'ris.* [From *obtu'ro*, *obtura'tum*, to "stop up."] A stopper-up of any cavity. Applied to two muscles and a nerve of the thigh.

Obtura'tor Ex-ter'nus.* A muscle which arises from the obturator foramen, etc., and is inserted into the root of the *trochanter major*. It rotates the thigh outwards.

Obtura'tor In-ter'nus.* A muscle formerly called *marsupialis*, or *bursalis*. Its origin and insertion are nearly the same as those of the *obturator externus*.

Obtura'tor Nerve. A nerve which comes principally from the second and third lumbar nerves, and descends into the pelvis.

Ob-tur-bi-na'tus.* [From *ob*, "inversely," and *tur'bo*, *tur'binis*, a "top."] Having the form of a top reversed.

Ob-tu-sa'tus.* [From *obtun'do*, *obtu'sum*, to "blunt," or "make dull."] Applied to leaves the summits of which are blunt, or obtuse.

Ob-tuse'. [**Obtu'sus;** from the same.] Blunt. A leaf is termed obtuse when its apex is an obtuse angle, or is rounded.

Ob-tu-sif'ĭ-dus.* [From *obtun'do*, to "make blunt, or obtuse," and *fin'do*, to "cleave."] Cleft into obtuse segments.

Ob-tu-sĭ-fo'lĭ-us.* [From *obtu'sus*, "blunt," and *fo'lium*, a "leaf."] Having obtuse leaves: obtusifo'lious.

Ob-tu-sil'o-bus.* [From *obtu'sus*, "dull," or "blunt," and *lo'bus*, a "lobe."] Having leaves divided into round or obtuse lobes: obtusil'obous.

Ob'verse. [**Obver'sum;** from *ob*, "against," "in the way," hence, "obvious," and *ver'to*, *ver'sum*, to "turn."] Literally, the "obvious side." Applied in Numismatics to the side of a coin which contains the head, or principal figure.

Ob'vo-lute. [**Obvolu'tus;** from *obvol'vo*, *obvolu'tum*, to "wrap about."] Enrolled one within another.

Oc'cĭ-dent. [**Oc'cidens;** from *oc'cido*, to "fall down," to "set."] Going down; declining, or setting.

Oc'cĭ-dent. [**Oc'cidens;** from the same.] Literally, the "setting." The west, or place of sunset.

Oc-cĭ-den'tal. [**Occidenta'lis;** from the same.] Belonging to the west; western.

Oc-cip'ĭ-tal. [**Occipita'lis.**] Belonging to the occiput.

Occip'ito-Fron-ta'lis.* [From *oc'ciput*, and *frons*, *fron'tis*, the "forehead."] The name of a muscle which arises from the transverse ridge of the occipital bone, passes over the upper part of the cranium, and is inserted into the *orbicularis palpebrarum* and the skin under the eyebrows.

Oc'çĭ-put,* gen. **Oc-cip'ĭ-tis.** [From *ob*, "against," or "opposite," and *ca'put*, the "head."] The back part of the head.

Oc-cluse'. [**Occlu'sus;** from *occlu'do*, *occlu'sum*, to "shut up;" from *ob*, "against," and *clau'do*, to "close."] Enclosed; shut up.

Oc-clu'sion. [**Occlu'sio, o'nis;** from the same.] A closing or shutting up; imperforation.

Oc-cult'. [From *occul'tus*, "hidden."] Hidden, as applied to diseases the causes and treatment of which are not understood, or to qualities of bodies which do not admit of any rational explanation.

Oc-cul-tā'tion. [**Occulta'tio, o'***nis;* from *occul'to, occulta'tum,* to "hide."] The eclipse of a star or planet by the intervening passage of the moon or another planet.

Oceanic, o-she-an'ik. [**Ocean'icus;** from *oce'anus,* the "ocean."] Living or growing in the ocean; pertaining to the ocean.

O-cel'late. [**Ocella'tus;** from *ocel'lus,* a "little eye."] Marked by spots resembling the pupil of the eye.

O-cel-lif'er-us.* [From *ocel'lus,* a "little eye," and *fe'ro,* to "bear."] Bearing spots resembling eyes: ocellif'erous.

O-cel'lus.* [Diminutive of *oc'ulus,* an "eye."] Applied to rounded spots of which the centre is of a different color from the circumference, giving some resemblance to the pupil of the eye.

Och-le'sis.* [Gr. ὄχλησις; from ὀχλέω, to "disturb by a mob, or crowd."] A general condition of disease produced by a vast number of sick persons under one roof.

Ochnaceæ,* ok-na'she-ē. [From *Och'na,* one of the genera.] A natural order of exogenous plants (trees or shrubs), found in tropical India, Africa, and America.

Och-o-pet'a-lus.* [From ὀχός, "capacious," and πέταλον, a "petal."] Having broad and ample petals.

Ochre, ō'kẹr. [**O'chra;** from ὠχρός, "pale," or "sallow."] An argillaceous earth, impregnated with iron, of a red or yellow color.

O'chre-a.* Literally, a "boot." A union of stipules around the stem of some plants.

O'chre-ate. [From *o'chrea,* a "boot."] Having tubular stipules, or *ochreæ,* as some leaves.

O-chrop'y̆-ra.* [From ὠχρός, "pale," or "sallow," and πῦρ, "fever."] A name sometimes applied to the yellow fever.

Oc'ta-gon. [**Octago'num;** from ὀκτώ, "eight," and γωνία, an "angle."] A plane figure having eight angles and sides.

Oc-tag'o-nal. [**Octago'nus.**] Belonging to an octagon, or having eight angles or sides.

Oc-ta-he'dral. [**Octahe'drus.**] Belonging to an octahedron, or having eight sides.

Oc-ta-hed'rĭ-cus.* The same as OCTAHEDRAL, which see.

Oc-ta-he'dron. [**Octahe'drum;** from ὀκτώ, "eight," and ἕδρα, a "base."] A solid figure having eight equal triangular faces.

Oc-ta'na.* [From *oc'to,* "eight."] An erratic intermittent fever which returns every eighth day.

Oc-tan'drĭ-a.* [From ὀκτώ, "eight," and ἀνήρ, a "man," or "male."] The eighth Linnæan class of plants, including those which have eight stamens in each flower.

Oc-tan'drous. [**Octan'drius;** from ὀκτώ, "eight," and ἀνήρ, a "man," or "male."] Having eight stamens: octan'drious.

Oc-ta'rĭ-us.* [From *octa'vus,* the "eighth."] The eighth part of a gallon, or sixteen fluidounces; a pint.

Oc'to-fid. [**Octof'idus;** from *oc'to,* "eight," and *fin'do,* to "cleave."] Presenting eight clefts, or incisions, which reach about half-way to the midrib.

Oc-tof'o-rus.* [From *oc'to,* "eight," and *fo'ris,* a "door," or "opening."] Having eight holes, or openings.

Octogynia. See OCTOGYNIOUS.

Oc-to-ġy̆n'ĭ-ous. [**Octogyn'ius;** from ὀκτώ, "eight," and γυνή, a "female."] Having eight pistils.

Octohedron. See OCTAHEDRON.

Oc-to-ner'vĭ-us.* [From *oc'to,* "eight," and *ner'vus,* a "nerve."] Having eight nerves. Applied to plants.

Oc-to-pet'a-lous. [**Octopet'alus;** from *oc'to,* "eight," and *pet'alum,* a "petal."] Having eight petals.

Oc-to-stem'o-nis.* [From ὀκτώ, "eight," and στήμων, a "thread," or "stamen."] Having eight free stamens.

Oc'u-lar. [**Ocula'ris;** from *oc'ulus,* the "eye."] Belonging to the eye.

Oc'ular Spec'tres. Imaginary objects floating before the eyes, and assuming the form of *muscæ volitantes,* etc.

Oc'u-late. [**Ocula'tus;** from *oc'ulus,* the "eye."] Having spots like eyes. Having very large eyes.

Oc'u-li,* gen. **Oc-u-lo'rum,** the plural of OCULUS, which see.

Oc'uli is also the genitive singular of OCULUS.

Oc'u-lĭ-form. [**Oculifor'mis;** from *oc'ulus,* the "eye."] Having the form of an eye.

Oc'u-list. [From *oc'ulus,* the "eye."] One skilled in diseases of the eye.

Oc'u-lus,* plural **Oc'u-li.** [From ὄκο; or ὄκκος, the "eye."] The organ of vision. See EYE.

Od. [From ὁδός, a "way," or "passage."] A term proposed by Reichenbach for the peculiar force or influence produced on the nervous system by all magnetic agents.

Od-ax-es'mus* [Gr. ὀδαξησμός, a "sharp or acrid biting"], also written **Odaxis'mus.*** A sensation of biting, or pricking, as that felt in the gums previous to cutting the teeth. Also applied to the bitten tongue, lip, or cheek, which occurs as a symptom, and one of the most pathognomonic character, of the epileptic seizure.

O-dax-et'ĭ-cus.* Belonging to *odaxesmus:* odaxet'ic.

Odaxismos. See ODAXESMUS.

-O'dēs. [Gr. -ώδης; from εἶδος, a "form," or "resemblance."] A terminal similar to *-oid,* or *-oides,* properly signifying *resemblance;* but sometimes denoting *fulness, much,* etc.

O'dic. [**Od'icus.**] Pertaining to OD, which see.

O-don'tạ-grạ.* [From ὀδούς, ὀδόντος, a "tooth," and ἄγρα, a "seizure."] Toothache arising from gout or rheumatism. Also, a kind of forceps, or pincers, for extracting teeth.

Od-on-tăl'ġĭ-ạ. [From ὀδούς, ὀδόντος, a "tooth," and ἄλγος, "pain."] Odontalgy. Violent pain in a tooth, usually from caries, by which the nerve is exposed to the cold air, etc.; toothache. A genus of the order *Phlegmasiæ,* class *Pyrexiæ,* of Cullen's Nosology.

Od-on-tăl'ġic. [**Odontal'gicus.**] Belonging to *odontalgia,* or toothache.

Odontia,* o-don'she-ạ, or o-don'te-ạ. [From ὀδούς, a "tooth."] A generic term employed by Dr. Good, comprising all morbid affections of the teeth. It is also applied in the same manner as ODONTALGIA, which see.

O-don'tic. [**Odon'ticus;** from ὀδούς, a "tooth."] Pertaining to the teeth.

O-don-tit'ĭ-cus.* Belonging to *odontitis.*

O-dọn-ti'tis, *idis.** [From ὀδούς, a "tooth."] Inflammation of a tooth.

O-don-to-bo-thri'tis, *idis.** [From *odontoboth'rium.*] Inflammation of an *alveolus,* or tooth-socket.

O-don-to-both'rĭ-um.* [From ὀδούς, a "tooth," and βοθρίον, a "little hole or cavity."] The same as ALVEOLUS, which see.

O-don-to'dēs.* [From ὀδούς, a "tooth."] Resembling teeth, or full of teeth.

O-don-toġ'e-nȳ. [**Odontoge'nia;** from ὀδούς, a "tooth," and γένω, to "be born," to "be produced."] That branch of Physiology which treats of the development of the teeth.

Od-on-tog'rạ-phȳ. [**Odontogra'phia;** from ὀδούς, a "tooth," and γράφω, to "write."] A description, or history, of the teeth.

O-don'toid. [**Odontoi'des;** from ὀδούς, a "tooth," and εἶδος, a "form."] Resembling a tooth.

Od-on-tol'ĭ-thos,* **Od-on-tol'ĭ-thus.*** [From ὀδούς, a "tooth," and λίθος, a "stone."] (Fr. *Tartre des Dents,* tartr dȧ dŏnᵍ.) The tartar, or stone-like incrustation, on the teeth.

Od-on-to-loġ'ĭ-cạl. [**Odontoloġ'icus.**] Belonging to odontology.

Od-on-tol'o-ġȳ. [**Odontolo'gia;** from ὀδούς, a "tooth," and λόγος, a "discourse."] A dissertation on the structure of the teeth; the science of the teeth.

Od-on-to-lox'ĭ-ạ.* [From ὀδούς, a "tooth," and λοξός, "slanting," or "oblique."] Irregularity, or obliquity, of the teeth.

Od-on-to-ne-cro'sis.* [From ὀδούς, a "tooth," and νεκρόω, to "deaden."] *Necrosis,* or deadness, of the tooth.

O-don-to-no-sol'o-ġȳ. [**Odontonosolo'gia;** from ὀδούς, a "tooth," νόσος, a "disease," and λόγος, a "discourse."] A treatise on the diseases of the teeth; also, that branch of medicine which treats of the diseases of the teeth.

O-don-to-pri'sis.* [From ὀδούς, a "tooth," and πρῖσις, a "sawing."] *Stridor dentium,* or grinding of the teeth.

Od-on-to'sis.* [From ὀδούς, a "tooth."] The formation, growth, or development of a tooth.

O-don-to-thĕr-ạ-pi'ạ.* [From ὀδούς, a "tooth," and θεραπεία, "medical treatment."] The treatment, or care, of the teeth.

O-do-rạ-men'tạ,* plural of *Odoramen'tum.* [From *o'dor,* an "odor."] Odoraments; substances employed in medicine on account of their odor.

Odoramentum. See ODORAMENTA.

O'do-rate. [**Odora'tus;** from *o'dor,* "smell," "fragrance."] Scented; having a strong odor.

Od-o-ra'tus.* [From *o'dor,* "smell," "fragrance."] The sense, also the act, of smelling.

O-do-rif'er-ant. The same as ODORIFEROUS, which see.

O-do-rif'er-ous. [**Odorif'erans, an'tis, Odorif'erus;** from *o'dor,* "fragrance," "odor," and *fe'ro,* to "bear," to "produce."] Having an agreeable odor. Producing or emitting odor.

Œconomia. See ECONOMY.

Œconomia Animalis. See ANIMAL ECONOMY.

Œconomia Vegetabilis. See VEGETABLE ECONOMY.

Œconomicus. See ECONOMICAL.

Œ-de'ma, atis.* [From οἰδέω, to "swell."] A swelling from effusion of serous fluid into the cellular substance.

Œd-e-mat'ic. [**Œdemat'icus.**] Nearly the same as ŒDEMATOUS.

Œ-dem-a-to'dēs.* [From *œde'ma*, a "swelling," and εἶδος, a "form."] Resembling œdema: œdem'atous.

Œ-dem'a-toid. [**Œdematoi'des;** from the same.] Resembling œdema.

Œ-dem'a-tous. [**Œdemato'sus;** from *œde'ma.*] Pertaining to œdema; of the nature of œdema.

Œil, ūl or uī. The French term for EYE, which see.

Œ-nan'thic. [**Œnan'thicus;** from οἶνος, "wine," and ἄνθος, a "flower."] Applied to a peculiar liquid, or ether, held to be the principle that gives wine its peculiar aroma, or flavor.

Œ-no'dēs.* [From οἶνος, "wine."] The same as VINOSUS.

Œ-no-ma'ni-a.* [From οἶνος, "wine," and μανία, "madness."] Excessive inclination for wine or intoxicating liquors. Also, wine-madness, or *mania a potu* resulting from the excessive use of wine.

Œ-soph-a-găl'ġi-a.* [From *œsoph'agus*, and ἄλγος, "pain."] Pain of the œsophagus: œsophagalgy.

Œ-soph-a-ġe'al, or es-o-fā'je-al. [**Œsophagæ'us.**] Belonging to the œsophagus.

Œsophage'al Cords. Two elongated cords, formed of the pneumogastric nerves, which descend along the œsophagus.

Œ-soph'a-ġis'mus.* [From *œsoph'agus.*] Used by some writers in the same manner as *œsophagitis;* by others, as *dysphagia;* by Vogel, for *œsophagospasmus.* Difficulty in swallowing, from spasmodic stricture of the œsophagus.

Œ-soph'a-ġi'tis, idis.* [From *œsoph'agus.*] Inflammation of the œsophagus.

Œ-soph-a-go-dўn'i-a.* [From *œsoph'agus*, and ὀδύνη, "pain."] Pain (spasmodic) of the œsophagus.

Œ-soph'a-gor-rha'ġi-a.* [From *œsoph'agus*, and ῥήγνυμι, to "burst forth."] Hæmorrhage from the œsophagus.

Œ-soph'a-go-spas'mus.* [From *œsoph'agus*, and *spas'mus*, a "contraction."] Cramp, or spasm, of the œsophagus. See ŒSOPHAGISMUS.

Œ-soph-a-gos-te-no'ma, atis.* [From *œsoph'agus*, and στένωμα, a "narrow place."] Constriction of the œsophagus.

Œ-soph-a-go-ste-no'sis.* The formation or progress of *œsophagostenoma.*

Œ-soph-a-got'o-mў. [**Œsophagoto'mia;** from *œsoph'agus*, and τέμνω, to "cut."] The operation of cutting into the œsophagus.

Œ-soph'a-gus.* [From οἴσω (the future of οἴω, another form for φέρω), to "bear," to "carry," and φάγημα, "food" (from φάγω, to "eat").] Literally, "that which carries or conveys the food." The membranous and muscular tube continued from the pharynx to the cardiac orifice of the stomach.

Œs'tru-al. [**Œstrua'lis.**] Belonging to the *œstrum*, or orgasm. Applied to the period during which conception takes place in the Mammalia, analogous to the menstrual period of the human female.

Œs-tru-ā'tion. [**Œstrua'tio, o'nis;** from *œs'trum.*] The state of being under influence of the *œstrum*, or orgasm; rutting.

Œs'trum,* or **Œs'trus.*** [From οἶστρος, the "gad-fly;" hence applied to the sting of passion.] Intense desire, or passionate impulse; usually applied to the orgasm, or pleasurable sensation, experienced during the indulgence of the appetites or passions, particularly of the sexual passion, termed more distinctively *œs'trum vene'reum*, or *œs'trum Ven'eris.*

Œuf, uf. The French word for "egg." See OVUM.

Of-fĭ-çi'na,* gen. **Of-fĭ-çi'næ.** A shop where goods are sold. In medical language, an apothecary shop.

Of-fĭ-çi'næ,* gen. **Of-fĭ-çi-na'rum,** the plural of OFFICINA, a "shop." It occurs in names like the following: *Camphora officinarum* (literally, the "camphor of the shops," or officinal camphor), *Saccharum officinarum* (the "sugar of the shops"), etc.

Of-fiç'i-nal. [**Officina'lis;** from *offici'na*, a "shop where goods are sold."] Applied to such medicines as are directed by the colleges to be prepared or kept in the shops.

-Oid, or **-I'dēs.** [From εἶδος, a "form," or "resemblance."] A terminal denoting resemblance to an object indicated by the word to which it is joined; as, *Al'kaloid*, or *Alkaloi'des*, "resembling an *alkali*;" *Cri'coid*, or *Cricoi'des* [from κρίκος, a "ring," or "circle"], "resembling a *ring* or *circle*," "in the form of a *ring*," etc.

Oil. [Lat. **O'leum**; Fr. *Huile*, wēl.] A term applied to various unctuous substances, obtained mostly from animals and vegetables. They are divided into two classes, fixed oils and volatile oils, the former of which give a permanently greasy stain to paper.

Oil of Tur'pen-tine. [**O'leum Terebin'thinæ.**] The oil obtained by distillation from the liquid resin of the *Pi'nus sylves'tris.*

Oil of Vit'ri-ol. A name for sulphuric acid.

Oil, Rock. A name for PETROLEUM, which see.

Oils, Fixed. [Lat. **O'lea Fix'a**; Fr. *Huiles Fixes*, wēl fēks.] A general term for oils which are not volatile; but commonly applied to vegetable oils of this description.

Oils, Vol'a-tile. [Lat. **O'lea Volatil'ia**, or **O'lea Destilla'ta**; Fr. *Huiles Volatiles*, wēl vo'lā'tēl'.] Oils found in aromatic vegetables, from which they are usually obtained by distillation. Hence they are termed "*distilled* oils" (olea *destillata*), and sometimes "essential oils," because they constitute the essence of the plant. See OLEA.

Ointment. See UNGUENTUM.

O-i-o-ca-lym'ma, a'tis,* or **O-i-o-ca-lyp'trum.*** [From ᾠόν, an "egg," and κάλυμμα, or καλύπτρα, a "covering."] The cortical membrane, or outer covering, of an egg.

Ol. = *O'leum.** "Oil."

Olacaceæ,* ol-a-ka'she-ē. [From *O'lax*, one of the genera.] A small natural order of tropical, or nearly tropical, trees and shrubs, found in the East Indies, Australia, and Africa.

O'le-a.* [Gr. ἐλαία, or ἐλάα.] An olive, or the olive-tree. A Linnæan genus of the class *Monandria*, natural order *Oleaceæ.*

O'le-a,* O-le-o'rum,* the plural of OLEUM, which see.

O'lea Eu-ro-pæ'a.* ("European Olive.") The systematic name of the olive-plant; also called *Olea sativa.*

O'lea Fix'a.* The Latin term for "Fixed Oils." See OILS, FIXED.

O'lea Vol-a-til'i-a.* The Latin term for "Volatile, or Distilled, Oils" See OILS, VOLATILE.

Oleaceæ,* o-le-a'she-ē. A natural order of exogenous trees and shrubs, found chiefly in temperate climates. It includes the Ash (*Frax'inus*), Lilac (*Syrin'ga*), and Olive (*O'lea*), from the fruit of which olive oil is procured.

O-le-ā'ceous. [**Olea'ceus.**] Resembling the *Olea*, or olive-tree.

O-le-ag'i-nous. [**Oleagino'sus**; from *o'leum*, "oil."] Oily; unctuous.

O'le-āte. [**O'leas, a'tis.**] A combination of oleic acid with a base.

O-le-cran-ar-thri'tis, idis.* [From *olecra'non*, an "elbow-joint," and *arthri'tis*, "inflammation of a joint."] Inflammation of the elbow-joint.

O-le-cran-ar-throc'a-cē.* [From *olecra'non*, an "elbow-joint," and *arthroc'ace*, "ulceration of the cavity of a bone."] Ulceration of the elbow-joint.

O-lec-ra'non,* or o-lek'ra-non. [From ὠλένη, the "ulna," and κράνον, the "head."] The humeral extremity of the *ulna*, on which we lean when resting on the elbow; also, the elbow itself.

O-lef'i-ant or **O'le-fi-ant Gas.** [From *o'leum*, "oil," and *fi'o*, to "become."] The hydruret of carbon, or heavy carburetted hydrogen gas; so named because, when mixed with chlorine, it forms a peculiar, oily-looking compound.

O-le'ic. [**Ole'icus**; from *olei'na.*] Applied to an acid obtained from olein.

O-le-if'er-ous. [**Oleif'erus**; from *o'leum*, "oil," and *fe'ro*, to "bear."] Bearing or producing oil.

O-le-i-ge'ni-um.* [From *o'leum*, "oil," and γεννάω, to "produce."] Applied to olefiant gas.

O'le-in, or **O'le-ine.** [**Olei'na**; from *o'leum*, "oil."] A simple oil entering into the constitution of the various fats and oils.

O-le-in'e-ous. [**Olei'neus.**] Synonymous with OLEACEOUS.

O'le-o-res'in, or **O'le-o-Res'in.** [**Oleoresi'na.**] A term for the native combinations of resins with essential oils, forming various balsamic and terebinthinate substances.—(MAYNE.) The term is applied in the U.S. Pharmacopœia (1860) to those fluid extracts (consisting mainly of volatile oil and resin) which are prepared by using ether as the menstruum.

Oleoresina, plural **Oleoresinæ.** See OLEORESIN.

O-le-o-sac'cha-rum.* [From *o'le-*

um, "oil," and *sac'charum,* "sugar."] A medicine composed of essential oil and sugar, mixed with each other to render the oil more easily diffusible in watery liquors.

Ol-e-rā'ceous. [**Olera'ceus;** from *o'lus, ol'eris,* a "pot-herb."] Of the nature of pot-herbs; esculent.

O'le-um,* plural **O'le-a.** [From *O'lea,* the "olive."] (Gr. ἔλαιον; Fr. *Huile,* wēl.) A fat, unctuous, combustible matter, solid or fluid, not soluble in water, and volatile in various degrees: oil.

O'leum A-mўg'da-læ.* ("Oil of Almond.") See Oleum Amygdalæ Dulcis.

O'leum Amyg'dalæ A-ma'ræ.* ("Oil of Bitter Almond.") The Pharmacopœial name (U.S. Ph.) for the oil obtained by distilling with water the kernels of the fruit of the *Amygdalus communis,* variety *amara.*

O'leum Amyg'dalæ Dul'cis,* or **O'leum Amyg'dalæ.*** ("Oil of Sweet Almond," or "Oil of Almond.") The Pharmacopœial name (U.S. Ph.) for the fixed oil obtained from the kernels of the fruit of the *Amygdalus communis,* variety *dulcis.*

O'leum Ber-ga'mĭ-i.* ("Oil of Bergamot.") The Pharmacopœial name (U.S. Ph.) for the volatile oil of the rind of the fruit of *Citrus limetta.*

O'leum Bu'bu-lum.* Neat's-foot oil. The Pharmacopœial name (U.S. Ph.) for the oil prepared from the bones of the *Bos domesticus.*

Oleum Cajuputi. See Cajuputi, Oleum.

O'leum Cam'pho-ræ.* ("Oil of Camphor.") The name given to the volatile oil obtained from *Cam'phora officina'rum.* It has been placed on the primary list of the Materia Medica of the U.S. Pharmacopœia for 1860.

O'leum Cam-pho-ra'tum.* The *Linimen'tum cam'phoræ.*

O'leum Cin-na-mo'mi.* ("Oil of Cinnamon," or "Oil of Ceylon Cinnamon.") The Pharmacopœial name ‖ for the volatile oil obtained from the bark of the *Cinnamo'mum Zeylan'icum.*

Oleum Crotonis. See Oleum Tiglii.

O'leum Jec'oris A-sel'li.* A name for cod-liver oil. See Oleum Morrhuæ.

O'leum Li-mo'nis.* ("Oil of Lemon.") The Pharmacopœial name ‖ for the volatile oil which is obtained from the rind of the fruit of the *Citrus Limonum.*

O'leum Li'ni.* ("Oil of Flax.") The Pharmacopœial name ‖ for the fixed oil obtained from the seeds of *Linum usitatissimum;* linseed oil.

O'leum Mor'rhu-æ.* ("Oil of the [*Gadus*] *Morrhua;*" Fr. *Huile de Morue,* wēl dẹh mo'rü'.) Cod-liver oil. The Pharmacopœial name ‖ for the fixed oil which is obtained from the liver of the *Gadus Morrhua.* Cod-liver oil is esteemed one of the most valuable remedies in the Materia Medica. It has been found especially useful in chronic rheumatism and gout, and in the various diseases connected with a scrofulous diathesis, including scrofulous affections of the joints, *Tabes mesenterica,* rickets, phthisis, etc.

O'leum Mў-ris'tĭ-çæ.* ("Oil of Nutmeg.") The Pharmacopœial name (U.S. Ph.) for the volatile oil of the kernels of the fruit of *Myristica moschata;* (Ed. Ph.) *Myristicæ oleum;* oil of nutmegs.

O'leum O-li'væ.* ("Oil of Olive," or "Olive Oil.") The Pharmacopœial name ‖ for the fixed oil obtained from the fruit of *O'lea Europæ'a.*

O'leum Riç'ĭ-ni.* ("Oil of Ricinus," or Castor Oil; Fr. *Huile de Ricin,* wēl dẹh rė̀'săɴᵍ'.) The Pharmacopœial name (U.S. Ph.) for the oil of the seeds of the *Ricinus communis;* (Lond. Ph.) *Ricini oleum.* See Castor Oil.

O'leum Ro'sæ.* ("Oil of Rose.") The Pharmacopœial name (U.S. Ph.) for the volatile oil of the petals of *Rosa centifolia;* (Ed. Ph.) *Rosæ oleum.*

O'leum Ses'a-mi.* ("Oil of Sesame.") Benne Oil. The Pharmacopœial name (U.S. Ph.) for the oil of the seeds of *Ses'amum In'dicum,* and of *Ses'amum orienta'le.*

O'leum Suc'cĭ-ni.* ("Oil of Amber.") The Pharmacopœial name (U.S. Ph.) for the volatile oil obtained by the destructive distillation of amber.

O'leum Tĕr-e-bin'thĭ-næ.* ("Oil of Turpentine.") The Pharmacopœial name ‖ for the volatile oil distilled from the turpentine of *Pinus palustris,* and other species of *Pinus;* the *Terebinthinæ oleum* of the London and Edinburgh Pharmacopœias.

O'leum Tĕr'ræ.* ("Oil of Earth.") A name for Petroleum, which see.

O'leum The-o-bro'mæ.* ("Oil of Theobroma," or Butter of Cacao.) The name applied to the concrete oil of the kernels of the fruit of the *Theobroma cacao.* It has been placed on the primary list of the Materia Medica of the U.S. Pharmacopœia for 1860.

O'leum Thy'mi.* ("Oil of Thyme.") The name given to the volatile oil obtained from the *Thy'mus vulga'ris.* It has been placed on the primary list of the Materia Medica of the U.S. Pharmacopœia for 1860.

O'leum Tig'lĭ-i.* ("Oil of Tiglium.") Croton Oil. The Pharmacopœial name (U.S. Ph.) for the oil of the seeds of *Croton tiglium.* The *O'leum Croto'nis* of the British Pharmacopœia.

Ol-fac'tion. [**Olfac'tio,** **o'nis;** from *olfa'cio, olfac'tum,* to "smell."] The exercise of the sense of smell.

Ol-fac'to-rỹ. [**Olfacto'rius;** from the same.] Belonging to the organ or sense of smell.

Olfac'tory Nerves. The first pair of nerves distributed on the pituitary or Schneiderian membrane of the nose.

Ol-fac'tus.* [From *olfa'cio, olfac'tum,* to "smell."] The sense of smell, or act of smelling.

O-lib'a-num.* [From ὀλίβανος, the "frankincense-tree."] Frankincense, believed to come from the *Boswellia serrata.*

Ol-ĭ-ga-can'thus.* [From ὀλίγος, "few," and ἄκανθα, a "thorn."] Having few thorns or spines.

Ol-ĭ-gæ'mĭ-a.* [From ὀλίγος, "little," and αἷμα, the "blood."] Poverty of the blood.

Ol-ĭ-gan'drous. [From ὀλίγος, "few," and ἀνήρ, a "man," or "male."] Having few stamens.

Ol-ĭ-gan'thus.* [From ὀλίγος, "few," and ἄνθος, a "flower."] Having but a small number of flowers.

Ol-ĭ-go-car'pus.* [From ὀλίγος, "few," and καρπός, "fruit."] Having few seeds or fruits.

Ol-ĭ-go-cho'lĭ-a.* [From ὀλίγος, "few," or "little," and χολή, "bile."] Want or deficiency of bile.

Ol-ĭ-go-chỹl'ĭ-a.* [From ὀλίγος, "few," or "little," and χυλός, "chyle."] Want or deficiency of chyle.

Ol-ĭ-go-chy'mĭ-a.* [From ὀλίγος, "few," or "little," and χυμός, "juice."] Want or deficiency of chyme.

Ol-ĭ-go-ga-lac'tĭ-a.* [From ὀλίγος, "few," or "little," and γάλα, "milk."] Want or deficiency of milk. See AGALACTIA.

Ol-ĭ-go-phỹl'lous. [**Oligophyl'lus;** from ὀλίγος, "few," or "small," and φύλλον, a "leaf."] Having few leaves, or those distant from each other.

Ol-ĭ-go-sper-mat'ĭ-cus.* Belonging to *oligospermia.*

Ol-ĭ-go-sper'mĭ-a.* [From ὀλίγος, "little," and σπέρμα, "seed."] Want or deficiency of semen.

Ol-ĭ-go-sper'mous. [**Oligosper'mus;** from the same.] Having few seeds; also, deficient in semen.

O-li'va.* [From *O'lea,* the "olive."] The olive-tree; also, the olive. See OLEA.

Olivæformis. See OLIVIFORMIS.

Olivaris. See OLIVARY.

Ol'ĭ-va-rỹ. [**Oliva'ris;** from the same.] Olive-shaped; like an olive.

Olive. See OLEA, and OLIVA.

Ol'ive Oil. A fixed oil expressed from the ripe fruit of the *Olea Europæa.*

Ol'ive, Spurge. The *Daphne mezereon* or *mezereum.*

Ol'ive-Tree. The *Olea Europæa.*

O-liv-ĭ-for'mis.* [From *oli'va,* an "olive."] Having the form of an olive: oliveform.

Ol. lini s. i. = *O'leum li'ni si'ne ig'ne.** (Literally, "linseed oil without fire.") "Cold-drawn linseed oil."

Ol-o-phlỹc'tis.* [From ὅλος, "whole," and φλύζω, to "boil."] A small hot eruption covering the whole body.

O-lop'ter-us.* [From ὁλός, "entire," and πτερόν, a "wing."] Having entire wings.

Om'a-gra.* [From ὦμος, the "shoulder," and ἄγρα, a "seizure."] Gout in the shoulder; pain of the shoulder.

Om-ar-thri'tis, idis.* [From ὦμος, the "shoulder," and *arthri'tis,* "inflammation of a joint."] Inflammation of a shoulder-joint.

O-ma'sum.* The third and smallest stomach of the *Ruminantia.*

O-men-ta'lis.* Belonging to the omentum: omental.

O-men-ti'tis, idis.* [From *omen'tum,* the "caul."] Inflammation of the omentum; *epiploïtis.*

O-men'to-çēle.* [From *omen'tum,* the "caul," and κήλη, a "tumor."] The same as EPIPLOCELE.

O-men'tu-lum.* [Diminutive of *omen'tum,* a "caul."] The OMENTUM MINUS, which see.

O-men'tum.* [Perhaps from *o'men,* a "sign," or "omen;" because the ancient soothsayers consulted it in order to form their prognostications.] A duplicature of the peritonæum, with more or less fat interposed; called also *epip'loön.*

Omen'tum Ma'jus.* ("Greater

Omentum.") This arises from the whole of the great curvature of the stomach, or as far as the spleen, descending over the intestines to the navel, and sometimes into the pelvis.

Omen'tum Mi'nus.* ("Smaller Omentum.") Arising posteriorly from the transverse fissure of the liver, it passes over the duodenum, small lobe of the liver (*lobulus Spigelii*), and pancreas, into the colon and small curvature of the stomach: also called *Omentum hepatico-gastricum* (*i.e.* the "omentum connected with the liver and stomach"). It is also termed *Omentulum.*

O-mi'tis, i*dis.** [From ὦμος, the "shoulder."] Inflammation of or in the shoulder.

Omn. alt. hor. = *Om'nibus alter'nis ho'ris.** "Every other hour."

Omn. bid. = *Om'ni bid'uo.** "Every two days."

Omn. bih. = *Om'ni biho'rio.** "Every two hours."

Omn. hor. = *Om'ni ho'râ.** "Every hour."

Omn. man. = *Om'ni ma'ne.** "Every morning."

Omn. noct. = *Om'ni noc'te.** "Every night."

Omn. quadr. hor. = *Om'ni quadran'te ho'ræ.** "Every quarter of an hour."

Om-niv'o-rous. [**Omniv'orus;** from *om'nis,* "all," and *vo'ro,* to "devour."] Applied to animals which take all kinds of food.

Om'o-Hy-o-i'de-us.* [From ὦμος, the "shoulder," and os *hyoi'des,* the "hyoid bone."] The name of a muscle which arises from the shoulder and is inserted into the *os hyoides.* It depresses that bone and the lower jaw.

Om-o-pha'ġi-a.* [From ὠμός, "crude," and φάγω, to "eat."] The eating of raw food.

O-moph'a-gus.* [From the same.] Living on raw food: omoph'agous.

Omoplate, o'mo'plåt'. [*I.e.* "shoulder-plate;" from ὦμος, the "shoulder," and πλατύς, "flat," or "broad."] The French term for SCAPULA, which see.

Om-o-to'ci-a.* [From ὠμός, "crude," "untimely," and τόκος, a "birth."] A miscarriage or untimely birth.

O-mot'o-cus.* [From the same.] Bringing forth untimely offspring; miscarrying.

Om'phal-el-co'sis.* [From ὀμφαλός, the "navel," and ἕλκωσις, "ulceration."] Ulceration of the umbilicus.

Om-phal'ic. [**Omphal'icus;** from ὀμφαλός, the "navel."] Belonging to the umbilicus, or navel.

Om-pha-li'tis, i*dis.** [From ὀμφαλός, the "navel."] Inflammation of the umbilicus, or its vessels.

Om'pha-lo-çele.* [From ὀμφαλός, the "navel," and κήλη, a "tumor."] Protrusion of a portion of bowel, or omentum, or both, at the umbilicus; *hernia umbilicalis; exomphalos.*

Om'pha-loid. [**Omphaloi'des;** from ὀμφαλός, the "navel," and εἶδος, a "form."] Resembling the navel.

Om-pha-lon'cus.* [From ὀμφαλός, the "navel," and ὄγκος, a "tumor."] A hard tumor or swelling of the navel.

Om-pha-lor-rha'ġi-a.* [From ὀμφαλός, the "navel," and ῥήγνυμι, to "burst forth."] Hæmorrhage from the umbilicus.

Om-pha-lor-rhex'is.* [From ὀμφαλός, the "navel," and ῥῆξις, a "breaking."] Rupture of the umbilical cord.

Om-pha-lor-rhœ'a.* [From ὀμφαλός, the "navel," and ῥέω, to "flow."] Applied to an effusion of lymph from the umbilicus.

Om-pha-lot'o-mў. [**Omphalo-to'mia;** from ὀμφαλός, the "navel," and τέμνω, to "cut."] Division of the umbilical cord from the umbilicus.

Onagraceæ,* on-a-gra'she-ē, or **On'-agræ.*** [From *On'agra,* one of the genera.] A natural order of exogenous plants, natives of Europe and the temperate parts of America. It includes the *Fuchsia* and *Epilobium.*

On'agræ.* The Jussieuan name of a natural order of plants. See ONAGRACEÆ.

O'nan-işm. [**Onanis'mus;** from *O'nan;* see Genesis xxxviii.] The same as *Masturbation* (as applied to males). See MASTURBATION.

On-co-lo'ġi-a.* [From ὄγκος, a "tumor," and λόγος, a "discourse."] A treatise on tumors; that branch of medicine which treats of boils or tumors.

On-co'sis.* [From ὄγκος, a "tumor."] The progress or formation of a boil or tumor.

On-cot'o-mў. [**Oncoto'mia;** from ὄγκος, a "tumor," and τέμνω, to "cut."] The cutting or opening of a boil, tumor, or abscess.

O-nei-ro-dўn'i-a.* [From ὄνειρον, a "dream," and ὀδύνη, "pain," or "distress."] Disturbance or restlessness of the imagination during sleep; nightmare. A genus of the order *Vesaniæ,* class *Neuroses,* of Cullen's Nosology.

Oneirodyn'ia Ac-ti'va.* Sleep-walking, or somnambulism.

Oneirodyn'ia Gra'vans.* Nightmare. See EPHIALTES, and INCUBUS.

Oneirogonorrhœa,* o-nī-ro-gon-or-rē'a. [From ὄνειρον, a "dream," γονή, "semen," and ῥέω, to "flow."] The same as ONEIROGONUS, which see.

O-nei-rog'o-nus.* [From ὄνειρον, a "dream," and γονή, "semen."] The emission of semen during sleep. See SPERMATORRHŒA DORMIENTIUM.

O-nei-rol'o-gy̆. [**Oneirolo'gia;** from ὄνειρον, a "dream," and λόγος, a "discourse."] The doctrine or theory of dreams; the science of dreams.

Onglade, ŏnᴳ'glåd'. The French term for PARONYCHIA, which see.

Ongle, ŏngl. The French term for NAIL, which see.

On'ion. The *Allium cepa.*

Onion, Sea. See SCILLA MARITIMA.

O-nis'cus A-sel'lus.* The wood-louse. An insect found in rotten wood. It was once regarded as a stimulant and diuretic, and employed in jaundice.

On'o-ma,* plural **O-nom'a-ta.** [Gr. ὄνομα.] A name.

O-nom-a-tol'o-gy̆. [**Onomatolo'gia;** from ὄνομα, a "name," and λόγος, a "discourse."] The science of names; nomenclature.

On-om-a-to-pœ'ia,* or **On-om-a-to-poi-e'sis.*** [From ὄνομα, a "name," and ποιέω, to "make."] The formation of names, or rather their creation in imitation of sounds or indication of appearances.

On-to-graph'ic. [**Ontograph'icus.**] Belonging to ontography.

On-tog'ra-phy̆. [**Ontogra'phia;** from ὤν, ὄντος, a "being," and γράφω, to "write."] A description of beings, their nature and essence.

On-to-log'i-cal. [**Ontolog'icus.**] Belonging to Ontology.

On-tol'o-gy̆. [**Ontolo'gia;** from ὤν, a "being," and λόγος, a "discourse."] The doctrine of beings, or of principles in the abstract. The science of existence, its ultimate laws, etc.; a branch of metaphysics.

O-ny̆ch'i-a.* [From ὄνυξ, the "nail" of the fingers or toes.] An abscess near the nail of the fingers; whitlow. See PARONYCHIA.

O-ny̆ch'i-cus.* Belonging to the nails.

On-y̆-chi'tis, *idis.** [From ὄνυξ, the "nail."] Inflammation of the nail of a finger or toe.

On-y̆-cho-cli'ne.* [From ὄνυξ, the "nail," and κλίνη, a "bed."] The "bed of the nail." An extremely sensitive portion of the finger or toe, lying immediately below the nail.

On-y̆-cho'dēs.* [From ὄνυξ, the "nail."] Having large nails.

On-y̆-cho-i'dēs.* [From ὄνυξ, the "nail," and εἶδος, a "form."] Like, or resembling, a nail; on'ychoid.

On-y̆-chon'o-sos,* or **On-y̆-chon'o-sus.*** [From ὄνυξ, the "nail," and νόσος, "disease."] Disease of the finger or toe nails.

On-y̆-cho-stro'ma.* [From ὄνυξ, the "nail," and στρῶμα, a "mattress," or "bed."] The same as ONYCHOLINE, which see.

O'ny̆x, *y̆chis.** [From ὄνυξ, a "nail."] A small collection of matter in the anterior chamber of the eye, or between the layers of the cornea. Also, a precious stone of the agate family, much prized for cameos. Named, perhaps, from the interchange of white and semi-transparent lines (or layers) resembling those sometimes occurring on the nail.

O-ny̆x'is.* [From ὄνυξ, the "nail."] A sinking or immersion of the nails into the flesh.

Ooides. See OVOID.

O'o-in. [**Ooi'na;** from ᾠόν, an "egg."] A substance resembling or constituting albumen, or white of egg.

O'o-lite. [**Ooli'tes;** from ᾠόν, an "egg," and λίθος, a "stone."] A name applied to those masses of rock which result from an accumulation of small round particles like the roe or eggs of a fish joined together, either immediately or by a visible cement.

O-o-lit'ic. [**Oolit'icus.**] Belonging to an oolite.

O. O. O. = *O'leum Oli'væ Op'timum.** "Best olive oil."

O-o-pho-ri'tis, *idis.** [From *ooph'orum.*] The same as OVARITIS, which see.

O-oph'o-ron,* or **O-oph'o-rum.*** [From ᾠόν, an "egg," and φέρω, to "bear."] The same as OVARY, which see.

O-paç'i-ty̆. [**Opa'citas, a'***tis;* from *opa'cus,* "dark," "shady."] Incapability of transmitting light; the reverse of transparency. Opacity is used to express any defect in the transparency of the cornea, from a slight film to an intense whiteness.

O'pal. [**Op'alus.**] The name of a precious stone.

O'pal, Preç'ious. A beautiful and rare mineral, characterized by its iridescent reflection of light. It consists of silica, with about ten per cent. of water. Common Opal resembles the preceding in some respects, but has no play of colors.

O-pa-lĕs'çence. [From *o'palus*, the "precious opal."] A kind of reflected milky light which some minerals exhibit.

O'pa-line. [**Opali'nus**; from the same.] Having the milky and bluish tint, with the reflection of light, of the opal.

O'pal-ized. [**Opaliza'tus**; from the same.] Converted into, or assuming the appearance of, the opal.

Op-e-rā'tion. [**Opera'tio, o**'*nis*; from *op'eror*, *opera'tus*, to "operate," to "work."] The performance of any of the greater acts of surgery, as amputation or excision of a limb or part, tying of arteries, etc.

O-per'cu-lar. [**Opercula'ris**; from *oper'culum*, a "lid."] That which closes a cavity in the manner of a lid. A term used by Owen for the diverging appendages of the tympano-mandibular arch.

O-per'cu-late. [**Opercula'tus**; from *oper'culum*, a "lid."] Having a lid, or cover.

O-per'cu-lĭ-form. [**Operculifor'mis**; from *oper'culum*, a "lid."] Having the form of an opercule, or lid.

O-per'cu-lum.* [From *ope'rio*, *oper'tum*, to "cover."] A lid, or cover. The cover of the peristome of mosses. Also, a bony formation which, with the *suboperculum* and *interoperculum*, closes the great opening of the gills of fishes: an opercule.

O-phi'a-sis.* [From ὄφις, a "serpent."] A term applied by Celsus to a variety of *Area* (or baldness) which spreads in a *serpentine* form round both sides of the head from the occiput.

O-phid'ĭ-an. [**Ophid'ius**; from ὄφις, a "serpent."] Belonging to a serpent, or resembling serpents.

Ophioglossaceæ,* o-fe-o-glos-sa'-she-ē. [From *Ophioglos'sum*, one of the genera.] "Adders' Tongues." A natural order of cryptogamic plants allied to ferns.

O-phĭ-og'ra-phy̆. [**Ophiogra'phia**; from ὄφις, a "serpent," and γράφω, to "write."] A description of serpents.

O-phĭ-o-i'dēs.* [From ὄφις, a "serpent," and εἶδος, a "form."] Resembling a serpent: o'phioid.

O-phĭ-oph'a-gous. [**Ophioph'agus**; from ὄφις, a "serpent," and φάγω, to "eat."] Eating serpents as food. Applied to certain birds.

O-phĭ-os'to-ma.* [From ὄφις, a "serpent," and στόμα, a "mouth."] The name of a genus of intestinal worms.

Oph-thăl'ma-gra.* [From ὀφθαλμός, the "eye," and ἄγρα, a "seizure."] Sudden pain of the eye, gouty in its nature or otherwise.

Oph-thăl-măl'ġĭ-a.* [From ὀφθαλμός, the "eye," and ἄλγος, "pain."] The same as Ophthalmodynia, which see.

Oph-thăl-măl'ġĭ-cus.* Belonging to *ophthalmalgia:* ophthalmalgic.

Oph-thăl-ma-tro'phĭ-a.* [From ὀφθαλμός, the "eye," and ἀτροφία, a "pining away."] Atrophy, or wasting away, of the eye.

Oph-thăl'mĭ-a.* [From ὀφθαλμός, the "eye."] (Fr. *Ophthalmie*, of'tâl'mè', or *Ophthalmite*, of'tâl'mèt'.) Inflammation of the eye. A genus of the order *Phlegmasiæ*, class *Pyrexiæ*, of Cullen's Nosology. It is nearly synonymous with Ophthalmitis. The following important varieties may be noticed.

Catar'rhal Ophthal'mia. [*Ophthal'mia Catarrha'lis*.] Arising from atmospheric causes, and popularly designated by the terms *cold*, or *blight*. The expression *ophthalmia mucosa* ("mucous ophthalmia") denotes the increased mucous discharge which accompanies it. It is seated in the conjunctiva.

Gonorrhœ'al Ophthal'mia. [*Ophthal'mia Gonorrho'ica*.] A very severe form of the disease, produced by the accidental introduction of gonorrhœal matter into the eye. See Gonorrhoblepharrhœa.

Ophthal'mia Neonato'rum.* ("Ophthalmia of New-born [Children]".) A kind of purulent ophthalmia which sometimes attacks infants soon after birth.

Pu'rulent Ophthal'mia. [*Ophthal'mia Purulen'ta*.] Also termed *Egyp'tian Ophthal'mia*, because it is common in Egypt. An acute form of ophthalmia, attended with a puriform secretion. This is the *blepharo-blennorrhœa*, *ophthalmo-blennorrhœa*, of Schmidt and Beer. This form of the disease is generally, if not always, contagious.

Oph-thăl'mic. [**Ophthal'micus**; from ὀφθαλμός, the "eye."] Belonging to, or connected with, the eye, or with ophthalmia.

Ophthalmic Ganglion. See Lenticular Ganglion.

Oph-thăl-mit'ic. [**Ophthalmit'icus.**] Belonging to *ophthalmitis*.

Oph-thăl-mi'tis, *idis.** [From ὀφθαλμός, the "eye."] Inflammation of the eye; more specially of the bulb or globe of the eye, with its membranes. Nearly synonymous with OPHTHALMIA.

Oph-thăl-mo-blen-nor-rhœ'a.* [From ὀφθαλμός, the "eye," βλέννα, "mucus," and ῥέω, to "flow."] Literally, a "flow of mucus from the eye:" usually applied to a gonorrhœal discharge from the eyelids. See OPHTHALMIA (GONORRHŒAL).

Oph-thăl-mo-car-çĭ-no'ma, *atis.** [From ὀφθαλμός, the "eye," and καρκίνωμα, a "cancerous tumor."] Cancer of the eye.

Oph-thăl'mo-çēle.* [From ὀφθαλμός, the "eye," and κήλη, a "tumor."] The same as OPHTHALMOPTOMA.

Oph-thăl-mo-çel'ĭ-cus.* Belonging to ophthalmocele: ophthalmocel'ic.

Oph-thăl-mo-dўn'ĭ-a.* [From ὀφθαλμός, the "eye," and ὀδύνη, "pain."] Violent pain in the eye, not the effect of inflammation.

Oph-thăl-mog'ra-phў. [**Ophthalmogra'phia;** from ὀφθαλμός, the "eye," and γράφω, to "write."] A description of the eye.

Oph-thăl-mol'o-ġў. [**Ophthalmolo'gia;** from ὀφθαλμός, the "eye," and λόγος, a "discourse."] A treatise on the eye. That part of Anatomy which treats of the eye.

Oph-thăl-mo-ma-cro'sis.* [From ὀφθαλμός, the "eye," and μακρός, "long," or "great."] Enlargement of the eyeballs.

Oph-thăl-mom'e-ter. [**Ophthalmom'etrum;** from ὀφθαλμός, the "eye," and μέτρον, a "measure."] An instrument for measuring the capacity of the chambers of the eye.

Oph-thăl-moph'thĭ-sis.* [From ὀφθαλμός, the "eye," and φθίσις, a "wasting."] Wasting, or diminution, of the eyeballs.

Oph-thăl-mo-ple'ġĭ-a.* [From ὀφθαλμός, the "eye," and πληγή, a "stroke," or "wound."] Paralysis of the muscles of the eyeball.

Oph-thăl-mop-to'ma, *atis.** [From ὀφθαλμός, the "eye," and πτῶμα, a "fall."] *Procidentia oculi*, or protrusion of the eyeball: usually caused by some tumor or abscess within the orbit. See OPHTHALMOCELE.

Oph-thăl-mop-to'sis.* The progress of *ophthalmoptoma*.

Oph-thăl-mor-rha'ġĭ-a.* [From ὀφθαλμός, the "eye," and ῥήγνυμι, to "burst forth."] Hæmorrhage from the eye or orbit.

Oph-thăl-mor-rhex'is.* [From ὀφθαλμός, the "eye," and ῥῆξις, a "breaking," or "bursting."] A bursting, or disruption, of the eyeball.

Oph-thăl-mor-rhœ'a.* [From ὀφθαλμός, the "eye," and ῥέω, to "flow."] An oozing (of blood) from the eye.

Ophthalmorrhœ'a Ex-ter'na.* Extravasation of blood beneath the eyelids.

Ophthalmorrhœ'a In-ter'na.* A term for extravasation of blood within the eye.

Oph-thăl'mo-scope. [**Ophthalmos'copus;** from ὀφθαλμός, the "eye," and σκοπέω, to "examine."] An instrument for facilitating examination of the eye.

Oph-thăl-mo-scop'ic. [**Ophthalmoscop'icus.**] Belonging to ophthalmoscopy.

Oph-thăl-mos'co-pў. [**Ophthalmosco'pia;** from ὀφθαλμός, the "eye," and σκοπέω, to "examine."] Examination, or inspection, of the eyes.

Opiane. See NARCOTINE.

O'pĭ-ate. [**Opia'tum;** from *o'pium*.] A medicine which causes sleep.

O'pĭ-i,* the genitive of OPIUM.

Op-is-thot-o-no-i'dēs.* [From *opisthot'onos*, and εἶδος, a "form."] Resembling *opisthotonos*.

Op-is-thot'o-nos.* [From ὄπισθε, "at the back," and τείνω, to "stretch," or "bend."] Bent or stretched backwards; a variety of tetanus.

O'pĭ-um.* [Gr. ὄπιον; from ὀπός, "juice."] The Pharmacopœial name ‖ of the concrete juice of the *Papa'ver somnif'erum*, obtained from incisions in the cortical part of its capsule. Good opium should yield at least seven per cent. of morphia by the officinal process. Opium is a stimulant narcotic. Taken in a moderate dose, its first effect is to increase the force and fulness of the pulse, to augment the temperature of the skin, to quicken the senses and give new energy to the intellectual faculties. This state of excitement gradually subsides, and is followed by a feeling of placid repose, which at length terminates in sleep. Some persons, however, are not affected by opium in the manner here described, but are rendered restless, and even delirious, by its action. When this narcotic has been taken in poisonous doses, the patient soon sinks into a profound lethargy or torpor, and death ensues, caused, it would seem, by a suspension of respiration from the want of due influence from the brain. As a medicine, opium (or its preparations) may be advantageously employed in a greater variety of affections than perhaps any other article in the Materia Medica. For allaying restlessness, assuaging pain, and producing sleep, it is an invaluable resource to the physician. Being a powerful antispasmodic, it may often be used with the greatest advantage in tetanus, colic, violent cough, especially of a nervous character, and other convulsive affections. Its influence in checking the secretions, renders it a most valuable remedy in diarrhœa, in catarrh attended with excessive expectoration, in diabetes, etc. But, if it is one of the most useful of medicines, it is also perhaps more than any other, liable to abuse; the habit of taking it, when not absolutely needed, is easily acquired, and is often followed by the most distressing and deplorable effects on both the body and the mind. See POISONS.

Op-o-bâl'sam. [**Opobal'samum;** from ὀπός, "juice," and *bal'samum.*] The most valued of the balsams; also called Balm of Gilead. It is obtained from the *Amyris Gileadensis*, otherwise called *A. opobalsamum.* The same as BALSAM OF MECCA, which see.

Op-o-del'doc. The camphorated soap-liniment.

O-po-i'dĭ-a Gal-ba-nif'e-ra.* The name of the plant to which the Dublin College has referred the gum-resin galbanum.

O-pop'o-nax, a'*cis.** [From ὀπός, "juice," and πάναξ, the "panacea herb."] A gum-resin obtained from a plant formerly called *Pastina'ca opop'onax*, now *Opop'onax chiro'nium.*

Opop'onax Chi-ro'nĭ-um.* A new name for the plant which affords *Opoponax;* formerly called *Pastinaca opoponax.*

Oppilatio (op-pe-la'she-o), **o'***nis.** [From *oppi'lo, oppila'tum*, to "obstruct."] Synonymous with OBSTIPATION, and CONSTIPATION, which see.

Op-po'nens Pol'lĭ-cis.* ("Opposing [Muscle] of the Thumb.") [From *oppo'no*, to "oppose," and *pol'lex, pol'licis*, the "thumb."] A muscle which arises from the annular ligament of the wrist, etc., and is inserted into the thumb. It brings the thumb inwards, thus opposing it to the fingers.

Op'po-site. [From *oppo'no, oppos'itum*, to "place against."] A term applied to leaves when two of them are situated at the same node, on opposite sides of the stem.

Op-pos'ĭ-tĭ-fo'lĭ-ous. [**Oppositifo'lius;** from *oppos'itus*, and *fo'lium*, a "leaf."] Having opposite leaves. Also, growing opposite a leaf. Applied to a peduncle or a tendril.

Op-pos'ĭ-tĭ-pen-na'tus.* [From *oppo'no, oppos'itum*, to "place against," and *penna'tus*, "feathery."] Applied to pennate leaves of which the folioles are opposite: oppositipen'nate.

Op-pres'sion. [**Oppres'sio, o'***nis;* from *op'primo, oppres'sum*, to "press down."] A sensation of weight on a part; the state of being oppressed.

Oppres'sion, Pre-cor'dĭ-al. A sense of weight experienced about the *præcordia*, or fore part of the chest.

Op'tic. [**Op'ticus;** from ὄπτω, to "see."] Relating to the organ of vision.

Op'tic Nerve. [**Ner'vus Op'ticus,** plural **Ner'vi Op'tici.**] The optic nerve forms the communication between the brain and the organ of vision. The expansion of its orbital extremity constitutes the retina. The optic nerves are also called the *Par secundum*, or "Second Pair," of the encephalic nerves, the olfactory being reckoned as the first.

Op'tic Thal'a-mus. [**Thal'amus Op'ticus.**] Each of two eminences in the anterior and internal part of the lateral ventricles of the brain; the bed of the optic nerve.

Op'tics. [**Op'tica;** from ὄπτω, to "see."] The branch of physical science which treats of the phenomena of light and vision, and of the instruments by the use of which the faculty of vision is aided and improved.

Opun'tia (o-pŭn'she-a) **Coc-cĭ-nel-lif'er-a.*** The Nopal, a cactaceous plant on which the cochineal insects feed. The natives in the Mexican State of Oajaca form plantations of the Nopal for the culture of these valuable insects, of which three crops are said to be collected annually.

Or, OR. The French term for GOLD, which see.

O'ra.* The plural of Os, a "mouth," which see.

O'ral. [**Ora'lis;** from *os, o'ris*, a "mouth."] Relating to the mouth, or uttered by the mouth; verbal.

Or'ange. [**Auran'tium.**] The fruit of the *Citrus aurantium.*

Or'ange, Sev'ille (sev'il). A variety of the *Citrus aurantium*.

Or-bic'u-lar. [**Orbicula'ris;** from *orbic'ulus*, diminutive of *or'bis*, an "orb," or "circle."] Shaped like an orb; circular in outline.

Or-bic-u-la're Os.* ("Orbicular Bone.") The small orbed bone of the ear articulating with the head of the *stapes*.

Or-bic-u-la'ris Oc'u-li.* ("Circular [Muscle] of the Eye.") The same as the ORBICULARIS PALPEBRARUM.

Orbicula'ris O'ris.* ("Circular [Muscle] of the Mouth.") A muscle constituting the substance of the lips; also termed *constric'tor o'ris, sphinc'ter labio'-rum*, or *oscula'tor*.

Orbicula'ris Păl-pe-bra'rum.* ("Circular [Muscle] of the Eyelids.") A muscle arising from the outer edge of the orbitar process and inserted into the nasal process of the superior maxillary bone. It shuts the eye.

Or-bic'u-late. [**Orbicula'tus;** from *orbic'ulus*, a "little circle, or round ball."] Round and flat. Applied to leaves. In Zoology, having the shell round, or orbicular.

Or-bic'u-lus.* [Diminutive of *or'-bis*, a "circle."] A little circle. See next article.

Orbic'ulus Cil-ĭ-a'ris.* ("Ciliary Circle.") The white circle formed by the ciliary ligament, marking the distinction between the choroid and iris.

Or'bit. [From *or'bita*, a "track," or "path," the "rut of a wheel."] The path described by a planet in its course round the sun, or by a moon round its primary planet. Also applied to the bony cavity in which the eyeball is located, the eye being compared to a wheel (*orbis*), and the socket to the rut or cavity into which the wheel has sunk.

Or'bĭ-tal. [**Orbita'lis;** from *or'-bita*, the "orbit of the eye."] Belonging to the orbit of the eye.

Or'bĭ-ta-rỹ. [**Orbita'rius,** or **Or-bita'ris;** from the same.] Relating to the orbit of the eye.

Or-bĭ-to-sphe'noid. [**Orbitosphe-noi'des;** from *or'bita*, the "orbit," and *sphenoi'des* os, the "sphenoid bone."] A term used by Owen for the orbital, or lesser, wing of the sphenoid bone.

Or-che-i'tis, idis.* [From ὄρχεα for ὄσχεον, the "scrotum."] Inflammation of the scrotum.

Or-chel'la.* The *Roccel'la Tincto'ria*, a plant of the order *Lichenes*, which yields the coloring matter called *orchil*, or *archil*.

Or'che-o-çēle.* The same as OSCHEOCELE.

Or-che-o-plas'tỹ. [**Orcheoplas'-tia;** from ὄρχεα, a term for the "scrotum," and πλάσσω, to "form."] The operation of removing fungous portions of the scrotum, and supplying their place with healthy flaps from the vicinity.

Orcheotomia. See ORCHOTOMY.

Or-chĭ-ăl'ġĭ-a.* [From ὄρχις, a "testicle," and ἄλγος, "pain."] Pain in the testicle.

Orchidaceæ,* or-ke-da'she-ē, or **Or'-chĭ-dēs.*** A natural order of endogenous herbaceous plants, found in all parts of the world except those regions which are excessively cold or dry. Some of them are parasitical. This order, which is more remarkable for beauty than utility, includes the *Or'chis* and the delightful aromatic known as Vanilla.

Orchidalgia. See ORCHIALGIA.

Or-chid'e-ous. [**Orchid'eus.**] Resembling the *Orchis*, or relating to the *Orchis*.

Or'chĭ-dēs,* the plural of *Or'chis*, forming the Jussieuan name of a natural order of plants. See ORCHIDACEÆ.

Orchidotomia. See ORCHOTOMY.

Orchids. The same as ORCHIDES.

Or-chil'la.* The same as ORCHELLA.

Or'chĭ-o-çēle.* [From ὄρχις, a "testicle," and κήλη, a "tumor."] Hernia of the testicle.

Or-chĭ-o-dỹn'ĭ-a.* [From ὄρχις, a "testicle," and ὀδύνη, "pain."] Pain, of a pungent character, in the testicle.

Or-chĭ-o-scir'rhus.* [From ὄρχις, a "testicle," and σκίῤῥος, an "indurated tumor."] Scirrhus, or incipient cancer, of the testicle.

Orchiotomia. See ORCHOTOMY.

Or'chis Mas'cu-la.* The Male Orchis; a plant from the tubers of which salep is procured.

Or-chit'ĭ-cus.* Belonging to *orchitis*: orchit'ic.

Or-chi'tis, idis.* [From ὄρχις, a "testicle."] Inflammation of the testicle; swelled testicle. The same as HERNIA HUMORALIS.

Or-chot'o-mỹ. [**Orchoto'mia;** from ὄρχις, a "testicle," and τέμνω, to "cut."] The operation of cutting out or removing a testicle by the knife; castration.

Or'dĕr. [**Or'do, Or'dinis.**] A division of a class, comprising genera varying in some respects from each other, but agreeing in essential characters. In Architecture, a system or assemblage of parts arranged according to some particular plan or style.

Or'dĭ-nēs,* gen. **Or'dĭ-num.** The plural of *Ordo.* See ORDER.

Or'do.* The Latin term for ORDER, which see.

Ore. [Probably from *æs, æ'ris,* "brass."] A mineral substance from which a metal is extracted; a native combination of a metal with some substance which disguises its metallic properties. Ores are termed *sulphurets* when combined with sulphur, *oxides* when combined with oxygen, and *salts* when combined with acids.

Or'gan. [**Or'ganum;** from ὄργανον, an "instrument," or "organ."] A part of an animal or vegetable capable of performing some act or office appropriate to itself.

Or-gan'ic. [**Organ'icus;** from the same.] Relating to, or acting by means of, organs; having an organized structure. Generally used to express the distinction between a disease of structure and one of function, the former being *organic,* the latter *functional.*

ORGAN'IC CHEM'ISTRY is that branch of Chemistry which treats of the properties and combinations of animal and vegetable substances.

ORGAN'IC FUNC'TIONS are those possessed by both animals and vegetables.

Organic Force. See VITAL FORCE.

Organ'ic Life. A term applied to that life which belongs properly to the organs necessary to vital existence. It is shared in common by both animals and vegetables, and is contradistinguished from *animal life,* comprising those functions which are peculiar to animals.

Organ'ic Mol'e-cules. [**Molec'ulæ Organ'icæ.**] A term applied by Spallanzani to certain floating bodies supposed to exist in the male semen, and which he regarded as primordial monads of peculiar activity existing through all nature and constituting the nutrient elements of living matter.

Organ'ic Re-mains'. The remains of plants and animals; that is, all organized bodies found in a fossil state.

Or'gan-ism. [**Organis'mus;** from ὄργανον, an "organ."] Organic structure; the living economy; the assemblage of the forces which act in organized beings.

Or-gan-i-zā'tion. [**Organiza'tio, o'nis;** from ὄργανον, an "organ."] The process by which an organized body is formed; also, the totality of the parts which constitute, and of the laws which regulate, an organized body.

Or'gan-īzed. [**Organiza'tus;** from ὄργανον, an "organ."] Having a defined structure; formed, or furnished, with organs, each of which has its proper function.

Or-ga-nog'e-ny̆. [**Organoge'nia;** from ὄργανον, an "organ," and γένεσις, "generation."] Originally, the formation, or growth, of organs; usually applied to a description of the organs of a living body.

Or-gan-o-graph'ĭ-cal. [**Organograph'icus.**] Relating to organography.

Or-ga-nog'ra-phy̆. [**Organogra'phia;** from ὄργανον, an "organ," and γράφω, to "write."] A description of the organs of some living body; the study of the organs or conspicuous parts of plants as to their external conformation, including Morphology (the study of forms).—(GRAY.)

Or-ga-no-log'ĭ-cal. [**Organolog'icus.**] Relating to organology.

Or-ga-nol'o-gy̆. [**Organolo'gia;** from ὄργανον, an "organ," and λόγος, a "speech."] That branch of Physiology which treats of the different organs of animals, but more particularly of those of the human body.

Organon, Organum. See ORGAN.

Or-ga-no-no'mĭ-a.* [From ὄργανον, an "organ," and νόμος, a "law."] A declaration of the laws which regulate the activity of the organism, or organic life: organon'omy.

Or-ga-no-nom'ĭ-cus.* Belonging to *organonomia.*

Or'gans of Re-pro-duc'tion. Applied in Botany to the flowers (consisting essentially of stamens and pistils).

Or'gans of Veg-e-tā'tion (in other words, the organs which are essential to vegetable life, or the life of the individual plant). This term includes the root, stem, and leaves, which are also called the *fundamental organs* of plants.

Or'gasm. [**Orgas'mus;** from ὀργάω, to "swell."] Eager desire or excitement, especially venereal; salacity. See ŒSTRUM.

Orgasm, Diseases affecting the. See ORGASTICA.

Or-gas'tĭ-ca.* [From *orgas'ticus.*] The name of an order of the class *Genetica* in Good's Nosology. It comprises diseases affecting the procreative power.

Or-gas'tĭ-cus.* Belonging to orgasm

Orgeat, or'zhat. (French pronunciation, OR'zhå'.) A sweetened emulsion of almonds with orange-flower water.

Or-ĭ-chal'cum.* [From ὄρος, a "mountain," and χαλκός, "brass."] Literally, "mountain brass." A peculiar kind of mixed metal in general use among the ancient Greeks and Romans. It is proved to have been composed of nearly the same ingredients as brass.

O'rĭ-ent. [**O'riens;** from *o'rior*, to "rise up," to "arise."] Literally, the "rising." Applied to that part of the heavens at which the sun arises and ascends above the horizon; eastern.

Or'ĭ-fice. [**Orific'ium;** from *os, o'ris*, a "mouth," and *fa'cio*, to "make."] A mouth or entrance to any cavity of the body; as the orifice of the stomach.

O-rig'a-num.* [Gr. ὀρείγανον.] A Linnæan genus of the class *Didynamia*, natural order *Labiatæ*. The Pharmacopœial name (Ed. and U.S. Ph.) of *Origanum vulgare*, or common marjoram.

Orig'anum Mar-jo-ra'na.* The sweet marjoram.

Orig'anum Vul-ga're.* The common marjoram.

Or'ĭ-gin. [From *ori'go, orig'inis*, a "source," "beginning."] Properly, the source or commencement of any thing. The commencement of a muscle from any part. Its attachment to the part it moves is called its *insertion*.

Or-le-a'na, Ter'ra.* A name for *annotto*.

Orme, ORM. The French for "elm." See ULMUS.

Or-nĭ-thich-ni'tis.* [From ὄρνις, ὄρνιθος, a "bird," and ἴχνος, a "path," or "track."] A name applied to the stone found in Massachusetts, marked with the track of birds' feet.

Or-nĭ-tho-ceph'a-lous. [**Ornithoceph'alus;** from ὄρνις, a "bird," and κεφαλή, a "head."] Having the appearance of a bird's head. Applied to parts of certain plants and shells.

Or-nĭ-tho-co'prus.* [From ὄρνις, a "bird," and κόπρος, "dung."] A name for GUANO, which see.

Or'nĭ-thoid. [**Ornithoi'des;** from ὄρνις, a "bird," and εἶδος, a "form."] Resembling a bird.

Or-nith'o-līte. [**Ornitholi'tes;** from ὄρνις, a "bird," and λίθος, a "stone."] Applied to the fossil remains of birds.

Or-nĭ-thol'ĭ-thus.* [From the same.] The petrifaction of birds.

Or-nĭ-tho-log'ĭ-cal. [**Ornitholog'icus.**] Relating to Ornithology.

Or-nĭ-thol'o-gy̆. [**Ornitholo'gia;** from ὄρνις, ὄρνιθος, a "bird," and λόγος, a "discourse."] The science which treats of the natural history and classification of birds.

Or-nĭ-tho-rhy̆n'chus.* [From ὄρνις, ὄρνιθος, a "bird," and ῥύγχος, a "beak."] A remarkable animal of Australia, having the body of a quadruped and a mouth which resembles the bill of a duck.

Or'nus.* [From ὀρεινός, "mountainous."] The Wild Ash. A Linnæan genus of the class *Polygamia*, natural order *Oleaceæ*.

Or'nus Eū-ro-pæ'a.* The tree which chiefly yields manna. Also named *Frax'inus or'nus*.

Orobanchaceæ,* or-o-ban-ka'she-ē. [From *Oroban'che*, one of the genera.] A natural order of exogenous herbaceous parasitical plants, found in Europe, Asia, and North America.

Or-o-bo-i'dēs.* [From ὄροβος, "pulse," and εἶδος, a "form."] Resembling pulse.

O-rog-no'sĭ-a.* [From ὄρος, a "mountain," and γνῶσις, "knowledge."] The science which treats of mountains, their origin, structure, etc.

O-ro-graph'ĭ-cal. [**Orograph'icus.**] Relating to orography.

O-rog'ra-phy̆. [**Orogra'phia;** from ὄρος, a "mountain," and γράφω, to "write."] A description of mountains.

Or-o-hy̆-drog'ra-phy̆. [**Orohydrogra'phia;** from ὄρος, a "mountain," ὕδωρ, "water," and γράφω, to "write."] A history of waters which flow from mountains, or of the waters and geognostic formations of a country.

O-ro-log'i-cal. [**Orolog'icus.**] Relating to orology.

O-rol'o-gy̆. [**Orolo'gia;** from ὄρος, a "mountain," and λόγος, a "discourse."] A dissertation on mountains. The science which treats of the structure, etc., of mountains.

Orontiaceæ,* o-ron-te-a'she-ē. [From *Oron'tium*, one of the genera.] A natural order of endogenous herbaceous plants, found in many tropical and temperate regions. It includes the *Cal'la palus'tris*, and *Ac'orus cal'amus*. Several of the genera are stimulant and tonic.

Or'pĭ-ment. [**Orpimen'tum;** *i.e. au'ri pigmen'tum*, "pigment of gold:" so named from its color.] Yellow sulphuret of arsenic, or king's yellow.

Or-rhor-rha'gĭ-a.* [From ὀῤῥός, "serum," and ῥήγνυμι, to "burst forth."] A sudden discharge or bursting forth of serum, as from the bowels in Asiatic cholera.

Or-rhor-rhœ'a.* [From ὀῤῥός, "serum," and ῥέω, to "flow."] A flow or discharge of serum; a watery discharge.

Or-rho-so'len, e'nis.* [From ὀῤῥός, "serum," and σωλήν, a "pipe."] A lymphatic vessel.

Or-rhy'men, enis,* or **Or-rho-hy'-men.*** [From ὀῤῥός, "serum," and ὑμήν, a "membrane."] A serous membrane.

Or-rhy-me-ni'tis, idis,* or **Or-rho-hy-me-ni'tis.*** [From *orrhy'men.*] Inflammation of a serous membrane.

Or-rhy-men-o-i'dēs.* [From *orrhy'men*, and εἶδος, a "form."] Resembling a serous membrane.

Orris Florentine. See IRIS FLORENTINA.

Or-tha-can'thus.* [From ὀρθός, "straight," or "right," and ἄκανθα, a "spine."] Having straight spines: orthacanthous.

Or-thar'thra-gra.* [From ὀρθός, "straight," or "right," "true," ἄρθρον, a "joint," and ἄγρα, a "seizure."] True or regular gout.

Or-thoc'la-dus.* [From ὀρθός, "straight," or "right," and κλάδος, a "branch."] Having straight or upright branches.

Or-tho-pæ-di'a.* [From ὀρθός, "straight," or "right," and παῖς, a "child."] The straightening, correcting, or curing deformities of children.

Or-tho-ped'ic. [**Orthopæ'dicus.**] Belonging to *orthopædia.*

Or-thop-nœ'a.* [From ὀρθός, "straight," or "right," and πνόη, "breathing."] Literally, "upright breathing." Quick and labored breathing, in which the person has to maintain an upright posture to allow of even this.

Or-thop-no'ĭ-cus.* Belonging to *orthopnœ'a.*

Or-thop'ter-us.* [From ὀρθός, "straight," and πτερόν, a "wing."] Straight-winged. Applied in the plural neuter (*Orthop'tera*) to an order of insects: orthop'terous.

Or-thos'to-mus.* [From ὀρθός, "straight," and στόμα, a "mouth."] Having the mouth or opening straight: orthostomous.

Or-thot'ro-pal, or **Or-thot'ro-pous.** [From ὀρθός, "straight," and τρέπω, to "turn."] A term applied to a straight ovule of a plant which has its radicle next to the hilum.

O-ry̆c-to-che'mĭ-a.* [From ὀρυκτός, "dug out," "fossil," and χημεία, "chemistry."] The chemical examination of fossils.

O-ry̆c-toġ'e-ny̆. [**Oryctoge'nia;** from ὀρυκτός, "fossil," and γεννάω, to "produce."] The generating or producing of fossils.

O-ry̆c-to-ġe-o-loġ'ĭ-cal. [**Oryctogeoloġ'icus.**] Belonging to oryctogeology.

O-ry̆c-to-ġe-ol'o-ġy̆. [**Oryctogeolo'gia;** from ὀρυκτός, a "fossil," or "mineral," γῆ, the "earth," and λόγος, a "discourse."] That branch of science which treats of the arrangement of minerals in the bosom of the earth.

O-ry̆c-tog-nos'tic. [**Oryctognos'ticus.**] Relating to oryctognosy.

O-ry̆c-tog'no-sy̆. [**Oryctogno'sia;** from ὀρυκτός, "fossil," and γνῶσις, "knowledge."] The same as ORYCTOLOGY.

O-ry̆c-to-graph'ĭ-cal. [**Oryctograph'icus.**] Belonging to oryctography.

O-ry̆c-tog'ra-phy̆. [**Oryctogra'phia;** from ὀρυκτός, "fossil," and γράφω, to "write."] A description of fossils or minerals.

O-ry̆c-to-loġ'ĭ-cal. [**Oryctoloġ'icus.**] Belonging to oryctology.

O-ry̆c-tol'o-ġy̆. [**Oryctolo'gia;** from ὀρυκτός, "fossil," and λόγος, a "discourse."] That department of Natural History which treats of fossil organic remains. This term is sometimes used to denote those parts of Mineralogy which have for their object the classification of minerals, their description, nomenclature, and arrangement.

O-ry̆c-tom'e-try̆. [**Oryctome'tria;** from ὀρυκτός, "fossil," and μετρέω, to "measure."] The science of measuring fossils.

O-ry̆c-to-zo-o-lo'ġĭ-a.* [From ὀρυκτός, "fossil," ζῶον, an "animal," and λόγος, a "discourse."] A treatise on animal fossils: oryctozoölogy.

O-ry̆c-to-zo-o-loġ'ĭ-cus.* Belonging to oryctozoölogia: oryctozoölogical.

O-ry'za.* A Linnæan genus of the class *Triandria*, natural order *Graminaceæ.* The rice-plant.

Ory'za Sa-ti'va.* The systematic name of the rice-plant.

O-ry-zo-i'dēs.* [From *ory'za*, "rice," and εἶδος, a "form."] Resembling the rice-plant.

Os,* genitive **O'ris,** plural **O'ra.** The mouth, or aperture by which food is received into the body, and in which, by its peculiar apparatus of nerves, muscles, bones, and teeth, taste, speech, respiration, suction, mastication, and deglutition are exercised or performed. Also applied to various apertures or openings of the body.

Os,* genitive **Os'sis,** nominative plural **Os'sa,** genitive **Ossium,** osh'e-um. [Gr. ὀστέον; Fr. *Os,* ō.] A bone. See BONE.

Os Coc'çy̆-ġis. See COCCYX.

Os Cribleux, ō krė'bluh'. The French term for the ETHMOID BONE.

Os de la Cuisse, ō d'lå kwėss. The French term for FEMUR, which see.

Os de l'Assiette, ō d'lå'se-ĕtt'. The French term for ISCHIUM, which see.

Os Ex-ter'num.* ("External Aperture.") The opening or entrance of the vagina. See OS INTERNUM.

Os Femoris. See FEMUR.

Os I-li'a-cum,* plural **Os'sa I-li'a-ca.** Another name for the *Os Innominatum.* See OSSA INNOMINATA.

Os Ilium. See ILIUM.

Os Innominatum. See OSSA INNOMINATA.

Os In-ter'num,* or **Os Tin'çæ.*** The orifice of the uterus or womb.

Os Ischii. See ISCHIUM.

Os Lachrymale. See UNGUIS OS.

Os Orbiculare. See ORBICULARE OS.

Os Pubis. See PUBIS, OS.

Os U'te-ri.* ("Mouth of the Uterus.") See UTERUS.

Os'che-al. [**Oschea'lis;** from ὄσχεον, the "scrotum."] Belonging to the scrotum.

Os-che-i'tis, i*dis.** [From ὄσχεον, the "scrotum."] Inflammation of the scrotum; also, the same as ORCHEITIS.

Os-chel-e-phan-ti'a-sis.* [From ὄσχεον, the "scrotum," and *elephanti'asis.*] Enormous enlargement of the scrotum.

Os'che-o-car-çĭ-no'ma, a*tis.** [From ὄσχεον, the "scrotum," and καρκίνωμα, a "cancer."] Cancer of the scrotum.

Os'che-o-çēle.* [From ὄσχεον, the "scrotum," and κήλη, a "tumor."] Tumor of the scrotum; also, scrotal hernia.

Os'cil-lăt-ing. [**Os'cillans;** from *oscil'lo, oscilla'tum,* to "oscillate," to "swing as a pendulum."] Applied to anthers attached, not by a fillet, but by a very small point towards the middle of their length, so that they are nearly balanced, and move from the slightest cause.

Os-cil-lā'tion. [**Oscilla'tio, o'***nis;* from the same.] A swinging motion to and fro; also, a tremulous or vibrating motion.

Os-cil'la-to-ry̆. [**Oscillato'rius;** from the same.] Swinging or moving like a pendulum. Applied to the arterial pulsation, etc.

Os'cĭ-tant. [**Os'citans;** from *os'cito, oscita'tum,* to "yawn."] Yawning; gaping; sleepy; sluggish.

Os-cĭ-tā'tion. [**Oscita'tio, o'***nis;* from the same.] The act of yawning.

Os'cu-late. [**Oscula'tus;** from *os'culum,* a "little mouth."] Having little mouths or suckers.

Os-cu-la'tor.* ("That which kisses;" from *os'culor, oscula'tus,* to "kiss:" so named because it contracts the mouth.) A name for the ORBICULARIS ORIS (Muscle), which see.

Os'cu-lum.* [Diminutive of *os,* a "mouth."] A little mouth or aperture.

Os'ma-zome. [**Osmazo'ma;** from ὀσμή, "odor," and ζωμός, "sauce."] A peculiar principle of muscular fibre, of a brownish-yellow color, which gives the rich agreeable taste and flavor to roasted meat, soups, etc.

Os'mĭ-um.* [From ὀσμή, an "odor."] A metal named from the peculiar odor which one of its oxides exhales. It is rare, and has not been applied to any use.

Os-mom'e-ter. [From ὠσμός, "impulsion," and μέτρον, a "measure."] An apparatus for exhibiting the osmotic force. It consists of a porous vessel filled with a saline solution and immersed in pure water.

Os-mo-met'ric. [**Osmomet'ricus.**] Belonging to osmometry.

Os-mom'e-try̆. [**Osmome'tria;** from ὀσμή, an "odor," and μετρέω, to "measure."] The estimating of the qualities of odoriferous substances.

Os'mose. [**Osmo'sis;** from ὠσμός, "impulsion."] The power or action by which liquids are impelled through a moist membrane, and other porous partitions, in experiments of endosmose and exosmose.

Os-phre-sĭ-ol'o-ġy̆. [**Osphresiolo'gia;** from ὄσφρησις, a "smelling," and λόγος, a "discourse."] A treatise on smelling.

Os-phy̆-ăl'ġĭ-a.* [From ὀσφύς, the "loin," and ἄλγος, "pain."] Pain in the hips and loins; sciatica.

Os-phy̆-ăl'ġĭ-cus.* Belonging to *osphyalgia:* osphyalgic.

Os-phy̆-ar-thri'tis, i*dis.** [From ὀσφύς, the "loin," and ἀρθρῖτις, "gout."] Strictly, gout of the loins or hip; but used for *Osphyitis,* or inflammation of the loins.

Os-phȳ-i'tis, idis.* [From ὀσφύς, the "loin."] Inflammation of the loins.

Os-phȳ-o-my-e-li'tis, idis.* [From ὀσφύς, the "loin," and μυελός, "marrow."] Lumbar *myelitis*, or inflammation of the spinal marrow in the region of the loins.

Os-phȳr-rheū'ma, atis.* [From ὀσφύς, the "loin," and ῥεῦμα, "rheumatism."] Rheumatism of the hip-joint.

Os'sa,* gen. **Ossium,** osh'e-ŭm, the plural of Os, a "bone."

Ossa Anonyma. See Ossa Innominata.

Os'sa Con-vo-lu'ta.* ("Convoluted Bones.") A name for the Turbinated Bones, which see.

Ossa Iliaca. See Ossa Innominata.

Os'sa In-nom-ĭ-na'ta.* [Plural of *Os Innomina'tum.*] "Unnamed Bones." The two large, irregularly shaped bones which, with the sacrum and *coccyx*, compose the cavity of the pelvis.

Os'sa La'ta* ("Broad Bones"), or **Os'sa Pla'na*** ("Flat Bones"). The flat or broad bones which protect important viscera, or form the walls of certain cavities, as the sternum and bones of the cranium.

Os'sa Lon'ga.* ("Long Bones.") The long or cylindrical bones occurring in the limbs.

Ossa Spongiosa. See Turbinated Bones.

Ossa Triquetra, Ossa Wormii. See Wormii, Ossa.

Osseous, osh'e-ŭs. [**Os'seus;** from *os*, a "bone."] Of the nature or quality of bone; bony.

Os'sĭ-cle. [**Ossic'ulum;** diminutive of *os*, a "bone."] A small bone.

Os-sic'u-la Au-di'tus.* The "small bones of hearing;" the *Malleus, Incus, Stapes*, and *Os orbiculare*, situated in the cavity of the tympanum.

Ossic'ula Ber-ti'ni.* ("Ossicles of Bertin.") See Bertin, Spongy Bones of.

Os-sic'u-lar. [**Ossicula'ris;** from *ossic'ulum*, "ossicle."] Having the form or appearance of ossicles.

Os-sic'u-late. [**Ossicula'tus;** from the same.] Provided with small bones.

Os-sif'er-ous. [**Ossif'erus;** from *os*, a "bone," and *fe'ro*, to "bear."] Bearing, or containing, bones.

Os-sif'ic. [**Ossif'icus;** from *os*, a "bone," and *fa'cio*, to "make."] Forming bone.

Os-sĭ-fĭ-cā'tion. [**Ossifica'tio, o'nis;** from the same.] The formation of bone or bony substance. For the distinction between ossification and calcification, see Petrifaction.

Ossium,* osh'e-ŭm. The genitive plural of *Os*, a "bone," signifying "of the bones:" *e.g. Fragil'itas os'sium*, "brittleness of the bones."

Os-tæ'mĭ-a.* [From ὀστέον, a "bone," and αἷμα, "blood."] Morbid fulness of blood in a bone.

Os-tăl'ġĭ-a.* [From ὀστέον, a "bone," and ἄλγος, "pain."] Pain in the bones.

Os-tăl-ġi'tis, idis.* [From ὀστέον, a "bone," and ἄλγος, "pain."] Inflammation of a bone, with excessive pain; also spelled *Ostealgitis.*

Osteæmia. See Ostæmia.

Os-te-al-lœ-o'sis.* [From ὀστέον, a "bone," and ἀλλοίωσις, an "alteration."] Metamorphosis of the substance of a bone, as the progress of *osteosarcoma;* also termed Osteometabole.

Os-te-an-a-ġen-ne'sis.* [From ὀστέον, a "bone," and ἀναγέννησις, "regeneration."] Renewal of bone.

Os-te-a-naph'ȳ-sis.* [From ὀστέον, a "bone," and ἀναφύω, to "produce."] Reproduction of bone.

Os-te-ar-throc'a-çe.* [From ὀστέον, a "bone," ἄρθρον, a "joint," and κάκη, "vice," "disease."] Cancer or caries of the bones of a joint.

Os'te-in, or **Os'te-ĭne.** [From ὀστέον, a "bone."] A name for bony tissue, or the animal matter of bone.

Os-te-i'tis, or **Os-ti'tis, i**dis.* [From ὀστέον, a "bone."] Inflammation of the substance of a bone.

Os-tem'brȳ-on, o'nis.* [From ὀστέον, a "bone," and ἔμβρυον, a "fœtus."] An osseous or hardened state of the substance of the embryo.

Os-tem-py-ē'sis.* [From ὀστέον, a "bone," and ἐμπύησις, "suppuration."] Abscess or suppuration within a bone.

Osteo-anabrosis. See Osteonabrosis.

Os'te-o-çēle.* [From ὀστέον, a "bone," and κήλη, a "tumor."] The osseous or cartilaginous substance found in old hernial sacs after reduction.

Os-te-o-col'la.* [From ὀστέον, a "bone," and κόλλα, "glue."] Bone-glue, or bone-cement; a name for a particular carbonate of lime found in Germany, formerly celebrated for promoting the reunion of fractured bones.

Os-te-o-den'tĭne. [From ὀστέον, a "bone," and *den'tine.*] A modification of the fundamental tissue of the teeth, in which the cellular basis is arranged in concentric layers around the vascular canals. It resembles both dentine and bone: hence the name.

Os-te-o-dyn'i-a.* [From ὀστέον, a "bone," and ὀδύνη, "pain."] Pain in a bone, especially chronic pain.

Os-te-o-ge-net'i-cus.* Bone-generating; belonging to *osteogenesis.*

Os-te-o-gen'ic. [**Osteogen'icus.**] The same as OSTEOGENETICUS.

Os-te-og'e-ny. [**Osteogen'esis,** or **Osteoge'nia;** from ὀστέον, a "bone," and γένεσις, "generation."] The formation or growth of bones.

Os-te-og'ra-phy. [**Osteogra'phia;** from ὀστέον, a "bone," and γράφω, to "describe."] A description of the bones.

Os'te-oid. [**Osteoi'des;** from ὀστέον, a "bone," and εἶδος, a "form."] Resembling bone. Applied by Virchow to "soft, uncalcified, osseous tissue;" that is, osseous tissue previous to the deposition of calcareous matter.

Os-te-ol'o-gy. [**Osteolo'gia;** from ὀστέον, a "bone," and λόγος, a "discourse."] That branch of Anatomy which treats of the bones.

Os-te-o'ma, *atis.** [From ὀστέον, a "bone."] A tumor of a bone: an osteome. See OSTEONCUS.

Osteomalacia,* os-te-o-ma-la'-she-a. [From ὀστέον, a "bone," and μαλακός, "soft."] The same as MOLLITIES OSSIUM, which see.

Ostéo-malacie, os'tā'o'mā'lā'sē'. The French term for MOLLITIES OSSIUM.

Os-te-o-me-tab'o-le.* [From ὀστέον, a "bone," and μεταβολή, a "change."] The same as OSTEALLŒOSIS.

Os-te-o-my-e-li'tis, *idis.** [From *osteomy'elon.*] Inflammation of the marrow of a bone.

Os-te-o-my'e-lon,* or **Os-te-o-my'e-lum.*** [From ὀστέον, a "bone," and μυελός, "marrow."] The marrow of bones.

Os'te-on-a-bro'sis,* or **Os'te-o-An-a-bro'sis.*** [From ὀστέον, a "bone," and ἀνάβρωσις, "consumption," or "absorption."] A term applied to the simple absorption of bone, such as occurs in the removal of the milk-teeth.

Os-te-on'cus.* [From ὀστέον, a "bone," and ὄγκος, a "tumor."] Tumor of a bone. See EXOSTOSIS.

Os'te-o-ne-cro'sis.* [From ὀστέον, a "bone," and νεκρωσις, "death."] *Necrosis,* or death, of a bone.

Os-te-o-pæ'di-on,* or **Os-te-o-pæ'di-um.*** [From ὀστέον, a "bone," and παῖς, παιδός, an "infant."] An ossified fœtus. See OSTEMBRYON.

Os-te-o-phy'ma, *atis.** [From ὀστέον, a "bone," and φῦμα, a "tumor," or "swelling."] The same as OSTEONCUS.

Os'te-o-phyte. [**Osteoph'yton,** or **Osteoph'ytum;** from ὀστέον, a "bone," and φύω, to "produce."] An osseous tumor. See OSTEONCUS.

Os-te-o-po-ro'sis.* [From ὀστεον, a "bone," and πόρος, a "passage," or "pore."] A morbid porosity of the bones.

Os'te-o-sar-co'ma.* [From ὀστέον, a "bone," and σάρξ, "flesh."] A fleshy, medullary, or cartilaginous mass growing within a bone, causing at first an enlargement, and at length partially absorbing it, or causing it to fracture.

Os'te-o-sar-co'sis.* The progress or formation of *osteosarcoma.*

Os'te-o-scen-o-gra'phi-a.* [From ὀστέον, a "bone," and σκηνογραφία, the "art of scene-painting."] The representation of the bones, or skeleton.

Os-te-o-scir'rhus.* [From ὀστέον, a "bone," and σκίῤῥος, an "indurated tumor."] Scirrhus of a bone.

Os-te-ō'sis.* The same as OSTEOGENY, which see.

Os'te-o-to-mis'ta.* [From ὀστέον, a "bone," and τέμνω, to "cut."] An instrument for breaking down the bones of the child in impracticable labors.

Os-te-ot'o-mus.* [From the same.] An instrument for cutting through bones; an osteotome.

Os-te-ot'o-my. [**Osteoto'mia;** from the same.] The part of Anatomy which relates to the dissection of bones.

Os-te-ot'o-phus.* [From ὀστέον, a "bone," and τόφος, a loose kind of stone.] A bony excrescence.

Ost-hex'i-a.* [From ὀστέον, a "bone," and ἕξις, a "habit."] Ossific diathesis; ossification.

Os-Tin'cæ.* The orifice of the womb. See UTERUS.

Ostitis. See OSTEITIS.

Os'ti-um.* [From *os, o'ris,* a "mouth."] Originally, a "door;" also, the "mouth of a river." Applied to any opening, but particularly to that between the auricle and ventricle of the heart.

Os'tium Ab-dom-i-na'le.* ("Abdominal Opening.") The orifice at the fimbriated extremity of the Fallopian tube,—the only place in the whole body where a serous membrane communicates with the exterior.

Os-tra-co-i'dēs.* [From ὄστρακον, a "shell," and εἶδος, a "form."] Resembling a shell: ostracoid.

Os-tra-co'sis.* [From ὄστρακον, a

"shell."] The desiccation and conversion of parts of bone, especially of the cranium, into a substance like oyster-shell.

Os'tre-a.* [Gr. ὄστρεον, from ὄστρακον, a "shell;" Fr. *Huître*, wētr.] The oyster; a genus of the *Ostracea*.

Os'trea E-du'lis.* ("Edible Oyster.") The common oyster, the shells of which are used medicinally.

Os-tre-ā'ceous. [**Ostrea'ceus;** from *os'trea*, an "oyster."] Having the form of a bivalve shell.

Os'tre-æ,* gen. **Os-tre-a'rum.** The plural of OSTREA, which see.

Os'trich. [Gr. στρουθός.] The largest known bird, and the type of the Cursorial or Struthious order. Ostriches abound in the sandy deserts of Arabia and Africa.

-Osus. A Latin termination usually denoting "fulness," or "abundance;" as, *vasculosus*, "full of vessels," or "abounding in vessels."

Os-U'te-ri.* ("Mouth of the Uterus.") See UTERUS.

O-tăl'ġĭ-a.* [From οὖς, ὠτός, the "ear," and ἄλγος, "pain."] Otal'gy; pain in the ear; ear-ache. It has been distinguished into *external* and *internal*, according as it affects the *meatus auditorius*, or the cavity of the tympanum. See OTITIS.

O-tăl'ġic. [**Otal'gicus.**] Belonging to *otalgia*.

O-ten'chȳ-tēs.* [From οὖς, ὠτός, the "ear," and ἐγχύω, to "pour in."] A syringe for the ears.

Oth-el-co'sis.* [From οὖς, the "ear," and ἕλκος, an "ulcer."] Suppuration of the ears.

Ot-ĭ-at'rics. [**Otiat'rica;** from οὖς, the "ear," and ἰατρικός, "belonging to medicine."] The consideration of the nature and principles of the treatment of the ear.

Ot'ĭ-cus.* [From οὖς, the "ear."] (Fr. *Otique*, o'tēk'.) Belonging to the ear; auricular. Applied to medicines, etc.

O-ti'tis, i*dis*.* [From οὖς, ὠτός, the "ear."] Inflammation of the ear. It is said to be *external* when confined chiefly to the *meatus auditorius; internal*, if the internal ear is effected.

Ot-o-blen-nor-rhœ'a.* [From οὖς, the "ear," βλέννα, "mucus," and ῥέω, to "flow."] Mucous discharge from the ear.

Ot-o-ca-tar'rhus.* [From οὖς, the "ear," and κατάῤῥοος, a "defluxion."] Catarrh of the ear.

Ot'o-crane. [**Otocra'nia;** from οὖς, the "ear," and κράνον, the "head."] The cavity for the reception of the osseous or cartilaginous immediate capsule of the labyrinth of the ear.

Ot-o-cra'nĭ-al. [**Otocrania'lis.**] Belonging to the *otocrane*.

Ot-o-dȳn'ĭ-a.* [From οὖς, the "ear," and ὀδύνη, "pain."] Pain, more especially chronic pain, in the ear.

Ot-o-dȳn'ĭ-cus.* Belonging to *otodynia*.

Ot-o-gan'glĭ-on,* or **Ot-o-gan'glĭ-um.*** [From οὖς, the "ear," and γαγγλίον, a "ganglion."] The auricular ganglion.

Ot-o-graph'ĭ-cal. [**Otograph'icus.**] Belonging to otography.

O-tog'ra-phȳ. [**Otogra'phia;** from οὖς, ὠτός, the "ear," and γράφω, to "write."] A description of the ear.

Ot-o-loġ'ĭ-cal. [**Otoloġ'icus.**] Belonging to otology.

O-tol'o-ġȳ. [**Otolo'gia;** from οὖς, ὠτός, the "ear," and λόγος, a "speech."] A treatise on the ear; the science of the ear.

Ot-o-neū-răl'ġĭ-a.* [From οὖς, the "ear," and *neural'gia*.] Nervous pain of the ear.

Ot-o-neū-răl'ġic. [**Otoneural'gicus.**] Belonging to *otoneuralgia*.

Ot-o-phleg'mo-ne.* [From οὖς, the "ear," and φλεγμονή, "inflammation."] The same as OTITIS.

Ot-o-pho'ne.* [From οὖς, the "ear," and φωνή, a "voice," a "sound."] An ear-trumpet.

Ot-o-plas'tic. [**Otoplas'ticus.**] Belonging to otoplasty.

Ot'o-plas-tȳ. [**Otoplas'tia,** or **Otoplas'tice;** from οὖς, the "ear," and πλάσσω, to "form."] An operation by which lesions of the ear are repaired by having recourse to a sound portion of the contiguous integument.

Ot-o-py-or-rhœ'a.* [From οὖς, ὠτός, the "ear," πύον, "pus," and ῥέω, to "flow."] Purulent *otorrhœa*, or a discharge of pus from the ear.

Ot-o-pȳ-o'sis.* [From οὖς, the "ear," and πύον, "pus."] Purulent discharge from the ear.

Ot-or-rha'ġĭ-a.* [From οὖς, the "ear," and ῥήγνυμι, to "burst forth."] A sudden discharge of blood from the ear.

Ot-or-rhaġ'ĭ-cus.* Belonging to *otorrhagia*.

Ot-or-rheū-ma-tis'mus.* [From οὖς, the "ear," and ῥευματισμός, "rheumatism."] Rheumatic pain of the ear; ear-ache.

Ot-or-rhœ'a.* [From οὖς, the "ear," and ῥέω, to "flow."] A flow or running from the ear.

Ot'o-scope. [**Otos'copus;** from οὖς, the "ear," and σκοπέω, to "examine," to "explore."] An instrument for listening to the sound of air passed through the tympanic cavity in certain morbid conditions of the ear.

Ot-o-scop'ic. [**Otoscop'icus.**] Belonging to the otoscope.

Otoscopium. See OTOSCOPE.

O-tos'te-al. [**Otostea'lis;** from οὖς, the "ear," and ὀστέον, a "bone."] Applied by Owen to the homologues of the ossicles of the ear.

O-tot'o-my̆. [**Ototo'mia;** from οὖς, the "ear," and τέμνω, to "cut."] Dissection of the ear.

Otto of Roses. See ATTAR OF ROSES.

Oulorrhagia. See ULORRHAGIA.

Ourology, or **Ourologia.** See UROLOGY.

Ouroscopia. See UROSCOPY.

-Ous. A terminal used in Chemistry, and denoting a smaller quantity of oxygen in a compound than in the corresponding one the name of which ends in *-ic*. Compare *nitric, nitrous, sulphuric, sulphurous*, etc.

Ov. = *O'vum.** "An egg."

O'va,* the plural of OVUM, which see.

Ovaire. See OVARIUM.

O'val. [**Ova'lis;** from *o'vum*, an "egg."] Broadly elliptical, resembling the longitudinal section of an egg; egg-shaped.

O-val-ĭ-fo'lĭ-us.* [From *ova'lis*, "oval," and *fo'lium*, a "leaf."] Having oval leaves: ovalifo'lious.

O-va-rĭ-ăl'ġĭ-a.* [From *ova'rium*, an "ovary," and ἄλγος, "pain."] Pain in the ovary.

O-va-rĭ-ăl'ġic. [**Ovarial'gicus.**] Belonging to *ovarialgia*.

O-va'rĭ-an. [**Ovaria'nus.**] Belonging to the ovary.

O-va-ri'tis, *idis.** [From *ova'rium*, an "ovary."] Inflammation of the ovary or its membranes.

O'va-ry̆. [**Ova'rium;** from *o'vum*, an "egg," or "ovule," and *-a'rium*, a termination signifying "the place of any thing." Compare HERBARIUM, etc.] Literally, "the place of the ova." (Fr. *Ovaire*, o'vêR'.) A flat, oval body, connected with the uterus by the broad ligament, one on each side, and containing a number of vesicles, or ova. Also, the germen, or lower part of the pistil. containing the ovules of plants.

O'vate. [**Ova'tus;** from *o'vum*, an "egg."] Egg-shaped; or resembling the longitudinal section of an egg. In reference to leaves, it has the latter meaning.

O-vat-ĭ-fo'lĭ-us.* [From *ova'tus*, "ovate," and *fo'lium*, a "leaf."] The same as OVALIFOLIUS, which see.

O'vĭ-duct. [**Oviduc'tus;** from *o'vum*, an "egg," and *duc'tus*, a "canal."] The Fallopian tube, which conveys the *ovum* from the ovary to the uterus. Also applied to the duct or canal which terminates in the *cloaca* of birds and certain other animals.

O'vĭ-form. [**Ovifor'mis;** from *o'vum*, an "egg."] Having the shape of an egg; egg-like.

O-vil'lus.* [From *o'vis*, a "sheep."] Belonging to the sheep. See ADEPS OVILLUS.

O-vi'nus.* [From the same.] Pertaining to sheep: o'vine.

O-vip'a-rous. [**Ovip'arus;** from *o'vum*, an "egg," and *pa'rio*, to "bring forth."] Bringing forth or producing eggs. Applied to animals which produce eggs, instead of bringing forth living young.

O-vĭ-po-sĭ'tion. [**Oviposi'tio,** *o'nis;* from *o'vum*, an "egg," and *po'no, pos'itum*, to "lay," to "place."] The act or process of depositing *ova* by the females of oviparous animals.

O-vĭ-pos'ĭ-tor.* [From the same.] A projecting apparatus formed by the last *annuli* of the abdomen in certain insects, for depositing their eggs.

O'vis,* plural **O'vēs.** Sheep. The name of a genus of domesticated animals.

Ovisac. See GRAAFIAN FOLLICLE.

O'void. [**Ovoi'des;** from *o'vum*, an "egg," and εἶδος, a "form."] Egg-shaped. Applied to s ids.

O-vo-vi-vip'a-rous. [**Ovovivip'arus;** from *o'vum*, an "egg," *vi'vus*, "living," and *pa'rio*, to "bring forth."] Applied to an oviparous animal in whose body the *ova* are hatched before they are brought forth. This phenomenon is observed in many reptiles (*e.g.* the viper), fishes, certain *Mollusca*, and various insects.

Ov'u-la,* the plural of *Ov'ulum*. See OVULE.

Ov-u-la'ris.* [From *ov'ulum*, an "ovule."] Resembling an egg. Applied to the grains of granulated rock, when of the size of a hen's egg.

Ov'u-late. [**Ovula'tus.**] Having or bearing ovules.

Ov-u-lā'tion. [**Ovula'tio, o'***nis;* from the same.] A kind of generation consisting in the formation and separation of a membranous sac filled with nutritious matter from the female, for the reception and nutrition of a germ separated from the male.

O'vule. [**Ov'ulum;** diminutive of *o'vum,* an "egg."] A little egg. Applied in Anatomy to the unimpregnated germ or *ovum;* also to the rudimentary seed of a plant, a small body formed in the ovary, which on being fertilized by pollen becomes a seed.

O'vum,* plural **O'vạ.** [Gr. ᾠόν; Fr. *Œuf,* uf.] Literally, "an egg." Applied to the vesicle of Baer, contained in the Graafian vesicle of the ovary of Mammalia. Also, the Pharmacopœial name (U.S. Ph.) for the egg of the *Phasianus gallus,* or common domestic fowl.

Ox. = *Ox'ymel.** See OXYMEL.

Ox-aç'id. [**Oxaç'idum;** from *oxyge'nium,* "oxygen," and *aç'idum,* an "acid."] Acids that contain oxygen, as distinguished from those formed with chlorine, etc.

Ox'ạ-lāte. [**Ox'alas, a'***tis.*] A combination of oxalic acid with a base.

Ox'ạ-lāt-ed. [**Oxala'tus;** from *ox'alas,* an "oxalate."] Applied to a base converted into a salt by combination with oxalic acid.

Ox-al'ic. [**Oxal'icus;** from *ox'alis,* "sorrel."] Belonging to wood-sorrel. Applied to a highly poisonous acid obtained from it, also from sugar and other substances. It is sometimes called acid or essence of sugar.

Oxalidaceæ,* ox-ạ-le-da'she-ē. A natural order of exogenous plants, found in all the hot and temperate parts of the world. It comprises *Ox'alis* (Sorrel), which contains nearly pure oxalic acid.

Ox'ạ-lis, i*dis.** [From ὀξύς, "sharp," "sour."] Sorrel. A Linnæan genus of the class *Decandria,* natural order *Oxalidaceæ.*

Ox'alis A-cet-o-sel'lạ.* The systematic name for the wood-sorrel.

Ox-ạ-lu'rāte. [**Oxalu'ras, a'***tis.*] A combination of oxaluric acid with a base.

Ox-ạ-lu'rĭ-ạ.* [From *ox'alas,* "oxalate," and *uri'na,* the "urine."] Applied to a condition in which the urine shows the presence of a quantity of oxalate of lime.

Ox-ạ-lu'ric. [**Oxalu'ricus;** from *oxalu'ria.*] Applied to an acid formed from parabanic acid when brought into contact with bases.

Ox-ĭ-chlo'rāte. [**Oxychlo'ras, a'***tis.*] A combination of oxichloric acid with a base.

Ox-ĭ-chlo'rīde. [**Oxychlo'ridum.**] Applied to phosgene gas, termed carbonic oxichloride.

Ox-i-dạ-bil'ĭ-tў. [**Oxydabil'itas, a'***tis;* from *ox'ydum,* an "oxide."] The capability of combining with oxygen.

Ox'ĭ-dạ-ble. [**Oxydab'ilis;** from the same.] Susceptible of combining with oxygen.

Ox'ĭ-dāt-ed. [**Oxyda'tus;** from the same.] Combined with oxygen.

Ox-ĭ-dā'tion. [**Oxyda'tio, o'***nis;* from the same.] The combining of a certain quantity of oxygen with metals or other substances.

Ox'īde. [**Ox'ydum,** or **Ox'idum.**] A compound of oxygen with a metal or other substance. It is usually applied to those compounds of oxygen which are not acids.

Ox'ĭ-doid. [**Oxydoi'des;** from *ox'ydum,* an "oxide," and εἶδος, a "form."] Resembling an oxide. Applied to oxidated bodies which are neither acids nor salifiable bases.

Ox-id'u-lāt-ed. [**Oxydula'tus;** from *oxyd'ulum.*] Having an inferior degree of oxidation.

Ox-id-u-lā'tion. [**Oxydula'tio, o'***nis;* from the same.] Inferior oxidation.

Ox'i-dum,* gen. **Ox'i-di.** See OXIDE.

Ox-im'e-ter. [**Oxym'etrum;** from *ox'ygen,* and μέτρον, a "measure."] A measurer of oxygen.

Ox-ī'o-dīne. Iodic acid, a white, transparent solid, obtained by boiling iodine with nitric acid.

Ox-u'rāte. [**Oxu'ras, a'***tis.*] A combination of oxuric acid with a base.

Ox-u'ric. [**Oxu'ricus;** from *ox'ygen,* and *u'ric.*] Applied to the superoxygenated uric acid of Vauquelin.

Ox'ў-ạ.* [Gr. ὀξύα.] A name for the *Fa'gus sylvat'ica,* or beech-tree.

Ox-ў-ạ-can'thus.* [From ὀξύς, "sharp," and ἄκανθα, a "thorn."] Having numerous sharp thorns.

Ox-ў-ad'e-nus.* [From ὀξύς, "sharp," and ἀδήν, a "gland."] Having pointed glands. Applied to certain plants.

Ox-ў-æs-the'sĭ-ạ.* [From ὀξύς, "sharp," and αἴσθησις, "sense," or "feeling."] A term for increased sensation. See OXYAPHE.

Ox-y'ạ-phe,* or **Ox-ў-a'phĭ-ạ.*** [From ὀξύς, "sharp," and ἁφή, "touch."]

Acute sense of touch; excessive sensibility of touch.

Ox-ȳ-blep'sĭ-a.* [From ὀξύς, "sharp," and βλέπω, to "see."] Acute sight. See OXYOPIA.

Ox-ȳ-car'pous. [**Oxycar'pus;** from ὀξύς, "sharp," and καρπός, "fruit."] Having acuminated fruit or capsules.

Ox-ȳ-coc'cos.* [From ὀξύς, "sour," or "sharp," and κόκκος, a "berry."] A name applied to the cranberry-plant (the *Vaccin'ium oxycoc'cos*, or *Oxycoc'cos palus'tris*), on account of the acidity of its fruit.

Ox-ȳd'u-lum.* [Diminutive of *ox'ydum*, an "oxide."] A body in an inferior degree of oxidation.

Oxydum. See OXIDE.

Ox'ȳ-ġen. [**Oxyge'nium;** from ὀξύς, "sharp," or "sour," and γεννάω, to "produce."] (Fr. *Oxygène*, ok'sè'zhĕn' or ok'se'zhån'.) An elementary substance universally diffused throughout nature, being a constituent of atmospheric air, water, most of the acids, and all bodies of the animal and vegetable kingdoms. It is a permanent gas when uncombined.

Oxygenabilis. See OXIDABLE.

Ox'ȳ-ġe-nāt-ed. [**Oxygena'tus.**] Combined with oxygen.

Ox-ȳ-ġe-nā'tion. [**Oxygena'tio, o'nis;** from *ox'ygen*.] Applied to every combination with oxygen: often confounded with oxidation, but distinct from it, as being of more general import.

Oxygène. See OXYGEN.

Ox-ȳ-ġe-nom'e-trum.* The same as OXYMETER, which see.

Ox'ȳ-mel, el'lis.* [From ὀξύς, "acid," and μέλι, "honey."] A mixture of vinegar and honey boiled to a syrup.

Ox-ȳ-mu'rĭ-āte. [**Oxymu'rias, a'tis.**] A combination of oxymuriatic acid with a base.

Oxymuriate of Lime. See CHLORIDE OF LIME.

Oxymuriate of Mercury. See CORROSIVE SUBLIMATE.

Ox-ȳ-mu-rĭ-at'ic Aç'id. [**Aç'idum Oxymuriat'icum.**] The name applied by Lavoisier to a substance supposed to be a compound of muriatic acid and oxygen, but ascertained by Sir H. Davy to be an elementary body, which he termed *Chlorine*.

Ox-ȳ-o'pĭ-a.* [From ὀξύς, "sharp," and ὤψ, the "eye."] Unusual acuteness of vision.

Ox-ȳ-pho'nĭ-a.* [From ὀξύς, "sharp," or "shrill," and φωνή, "voice."] A shrill or squalling voice; a symptom attendant on certain morbid conditions of the larynx.

Ox-ȳ-phȳl'lus.* [From ὀξύς, "sharp," and φύλλον, a "leaf."] Having acuminated leaves.

Ox-ȳ-sac'cha-rum.* [From ὀξύς, "sharp," "sour," and *sac'charum*, "sugar."] A mixture of vinegar and sugar. When it contains squills, it is termed *Oxysac'charum scillit'icum*.

Ox'ȳ-sal, alis.* [From *ox'ygen*, and *sal*, a "salt."] An oxysalt. See OXYSALTS.

Ox'ȳ-salts. Applied to certain combinations in which oxygen is found both in the acid and base.

Ox-ȳ-sul'pho-sal.* A combination of an oxysalt and sulphosalt.

Ox-ȳt'o-cus.* [From ὀξύς, "sharp," "quick," and τόκος, "childbirth."] "Accelerating parturition." Applied to ergot.

Ox-ȳ-u'rus.* [From ὀξύς, "sharp," and οὐρά, the "tail."] A genus of *entozoa*.

Oxyu'rus Ver-mic-u-la'ris.* Formerly, the *As'caris Vermicula'ris;* called "*Thread-Worm*" (from its resemblance to a piece of thread), and also *Maw-Worm*. A species of small worm, about half an inch in length, having a tail tapering to a sharp point. It is usually found in the rectum, often occasioning an intolerable itching in the anus. The best treatment for this distressing complaint appears to consist in injections containing oil of turpentine. Injections of whale oil have also been found serviceable.

Oyster. See OSTREA.

Oys'ter Shells. The *Testæ ostrearum*, or shells of the *Ostrea edulis*.

O-zæ'na.* [From ὄζη, a "stench."] (Fr. *Ozène*, o'zĕn' or o'zån'.) A foul, stinking ulcer in the inside of the nostrils, discharging a purulent matter, and sometimes accompanied by caries of the bones.

O'ze.* [Gr. ὄζη.] A bad smell from the mouth. The same as OZOSTOMIA.

Ozène. See OZÆNA.

O'zone. [From ὄζη, a "stench."] A gaseous substance, the true nature of which is not well known. It is supposed to be a peculiar modification of oxygen. Perhaps a combination of nitrogen and oxygen, or of oxygen and hydrogen, in new proportions.

Oz-o-sto'mĭ-a.* [From ὄζη, a "stench," and στόμα, a "mouth."] The same as OZE, which see.

P.

P. An abbreviation for *pugil'lus,** a "handful," or *pars,** a "part" or "parts;" also, for *pul'vis,** "powder," *pon'dere,** "by weight," *pil'ula,** "pill."

Pab'u-lum.* [From *pas'co,* to "feed."] Food; aliment; sustenance.

Pac-chĭ-o'nĭ-æ, Glan'du-læ.* Certain small, oval-shaped, fatty eminences under the *dura mater* and along the sides of the longitudinal sinus.

Pa-chom'e-trum.* [From παχύς, "thick," and μέτρον, a "measure."] An instrument for measuring the thickness of the glass of mirrors.

Pach-u-lo'sis.* [From παχυλός, "somewhat thick or coarse."] Proposed by E. Wilson as a term for a chronic affection in which the skin is secondarily involved, particularly that of the lower extremities, and the epidermis is produced in abnormal quantity.

Pach-ȳ-æ'ma, atis.* [From παχύς, "thick," and αἷμα, "blood."] Thick or curdled blood.

Pach-ȳ-æ'mĭ-a.* [From the same.] Thickening of the blood.

Pach-ȳ-æm'ĭ-cus.* Belonging to *pachyæmia:* pachyem'ic.

Pach-ȳ-æ'mus.* [From *pachyæ'ma,* "thick blood."] Having thick blood.

Pach-ȳ-bleph-a-ro'sis.* The formation or progress of *pachyblepharum.*

Pach-ȳ-bleph'a-rum.* [From παχύς, "thick," and βλέφαρον, the "eyelid."] A thickening of the eyelid, particularly towards the border, from obstruction of the Meibomian glands.

Pach-ȳ-car'pus.* [From παχύς, "thick," and καρπός, "fruit."] Having thick fruit.

Pach-ȳ-der'ma-ta,* or **Pach'ȳ-derms.** [From παχύς, "thick," and δέρμα, the "skin."] An order of Mammalia, many of which are remarkable for the thickness of their skins. It includes the rhinoceros, the elephant, the tapir, horse, and hog.

Pach-ȳ-der'ma-tous. [**Pachyder'matus;** from the same.] Thick-skinned. Applied to an order of animals.

Pach-ȳ-me'nĭ-a.* [From παχύς, "thick," and ὑμήν, a "membrane."] A thickening of the skin.

Pach-ȳ-men'ĭ-cus.* Belonging to *pachymenia.*

Pach-ȳ-phȳl'lus.* [From παχύς, "thick," and φύλλον, a "leaf."] Having thick leaves.

Pach-ȳ-po'mus.* [From παχύς, "thick," and πῶμα, an "operculum."] Having a thick operculum. Applied to certain plants.

Paci'ni (på-chee'nè), **Cor'pus-çles of,** or **Pa-çin'ĭ-an Bod'ies.** [**Cor'pora** (or **Corpus'cula**) **Pacinia'næ.**] Numerous, small, pedunculated, whitish bodies, in union with the filaments of the cutaneous nerves of the palm of the hand and sole of the foot: also found on other nerves of the cerebral and spinal systems, and on the great sympathetic or internal ganglionic nerve.

Pæd-ar-throc'a-çe.* [From παῖς, a "child," ἄρθρον, a "joint," and κάκη, "vice," "disease."] Scrofulous necrosis of the joints in children. Sometimes applied to Spina Ventosa, which see.

Pæd-a-tro'phĭ-a.* [From παῖς, a "child," and ἀτροφία, a "wasting."] Atrophy of children.

Pæd-a-troph'ĭ-cus.* Belonging to *pædatrophia.*

Pæ-dĭ-aph'tha.* [From παιδίον, a "little child," and *aph'tha.*] The *aphtha,* or thrush, of infants.

Pæ-dĭ-a-trī'a.* [From παῖς, a "child," and ἰατρεία, a "healing."] The treatment of diseases of children.

Pæ-dĭ-at'rĭ-cus.* Belonging to *pediatria.*

Pæ-dom'e-trum.* [From παῖς, a "child," and μέτρον, a "measure."] An instrument for ascertaining the length and other dimensions of infants: a pedom'eter.

Pæ-don-o-so-lo'gĭ-a.* [From παῖς, παιδός, a "child," νόσος, a "disease," and λόγος, a "discourse."] A consideration of the diseases of children: pædonosol'ogy.

Pæ-don'o-sus.* [From παῖς, a "child," and νόσος, "disease."] A disease peculiar to childhood.

Pæ-doph'thĭ-sis.* [From παῖς, a "child," and φθίσις, a "wasting."] *Tabes,* or wasting, in children.

Pæd-o-tro'phĭ-um.* [From παῖς, a "child," and τρέφω, to "nourish."] An orphan or foundling hospital.

Pag'ĭ-na.* Literally, a "page." Applied in Botany to the surface of a leaf.

Paī'dĭ-cus,* or **Pæd'ĭ-cus.*** [From παῖς, a "child."] Pertaining to children

Painter's Colic. See COLICA PICTONUM.

Palæontographia. See PALEONTOGRAPHY.

Palæontologia. See PALEONTOLOGY.

Pa-læ-o-sau'rus.* [From παλαιός, "ancient," and σαῦρος, a "lizard."] A fossil lizard.

Pa-læ-o-the'rĭ-um.* [From παλαιός, "ancient," and θηρίον, a "beast."] The fossil relics of a group of pachydermatous animals found in the gypsum-quarries near Paris, and in various parts of France. Ten or eleven species are recognized, varying from the size of a rhinoceros to that of a hog.

Palæozoologia. See PALEOZOOLOGY.

Palais. See PALATUM.

Palate. See PALATUM.

Palate, Hard. See PALATUM DURUM.

Palate, Soft. See PALATUM MOLLE.

Pal'a-tīne. [**Palati'nus;** from *pala'tum* du'rum, the "hard palate."] Relating to the palate-bone. Applied to the palate-bone itself.

Pal-a-tor'rha-phy̆. [**Palatorrha'phia;** from *pala'tum,* the "palate," and ῥαφή, a "suture."] The operation of uniting by suture the cleft palate; nearly synonymous with STAPHYLORRHAPHY.

Pa-la'tum.* (Fr. *Palais,* på'lå'.) The roof of the mouth, or palate. In Botany, an inward projection of the lower lip of a personate corolla.

Pala'tum Du'rum.* ("Hard Palate.") The fore part of the roof of the mouth, formed by the palate-bone.

Pala'tum Mol'le* ("Soft Palate"), called also the **Ve'lum Pala'ti*** ("Veil, or Curtain, of the Palate"). The soft, movable septum, or fleshy membrane, attached to the posterior part of the palate, and situated between the mouth and the pharynx.

Pa'le-a.* [From *Pa'les,* the goddess of pasturage.] Chaff; one of the inner bracts or glumes of grasses, or one of the bracts on the receptacle of *Compositæ.*

Pā-le-ā'ceous. [**Palea'ceus;** from *pa'lea,* "chaff."] Chaffy; of the nature or appearance of chaff.

Pa'le-ar.* [From *pa'lea,* "chaff," also the "wattles" of a fowl.] The dewlap of oxen: named on account of its supposed resemblance to the wattles of a fowl. See next article.

Pa'lear Lax'um.* [From *lax'us,* "loose."] The dewlap (which is so named because when the animal grazes it laps the dew), more especially the loose portion of it; the thick membranous fold which hangs from the throat of the ox.

Pā'le-ĭ-form. [**Paleifor'mis;** from *pa'lea,* "chaff."] Having the appearance of chaff.

Pā-le-ol'o-ġy̆. [**Palæolo'gia;** from παλαιός, "ancient," and λόγος, a "discourse."] A discourse on antiquities, or the science of antiquities.

Pā-le-on-to-graph'ĭ-cal. [**Palæontograph'icus.**] Belonging to palæontography.

Pā-le-on-tog'ra-phy̆. [**Palæontogra'phia;** from παλαιός, "ancient," ὄντα, "beings," and γράφω, to "write."] A description or history of organized beings, of which the fossil remains alone are extant.

Pā-le-on-to-loġ'ĭ-cal. [**Palæontolog'icus.**] Belonging to paleontology.

Pā-le-on-tol'o-ġy̆. [**Palæontolo'gia;** from παλαιός, "ancient," ὄντα, "beings," and λόγος, a "discourse."] The science which treats of fossil organic remains.

Pā-le-o-phy̆-tol'o-ġy̆. [**Palæophytolo'gia;** from παλαιός, "ancient," φυτόν, a "plant," and λόγος, a "discourse."] The science which treats of fossil remains of plants.

Pā-le-o-zo'ic. [**Palæozo'icus;** from παλαιός, "ancient," and ζῶον, an "animal."] Belonging to fossil animals. Applied to the fossiliferous strata of earlier date than the carboniferous system and the mountain limestone.

Pā-le-o-zo-ol'o-ġy̆. [**Palæozoolo'gia;** from παλαιός, "ancient," and *zoolo'gia,* the "science of animals."] That branch of science which treats of the fossil remains of animals.

Pal'imp-sest. [**Palimpses'tus;** from πάλιν, "again," and ψάω, to "rub," to "erase."] The name given to parchment from which one writing was erased to make room for another. Palimpsests were used in the time of Cicero, who mentions them in one of his letters.

Pal-la'dĭ-um.* [From *Pal'las, Pal'ladis,* the name of a planet; see TELLURIUM.] A ductile, malleable, and very hard metal, found associated with platinum, which it resembles in color and lustre. Its specific gravity is about 11.8.

Pal'lĭ-āte. [From *pal'lio, pallia'tum,* to "hide," or "cloak" (from *pal'lium,* a "cloak").] Originally, to "cloak," or "hide," as a fault: hence, to soften, or mitigate. See next article.

Pal'lĭ-a-tīve. [**Palliati'vus;** from

the same.] Relieving, but not radically curative; assuaging; mitigating.

Pal-lĭ-dĭ-flo'rus.* [From *pal'lidus,* "pale," and *flos,* a "flower."] Having flowers of a pale tint.

Pal'lor.* [From *pal'leo,* to "be pale."] Paleness; loss of color.

Palm Oil. [**O'leum Pal'mæ.**] The product of a species of palm-tree, called *Elais Guineensis.*

Pal'ma,* gen. **Pal'mæ.** [Gr. παλάμη.] The palm of the hand; likewise, the hand itself. (See THENAR.) Also, a palm-tree.

Pal'ma Chris'ti.* A name for the *Riç'inus commu'nis,* or castor-oil plant.

Palmaceæ,* pal-ma'she-ē [from *Pal'ma,* a "palm-tree"], or **Pal'mæ.*** A natural order of endogenous trees of great beauty and value, which impart a peculiar character of grandeur to tropical landscapes. They are found mostly between 35° South and 40° North latitude. Among the products of this order are palm wine, palm oil, sugar, sago, dates, cocoanuts, timber, thread, and the intoxicating betel-nut. According to Humboldt, it also produces flour and salt. It includes the *Phœnix* (Date Palm), *Elais, Cocos,* and other kinds of palm.

Pal-mā'ceous. [**Palma'ceus;** from *Pal'ma,* the "palm-tree."] Resembling the palm-tree.

Pal'mæ,* the plural of *Pal'ma,* forming the Jussieuan name of a natural order of plants. See PALMACEÆ.

Păl'mar. [Lat. **Palma'ris,** from *pal'ma,* "palm;" Fr. *Palmaire,* pâl'mêR'.] Belonging to the palm of the hand.

Pal'mar Arch. Applied to each of two arches formed by the natural distribution of the blood-vessels in the palm of the hand; the *deep,* formed by the radial artery; and the *superficial,* by the ulnar artery.

Pal-ma'ris Bre'vis.* ("Short Palmar [Muscle].') A muscle arising from the annular ligament of the wrist, and the palmar aponeurosis, and inserted into the integuments of the palm of the hand. It is sometimes called *palmaris cutaneus,* or "cutaneous palmar [muscle]."

Palma'ris Lon'gus.* ("Long Palmar [Muscle].") A muscle arising from the inner condyle of the os humeri and spread out into the *palmar aponeurosis,* which is finally attached to the roots of all the fingers. It is a flexor of the wrist.

Palma'ris Mag'nus.* ("Large Palmar [Muscle].") A muscle which arises from the internal condyle of the humerus, and is inserted into the second metacarpal bone. It bends the hand and forearm.

Păl'mate. [**Palma'tus;** from *pal'ma,* the "hand."] Shaped like a hand; resembling a hand with the fingers spread. A palmate leaf is lobed or divided so that the sinuses all point to the apex of the petiole, as the leaves of the maple.

Păl'māte. [**Pal'mas, a'***tis.*] A combination of palmic acid with a base.

Pal'mate-ly Com'pound. The same as DIGITATE.

Pal'mately-Lobed. [**Palmati-loba'tus;** from *palma'tus,* "palmate," and *loba'tus,* "lobed."] Applied to palmately-veined leaves which are lobate.

Pal'mately-Part'ed. [**Palmati-parti'tus;** from *palma'tus,* "palmate," and *parti'tus,* "parted."] Parted as palmately-veined leaves the sinuses of which reach almost to the base.

Pal'mately-Veined. The same as RADIATED-VEINED, which see.

Păl-mat'ĭ-fid. [**Palmatif'idus;** from *palma'tus,* "palmate," and *fin'do,* to "cleave."] Palmately-cleft. Applied to leaves.

Pal-mat-ĭ-flo'rus.* [From *palma'tus,* "palmate," and *flos,* a "flower."] Applied to heads composed of flowers with palmated corols.

Pal-ma-tĭ-fo'lĭ-ous. [**Palmatifo'lius;** from *palma'tus,* "palmate," and *fo'lium,* a "leaf."] Having palmated leaves.

Pal-mat'ĭ-form. [**Palmatifor'mis;** from *palma'tus,* "palmate."] Having the form (or resemblance) of something palmate; somewhat palmate.

Păl-mat'ĭ-sect. [**Palmatisec'tus;** from *palma'tus,* "palmate," and *sec'tus,* "cut."] Palmately-divided. Applied to a palmately-veined leaf when the incisions reach to the base.

Palmatus. See PALMATE.

Pal-mic'o-lus.* [From *pal'ma,* the "palm-tree," and *co'lo,* to "inhabit."] Growing on the palm-tree. Applied to plants.

Pal-mif'er-ous. [**Palmif'erus;** from *pal'ma,* a "palm-tree," and *fe'ro,* to "bear."] Bearing palms.

Pal-mĭ-fo'lĭ-us.* The same as PALMATIFOLIOUS, which see.

Pal-mĭ-for'mis.* The same as PALMATIFORMIS, which see.

Pal-mĭ-ner'vis.* [From *pal'ma,* a "palm," or "hand," and *ner'vus,* a "nerve."] A term sometimes applied to radiated-veined leaves: palminer′-vate.

Păl′mĭ-ped. [**Pal′mipes, p′e***dis;* from *pal′ma,* a "palm," or "hand," and *pes,* a "foot."] Having palmated feet; web-footed.

Pal-mip′e-dēs.* [The plural of PAL′MIPES, which see.] A name for an order of birds; also called NATATORES.

Păl′mu-lạ.* [Diminutive of *pal′ma,* a "palm."] Literally, "a little hand," or "little palm." Applied to the flat broad end of a rib, like the leaf of a palm: pal′mule. Also, the *Dactylus,* or date.

Pal-mu-la′tus.* [From *pal′mula.*] Having palmulẹs.

Palo de Vaca, på′lo då vå′kå. ("Cow-tree.") The Spanish name of the *Galactoden′dron U′tile,* a tree which produces an agreeable and nutritious milky sap, called *vegetable milk.* It is a native of Venezuela.

Pal-pa′lis,* Pal-pa′tus.* [From *pal′pus,* a "feeler."] Having *palpi:* pal′pal: pal′pate.

Pal-pā′tion. [**Palpa′tio, o′***nis;* from *pal′po, palpa′tum,* to "handle gently," to "feel."] Examination by the hand, or touch. See EXPLORATION.

Păl′pe-brạ,* plural **Păl′pe-bræ.** (Fr. *Paupière,* pō′pe-ėr′.) The eyelid.

Păl′pe-bræ,* gen. **Păl-pe-bra′rum,** the plural of PALPEBRA, which see.

Păl′pe-brạl. [**Palpebra′lis.**] Belonging to the eyelid.

Pal′pe-brate. [**Palpebra′tus;** from *pal′pebra,* the "eyelid."] Having *palpebræ.*

Păl′pi,* gen. **Păl-po′rum,** the plural of PALPUS, which see.

Pal-pif′er-ous. [**Palpif′erus;** from *pal′pus,* a "feeler," and *fe′ro,* to "bear."] Bearing or having *palpi.*

Păl′pĭ-form. [**Palpifor′mis;** from *pal′pus,* a "feeler."] Having the form of a *palpus.*

Pal-pĭg′er-us.* [From *pal′pus,* a "feeler," and *ge′ro,* to "bear."] The same as PALPIFEROUS, which see.

Pal-pĭ-tā′tion. [**Palpita′tio, o′***nis;* from *pal′pito, palpita′tum,* to "throb."] Convulsive motion of a part. Applied especially to the rapid action of the heart. A genus of the order *Spasmi,* class *Neuroses,* of Cullen's Nosology.

Păl′pus,* plural **Păl′pi.** [From *pal′po,* to "feel," or "touch."] A feeler. Applied to the articulated filaments attached to the jaws or lower lip of certain *Crustaceæ, Arachnides,* and *Insecta,* apparently employed by the animal in recognizing its food. The *palpus* must not be confounded with the *antenna,* also termed a feeler. See ANTENNA.

Palsy. See PARALYSIS.

Pa-lu-dic′o-lus.* [From *pa′lus, palu′dis,* a "marsh," or "stagnant water," and *co′lo,* to "inhabit."] Growing or living on the margins of ponds in marshy grounds.

Pạ-lu′dose. [**Paludo′sus;** from *pa′lus,* a "marsh," or "stagnant water."] Marshy, or fenny; growing or living in marshes.

Pạ-lus′trine. [From the same.] The same as PALUDOSE, which see.

Pam-pin′ĭ-form. [**Pampinifor′-mis;** from *pam′pinus,* a "tender shoot," or "tendril of a vine."] Having the appearance of a tendril.

Pan-ạ-çe′ạ.* [Gr. πανάκεια; from πᾶς, "all," and ἀκέομαι, to "cure."] A pretended remedy for every disease.

Panacea Lapsorum. See ARNICA MONTANA.

Pạ-nā′do, or **Pạ-nā′dạ.** [From *pa′nis,* "bread."] Bread boiled in water to a pulpy consistence.

Pa′nax.* Ginseng. The Pharmacopœial name (U.S. Ph.) for the root of the *Pa′nax quinquefo′lium.* It is an aromatic stimulant, and is prized by the Chinese for its supposed power of increasing virility.

Pan′cre-as, a*tis.** [From πᾶς, παντός, "all," and κρέας, "flesh."] A long, flat, glandular viscus in the epigastric region, somewhat resembling a dog's tongue. The sweet-bread in the lower animals.

Pan-cre-ạ-tăl′gĭ-ạ.* [From πάγκρεας, the "pancreas," and ἄλγος, "pain."] Pain in the pancreas: pan′creatalgy.

Pan-cre-at′ic. [**Pancreat′icus.**] Belonging to the pancreas.

Pancreat′ic Duct. The duct formed by the union of the numerous excretory ducts proceeding from the lobules of the pancreas.

Pancreat′ic Juice. The peculiar fluid secreted by the pancreas.

Pan-cre-ạ-ti′tis, i*dis.** [From *pan′creas.*] Inflammation of the pancreas.

Pan-cre-ạ-ton′cus.* [From πάγκρεας, and ὄγκος, a "tumor."] A hard tumor of the pancreas.

Pandanaceæ,* pan-dạ-na′she-ē. [From *Pan′danus,* one of the genera.] A natural order of endogenous trees or shrubs, found in tropical regions. It includes the *Carludovi′ca,* from the leaves of which Panama hats are made.

Pan-de′mĭ-ạ.* [From πᾶς, "all,"

and δῆμος, the "people."] A disease which affects the people of a country generally. See EPIDEMIC.

Pan-dem'ic. [**Pandem'icus;** from the same.] The same as EPIDEMIC.

Pan-dic-u-lā'tion. [**Pandicula'tio, o'nis;** from *pandic'ulor, pandicula'tus,* to "stretch," to "yawn."] The act of yawning or gaping.

Pan-du'rĭ-form. [**Pandurifor'mis;** from *pandu'ra,* a "musical instrument," a "violin"?] Resembling a violin: fiddle-shaped.

Pangiaceæ,* pan-je-a'she-ē. [From *Pan'gium,* one of the genera.] A small natural order of exogenous trees, found in the hotter parts of India. They are all poisonous.

Pan'ĭ-cle. [**Panic'ula;** diminutive of *pa'nus,* the "woof wound on the quill in the shuttle."] A form of inflorescence; a raceme the branches of which bear each more than one flower.

Pa-nic'u-late. [**Panicula'tus.**] Having panicles.

Pan-ic-u-lĭ-for'mis.* [From *panic'ula,* a "panicle."] Having the form of a panicle.

Pa'nis.* (Fr. *Pain,* pănᴺᴳ.) A Latin term signifying "bread." It occurs in the following phrases:—*Pa'nis tritiç'eus,* "wheaten bread;" *mi'ca pa'nis,* a "crumb of bread;" *pa'nis tos'tus,* "toasted bread," for making toast-water; *pa'nis furfura'ceus,* "bran-bread;" *pa'nis biscoc'tus* (*i.e.* "twice-baked"), "biscuit;" *pa'nis nau'ticus,* "sea bread or biscuit."

Pan-nic'u-lus.* [Diminutive of *pan'nus,* "cloth."] A pan'nicule. Originally, a "small cloth," or "piece of cloth." Usually applied to a membrane or covering; but sometimes to a disease of the eye. See PANNUS.

Pannic'ulus Ad-ĭ-po'sus.* Adipose membrane.

Pannic'ulus Cor'dis.* ("Covering of the Heart.") See PERICARDIUM.

Pan'nĭ-form. [**Pannifor'mis;** from *pan'nus,* "cloth."] Applied to parts of a spongy, thick substance, as certain lichens.

Pan'nus,* or **Pan'num.*** [From πῆνος, a "web of cloth."] Literally, a "cloth," or "rag." Sometimes applied to an irregular mark on the skin; also to a thick membranous excrescence, stretching over the cornea. A tent for a wound, or soft rag for covering a wound.

Pan'nus Ves-ĭ-ca-to'rĭ-us.* ("Blistering Cloth.") Prepared by digesting powder of cantharides in sulphuric ether, evaporating, and spreading the oily mass which remains, melted with twice its weight of wax, on cloth prepared with waxed plaster.

Pan-ta-mor'phĭ-a.* [From πᾶς, παντός, "all," and ἀμορφία, "shapelessness."] Complete deformity.

Pan-ta-mor'phĭ-cus.* Belonging to *pantamorphia:* pantamorphic.

Pan-ta-nen-çe-pha'lĭ-a.* [From πᾶς, "all," and *anencepha'lia,* a "deficiency of brain."] Total absence of brain in a monster-fœtus.

Pan-ta-tro'phĭ-a.* [From πᾶς, "all," and ἀτροφία, "want of nourishment."] Complete innutrition.

Pan-tat'ro-phus.* [From πᾶς, "all," and ἄτροφος, "without nourishment."] Totally without nutrition.

Pan-zo-o'tĭ-a.* [From πᾶς, "all," and ζῶον, an "animal."] See EPIZOOTY.

Pa-pa'ver, eris.* (Fr. *Pavot,* pȧ'vo'.) The Poppy. A Linnæan genus of the class *Polyandria,* natural order *Papaveraceæ.* Also, the Pharmacopœial name ‖ for the capsules of the *Papaver somniferum.*

Papa'ver Al'bum.* Another name for the *Papaver somniferum.*

Papa'ver Er-rat'ĭ-cum.* Another name for the *Papaver rhœas.*

Papa'ver Rhœ'as.* The red corn poppy. The juice possesses narcotic properties; but it is little used as a medicine.

Papa'ver Som-nif'er-um.* The white poppy, from which opium is obtained.

Papaveraceæ,* pa-pav-e-ra'she-ē. A natural order of exogenous plants (herbs or shrubs), nearly two-thirds of which are natives of Europe. They are generally narcotic. The order includes the *Papa'ver* (Poppy), *Argemo'ne,* and *Sanguina'ria* (Blood-root). Opium is the inspissated juice of the *Papa'ver somnif'erum.*

Pa-pav-e-rā'ceous. [**Papavera'ceus;** from *papa'ver,* a "poppy."] Resembling the poppy. Applied to an order of plants. See PAPAVERACEÆ.

Pa-pav'e-rāte. [**Papav'eras, a'tis.**] A combination of papaveric acid with a base. The same as MECONATE.

Pa-pav'er-in. [**Papaveri'na;** from *papa'ver,* a "poppy."] A new base discovered in opium.

Pa-paw'. The *Car'ica Papa'ya,* a tree with a milky juice, containing fibrin in such abundance that the juice bears a remarkable resemblance to animal matter.—(HOBLYN.) The juice and seed are considered to possess anthelmintic properties.

Papayaceæ,* pa-pa-ya'she-ē. A natural order of exogenous trees and shrubs, natives of tropical and temperate regions. It includes the *Car'ica Papa'ya* (Papaw), the fruit of which is eatable when cooked, and is used as a vermifuge.

Pa-pil-ĭ-o-nā'ceous. [**Papilio-na'ceus;** from *papil'io,* a "butterfly."] Resembling a butterfly, as the flowers of leguminous plants. Applied to a form of polypetalous corolla with five dissimilar petals, as in the pea.

Pa-pil'la,* plural **Pa-pil'læ.** [From *pap'ula,* a "pimple."] Originally, a "pimple." Usually applied to the minute eminences on various surfaces of the body, consisting of the terminations of nerves with their accompanying vessels, as the *papillæ* of the tongue.

Pa-pil'læ,* gen. **Pap-il-la'rum,** the plural of PAPILLA, which see.

Papil'læ Cir-cum-val-la'tæ.* Situated on the dorsum of the tongue, near its root, and forming a row on each side which meets its fellow at the middle line, like the two branches of the letter A. They resemble cones attached by the apex to the bottom of a cup-shaped depression, and are hence named *calyciformes.* This cup-shaped cavity forms a kind of fossa around the papillæ, and hence they are called *circumvallatæ* (*i.e.* "fortified around").

Papil'læ Med-ul-la'rēs.* ("Medullary Papillæ.") Small eminences on the *Medulla oblongata.*

Papil'læ Re'nis.* ("Papillæ of the Kidney.") Applied to the apices of the *Tubuli uriniferi* of the kidney, arranged into eight or ten conical *fasciculi;* called also papillary caruncles.

Pap'il-la-ry̆. [**Papilla'ris;** from *papil'la.*] Belonging to the nipple.

Pap'illary Ca-run'cles. A name for the *Papillæ renis.*

Pap'il-late. [**Papilla'tus;** from *papil'la.*] In Botany, bearing small, soft projections.

Pap-il-lif'er-ous. [**Papillif'erus;** from *papil'la,* and *fe'ro,* to "bear."] Bearing *papillæ.*

Pa-pil'lĭ-form. [**Papillifor'mis;** from *papil'la.*] Resembling a *papilla.*

Pap-il-lo'ma,* plural **Pap-il-lom'a-ta.** [From the same.] The name of a tumor arising on the skin, or surface of the body, from a morbid transformation of the *papillæ.* The *wart* is an example of this kind.

Pap-il-lose'. [**Papillo'sus;** from the same.] The same as PAPILLATE.

Pap-pif'er-us.* [From *pap'pus,* "down," and *fe'ro,* to "bear."] Bearing down, wool, or hair: pappif'erous.

Pap-pĭ-for'mis.* [From *pap'pus,* "down."] Having the appearance of a tuft of wool or small feather.

Pap-pose'. [**Pappo'sus;** from the same.] Having a pappus; downy.

Pap'pus.* [Gr. πάππος, "down of thistles," etc.] The first downy beard on the cheek or chin. Also, a tuft of hairs attached to the seed of certain plants.

Pap'u-la,* plural **Pap'u-læ.** [Diminutive of *pa'pa,* a "teat."] A pimple; a round protuberance, soft and full of an aqueous fluid, formed by a little pocket of the epidermis. A small, acuminated, inflamed elevation of the skin; a wheal. Applied in the plural to an order of Willan's arrangement of skin-diseases.

Pap-u-lif'er-ous. [**Papulif'erus;** from *pap'ula,* a "pimple," and *fe'ro,* to "bear."] Bearing or having *papulæ.*

Pap'u-lous. [**Papulo'sus;** from *pap'ula,* a "pimple."] Pertaining to pimples; covered with pimples.

Pap-y̆-rā'ceous. [**Papyra'ceus;** from *Papy'rus,* an Egyptian plant; also, "paper."] Resembling papyrus or paper; having some analogy to paper in thickness and consistence. Applied to many shells.

Pa-py'ri,* the plural of PAPYRUS. The name given to the written scrolls made of the papyrus, found in Egypt, Herculaneum, etc.

Pa-py'rus,* plural **Pa-py'ri.** The *Cype'rus Papy'rus.* A cyperaceous plant, whose soft, cellular flower-stem afforded the most ancient material of which paper was made. It was abundant in the valley of the Nile. See PAPYRI.

Par Nervo'rum.* ("Pair of Nerves.") See PARIA NERVORUM.

Par No'num.* ("Ninth Pair.") An encephalic nerve which sends filaments to the pharynx and portions of the neck, but especially to the tongue, whence it has been variously termed the *lingual, gustatory,* and *hypoglossal* nerve.

Par Octavum. See PNEUMOGASTRIC.

Par Primum. See OLFACTORY NERVES.

Par Quartum. See PATHETIC.

Par Quintum. See TRIGEMINI.

Par Secundum. See OPTIC NERVE.

Par Septimum. See SEVENTH PAIR.

Par Sextum. See SIXTH PAIR.

Par Tertium. See MOTORES OCULORUM.

Par Va'gum.* (The "Wandering Pair.") A name of the eighth pair of nerves. See PNEUMOGASTRIC.

Pa'ra (*παρά*). A Greek preposition, signifying "from or by the side of;" "near;" "beyond." When combined with other words, it often signifies "amiss," or "wrong."

Păr-a-blas'ta.* [From *παρά*, "beside," "from the side of," and *βλάστη*, an "offshoot."] A sucker or offshoot. Also, disease with anatomical conversion or alteration: a parablast.

Păr-a-blep'sis.* [From *παρά*, "amiss," and *βλεψίς*, a "looking," "vision."] False vision.

Pa-rab'o-la.* [Gr. *παραβολή*; from *παραβάλλω*, to "throw beside," to "place side by side."] One of the conic sections, formed by the intersection of a cone with a plane parallel to one of its sides. It is the curve which would be described by a projectile in a vacuum.

Păr-a-bys'ma, atis.* [From *παραβύω*, to "stuff."] Turgescence of a part.

Păr-a-bys'ti-a.* [From the same.] A stuffing in or insertion.

Păr-a-çen-te'sis.* [From *παρακεντέω*, to "pierce at the side."] The operation of tapping the thorax, abdomen, etc., to discharge the fluid, as in *hydrothorax*, *ascites*, *empyema*, etc.

Păr-a-cu'sis.* [From *παρά*, "amiss," "wrong," and *ἀκούω*, to "hear."] Depraved or defective hearing. A genus of the order *Dysæsthesiæ*, class *Locales*, of Cullen's Nosology.

Paracu'sis I-mag-i-na'ri-a.* The hearing of imaginary sounds, not existing without, but excited within the ear.

Paracu'sis Im-per-fec'ta.* Deafness, or inability to hear sounds as usual.

Păr-a-çy-e'sis.* [From *παρά*, "beyond," and *κύησις*, "pregnancy."] Preternatural or morbid pregnancy.

Păr-æs-the'si-a,* or **Par-æs-the'sis.*** [From *παρά*, "amiss," "wrong," and *αἴσθησις*, "sensation."] Morbid or depraved sensation.

Păr'af-fin, or **Păr'af-fine.** [**Paraffi'na;** from *pa'rum*, "little," and *affi'nis*, "related," or "inclined to unite."] A white, crystalline substance, without taste or smell, obtained from petroleum, wood-tar, and other materials. It is solid at the common temperatures, is soluble in alcohol and ether, but resists the action of acids, alkalies, etc. It receives its name from its little affinity for other substances. It is used for making candles, and for various other purposes for which wax is employed.

Păr-a-geu'sis,* or **Par-a-geu'si-a.*** [From *παρά*, "amiss," and *γεύω*, to "taste."] Morbid or depraved taste.

Păr-a-guay' Tea. The product of the *Ilex Paraguayen'sis*, a plant growing in South America. The leaves have a balsamic odor and a bitter taste, which is disagreeable to those unaccustomed to it. They are said to contain a principle identical with the caffein of coffee and tea.

Păr'al-lax. [**Parallax'is;** from *παράλλαξις*, a "change," a "difference."] Literally, a "change." A change of place, or of aspect. The term is used to denote the difference between the apparent place of a celestial body and its true place, or that in which it would be seen if the observer were placed at the centre to which the motion is referred.—(BRANDE.)

Păr'al-lel. [**Paralle'lus;** from *παρά*, "beside," and *ἀλλήλων*, "each other."] Having the same direction, and equally distant from each other in all their extent, as parallel lines.

Păr-al-lel-i-ner'vis,* or **Păr-al-lel-i-ner'vi-us.*** [From *paralle'lus*, "parallel," and *ner'vus*, a "nerve."] Applied to leaves of which the nerves are parallel, or nearly so, as in all endogenous plants.

Păr-al-lel'o-gram. [**Parallelogram'ma;** from *παράλληλος*, "equally distant," and *γραμμή*, a "line."] Any quadrilateral figure whose opposite sides are parallel.

Par'allel-Veined. [**Parallelivenо'sus;** from *paralle'lus*, "parallel," and *ve'na*, a "vein."] Applied to leaves which are marked by parallel veins running from the base to the apex. Such leaves are characteristic of endogenous plants.

Paralysé. See PARALYTIC.

Paralysie. See PARALYSIS.

Pa-ral'y-sis.* [From *παραλύω*, to "loosen," also, to "disable."] (Fr. *Paralysie*, pȧ'rȧ'le'zē'.) Palsy. A disease characterized by loss or great diminution of the power of voluntary motion, affecting any part of the body. A genus of the order *Comata*, class *Neuroses*, of Cullen's Nosology.

Paral'ysis Ag'i-tans.* The "shaking palsy."

Paral'ysis Hem-i-pleg'i-ca.* Palsy of one half or side of the body. See HEMIPLEGIA.

Paral'ysis Par-a-pleg'i-ca.* Palsy of one half (usually the lower part) of the body. See PARAPLEGIA.

Paral'ysis Partia'lis* (par-she-a'-lis). "Partial Paralysis." Palsy of some particular muscle or nerve.

Paral'ysis Ven-e-na'ta.* Palsy from the effects of some poison.

Păr-a-lўt'ic. [Lat. **Paralyt'icus;** Fr. *Paralysé*, på'rå'lè'zå', or *Paralytique*, på'rå'lè'tèk'.] Belonging to paralysis, or affected with paralysis.

Păr-a-me'nĭ-a.* [From παρά, "amiss," and μῆνες, the "menses."] Disordered menstruation.

Păr-a-mor'phĭ-a.* [From παρά, "amiss," and μορφή, "form."] Morbid structure. Applied to organic diseases.

Păr-a-ne-phri'tis, idis.* [From *paran'ephrus.*] Inflammation of the suprarenal capsules.

Pa-ran'e-phrus.* [From παρά, "beside," and νεφρός, the "kidney."] A name for the suprarenal capsule.

Păr-a-phi-mo'sis.* [From παρά, "amiss," and φιμόω, to "bridle."] A disorder in which the prepuce is constricted behind the *glans penis* and cannot be drawn forward.

Păr-a-phi-mot'ĭ-cus.* Belonging to *paraphimosis.*

Păr-a-pho'nĭ-a.* [From παρά, "amiss," or "wrong," and φωνή, the "voice."] Change or alteration of the voice; bad voice. A genus of the order *Dyscinesiæ* of Cullen's Nosology.

Păr-a-plec'tĭ-cus,* or **Par-a-plec'-tus.*** [From παρά, "amiss," and πλήσσω, to "strike."] Paraplectic; stricken on one side; paralyzed; also, frenzy-stricken.

Păr-a-ple'gĭ-a.* [Gr. παραπληγία, a "benumbing of parts;" from παρά, "amiss," "wrong," and πλήσσω, to "strike."] A paralytic stroke affecting one-half of the body, either the upper or lower, usually the lower; also termed *Paralysis paraplegica.*

Păr-a-pleg'ic. [**Parapleg'icus.**] Belonging to *paraplegia.*

Păr-a-poph'ў-sis,* plural **Par-a-poph'ў-sēs.** [From παρά, "near," "beside," and ἀποφύω, to "be arisen from."] Applied by Owen to the homologues of the lower transverse process of a vertebra.

Pa-rap'sis.* [From παρά, "amiss," or "wrong," and ἅψις, "touch."] A generic term applied by Dr. Good to the various forms of morbid or defective sense of touch.

Păr-a-se-le'nĭ-a,* or **Păr-a-se-le'-ne.*** [From παρά, "beside," and σελήνη, the "moon."] A luminous phenomenon consisting in the appearance of one or more images of the moon.

Păr'a-site. [Lat. **Parasi'ta;** Gr. παράσιτος, "one who lives at another's expense."] Applied to a vegetable, or animal, that draws its sustenance from others; the one living on or in the bodies of other animals, the other fixing its roots into other plants.

Păr-a-sit'ĭ-cal. [**Parasit'icus;** from *parasi'tus*, a "sponger," or "parasite."] (Fr. *Parasitaire*, på'rå'zè'têr'.) Belonging to a parasite: parasitic.

Păr-a-si'tus.* [Gr. παράσιτος, a "sponger," or "parasite."] Applied in the plural neuter (*Parasi'ta*) to an order of insects, from their parasitical habits.

Păr-a-spa'dĭ-a.* [From παρά, "from the side," and σπάω, to "draw."] An opening of the urethra upon one side of the penis.

Pa-ras'ta-dus.* [From παραστάς, a "series of pillars."] Applied to the sterile filaments between petals and stamens.

Păr-as-ta-ti'tis.* The same as PROSTATITIS, which see.

Păr-a-ste'mon, onis.* [From παρά, "amiss," and στήμων, a "stamen."] An altered and sterile stamen.

Păr-a-sty'lus.* [From παρά, "near," and στῦλος, a "pillar."] Applied to parts of the flower which resemble pistils but do not fulfil their functions: a par'-astyle.

Păr-a-sўs'to-lē.* [From παρά, "amiss," and συστολή, a "contracting."] An unusual interval between the pulsations, or between the systole and diastole of the heart and arteries.

Păr-at'o-mous. [**Parat'omus;** from παρά, "beside," and τέμνω, to "cut."] Applied to the cleavage of minerals when the planes are parallel with those of the fundamental figure, or are inclined to the axis.

Pa-rec'ta-ma, atis.* [From παρεκτείνω, to "stretch out."] Excessive extension.

Păr-ec-tam'ĭ-cus.* Belonging to *parectama:* parectamic.

Pa-rec'ta-sis.* [From the same.] A stretching out; extension.

Păr-e-gor'ic. [**Paregor'icus;** from παρηγορέω, to "encourage," to "soothe," or "assuage."] Mitigating or assuaging pain.

Păregor'ic E-lix'ir. The *Tinctura opii camphorata.* Also formerly applied to the *Tinctura opii ammoniata.*

Pareira (Sp.), på-rā'rå, or **Parei'ra Bra'va.** The Pharmacopœial name ‖ of the root of *Cissampelos pareira.*

Pareira Brava, på-rā'rå brå'vå. The Spanish name for the root of *Cissampelos pareira.*

Păr-en-çeph-a-li'tis, *idis.** [From *parenceph'alis,* the "cerebellum."] Inflammation of the cerebellum.

Pa-ren'chy̆-ma, *atis.** [From παρεγχέω, to "pour in beside."] Originally applied to the mass of tissue lying between the vessels of any organ or part. This mass was supposed to be the result of an effusion of blood or other fluid. Now applied to the connecting tissue of the viscera, considered as distinct from the vessels, ducts, nerves, etc. In Botany it denotes soft, cellular tissue, such as that which forms the green pulp of leaves, and the outer bark of stems.

Pa-ren-chy̆-mat'ic. [**Parenchymat'icus.**] Belonging to parenchyma.

Păr-en-chy̆m-a-ti'tis, *idis.** [From *paren'chyma.*] Inflammation of the parenchyma.

Păr-en-chy̆m'a-tous. [**Parenchym'atus,** or **Parenchymato'sus;** from the same.] Applied to parts or organs formed of parenchyma.

Pa-ren-chy̆m-ep-a-ti'tis, *idis.** [From *paren'chyma,* and *hepati'tis,* "inflammation of the liver."] Parenchymatous inflammation of the liver.

Par-ep-ĭ-thym'ĭ-a.* [From παρά, "amiss," and ἐπιθυμία, a "longing."] Morbidly changed or depraved desires.

Păr'e-sis.* [From παρίημι, to "relax."] The paralysis of a part from debility.

Pa-ret'ic. Belonging to paresis.

Par-he'lĭ-on.* [From παρά, "near," and ἥλιος, the "sun."] A mock-sun. A meteor consisting in the simultaneous appearance of one or more faint images of the sun. They are often tinted with prismatic colors.

Păr'ĭ-a Ner-vo'rum.* ("Pairs of Nerves.") An appellation especially applied to the cranial or encephalic nerves, of which there are reckoned nine pairs according to some anatomists, and twelve pairs according to others. The first pair is the olfactory, the second the optic, the third the oculo-motor, and so on. The *portio mollis* of the seventh pair, is by some writers reckoned as the eighth pair; so the two portions of the pneumogastric, or eighth pair (proper), are considered as two pairs. In like manner, the accessory nerve of Willis, usually reckoned as belonging to the eighth pair, is counted as the eleventh; while the ninth pair (proper) becomes the twelfth.

Pa'rĭ-ēs,* plural **Pa-ri'e-tēs.** The sides or walls of any cavity or organ are termed its *parietes.*

Pa-rī'e-tal. [**Parieta'lis;** from *pa'ries,* a "wall."] Belonging to the *parietes* or walls of any cavity, organ, etc.

Pari'etal Bones. [**Os'sa Parieta'lia.**] The two quadrangular bones forming the transverse arch of the cranium.

Pa-ri'e-tēs,* gen. **Pa-ri'e-tum,** the plural of Paries, which see.

Păr-ĭ-pen'nate, or **Păr-ĭ-pin'nate.** [**Paripenna'tus;** from *par,* "equal," and *pen'na,* a "feather," or "quill."] Applied to a pennate leaf which has an even number of leaflets, and has none on the very apex of the petiole.

Paripinnate. See Paripennate.

Păr-isth-mi'tis.* [From παρά, "near," and ἰσθμός, the "fauces."] Inflammation about the throat. The *squincy,* or *squinancy,* of the old writers, and the quinsy, *cynanche,* or *angina,* of the moderns.

Păr-oc-cip'ĭ-tal. [**Paroccipita'lis;** from παρά, "by the side of," or "near," and *occipita'le* os, the "occipital bone."] Proposed by Owen for the elements of the occipital segment of the cranium, below the supraoccipital.

Păr-o-dy̆n'ĭ-a.* [From παρά, "amiss," or "wrong," and ὀδύνη, "pain."] Morbid labor. The name of a genus in Good's Nosology.

Pa-rom'pha-lo-çēle.* [From παρά, "near," ὀμφαλός, the "navel," and κήλη, a "tumor."] Hernia near the navel.

Păr-o-nīr'ĭ-a.* [From παρά, "amiss," and ὄνειρος, a "dream."] A generic term applied by Dr. Good to morbid dreams, including somnambulism, nocturnal pollution, etc.

Păr-o-ny̆ch'ĭ-a.* [From παρά, "near," and ὄνυξ, the "nail."] (Fr. *Onglade,* ôɴᴳ'glåd'.) A collection of pus, or an abscess, in the fingers; the disease termed whitlow. The term was originally applied to a tumor situated near or under the nail.

Păr-o-ny̆ch'ĭ-cus.* Belonging to *paronychia.*

Pa-rop'sis.* [From παρά, "amiss," and ὄψις, "vision."] A generic term applied by Dr. Good to disorders of the sense of vision; false-seeing.

Păr-os'mis.* [From παρά, "amiss," or "wrong," and ὀσμή, "smell."] Morbid or depraved smell. The name of a genus in Good's Nosology.

Pa-ros'tĭ-a.* [From παρά, "amiss," or "wrong," and ὀστέον, a "bone."] Defective ossification.

Parotia,* pa-ro'she-a. [From *paro'tis*, the "parotid gland."] The same as PAROTITIS, which see.

Pa-rot'id. [**Parotide'us,** or **Parotidæ'us;** from παρά, "near," and οὖς, ὠτός, the "ear."] Situated near the ear. Applied to a gland.

Parot'id Duct. [**Ductus Parotide'us.**] See PAROTID GLAND.

Parot'id Gland. [**Glan'dula Parotide'a** (or **Parotidæ'a**), or **Paro'tis.**] The large, conglomerate, salivary gland under the ear. Its secretions are discharged through the parotid duct into the mouth, opposite the second superior molar tooth.

Parotide. See PAROTIS.

Parotidean Plexus. See PES ANSERINUS.

Par-ot-ĭ-don'cus.* [From παρωτίς, the "parotid gland," and ὄγκος, a "tumor."] Tumor or swelling of the parotid gland, commonly termed the mumps. See PAROTITIS.

Par-ot-ĭ-do-scir'rhus.* [From παρωτίς, the "parotid gland," and σκίρρος, an "induration."] Scirrhous hardening of one or both parotid glands.

Pa-ro'tis, idis.* [From παρά, "near," and οὖς, ὠτός, the "ear."] (Fr. *Parotide*, på'ro'tėd'.) The parotid gland, situated under the ear.

Păr-o-ti'tis, idis.* [From *paro'tis*, the "parotid gland."] Inflammation of the parotid gland, popularly termed the mumps; also called *Cynan'che parotide'a.*

Păr'ox-ÿsm. [**Paroxys'mus;** from παροξύνω, to "aggravate."] An evident increase of symptoms, which after a certain time decline; a periodical fit or attack.

Part. aff. = *Par'tem affec'tam.** "The part affected."

Part. dolent. = *Par'tem dolen'tem.** "The part in pain."

Par-the-no-gen'e-sis.* [From παρθένος, a "virgin," and γένω, to "be born."] The successive production of procreating individuals from a single ovum. In Botany, the formation of a perfect seed without the agency of pollen.

Par'tial Pe'tĭ-ole. The stalk of a leaflet of a pinnate leaf.

Par'tial Um'bel. A part of a compound umbel; an umbellet.

Par'tĭ-cle. [**Partic'ula;** diminutive of *pars*, a "part."] An atom; a corpuscle; the minutest part into which a body can be mechanically divided.

Par'tīte. [From *par'tio, parti'tum*, to "part," or "divide."] Parted, or divided, as leaves the incisions or sinuses of which reach almost to the midrib.

Par-tu'rĭ-ent. [**Partu'riens, en'tis;** from *partu'rio*, to "travail," to "bring forth."] Bringing forth; child-bearing.

Par-tu-rĭ-fā'cient. [From *partu'rio*, to "bring forth," and *fa'cio*, to "cause."] A medicine which facilitates parturition.

Par-tu-rĭ'tion. [**Parturi'tio, o'nis;** from *partu'rio, parturi'tum*, to "bring forth."] (Fr. *Accouchement*, å'koosh'mŏnᵍ'.) Expulsion of the fœtus from the uterus. Also, the state of being in childbed.

Par'tus.* [From *pa'rio, par'tum*, to "bring forth."] The act of bringing forth young, otherwise called labor; also, the young when brought forth; the birth.

Part. vic. = *Parti'tis viç'ibus.** "In divided doses."

Pa-ru'lis, idis.* [From παρά, "near," or "by the side of," and οὖλον, the "gum."] Gum-boil. Inflammation, boil, or abscess of the gums.

Pa-ru'rĭ-a.* [From παρά, "amiss," and οὐρέω, to "pass urine."] Mismicturition, or difficulty in passing urine.

Par-Vagum. See PNEUMOGASTRIC.

Par-vĭ-flo'rus.* [From *par'vus*, "small," and *flos*, a "flower."] Having small flowers.

Par-vĭ-fo'lĭ-us.* [From *par'vus*, "small," and *fo'lium*, a "leaf."] Having small leaves.

Pas'sa.* [Nominative singular feminine of *pas'sus*, "dried in the sunshine."] Applied to *uva*, to signify a dried grape or raisin. See PASSUS.

Pas'ser,* plural **Pas'ser-ēs.** A sparrow. Applied to an order of birds. See PASSERES.

Pas'ser-ēs* [the plural of PASSER, a "sparrow"], otherwise termed **Pas-se-ri'næ.*** The name of an order of birds of the sparrow kind. They form the most extensive and varied order of birds.

Passerine. See PASSERINUS.

Pas-se-ri'nus.* [From *pas'ser*, a "sparrow."] Belonging to the sparrow. Applied in the plural (*Passeri'næ*) to an order of birds otherwise termed *Passeres:* pas'serine.

Passifloraceæ,* pas-se-flo-ra'she-ē, or **Passiflo'reæ.*** A natural order of exogenous twining plants with showy flowers, abundant in South America and the West Indies. It includes the *Passiflo'ra* (Passion Flower), the fruit of which is edible.

Pas-sĭ-flo're-æ.* The Jussieuan name of a natural order of plants. See PASSIFLORACEÆ.

Pas'sio (pash'e-o) **Hȳs-ter'ĭ-cạ.*** *Hysteria*, or hysterics.

Passio Iliaca. See ILIAC PASSION.

Passion, Ungovernable. See EMPATHEMA.

Pas'sĭve Mo'tion. Applied to motion caused not by the patient himself, but gently by another person.

Pas'su-lạ.* [Diminutive of *pas'sa*, "dried in the sun," *u'va*, a "grape," being understood.] A little dried grape; a raisin.

Pas'sula Ma'jor.* ("Larger Raisin.") The systematic name of the dried fruit of the *Vitis vinifera;* a raisin.

Pas-su-la'tus.* [From *pas'sula*, a "raisin."] Pas'sulate. Applied to certain medicines of which raisins formed the chief ingredient.

Pas'sus.* [From *pan'do, pan'sum* or *pas'sum*, to "spread out" for drying.] Dried by exposure to the sun. See PASSA, and PASSULA.

Pas'til. [**Pastil'lum;** diminutive of *pas'ta*, a "lozenge."] A little lump like a lozenge; a troch.

Pas-tĭ-na'cạ.* The Parsnip. A Linnæan genus of the class *Pentandria*, natural order *Umbelliferæ*.

Pastina'ca O-pop'o-nax.* The plant formerly stated to afford *Opoponax*, now referred to the *Opoponax chironium*.

Pâte Arsénicale, pât aR'sà'nè'kål'. ("Arsenical Paste.") An application for cancers, consisting of seventy parts of cinnabar, twenty-two of dragon's blood, and eight of arsenious acid.

Pạ-tel'lạ,* gen. **Pạ-tel'læ.** [Diminutive of *pat'ina*, a "pan."] The knee-pan, or knee-cap; also termed **Mo'lạ,*** and **Rot'u-lạ.*** (Fr. *Rotule*, ro'tül'.) In Botany, a plain receptacle, having a distinct border of the *thallus*. Also, a genus of the *Gasteropoda Mollusca*, inhabiting a univalve shell; a limpet.

Pat-el-la'tus.* [From *patel'la*, a "little dish, or platter."] Applied to a polypus which forms an expansion almost orbicular.

Pa-tel'lĭ-form. [**Patellifor'mis;** from *patel'la*, the "knee-pan."] Having the form of a knee-pan, or patella.

Pa-tel'lu-lạ.* [Diminutive of *patel'la*, the "knee-pan."] Applied in Botany to a sessile receptacle, orbicular, and surrounded by a proper border, not produced by the *thallus*.

Pạ-the'mạ,* plural **Pạ-them'ạ-tạ.** [From πάθος, "affection."] Affection, suffering, or disease. Passion, or an instinctive feeling become extreme and exclusive.

Pạ-them-ạ-to-loġ'ĭ-cạl. [**Pathematoloġ'icus.**] Belonging to pathematology.

Pạ-them-ạ-tol'o-ġȳ. [**Pathematolo'gia;** from *pathe'ma*, "affection of body or mind," and λόγος, a "discourse."] The doctrine (or science) of the passions or affections of the mind. Also, the same as PATHOLOGY.

Pạ-them'ic. [**Pathem'icus.**] Belonging to *pathema*.

Pạ-thet'ic. [**Pathet'icus;** from πάθος, "affection."] Belonging to the feelings, or passions. Applied to the superior oblique muscle of the eye; also, to the fourth pair of nerves. See next article.

Pạ-thet'ic Nerves. [**Ner'vi Pathet'ici.**] The fourth pair of nerves, or *Trochleato'res:* so called because the eyes express the feelings or passions by means of them.

Path-o-ġen'e-sis.* [From πάθος, "affection," or "disease," and γένεσις, "generation."] The origin, production, or generation of disease.

Path-o-ġe-net'ĭ-cus.* Belonging to *pathogenesis:* pathogenet'ic.

Path-o-ġen'ic, Path-o-ġen'ĭ-cạl. [**Pathogen'icus.**] Belonging to pathogeny. Applied to substances, *effluvia*, *miasmata*, etc., which produce disease.

Pạ-thog'e-nȳ. [**Pathoge'nia;** from πάθος, "affection," or "disease," and γένω, to "be born," to "be produced."] That branch of Pathology which treats of the causes and development of diseases.

Pạ-thog-no-mon'ic. [**Pathognomon'icus;** from πάθος, "affection," or "disease," and γινώσκω, to "know."] Applied to the peculiar characteristic symptoms of a disease.

Path-o-graph'ĭ-cạl. [**Pathograph'icus.**] Belonging to pathography.

Pạ-thog'rạ-phȳ. [**Pathogra'phia;** from πάθος, "affection," or "disease," and γράφω, to "write."] A description or history of diseases.

Path-o-loġ'ĭ-cạl. [**Patholoġ'icus.**] Belonging to pathology.

Pạ-thol'o-ġȳ. [**Patholo'gia;** from

πάθος, an "affection," or "disease," and λόγος, a "discourse."] The doctrine or consideration of diseases. That branch of medical science which treats of diseases, their nature and effects. It is distinguished into Medical and Surgical Pathology.

Pat'u-lous. [**Pat'ulus;** from *pa'teo,* to "be open."] Open; broad; spreading. Applied to certain parts of plants.

Pau-cĭ-den'tate. [**Paucidenta'tus;** from *pau'ci,* "few," "little," and *dens,* a "tooth."] Slightly dentated.

Pau-cĭ-flo'rous. [**Pauciflo'rus;** from *pau'ci,* "few," and *flos,* a "flower."] Having few flowers.

Pau-cĭ-fo'lĭ-ous. [**Paucifo'lius;** from *pau'ci,* "few," and *fo'lium,* a "leaf."] Having few leaves, or folioles.

Pau-cĭ-ju-ga'tus,* Pau-cij'u-gus.* [From *pau'ci,* "few," and *ju'gum,* a "yoke," or "pair."] Applied to a compound leaf formed of but three or four pairs of folioles: paucij'ugate; paucij'ugous.

Pau-cĭ-ner'vate. [**Paucinerva'tus, Pauciner'vius;** from *pau'ci,* "few," and *ner'vus,* a "nerve."] Having but few nerves, or slightly veined.

Pau-cĭ-ra-dĭ-a'tus.* [From *pau'ci,* "few," and *ra'dius,* a "ray."] Applied to the umbel when it contains but a small number of rays.

Pau-cĭ-se-rĭ-a'tus.* [From *pau'ci,* "few," and *se'ries,* a "row," or "order."] Divided into a small number of series.

Paul-lin'ĭ-a Sor'bĭ-lis.* A Brazilian plant from which an extract called *Paullinia,* or *Guarana,* is procured. It is recommended as a tonic.

Paunch. The stomach. Applied especially to the first and greatest stomach of the *Ruminantia.*

Paupière, pō'pe-ĕr'. The French term for "eyelid." See PALPEBRA.

Pav'o-nine. [**Pavoni'nus;** from *pa'vo, pavo'nis,* the "peacock."] Having eye-like spots resembling those seen on the peacock's tail.

Pavot, på'vo'. The French name for "poppy." See PAPAVER.

Peach. (Fr. *Pêche,* pĕsh or påsh.) The *Malum Persicum,* or fruit of the *Amygdalus Persica.*

Peach-Tree. The *Amyg'dalus Per'sica.*

Pear. The fruit of the *Pyrus communis.*

Pearl. [Lat. **Margari'ta;** Fr. *Perle,* pĕRl.] A highly prized substance found within the shells of certain bivalve mollusks, formed, as it would appear, by the deposition of calcareous matter round some nucleus. A pure pearl is generally spherical, and has a white or yellowish-white color, with a peculiar lustre and iridescence, and consists of alternating concentric layers of membrane and carbonate of lime. The most valuable pearls are obtained from the pearl oyster of Ceylon.

Pearl'-ash. [Named from its white, pearly color.] A purer carbonate of potassa, prepared by dissolving potash and allowing the impurities to subside.

Pearl Barley. See HORDEUM.

Pearl-White. The subnitrate or trisnitrate of bismuth; flake-white. See BISMUTHUM ALBUM.

Pēat. The natural accumulation of vegetable matter from the decaying roots of grass, etc., mostly occurring on the surface of a bog or moor. When dried, it is used as fuel.

Pec'ten,* gen. **Pec'tĭ-nis.** A Latin word signifying a "comb;" also, the "pubes." Commonly applied to the *os pubis,* which is a distinct bone in the fœtal pelvis.

Pec'tic. [**Pec'ticus;** from πηκτίς, a "coagulum."] Applied to an acid which is found in many kinds of fruits, and has the property of forming jelly.

Pec'tin. [From the same.] A principle which forms the base of vegetable jelly.

Pec-tĭ-næ'us.* [From *pec'ten,* the "*os pubis.*"] Belonging to the *pecten,* or *os pubis:* pectine'al. See PECTINALIS.

Pec-tĭ-na'lis,* or **Pec-tĭ-næ'us.*** [From the same.] Belonging to, or connected with, the *os pubis.* Also, the name of a long, flat muscle arising from the pectineal line of the *os pubis,* and inserted into the line leading from the *trochanter minor* to the *linea aspera.*

Pec'tĭ-nate. [**Pectina'tus;** from *pec'ten,* a "comb."] Having the appearance of a comb. A pinnatifid leaf with regular close and narrow incisions, is called pectinate.

Pectinated Muscles. See MUSCULI PECTINATI.

Pectineus, or **Pectineal.** See PECTINALIS.

Pec'tĭ-nĭ-bran-chĭ-a'ta.* [See next article.] A name given by Cuvier to his sixth order of *Gasteropoda.* It includes almost all the spiral univalve shells.

Pec'tĭ-nĭ-bran-chĭ-a'tus.* [From *pec'ten,* a "comb," and *branchia'tus,* "having *branchiæ*."] Having comb-like *branchiæ*: pectinobranchiate.

Pec-tĭ-nif'er-ous. [**Pectinif'erus;** from *pec'ten*, a "comb," and *fe'ro*, to "bear."] Bearing or having combs. Applied to birds.

Pec-tĭ-nĭ-fo'lĭ-us.* [From *pec'ten*, a "comb," and *fo'lium*, a "leaf."] Having pectinated leaves.

Pec'tĭ-nĭ-form. [**Pectinifor'mis;** from *pec'ten*, a "comb."] Resembling a comb.

Pec-tĭ-no-i'dēs.* [From *pec'ten*, a "comb," and εἶδος, a "form."] Resembling one of the shells termed *Pecten;* like a comb: pectinoid.

Pec'to-ra,* the plural of PECTUS, which see.

Pec'to-ral. [**Pectora'lis;** from *pec'tus*, *pec'toris*, the "breast."] Belonging to the breast, or chest. In Ichthyology, applied to those fins which correspond to the anterior extremities of quadruped animals, and are termed pectorals.

Pectoralia. See PECTORALS.

Pectoralis. See PECTORAL.

Pec-to-ra'lis Ma'jor.* ("Greater Pectoral [Muscle].") A muscle arising from half the clavicle, all the edge of the sternum, and the cartilages of the three lower true ribs, and inserted into the outer border of the bicipital groove of the humerus. It moves the arm forwards, etc.

Pectora'lis Mi'nor.* ("Lesser Pectoral [Muscle].") A muscle arising from the third, fourth, and fifth ribs, and inserted into the coracoid process of the scapula. It draws the shoulder-bone forwards and downwards, and elevates the ribs.

Pec'to-rals. [**Pectora'lia;** from *pectora'lis*, "pectoral."] Medicines which relieve disorders of the chest.

Pectoriloquia. The same as PECTORILOQUY, which see.

Pec-to-ril'o-quism. [**Pectoriloquis'mus;** from *pec'tus*, the "breast," and *lo'quor*, to "speak."] The same as PECTORILOQUY.

Pec-to-ril'o-quy. [**Pectorilo'quium,** or **Pectorilo'quia;** from the same.] A form or condition of disease in which the voice of the patient seems to issue from the breast through the stethoscope: also termed Pectoriloquism.

Pec'tus,* gen. **Pec'to-ris.** That part between the neck and abdomen; the breast, or chest. The inferior surface of the thorax of insects, divided according to its segments into the *antepectus*, *mediopectus*, and *postpectus*.

Pedaliaceæ,* pe-da-le-a'she-ē. A natural order of exogenous herbaceous plants, found within the tropics, especially in Africa. It includes the *Peda'lium* and *Ses'amum*.

Pe'date. [**Peda'tus;** from *pes*, *pe'dis*, a "foot."] A term applied to a palmate leaf, the lateral lobes of which are each cleft into two or more segments.

Pe-dat'ĭ-fid. [**Pedatif'idus;** from *pes*, *pe'dis*, a "foot," and *fin'do*, to "cleave."] Applied to leaves which are divided in a pedate manner nearly halfway to the base.

Pedatus. See PEDATE.

Pe'dēs,* gen. **Pe'dum,** the plural of PES, which see.

Pe-dĭ-ăl'gĭ-a.* [From πέδιον, the "bones of the foot," or foot itself, and ἄλγος, "pain."] Neuralgic affection in the foot.

Ped'ĭ-cel. [**Pedicel'lus;** diminutive of *pedic'ulus*, a "flower-stalk."] The stalk of each particular flower in a cluster or raceme of flowers; a partial peduncle; a pedicle. Also, the second joint of the antennæ of insects.

Ped'ĭ-cel-late. [**Pedicella'tus;** from *pedicel'lus*, a "pedicel."] Having a pedicel.

Ped'ĭ-cle. The same as PEDICEL, which see.

Pe-dic'u-lar. [**Pedicula'ris.**] Belonging to the *pediculus*.

Pe-dic'u-late. [**Pedicula'tus;** from *pedic'ulus*, a "foot-stalk."] Having foot-stalks.

Pe-dic-u-lā'tion. [**Pedicula'tio, o'nis;** from *pedic'ulus*, a "louse."] A state of disease in which lice are constantly breeding on the skin. See PHTHIRIASIS.

Pe-dic'u-lus.* [Diminutive of *pes*, a "foot."] The foot-stalk of a flower and of fruits. Also, a genus of parasitic animals; the louse (Fr. *Pou*, poo).

Pedic'ulus Pu'bis* ("Louse of the Pubes"), or **Mor'pĭ-o.*** Vulgarly, "crab-louse." A species of louse found chiefly on the pubes, distinguished by the cheliform structure of its legs. It causes intolerable itching, and frequently induces local prurigo. Dusting the part with calomel mixed with starch powder, and attention to cleanliness, will nearly always be found efficacious in cases of this kind.

Pe-dif'er-ous. [**Pedif'erus;** from

pes, a "foot," and *fe'ro*, to "bear."] Bearing feet.

Ped-ĭ-lu'vĭ-um.* [From *pes*, a "foot," and *la'vo*, to "wash."] A bath for the feet: a foot-bath.

Ped-ĭ-păl'pus.* [From *pes*, a "foot," and *pal'pus*, a "feeler."] Applied in the plural (*Pedipăl'pi*) to a family of *Arachnides* having palpi in the form of a claw or arm.

Pe'dis,* the genitive of Pes, which see.

Pe-dun'cle. [**Pedun'culus**; diminutive of *pes*, a "foot."] The foot-stalk which supports a flower, or a cluster of flowers. The foot-stalk of each flower of a cluster is called a partial peduncle, or a pedicel.

Pe-dun'cu-late. [**Peduncula'tus**; from *pedun'culus*, a "foot-stalk."] Having, or growing on, a peduncle.

Pe-lā'ġĭ-an. [**Pelagia'nus**; from πέλαγος, the "deep sea."] Pertaining to the sea.

Pe-laġ'ic. [**Pelaġ'icus**; from the same.] Belonging to the deep sea.

Pe-lā'ġĭ-ous. [**Pela'gius.**] The same as Pelagic, which see.

Pel'la-gra.* [From *pel'lis*, a "skin," and ἄγρα, a "seizure."] A disease common in certain parts of Italy, beginning by a shining red spot on some part of the head or body; termed also *Elephantiasis Italica.*

Pel'lĭ-cle. [**Pellic'ula**; diminutive of *pel'lis*, a "skin."] A very thin skin; a film on the surface of fluids; slender membranous productions, etc.

Pel-lic'u-lar. [**Pellicula'ris.**] Relating to a pellicle.

Pel'lis.* [From πέλλα, a "hide."] The *Cutis*, or skin.

Pel'lĭ-to-rȳ of Spain. The Anthemis Pyrethrum, which see.

Pel-lu'cid. [**Pellu'cidus**; from *per*, "through," and *lu'ceo*, to "shine."] Translucent; pervious to light, or semitransparent.

Pel'o-sin, or **Pel'o-sine.** A colorless substance extracted from the root of the *Cissam'pelos parei'ra.* It is a powerful base, forming salts with several acids.

Pel'ta.* [From πέλτη, a "shield."] A variety of the *calyculus*, oblong, flat, and obtuse, found in the lichens.

Pel-ta'lis.* [From *pel'ta*, a "shield."] Belonging to a shield; also, scutiform.

Pel'tate. [**Pelta'tus**; from *pel'ta*, a "shield."] Shield-shaped. Applied to roundish leaves, the petioles of which are attached to a point near the centre.

Pel-tĭ-fo'lĭ-us.* [From *pel'ta*, a "shield," and *fo'lium*, a "leaf."] Having peltate leaves: peltifo'lious.

Pel'tĭ-form. [**Peltifor'mis**; from *pel'ta*, a "shield."] Formed like a shield.

Pel-to-i'dēs.* [From *pel'ta*, a "shield," and εἶδος, a "form."] Resembling a shield: peltoid.

Pel'vic. [**Pel'vicus.**] Belonging to the pelvis.

Pel'vĭ-form. [**Pelvifor'mis**; from *pel'vis*, a "basin."] Having the form of a basin.

Pel-vim'e-ter. [**Pelvim'etrum**; from *pel'vis*, a "basin," and μέτρον, a "measure."] An instrument used in obstetrics for measuring the capacity of the pelvis.

Pel-vĭ-ot'o-mȳ. [**Pelvioto'mia**; from *pel'vis*, a "basin," and τέμνω, to "cut."] Section of the bones of the pelvis. See Sigaultian Operation.

Pel'vis.* (Fr. *Bassin*, bâs'săNᵍ'.) Literally, "a basin." The osseous cavity forming the lowest part of the trunk. It is bounded behind by the sacrum and coccyx, at the sides and in front by the ossa innominata. See Sinus.

Pem-phĭ-go-i'dēs.* [From *pem'phigus*, and εἶδος, a "form."] Resembling *pemphigus*: pemphigoid.

Pem'phĭ-gus,* or pem-fi'gŭs. [From πέμφιξ, a "blister."] (Fr. *Fièvre Bulleuse*, fe-ĕvR' bül'luz'.) An eruption of vesicles from the size of a pea to a walnut, generally accompanied by fever; vesicular fever, or *Febris bullosa.* A genus of the order *Exanthemata*, class *Pyrexiæ*, of Cullen's Nosology.

Penæaceæ,* pe-ne-a'she-ē. [From *Penæ'a*, one of the genera.] A natural order of exogenous evergreen shrubs, natives of the Cape of Good Hope.

Pen-du-lĭ-flo'rus.* [From *pen'dulus*, "hanging," or "pendulous," and *flos*, a "flower."] Having pendant flowers.

Pen-du-lĭ-fo'lĭ-us.* [From *pen'dulus*, "hanging," and *fo'lium*, a "leaf."] Having pendant leaves.

Pen-ĭ-cil'late. [**Penicilla'tus**; from *penicil'lus*, a "painter's brush."] Tipped with a brush of hairs like a camel's-hair pencil.

Pen-ĭ-cil'lĭ-form. [**Penicillifor'mis**; from *penicil'lus*, a "painter's brush."] Resembling a hair-pencil.

Pen-ĭ-cil'lum,* **Pen-ĭ-cil'lus.*** [Diminutive of *penic'ulum*, a "brush."] Applied to the arrangement of minute ramifications of the *Vena portæ*, composing the small glands or glandiform bodies which form the substance of the liver, because resembling a hair-pencil. In Surgery, a tent or pledget of charpie, or soft sponge, etc. See PANNUS.

Pe'nis,* gen. the same. [Gr. πέος.] The *Mem'brum viri'le*, or chief organ of generation in man, permeated by the urethra. It consists of two principal portions: the *Cor'pus caverno'sum* (or *Cor'pora caverno'sa*) and the *Cor'pus spongio'sum*, also called *Cor'pus spongio'sum ure'thræ* ("Spongy Body of the Urethra"), because it surrounds the urethra. See CORPORA CAVERNOSA, and CORPUS SPONGIOSUM.

Pennate. See PINNATE.

Pen-na-tif'er-us.* [From *pen'na*, a "feather," and *fe'ro*, to "bear."] Bearing feathers, or appendages like feathers. Applied to certain animals.

Pen-nat'ĭ-fid. [**Pennatif'idus.**] See PINNATIFID.

Pen-nat-ĭ-fo'lĭ-us.* [From *penna'tus*, "pinnate," and *fo'lium*, a "leaf."] Having pinnate leaves.

Pen-nat-ĭ-par-ti'tus.* [From *penna'tus*, "pinnate," and *par'tio, parti'tum*, to "part."] Pinnately-parted, as feather-veined leaves the sinuses of which reach almost to the midrib: pennatipartite.

Pen-nat'ĭ-sect-ed, or **Pin-nat'ĭ-sect.** [**Pennatisec'tus**; from *penna'tus*, "pinnate," and *se'co, sec'tum*, to "cut."] Applied to feather-veined leaves with sinuses which reach quite to the midrib: pinnately-divided.

Pen-nat-ĭ-stip-u-la'tus.* Applied to a plant that has pinnatifid stipules.

Pen-nif'er-ous. [**Pennif'erus**; from *pen'na*, a "feather," and *fe'ro*, to "bear."] Bearing quills, or feathers; covered with feathers.

Pen'nĭ-form. [**Pennifor'mis**; from *pen'na*, a "feather."] Having the form of a feather.

Pen-nĭ-ner'vis.* [From *pen'na*, a "feather," and *ner'vus*, a "nerve."] Having nerves or veins disposed like a feather; pinnately-nerved.

Pen-nĭ-ve'nĭ-us.* [From *pen'na*, a "feather," and *ve'na*, a "vein."] Feather-veined. A term applied to leaves the veins of which proceed from a midrib. See PINNATELY-VEINED.

Pen'nu-la.* [Diminutive of *pen'na*, a "feather."] A small feather with a short stem: a pen'nule.

Pennyroyal. See MENTHA PULEGIUM.

Pen-ta-car'pel-la-rў. [From πέντε, "five," and καρπός, "fruit."] Composed of five carpels.

Pen-ta-chæ'nĭ-um,* or **Pen-ta-chai'nĭ-um.*** [From πέντε, "five," and χαίνω, to "open."] A simple fruit formed by an ovary adherent to the calyx, which at maturity separates into five lobes, like the fruit of the *Araliaceæ*.

Pen-ta-chot'o-mous. [**Pentachot'omus**; from πενταχῆ, "in five ways or parts," and τέμνω, to "cut."] Applied to cymes where each terminal flower has under it five bracts, and gives origin to as many branches.

Pen'ta-gon. [**Pentago'num**; from πέντε, "five," and γωνία, an "angle."] A plane figure, having five angles and sides. A regular pentagon has five equal sides.

Pen-tag'o-nal. [**Pentago'nus.**] Belonging to a pentagon; five-cornered.

Pen-ta-ġўn'ĭ-a.* [From πέντε, "five," and γυνή, a "woman," or "female."] A Linnæan order of plants, comprising those which have five pistils in each flower.

Pen-ta-ġўn'ĭ-ous. [**Pentagyn'ius**; from the same.] Having five pistils.

Pen-taġ'ў-nous. The same as PENTAGYNIOUS, which see.

Pen-tam'e-rous. [From πέντε, "five," and μέρος, a "part."] Consisting of five parts or five organs of each kind. Applied to a flower which has five petals, five stamens, etc.

Pen-tan'drĭ-a.* [From πέντε, "five," and ἀνήρ, a "man," or "male."] The fifth class in the Linnæan system of plants, comprising those which have five stamens in each flower.

Pen-tan'drous. [**Pentan'drius**; from the same.] Having five stamens.

Pen-ta-pet'a-lous. [**Pentapet'alus**; from πέντε, "five," and πέταλον, a "petal."] Applied to a corol composed of five petals.

Pen-ta-phўl-lo-i'dēs.* [From *pentaphyl'lum*, the "cinquefoil," and εἶδος, a "form."] Resembling the cinquefoil.

Pen-ta-phўl'lous. [**Pentaphyl'lus**; from πέντε, "five," and φύλλον, a "leaf."] Having five leaves; five-leaved.

Pen-tap'ter-ous. [**Pentap'terus**; from πέντε, "five," and πτερόν, a "wing."] In Botany, having five expansions in form of wings; five-winged.

Pen-ta-sep'a-lous. [**Pentasep'alus**; from πέντε, "five," and *sep'alum*, a "sepal."] Applied to a calyx composed of five sepals.

Pen-ta-sper'mous. [**Pentasper'-**

mus; from πέντε, "five," and σπέρμα, a "seed."] Having five seeds.

Pen-tas'tĭ-chous. [**Pentas'tichus;** from πέντε, "five," and στιχη, a "row."] Disposed in five rows, or in five vertical ranks. Applied to leaves.

Pen-ta-sty'lus.* [From πέντε, "five," and στῦλος, a "pillar."] Applied to an ovary which bears five styles.

Pe-num'bra.* [From *pe'ne*, "almost," and *um'bra*, a "shade."] A faint shadow, or the edge of a perfect shadow; that portion of space which in an eclipse of the sun is partly, but not entirely, deprived of light; situated between the perfect shadow, where the light is wholly intercepted, and the full light.

Pe-o-to'mĭ-a.* [From πέος, the "penis," and τέμνω, to "cut."] Amputation of the penis: peot'omy.

Pe'po.* A pumpkin. Also, a general term applied to such fruits as the melon, cucumber, and gourd; being a modification of the berry. Likewise, the Pharmacopœial name for the seeds of the *Cucur'bita Pe'po*. They have been assigned a place on the primary list of the Materia Medica of the U.S. Pharmacopœia for 1860. These seeds have recently acquired a high reputation as a remedy against the tape-worm. The pulp of the pumpkin has also been administered with similar effect. The dose of the seeds is about two ounces; deprived of their outer covering, they may be beaten into a paste with sugar, and taken, fasting, followed in an hour or two by a free dose of castor oil.

Pepper. See PIPER.

Pepper, Cayenne, or **Pepper, Guinea.** See CAPSICUM ANNUUM.

Pepper, Jamaica. See MYRTUS PIMENTA.

Pep'per-mint. The MENTHA PIPERITA, which see.

Pep'sin. [**Pepsi'na;** from πέπτω, to "digest."] A supposed substance concerned in the process of digestion.

Pep'tic. [**Pep'ticus;** from the same.] Digestive; promoting digestion.

Per. A Latin particle signifying "through," "by;" also, "thoroughly." It is often *intensive*, being equivalent to "very." In Chemistry, it forms a prefix denoting an oxide containing the largest quantity of oxygen that can exist in any oxide formed by the same materials; also applied to acids which contain still more oxygen than those whose names end with *-ic*, as *perchloric* acid.

Per In-for-tu'nĭ-um.* ("By Misadventure.") Applied in medical jurisprudence to excusable homicide, or death from a lawful act done without intention of hurt.

Per'a-cute. [**Peracu'tus;** from *per*, intensive, and *acu'tus*, "acute."] Extremely severe; very acute.

Per-chlo'rāte. [**Perchlo'ras, a'tis.**] A combination of perchloric acid and a base. Applied to the oxichlorates.

Per-chlo'rāt-ed E'ther. The name of a fluid obtained by directly combining chlorine with olefiant gas, or by causing certain chlorides to react upon that gas.

Per-chlo'rīde of For'mȳle. The same as CHLOROFORM, which see.

Percolate. See next article.

Per-co-lā'tion. [**Percola'tio, o'nis;** from *per*, "through," and *co'lo, cola'tum*, to "strain."] Filtration. Also applied to animal secretions, the glands being compared to strainers or filters. Used in Pharmacy in the same sense as DISPLACEMENT (which see). See also the U.S. Pharmacopœia, pp. 3, 4, 5, 6. The filtered liquid is termed a *per'colate*.

Per-co-lā'tor. An instrument by means of which percolation is performed. See U.S. Pharmacopœia, pp. 4 and 5.

Per-cus'sion. [**Percus'sio, o'nis;** from *percu'tio, percus'sum*, to "strike," to "shock."] The act of striking any part of the body with the fingers, or an instrument, to ascertain its condition.

It is distinguished into—1. *Direct Percussion*, which consists in striking the surface of the chest, etc., with one or more fingers, and observing the degree and quality of the sounds produced. 2. *Mediate Percussion*, in which case a piece of ivory or leather, called a *pleximeter*, or the second phalanx of the forefinger of the left hand, is struck by the fingers of the right hand. See EXPLORATION.

Pe-ren'nĭ-al. [**Peren'nis;** from *per*, "through," and *an'nos*, "years."] Lasting through more than two years; also, perpetual; permanent.

Pe-ren'nĭ-bran'chĭ-ate. [**Perennibranchia'tus;** from *peren'nis*, "perennial," and *bran'chiæ*, "gills."] Having *branchiæ* persistent during life.

Per'fect Flow'er. A term applied to flowers which have both stamens and pistils.

Per'fect Num'ber. A number which is equal to the sum of all its divisors, as 6, 28, etc. Thus, the divisors of 6 are 1, 2, and 3, which added together make 6.

Per-fo'lĭ-ate. [**Perfolia'tus;** from *per*, "through," and *fo'lium*, a "leaf."]

Leaves are called perfoliate when the stem appears to pass through them. These in some cases originate in the union of the bases of a pair of opposite sessile leaves.

Per'fo-rans.* [From *per*, "through," and *fo'ro, fora'tum*, to "bore."] A designation of the *flex'or digito'rum profun'dus* muscle, from its perforating the tendon of the *flexor sublimis*.

Per'fo-rāt-ing. [From the same.] Piercing; passing through.

Per-fo-rā'tion. [**Perfora'tio, o'***nis;* from the same.] The application of the trepan or trephine.

Per'fo-rā-tor. [**Perforato'rium;** from the same.] An instrument for boring into the cranium.

Per-fo-ra'tus.* [From the same.] Perforated, or pierced through. A term applied to the *coraco-brachialis* muscle, from its being perforated by the external cutaneous nerve; also to the *flexor digitorum communis sublimis*, from its tendon being perforated by the tendon of the *flexor profundus*.

Per-fri-cā'tion. [**Perfrica'tio, o'***nis;* from *per*, "through," and *fri'co, fric'tum* or *frica'tum*, to "rub."] Inunction, or rubbing in through the pores of the skin any unctuous or oily substance.

Per-ga-me'ne-ous, or **Per-ga-men-tā'ceous.** [**Pergame'neus,** or **Pergamenta'ceus;** from *pergamen'ta*, "parchment."] Like parchment.

Peri (περί). A Greek preposition usually signifying "around," or "about," "near;" it is sometimes *intensive*, being equivalent to "very."

Pĕr'ĭ-anth. [**Perian'thium;** from περί, "about," and ἄνθος, a "flower."] The calyx and corolla taken together, or the whole floral envelope, whatever it may consist of, is sometimes called the perianth. Also termed PERIGONIUM.

Pĕr-ĭ-an'the-us.* Provided with a perianth: perian'theous.

Péricarde. See PERICARDIUM.

Pĕr-ĭ-car'dĭ-ac, or **Pĕr-ĭ-car-di'a-cal.** [**Pericardi'acus.**] Belonging to the pericardium.

Pĕr-ĭ-car-dit'ic. [**Pericardit'icus.**] Belonging to *pericarditis*.

Pĕr-ĭ-car-di'tis, *idis.** [From *pericar'dium.*] Inflammation of the pericardium.

Pĕr-ĭ-car'dĭ-um.* [From περί, "about," and καρδία, the "heart."] (Fr. *Péricarde*, pà'rè'kaRd'.) The membranous bag which contains the heart.

Pĕr'ĭ-carp. [**Pericar'pium;** from περί, "about," and καρπός, "fruit."] A seed-vessel; a ripened ovary. The pericarp and the contained seeds together constitute the *fruit* in the botanical sense of the term. It consists of an epicarp, endocarp, and mesocarp, which last in fleshy fruits is called sarcocarp.

Pĕr-ĭ-car'pic, or **Pĕr-ĭ-car'pĭ-al.** [**Pericarpia'lis.**] Belonging to a pericarp.

Pĕr-ĭ-chæ'tĭ-um.* [From περί, "about," and χαίτη, a "hair."] A scaly sheath investing the fertile flower and base of the foot-stalk of some mosses.

Pĕr-ĭ-chon-drĭ-o-dȳn'ĭ-a.* [From *perichon'drium*, and ὀδύνη, "pain."] Pain of the *perichondrium.*

Pĕr-ĭ-chon-drit'ĭ-cus.* Belonging to *perichondritis.*

Pĕr-ĭ-chon-dri'tis, *idis.** [From *perichon'drium.*] Inflammation of the *perichondrium.*

Pĕr-ĭ-chon'drĭ-um.* [From περί, "about," and χόνδρος, a "cartilage."] A membrane forming the immediate covering of cartilages.

Pĕr-ĭ-clin'ĭ-um.* [From περί, "around," and κλίνη, a "bed."] The involucre of the *Compositæ;* the collection of bracts which surround an assemblage of syngenesious flowers.

Pĕr-ĭ-co-rol'le-us.* [From περί, "around," and *corol'la.*] Applied in the plural feminine (*Pericorol'leæ*) to a Jussieuan division of the *Monopetaleæ*, including dicotyledonous plants with perigynous corols.

Pĕr-ĭ-cra'nĭ-um.* [From περί, "around," and κρανίον, the "cranium."] The membrane immediately covering the bones of the cranium.

Pĕr-ĭ-des-mi'tis, *idis.** [From *peri-des'mium.*] Inflammation of the *peridesmium.*

Pĕr-ĭ-des'mĭ-um.* [From περί, "around," and δέσμιον, a "band."] The membrane which covers the ligaments.

Pĕr-ĭ-did'ȳ-mis.* [From περί, "about," and δίδυμος, a "testicle."] The serous coat which covers the testes.

Pe-rid'ĭ-um.* [Diminutive of πήρα, a "leathern pouch."] The round, membranous, dry case of the seeds of some angiospermatous mushrooms. The envelope of fruit.

Pĕr'ĭ-gee. [**Perigæ'um;** from περί, "about," or "near," and γῆ, the "earth."] That point of the moon's orbit which is nearest to the earth.

Pĕr-ĭ-glot'tis, *idis.** [From περί,

"about," and γλῶττα, the "tongue."] The villous membrane covering the tongue.

Pĕr-ĭ-go'nĭ-um,* or **Pĕr'ĭ-gōne.** [From περί, "around," and γονή, a "seed," or "fruit."] The same as PERIANTH, which see.

Pĕr-ĭ-ġȳn'ĭ-um.* [From περί, "around," and γυνή, a "woman," or "female."] The urceolate body formed in the genus *Carex* by two bracts, which become confluent at their edges and enclose the pistil.

Pe-riġ'ȳ-nous. [**Periġ'ynus;** from the same.] Applied to stamens when situated around the ovary; adnate to the base of the ovary, or to the calyx.

Pĕr-ĭ-he'lĭ-on.* [From περί, "about," or "near," and ἥλιος, the "sun."] That point in the orbit of a planet or comet which is nearest to the sun.

Pĕr'ĭ-lȳmph. [From περί, "around," and *lym'pha*, "water," or "watery fluid:" so named because poured around in the canals of the ear.] See COTUNNIUS, WATER OF.

Pe-rim'e-ter. [**Perim'etron,** or **Perim'etrum;** from περί, "around," and μέτρον, a "measure."] The line which bounds any plane figure. When applied to a circular ellipse, it is equivalent to the circumference.

Pĕr-ĭ-me'trĭ-a.* [From περί, "around," and μετρέω, to "measure."] The measuring of the circumference or of all the sides of any plane figure: perim'etry.

Pĕr-ĭ-mȳs'ĭ-um.* [From περί, "around," and μῦς, a "muscle."] The delicate membrane immediately covering the muscles. Also termed *vagi'na muscula'ris*, or "muscular sheath."

Pĕr-ĭ-næ'o-çēle.* [From περίναιον, the "perinæum," and κήλη, a "tumor."] Hernia, or rupture, in the perinæum.

Pĕr-ĭ-næ'um,* or **Pĕr-ĭ-ne'um.** [Etymology uncertain.] (Fr. *Périnée*, pȧ'rē'nȧ'.) The space between the anus and the genital organs. Applied by some writers to the entire space between the *Os coccygis* and the arch of the pubis.

Pĕr-ĭ-næ'us.* The same as PERINEAL, which see.

Pĕr-ĭ-ne'al, or **Per-ĭ-næ'al.** [**Pĕrinæa'lis.**] Belonging to the perinæum.

Périnée. See PERINÆUM.

Pĕr-ĭ-ne-phri'tis.* [From περί, "around," and νεφρός, a "kidney."] (Fr. *Phlegmon périnéphrétique*, flĕg'mōɴɢ' pȧ'-rē'nȧ'fʀȧ'tēk'.) Inflammation of the peritonæal covering of the kidney.

Pĕr-ĭ-ne'phrĭ-um,* or **Pĕr-ĭ-ne'phrus.*** [From περί, "around," and νεφρός, the "kidney."] The membrane immediately enveloping the kidney.

Perineum. See PERINÆUM.

Pĕr-ĭ-neū'rĭ-on,* or **Pĕr-ĭ-neū'rĭ-um.*** [From περί, "around," and νεῦρον, a "nerve."] The *theca* or membranous covering of a nerve; the neurilemma.

Périnèvre, pȧ'rē'nĕvʀ'. [From περί, "around," and νεῦρον, a "nerve."] A French term for NEURILEMMA, which see.

Pe'rĭ-od. [**Peri'odus;** from περί, "around," and ὁδός, a "way," or "journey."] Literally, a "journeying round," a "circuit." The time in which one of the heavenly bodies describes its orbit; hence, a stated time. The space of time during which a disease prevails from its access to its declension.

Pe-rĭ-od'ĭ-cal. [**Period'icus;** from *peri'odus*, a "period."] Coming round or returning at certain, or stated, times.

Pĕr-ĭ-o-diç'ĭ-tȳ. [**Periodiç'itas;** from *period'icus*, "periodical."] The tendency of certain phenomena to recur at stated times, as, for example, the paroxysms of an intermittent, the *catamenia*, the budding of plants, etc.

Pe-rĭ-o-don-ti'tis, *idis.** [From περί, "about," and ὀδούς, a "tooth."] Inflammation of the lining membrane of the socket of a tooth.

Pe-rĭ-od'o-scope. [**Periodos'copus;** from περίοδος, a "period," and σκοπέω, to "observe."] An instrument for determining the date of menstruation, labor, etc., and for other calculations.

Pe-ri'o-dus Lu-na'ris.* ("Lunar Period.") The catamenial or menstrual period.

Pĕr-ĭ-or'bĭ-ta.* [From περί, "around," and *or'bita*, the "orbit."] The lining membrane of the orbit or socket of the eye; the periosteum of the orbit.

Périoste. See PERIOSTEUM.

Pĕr-ĭ-os-te-ĭ'tis.* The same as PERIOSTITIS, which see.

Pĕr-ĭ-os'te-um.* [From περί, "around," and ὀστέον, a "bone."] (Fr. *Périoste*, pȧ'rē'ost'.) The thin, delicate membrane forming the immediate covering of the bones.

Pĕr-ĭ-os-ti'tis, *idis.** [From *perios'teum*.] Inflammation of the periosteum.

Pĕr-ĭ-os-to'ma, *a'tis.** [From περί, "around," and *osto'ma*, an "osseous tumor."] A morbid osseous formation surrounding a bone: a periostome.

Pĕr-ĭ-os-to'sis.* The progress or formation of *periostoma*.

Pĕr-ĭ-pet'a-lous. [**Peripet'alus;** from περί, "around," and πέταλον, a "petal."] Surrounding the petals.

Pĕr-ĭ-pha-ci'tis, idis.* [From *periph'acus.*] Inflammation of the capsule of the eye; circumfused inflammation of the lens.

Pe-riph'a-cus.* [From περί, "around," and φακός, a "lentil," and hence a "lens."] The capsule of the lens of the eye.

Pe-riph'e-ral. [From *periphe'ria*, the "periphery."] Belonging to the periphery of any roundish substance. Applied by Dr. Barclay as meaning "towards the circumference."

Pĕr-ĭ-phĕr'ic, or **Pĕr-ĭ-phĕr'ĭ-cal.** [**Peripher'icus.**] Relating to the periphery, or situated around the periphery of an organ.

Peripher'ic Im'pul-ses. A term applied by Naumann to the influence which is transmitted from the nerves of any particular part of the body to the centres of the nervous system (*i.e.* the brain and the spinal cord).

Pe-riph'e-rȳ. [**Periphe'ria;** from περί, "about," and φέρω, to "carry."] The circumference of a circle, ellipse, or other similar figure.

Pĕr-ĭ-phȳl'lum.* [From περί, "around;" and φύλλον, a "leaf."] Applied in the plural (*periphyl'la*) to the scales around the ovary of the *Graminaceæ.*

Pĕr-ip-neū-mo'nĭ-a No'tha.* ("Spurious or Bastard Peripneumony.") A name applied to a variety of acute bronchitis.

Pĕr-ip-neū-mon'ic. [**Peripneumon'icus.**] Belonging to peripneumony.

Peripneumonitis. See PNEUMONIA.

Pĕr-ip-neū'mo-nȳ. [**Peripneumo'nia;** from περί, "around," or "near," and πνεύμων, the "organs of breathing;" hence, perhaps, the principal air-passages.] Inflammation of the substance of the lungs, being that part which surrounds the air-passages. See PNEUMONIA.

Pĕr'ĭ-sperm. [**Perisper'mium,** or **Perisper'mum;** from περί, "around," or "near," and σπέρμα, a "seed."] The albumen of the seed of plants.

Pĕr-ĭ-sper'mate. [**Perisper'matus,** or **Perisper'micus.**] Provided with a perisperm: perisper'mic.

Pĕr-ĭ-sta'chȳ-um.* [From περί, "around," or "near," and σταχύς, a "spike," or "ear."] Applied to the glume of the *Graminaceæ.*

Pĕr-ĭ-stăl'tic. [**Peristal'ticus;** from περιστέλλω, to "contract."] Applied to the peculiar movement of the intestines, like that of a worm in its progress (hence also named *vermicular motion*), by which they gradually propel their contents; applied by M. Hall to all the movements of the heart, stomach, intestines, uterus, etc., which movements are not directly dependent on the spinal marrow.

Pĕr-ĭ-sta-min'e-us.* [From περί, "around," and *sta'men.*] Applied in the plural feminine (*peristamin'eæ*), in the Jussieuan system, to dicotyledonous, apetalous plants, in which the stamens are perigynous.

Pĕr-ĭ-sta-min'ĭ-us.* The same as PERISTAMINEUS.

Pĕr-ĭ-staph-ȳ-li'nus.* [From περί, "around," and σταφυλή, the "uvula."] Belonging to, or connected with, the uvula: peristaphyline. A term applied to two muscles of the palate, the *externus*, or *circumflexus palati*, and the *internus*, or *levator palati mollis.*

Pĕr-ĭ-staph'ȳ-lo Phăr-ȳn-ġe'us* [from φάρυγξ, the "pharynx"]. The first, or upper, portion of the *palato-pharyngeus* muscle; the second, or middle, portion is termed *pharyngo-staphylinus;* the third, or lower, portion, *thyro-staphylinus.*

Pĕr-ĭ-stem'o-nis.* [From περί, "around," and στήμων, a "stamen."] The same as PERISTAMINEUS, which see.

Pe-ris'to-ma, a'tis.* [From περί, "around," and στόμα, a "mouth."] The margin or circumference of a mouth, or of a mouth-like opening: a peristome.

Pĕr'ĭ-stome. [**Peristo'mium;** from the same.] The fringe of rigid processes around the mouth of the spore-case or *theca* of certain mosses.

Pĕr-ĭ-stom'ic. [**Peristom'icus.**] Belonging to a peristome.

Pĕr'ĭ-stȳle. [**Peristy'lus;** from περί, "around," and στῦλος, a "pillar."] A range of columns around an edifice. Also, a series of stamens inserted around the ovary.

Pĕr-ĭ-sȳs'to-le.* [From περί, "around," or "near," and συστολή, "contraction."] The instant of time between the contraction and dilatation of the heart, perceptible, it is said, only in the dying.

Péritoine. See PERITONÆUM.

Pe-rit'o-mous. [From περί, "around," and τέμνω, to "cut."] Applied in Mineralogy to cleavage parallel to the axis and in more than one direction.

Pĕr-ĭ-to-næ'um,* or **Pĕr-ĭ-to-ne'-um.** [From περιτείνω, to "stretch around," or "stretch all over."] (Fr. *Péritoine*, pȧ'rè'twȧN'.) A strong serous membrane investing the entire parietes and viscera of the abdomen.

Pĕr-ĭ-to-ni'tis, idis.* [From *peritonæ'um.*] Inflammation of the peritonæum lining the parietes of the abdomen; when it attacks that investing any of the viscera, the disease usually takes the name of the viscus, as *enteritis, gastritis, hepatitis, nephritis*, etc.

Pĕr-ĭ-tre'mạ, atis.* [From περί, "around," and τρῆμα, a "hole."] The per'itreme. In Entomology, a small piece of hornlike substance surrounding the stigmatic opening along the anterior border of the *episternum*, or *sternum*, of the *Hexap'oda*.

Pe-rit'ro-pạl, or **Pĕr-it'ro-pous.** [From περί, "around," and τρέπω, to "turn."] Horizontal to the axis of the fruit. Applied to an embryo of a plant.

Pĕr-ĭ-zo'mạ.* [From περί, "around," and ζώννυμι, to "gird."] Literally, a "girdle," a "truss." A name for the diaphragm.

Per'kin-ism. A mode of treatment first employed by Dr. Perkins, of Norwich, Connecticut. It consists in applying to the diseased part, the extremities of two metallic rods, made of different metals, and called *Metallic Tractors*. The success obtained was probably through the influence of the imagination.

Per'late. [**Perla'tus;** from the Italian and Spanish *per'la*, a "pearl."] "Pearled." Applied to leaves raised from small, round, firm eminences; also to the expansions of lichens provided with round tubercles, compared to an embroidery of small pearls; and sometimes to plants of which the white flowers are disposed in small oblong bunches.

Perle, pêRl. The French name for PEARL, which see.

Permanent. See PERSISTENT.

Per-man-gan'ic Aç'id. A name proposed for the compound previously called manganesic acid.

Per-me-ạ-bil'ĭ-tў. [**Permeabil'itas, a'***tis;* from *per*, "through," and *me'o*, to "pass."] That property of certain bodies which permits others to pass through their pores.

Per'me-ạ-ble. [**Permeab'ilis;** from the same.] Per'vious; that may be permeated; that possesses permeability.

Per-mis'tion. [**Permis'tio, o'***nis*, or **Permix'tio, o'***nis;* from *per*, "through," or "thorough," and *mis'ceo*, *mis'tum* or *mix'tum*, to "mix."] A complete mingling or mixture.

Per'mu-tate. [**Permuta'tus;** from *permu'to*, *permuta'tum*, to "change," or "interchange."] Applied to flowers in which the abortion of the sexual organs causes a remarkable change in the floral teguments, as in many double flowers.

Per-niç'ious [from *perniç'ies*, "destruction"] **Fe'ver.** A name applied by Dr. Wood to a form of congestive intermittent, on account of its great fatality.

Per'nĭ-o, o'*nis.** [From πτέρνα, the "heel."] A kibe or chilblain.

Per'nio Sim'plex.* ("Simple Chilblain.") Chilblain in which the cuticle is unbroken.

Pĕr-o-næ'us,* or **Pĕr-o-ne'us.*** [From περόνη, the "fibula."] Perone'al. Belonging to or connected with the fibula.

Peronæ'us (or **Perone'us**) **Bre'vis.*** ("Short Peronæal [Muscle].") A muscle of the leg, situate below the *peronæus longus*. It is attached above to the outer surface of the fibula.

Peronæ'ụs Lon'gus.* ("Long Peronæal [Muscle].") A muscle placed at the outer part of the leg, and under the sole of the foot.

Peronæ'us Ter'tius.* ("Third Peronæal [Muscle].") A muscle arising from the lower third of the fibula, and inserted into the outer metatarsal bone.

Pĕr'o-ne.* [Gr. περόνη.] The fibula, or external bone of the leg.

Péroné, pȧ'ro'nȧ'. The French term for FIBULA, which see.

Pĕr-o-ne'ạl. Belonging to the fibula. See PERONÆUS.

Peroneus. See PERONÆUS.

Per. op. emet. = *Perac'tâ operatio'ne emet'ici.** "When the operation of the emetic is finished."

Per-ox'ĭ-dāt-ed. [**Peroxyda'tus.**] Applied to a metal, or other simple body, in the state of a peroxide.

Per-ox'īde. [**Perox'ydum;** from *per*, "intensive," and *ox'ydum*, an "oxide."] The compound which results from the combination of a simple body with the maximum of oxygen.

Pĕr'rў. [**Vi'num Pyra'ceum.**] [From the French *Poire*, a "pear."] A vinous liquor made from pears, in the same way as cider is made from apples.

Per'sĭ-cạ.* [From *Per'sia*, its native country.] The peach-tree, or the *Amyg'dalus Per'sica*.

Per-sis'tent. [**Persis'tens;** from

persis'to, to "continue," to "persevere."] Constant; permanent; remaining, as the leaves of evergreens through the winter, and the calyx of many plants until the fruit is formed.

Per'so-nate. [**Persona'tus;** from *perso'na*, a "character in a drama," a "mask."] Masked; disguised. Applied to certain flowers.

Per-spe-cil'lum.* [From *per*, "through," and *spe'cio*, to "behold."] An eye-glass; in the plural (*perspecil'la*) spectacles.

Per-spi-rā'tion. [**Perspira'tio, o'nis;** from *perspi'ro, perspira'tum*, to "breathe through."] The fluid secreted by the extremities of the cutaneous arteries on the surface of the body; sweat. See DIAPHORESIS, HIDROSIS, SUDATION, and SUDOR.

Perspiration, Diminished. See ADIAPHORESIS, ADIAPNEUSTIA, and ANIDROSIS.

Perspira'tion, In-sen'sĭ-ble. The same as TRANSPIRATION, which see.

Perspiration, Morbid. See EPHIDROSIS.

Perspiration, Obstructed. See ADIAPHORESIS, and ANIDROSIS.

Perturba'tio (per-tur-ba'she-o) **Crit'ĭ-ca.*** A critical disturbance or excitement of the organism, forming the crisis of a disease.

Per-tur-bā'tion. [**Perturba'tio, o'nis;** from *per*, "very," or "greatly," and *tur'bo, turba'tum*, to "disturb."] In Pathology, excessive restlessness or disquiet. Applied in Astronomy to the deviation of a celestial body from the elliptic orbit which it would describe if acted upon by no other attractive force than that of the sun or central body around which it revolves.—(BRANDE.)

Per-tuse'. [**Pertu'sus;** from *pertun'do, pertu'sum*, to "pierce."] Pierced with large holes distributed irregularly. Applied to certain parts of plants.

Per-tus'sis.* [From *per*, intensive, and *tus'sis*, a "cough."] (Fr. *Toux convulsive*, too kôɴ'vül'sêv', and *Coqueluche*, kôk'lüsh'.) Hooping-cough. A contagious disease characterized by a convulsive strangulating cough, with hooping, returning by fits which are usually terminated by vomiting. A genus of the order *Spasmi*, class *Neuroses*, of Cullen's Nosology.

Pĕr-u-if'er-us.* [From *Peruvia'nus*, "Peruvian," and *fe'ro*, to "bear."] Literally, "bearing what is Peruvian:" as, *Myrospermum Peruiferum*, the "*Myrospermum* which produces the Peruvian [Balsam]."

Pĕr'u-late. [**Perula'tus.**] Having bud-scales (*perulæ*).

Pĕr'ule. [**Per'ula;** diminutive of *pe'ra*, a "shepherd's pouch."] In Botany, a kind of sac formed by the prolonged, adherent bases of two lobes of the perigone of certain *Orchideæ;* also, the envelope of buds of trees of cold climates; a bud-scale.

Peruvian Balsam. See BALSAM OF PERU.

Peruvian Bark. See CINCHONA.

Pe-ru-vĭ-a'nus.* Belonging to Peru: Peru'vian.

Per-vĭ-ġil'ĭ-um.* [From *per*, intensive, and *vig'ilo*, to "watch."] Disinclination to sleep; watching; vigilance.

Pĕs,* gen. **Pe'dis.** [From πούς, a "foot."] (Fr. *Pied*, pe-à'.) The foot; the base on which the body rests when standing. It consists of the *tarsus, metatarsus*, and toes; with their blood-vessels, nerves, tendons, sheaths, and integuments.

Pes An-se-ri'nus.* ("Goose-Foot.") The distribution of the facial nerve, so called from a fancied resemblance; the parotidean plexus.

Pes Equinus. See TALIPES EQUINUS.

Pes Hip-po-cam'pi.* ("Foot of the Hippocampus.") Properly, the *anterior* part of the *hippocampus*, but often used as synonymous with *hippocampus*.

Pĕs'sa-rȳ. [**Pessa'rium;** from πεσσός, an "oval-shaped stone."] (Fr. *Pessaire*, pĕs'sêʀ'.) An instrument in the form of a ring, or ball, for introduction into the vagina, to prevent or remedy the prolapse of the uterus.

Peste. See PESTIS.

Pĕs-tif'er-ous. [**Pes'tifer;** from *pes'tis*, a "plague," and *fe'ro*, to "bear," or "produce."] Producing or causing pestilence.

Pĕs'tĭ-lence. [**Pestilen'tia,** and **Pes'tis.**] A contagious or infectious disease which is epidemic, or endemic, and fatal; a plague.

Pĕs-tĭ-len'tial, or **Pĕs'tĭ-lent.** [**Pestilentia'lis.**] Pertaining to pestilence; producing the plague, or pestilence.

Pĕs'tis.* (Fr. *Peste*, pĕst.) The plague, a disease characterized by typhus fever, great prostration of strength, buboes, carbuncles, *petechiæ*, hæmorrhage, and sometimes by diarrhœa A genus of the order *Exanthemata*, class *Pyrexiæ*, of Cullen's Nosology.

Pes'tle. [**Pistil'lum.**] An instrument to pound with in a mortar.

Pet'al. [Lat. **Pet'alum;** Gr. πέταλόν, an "expanded leaf."] A flower-leaf; a leaf of a corolla.

Pet-a-lan'thus.* [From πέταλον, a "petal," and ἄνθος, a "flower."] Having flowers with petals.

Pe-tal'i-form. [**Petalifor'mis;** from πέταλον, a "petal."] Shaped like a petal; petaloid.

Pet-a-lo'dēs.* [From πέταλον, a "petal," and εἶδος, a "form."] Resembling petals; also, having petals, or the appearance of petals.

Pet-a-lo'de-us.* The same as Petalodes, which see.

Pet'a-loid. [**Petaloi'des;** from πέταλον, a "petal," and εἶδος, a "form."] Resembling a petal.

Pet'a-lous. Having petals.

Pe-te'chi-a,* plural **Pe-te'chi-æ.** [From *pete'chio*, a "flea-bite."] A small red or purplish spot, like a flea-bite.

Pete'chiæ si'ne Fe'bre.* ("Petechiæ without Fever.") A term applied to *purpura simplex*, or petechial scurvy.

Pe-te'chi-al, or pe-tek'e-al. [**Petechia'lis.**] Belonging to *petechiæ*.

Pe-ti-o-lā'ceous. [**Petiola'ceus;** from *peti'olus*, a "petiole."] Applied to buds when the bases of the petioles, dilated into shells, form the investiture of the young shoot.

Pet'i-o-lar. [**Petiola'ris.**] Belonging to a petiole, or borne on a petiole.

Pet'i-o-late. [**Petiola'tus.**] Provided with a petiole.

Pet-i-o-lā'tion. [**Petiola'tio, o'***nis.*] The state of leaves provided with a petiole.

Pet'i-ole. [**Peti'olus;** diminutive of *pes*, a "foot."] The foot-stalk of a leaf; a leaf-stalk.

Pet-i-ol'u-late. [**Petiolula'tus.**] Applied to a foliole borne upon a petiolule.

Pet'i-o-lule. [**Petiol'ulus;** diminutive of *peti'olus*, a "petiole."] The particular petiole of each foliole in a compound leaf.

Petit Argent, peh-tē' tar'zhŏng'. A French term for Platinum, which see.

Petit (peh-tē'), **Ca-năl' of.** A small triangular canal, between the layers of the hyaloid membrane that enclose the crystalline lens: discovered by Petit.

Petite Vérole, peh-tēt' vā'rol'. A French name for "small-pox." See Variola.

Petit Mal, peh-tē' mål. A French term for the slighter form of epilepsy.

Petiveriaceæ,* pet-e-ve-re-a'she-ē. [From *Petive'ria*, one of the genera.] A small natural order of exogenous West Indian or tropical plants (herbs or undershrubs).

Pe-tral'o-ġy̆. [**Petralo'gia;** from πέτρα, a "rock," and λόγος, a "discourse."] The science which treats of the nature of rocks.

Petrelæum. See Petroleum.

Pet-ri-fac'tion. [From *pe'tra*, a "rock," and *fa'cio*, to "make."] The act of petrifying, or converting into stone. Also applied to a body changed into stone. The term petrifaction is applied by Virchow to the change which takes place when any soft part of the body assumes the form or appearance of bone by absorbing calcareous matter. In this sense, it is synonymous with *calcification*, and must not be confounded with *ossification*, which denotes the formation of actual bone.

Petrification. See Petrifaction.

Pet-ro-graph'i-cal. [**Petrograph'icus.**] Belonging to petrography.

Pe-trog'ra-phy̆. [**Petrogra'phia;** from πέτρα, a "rock," and γράφω, to "write."] A description of rocks; or the art of writing on stone.

Pe-tro'le-um.* [From *pe'tra*, a "rock," and *o'leum*, "oil."] "Rock oil." A bituminous liquid substance that flows between rocks, or issues from the earth. The Pharmacopœial name (Lond. and Ed. Ph.) for the *Petroleum Barbadense*.

Petro'leum Bar-ba-den'se.* A kind of tar found in some parts of England and Scotland; mineral tar; termed also *Bitumen Barbadense*.

Pet'ro-lin, or **Pet'ro-line.** [**Petroli'na.**] A substance obtained by distillation from petroleum.

Pet-ro-mas'toid. [From πέτρα, a "rock," and *mastoi'des*.] Applied by Owen to the homologues of the mastoid process in certain *mammalia*.

Pe-troph'i-lus.* [From πέτρα, a "rock," and φιλέω, to "love."] Literally, "loving rocks." Growing in rocky or stony places: petroph'ilous.

Pe-tro'sal. [**Petro'sus;** from πέτρα, a "rock."] Belonging to the petrous portion of the temporal bone.

Petro'sal Si'nus. Applied to each of two sinuses of the dura mater, the *superior* and *inferior*, leading from the cavernous sinus backwards to the lateral sinus: so named because they are adjacent to the petrous bone.

Pet-ro-se-li'num.* [From πέτρα, a "rock," and σέλινον, "parsley:" named because it grows among stony places.] Parsley. A Linnæan genus of the class *Pentandria,* natural order *Apiaceæ.* Also, the Pharmacopœial name (U.S. Ph.) for the root of *Petroseli'num sati'vum.* See APIUM PETROSELINUM.

Petroseli'num Sa-ti'vum.* The systematic name of the common parsley-plant. Also called APIUM PETROSELINUM.

Petroseli'num Vul-ga're.* Another name for PETROSELINUM SATIVUM, which see.

Pe'trous. [**Petro'sus;** from πέτρα, a "rock."] Belonging to, or resembling, a rock or stone. See PETROSAL.

Pew'ter. [Old French, *Peautre,* pō′t'r; modern French, *Étain,* à'tăNᵍ'.] An alloy of tin and lead, to which antimony and copper in small proportions are sometimes added.

Pey'er's Glands [Peye'ri Glan'dulæ], or **Pey'er's Patch'es.** *The glandulæ aggregatæ,* or assemblages of minute glands on the internal surface of the intestines, first noticed by Peyer. According to Virchow, "a Peyer's Patch is nothing more than a lymphatic gland spread out as it were upon the surface."

Pha-ci'tis, i*dis.** [From φακός, the "lentil;" also, the "lens of the eye."] Inflammation of the crystalline lens.

Phac-o-cys'ta,* or **Phac-o-cys'te.*** [From φακός, a "lentil," and κύστη or κύστις, a "bag."] The capsule of the crystalline lens.

Phac-o-cys-tec'to-me.* [From *phacocys'ta,* and ἐκτομή, a "cutting out."] Rognetta's operation for cataract by cutting out a part of the capsule.

Phac-o-cys-tec'to-mus.* The instrument used in the operation of phacocystectomy: a phacocystectome.

Phac-o-cys-ti'tis, i*dis.** [From *phacocys'ta.*] Inflammation of the capsule of the crystalline lens.

Pha-co-i'dēs.* [From φακός, a "lentil," and εἶδος, a "form."] Resembling a lentil in form.

Phacomalacia,* fak-o-ma-la'she-a. [From φακός, a "lentil," or "lens," and μαλακία, "softness."] Softening of the crystalline lens.

Phac-o-plas'ma, a*tis.** [From φακός, a "lentil," and πλάσμα, "any thing moulded."] A cataplasm, or poultice, of lentils; also applied to a poultice of linseed meal.

Phæn-o-car'pus.* [From φαίνομαι, to "appear," and καρπός, "fruit."] Having fruits very apparent.

Phæ-nog'a-mous. [**Phænoga'mius;** from φαίνω, to "appear," and γάμος, "marriage."] Having stamens and pistils distinctly developed; having manifest flowers. See PHANEROGAMUS.

Phænomenon. See PHENOMENON.

Phæ-nom'e-no-sco'pi-a.* [From *phænom'enon,* and σκοπέω, to "examine."] The observation and examination of (morbid) phenomena.

Phag-e-dæ'na.* [From φάγω, to "eat," or "eat away."] A malignant ulcer which spreads very rapidly.

Phagedæ'na Gan-gre-no'sa.* Hospital gangrene.

Phag-e-den'ic. [**Phagedæn'icus.**] Belonging to *phagedæna.*

Pha-lan'ga-gra,* **Pha-lan-gar-thri'tis, i***dis.** [From *pha'lanx,* ἄγρα, a "seizure," and *arthri'tis,* "gout."] Gout of the finger or toe.

Pha-lan'gēs,* the plural of PHALANX, which see.

Pha-lan'gic. [**Phalan'gicus.**] Belonging to the *phalanges.*

Phal'anx* or fā'lanks, plural **Pha-lan'gēs.** [Gr. φάλαγξ, a "battalion."] Applied in the plural to the small bones of the fingers and toes. In Botany, it signifies bundles of adelphous or clustered stamens.

Phal-lăl'gi-a.* [From φαλλός, the "*membrum virile,*" or "penis," and ἄλγος, "pain."] Pain in the *membrum virile.*

Phal-la-neu-rys'ma, a*tis.** [From φαλλός, the "*membrum virile,*" or "penis," and ἀνεύρυσμα, a "widening," also "aneurism."] Aneurism of the penis.

Phal-lo-blen-nor-rhœ'a.* [From φαλλός, the "penis," and *blennorrhœ'a.*] Chronic *blennorrhœa,* or gleet.

Phal-lo-car-ci-no'ma, a*tis.** [From φαλλός, the "penis," and καρκίνωμα, "cancer."] Cancer of the penis.

Phal-lo-i'dēs.* [From φαλλός, the "penis," and εἶδος, a "form."] Resembling a penis.

Phal-lon'cus.* [From φαλλός, the "penis," and ὄγκος, a "tumor."] A morbid swelling of the penis.

Phal-lor-rha'gi-a.* [From φαλλός, the "penis," and ῥήγνυμι, to "burst forth."] A bursting forth of blood from the penis.

Phal-lor-rhœ'a.* [From φαλλός, the "penis," and ῥέω, to "flow."] A flow from the penis (or urethra). Another term for gonorrhœa.

Phan-er-an-the'rus,* **Phan-e-ran'thus.*** [From φανερός, "evident," ἀνθηρός, an "anther," and ἄνθος, a "flower."] Having anthers on the outside: phaneranthe'rous.

Phan-e-rog'a-mous. [**Phanerog'-amus, Phaneroga'mius**; from φανερός, "manifest," "conspicuous," and γάμος, "marriage," or "union."] Having manifest or conspicuous flowers. A term applied to a grand division of plants, called also *flowering*, or *phænogamous*, plants.

Phan-tas'ma, a*tis*.* [From φαντάζω, to "make appear."] Phantasm. An apparition; an imaginary representation of objects not really present, the effect of disease of the eye or brain; phantasy.

Phan-tas-mat'ic. [**Phantasmat'-icus.**] Pertaining to phantasma.

Phan'tom. [**Phanto'ma, a***tis;* from φαντάζω, to "make visible."] The same as PHANTASMA. Also, the small effigy of a child employed to illustrate the progress of labor.

Phar-bi'tis Nil.* A convolvulaceous tropical plant with purgative seeds, which may be substituted for jalap.

Phar-ma-çeū'tic. [**Pharmaceu'-ticus**; from φαρμακεύω, to "use medicines."] Belonging to pharmacy.

Phar-ma-çeū'tics. [**Pharmaceu'-tica**; from the same.] The science of preparing medicines.

Phar-ma-ceū'tist. One skilled in pharmacy; a druggist.

Phar'ma-cist. The same as PHARMACEUTIST.

Phar-ma-co-dȳ-nam'ics. [**Pharmacodynam'ica**; from φάρμακον, a "medicine," also "poison," and δύναμις, "power."] That branch of Materia Medica which treats of the power or effects of medicines and poisons.

Phar-ma-cog'no-sȳ. [From φαρμακον, a "medicine," and γνῶσις, "knowledge."] That branch of Pharmacology which treats of simples or unprepared medicines.

Phar-ma-co-loġ'ĭ-cal. [**Pharmacoloġ'icus.**] Of, or belonging to, Pharmacology.

Phar-ma-col'o-ġȳ. [**Pharmacolo'gia**; from φάρμακον, a "medicine," and λόγος, a "discourse."] A treatise on the art or science of preparing medicines; that branch of science which treats of medicines; pharmacy.

Phar'ma-con.* [Gr. φάρμακον.] A medicine; a drug; also, a poison.

Phar-ma-co-pœ'ia.* [From φάρμακον, a "medicine," and ποιέω, to "make."] A book containing directions for compounding or preparing medicines.

Phar-ma-co-pœ'ial. [**Pharmacopœia'lis.**] Of, or belonging to, a pharmacopœia.

Phar'ma-cȳ. [**Pharma'cia**; from φάρμακον, a "medicine."] The art of preparing medicines to be used in the treatment of diseases; the trade of a druggist.

Phăr-ȳn-găl'ġĭ-a.* [From φάρυγξ, the "throat," or "pharynx," and ἄλγος, "pain."] Pain in the pharynx.

Phăr-ȳn-găl'ġĭ-cus.* Belonging to *pharyngalgia*.

Phăr-ȳn-ġe'al. [**Pharynge'us**; from φάρυγξ, the "pharynx."] Belonging to the pharynx.

Pha-rȳn-ġem-phrax'is.* [From φάρυγξ, the "pharynx," and ἔμφραξις, a "stoppage."] A stoppage or obstruction in the pharynx.

Phăr-ȳn-ġis'mus.* [From φάρυγξ, the "pharynx."] Spasm of the muscles of the pharynx.

Phăr-ȳn-ġi'tis, i*dis*.* [From φάρυγξ, the "pharynx."] Inflammation of the pharynx; also termed *Cynan'che pharynge'a.*

Pha-rȳn'go-dȳn'ĭ-a.* [From φάρυγξ, the "pharynx," and ὀδύνη, "pain."] Pain, spasmodic or chronic, of the pharynx.

Phăr-ȳn-gol'o-ġȳ. [From φάρυγξ, the "pharynx," and λόγος, a "discourse."] That part of Anatomy which treats of the pharynx.

Pha-rȳn'go-pĕr-is'to-le.* [From φάρυγξ, the "pharynx," περί, "around," and στέλλω, to "set," to "arrange;" also, to "bind."] Contraction or constriction of the pharynx. See PHARYNGOSTENIA.

Pha-rȳn'go-ple'ġĭ-a.* [From φάρυγξ, the "pharynx," and πληγή, a "stroke."] A paralysis of the muscles of the pharynx.

Pha-rȳn-gor-rha'ġĭ-a.* [From φάρυγξ, the "pharynx," and ῥήγνυμι, to "burst forth."] A bursting forth or sudden discharge (of blood) from the pharynx.

Pha-rȳn-go-spas'mus.* [From φάρυγξ, the "pharynx," and σπασμός, a "convulsion."] Spasm of the pharynx.

Pha-rȳn-go-ste'nĭ-a.* [From φάρυγξ, the "pharynx," and στένος, a "strait," or "difficulty."] Contraction of the pharynx, like *pharyngoperistole.*

Pha-rȳn'go-tome. [**Pharyngot'-omus**; from φάρυγξ, the "pharynx," and τέμνω, to "cut."] An instrument invented by Petit for scarifying the tonsils and opening abscesses about the fauces.

Phăr-ўn-got'o-mў. [**Pharyngoto'mia;** from the same.] The operation of cutting into the pharynx.

Phăr'ўnx.* [Gr. φάρυγξ.] The common opening or passage of the gullet and windpipe: in other words, the musculo-membranous sac at the back of the mouth and upper part of the œsophagus.

Phase. [Lat. **Pha'sis;** Gr. φάσις, an "appearance."] Applied in Astronomy to the appearance or shape which the moon and some of the planets present, such as gibbous, horned, halved, and round, or full.

Pha-sĭ-an'ĭ-dæ.* [From *phasia'nus,* a "pheasant."] The name of a family of gallinaceous birds, of which the pheasant is the type.

Pha-sĭ-a'nus.* [Named from the river *Phasis,* in Colchis or Pontus, from which it is supposed to have been brought into Europe.] The pheasant. A genus of the order *Gallinaceæ.*

Phasia'nus Col'chĭ-cus.* ("Colchican Pheasant.") The systematic name of the common pheasant, the flesh of which is delicate and easy of digestion.

Phasia'nus Gal'lus.* The systematic name of the common domestic fowl; also called *Gallus domesticus.*

Phat-nor-rha'ġĭ-a.* [From φάτνη, the "socket of a tooth," and ῥήγνυμι, to "break or burst forth."] A sudden discharge of blood from an *alveolus,* or tooth-socket.

Phen-go-pho'bĭ-a.* [From φεγγός, "light," and φόβος, "fear."] A fear or intolerance of light.

Phen'ĭ-cin, or **Phen'ĭ-cĭne.** [**Phœnici'na;** from φοίνιξ, "purple."] A name given by Crum to the substance otherwise named *Indigo-carmina,* which he discovered.

Phe-nom'e-no-graph'ĭ-cal. [**Phænomenograph'icus.**] Belonging to phenomenography.

Phe-nom-e-nog'ra-phў. [**Phænomenogra'phia;** from *phænom'enon,* and γράφω, to "write."] A history of morbid phenomena.

Phe-nom-e-nol'o-ġў. [**Phænomenolo'gia;** from *phænom'enon,* and λόγος, a "discourse."] The science which treats of the symptoms or phenomena of disease.

Phe-nom'e-non. [**Phænom'enon,** or **Phænom'enum;** from φαίνομαι, to "appear."] An appearance: any thing remarkable.

Phī'al, or **Vī'al.** [**Phi'ala;** from φιάλη, a "shallow cup, or bowl."] A small glass bottle for containing liquid medicines.

Philadelphaceæ,* fil-a-del-fa'she-ē. A small natural order of exogenous shrubs, natives of India, Japan, and North America. It includes the *Philadel'phus* (Syringa, or Mock-Orange).

Phĭ-los'o-pher's Stone. [**La'pis Philosopho'rum.**] An imaginary substance which, according to the opinion of the alchemists, had the power to transmute base metals into gold.

Phĭ-los'o-phў. [**Philoso'phia;** from φιλέω, to "love," and σοφία, "wisdom."] The knowledge of things, natural and moral, founded upon reason and experience. The science of causes and principles. It is sometimes employed to signify the sum total of systematic human knowledge.

Phil'tre, or **Phil'ter.** [From φιλέω, to "love."] A love-potion; a medicine often used by the ancients for the purpose of inspiring love.

Philydraceæ,* fil-e-dra'she-ē. [From *Phily'drum,* one of the genera.] A small natural order of endogenous herbaceous plants, found in China and New Holland.

Phi-mo'sis.* [From φιμόω, to "muzzle," to "bind."] A constriction of the extremity of the prepuce, so that it cannot be drawn back to uncover the glans.

Phi-mot'ĭ-cus.* Belonging to *phimosis:* phimotic.

Phleb-ec-ta'sĭ-a,* or **Phle-bec'ta-sis.*** [From φλέψ, a "vein," and ἐκτείνω, to "extend."] Terms for *varix,* an enlarged or swelled vein.

Phleb-ec-to'pĭ-a.* [From φλέψ, a "vein," and ἔκτοπος, "out of place."] The abnormal situation of a vein, from original malformation or the pressure of a tumor.

Phle-bī'tis, *idis.** [From φλέψ, a "vein."] Inflammation of a vein. It is distinguished by a hard, cord-like line, tender or painful on being touched, extending along the course of a vein or veins, from an incision or wound.

Phlebi'tis, U'ter-ĭne. A term for puerperal fever.

Phle-bo'dēs.* [From φλέψ, a "vein," and εἶδος, a "form."] Resembling a vein; also, having veins.

Phle-bog'ra-phў. [**Phlebogra'-**

phia. from φλέψ, a "vein," and γράφω, to "write."] A description, or history, of the veins.

Phle-bo-i'dēs.* [From φλέψ, a "vein," and εἶδος, a "form."] Resembling a vein: phle'boid.

Phleb'o-lite. [**Phleboli'tes;** from φλέψ, a "vein," and λίθος, a "stone."] Literally, "vein-stone." Applied to small, fibrous, dense bodies sometimes found loose in the veins.

Phle-bol'o-ġy̆. [**Phlebolo'gia;** from φλέψ, a "vein," and λόγος, a "discourse."] A treatise on the veins; the anatomy of the veins.

Phleb'o-me-tri'tis, idis.* [From φλέψ, a "vein," and *metri'tis*, "inflammation of the womb."] Venous *metritis*, or inflammation of the veins of the womb.

Phleb-or-rha'ġĭ-a.* [From φλέψ, a "vein," and ῥήγνυμι, to "burst forth."] Sudden discharge of blood from the rupture of a vein: phlebor'rhagy.

Phleb-or-rhex'is.* [From φλέψ, a "vein," and ῥῆξις, a "breaking," or "bursting."] The bursting, or rupture, of a vein.

Phleb-o-sçe-nog'ra-phy̆. [**Phleboscenogra'phia;** from φλέψ, a "vein," σκηνή, a "scene," and γράφω, to "write."] An illustrated description of the veins. See PHLEBOGRAPHY.

Phleb-o-tom'ĭ-cal. [**Phlebotom'icus.**] Belonging to phlebotomy.

Phle-bot'o-my̆. [**Phleboto'mia;** from φλέψ, a "vein," and τέμνω, to "cut."] The operation of opening a vein; venesection; blood-letting.

Phlegm, flĕm. [Gr. φλέγμα; from φλέγω, to "burn."] Originally, "inflammation," but afterwards applied to certain humors supposed to be the cause of inflammation, and also of diseases unattended with inflammation. One of the four natural humors of the ancients. A name given by the old chemists to a watery distilled liquor, as distinguished from a spirituous liquor. In popular language, the thick viscid mucus secreted by the lungs.

Phlegmasia,* fleg-ma'she-a, plural **Phlegmasiæ,** fleg-ma'she-ē. [From φλέγω, to "burn."] Phleg'masy. Inflammation accompanied by fever. In the plural, inflammations with fever. An order of the class *Pyrexiæ* of Cullen's Nosology.

Phleg-ma-sit'ĭ-cus.* Of or belonging to *phlegmasia*, or inflammation; inflammatory.

Phlegmatia,* fleg-ma'she-a. [From φλέγμα, "phlegm," a "watery humor."] Dropsical swelling.

Phlegma'tia Do'lens.* ("Painful Phlegmatia.") White-leg. A disease sometimes occurring in women soon after delivery, characterized by pain, increasing to an excruciating degree, along the thigh and leg to the foot, each part gradually becoming much swelled and very tense.

Phleg-mat'ic. [**Phlegmat'icus.**] Relating to phlegm; abounding in phlegm; dull; sluggish.

Phleg'mon. [**Phleg'mone;** from φλέγω, to "burn."] A bright red inflammation.

Phleg'mo-noid. [**Phlegmonoi'des;** from φλεγμονή, a "tumor," and εἶδος, a "form."] Resembling phlegmon.

Phlegmonosus. See PHLEGMONOUS.

Phleg'mo-nous. [**Phlegmono'des;** from φλεγμονή, "tumor," or "inflammation."] Of the nature of phlegmon; pertaining to phlegmon.

Phlœ-o-ri'zin, written also **Phlorid'zin,** or **Phlo-rid'zine.** [From φλοιός, "bark," and ῥίζα, a "root."] A peculiar substance discovered in the bark of the root of the apple, pear, and cherry tree.

Phlo-ġis'tic. [**Phlogis'ticus.**] Belonging to the supposed principle named phlogiston; also, synonymous with "inflammatory."

Phlo-ġis'tĭ-cāt-ed Air, or **Phlogis'ticated Gas.** A term for nitrogen.

Phlo-ġis'ton.* [From φλογίζω, to "burn."] An imaginary principle by which Stahl and the chemists of his school accounted for the phenomena of combustion. They supposed the matter of fire existing in combustible bodies to be expelled in the process of combustion. By some, phlogiston was thought to be identical with hydrogen; while oxygen was termed *dephlogisticated* air, that is, air destitute of phlogiston (or the principle of inflammability).

Phlo-gos'ic. [**Phlogos'icus;** Fr. *Phlogosique*, flo'go'zėk'.] In Pathology, belonging to *phlogosis*. Applied in Geology to an order of pyrogenous earths, comprehending the PSEUDO-VOLCANIC, which see.

Phlo-go'sis.* [From φλογόω, to "inflame."] Inflammation: some writers apply it to erysipelatous inflammation. A genus of the order *Phlegmasiæ*, class *Pyrexiæ*, of Cullen's Nosology.

Phlo-got'ic. [**Phlogot'icus.**] Belonging to *phlogosis;* inflammatory.

Phlo-got'ĭ-ca.* [From *phlogot'icus,* "inflammatory."] The name of an order in Dr. Good's Nosology, comprising the various forms of inflammation.

Phloridzin. See PHLŒORIZIN.

Phlȳc-tæ'na.* [From φλύω, to "bubble up."] A pellucid vesicle coning a serous fluid.

Phlȳc-tæ-no'dēs.* [From *phlyctæ'na.*] Having or resembling *phlyctæna.*

Phlȳc-tæn'u-la.* [Diminutive of *phlyctæ'na.*] A little vesicle; applied to such as occur in scrofulous inflammation of the conjunctiva, filled with a thin, colorless fluid.

Phlȳc'te-noid. [**Phlyctænoi'des;** from *phlyctæ'na,* and εἶδος, a "form."] Resembling *phlyctæna.*

Phlȳc'tis, idis.* [From φλύζω, to "boil."] The same as PHLYCTÆNA, which see.

Phly'sis.* [From φλύζω, or φλύω, to "boil," to "swell up."] A generic term applied by Dr. Good to the different forms of whitlow.

Phly-zā'cious. [**Phlyza'cius.**] Belonging to a *phlyzacium.*

Phlyzacium,* fli-za'she-um. [From φλύζω, to "boil," to "swell up."] Applied by Willan to a small pustule containing pus, raised on a round, hard, inflamed base, and terminating in a dark-colored scab.

Phœnicina. See PHENICIN.

Phœn-ĭ-cis'mus.* [From φοῖνιξ, "red."] A name given to RUBEOLA, which see.

Phœn-ĭ-cis'tĭ-cus.* Belonging to *phœnicismus.*

Phœn-ĭ-cop'ȳ-rus.* [From φοῖνιξ, a "purple-red," and *py'rum,* a "pear."] Having pyriform and red fruit.

Phœ'nix Dac-tȳ-lif'e-ra.* The systematic name of the date palm-tree.

Phœn-o-di'na,* or **Phœn'o-dīne.** [From *phœno'des,* "of a blood-color."] A term for the *Cruor sanguinis,* or blood clot; also used for *hæmatina.*

Phœn-o-din'ĭ-cus.* Belonging to *phœnodi'na:* phenodinic.

Pho-nā'tion. [**Phona'tio, o'nis;** from φωνή, the "voice."] The formation of the voice; also, the physiology of the voice.

Pho-net'ic. [**Phonet'icus;** from φωνή, the "voice."] Pertaining to the voice; pertaining to, or representing, articulate sounds.

Phon'ic. [**Phon'icus;** from the same.] Sometimes the same as PHONETIC. In Physics, the point or place in which is situated either the person who speaks, or the body which emits the sound, is called the *phonic centre.*

Phon'ĭ-ca.* [From *phon'icus,* "pertaining to sound."] Diseases affecting the vocal avenues. The name of an order in Good's Nosology.

Phon'ics. [From the same.] The doctrine or science of sounds. Sometimes employed in the same manner as ACOUSTICS.

Phon-o-camp'sis.* [From φωνή, the "voice," and κάμψις, a "bending," or "reflecting."] In Physics, a throwing back, or reflecting, of sound; echo.

Phon-o-camp'tic. [**Phonocamp'ticus.**] Belonging to *phonocampsis;* able, or adapted, to reflect sounds. The *phonocamptic centre* is the situation where the ear is placed in order to receive reflected sounds.

Phon-o-camp'tĭ-ca.* [From *phonocamp'sis,* an "echo."] That branch of Physics which treats of the reflection of sound: phonocamp'tics.

Phon-o-chor'dæ.* [From φωνή, a "voice," and *chor'dæ,* "chords."] The *Chordæ vocales,* or vocal chords.

Pho-nog'ra-phȳ. [**Phonogra'phia;** from φωνή, "voice," or "sound," and γράφω, to "write."] The art of writing words according to their pronunciation or sound. Also, a description of the voice or of sound.

Pho-nol'o-ġȳ. [**Phonolo'gia;** from φωνή, "voice," or "sound."] The science which treats of the modifications of the voice, or of the distinctive character of different articulate sounds.

Phos'ġēne. [**Phos'genus;** from φῶς, "light," and γένω, to "be born."] Literally, "born of light." Applied to chloro-carbonic gas, because it is produced by the action of the solar rays upon a mixture of equal parts of chlorine and carbonic oxide gas.

Phosgene Gas. See PHOSGENE, and PHOTOGENE GAS.

Phos'phāte. [**Phos'phas, a'tis.**] A salt formed of phosphoric acid and a base.

Phos'phate of Lime. [**Cal'cis Phos'phas, a'tis.**] A combination of phosphoric acid and lime, forming the solid, or earthy, portion of bones.

Phosphate of Soda. See SODÆ PHOSPHAS.

Phos'phāt-ed. [**Phospha'tus;**

from *phos'phas*, a "phosphate."] Applied to a base converted into a phosphate by combination with phosphoric acid.

Phos-phat'ic. [**Phosphat'icus.**] Belonging to, or containing, a phosphate.

Phos'phite. [**Phos'phis, i'tis.**] A combination of phosphorous acid with a base.

Phos'pho-rāt-ed. [**Phosphora'tus**; from *phos'phorus.*] Combined, or impregnated, with phosphorus.

Phosphore. See PHOSPHORUS.

Phos-pho-rĕs'çence. [**Phosphorescen'tia**; from *phos'phorus.*] The quality of becoming luminous at the ordinary temperature in the dark. A luminous appearance presented by many vegetable and animal substances, such, for example, as phosphorescent (decaying) wood, the glow-worm, jelly-fish, etc.

Phos-pho-rĕs'çent. [**Phosphores'cens**; from the same.] Emitting light without heat, like phosphorus. See PHOSPHORESCENCE.

Phos-phor'ic. [**Phosphor'icus**; from the same.] Applied to an acid of the third degree of oxidation of phosphorus.

Phos'pho-rous. [**Phosphoro'sus**; from the same.] Applied to an acid which contains one equivalent of phosphorus and three of oxygen.

Phos-pho-ru'rĭ-a.* [From *phos'phorus*, and οὖρον, the "urine."] The presence of phosphorus in the urine. See PHOTURIA.

Phos'pho-rus.* [Gr. φωσφόρος, the "day-star;" from φῶς, "light," and φέρω, to "bring."] (Fr. *Phosphore*, fos'for'.) Originally, the "day-star." A translucent, nearly colorless substance, resembling wax, without taste, but having a peculiar smell. It is extremely inflammable, and should be kept under water and protected from the light. When exposed to the air, it emits white fumes which are luminous in the dark. It has been placed on the primary list of the Materia Medica of the U.S. Pharmacopœia for 1860. In nature it is always found in combination with oxygen, *i.e.* in the state of phosphoric acid. Phosphorus, in small doses, acts as a powerful general stimulant; in large doses, it is an irritant poison.

Phosphorus, Baldwin's. See HOMBERG'S PHOSPHORUS.

Phosphorus of Canton. See CANTON'S PHOSPHORUS.

Phos'phu-ret. [**Phosphure'tum**; from *phos'phorus.*] A combination of phosphorus with a combustible body, or a metallic oxide.

Phos'phu-ret-ed. The same as PHOSPHORATED, which see.

Phosphuria. See PHOTURIA.

Pho-tăl'gĭ-a.* [From φῶς, φωτός, "light," and ἄλγος, "pain."] Pain arising from too much light: photalgy.

Phot'ĭ-ca.* [From φῶς, φωτός, "light."] The doctrine of the nature and appearance of light: phot'ics.

Phot'ĭ-cus.* Of or belonging to light: photic.

Pho-to-camp'sis.* [From φῶς, φωτός, "light," and κάμψις, a "bending."] Refraction of the rays of light.

Pho-to-dȳs-pho'rĭ-a.* [From φῶς, φωτός, "light," and *dyspho'ria*, "restlessness."] Intolerance of light.

Pho'to-ġēne Gas. The same as PHOSGENE, which see.

Pho-to-ġen'ic. [**Photogen'icus**; from φῶς, φωτός, "light," and γένω, to "be born or produced."] Produced or created by the light, as photographic pictures.

Pho-to-graph'ic, or **Pho-to-graph'ĭ-cal.** [**Photograph'icus.**] Belonging to photography; photogenic.

Pho-tog'ra-phȳ. [**Photogra'phia**; from φῶς, φωτός, "light," and γράφω, to "delineate."] The production of the images of objects by the action of light on metal, paper, glass, etc., prepared for the purpose by chemical agencies. This art is sometimes called, from the name of M. Daguerre, the inventor, *daguerreotype*, which term is also applied to a picture or representation thus produced.

Pho-to-loġ'ĭ-cal. [**Photoloġ'icus.**] Belonging to photology.

Pho-tol'o-ġȳ. [**Photolo'gia**; from φῶς, φωτός, "light," and λόγος, a "discourse."] The science or doctrine of light.

Pho-tom'e-ter. [**Photom'etrum**; from φῶς, "light," and μέτρον, a "measure."] An instrument by which to ascertain the comparative intensity of light.

Pho-to-met'rĭ-cal. [**Photomet'ricus.**] Belonging to photometry.

Pho-tom'e-trȳ. [**Photome'tria**; from φῶς, φωτός, "light," and μετρέω, to "measure."] The science which treats of the measurement of light. Also, the act of measuring light.

Pho-ton'o-sos,* **Pho-ton'o-sus.*** [From φῶς, "light," and νόσος, "disease."] Applied to any disease arising from exposure to a glare of light, as snow-blindness, sun-stroke, etc.

Pho-to-pho'bi-a.* [From φῶς, "light," and φόβος, "fear."] A dread or intolerance of light.

Pho-to-phob'i-cus.* Belonging to *photophobia:* photopho'bic.

Pho-top'sy̆. [**Photop'sia;** from φῶς, "light," and ὄψις, "sight."] An appearance or sense of light from internal causes.

Pho-tor-rhex'is.* [From φῶς, "light," and ῥῆξις, a "breaking."] Refraction of the rays of light.

Pho'to-sphere. [**Photosphæ'ra;** from φῶς, "light," and σφαῖρα, a "sphere."] The "Sphere of Light." The luminous atmosphere of the sun.

Pho-tu'ri-a.* [From φῶς, "light," and οὖρον, the "urine."] Urine which has a luminous appearance as it passes from the urethra; luminous urine.

Phrag'ma, atis.* [From φράσσω, to "enclose."] Applied in Botany to a spurious dissepiment of a pericarp.

Phrag'mo-cone. [**Phragmoco'nus;** from φράσσω, to "divide," and κῶνος, a "cone."] The cone of the Belemnite, which is divided into chambers.

Phrénésie. See Phrenitis.

Phren'ic. [**Phren'icus;** from φρήν, the "diaphragm."] Belonging to the diaphragm.

Phren'i-ca.* [From φρήν, the "diaphragm," or parts adjacent to the heart (supposed by the ancients to be the seat of the intellect, as well as of the feelings): hence, the "mind."] Medicines which affect the mental faculties; also, the name of an order in Dr. Good's Nosology, comprising diseases affecting the intellect.

Phre-nit'ic, or **Phre-net'ic.** [**Phrenit'icus.**] Belonging to *phrenitis.*

Phre-ni'tis, idis.* [From φρήν, the "mind."] (Fr. *Phrénésie,* frà'nà'zè'.) Inflammation of the brain; phrenzy. A genus of the order *Phlegmasiæ,* class *Pyrexiæ,* of Cullen's Nosology.

Phren-o-log'i-cal. [**Phrenolog'icus.**] Belonging to Phrenology.

Phre-nol'o-gy̆. [**Phrenolo'gia;** from φρήν, the "mind," and λόγος, a "discourse."] A treatise on the faculties of the human mind, and the organs by which they are said to manifest themselves. Usually applied to the science (if so it may be called) which treats of the faculties and propensities of the human mind, as dependent on the development of brain. Each different faculty is supposed to reside in a particular part of the brain, which part is termed the organ of the faculty to which it is appropriated.

Phreno-Magnetism, Phreno-Mesmerism. See Mesmero-Phrenology.

Phrenzy. See Phrenitis.

Phtheiriasis. See Phthiriasis.

Phthiriasis,* the-ri'a-sis. [From φθείρ, a "louse."] A disease in which lice are bred on different parts of the body; called also *Mor'bus pedicula'ris,* or "lousy disease." See Pediculation.

Phthis'i-cal. [**Phthis'icus.**] Belonging to *phthisis;* consumptive.

Phthisicus. See Phthisical.

Phthisie. See Phthisis Pulmonalis.

Phthis-i-ol'o-gy̆. [**Phthisiolo'gia;** from φθίσις, "consumption," and λόγος, a "discourse."] A dissertation or treatise on *phthisis,* or consumption; that branch of Pathology which treats of consumption.

Phthisis,* ti'sis. [From φθίω, to "consume."] Pulmonary consumption, characterized by emaciation, debility, cough, hectic fever, and purulent expectoration.

Phthi'sis Pul-mo-na'lis.* (Fr. *Phthisie,* tè'zè'.) See Pulmonary Consumption.

Phthoe,* tho'ē. [From φθίνω, to "corrupt."] Ulceration of the lungs.

Phy̆-cog'ra-phy̆. [**Phycogra'phia;** from φῦκος, a "fucus," or "sea-weed," and γράφω, to "write."] A history or description of the *Fuci.*

Phy-co-i-da'tus.* [From φῦκος, a "fucus," and εἶδος, "resemblance."] Applied in the plural neuter (*Phycoida'ta*) by Lingbye to a section of the *Hydrophyta* (aquatic plants).

Phy̆-col'o-gy̆. [**Phycolo'gia;** from φῦκος, a "fucus," or "sea-weed," and λόγος, a "discourse."] That part of Botany which treats of the *Fuci.*

Phy̆l-lan'thus.* [From φύλλον, a "leaf," and ἄνθος, a "flower."] Having flowers upon the leaves, with their peduncles adherent to the principal nervure of the leaves: phyllan'thous.

Phy̆l'le-rin. [**Phylleri'na.**] An alkaloid substance obtained from the *Phylleria latifolia.*

Phy̆l-le-ry̆th'rin. [**Phylleryth-ri'na;** from φύλλον, a "leaf," and ἐρυθρός, "red."] The same as Erythrophyll, which see.

Phȳl-lo'dēs.* [From φύλλον, a "leaf," and εἶδος, "resemblance."] Having leaves; resembling leaves.

Phȳl-lo'dĭ-um.* [From the same.] A petiole which dilates so much as to resemble a leaf.

Phȳl-loğ'e-nous. [**Phylloğ'enus;** from φύλλον, a "leaf," and γένω, to "be born," to "grow."] Growing upon leaves.

Phȳl'loid. [**Phylloi'des;** from φύλλον, a "leaf," and εἶδος, a "form."] Resembling a leaf.

Phȳl-lo-phe'in. [**Phyllophæi'na;** from φύλλον, a "leaf," and φαιός, "dusky."] The dusky or brown coloring matter of leaves.

Phȳl-los'po-rus.* [From φύλλον, a "leaf," and σπορά, "seed."] Having the seed in or under the leaf.

Phȳl-lo-tax'is,* or **Phȳl-lo-tax'ȳ.** [From φύλλον, a "leaf," and τάξις, "arrangement."] The arrangement of leaves on the stem. It is a curious fact that the course of development in growing plants is universally spiral. A complete circuit around a stem formed by the spiral line drawn from any leaf to the leaf which is exactly over it, is called a *cycle*.

Phyl-lox-an'thin. [**Phylloxanthi'na;** from φύλλον, a "leaf," and ξανθός, "yellow."] The yellow coloring matter of the leaf of a plant.

Phy'ma, a'is,* plural **Phy'ma-ta.** [From φύω, to "produce."] A tubercle on any external part of the body; also, a genus of Willan's arrangement of cutaneous diseases.

Phy-mat'ic. [**Phymat'icus.**] Belonging to *phyma*.

Phy-ma-to'dēs.* [From *phy'ma.*] Resembling or having *phymata.*

Phȳ'ma-toid. [**Phymatoi'des;** from φῦμα, a "growth," a "tumor," and εἶδος, a "form."] Resembling a tumor.

Phy-ma-to'sis.* [From φῦμα, a "growth," a "tumor."] The formation or progress of tubercular disease.

Phȳs-co'nĭ-a.* [From φύσκων, "big-bellied."] Enlargement of the abdomen, marked by a tumor occupying one part of it, of slow growth, and neither sonorous nor fluctuating. A genus of the order *Intumescentiæ*, class *Cachexiæ*, of Cullen's Nosology.

Phȳs-con'ĭ-cus.* Belonging to *physconia.*

Phȳ-se'ter, e'ris.* [From φυσάω, to "blow."] A "blower;" the spermaceti whale; also called by its Biscayan name of *Cachalot*. A genus of the class *Mammalia*, order *Cetacea*.

Physe'ter Mac-ro-çeph'a-lus.* The systematic name for the species of whale principally affording spermaceti and ambergris.

Phȳs-ĭ-at'rĭ-ca.* [From φύσις, "nature," and ἰατρεία, "medical treatment."] The doctrine or science which treats of the healing powers of nature: physiatrics.

Phȳs-ĭ-at'rĭ-cus.* Belonging to *physiatrica:* physiat'rical.

Phȳs'ic. [From φυσικός, "pertaining to nature," "natural," or "according to the laws of nature."] Applied to the science of medicine, and to medicines employed in the cure of diseases.

Phȳs'ĭ-cal. [**Phys'icus;** from φύσις, "nature."] Belonging to nature; nearly synonymous with *natural*.

Phȳ-sĭ'çian. [From the same.] (Fr. *Médecin*, mād'säɴᴳ'.) A doctor of medicine or physic; one who has been authorized by an incorporated institution to practise medicine.

Phȳs'ics. [**Phys'ica;** from the same.] In its most extensive signification, that science which treats of the nature, laws, etc. of the entire material universe.

The objects of physical science may be studied in three different points of view: they may be examined in relation to their different properties, with respect to their constituent parts, and in regard to their appearance and exterior qualities. These three distinct views give rise to the three great divisions of natural science, namely, Natural Philosophy (or Physics, in a more restricted sense), Chemistry, and Natural History. Natural Philosophy has for its object the properties of bodies, Chemistry studies their elementary principles, and Natural History observes their physiognomy and external characteristics.

Phȳs-ĭ-oğ'e-nȳ. [**Physioge'nia;** from φύσις, "nature," and γένω, to "be born," to "be produced."] The production of things by nature.

Phys-ĭ-og-no-mon'ĭ-ca.* [From φυσιογνωμονέω, to "judge of a man by his features."] The doctrine of judging by the looks or features of the countenance: physiognomon'ics.

Phȳs-ĭ-og-nom'o-nȳ. [**Physiognomo'nia.**] See PHYSIOGNOMY.

Phȳs-ĭ-og'no-mȳ. [**Physiogno'mia;** from φυσιογνωμονέω, to "judge of a man by his features."] The art of judging of the moral and intellectual character by examining the features of the countenance. Also, the study of diseases from an examination of the features or general appearance of the countenance.

Phȳs-ĭ-og'ra-phȳ. [**Physiogra'phia;** from *φύσις*, "nature," and *γράφω*, to "write."] A description of objects which together constitute nature.

Phȳs-ĭ-o-loġ'ĭ-cal. [**Physioloġ'icus.**] Belonging to Physiology.

Phȳs-ĭ-ol'o-ġȳ. [**Physiolo'gia;** from *φύσις*, "nature," and *λόγος*, a "discourse."] The doctrine of vital phenomena, or the science of the functions of living bodies, is divided, according to the two great classes of organized beings, into *animal* and *vegetable* physiology. Animal physiology is by some writers divided into three branches: namely, the physiology of the *sanguineous*, of the *nervous*, and of the *muscular* system. These three systems, which have been termed the *tripod of life*, are intimately linked or mingled together; and they can only be properly studied by keeping constantly in view their relations to each other.

Physiol'ogy, Gen'e-ral. That which regards the general laws of life.

Physiol'ogy, Speç'ial, treats of the nature and functions of particular organs, as of the heart, the lungs, the liver, the kidneys, etc.

Physiology, Vegetable. See VEGETABLE PHYSIOLOGY.

Phȳs-ĭ-on'o-mȳ. [**Physiono'mia;** from *φύσις*, "nature," and *νόμος*, a "law."] The doctrine of the laws of nature.

Phȳs-o-car'pus.* [From *φῦσα*, "wind," and *καρπός*, "fruit."] Having fruit containing air, as the pods of certain plants.

Phȳs-o-col'ĭ-ca.* [From *φῦσα*, "wind," and *col'ica*, the "colic."] Flatulent colic.

Phȳs-o-me'tra.* [From *φῦσα*, "wind," and *μήτρα*, the "womb."] Tympany, or windy swelling of the womb. A genus of the order *Intumescentiæ*, class *Cachexiæ*, of Cullen's Nosology.

Phy-tan-a-to'mĭ-a.* [From *φυτόν*, a "plant," and *anato'mia*, "anatomy."] The anatomy of vegetables.

Phȳt-e-rȳth-ri'na.* [From *φυτόν*, a "plant," and *ἐρυθρός*, "red."] The red coloring matter in plants. See ERYTHROPHYLL.

Phȳ-tiph'a-gous. The same as PHYTOPHAGOUS, which see.

Phȳ-tiv'o-rous. [**Phytiv'orus;** from *φυτόν*, a "plant," and *vo'ro*, to "devour."] Plant-devouring. The same as PHYTOPHAGOUS.

Phy-to-che'mĭ-a.* [From *φυτόν*, a "plant," and *che'mia*, "chemistry."] The chemistry of plants; or vegetable chemistry.

Phȳ-to-chem'ĭ-cal. [**Phytochem'icus.**] Belonging to *phytochemia*.

Phȳ-toġ'e-nȳ, or **Phy-to-ġen'e-sis.*** [**Phytogene'sia;** from *φυτόν*, a "plant," and *γένω*, to "be born."] Germination, the commencement of vegetation; also, the doctrine or science of the generation of plants.

Phȳ-to-ġe-og'ra-phȳ. [**Phytogeogra'phia;** from *φυτόν*, a "plant," *γῆ*, the "earth," and *γράφω*, to "write."] Geographical Botany; or that part of Botany which treats of the geographical distribution of plants.

Phȳ-to-graph'ĭ-cal. [**Phytograph'icus.**] Belonging to phytography.

Phȳ-tog'ra-phȳ. [**Phytogra'phia;** from *φυτόν*, a "plant," and *γράφω*, to "write."] A description of plants. Descriptive Botany; or that part of Botany which treats of the rules to be observed in describing and naming plants.

Phȳ'toid. [**Phytoi'des;** from *φυτόν*, a "plant," and *εἶδος*, a "form."] Resembling a plant.

Phytolaccaceæ,* fi-to-lak-ka'she-ē. A natural order of exogenous plants (herbs or under-shrubs), natives of Africa, India, and America. It includes *Phytolac'ca* (Poke).

Phy-to-lac'çæ Bac'ca,* or **Phytolac'cæ Bac'çæ.*** ("Poke Berry," or "Poke Berries.") The Pharmacopœial name (U.S. Ph.) for the berries of the *Phytolacca decandra*.

Phytolac'cæ Ra'dix.* ("Poke Root.") The Pharmacopœial name (U.S. Ph.) for the root of the *Phytolacca decandra*.

Phȳ'to-līte. [**Phytoli'tes;** from *φυτόν*, a "plant," and *λίθος*, a "stone."] A petrified or fossil plant.

Phȳ-to-loġ'ĭ-cal. [**Phytoloġ'icus.**] Belonging to phytology.

Phȳ-tol'o-ġȳ. [**Phytolo'gia;** from *φυτόν*, a "plant," and *λόγος*, a "discourse."] A treatise on plants, or the science of plants. Botany in general.

Phy'ton. A term applied by some to a simple plant-element, such as, first, the radicle of the embryo, secondly, the joint of stem and leaf; and so on. (See GRAY'S Structural and Systematic Botany.)

Phy-toph′a-gous. [**Phytoph′agus**; from φυτόν, a "plant," and φάγω, to "eat."] Subsisting on the leaves of trees and plants.

Phy-to-phys-i-ol′o-gy. [**Phytophysiolo′gia**; from φυτόν, a "plant," and *physiolo′gia*, "physiology."] The doctrine of the internal economy of plants.

Phy-tot′o-my. [**Phytoto′mia**; from φυτόν, a "plant," and τέμνω, to "cut."] The dissection of vegetables. Vegetable anatomy; the study of the minute structure of plants as revealed by the microscope.

Phy-to-tro′phi-a.* [From φυτόν, a "plant," and τροφή, "nourishment."] The nutrition of plants, and the consideration of the best means for promoting it.

Phy-to-zo′on,* or **Phy-to-zo′um.*** [From φυτόν, a "plant," and ζῶον, an "animal."] A term applied by some naturalists to such animals as polypi and corallina; a zoophyte.

Pi′a Ma′ter.* ("Tender Mother.") (Fr. *Pie Mère*, pè mêR.) The most internal of the three membranes of the brain. See DURA MATER.

Pi-ar-hæ′mi-a.* [From πῖαρ, "fat," and αἷμα, "blood."] The presence of fat in the blood.

Pi′ca.* A term applied to depraved appetite, or desire for varied and unnatural food, common in *chlorosis*, pregnancy, etc. A genus of the order *Dysorexiæ*, class *Locales*, of Cullen's Nosology.

Pi′ce-a.* [From *pix*, *pi′cis*, "pitch;" Gr. πίττα, or πίσσα, the "pitch-tree."] A name for the *Pinus abies*.

Pi′ce-us.* Belonging to pitch, or tar: pi′ceous.

Picræna Excelsa. See QUASSIA.

Pic′rin, or **Pic′rine.** [From πικρός, "bitter."] A bitter substance procured from *Digita′lis purpu′rea*, and said to be identical with digitalin.

Pic′ro-mel, el′lis.* [From πικρός, "bitter," and μέλι, "honey."] A substance having a bitter and sweetish taste. The characteristic principle of bile.

Pic-ro-tox′ic. [**Picrotox′icus.**] Applied to salts of which picrotoxin forms the base.

Pic-ro-tox′in, or **Pic-ro-tox′ine.** [**Picrotoxi′na**; from πικρός, "bitter," and τοξικόν, "poison."] The poisonous principle of the *Cocculus Indicus*.

Pied, pe-à′. The French word for "foot." See PES.

Pie Mère. See PIA MATER.

Pierre, pe-êR. The French term for CALCULUS, which see.

Pierre d'Aimant, pe-êR dà′mòNᵍ′. A French term for MAGNET, which see.

Pig′ment. [**Pigmen′tum**; from *pin′go*, to "paint."] Any color used by painters.

Pig′ment. A black amorphous substance, found normally in the skin, etc., and abnormally in various other parts of the body. See MELANÆMIA.

Pig-men′tum Ni′grum.* A black or dark pigment which covers the internal surface of the choroid membrane of the eye.

Pil. = *Pil′ula*,* or *pil′ulæ*.* A "pill," or "pills."

Pi-la′re Ma′lum.* ("Hair Disease.") See TRICHOSIS.

Pil′e-ate. [**Pilea′tus**; from *pi′leus*, a "hat."] Having a hat or a cap.

Pil-e-i-for′mis.* [From the same.] Having the form of a hat: pil′eiform.

Piles. (Fr. *Hémorrhoïdes*, à′me′ro′-èd′.) A disease of the veins at the extremity of the rectum, around the anus, assuming a knotted or clustered condition; hemorrhoids. See HÆMORRHOIS.

Pil′e-us.* [From πῖλος, a "hat," or "cap."] The cap or orbicular expansion of a mushroom.

Pi′li,* gen. **Pi-lo′rum**, the plural of PILUS, which see.

Pi′li Con-gen′i-ti.* ("Congenital Hairs.") A term for the hair of the head, eyebrows, and eyelids, because it exists at birth.

Pi′li Post-gen′i-ti.* ("Postgenital Hairs.") That hair which grows on certain parts after birth, at puberty, for example.

Pi-lif′er-ous. [**Pilif′erus**; from *pi′lus*, "hair," and *fe′ro*, to "bear."] Bearing hair, or covered with hair.

Pi′li-form. [**Pilifor′mis**; from *pi′lus*, "hair."] Having the appearance of hairs.

Pi-lig′er-ous. [**Pilig′erus**; from *pi′lus*, "hair," and *ge′ro*, to "bear."] The same as PILIFEROUS, which see.

Pi′line. [From *pi′lus*, "hair."] A kind of cloth composed of a mixture of sponge and wool, felted together so as to form an even and soft fabric, and afterwards rendered water-proof by a coating of caoutchouc; employed as a substitute for poultices and fomentation cloths.

Pill. See PILULA.

Pil-li-o-cau′si-a.* A modern name (of uncertain etymology) for the old composition called *Hi'era pi'cra*, or holy bitter; vulgarly rendered "Pillicoshy."

Pil-o-car'pus.* [From *pi'lus*, "hair," and καρπός, "fruit."] Having fruit covered with hair.

Pilon. See PILUM.

Pi-lo'rum,* the genitive plural of PILUS, a "hair." See next article.

Pilo'rum Ar-rec-to'rēs.* ("Raisers of the Hairs.") A name applied to the minute muscles of the skin, whose action produces the appearance termed *cu'tis anseri'na*, or "goose-skin." They are supposed also to raise the hairs when one is seized with horror or fright.

Pī-lose'. [**Pilo'sus;** from *pi'lus*, "hair."] Hairy, as distinguished from woolly or downy,—*i.e.* having distinct and straight, but not rigid, hairs.

Pil'u-la,* plural **Pil'u-læ.** [Diminutive of *pi'la*, a "ball."] A pill. A small round form of dry medicine, of the size of a pea, or less, which can be swallowed whole.

Pil'u-læ,* gen. **Pil-u-la'rum,** the plural of PILULA, which see.

Pil'ulæ Al'o-ēs.* ("Pills of Aloes.") Take of Socotrine aloes, in fine powder, soap, in fine powder, each a troyounce. Beat them together with water, so as to form a pilular mass, to be divided into two hundred and forty pills.

Pil'ulæ Al'oes et As-sa-fœt'ĭ-dæ.* ("Pills of Aloes and Assafœtida.") Take of Socotrine aloes, in fine powder, assafœtida, soap, in fine powder, each half a troyounce. Beat them together with water, so as to form a pilular mass, to be divided into one hundred and eighty pills.

Pil'ulæ Al'oes et Mas'tĭ-chēs.* ("Pills of Aloes and Mastic.") Take of Socotrine aloes, in fine powder, a troyounce and a half; mastic, in fine powder, red rose, in fine powder, each half a troyounce. Beat them together with water, so as to form a pilular mass, to be divided into four hundred pills.

Pil'ulæ Al'oes et Mȳr'rhæ.*("Pills of Aloes and Myrrh.") Take of Socotrine aloes, in fine powder, two troyounces; myrrh, in fine powder, a troyounce; saffron, in fine powder, half a troyounce; syrup, a sufficient quantity. Beat the whole together, so as to form a pilular mass, to be divided into four hundred and eighty pills.

Pil'ulæ An-tĭ-mo'nĭ-i Com-pos'ĭ-tæ.* ("Compound Pills of Antimony.") Plummer's Pills. Take of sulphurated antimony, mild chloride of mercury, each one hundred and twenty grains; guaiac, in fine powder, molasses, each half a troyounce. Rub the sulphurated antimony first with the mild chloride of mercury, and afterwards with the guaiac and molasses, so as to form a pilular mass, to be divided into two hundred and forty pills.

Pil'ulæ As-sa-fœt'ĭ-dæ.* ("Pills of Assafœtida.") Take of assafœtida, a troyounce and a half; soap, in fine powder, half a troyounce. Beat them together with water, so as to form a pilular mass, to be divided into two hundred and forty pills.

Pil'ulæ Ca-thar'tĭ-cæ Com-pos'ĭ-tæ.* ("Compound Cathartic Pills.") Take of compound extract of colocynth, half a troyounce; extract of jalap, in fine powder, mild chloride of mercury, each one hundred and eighty grains; gamboge, in fine powder, forty grains. Mix the powders together; then with water form a pilular mass, to be divided into one hundred and eighty pills.

Pil'ulæ Co-pai'bæ.* ("Pills of Copaiba.") Take of copaiba, two troyounces; magnesia, recently prepared, sixty grains. Mix them together, and set the mixture aside until it concretes into a pilular mass, to be divided into two hundred pills.

Pil'ulæ Fer'ri Car-bo-na'tis* ("Pills of Carbonate of Iron") are composed of eight parts of sulphate of iron and nine parts of carbonate of soda, with sugar, honey, and water in sufficient quantity. For particular directions respecting the mode of preparation, see U.S. Pharmacopœia, page 254.

Pil'ulæ Fer'ri Com-pos'ĭ-tæ.* ("Compound Pills of Iron.") Take of myrrh, in fine powder, one hundred and twenty grains; carbonate of soda, sulphate of iron, each sixty grains; syrup, a sufficient quantity. Rub the myrrh first with the carbonate of soda, and afterwards with the sulphate of iron, until they are thoroughly mixed; then beat them with syrup, so as to form a pilular mass, to be divided into eighty pills.

Pil'ulæ Fer'ri I-od'ĭ-di* ("Pills of Iodide of Iron") are composed of four parts of iodine, two parts of metallic iron (in the form of wire cut in pieces), and one part of reduced iron, with sugar, marshmallow, gum arabic, and water, in sufficient quantity. For particulars respecting the preparation, see U.S. Pharmacopœia, page 256.

Pil'ulæ Gal'ba-ni Com-pos'i-tæ.* ("Compound Pills of Galbanum.") Take of galbanum, myrrh, each three hundred and sixty grains; assafœtida, one hundred and twenty grains; syrup, a sufficient quantity. Beat them together, so as to form a pilular mass, to be divided into two hundred and forty pills.

Pil'ulæ Hy-drar'gy-ri* ("Pills of Mercury, or Mercurial Pills"), commonly called **Blue Pills.** Take of mercury, a troyounce; confection of rose, a troyounce and a half; liquorice-root, in fine powder, half a troyounce. Rub the mercury with the confection until the globules cease to be visible; then add the liquorice-root, and beat the whole into a pilular mass, to be divided into four hundred and eighty pills.

Pil'ulæ O'pi-i.* ("Pills of Opium.") Take of opium, in fine powder, sixty grains; soap, in fine powder, twelve grains. Beat them together with water, so as to form a pilular mass, to be divided into sixty pills.

Pil'ulæ Quin'i-æ Sul-pha'tis.* ("Pills of Sulphate of Quinia.") Take of sulphate of quinia, a troyounce; gum arabic, in fine powder, one hundred and twenty grains; clarified honey, a sufficient quantity. Mix the sulphate of quinia and gum arabic; then beat them with clarified honey, so as to form a pilular mass, to be divided into four hundred and eighty pills.

Pil'ulæ Rhe'i.* ("Pills of Rhubarb.") Take of rhubarb, in fine powder, three hundred and sixty grains; soap, in fine powder, one hundred and twenty grains. Beat them together with water, so as to form a pilular mass, to be divided into one hundred and twenty pills.

Pil'ulæ Rhe'i Com-pos'i-tæ.* ("Compound Pills of Rhubarb.") Take of rhubarb, in fine powder, a troyounce; Socotrine aloes, in fine powder, three hundred and sixty grains; myrrh, in fine powder, half a troyounce; oil of peppermint, half a fluidrachm. Beat them together with water, so as to form a pilular mass, to be divided into two hundred and forty pills.

Pil'ulæ Sa-po'nis Com-pos'i-tæ.* ("Compound Pills of Soap.") Take of opium, in fine powder, sixty grains; soap, in fine powder, half a troyounce. Beat them together with water, so as to form a pilular mass. This is a convenient preparation for administering opium in a pilular and readily soluble form, in fractions of a grain. The name seems to have been intended to conceal the character of the medicine from the patient.

Pil'ulæ Scil'læ Com-pos'i-tæ.* ("Compound Pills of Squill.") Take of squill, in fine powder, sixty grains; ginger, in fine powder, ammoniac, in fine powder, each one hundred and twenty grains; soap, in fine powder, one hundred and eighty grains; syrup, a sufficient quantity. Mix the powders; then beat them with syrup, so as to form a pilular mass, to be divided into one hundred and twenty pills.

Pil'u-lar. [**Pilula'ris;** from *pil'ula*, a "pill."] Pertaining to a pill.

Pilule. See PILULA.

Pil-u-li-flo'rus.* [From *pil'ula*, a "little ball," and *flos*, a "flower."] Having flowers united into capitules of a round form.

Pi'lum.* (Fr. *Pilon*, pè'lȯɴᵍ'.) A pestle; an instrument for breaking substances in a mortar.

Pi'lus,* plural **Pi'li.** [From πῖλος, "felt."] A hair. *Pilus* is usually applied to the hairs considered individually, while *capillus* signifies, properly, a "head of hair."

Pi-mel'a-den, en*is*.* [From πιμελή, "fat," and ἀδήν, a "gland."] A sebaceous gland.

Pim-e-li'tis, i*dis*.* [From πιμελή, "fat."] Inflammation of the adipose tissue.

Pim-e-lo'dēs.* [From the same.] Fatty, or full of fat.

Pim-e-lo'sis.* [From the same.] Fatness, or obesity.

Pi-men'ta.* Pimento. The Pharmacopœial name ‖ of the unripe berries of the *Euge'nia pimen'ta;* otherwise called the *Myr'tus pimen'ta.*

Pim-pi-nel'la.* A Linnæan genus of the class *Pentandria*, natural order *Umbelliferæ*, or *Apiaceæ*.

Pimpinel'la A-ni'sum.* The systematic name of the plant commonly known as Anise; otherwise called *Ani'sum vulga're.*

Pimple. See PAPULA.

Pin and Web. An old popular name for an opacity of the cornea. See ALBUGO, and LEUCOMA.

Pinaceæ,* pi-na'she-ē. [From *Pi'nus*, one of the genera.] A synonym of a natural order of plants. See CONIFERÆ.

Pinch'beck. An alloy of copper, brass, and zinc, made in imitation of gold. It is sometimes called *tom'bac*, or *sim'ilor*.

Pinck-ne'ya Pu'bens.* The plant which produces the GEORGIA BARK, which see.

Pine. See PINUS.

Pin'e-al. [**Pinea'lis;** from *Pi'nea*, a "pine-tree."] Belonging to, or like the fruit of, a pine-tree.

Pin'eal Gland. [**Cona'rium.**] A small substance, about the size of a pea, situated above the *tuber'cula quadrigem'-ina* of the brain. Descartes supposed it the seat of the soul.

Pin-guec'u-la.* [From *pin'guis*, "fat."] A tumor near the edge of the cornea, apparently, but not really, adipose.

Pin-gued'ĭ-nous. [**Pinguedino'-sus;** from *pingue'do, pingued'inis*, "fat."] Fatty; greasy; unctuous.

Pin-gue'do,* gen. **Pin-gued'ĭ-nis.** Another term for "fat." See ADEPS.

Pin-gue-fo'lĭ-us.* [From *pin'guis*, "fat," and *fo'lium*, a "leaf."] Having thick and fleshy leaves.

Pi'nic. [**Pin'icus;** from *Pi'nus*, the "pine-tree."] Belonging to the pine or fir tree. Applied to an acid.

Pin-ĭ-fo'lĭ-us.* [From *Pi'nus*, the "pine-tree," and *fo'lium*, a "leaf."] Having linear or coriaceous leaves, like those of the fir.

Pink Dye. A dye made by macerating safflower and carbonate of potash in spirit of wine and water, and then adding distilled water, or lemon-juice.

Pink Root. One of the common names of *Spige'lia Marilan'dica*.

Pin'na.* (Literally, a "wing," or "feather.") The *ala*, or lower cartilage of either side of the nose. Also, the broad portion of the external ear. In Botany, one of the primary divisions of a pinnately-compound leaf. Also, the fin of a fish.

Pin'nate, or **Pin'năt-ed.** [**Pinna'-tus;** from *pin'na*, a "feather."] Feather-shaped. This term is applied to a compound leaf with several pairs of leaflets arranged along the sides of a common petiole.

Pinnately-Parted. See PENNATIPARTITUS.

Pin-nate'lȳ-Veined. [**Pennive'-nius.**] Having veins all proceeding from a midrib; feather-veined. Applied to leaves.

Pin-nat'ĭ-fid. [**Pinnatif'idus;** from *pin'na*, a "feather," and *fin'do*, to "cleave."] Pinnately-cleft, as feather-veined leaves which are marked with sinuses or incisions reaching nearly half-way to the midrib.

Pin-nat'ĭ-pēs, p'edis.* [From *pin-na'tus*, "feathered," and *pes*, a "foot."] Having the toes bordered by membranes: pinnatipede. Applied to certain birds.

Pinnatisect. See PENNATISECTED.

Pinnatus. See PINNATE.

Pin'nu-late. [**Pinnula'tus;** from *pin'nula*.] Subdivided into leaflets. In Ichthyology, having small fins.

Pin'nule. [**Pin'nula;** diminutive of *pin'na*, a "fin," or "pinion."] A little leaflet; the secondary division of a pinnately-compound leaf. Also, a little fin.

Pint. [Lat. **Octa'rius;** Fr. *Pinte*, PĂNT.] A liquid measure containing sixteen fluidounces, the eighth part of a gallon.

Pin'ta.* Blue stain. A disease which prevails in Mexico, and which appears to be a variety of *Pityriasis nigra*.

Pi'nus.* [Gr. πίνυς.] A Linnæan genus of trees of the class *Monœcia*, natural order *Coniferæ*.

Pi'nus A'bĭ-ēs.* The spruce fir-tree, the tops of which are used for making spruce beer.

Pi'nus Băl-sa'me-a.* The tree which affords Canadian balsam.

Pi'nus La'rix,* otherwise called **La'rix Eu-ro-pæ'a,*** and **A'bĭ-ēs La'-rix.*** (Fr. *Mélèze*, mā̀'lĕz' or mā̀'lāz'.) The larch tree, from which is obtained the Venice turpentine.

Pi'nus Pa-lus'tris.* ("Swamp Pine.") One of the trees from which turpentine is obtained.

Pi'nus Pi'ce-a.* ("Pitch Pine.") The silver fir, from which the Strasburg turpentine is obtained.

Pi'nus Pi-nas'ter.* The Pinaster, or cluster pine, a tree which yields Bordeaux turpentine, galipot, tar, and pitch.

Pi'nus Sȳl-ves'tris.* ("Forest Pine.") The Scotch fir tree, which yields the common turpentine, white and yellow resin, tar, or common pitch.

Pi'per, er'is.* Black Pepper. The Pharmacopœial name ‖ for the berries of *Piper nigrum*.

Pi'per Al'bum.* ("White Pepper.") It is obtained from the same tree as is black pepper. Also called *Leucopiper*. White pepper is the ripe berry deprived of its skin. It is less active than black pepper, and is little used. See PIPER NIGRUM.

Pi'per Ar-o-mat'ĭ-cum.* ("Aromatic Pepper.") A name for the *Piper nigrum*.

Pi'per Bra-sil-ĭ-a'num.* ("Brazilian Pepper.") The produce of the *Capsicum annuum.*

Pi'per Cu-be'bạ.* The plant the dried fruit or berries of which are termed cubebs. See CUBEBA.

Pi'per Guin-e-en'se,* Pi'per His-pan'ĭ-cum,* or **Pi'per In'dĭ-cum.*** ("Guinea Pepper," "Spanish Pepper," or "Indian Pepper.") The produce of the *Capsicum annuum.*

Pi'per Jạ-mai-çen'se.* ("Jamaica Pepper.") The *Myrtus pimenta,* or allspice.

Pi'per Lon'gum.* ("Long Pepper.") The Pharmacopœial name (Lond. and Ed. Ph.) for the immature fruit, or dried spikes, of long pepper.

Pi'per Me-thỹs'tĭ-cum* [from μεθύω, to "be intoxicated."] The Ava (or Cava) plant of the Sandwich Islands. An intoxicating drink is obtained from its roots.

Pi'per Ni'grum.* ("Black Pepper.") The Pharmacopœial name (Lond. and Ed. Ph.) for the dried unripe berries of black pepper.

Piperaceæ,* pip-e-ra'she-ē. A natural order of exogenous plants (shrubs or herbs), found in the hotter parts of the world. They are generally pungent aromatics, and in some cases powerful narcotics. It includes *Pi'per ni'grum* (Black Pepper).

Pip-e-rā'ceous. [**Pipera'ceus;** from *pi'per,* "pepper."] Belonging to the genus *Piper.*

Pip'e-rin. [**Piperi'na;** from *pi'per,* "pepper."] A fatty resinous substance, the active principle of black pepper.

Pis'çēṡ.* Fishes: the name of the fourth great subdivision of vertebrate animals, or the class of fishes, characterized by a branchial respiration, a bilocular heart, and a covering of scales.

Pis-çid'ĭ-ạ Er-ỹ-thri'nạ.* Jamaica Dogwood. A West Indian tree, of the Linnæan class *Diadelphia,* natural order *Leguminosæ.* A tincture of the bark is powerfully narcotic and diaphoretic, and is used for removing the pain of carious teeth.

Pis-çiv'o-rous. [**Pisciv'orus;** from *pis'cis,* a "fish," and *vo'ro,* to "devour."] Fish-devouring; synonymous with *Ichthyophagous.*

Pis-ĭ-for'mis.* [From *pi'sum,* a "pea."] Resembling a pea: pi'siform.

Pis'mire. The *Formica rufa.*

Pistacia,* pis-ta'she-ạ. [Gr. πιστάκια.] The fruit of the pistachio-tree. A Linnæan genus of the class *Diœcia,* natural order *Terebinthaceæ,* or *Anacardiaceæ.*

Pista'cia Len-tis'cus.* The shrub which yields mastic, or mastick. See MASTIC.

Pista'cia Tĕr-e-bin'thus.* The tree which yields Chian or Cyprus turpentine.

Pista'cia Ve'rạ.* ("True Pistacia.") A tree which yields the pistacia-nut and a fixed oil, which is used to form an excellent emulsion in irritation of the urethra.

Pistiaceæ,* pis-te-a'she-ē. [From *Pis'tia,* one of the genera.] A synonym of a natural order of plants. See LEMNACEÆ.

Pis'til. [**Pistil'lum;** from *pin'so, pis'tum,* to "bray," or "bruise."] Literally, a "pestle:" so named from the resemblance in form. A pointal; the female organ of generation in plants; the ovule-bearing organ of a flower. The pistils and stamens are the essential organs of a flower.

Pis-til-la'ris.* [From *pistil'lum,* a "pistil."] Pertaining to a pistil.

Pis'til-late. [From the same.] Furnished with pistils, or with pistils only.

Pis-til-lif'er-ous. [**Pistillif'erus;** from *pistil'lum,* a "pistil," and *fe'ro,* to "bear."] Bearing or having pistils.

Pis-til'lĭ-form. [**Pistillifor'mis;** from *pistil'lum,* a "pestle."] Having the form of a pestle.

Pis-til'lum.* A pestle; also, the same as PISTIL, which see.

Pi'sum.* (Fr. *Pois,* pwå.) The pea. A Linnæan genus of the class *Diadelphia,* natural order *Leguminosæ.*

Pit. The depression made by the pressure of the finger on any part of the body in an œdematous state. Also applied to the cavities or depressions left on the skin after a severe attack of the small-pox.

Pit of the Stom'ach. [**Scrobic'ulus Cor'dis.**] The hollow part over the region of the stomach, and between the cartilages of the false ribs.

Pitch. See PIX.

Pitch, Jew's. A name for *Asphaltum,* or *Bitumen Judaicum.*

Pitch-Tree. See PINUS.

Pitch'er Plant. A plant of which the petiole is dilated and hollowed out like a pitcher, the *lamina* (or blade of the leaf) being articulated to it and closing the orifice. The pitcher is called *ascid'ium,* and the lid *oper'culum.* An example is found in the *Nepenthes.*

Pitcher-Shaped. See ASCIDIATE, and URCEOLATE.

Pith. [**Medul'la.**] The soft, spongy cellular tissue constituting the central portion of an exogenous stem or branch.

Pit'ta-cal. [From πίττα, "pitch," and κάλος, "beautiful."] A beautiful blue coloring matter discovered in the oil of tar.

Pit'ted Tis'sue. A name of a modification of cellular vegetable tissue, having its sides marked by pits sunk in the substance of the membrane.

Pittosporaceæ,* pit-to-spo-ra'she-ē. A natural order of exogenous plants (trees or shrubs), mostly natives of Australia. It includes the *Pittos'porum.*

Pit-u-i'ta.* [From πήττω, or πήσσω, to "congeal."] Phlegm; viscid and glutinous mucus.

Pit-u'ĭ-ta-rȳ. [**Pituita'rius;** from *pitui'ta,* "phlegm."] Belonging to phlegm.

Pituitary Body. See PITUITARY GLAND.

Pitu'itary Gland. The small glandular body which rests on the *Sella Turcica.* Its functions are unknown.

Pitu'itary Mem'brane. The SCHNEIDERIAN MEMBRANE, which see.

Pit-ȳ-ri'a-sis.* [From πίτυρα, "scurf," or "dandriff."] A skin-disease in which irregular patches of small thin scales repeatedly form and separate, unattended with inflammation, and never collecting into crusts. A genus of the order *Squamæ* of Willan's classification.

Pix,* gen. **Pi'cis.** [From πίσσα, "pitch."] The Pharmacopœial name (Lond. Ph., 1851) for a dry bitumen prepared from liquid pitch; black pitch.

Pix Ar'ĭ-da.* ("Dry Pitch.") The Pharmacopœial name (Ed. Ph.) for pitch from various species of *Pinus abies.*

Pix Bur-gun'dĭ-ca.* ("Burgundy Pitch.") The Pharmacopœial name ‖ of a concrete resinous exudation from the *Abies excelsa.*

Pix Can-a-den'sis* ("Canada Pitch"), or **Hem'lock Pitch.** The Pharmacopœial name (U.S. Ph.) for the prepared concrete juice of the *Abies Canadensis.*

Pix Liq'uĭ-da.* ("Liquid Pitch.") Tar. The Pharmacopœial name ‖ of tar, obtained from the *Pinus palustris,* the *P. sylvestris,* and various other species of *Pinus* and *Abies.*

Pix Ni'gra.* ("Black Pitch.") Common pitch; inspissated tar.

Pla-ce'bo.* [The future tense of *pla'ceo,* to "please," or "soothe."] "I will please, or soothe." Applied to a medicine given rather to please than benefit the patient.

Pla-cen'ta.* [From πλακοῦς, a "cake."] A circular, flat, vascular, flesh-like substance in the impregnated uterus, forming the principal medium by which the communication is preserved between the mother and child. In Botany, that portion of the ovary to which the ovules or seeds are attached.

Placen'ta Præ'vĭ-a* [from *præ'vius,* "going before," or "foremost"]. Applied to those obstetrical cases in which the placenta is situated internally over the mouth of the womb, often proving a cause of excessive hæmorrhage.

Pla-cen'tæ,* the plural of PLACENTA, which see.

Placentæformis. See PLACENTIFORM.

Pla-cen'tal. [**Placenta'lis.**] Belonging to the placenta.

Pla-cen-ta'rĭ-um.* The same as the PLACENTA (of plants), which see.

Plaç-en-tā'tion. [**Placenta'tio, o'nis;** from *placen'ta,* a "cake."] The manner in which the seeds are attached to the pericarp; the arrangement of placentæ.

Pla-cen'tĭ-form. [**Placentifor'mis;** from *placen'ta,* a "cake."] Resembling a cake; nearly the same as quoit-shaped.

Plaç-en-ti'tis, idis.* [From *placen'ta,* a "cake."] Inflammation of the placenta.

Pla-cen'tu-la.* [Diminutive of *placen'ta.*] A little placenta: a placentule.

Plad-a-ro'sis.* [From πλαδαρός, "wet," or "soft."] A fungous and flaccid tumor within the eyelid.

Plague. See PESTIS.

Plaited. See PLICATE.

Plane. [From *pla'nus,* "smooth," "flat," or "plane."] A plain surface, all the points of which lie even between its bounding lines.

Plan'et. [**Plane'ta;** from πλανήτης, "wandering."] A star or heavenly body which, with a telescope of sufficient power, exhibits a round and well-defined disk, and revolves around the sun in an elliptic orbit. The planets are so named because they are constantly changing their apparent position in relation to the fixed stars, among which they seem to wander.

Plan'e-ta-rȳ. [**Planeta'rius;** from

plane'ta, a "planet."] Belonging to planets.

Pla-net'ic. [**Planet'icus;** from *plane'ta,* a "planet."] Belonging to a planet; wandering; erratic.

Plan-ĭ-flo'rus.* [From *pla'nus,* "flat," and *flos,* a "flower."] Having flat flowers: planiflo'rate.

Plan-ĭ-fo'lĭ-ous. [**Planifolia'tus;** from *pla'nus,* "flat," or "plane," and *fo'lium,* a "leaf."] Having flat or plane leaves.

Pla̧-no'dĭ-a̧.* [From πλανάομαι, to "wander," and ὁδός, a "way."] A false passage, as is sometimes made in stricture of the urethra by a bougie, sound, or catheter.

Plan'ta̧.* The inferior surface or sole of the foot. Also, a plant, or vegetable.

Plantaginaceæ,* plan-taj-e-na'-she-ē. A natural order of exogenous herbaceous plants, found in all parts of the world. It includes *Planta'go* (Plantain, or Ribwort).

Plan'ta̧r. [**Planta'ris;** from *plan'ta,* the "sole of the foot."] Belonging to the sole of the foot.

Plan-ta'ris.* [See Plantar.] The name of a muscle arising from the external condyle of the femur, and inserted into the inside of the *os calcis.* It extends the foot.

Plan'tĭ-grade. [**Plantig'radus;** from *plan'ta,* the "sole of the foot," and *gra'dior,* to "go," or "walk."] Applied to Man and certain other mammalia that walk on the sole of the foot.

Plan-tiv'o-rous. [**Plantiv'orus;** from *plan'ta,* a "plant," and *vo'ro,* to "devour."] The same as Phytivorous.

Pla̧-nu'rĭ-a̧.* [From πλανάομαι, to "wander," and οὖρον, the "urine."] The discharge of urine through an unusual or unnatural passage: plan'ury.

Pla'nus.* Flat, or level. Applied to the orbital portion (*Os planum*) of the ethmoid bone.

Plas'ma̧, a*tis.** [From πλάσσω, to "form."] A tenacious, plastic liquid, forming the coagulating portion of the blood; that in which the blood-corpuscles float; the *Liquor sanguinis.*

Plaster. See Emplastrum.

Plas'ter of Par'is. A common name for gypsum, or sulphate of lime: so called from its having been originally procured from Mont Martre, in the immediate vicinity of Paris.

Plas'tic. [**Plas'ticus;** from πλάσσω, to "form."] Forming, or having power to form. Also, capable of being formed or moulded as clay.

Plas-tiç'ĭ-tȳ. [**Plastiç'itas, a'***tis;* from *plas'ticus,* "plastic."] The quality of being plastic.

Platanaceæ,* plat-a̧-na'she-ē. A natural order of exogenous trees and shrubs, natives of North America, Barbary, and the Levant. It consists of one genus, the *Plat'anus,* several species of which are cultivated for their noble appearance. They are known as the Plane-tree, Sycamore, or Buttonwood.

Pla-teĭ-as'ma̧,* or **Pla-tĭ-as'mus.*** [From πλατύς, "broad."] A defect in speech characterized by the vulgar term "blobber-lipped," and observed in persons with very thick and broad lips.

Platina. See Platinum.

Plat'i-nāte. [**Plati'nas, a'***tis.*] A combination in which platinic oxide acts the part of an acid.

Pla̧-tin'ic. [**Platin'icus.**] Belonging to platinum.

Plat'ĭ-num,* or **Plat'ĭ-na̧.*** [Spanish diminutive of *pla'ta,* "silver;" Fr. *Platine,* plå'tèn', or *Petit Argent,* pȩh-tè' taʀ'zhŏɴɢ'.] A valuable, rare, and exceedingly ductile metal, which is the heaviest substance known. Its specific gravity is 21.5. It undergoes no change from air or moisture, and is not soluble in any of the pure acids. It may, however, be dissolved by nitro-muriatic acid. In color it resembles silver.

Plat'inum, Spon'gy, has the remarkable property of being ignited by contact with hydrogen gas.

Plat-ȳ-car'pous. [**Platycar'pus;** from πλατύς, "broad," and καρπός, "fruit."] Having broad fruit.

Plat-ȳ-çeph'a̧-lous. [**Platyceph'-alus;** from πλατύς, "broad," and κεφαλή, the "head."] Having a flat or broad head. Applied to a species of mushrooms; also to certain animals.

Plat-ȳ-glos'sus.* [From πλατύς, "broad," and γλῶσσα, the "tongue."] Having a broad tongue. The *Heliopsis platyglossa* has the corols of its corona prolonged into a very broad tongue.

Pla̧-tȳl'o-bus.* [From πλατύς, "broad," and λόβος, a "lobe."] Having broad lobes or segments.

Plat-ȳ-lo'mus.* [From πλατύς, "broad," and λῶμα, a "frame or edge."] Having broadly margined leaves.

Plat'ȳ-pēs, p'*edis.** [From πλατύς, "broad," and *pes,* a "foot."] Having the foot or *stipes* dilated at its base. Applied to plants.

Plat-y̆-pet'a-lus.* [From πλατύς, "broad," and πέταλον, a "petal."] Having broad petals: platypetalous.

Plat-y̆-phy̆l'lus.* [From πλατύς, "broad," and φύλλον, a "leaf."] Having broad leaves: platyphyllous.

Plat-y̆-sil'ĭ-quus.* [From πλατύς, "broad," and *sil'iqua*, a "pod."] Having flat, broad siliques.

Pla-tȳs'ma, atis.* [Gr. πλάτυσμα, a "broad sheet;" from πλατύνω, to "dilate."] An expansion, or dilatation.

Platys'ma My-o'dēs.* The broad, thin, subcutaneous muscle on the side of the neck.

Pled'get. (Fr. *Plumaceau*, plü'mȧ'sō'.) A small compress or piece of lint rolled up into an oval or orbicular form.

Pleiocene. See PLIOCENE.

Pleī-o-phy̆l'lus.* [From πλείων, "more," "many," and φύλλον, a "leaf."] Bearing a great number of leaves.

Pleis'to-çēne. [From πλεῖστος, "most," and καινός, "recent."] The most recent or uppermost of the tertiary strata, containing the largest proportion of recent (or living) species of shells.

Plenck's So-lu'tion. Mercury suspended in water by being rubbed for a considerable time with gum arabic.

Plen. riv. = *Ple'no ri'vo.** "In a full stream."

Ple'o-naṡm. [Pleonas'mus; from πλεονασμός, a "magnifying," or "exaggeration."] A faulty formation, with an overgrowth, or over-number, of parts. Also, a redundant phrase.

Ple-o-nec'tĭ-cus.* Belonging to *pleonexia*. Applied to a form of insanity.

Ple-o-nex'ĭ-a.* [Gr. πλεονεξία, "greediness."] Greediness, grasping selfishness, overbearing temper or arrogance, regarded as mental disease.

Ple-sĭ-o-mor'phous. [Plesiomor'phus; from πλησίος, "near," and μορφή, "form."] Nearly of the same form.

Ples'ser. [From πλήσσω, to "strike."] The same as PLEXOR.

Ples-sim'e-ter. [From πλήσσω, to "strike," and μέτρον, a "measure."] The same as PLEXIMETER, which see.

Ple-tho'ra* or pleth'o-ra. [From πλήθω, to "be full."] Excessive fulness of the vessels; repletion; also, a fulness or plumpness of body.

Ple-thŏr'ic. [Plethor'icus.] Relating to plethora; full of blood.

Pleū'ra.* [Gr. πλευρά, the "side," also, a "rib;" Fr. *Plèvre*, plĕvR or plȧvR.] A serous membrane, divided into two portions by the *mediastinum*, lining the right and left cavities of the thorax, and by its continuation reflected over each lung.

Pleu'ra Cos-ta'lis,* Pleu'ra Pa-ri-e-ta'lis.* That portion of the pleura which lines the ribs or *parietes* of the thorax.

Pleu'ra Pul-mo-na'lis.* ("Pleura of the Lungs.") That portion of the pleura which invests the lungs.

Pleū'ral. The same as PLEURIC, which see.

Pleū-răl'gĭ-a.* [From πλευρά, the "side," or "rib," and ἄλγος, "pain."] Pain in the pleura, or side: pleuralgy. See PLEURODYNIA.

Pleū-ra-po-phȳs'ĭ-al. [Pleurapophysia'lis.] Belonging to *pleurapophysis*.

Pleū-ra-poph'y̆-sis.* [From πλευρά, the "side," or "rib," and ἀποφύω, to "be born from."] Applied by Owen to the homologues of the costal process, or lateral part on each side of a vertebra.

Pleū-ra-pos-te'ma, atis.* [From *pleu'ra*, and ἀπόστημα, an "aposteme."] An aposteme, or abscess, in the pleura.

Pleū-rar-throc'a-çe.* [From *pleurar'thron*, and κακός, "evil."] Caries of a rib-joint.

Pleū-rar'thron,* or **Pleū-rar'-thrum.*** [From πλευρά, the "side," or "rib," and ἄρθρον, a "joint."] The articulation of a rib.

Pleū-ren'chy̆-ma.* [From πλευρά, the "side," and ἔγχυμα, any thing poured in, an "infusion."] A term applied by Lindley to woody tissue, or WOODY FIBRE, which see.

Pleurésie. See PLEURISY.

Pleū'ric. [Pleu'ricus.] Belonging to the pleura, etc.

Pleū'rĭ-sy̆. The same as PLEURITIS, which see.

Pleū-rit'ic. [Pleurit'icus.] Belonging to *pleuritis*, or pleurisy.

Pleū-ri'tis, idis.* [From *pleu'ra*.] (Fr. *Pleurésie*, pluh'rȧ'zē'.) Inflammation of the pleura: pleu'risy.

Pleū-ro-car'pus,* or **Pleū-ro-car'-pe-us.*** [From πλευρά, the "side," and καρπός, "fruit."] Applied in the plural masculine (*Pleurocar'pi*) to a division of the *Musci Calypteratæ*, in which the fruit is lateral upon the stem or branches.

Pleū-ro-dy̆n'ĭ-a.* [From πλευρά, the "side," and ὀδύνη, "pain."] External (rheumatic) pain in the side.

Pleū-ro-nec'tēs.* [From πλευρά, and

νήκτης, a "swimmer."] Literally, "swimming on the side." Applied to the sole fish.

Pleuronec'tes So'le-a.* The systematic name of the sole.

Pleū-ror-rhœ'a.* [From πλευρά, and ῥέω, to "flow."] An exudation from, or collection of fluid within, the pleura.

Pleū-ror-thop-nœ'a.* [From *pleu'ra*, ὀρθός, "upright," and πνέω, to "breathe."] A term for *Pleuritis*, in which the patient can only breathe when sitting erect.

Pleū-ro-spas'mus.* [From πλευρά, the "side," and σπασμός, a "spasm."] Cramp in the side: pleu'rospasm.

Pleū-ro-thot'o-nos.* [From πλευρόθεν, "from the side," and τείνω, to "bend."] Bent or stretched from one side. Applied to a variety of *Tetanus*.

Plèvre, plĕvr, or **Pleure,** plur. The French term for Pleura, which see.

Plex-im'e-ter. [**Plexim'etrum;** from πλῆξις, a "stroke," and μέτρον, a "measure."] A flat piece of ivory, or a circular piece of sole-leather, by means of which *mediate percussion* is performed. See Percussion.

Plex-i-met'ric. [**Pleximet'ricus.**] Belonging to the pleximeter.

Plexiometrum. See Pleximeter.

Plex'us.* [From *plec'to*, *plex'um*, to "knit," or "weave."] (Fr. *Lacis*, lå'sè'.) A network. The intertwining and intercrossing of the vessels and nerves of the system, but more especially of the latter.

Plexus Axillaris. See Axillary Plexus.

Plexus Cardiacus. See Cardiac Plexus.

Plexus Choroides. See Choroid Plexus.

Plex'us Pam-pin-ĭ-for'mis.* The plexus of blood-vessels about the spermatic cord. Also termed *Corpus pampiniforme*, or "tendril-like body." See Pampiniform.

Plex'us Pul-mon'ĭ-cus.* ("Pulmonic Plexus.") Formed by the union of the eighth pair of nerves with the great sympathetic.

Plex'us Re-tic-u-la'ris.* The network of vessels situated below the *Fornix* of the brain.

Plexus Solaris. See Solar Plexus.

Pli'ca.* [From *pli'co*, to "plait."] Knitted or plaited hair. A disease in which the hair becomes inextricably knitted and glued together. Also termed *Trichoma, Trichia, Trichiasis.*

Pli'ca Po-lon'ĭ-ca.* ("Polish Plica.") Another name for the disease termed *plica*, because prevalent in Poland.

Pli'ca Sem-ĭ-lu-na'ris.* [From *sem'i*, "half," and *lu'na*, a "moon."] A slight duplicature of the conjunctiva on the outer side of the *caruncula lachrymalis;* the rudiment of the third lid of animals. More fully developed, it becomes the *membra'na nic'titans* of birds.

Plī'cate. [**Plica'tus;** from *pli'co*, *plica'tum*, to "plait," or "knit."] Folded; plaited.

Pliç-ĭ-den'tĭne. [From *pli'ca*, a "fold," and *dens*, *den'tis*, a "tooth."] A modification of the fundamental tissue of teeth, in which, on a transverse section, the dentine exhibits sinuous wavings diverging from the central pulp-cavity of the tooth.

Plī-çif'er-ous. [**Plicif'erus;** from *pli'ca*, a "plait," a "fold," and *fe'ro*, to "bear."] Bearing or having folds. Applied to parts of plants.

Plī'o-çēne. [From πλείων, "more," and καινός, "recent."] A geological term applied to the most modern of the divisions of the tertiary epoch, because the greater part of its fossil Testacea are referable to recent species.

Plo-ca'rĭ-a Can'dĭ-da.* Ceylon Moss; an algaceous plant, abounding in mucilage and starchy matter, and yielding a decoction and a jelly employed in pharmacy.

Plomb, plôno. The French term for Lead, which see.

Plug'ging. A term for the operation of filling the cavity in a carious tooth, in order to exclude the air, and thus prevent toothache. Also applied to the operation of inserting pieces of rag, sponge, or the like, into the vagina, in cases of severe uterine hæmorrhage, to act as a plug for preventing the farther escape of blood, so that the *coagula* then formed will mechanically and effectually stop the mouths of the bleeding vessels. See Tampon. Applied also to an analogous operation on the nostrils, in *epistaxis.*

Plum. [**Pru'num.**] The fruit of the *Prunus domestica;* when dried and preserved, it is called a Prune, or French plum.

Plumaceau, plü'må'sō'. The French term for Pledget, which see.

Plumbaginaceæ,* plum-baj-e-na'-she-ē. A natural order of exogenous plants, found in many temperate, cold, and tropical regions. It includes *Plumba'go*, and *Stat'ice*, which is a powerful astringent. Some species are extremely caustic.

Plum-ba'go.* Graphite, or black lead. A combination of carbon with a minute quantity of iron, used in forming lead-pencils, and for a variety of other purposes.

Plum'bāte. [**Plum'bas, a'***tis*.] A combination of plumbic oxide with another oxide, with regard to which it acts the part of an acid.

Plum'bi A-çe'tas* ("Acetate of Lead"), or **Su'gar of Lead.** The Pharmacopœial name ‖ for a substance in colorless crystals which effloresce on exposure to the air. It is dissolved by distilled water with a slight turbidness, which is removed by the addition of distilled vinegar. Acetate of lead, in medicinal doses, is a powerful astringent and sedative, and is often given in hæmorrhages and in diarrhœa, with the most beneficial results. In over-doses, however, it is an irritant poison. In minute doses long continued, it sometimes produces lead colic (*colica pictonum*) and a species of paralysis, termed *lead palsy*.

Plum'bi Car-bo'nas* ("Carbonate of Lead"), or **White Lead.** The Pharmacopœial name ‖ for a white substance in powder or pulverulent masses, insoluble in water, but soluble with effervescence in dilute nitric acid. It is used as an external application to excoriated and inflamed surfaces. See POISONS.

Plum'bi Ni'tras.* ("Nitrate of Lead.") The Pharmacopœial name for a substance in white, nearly opaque, octahedral crystals, permanent in the air, and of a sweet, astringent taste. It is soluble in cold water and in alcohol. It is used as a disinfectant, and as an application to putrid and indolent ulcers.

Plum'bi Ox'ĭ-dum* ("Oxide of Lead"), or **Plum'bi Ox'idum Sem-ĭ-vit're-um*** ("Semi-vitreous Oxide of Lead"); also termed **Lith'arge.** The Pharmacopœial name (U.S. Ph.) for a substance in small yellowish or orange-colored scales, insoluble in water, but almost wholly soluble, with slight effervescence, in dilute nitric acid. Litharge is used in the preparation of the *Emplastrum Plumbi*, which forms the base of many other plasters.

Plum'bic. [**Plum'bicus;** from *plum'bum*, "lead."] Belonging to lead.

Plum'bic Aç'id. The same as peroxide of lead.

Plum-bo'sus.* [From *plum'bum*, "lead."] Leaden, or like lead.

Plum'bum,* gen. **Plum'bi.** (Fr. *Plomb*, plōNº.) The Latin term for LEAD, which see.

Plu'mĭ-form. [**Plumifor'mis;** from *plu'ma*, a "feather."] Like a plume, or feather.

Plum'mer's Pills. The *Pil'ulæ Calomel'anos Compos'itæ* ("Compound Calomel Pills") of the Pharmacopœias.

Plu-mose', or **Plu'mous.** [**Plumo'sus;** from *plu'ma*, a "feather."] Having feathers, or resembling feathers; feathered.

Plu'mule. [**Plu'mula;** diminutive of *plu'ma*, a "feather."] The bud or growing point of the embryo, above the cotyledons; the ascending axis of the embryo of a plant. See GEMMULE.

Plu-mu-lĭ-for'mis.* [From *plu'mula*, a "plumule."] Having the appearance of a small feather: plu'muliform.

Plu-rĭ-flo'rous. [**Pluriflo'rus;** from *plu'res*, "more," or "many," and *flos*, a "flower."] Having many, or several, flowers.

Plu-ril'o-bus.* [From *plu'res*, "more," or "many," and *lo'bus*, a "lobe."] Formed of many lobes.

Plu-rĭ-loc'u-lar. [**Pluriloculа'ris;** from *plu'res*, "more," or "many," and *loc'ulus*, a "cell."] Having many, or several, cells. Applied to the ovary of certain plants.

Plu-rĭ-par'tīte. [**Pluriparti'tus;** from *plu'res*, "more," or "many," and *par'tio*, *parti'tum*, to "divide."] Applied to a calyx when it presents many incisions extended almost to its base.

Plu-rĭ-pet'a-lus.* [From *plu'res*, "more," or "many," and *pet'alum*, a "petal."] The same as POLYPETALOUS, which see.

Plu-rĭ-se'rĭ-ate. [**Pluriseria'tus;** from *plu'res*, "more," or "many," and *se'ries*, an "order," or "row."] Disposed in many rows.

Plu-rĭ-văl'vis.* [From *plu'res*, "more," or "many," and *val'va*, a "valve."] Plu'rivalve. Applied to a capsule composed of many valves.

Plu-to'nĭ-an. [**Plutonia'nus;** from *Plu'to*, *Pluto'nis*, the god of *Ha'des*, or the infernal regions.] A term applied to rocks of igneous formation, and to a theory proposed by Hutton, that unstratified crystalline rocks were formed by igneous fusion.

Plu-ton'ic. [**Pluton'icus;** from the same.] The same as PLUTONIAN.

Plu'to-nism. [**Plutonis'mus;**

from the same.] A hypothesis which attributes to subterranean fires the constitution of the principal beds, or, at least, of the crust, of the globe. The Plutonian theory of Geology, also called Huttonian theory. See PLUTONIAN.

Plu'vi-al. [**Pluvia'lis;** from *plu'via*, "rain."] Pertaining to rain.

Plu-vi-om'e-ter. [From *plu'via*, "rain," and *μέτρον*, a "measure."] A rain-gauge; a vessel in which the rain is caught as it falls, and measured.

Pneū-mar-thro'sis.* (*P* silent, and so in all the subsequent words beginning with *pn.*) [From *πνεῦμα*, "air," and *ἄρθρον*, a "joint."] A secretion of air within the joints, which disappears spontaneously, and frequently in the course of a few days, and even a few hours.

Pneū-mat'ic. [**Pneumat'icus;** from *πνεῦμα*, "air," or "breath."] Pertaining to air (or gas), or to pneumatics.

Pneumat'ic Trough. A trough of a particular construction, for collecting gases under water (or quicksilver), so as to exclude atmospheric air; also called Hydropneumatic Trough: but this latter term is only applicable to a pneumatic trough with water,—not to one containing quicksilver.

Pneū-mat'ĭ-cạ.* [From *pneumat'icus*, "pertaining to air, or respiration."] The name of a class in Good's Nosology, comprising diseases of the respiratory function.

Pneū-mat'ĭ-ci.* [Masculine plural of *pneumat'icus*, "pneumatic."] "Pneumatic [Physicians]." A sect or school (founded by Athenæus) who imagined that there existed an immaterial principle or element, which they called *pneuma*, on which they conceived health and disease to depend.

Pneū-mat'ics. [**Pneumat'ica;** from *πνεῦμα*, "air," or "breath."] The science which treats of the mechanical properties of elastic fluids, and particularly of atmospheric air.

Pneumatocele,* nu'mạ-to-sēl. [From *πνεῦμα*, "air," or "breath," and *κήλη*, a "tumor."] Any kind of hernia filled with flatus.

Pneū'mạ-to-che'mĭ-ạ.* [From *πνεῦμα*, "air," or "breath," and *che'mia*, "chemistry."] Pneumatic chemistry. That branch of chemistry which treats of airs or gases.

Pneū'mạ-to-chem'ĭ-cạl. [**Pneumatochem'icus.**] Belonging to pneumatic chemistry. The pneumato-chemical apparatus, invented by Priestley, is a tub full of water arranged so that it will permit of gases being easily collected.

Pneū'mạ-to-chy-mif'er-us.* [From *πνεῦμα*, "air," or "breath," *χυμός*, "juice," or "sap," and *fe'ro*, to "bear."] Applied to the *tracheæ* of vegetables when composed of two tubes, the one straight and full of air, the other rolled into a spiral form and full of liquid.

Pneū'mạ-to-dȳsp-nœ'ạ.* [From *πνεῦμα*, "air," or "breath," and *dyspnœ'a*, "difficult breathing."] Emphysematous *dyspnœa.*

Pneū-mạ-tol'o-ġȳ. [**Pneumatolo'gia;** from *πνεῦμα*, "air," "breath," or "spirit," and *λόγος*, a "discourse."] The science which treats of spirit or of spiritual substances.

Pneū-mạ-tom'e-ter. [**Pneumatom'etrum;** from *πνεῦμα*, "breath," and *μέτρον*, a "measure."] An instrument for measuring the quantity of air inhaled at a single inspiration.

Pneū-mạ-toph'o-rus.* [From *πνεῦμα*, "air," or "breath," and *φέρω*, to "bear."] Applied to tubes in plants, full of air, which is conducted to the centre of the spiral tube of the *tracheæ.*

Pneū-mạ-to'sis.* [From *πνευματόω*, to "distend with wind."] Windy swelling. A genus of the order *Intumescentiæ*, class *Cachexiæ*, of Cullen's Nosology. Also termed *Emphysema.*

Pneumatothorax. See PNEUMOTHORAX.

Pneū-mo-gas'tric. [**Pneumogas'tricus;** from *πνεύμων*, a "lung," or the "lungs," and *γαστήρ*, the "belly," or "stomach."] Belonging to the lungs and stomach.

Pneumogas'tric Nerves. [**Ner'vi Pneumogas'trici.**] The *par vagum*, or eighth pair of nerves, distributed to the lungs and the stomach.

Pneū-mog'rạ-phȳ. [**Pneumogra'phia;** from *πνεύμων*, a "lung," or the "lungs," and *γράφω*, to "write."] An anatomical description of the lungs.

Pneū-mo-hæm-or-rha'ġĭ-ạ.* [From *πνεύμων*, the "lungs," and *hæmorrha'gia*, a "hæmorrhage."] A term proposed by Andral to denote pulmonary apoplexy, the term apoplexy having been originally applied to a determinate group of symptoms, and not to any particular form of lesion.

Pneū-mol'o-ġȳ. [**Pneumolo'gia;** from *πνεύμων*, the "lungs," and *λόγος*, a "discourse."] A treatise on the lungs; the science of the lungs.

Pneū-mo-næ'mĭ-ạ.* [From *πνεύμων*,

the "lungs," and αἷμα, "blood."] Congestion of blood in the lungs.

Pneū-mo-năl'ġī-ą.* [From πνεύμων, the "lungs," and ἄλγος, "pain."] Pain of the lungs: pneumonal'gy.

Pneū-mo'nĭ-ą.* [Gr. πνευμονία, a "disease of the lungs;" Fr. *Inflammation des poumons*, ăNᵍ'flâm'mâ'se-ôNᵍ' dȧ poo'-môNᵍ'.] Inflammation of the lungs. A genus of the order *Phlegmasiæ*, class *Pyrexiæ*, of Cullen's Nosology. The symptoms of this disease are fever, accompanied with pain in the thorax, which is aggravated by coughing, a quick and hard pulse, with more or less difficulty of breathing.

Pneū-mon'ic. [From πνεύμων, the "lungs."] Belonging to the lungs; pulmonary.

Pneū-mo-ni'tis, i*dis.** [From πνεύμων, the "lungs."] Inflammation of the lungs; also termed *pneumonia* and *peripneumonia*. See PNEUMONIA.

Pneū-mon-o-dy̆n'ĭ-ą.* [From πνεύμων, the "lungs," and ὀδύνη, "pain."] Pain of the lungs. See PNEUMONALGIA.

Pneū-mon-œ-de'mą, a*tis.** [From πνεύμων, the "lungs," and *œde'ma*.] *Œdema*, or dropsical condition, of the substance of the lungs.

Pneū-mon-o-gas'trĭ-cus.* The same as *Pneumogastricus*. See PNEUMOGASTRIC.

Pneū-mo-nom'e-ter. [**Pneumonom'etrum.**] The same as PNEUMATOMETER, which see.

Pneū'mo-Pĕr-ĭ-car'dĭ-um.* [From πνεῦμα, "air," and περικάρδιον, the "pericardium."] A name applied to an effusion of air into the cavity of the pericardium.

Pneū-mo-tho'rax,* or **Pneū-mą-to-tho'rax, a'***cis.** [From πνεῦμα, "air," or "breath," and θώραξ, the "chest."] An accumulation of air in the chest, or thorax.

Pock. A pustule of variola; also applied to *varicella*, or the chicken-pox.

Poc-u-la'ris.* [From *poc'ulum*, a "cup," or "bowl."] Belonging to a cup: poc'ular. See SINUS POCULARIS.

Poc'u-lĭ-form. [**Poculifor'mis;** from *poc'ulum*, a "cup," or "bowl."] Having the form of a cup; deep cup-shaped.

Poc'u-lum Di-oġ'e-nis.* ("Cup of Diogenes.") The hollow of the hand. See DIOGENES' CUP.

Pod. A legume, follicle, or any sort of capsule.

Pod'ą-grą.* [From πούς, ποδός, the "foot," and ἄγρα, a "seizure."] Gout in the joints of the foot. A genus of the order *Phlegmasiæ*, class *Pyrexiæ*, of Cullen's Nosology. The following forms of this disease may be noticed.

REG'ULAR GOUT. [*Pod'agra* (or *Arthri'tis*) *Regula'ris*.] Violent inflammation, remaining for a few days, and gradually receding with swelling, itching, and desquamation of the part.

ATON'IC GOUT. [*Pod'agra* (or *Arthri'tis*) *Aton'ica*.] Accompanied with atony of the stomach, or other internal part, with the usual inflammation of the joints, or with slight and temporary pains; with dyspepsia and other symptoms of atony often alternating with each other.

RET'ROGRADE GOUT. [*Pod'agra* (or *Arthri'tis*) *Retrog'rada*.] Also termed RETROCEDENT GOUT. Characterized by inflammation of the joints suddenly disappearing, and atony of some internal part immediately following.

ABER'RANT GOUT. [*Pod'agra Aber'rans*, or *Arthri'tis Errat'ica*.] Passing from one part to another, but usually attended with inflammation of some internal organ.

Po-dag'ric. [**Podag'ricus.**] Belonging to *podagra*.

Po-dăl'ġī-ą.* [From πούς, ποδός, the "foot," and ἄλγος, "pain."] Pain in the foot, as from gout, rheumatism, or the like.

Pod-ą-nen-çe-pha'lĭ-ą.* [From πούς, ποδός, the "foot," and *anencepha'lia*, "absence of brain."] The condition of a monster-fœtus without a brain, the cephalic extremity being supported by a pedicle. The term is also used for PODENCEPHALIA.

Pod-ar-thri'tis, i*dis.** [From πούς, a "foot," and *arthri'tis*, "inflammation of the joints."] Inflammation of the joints of the foot.

Pod-en-çe-pha'lĭ-ą.* [From *podenceph'alus*.] A term for the condition of a *podenceph'alus*.

Pod-en-çeph'ą-lus.* [From πούς, a "foot," and ἐγκέφαλος, the "brain."] A monster-fœtus, the brain of which, without a cranium, hangs by a pedicle.

Podetium,* po-de'she-ŭm. [Diminutive of πούς, a "foot."] The peculiar footstalk of the tubercles in cup-lichens.

Pod-o-car'pus.* [From πούς, a "foot," and καρπός, "fruit."] Applied to a plant the ovary of which is borne upon a pedicel: a podocarp.

Pod-o-çeph'ą-lus.* [From πούς, a "foot," and κεφαλή, the "head."] Having flowers united into heads: podocephalous.

Pod-œ-de'ma, a*tis*.* [From πούς, a "foot," and *œde'ma*, a "swelling."] *Œdema* of the feet.

Pod-o-phȳl'lin. [Podophylli'na.] A resinous principle of a yellow (or yellowish) color, found in the root of the *Podophyllum peltatum*. This is a medicine of great power, operating, in doses of from two to five grains, as a drastic purgative. In smaller doses it is said to act as an alterative and cholagogue. It is asserted by some of the Eclectics that, as a remedial agent, podophyllin may in all cases be substituted for mercury, and that in some instances it has even produced salivation.

Pod-o-phȳl'lum.* The Pharmacopœial name ‖ for the rhizoma of the *Podophyllum peltatum*, or May-apple. It is an active and certain cathartic, resembling jalap in its operation.

Po-dop'ter-us.* [From πούς, a "foot," and πτερόν, a "wing."] Having peduncles with expansions in the form of wings: podop'terous.

Pod'o-sperm. [**Podosper'ma, a***tis;* from πούς, a "foot," and σπέρμα, a "seed."] The stalk of a seed; the funiculus by which the ovule adheres to the placenta of a plant.

Podostemaceæ,* po-dos-te-ma'-she-ē. [From *Podoste'mon*, one of the genera.] A natural order of exogenous, aquatic, herbaceous plants, found in South America.

Pod-o-the'ca.* [From πούς, ποδός, a "foot," and θήκη, a "receptacle."] Applied to a preparation of the cuticle of the foot.

Pœ-cil-ĭ-a'nus.* [From ποικίλος, "many-colored," "varied."] Applied by Brongniart to rocks having varied or chequered coloration.

Pœ-ci-lop'o-dus.* [From ποικίλος, "many-colored," and πούς, a "foot."] Having dissimilar feet. Applied to an order of *Crustacea*.

Poignet (Fr.), pwån'yå'. See WRIST.

Poil, pwål. The French term for HAIR, which see.

Poin'tal. Another name for PISTIL.

Pointed. See ACUMINATE.

Point'ing. The conical softish projection, of a light-yellow color, observable in an abscess when nearly ripe.

Pois, pwå. The French name for "pea." See PISUM.

Poi'son. [Lat. **Tox'icum,** or **Vene'num;** Fr. *Poison*, pwå'zôNG'.] An animal, vegetable, or mineral substance which, when applied externally, or taken into the stomach, or circulatory system, operates such a change in the animal economy as to produce disease or death. These substances may be divided into two great classes, namely, *Inorganic poisons*, comprising those which exist native, as certain poisonous ores, gases, etc., and those which are produced by chemical operations; and *Organic poisons*, or those which are the result of vital action in animals or plants.

Viewed, however, with reference to their effect on the animal system, they may be arranged under the three following heads:—

1. *Irritant poisons*, or those which produce irritation, or inflammation, as the mineral acids, oxalic acid, the caustic alkalies, antimony, arsenic, baryta, the salts of copper, some of the compounds of lead, nitrate of silver, the salts of zinc, cantharides, iodine, phosphorus, etc. A distinction is sometimes drawn between *irritant* and *corrosive* poisons; but the difference appears to be, at least in some cases, one of *degree* rather than of *kind*. Thus, one of the more powerful mineral acids in a concentrated form, would be a corrosive poison, but in a diluted form, only an irritant poison.

2. *Narcotic poisons*, or such as produce stupor or delirium, as opium, hyoscyamus, etc.

3. *Sedative poisons*, or those which directly reduce the vital powers, as hydrocyanic acid, cyanide of potassium, sulphuretted hydrogen and other of the poisonous gases.

4. *Acro-narcotic* and *Acro-sedative poisons*, including those which produce sometimes irritation, sometimes narcotism (or sedation), or both together. They are chiefly derived from the vegetable kingdom. Stramonium or belladonna will furnish an example of the acro-narcotic, and aconite of the acro-sedative, poisons.

TREATMENT.—It is not deemed necessary to enter here into a minute consideration of the symptoms caused by the various kinds of poison. In fact, the symptoms produced by many different substances so nearly resemble each other that, without other data, they would be wholly insufficient for determining the character of the poison. But some assistance towards forming a correct diagnosis will undoubtedly be furnished by a knowledge even of the general properties of the various poisons. With respect, however, to the more important articles of this class, such as the mineral acids, the caustic alkalies, arsenic, and several of the other metals, it has been deemed important to describe the most usual and characteristic symptoms.

Acids.—Most of the mineral acids, as well as oxalic acid, are corrosive poisons: if taken into the stomach, they cause an extremely sour, acrid taste, with a sense of burning in the throat, and an excruciating burning pain in the stomach. The matter vomited causes effervescence with chalk, or other forms of carbonate of lime. The proper treatment in such cases is to administer chalk, or magnesia, made into a thin paste with water. In case these substances are not at hand, the plaster of the apartment may be beaten to powder and made into paste. As antidotes for nitric and oxalic acids, lime and magnesia only are admissible; for acetic, citric, muriatic, sulphuric, and tartaric acids, the carbonates of potash and soda may also be used. The effects of hydrocyanic (or prussic) acid are usually so rapid as to render medical treatment of no avail. When death does not follow instantaneously, cold affusions or a cold *douche* on the head will often prove extremely beneficial. Ammonia may also be administered with advantage.

Alkalies.—In cases of poisoning with the caustic alkalies, there is an extremely harsh, acrid taste, with intense burning or smarting in the throat, caused by the destruction of its lining membrane, accompanied with great difficulty or pain in swallowing. The matter vomited will turn vegetable blues to green, or turmeric to brown. The proper antidotes are the fluid fixed oils, as sweet oil, linseed oil, castor oil, etc., or the mild vegetable acids, as vinegar, lemon-juice, etc.

Antimony.—In cases of poisoning with the preparations of antimony, there is usually vomiting, which should be facilitated, and rendered as free as possible, by copious draughts of warm or tepid water, or by tickling the fauces with one's finger or with a feather, etc. This is to be followed by astringent drinks, such as the infusion of galls, oak bark, Peruvian bark, dogwood (*Cornus Florida*), etc.

Arsenic.—When any of the soluble compounds of arsenic have been taken, there is an intense burning pain in the stomach and bowels, accompanied by violent vomiting, a sense of dryness and tightness in the throat, with an incessant desire for drink. The eyes are red and sparkling, and the countenance expresses extreme suffering and anxiety. Frequently there are nervous tremors, and other symptoms showing that the nervous system is powerfully affected. In rare instances arsenic has been known to produce coma and other symptoms closely resembling narcotic poisoning. For the treatment of cases of poisoning with arsenious acid, the hydrated sesquioxide (or peroxide) of iron, made into a paste with water, is the best, if not the only efficient, antidote. But even this remedy has been found to be of little avail when the arsenic has been swallowed in a solid state. (See ARSENIC.) Hydrate of magnesia has also been found useful, it is said, when the poison has been taken in solution.

For Fowler's Solution (*Liquor arsenicalis*), lime-water is a good antidote. In case the other preparations of arsenic have been taken, an emetic of sulphate of zinc should be administered, followed by a copious use of demulcent drinks, such as flaxseed or slippery-elm tea, milk, farinaceous decoctions, etc.

Baryta.—The symptoms are similar to those produced by the corrosive metals. The sulphates of soda and magnesia are efficacious antidotes for the salts of baryta.

Copper.—In cases of poisoning with the salts of copper (which are corrosive poisons), the best antidotes are the white of eggs and metallic iron (in the form of filings or raspings). Vinegar should be carefully avoided, as likely to dissolve the solid or insoluble compounds that may have been formed by the salts of copper with animal or vegetable substances.

Iron.—For poisoning with the sulphate of iron (or copperas), carbonate of soda, and mucilaginous drinks, are the proper remedies.

Lead.—For the soluble salts of lead, such as the acetate (sugar of lead), the best antidotes are sulphate of magnesia (Epsom salts) and phosphate of soda. For lead in any form insoluble in water (white lead, for example), very dilute sulphuric acid should be administered. Strychnia has been recommended for paralysis resulting from lead.

Mercury.—For the poisonous compounds of mercury (such as corrosive sublimate, the cyanide and nitrate of mercury, red and white precipitates, etc.), the white of eggs beaten up with water, or milk, should be promptly and freely given; or, if these articles should not be at hand, flour made into a paste may be used as a substitute.

Silver.—For nitrate of silver (or lunar caustic), common salt is an excellent antidote.

Tin and *Zinc.*—For the poisonous compounds of tin and zinc, milk and the white of eggs will serve as antidotes. When the sulphate or acetate of zinc has been taken, vomiting should be promoted by plentiful draughts of warm water.

Gases.—Among the other most important inorganic poisons may be numbered the poisonous gases, including carbonic acid gas, carbonic oxide, carburetted and sulphuretted hydrogen, the vapor of ether, and chlorine. In cases of poisoning with these, the best remedy is fresh air: if there should be stupor, cold affusions may be applied to the head, and the vital powers quickened by artificial respiration, and by the use of a galvanic apparatus. For the poisonous effects of carbonic acid gas, the inhalation of oxygen is the best antidote. A cautious inhalation of ammonia may prove useful in cases of poisoning with chlorine.

For *Iodine*, the best antidote is starch; when this is not at hand, flour, which contains starch, may be substituted.

The poisonous effects of *creasote* may be counteracted or mitigated by the prompt administration of albumen in some form. In cases of poisoning with *phosphorus*, the chief reliance must be on some prompt emetic, which should be followed by mucilaginous drinks. If the phosphorus should have been taken in a solid form, the fluid oils should be carefully avoided, on account of their solvent property.

Organic Poisons.—Those found in the vegetable kingdom are to be treated according to their character. If vomiting has been produced by their action, this may be facilitated, or rendered more free, by plentiful draughts of warm water. But if the taking of the poison has been followed by insensibility, some active emetic, such as sulphate of zinc, should be administered, or, in extreme cases, recourse must be had to the stomach-pump. In the case of opium, and similar narcotics, copious affusions of cold water on the head have sometimes proved of great advantage. A strong infusion of coffee has been found beneficial in counteracting the subsequent effects of an over-dose of opium. The remarkable antagonism existing between belladonna and opium, has sometimes, it is stated, been used with the greatest advantage, each having, in its turn, been made to act as an antidote to the other. In like manner, it is said, opium and stramonium may be used mutually to counteract each other. Tannin is the proper antidote for strychnia, but, to be successful, it should be greatly in excess; in the proportion of not less than 25 or 30 of the antidote to 1 of the poison.

Animal Poisons may be properly ranked under two heads:—

1. Those taken into the stomach by mistake as food; such are the various kinds of poisonous fish, which should be treated on the same principles as the vegetable poisons, that is, by emetics, copious draughts of warm water, etc., followed, perhaps, by an active purgative, in order to remove any deleterious matter which may have lodged in the intestines. If *cantharides* should have been taken, vomiting should be excited by copious draughts of sweet oil, linseed tea, milk, etc.

2. The poisonous secretions of the various venomous animals, used by them as a weapon of defence. As such poisons are not taken into the stomach, but introduced into the system through a wound, an altogether different plan of treatment is required. A cupping-glass should be promptly placed over the wound, and the air exhausted, for the purpose of extracting the venom. At the same time, if practicable, a moderately tight ligature should be applied above the bite or sting, in order to prevent the virus from diffusing itself through the system. If a cupping-glass cannot be procured, the poison may be extracted by sucking, in which case, it is scarcely necessary to remark, care should be taken not to swallow the saliva. In cases of poisoning from venomous serpents, the alkalies, especially ammonia, applied to the wound and taken internally, are said, in some instances, to have proved extremely beneficial. The application of clay or mud to the part, by excluding the air, tends to obstruct the activity of the poison. From several cases recently reported, it would appear that by far the most efficient antidote for the venom of serpents, is the compound

known as Bibron's Antidote. A common formula for its preparation is the following:—Take of bromine two drachms and a half; iodide of potassium, two grains; corrosive sublimate, one grain; dilute alcohol, thirty fluidrachms. Mix. Dose, one fluidrachm, diluted with a tablespoonful of wine or brandy, to be repeated *pro re natâ*. For hydrophobia, after the poison has once been received into the system, there is no antidote known. As soon as possible after the wound has been inflicted, the bitten part should be completely cut out, and free bleeding promoted by immersing the wound in warm water; the surface should afterwards be burned with actual cautery, or with some efficient caustic.

Poi'son-Lau'rel. The *Prunus laurocerasus.*

Poi'son-Oak. A popular name for the *Rhus toxicodendron.*

Poitrine, pwå'trėn'. The French name for the chest or thorax. See THORAX.

Poivre de Jamaique, pwåvʀ dęh zhå'mĕk'. ("Jamaica Pepper.") The French name for "allspice." See MYRTUS PIMENTA.

Po'lar. [**Pola'ris;** from *po'lus*, a "pole."] Pertaining to the pole, or near the pole.

Po'lar Cir'cles. Those which circumscribe the poles,—the northern or Arctic, the southern or Antarctic.

Po-lăr'ĭ-tў. [**Polar'itas, a'***tis;* from *po'lus*, a "pole."] The property of the magnet in pointing to the poles. That property which disposes the particles of many kinds of bodies to arrange themselves in certain determinate directions, or point, as it were, to given poles. *Magnetic polarity* is the tendency of a magnet, when freely and horizontally suspended, to point to the magnetic poles of the earth.

Po-lar-ĭ-zā'tion of Light. Light which has undergone certain reflections or refractions, or been subjected to the action of material bodies in any one of a great number of ways, acquires a certain modification, in consequence of which it no longer presents the same phenomena of reflection and transmission as light which has not been subjected to such action. This modification is termed *polarization of light.*—(BRANDE.) One form of this polarization is exhibited in the phenomenon known as *double refraction.*

Pol-e-mo'nĭ-ą,* the plural of *Polemo'nium*, forming the Jussieuan name of a natural order of plants. See POLEMONIACEÆ.

Polemoniaceæ,* pol-e-mo-ne-a'-she-ē. A natural order of exogenous, herbaceous plants, abundant in North and South America. It includes the *Phlox*, and *Polemonium*, one species of which is the Greek Valerian.

Poles. [**Po'li,** plural of *po'lus.*] The extremities of the axis of a sphere; specially applied to those of the earth, termed the North and South Poles.

Po-lĭ-a'ter.* [From πολίς, a "city," and ἰατρός, a "physician."] A physician who practises his profession in a city by the appointment of the government.

Pol-ĭ-ti'ą.* [Gr. πολιτεία, the "government, or civil polity, of a state."] The polity by which a city or town is governed: police.

Politi'a Med'ĭ-cą.* The medical police of a town or city.

Pol'len, *inis.** Originally, fine flour. Applied to the powdery substance contained in the anthers of flowers, constituting the fecundating principle in phanerogamous plants.

Pol'len Tube. A tubular process, or extremely minute tube, which grows or sprouts from the grain of pollen when the latter comes in contact with the stigma. It is supposed to convey the fertilizing influence down the style to the ovule.

Pol'lex,* gen. **Pol'lĭ-cis.** [From *pol'leo*, to "be strong;" because it is stronger than the fingers.] (Fr. *Pouce*, pooss.) The thumb. Also applied to the great toe.

Pol-lin'ĭ-ą.* [From *pol'len.*] A term applied to the granular or waxy masses of pollen found in the *Orchidaceæ.*

Pol-lĭ-nif'er-ous. [**Pollinif'erus;** from *pol'len*, and *fe'ro*, to "bear."] Bearing, or containing, pollen.

Pol'lĭ-nin. [**Pollini'na.**] A peculiar and highly combustible substance obtained from the pollen of tulips.

Pollu'tio (pol-lu'she-o) **Di-ur'ną.*** ("Diurnal Pollution.") The same as SPERMATOCLEMMA, which see.

Pol-lu'tion. [**Pollu'tio, o'***nis;* from *pol'luo, pollu'tum*, to "defile."] (Fr. *Souillure*, swė'yüʀ'.) The emission of semen without coition. It may be voluntary (then termed *masturbation*, or *onanism*), or involuntary. Involuntary pollution is sometimes the result of weakness caused by masturbation. When it occurs in sleep, it is called *gonorrhœa dor-*

mientium, or SPERMATORRHŒA DORMIENTIUM, which see.

Pol-y̆-a-can'thus.* [From πολύς, "many," and ἄκανθα, a "thorn."] Having many spines or thorns: polyacanthous.

Pol-y̆-a-del'phi-a.* [From πολύς, "many," and ἀδελφός, a "brother."] Literally, "having many brotherhoods, companies, or sets." The eighteenth class in the Linnæan system of plants, comprising those whose stamens are united by their filaments into three or more sets.

Pol-y̆-a-del'phous. [**Polyadel'phius**, or **Polyadel'phus**; from the same.] Having the filaments in several sets: polyadel'phious. See POLYADELPHIA.

Pol-y̆-ad'e-nus.* [From πολύς, "many," and ἀδήν, a "gland."] Bearing many glands: polyadenous.

Pol-y̆-an'dri-a.* [From πολύς, "many," and ἀνήρ, a "man," or "male."] The thirteenth class in the Linnæan system of plants, comprising those which have twenty or more stamens inserted on the receptacle.

Pol-y̆-an'drous. [**Polyan'drius**, or **Polyan'drus**; from the same.] Having many hypogynous stamens: polyan'drious.

Pol-y̆-an'thous. [**Polyan'thus**; from πολύς, "many," and ἄνθος, a "flower."] Bearing many flowers.

Pol-y̆-car'pic. [**Polycar'picus**; from πολύς, "many," and καρπός, "fruit."] Bearing fruit many times, that is, year after year.

Pol-y̆-car'pous. [**Polycar'pus**; from the same.] Having, or bearing, much fruit.

Pol-y̆-çeph'a-lous. [**Polyceph'alus**; from πολύς, "many," and κεφαλή, the "head."] Having many heads. Applied to plants.

Pol-y̆-çe-ra'tus.* [From πολύς, "many," and κέρας, a "horn."] Applied to a plant of which the fruits resemble a bundle of small horns. In Zoology, having many horns.

Pol'y̆-chrĕst. [**Polychres'tos**, or **Polychres'tus**; from πολύς, "many," and χρηστός, "useful."] Having many uses or virtues. Also, a substance possessing many virtues.

Pol-y̆-chro-mat'ic. [**Polychromat'icus**; from πολύς, "many," and χρῶμα, "color."] Of various colors; many-colored.

Po-ly̆c'la-dous. [**Polyc'ladus**; from πολύς, "many," or "much," and κλάδος, a "branch."] Much branched. Applied to plants.

Pol-y̆-clo'nos,* or **Pol-y̆-clo'nus.*** [From πολύς, "many," and κλών, a "branch."] Having many branches.

Pol-y̆-coc'cous. [**Polycoc'cus**; from πολύς, "many," and κόκκος, a "kernel," or "berry."] Having many or several *cocci* (closed cells or carpels).

Pol-y̆-cot-y̆-le'don.* [From πολύς, "many," and κοτυληδών, a "cotyledon."] A plant that has several, or more than two, cotyledons.

Pol-y̆-cot-y̆-led'o-nous. [From the same.] Having several, or more than two, cotyledons.

Pol-y̆-dip'si-a.* [From πολύς, "much," and δίψη, "thirst."] Excessive thirst. A genus of the order *Dysorexiæ*, class *Locales*, of Cullen's Nosology.

Polyedron. See POLYHEDRON.

Po-ly̆g'a-la.* [From πολύς, "much," and γάλα, "milk:" named from the abundant milky juice found in some of the species.] Milkwort. A Linnæan genus of the class *Diadelphia*, natural order *Polygalaceæ*.

Polyg'ala Ru-bel'la.* Bitter Polygala. The Pharmacopœial name (U.S. Ph.) for the root and herb of *Polygala rubella*.

Polyg'ala Sen'e-ga.* The rattlesnake-root, or Seneka snake-root. See SENEGA.

Polygalaceæ,* pol-e-ga-la'she-ē, or **Pol-y̆-ga'le-æ.*** A natural order of exogenous plants (herbs or shrubs), with tonic, astringent, or nephritic properties. It includes *Polygala senega* (Snake-root).

Pol-y̆-ga-lac'ti-a.* [From πολύς, "much," and γάλα, "milk."] Excessive secretion, or an overflow, of milk.

Pol-y̆-ga'le-æ.* The Jussieuan name of a natural order of plants. See POLYGALACEÆ.

Pol-y̆-gal'ic. [**Polygal'icus**; from *Polyg'ala*.] Applied to an acid discovered in the *Polygala senega*, and other species.

Po-ly̆g'a-lin. [**Polygali'na.**] A bitter alkaline principle discovered in several species of *Polygala*.

Pol-y̆-ga'mi-a.* [From πολύς, "many," and γάμος, a "marriage."] A Linnæan class of plants, including those which have staminate, pistillate, and perfect flowers either on the same or on different plants.

Po-ly̆g'a-mous. [**Polyga'mius**, or **Polyg'amus**; from the same.]

Having both perfect and separated flowers: polyga'mious. See POLYGAMIA.

Pol-ў-gas'trĭ-ca.* [From πολύς, "many," and γαστήρ, a "stomach."] The first class of the *Diploneura*, or *Helminthoida*, consisting of minute, transparent, soft, aquatic animals, with numerous stomachs, or cæca, communicating with an internal alimentary cavity. They are without perceptible nerves or muscles, and move by external vibratile cilia.

Po-lў-ġen'ic. [**Polygen'icus;** from πολύς, "many," and γένω, to "be born," to "be produced."] Applied to a rock which owes its origin to fragments of several different rocks united by calcareous cement.

Pol'ў-gon. [**Polygo'num;** from πολύς, "many," and γωνία, an "angle."] A plane figure having more than four angles, and, consequently, more than four sides. If the sides are equal, it is called a regular polygon.

Polygonaceæ,* po-lig-o-na'she-ē. A natural order of exogenous plants, mostly herbaceous, natives of nearly all parts of the world. The roots are universally nauseous and purgative. It includes the *Polyg'onum* (Buckwheat,) *Ru'mex* (Dock), and *Rheum* (Rhubarb).

Po-lўg'o-nal. [**Polygo'nus.**] Belonging to a polygon.

Pol-ў-go-na'tus.* [From πολύς, "many," and γόνυ, a "knee;" also, a "joint," as of grasses.] Polyg'onate. Applied to certain plants and insects.

Po-lўg'o-num.* [From the same.] A Linnæan genus of the class *Octandria*, natural order *Polygonaceæ*.

Polyg'onum Bis-tor'ta.* The plant commonly known as bistort. The root is astringent.

Pol-ў-ġўn'ĭ-a.* [From πολύς, "many," and γυνή, a "woman," or "female."] An order in the Linnæan system of plants, including those which have many pistils, or more than twelve pistils.

Pol-ў-ġўn'ĭ-ous. [**Polygyn'ius,** or **Polyġ'ynus;** from the same.] Having many pistils.

Pol-ў-he'dral, or **Pol-ў-he'dric.** [**Polyhe'drus.**] Belonging to a polyhedron.

Pol-ў-he'dron. [**Polyhe'drum;** from πολύς, "many," and ἕδρα, a "base."] A solid figure contained by many sides or planes; a solid bounded by polygons.

Pol-ў-mor'phous. [**Polymor'phus;** from πολύς, "many," and μορφή, "shape."] Having many forms; various in form.

Pol-ў-neū'rus.* [From πολύς, "many," and νεῦρον, a "nerve."] Applied to a leaf the lateral nervures of which are very numerous.

Pol-ў-o'pĭ-a.* [From πολύς, "many," and ὄπτομαι, to "see."] An affection of the organs of sight, in which the objects are multiplied; multiple vision: polyo'py.

Pol'ў-pa-rў. [**Polypa'rium;** from *pol'ypus*, a "polype."] Applied to the habitation of a number of polypi.

Polype. See POLYPUS.

Pol-ў-pet'a-lous. [**Polypeta'leus,** or **Polypet'alus;** from πολύς, "many," and πέταλον, a "petal."] Having many petals, or distinct petals: polypeta'leous.

Pol'ў-phore. [From πολύς, "many," and φέρω, to "bear."] A common receptacle of many carpels, as in the Strawberry.

Pol-ў-phўl'lous. [**Polyphyl'lus;** from πολύς, "many," and φύλλον, a "leaf."] Having many leaves.

Pol'ў-pi,* gen. **Pol-ў-po'rum.** The plural of POLYPUS, which see.

Pol-ў-pif'er-ous. [**Polypif'erus;** from *pol'ypus*, a "polype," and *fe'ro*, to "bear."] Bearing polypi.

Pol'ў-pĭ-form. [**Polypifor'mis;** from *pol'ypus*, a "polype."] Having the form or appearance of a polypus.

Polypodiaceæ,* pol-e-po-de-a'-she-ē. A natural order of cryptogamous plants, including *Polypo'dium*, and many other kinds of ferns.

Pol-ў-po'dĭ-um.* [From πολύς, "many," and πούς, a "foot."] A Linnæan genus of the class *Cryptogamia*, order *Filices*, or *Polypodiaceæ*.

Polypo'dium Fi'lix Mas.* Another name for the *Aspidium filix mas*, or male fern.

Pol'ў-pous, or **Pol'ў-pal.** [**Polypo'sus;** from *pol'ypus*.] Having polypi, or many tumors like a polypus.

Pol'ў-pus.* [From πολύς, "many," and πούς, a "foot."] A tumor in the nose, uterus, or vagina; from its having numerous ramifications, like legs or feet. Also, an animal of the *Radiata*, characterized by a fleshy body of a conical or cylindrical form, commonly fixed at one extremity, having at the other the mouth, surrounded by several arms or tentacles: a polype.

Pol-ў-rhī'zous, or **Pol-ў-rhī'zal.** [**Polyrhi'zus;** from πολύς, "many," and ῥίζα, a "root."] Having many roots.

Pol-ў-sar'çĭ-a.* [From πολύς, "much,"

and σάρξ, "flesh."] An increased bulk of body beyond what is healthy; obesity. A genus of the order *Intumescentiæ*, class *Cachexiæ*, of Cullen's Nosology.

Pol-ȳ-sar'cous. [**Polysar'cus;** from the same.] Having much flesh; obese.

Pol-ȳ-sep'a-lous. [**Polysep'alus:** from πολύς, "many," and *sep'alum*, a "sepal."] Having two or more distinct sepals. Applied to a calyx.

Pol-ȳ-sper'mous. [From πολύς, "many," and σπέρμα, a "seed."] Having many seeds.

Pol-ȳs'po-rous. [**Polys'porus;** from πολύς, "many," and σπόρα, a "seed."] Containing many spores. See SPORE.

Pol-ȳ-sta'chȳ-us.* [From πολύς, "many," and στάχυς, an "ear."] Having many spikes or ears.

Pol-ȳ-ste'mo-nous. [**Polyste'monis;** from πολύς, "many," and στήμων, a "stamen."] Having many stamens.

Pol-ȳ-stig'mous. [**Polystig'mus;** from πολύς, "many," and στίγμα, a "stigma."] Having many stigmas in each flower.

Pol-ȳ-stȳ'lous. [**Polysty'lus;** from πολύς, "many," and στῦλος, a "pillar," or "style."] Having many styles.

Pol-ȳ-tech'nic. [**Polytech'nicus;** from πολύς, "many," and τέχνη, "art."] Pertaining to many, or several, arts and sciences. A polytechnic school is an institution in which many arts or sciences are taught. The first school bearing this name was founded in Paris in 1794.

Pol-ȳ-thal'a-mous. [**Polythal'amus;** from πολύς, "many," and θάλαμος, a "chamber."] Applied to a univalve shell divided into many apartments.

Po-lȳt'ri-chus.* [From πολύς, "many," or "much," and θρίξ, "hair."] Having abundant hair.

Po'ma,* gen. **Po-mo'rum,** the plural of POMUM, which see.

Pomaceæ,* po-ma'she-ē. [From *po'mum*, a Latin term for an "apple," or other fruit.] A natural order of exogenous trees and shrubs, natives of many temperate regions, but not found in the southern hemisphere. It includes the Apple, the Pear (*Pyrus*), the Quince (*Cydonia*), and Plum (*Prunus*). Some botanists consider *Pomaceæ* as a division of the order *Rosaceæ*.

Po-mā'ceous. [**Poma'ceus;** from *po'mum*, an "apple," or other fruit.] Resembling the apple, or of the nature of an apple.

Pome. [**Po'ma;** from *po'mum*, an "apple," or other fruit.] A fleshy fruit, composed of two or more carpels, usually more or less involved in a pulpy expansion of the receptacle or disk, and the whole invested by the thickened and succulent tube of the calyx; as the apple. —(GRAY.)

Pomegranate, pŭm'gran-at. [From *po'mum*, an "apple," or other fruit, and *grana'tus*, "having grains."] The fruit of the *Punica granatum*.

Po-mif'er-ous. [**Pomif'erus;** from *po'mum*, an "apple," or other fruit, and *fe'ro*, to "bear."] Bearing pomes.

Pom'ĭ-form. [**Pomifor'mis;** from *po'mum*, an "apple," or other fruit.] Having the form of an apple.

Pomme de Terre, pomm dẹh têR. The French name for POTATO, which see.

Po-mol'o-ġȳ. [**Pomolo'gia;** from *po'mum*, an "apple," or other fruit, and λόγος, a "discourse."] A treatise on fruits; the science of fruits, or the art of cultivating fruits; the department of Botany relating to fruits.

Pom-phol-ȳ-go'dēs.* [From *pom'pholyx*.] Resembling or having *pompholyx*.

Pom'pho-lȳx, *ygis.** [From πομφός, a "bladder."] A small vesicle or bladder especially containing water; also, a skin-disease in which there is an eruption of *bullæ* without inflammation round them, and unattended by fever.

Po'mum,* plural **Po'ma.** An apple, or larger fruit. Originally, a general name of fruit which grows on trees; as the apple, pear, etc. See POME.

Po'mum A-da'mi.* ("Adam's Apple.") The anterior part of the thyroid cartilage, forming an angular projection on the fore part of the neck.

Pon-der-a-bil'ĭ-tȳ. [**Ponderabil'itas, a'tis;** from *pon'dero*, to "weigh."] The property of having weight.

Pon'der-a-ble. [From *pon'dus, pon'deris*, "weight."] That may be weighed. A term applied to bodies having weight.

Pons Hep'a-tis.* ("Bridge of the Liver.") A portion of the substance of the liver which passes from one lobe to the other, frequently converting the lower half of the longitudinal fissure into a true canal.

Pons Ta-ri'ni.* ("Bridge of Tarinus.") A cineritious substance between the *corpora albicantia* of the brain, connecting the crura, and forming part of the floor of the third ventricle. The fossa, at the bottom of which it is placed, is called *Lo'cus perfora'tus posti'cus.*

Pons Va-ro'li-i.* ("Bridge of Varolius") The square portion of medullary substance connecting the cerebrum, cerebellum, and *Medulla oblongata*, first described by Varolius; otherwise termed the *Corpus annulare, Processus annularis, Tuber annulare,* and *Tuberculum annulare.*

Pontederaceæ,* pon-te-de-ra'she-ē. A natural order of endogenous aquatic plants, found in America, India, and tropical Africa. It includes the *Ponte-de'ria.*

Pop'les, litis.* [From *post,* "behind," and *pli'co,* to "fold."] (Fr. *Jarret,* zhå'rå'.) The ham, or back part of the knee-joint.

Pop-li-tæ'us.* ("Popliteal [Muscle].") [From *pop'les, pop'litis,* the "ham."] A muscle arising from the external condyle of the femur, and inserted into the superior triangular surface at the back of the tibia. It bends the thigh and leg.

Pop-li-te'al. [**Poplitæ'us;** from the same.] Belonging to the ham.

Poplite'al Space. A somewhat oval space, of considerable depth, behind the knee-joint.

Poppy. See Papaver.

Pop'py, Red Corn. The *Papaver rhœas.*

Pop'py, White. A name for the *Papaver somniferum.*

Pop'u-lin. [**Populi'na.**] A name given to an alkali found in the bark of the *Pop'ulus trem'ula,* or aspen-tree.

Por-cel-lā'ne-ous. [**Porcella'neus,** or **Porcella'nus;** from *porcella'na,* a "porcelain vessel."] Belonging to porcelain.

Pore. [**Po'rus;** from πόρος, a "passage."] A small opening at the extremity of a vessel at the surface of an organized body. Also, a small interstice between the particles of matter which compose bodies. It appears that pores exist in all bodies, even the most dense.

Po-rif'e-ra.* [From *po'rus,* a "pore," and *fe'ro,* to "bear."] A term applied to a group of polypi. Also employed by Dr. Grant to designate a class of organized bodies, including the marine and fresh-water sponges.

Po'ri-form. [**Porifor'mis;** from *po'rus,* a "pore."] Having the form of simple pores.

Por-nog'ra-phy̆. [**Pornogra'phia;** from πόρνη, a "prostitute," and γράφω, to "write."] A history or description of prostitution.

Po-ro'ma, atis.* [Gr. πωρῶμα; from πῶρος, a kind of stone.] A callus, or hardened part. See Porosis.

Por-o-phy̆l'lus.* [From πόρος, a "pore," and φύλλον, a "leaf."] Having leaves sprinkled with transparent points like pores, as the *Bœbera porophyl'la:* porophyl'lous.

Po-ro'sis.* [From πωρόω, to "turn to stone," to "harden." See Poroma.] The progress or formation of *Poroma,* or the process by which the extremities of fractured bones are reunited by a callus.

Po-ros'i-ty̆. [**Poros'itas, a'tis;** from *po'rus,* a "pore."] The property or quality of having pores or interstices between the particles.

Po'rous. [**Poro'sus;** from *po'rus,* a "pore."] Having pores, or full of pores.

Por'phy̆-ra.* [From πορφύρα, "purple."] A name for Purpura, which see.

Por-phy̆-ris'ma, atis.* [From πορφύρα, "purple."] A name for Scarlatina, which see.

Por'phy̆-ry̆. [From the same.] An extremely hard stone of a reddish or purple color, more or less variegated, being of all varieties of shade from violet to a claret color. It is susceptible of a high polish. It belongs to the igneous rocks.

Por-rig'i-nous. [**Porrigino'sus.**] Having *porrigo.*

Por-ri'go, g'inis.* [From *por'rum,* a "leek."] (Fr. *Teigne,* tēñ or tåñ.) Ringworm of the scalp; scald-head: also termed *Favus* and Tinea, which see.

Porrum. See Allium Porrum.

Por'ta.* [From *por'to,* to "carry."] Literally, a "door," or "gate." Applied to that part of the liver where its vessels enter.

Por'tal Cir-cu-lā'tion. A subordinate part of the venous circulation, in which the blood makes an additional circuit before it joins the rest of the venous blood. There are in the vertebrate classes of animals two portal circulations, one of the liver, and the other of the kidneys. The former exists in all the Vertebrata; the latter, only in reptiles, Amphibia, and fishes.

Por'tal Vein. [**Ve'na Por'tæ.**] A vein originating from all the organs within the abdomen, except the kidneys and bladder, and the uterus in the female. It has two principal trunks, the splenic and superior mesenteric veins.

Port-caus'tic. [From *por'to,* to

"carry," and *caus'ticum*, "caustic."] A small cylindrical instrument for carrying some caustic substance in the pocket.

Por'ter. An infusion of malt and hops, owing its dark color to high-dried, or charred, malt.

Por'tio (por'she-o) **Du'ra.*** ("Hard Portion.") The hard branch of the seventh pair of nerves; the facial nerve.

Por'tio Mol'lis.* ("Soft Portion.") The soft branch of the seventh pair of nerves; the auditory or acoustic nerve.

Port'land Stone. A granular limestone, belonging to the upper part of the oolite formation, and abounding in the island of Portland, on the southern coast of England.

Portulacaceæ,* por-tu-la-ka'she-ē, or **Portulaceæ,*** por-tu-la'she-ē. A natural order of exogenous succulent plants, found in dry places in South America and South Africa. It includes *Portula'ca*, one species of which is common Purslane.

Po'rus.* [Gr. πῶρος, "tuff-stone," "tufa."] The thick, hard skin, or brawn; callus.

Po'rus.* [Gr. πόρος, a "ford," a "ferry," or "passage."] A duct; a pore. See PORE.

Po'rus Op'ti-cus.* ("Optic Pore.") A dark point in the centre of the optic nerve, through which the central artery passes. See PUNCTUM CÆCUM.

Pos'i-tive El'e-ments. A term applied to the plates of zinc in the galvanic pile; the zinc or most oxidizable metal being in such combinations always found to be positively, and the copper (or silver), the least oxidizable, negatively, electrical.

Pos-i-tiv'i-ty. [**Positiv'itas, a'tis.**] The state of a body which manifests the phenomena of positive electricity.

Po-sol'o-gy. [From πόσος, "how much," and λόγος, a "discourse."] That branch of medicine which treats of quantity, or doses. See DOSE.

Pos'set. [**Posse'tum.**] A preparation peculiar to the English; being milk heated to boiling, and then curdled with wine, treacle, or an acid.

Post-di-lu'vi-an. [**Postdiluvia'nus;** from *post*, "after," and *dilu'vium*, the "deluge."] Applied to the earths deposited by rivers or temporary floods, etc., posterior to the great catastrophe called the Deluge.

Pos-te'ri-or Au'ris.* ("Posterior [Muscle] of the Ear.") A muscle situated behind the ear, and consisting of one or more bundles of fleshy fibres; sometimes called *musculi retrahentes auriculam* (muscles which draw back the auricle).

Pos-thi'tis, idis.* [From πόσθη, the "prepuce."] Inflammation of the membrane of the *glans penis*. The same as BALANITIS, which see.

Post-Mor'tem.* ("After Death.") Applied to the examination of a dead body.

Post Par'tum.* [From *post*, "after," and *par'tus*, the "time of travail."] "After or subsequent to childbirth." Applied to hæmorrhage or any other occurrence ensuing after parturition.

Post. sing. sed. liq. = *Post sin'gulas se'des liq'uidas.** "After every loose stool."

Pot. = *Po'tio.** "A potion."

Pot'ash. [**Potas'sa.**] The vegetable alkali also termed *Kali;* properly, an hydrated protoxide of potassium.

Po-tas'sa.* A Latinized form of the word "potash."

Potas'sa Fu'sa.* ("Fused Potash.") The hydrate of potash; also called *Lapis infernalis*. Prepared by evaporating a solution of potash to dryness in an iron vessel. It is a powerful caustic, and is employed for forming issues, etc.

Po-tas'sæ Bi-chro'mas.* ("Bichromate of Potash.") The name applied to a substance in orange-red, anhydrous, tabular crystals, soluble in ten parts of cold, and in much less of boiling, water, forming a solution having an acid reaction. It has been placed on the primary list of the Materia Medica of the U.S. Pharmacopœia for 1860. In small doses it is an alterative; in large doses, an irritant poison. Externally it is used as a caustic.

Potas'sæ Bi-tar'tras* ("Bitartrate of Potash"), or **Cream of Tar'tar.** The Pharmacopœial name for a substance which is dissolved sparingly by water, but freely by a hot solution of potassa, which deposits it again upon the addition of an acid. It is a cathartic, diuretic, and refrigerant.

Potas'sæ Car-bo'nas Im-pu'ra or **Im-pu'rus.*** ("Impure Carbonate of Potash.") The Pharmacopœial name (U.S. Ph.) for the substance known in commerce by the name of "pearlash."

Potas'sæ Chlo'ras.* ("Chlorate of Potash.") The Pharmacopœial name ‖ of a substance in colorless, tabular crystals, which have a pearly lustre, and are wholly soluble in distilled water. Chlorate of potash is an arterial sedative.

It is said to be a most valuable remedy in stomatitis caused by the use of mercury.

Potas'sæ Ni'tras.* ("Nitrate of Potash.") Nitre or Saltpetre. The Pharmacopœial name ‖ of a substance in colorless prismatic crystals, unalterable in the air, and wholly soluble in water. It is a refrigerant, diuretic, and diaphoretic.

Potas'sæ Per-man'ga-nas.* ("Permanganate of Potash.") The name applied to a substance in needle-shaped crystals of a deep purple color. It is soluble in sixteen parts of cold water, with the exception of a scanty, brown matter. It has been placed on the primary list of the Materia Medica of the U.S. Pharmacopœia for 1860. It is used as an escharotic.

Potas'sæ Sul'phas.* ("Sulphate of Potash.") The Pharmacopœial name ‖ of a substance in hard, colorless crystals, unalterable in the air, sparingly soluble in cold water, and insoluble in alcohol.

Po-tas'si-cus.* [From *potas'sium.*] Belonging to potassium: potassic.

Po-tas'si-i Fer-ro-çy̆-an'i-dum.* ("Ferrocyanide of Potassium.") Also termed the **Ferrocyan'uret of Potas'sium.** The Pharmacopœial name (U.S. Ph.) for a substance in crystals of a lemon-yellow color, wholly soluble in water. It is chiefly used in the preparation of hydrocyanic acid, Prussian blue, etc.

Potassium,* po-tash'e-ŭm. A very remarkable metal, discovered by Davy in 1807. It is the base of potash. One of the striking peculiarities of potassium is its low specific gravity (.865), it being the lightest known solid; another is its intense affinity for oxygen. in consequence of which it takes fire when thrown upon water.

Po-tā'to. [Span. *Batata,* bå-tå'tå; Fr. *Pomme de Terre,* pomm dęh têr.] The common name for the root (tuber) of the *Sola'num tubero'sum.*

Poten'tial (po-ten'shal) **Cau'te-rȳ.** [**Caute'rium Potentia'le.**] See CAUTERY, POTENTIAL.

Po-ten-til'la.* [From *po'tens,* "powerful."] The wild tansy. A Linnæan genus of the class *Icosandria,* natural order *Rosaceæ.*

Potentil'la Tor-men-til'la.* The systematic name of the tormentil plant.

Po'tion. [**Po'tio, o'nis;** from *po'to, pota'tum* or *po'tum,* to "drink."] A medicinal mixture to be taken as a drink. See DRAUGHT.

Po-to-ma'ni-a.* [From *po'to, po'tum,* to "drink," and μανία, "madness."] Drink-madness. The same as MANIA A POTU, which see.

Pot-Pour'ri, pot poo'ree. Literally, a "medley," a "hotch-potch." A mixture of fragrant flowers, roots, gums, etc., either mixed together dry or preserved with salt.

Pou, poo. The French name for "louse." See PEDICULUS.

Pouce, pooss. The French name for the "thumb." See POLLEX.

Pouch. See SACCULUS.

Poudre, poodr. The French name for "powder." See PULVIS.

Poudre de Chypre, poodr dęh shēpr. See ABELMOSCHUS.

Pouls, poo. The French term for "pulse." See PULSUS.

Poultice. See CATAPLASM.

Poumon, poo'mōng'. The French term for LUNGS, which see.

Pou'part's (poo'parts) **Lig'a-ment.** That portion of the inferior thickened edge of the tendon of the *Obliquus externus abdominis* muscle, stretching from the anterior superior spinous process of the ilium to the spine of the *os pubis;* the crural arch.

Pourpre, poorpr. The French term for PURPURA, which see.

Powder. See PULVIS.

Powder of Faynard. See FAYNARD'S POWDER.

Pox. The vulgar name for syphilis: formerly called *great pox,* to distinguish it from variola, or *small-pox.*

Prac'tice. [Gr. πρακτική; from πράσσω, to "do," to "conduct business."] A general term for the extent of business, as well as the performance of the duties, of a medical practitioner, physician, surgeon, or apothecary.

Præ. A Latin preposition signifying "before," or "beforehand."

Præ-cor'di-a, *o'rum.** [From *præ,* "before," and *cor, cor'dis,* the "heart."] The fore part of the thoracic region.

Præfloratio. See ÆSTIVATION.

Præputium. See PREPUCE.

Prævia. See PLACENTA PRÆVIA.

P. rat. æt. = *Pro ratio'ne æta'tis.** "According to the age of the patient."

Pre-cip'i-tant. [**Præcip'itans;** from *præcip'ito, præcipita'tum,* to "cast down."] Literally, "casting down," or "precipitating." Applied to the substance by the addition of which a precipitate is formed.

Pre-cip'i-tate. [**Præcipita'tum;**

from the same.] The substance which sinks to the bottom in the process of precipitation.

Precip'itate, Red. The red oxide of mercury. See HYDRARGYRI OXIDUM RUBRUM.

Precip'itate, White. A compound formed by the union of ammonia with a solution of chloride of mercury.

Pre-cip-i-tā'tion. [**Præcipita'tio, o'**nis; from *præcip'ito, præcipita'tum,* to "cast down."] The process of precipitating a substance held in solution by the addition of another substance: thus, when an acid and oxide are united in solution, if an alkali be added having a greater affinity for the acid, it will combine with it, and the oxide will be precipitated. The oxide is named the *precipitate,* the alkali the *precipitant.*

Precocity, Genital. See PRŒOTIA.

Pre-cur'sor. [**Præcur'sor;** from *præ,* "before," and *cur'ro, cur'sum,* to "run."] Literally, a "forerunner." Applied to symptoms which precede, or indicate the approach of, a disease.

Pre-dis-po'sing. [**Prædispo'nens;** from *præ,* "before," or "beforehand," and *dispo'no, dispos'itum,* to "dispose."] Applied to the peculiar condition or habit of body, temperament, or structure of a part, which renders a person susceptible of disease; and this peculiar condition, structure, etc. is said to be the predisposing cause of the disease.

Pre-dis-po-sĭ'tion. [**Prædisposi'tio, o'**nis; from the same.] Any state of the system which disposes to the action of disease.

Pre-flo-rā'tion. [**Præflora'tio, o'**nis; from *præflo'reo,* to "blossom before the time."] The same as ÆSTIVATION, which see.

Pre-fo-lĭ-ā'tion. [**Præfolia'tio, o'**nis; from *præ,* "before," and *fo'lium,* a "leaf."] The manner in which the leaves are disposed in the bud before evolution. The same as VERNATION.

Pre-fron'tal. [**Præfronta'lis;** from *præ,* "before," and *fronta'le* os, the "frontal bone."] Applied by Owen to the middle part of the ethmoid bone.

Preg'nan-cy̆. [**Prægnan'tia;** from *præg'nans,* literally, "previous to bringing forth."] (Fr. *Grossesse,* gRo'-sĕss'.) The state of being with young or with child. See GRAVIDITY.

Pregnancy, Morbid. See PARACYESIS.

Preg'nant. [**Præg'nans.** See PREGNANCY.] With young or with child.

Pre-hen'sĭle. [**Prehensi'lis;** from *prehen'do, prehen'sum,* to "take," to "lay hold on."] Capable of laying hold on a thing; adapted to the act of grasping.

Pre-hen'sion. [**Prehen'sio, o'**nis; from the same.] The act of grasping or taking hold; a seizure.

Pre-ma-ture' Lā'bor. That which takes place during the last three months of the natural term, but before its completion.

Pre-max'il-la-ry̆. [**Præ-maxilla'ris;** from *præ,* "before," and *maxilla're* os, the "maxillary bone."] Applied by Owen to the front part of the superior maxilla.

Premières Voies, prẹh-me-êR' vwå. The French term for PRIMÆ VIÆ, which see.

Pre-mo'lar. [From *præ,* "before," and *mola'ris,* "molar."] A term applied to the first two pairs of molar teeth in each jaw; also called bicuspids.

Pre-morse'. [**Præmor'sus;** from *præmor'deo, præmor'sum,* to "bite off."] Ending abruptly, as if bitten off. Applied to parts of plants.

Pre-o-per'cu-lar. [**Præopercula'ris;** from *præ,* "before," and *opercula'ris,* "opercular."] Applied by Owen to the first or proximal segment of the radiated appendage of the tympano-mandibular arch in fishes.

Pre'puce. [**Præpu'tium;** from *præ,* "before," and πόσθη, the "virile member."] The membranous or cutaneous fold which covers the *glans penis;* also, a similar covering for the *glans clitoridis:* the foreskin.

Pres-by̆-o'pĭ-a.* [From πρέσβυς, an "old man," and ὤψ, the "eye."] The opposite of near-sightedness. A defect of vision, common to persons advanced in years, by which objects are seen imperfectly when near, but clearly when a little removed.

Pre-scrip'tion. [**Præscrip'tio, o'**nis; from *præscri'bo, præscrip'tum,* to "write before," to "order," to "prescribe."] A formula, or writing of medicines to be exhibited; a *recipe.*

Preś-en-tā'tion. [**Presenta'tio, o'**nis; from *præsen'to, præsenta'tum,* to "present."] The particular position of the child in the passages at birth, as arm-presentation, foot-presentation, etc.

Pre-sphe'noid. [**Præsphenoi'des;** from *præ,* "before," and *sphenoi'des* os, the "sphenoid bone."] Applied by Owen to the anterior part of the base of the sphenoid bone.

Preternatural Combustion. See SPONTANEOUS COMBUSTION.

Pre-tÿm-pan'ic. [**Prætympan'icus;** from *præ*, "before," and *tympan'icus*, "tympanic."] Applied by Owen to the anterior subdivision of the tympanic pedicle which supports the mandible in fishes.

Prī'a-pism. [**Priapis'mus;** from πρίαπος, the "virile member."] Continual (morbid) erection of the penis.

Prickle. See ACULEUS.

Prickly. See ACULEATE.

Pri'mæ Vi'æ.* (Fr. *Premières voies*, preh-me-êR' vwå.) "First or Primary Passages." The stomach and intestines: so named in reference to their importance.

Pri-ma'lĭ-a.* [From *pri'mus*, "first:" because it includes those growths which are the first, or lowest, in the scale of creation.] A term recently applied to a proposed division or kingdom of organized bodies, including those of which "the structure is exclusively cellular without vascularity," and which possess simply the power or function of reproduction, without any organs appropriated to respiration or circulation.

This kingdom is intended to include the following sub-kingdoms. 1. *Algæ* (Sea-weeds). 2. *Lichenes* (Lichens). 3. *Fungi*. 4. *Spongiæ* (Sponges). 5. *Conjugata* (Infusoria).

In accordance with this view, all organized bodies may be distributed into three kingdoms, namely:—

1. *Primalia*, possessing simply the power of reproduction by cell-development.

2. *Vegetabilia* ("Vegetables"), in which to the function of reproduction are added those of respiration and circulation.

3. *Animalia* ("Animals"), possessing, in addition to the functions of reproduction, respiration, and circulation, the power of voluntary motion and perception or sensation. (An interesting memoir on this subject, by Messrs. Wilson and Cassin, may be found in the Proceedings of the Academy of Natural Sciences of Philadelphia, May, 1863.)

Prī'ma-ries. The ten elastic quills attached to the hand or third portion of the wing of birds.

Prī'ma-rÿ. [**Prima'rius;** from *pri'mus*, "first."] Primitive; original; principal. Primary planets are those planets that revolve around the sun as their centre, in contradistinction to the satellites, or secondary planets.

PRI'MARY ROCKS are the igneous or crystalline rocks, as granite and the metamorphic strata, which contain no organic remains.

PRI'MARY COL'ORS are those which by their union constitute white light. Newton supposed them to be seven: red, orange, yellow, green, blue, indigo, and violet. According to Brewster, there are but three, red, blue, and yellow, which by their various combinations produce all the others.

Pri-ma'tēs.* [From *pri'mus*, "first."] Originally, the "chief persons or individuals" of a city or kingdom. Applied by Linnæus to the first order of animals in his system, including man and the monkey.

Prī-mĭ-ge'nĭ-ous. [**Primig'enus;** from *pri'mus*, "first," and *ge'no*, to "beget."] First-born; primitive.

Prī'mĭne. [**Primi'na;** from *pri'mus*, "first."] The exterior of the two membranes which envelop the ovule of plants.

Pri-mip'a-ra.* [From *pri'mus*, "first," and *pa'rio*, to "bring forth."] A woman who has brought forth her first child.

Pri-mip'a-rus.* [From the same.] Belonging to a first birth: primip'arous.

Primitiæ (pri-mish'e-ē), **a'rum.*** [From *pri'mus*, "first."] The waters which usually escape before the birth of the child.

Prim'ĭ-tĭve Earths. These are nine: *Baryta*, *Strontia*, *Lime*, *Magnesia*, *Alumina* or Clay, *Silica*, *Glucina*, *Zirconia*, *Yttria*; to which a tenth, *Florina*, has lately been added.

Prim'itive Rocks. The same as PRIMARY ROCKS, which see.

Pri-mor'dĭ-al. [**Primordia'lis.** See PRIMORDIUM.] First in order; original. Applied to the first leaves which are produced after the seminal leaves.

Pri-mor'dĭ-um.* [From *pri'mus*, "first," and *or'dium*, a "beginning."] Literally, "first beginning or origin." Applied to the germ of the future bird in the egg, or to any germ.

Primulaceæ,* prim-u-la'she-ē. A natural order of exogenous herbaceous plants, common in the northern and colder parts of the world, and remarkable for their beauty. It comprises the Cowslip (*Prim'ula ve'ris*), Primrose (*Prim'ula Auric'ula*), and *Cyc'lamen*, a drastic purgative.

Prince's Met'al, or **Prince Ru'pert's Met'al.** An alloy of copper and zinc.

Pri'nos.* Black Alder. The Pharmacopœial name (U.S. Ph.) for the bark of the *Pri'nos verticilla'tus.*

Prism. [**Pris'ma, a***tis;* from πρίζω, to "cut with a saw."] A solid figure contained by several planes, of which the two ends are equal, similar, and parallel, and all the sides parallelograms. Prisms take particular names from the figures of their ends, or opposite, equal, and parallel sides, which may be triangles, squares, pentagons, hexagons, etc.: thus, we have triangular prisms, square prisms, and so on. In Dioptrics, a prism is a piece of glass, or other diaphanous substance, in the form of a triangular prism, employed to separate a ray of light into its constituent parts or colors by refraction.

Pris-mat'ic. [**Prismat'icus.**] Belonging to a prism.

Prismat'ic Spec'trum. [**Spec'trum Prismat'icum.**] See SPECTRUM.

Pris'ma-toid. [**Prismatoi'des;** from *pris'ma,* a "prism," and εἶδος, a "form."] Resembling a prism.

Privities. See NATURALIA.

P. r. n. = *Pro re na'tâ.** "According as circumstances may require." See PRO RE NATA.

Pro. [Gr. πρό, "before," "forwards," "forth."] A Latin preposition signifying "before," "for," "forth," "forwards," "according to," or "on account of."

Pro re na'tâ.* ("According to the circumstances [*i.e.* symptoms, etc.] arising" or occurring.) A Latin phrase often added to prescriptions, to signify that the dose or application is to be repeated or discontinued as occasion may require.

Pro'bang. [Supposed to be from *pro'bo,* to "prove," or "try."] A slender piece of whalebone with a portion of ivory or sponge at its extremity, for pushing down into the stomach bodies which may have lodged in the œsophagus.

Probe. [From *pro'bo,* to "prove," or "try."] (Lat. **Specil'lum,** and **Sty'lus;** Fr. *Stylet,* stè'là'.) An instrument for trying the depth and extent of wounds, etc.

Prob'lem. [**Proble'ma, a***tis;* from προβάλλω, to "lay before."] A difficulty or proposition to be discussed; a question proposed for solution.

Pro-bos-çid'i-ans. [**Proboscidia'na;** from *probos'cis.*] The name of a family of pachydermatous mammals having a proboscis, including the elephant.

Pro-bos-çi-dif'er-us.* [From *probos'cis,* and *fe'ro,* to "bear."] Bearing or having a proboscis: proboscidiferous.

Pro-bos'çis, i*dis.** [From πρό, "before," and βόσκω, to "feed."] The prehensile organ formed by a prolongation of the nose, of which a trunk of an elephant is an example. Also, the fleshy or membranous organ constituting a sort of sucker in certain of the *Suctoria,* etc.

Proç'ess. [**Proces'sus;** from *proce'do, proces'sum,* to "proceed," "to go forth."] (Fr. *Procès,* PRO'sà'.) A projecting point or eminence of a bone; also, similar objects in the soft parts; a protuberance; any projection from a surface. See PROTUBERANCE.

Proç'ess. [From the same.] (Fr. *Procédé,* PRO'sà'dà'.) The method of proceeding in a chemical or other operation.

Pro-ces'sus a Cĕr-e-bel'lo ad Tes'tes.* The name of two cords which pass from the cerebellum to the nates and testes of the brain. They are the superior peduncles.

Pro-chei'lum,* or **Pro-chei'lon.*** [From πρό, "before," and χεῖλος, a "lip."] The same as PROLABIUM, which see.

Procidentia,* pros-e-den'she-a. [From *proç'ido,* to "fall forward," to "fall down."] The falling down of some organ or part, as the anus, eye, uterus, etc. See PROLAPSUS.

Prociden'tia U'te-ri.* A "falling down of the womb," which descends into the vagina, owing to the relaxation of its connections; when it protrudes through the external parts, the displacement is termed *Prolapsus uteri.*

Pro-cliv'i-tў. [**Procliv'itas, a***'tis;* from *pro,* "forwards," and *cli'vus,* "sloping," or "inclining."] Inclination, or disposition; tendency; propensity.

Pro-çœ'li-us.* [From πρό, "before," and κοιλία, the "belly."] Having a swollen or prominent belly.

Proc'ta-gra.* [From πρωκτός, the "anus," and ἄγρα, a "seizure."] Pain of the anus or rectum.

Proc-tăl'ġi-a.* [From πρωκτός, the "anus," and ἄλγος, "pain."] Nervous pain of the anus or rectum: proctalgy.

Proc-ta-tre'si-a.* [From πρωκτός, the "anus," and *atre'sia,* "imperforation."] Imperforation of the anus.

Proc'ti-ca.* [From πρωκτός, the "anus."] A generic term applied by Dr. Good to diseases of the anus and rectum.

Proc-tit'i-cus.* Belonging to *proctitis.*

Proc-ti'tis, i*dis.** [From πρωκτός, the "anus."] Inflammation of the anus, or of the rectum.

Proc'to-çēle.* [From πρωκτός, the "anus," and κήλη, a "tumor."] Hernia, or *prolapsus*, of the anus.

Proc-to-çȳs-to-to'mĭ-ą.* [From πρωκτός, the "anus," and *cystoto'mia*, a "cutting into the bladder."] Proctocystot'omy. The recto-vesical section for calculus.

Proc-to-dȳn'ĭ-ą.* [From πρωκτός, the "anus," and ὀδύνη, "pain."] Spasmodic pain of the anus or rectum.

Proc-top-to'mą, *atis*.* [From πρωκτός, the "anus," and πτῶμα, a "fall."] A fall, or prolapse, of the anus.

Proc-top-to'sis.* The progress or formation of *proctoptoma*.

Proc-tot'o-mȳ. [**Proctoto'mia;** from πρωκτός, the "anus," and τέμνω, to "cut."] The cutting of the anus or rectum, as in imperforate anus; the operation for *fistula in ano*, etc.

Pro-cum'bent. [**Procum'bens;** from *procum'bo*, to "lie down flat," to "lean upon."] Lying on the ground; trailing. Applied to plants.

Pro'drome. [**Prod'romus;** from πρόδρομος, "running before."] A forerunner. Applied to some affections which indicate the supervention of another disease, as vertigo is sometimes said to be a prodrome or precursor of apoplexy.

Pro-e-gu'me-nąl, or **Pro-e-gu'me-nous.** [**Proëgu'menus;** from προηγέομαι, to "lead the way."] That which precedes: predisposing.

Prœ-o'tĭ-ą,* or pre-o'she-ą. [From πρωΐ, "early," "prematurely."] A generic term applied by Dr. Good to the different forms of sexual (or genital) precocity.

Pro-flu'vĭ-ą.* [Plural of *proflu'vium*, a "flux."] Fluxes with fever; an order of the class *Pyrexiæ* of Cullen's Nosology.

Pro-found'. [**Profun'dus;** from *pro'cul a fun'do*, "far from the bottom."] Deep. Applied to vessels, nerves, muscles, etc., from their relative situation as to others.

Profusio,* pro-fu'zhe-o. [From *pro*, "forth," and *fun'do, fu'sum*, to "pour."] A loss of blood. A genus of the order *Apocenoses*, or increased secretions, of Cullen's Nosology.

Prog-nā'thous. [From πρό, "forth," or "forward," and γνάθος, a "jaw."] A term applied to a head or cranium in which the jaw projects much farther forward than the forehead.

Prog-no'sis.* [From πρό, "before," and γιγνώσκω, to "know."] The knowledge of a disease, drawn from a consideration of its signs and symptoms.

Prog-nos'tic. [From the same.] Applied to the symptoms from a consideration of which a prognosis of any particular disease is formed.

Pro-la'bĭ-um.* [From *pro*, "before," and *la'bium*, a "lip."] The extreme prominent part of the lip. Also termed Procheilum.

Pro-lap'sus.* [From *prola'bor, prolap'sus*, to "slip or fall forth," to "fall down."] (Fr. *Chute*, shüt.) A protrusion, as well as falling down, of a part of some viscus, so as to be partly external or uncovered. Applied to the anus, uterus, etc. A genus of the order *Ectopiæ*, class *Locales*, of Cullen's Nosology.

Prolap'sus A'ni,* or **Prolap'sus Rec'tĭ.*** ("Prolapse of the Anus or of the Rectum.") A falling down of the extremity of the rectum, occurring at any period of life.

Prolap'sus Ir'ĭ-dis* [from *i'ris*]. A prolapse or protrusion of the iris through a wound of the cornea.

Prolap'sus U'te-ri.* ("Prolapse of the Uterus.") Protrusion of the womb beyond or at the vulva.

Prolate Spheroid. See Spheroid.

Pro-lif-er-ā'tion. [**Prolifera'tio;** see Proliferous.] Literally, the development of new branches, flowers, etc., from the older ones; more especially applied to the appearance of buds or flowers on a part of a plant which does not usually produce them. Applied in a similar manner to both normal and morbid growths, etc., in the animal economy.

Pro-lif'er-ous. [From *pro'les*, "offspring," and *fe'ro*, to "bear," or "produce."] Producing buds, branches, and flowers from older ones, or from unusual places. See Proliferation.

Pro-me'the-ąn. [From *Prome'theus*, who is fabled to have stolen fire from heaven in a hollow reed (or tube).] A small glass tube or bulb filled with concentrated sulphuric acid, and surrounded with an inflammable mixture, which it ignites on being pressed, affording an instantaneous light.

Prom'ĭ-nence. [**Prominen'tia;** from *promin'eo*, to "jut out," to "stand out."] The state of being prominent. Also, a projection, protuberance, or eminence.

Prom'on-to-rȳ. [**Promonto'ri-um;** from *pro*, "forwards," and *mons*, a "mountain."] A point of high land extending into the sea; a headland. Applied to a small projection at the inner wall of the cavity of the tympanum.

Prom'ontory of the Sa'crum. [**Promonto'rium Os'sis Sa'cri.**] Applied to the superior or projecting portion of the sacrum when *in situ* in the pelvis.

Pro-nā'tion. [**Prona'tio, o'***nis;* from *pro'nus,* "having the face downward," "prone."] The act of turning the palm of the hand downwards.

Pro-na'tor, o'r*is.** [From the same.] Applied to certain muscles used in the act of pronation.

Prona'tor Quad-ra'tus.* ("Square Pronator [Muscle].") A muscle arising from the edge of the ulna, and inserted into the edge of the radius. This muscle and the *pronator teres* turn the radius and the hand inwards.

Prona'tor Te'rēs.* ("Round Pronator [Muscle].") A muscle arising from the inner condyle of the humerus and the coronoid process of the ulna, and inserted into the middle of the radius.

Proof Spirit. See Spiritus Tenuior.

Prop. See Fulcrum.

Pro-pa'go, ġ'*inis.** A Latin word signifying a cutting, shoot, or stock of a vine or other plant, by setting which in the soil, new vines, etc. are produced. In Anatomy, the smaller branches of vessels and nerves have been called *propaġ'ines.*

Proph-ȳ-lac'tic. [**Prophylac'ticus;** from πρό, "before," or "beforehand," and φυλάσσω, to "guard."] Belonging to *prophylaxis.* Applied to any means used for the preservation of health or prevention of disease.

Proph-ȳ-lax'is.* [Gr. προφύλαξις; from the same.] Literally, "caution," or "providence." The art of guarding against disease; the observation of the rules necessary to the preservation of health or prevention of disease.

Prop'o-lis.* [From πρό, "before," and πόλις, a "city."] Literally, a "suburb or outwork of a city." Bee-bread; a resinous substance collected by bees from the buds of trees, and used by them to line the cells of a new comb, or to stop crevices, and thus to defend their dwelling against the cold or other enemies.

Pro-por'tions, Def'ĭ-nĭte. A term applied to the proportions in which chemical substances which have a strong attraction for each other mutually combine: thus, if sulphuric acid be saturated with caustic potash, it will be found that they always combine in the proportion of forty of the acid to forty-eight of the alkali. See Equivalents.

Pro Re Nata. See Pro, etc.

Pros (πρός). A Greek preposition, usually signifying, when combined with other words, "to," or "in addition to."

Pro-sec'tor, o'r*is.** [From *pro,* "for," and *se'co, sec'tum,* to "cut."] Properly, one who cuts or dissects for another: one who prepares the subject for the lecturer on anatomy.

Pros-en'ehȳ-mạ.* [From πρός, "in addition to," and *en'chyma,* "that which is poured or deposited within." See Parenchyma.] A name applied to certain vegetable tissues.

Pros-o-păl'ġĭ-ạ.* [From πρόσωπον, the "face," or "countenance," and ἄλγος, "pain."] Pain in the face, or neuralgia of the face.

Pro-so'po-lo'ġĭ-ạ.* [From πρόσωπον, the "face," and λόγος, a "discourse."] A dissertation on the countenance; the science of physiognomy: prosopol'ogy.

Pro-so'po-man-ti'ạ.* [From πρόσωπον, the "face," and μαντεία, "prophesying."] Prognosis from examination of the countenance.

Pro-so'po-neū-răl'ġĭ-ạ.* [From πρόσωπον, the "face," and *neural'gia.*] Neuralgia, or pain in the nerves of the face.

Pros-tạ-tăl'ġĭ-ạ.* [From *pros'tata glan'dula,* the "prostate gland," and ἄλγος, "pain."] Pain in the prostate gland.

Pros-tạ-taux'e.* [From *pros'tata glan'dula,* the "prostate gland," and αὔξη, "increase."] Enlargement of the prostate gland.

Pros'tate. [**Pros'tatus;** from πρό, "before," and ἵστημι, to "stand."] Applied to the large heart-shaped gland below the neck of the urinary bladder, and behind the bulb of the urethra.

Pros-tat'ic. [**Prostat'icus.**] Belonging to the prostate gland.

Pros-tạ-ti'tis, i*dis.** Inflammation in the prostate gland.

Pros'the-sis.* [From πρός, "to," or "in addition to," and τίθημι, to "put," or "place."] In Surgery, the addition of an artificial part to replace that which has been lost or destroyed, as, for example, an artificial eye. See Rhinoplastic.

Pros'trate. [**Prostra'tus;** see Prostration.] Lying at length; abject;

lying flat on the ground. Applied to certain plants.

Pros-trā'tion. [**Prostra'tio, o'***nis*; from *proster'no, prostra'tum*, to "cast or beat down," to "lay flat."] Extreme feebleness, or exhaustion, the effect of disease; dejection.

Pro'te-an. [From *Pro'teus*, a Grecian deity who possessed the power of changing himself into the most diverse and opposite appearances.] Assuming many different forms.

Pro'te-ĭ-form. [**Proteifor'mis;** from the same.] Changing its form.

Pro'te-in, or **Pro'te-ĭne.** [**Protei'na;** from πρωτεύω, to "be first."] A definite compound of oxygen, hydrogen, carbon, and nitrogen, forming the basis of the most important constituents of animal fibrin, albumen, casein, gluten, and legumen.

Pro-te-ĭ-nā'ceous Prin'cĭ-ples. A term applied to albuminous alimentary principles, from their yielding *protein*. Their composition is identical with that of the constituents of blood.

Prot-e-ran'thous. [From πρότερος, "earlier," and ἄνθος, a "flower."] Applied to plants of which the flowers are produced earlier than the leaves.

Pro-tho'rax, a'*cis*.* [From πρό, "before," and θώραξ, the "chest."] The anterior segment of the thorax in insects.

Pro'to-. [From πρῶτος, "first."] A prefix denoting the first degree of combination. See PROTOXIDE.

Pro'to-Com'pound. A binary compound of single equivalents of salt-radical and basyl.

Pro-to-phȳl'lum.* [From πρῶτος, "first," and φύλλον, a "leaf."] A seminal leaf: a pro'tophyl.

Pro'to-phȳte. [**Protoph'ytum;** from πρῶτος, "first," and φύτον, a "plant."] Applied to the *Algæ*, Lichens, etc., regarded as the first productions of the vegetable kingdom. See PRIMALIA.

Pro-top'la-sis.* [From πρῶτος, "first," and πλάσις, a "moulding."] The primary formation of a thing.

Pro-to-plas'ma, a'*tis*.* [From πρῶτος, "first," and πλάσσω, to "form."] The nitrogenous substance from which the cell-nucleus is formed.

Pro'to-plast. [**Protoplas'ta;** from the same.] A primary formation.

Pro-tox'ĭ-dāt-ed. [**Protoxyda'tus.**] Converted into a protoxide.

Pro-tox'ĭde. [**Protox'ydum;** from *pro'to-*, and *ox'ydum*, an "oxide."] When there are several different oxides of the same substance, the protoxide is that which is the first in the scale, or which has the smallest quantity of oxygen.

Protruding. See EXSERTED.

Pro-tu'be-rance. [**Protuberan'tia;** from *pro*, "forth," and *tu'ber*, a "swelling."] A swelling; an apophysis; a process.

Proud Flesh. A popular term for Fungus; commonly applied to any redundant growth of healthy granulation.

Prox'ĭ-mad. The same as PROXIMAL, used adverbially.

Prox'ĭ-mal. [From *prox'imus*, the "nearest."] Applied by Dr. Barclay as meaning towards the end nearest the trunk, when treating of the aspects of the four extremities.

Prox'ĭ-mate [from *prox'imus*, "next," or "nearest"] **Cause.** Literally, the "cause which is next" to the disease itself. That which occurs immediately after the exciting cause of any disease, being that particular condition of the system (or of an organ) in which the disease consists.

Prox'imate Prin'cĭ-ples. Distinct compounds which exist ready formed in animals and vegetables, such as albumen, gelatine, etc., in the former, and sugar, gum, starch, etc., in the latter.

Prox. luc. = *Prox'imâ lu'ce*.* "The day before."

Pru-i'na.* [From πρωϊνός, "belonging to the morning."] Hoar-frost. Also, "bloom," or the flour-like substance observed on ripe fruit, especially plums.

Pru'ĭ-nate, Pru'ĭ-nose. [**Pruina'tus,** or **Pruino'sus.**] Appearing as if frosted over, or covered with flour, like certain fruits.

Prune. [**Pru'num.**] The dried fruit of the *Prunus domestica*. See PRUNUM.

Pru'nĭ-form. [**Prunifor'mis;** from *pru'num*, a "plum."] Having the appearance of a plum; plum-shaped.

Pru'nin. [**Pruni'na;** from *pru'nus cer'asus*, the "cherry-tree."] The same as *Cerasin*. See TRAGACANTHIN.

Pru'num.* [From *Pru'nus*, a "plum-tree."] A plum, or prune. The Pharmacopœial name ‖ of the prepared fruit of the *Prunus domestica*. It is nutritious and laxative.

Pru'num Gal'lĭ-cum.* ("French Plum.") Another name for the prune. See PRUNUM.

Pru'nus.* [From προύνη, the "plum-tree."] A Linnæan genus of the class *Icosandria*, natural order *Drupaceæ*.

Pru'nus Do-mes'tĭ-ca.* ("Domestic Plum.") The plum, or damson-tree, the dried fruit of which constitutes the prune.

Pru'nus Lau'ro-Cĕr'a-sus.* The cherry-tree laurel, or poison-laurel. It is a nervous sedative, and is used for the same purposes as PRUSSIC ACID.

Pru'nus Vir-gin-i-a'na.* Wild-cherry Bark. The Pharmacopœial name (U.S. Ph.) for the bark of *Cer'asus Serot'ina* (of Decandolle). This valuable remedy combines the virtues of a tonic, with the property of allaying irritation and nervous excitability. It has been given with excellent effect in incipient phthisis and scrofulous affections accompanied with hectic fever.

Pru-ri'go, g'inis.* [From *pru'rio*, to "itch."] A papular eruption affecting the whole surface of the skin, or confined to some particular part or organ, accompanied with a sense of constant itching. Also termed *Pruritus*.

Pru-ri'tus.* [From the same.] An intense degree of itching. Also, the same as PRURIGO, which see.

Prus'sian Blue. A well-known pigment of a rich blue color: so called because it was discovered by Diesbach, a Prussian chemist. It has generally been considered as a ferrocyanate of the peroxide of iron; but, according to Berzelius, it is a double cyanuret,—that is, a ferrocyanuret of the sesquicyanuret of iron.

Prussiate, prŭsh'e-āt. [**Prus'sias, a'tis.**] A combination of prussic acid with a base.

Prus'siate of Pot'ash. Another name for ferrocyanide or ferrocyanuret of potassium, a substance occurring in the form of yellow crystals. It is much used as a test of the presence of metals, and especially of iron, the peroxide of which it throws down from its solutions in the state of Prussian blue. See POTASSII FERROCYANIDUM.

Prus'sic Aç'id. [**Aç'idum Prus'sicum.**] A common name applied to hydrocyanic acid, because it was formerly supposed to be an ingredient in Prussian blue. This acid is a nervous sedative, and the most deadly poison known, a single drop being sufficient in some cases to destroy life; yet minute doses of the dilute acid are sometimes administered with advantage in pulmonary affections.

Prus'sin. [**Prussi'na;** from *Prussian* blue.] Another name for *cyanogen*.

Psa'lis, idis.* [Gr. ψαλίς, an "arch," or "vault."] Also termed **Cor'pus Psaloi'des*** ("arch-like body"), and **For'nix Cĕr'ebri*** ("vault of the brain"). See FORNIX.

(☞ In all words beginning with *ps*, the *p* is silent.)

Psal-lo-i'dēs.* [From ψάλλω, to "play on a stringed instrument," and εἶδος, a "form."] Resembling a psalter, harp, or *cithara*: psalloid.

Psa-lo-i'dēs.* [From ψαλίς, an "arch," or "vault," and εἶδος, a "form."] Resembling an arch: psa'loid. See PSALIS.

Psalterium. See LYRA.

Psam-mo'dēs.* [From ψάμμος, "sand."] Sandy, or full of sand. See SABULOUS.

Psel-lis'mus.* [From ψελλίζω, to "stammer."] Hesitation of speech; stammering; bad utterance. A genus of the order *Dyscinesiæ*, class *Locales*, of Cullen's Nosology.

Pseū-dæs-the'si-a,* or **Pseū-dæs-the'sis.*** [From ψευδής, "false," and αἰσθάνομαι, to "feel."] (Fr. *Pseudesthésie*, sŭh'dĕs'tà'zè'.) False or imaginary feeling or sensation; imaginary sense of touch in organs that have been long removed, as often experienced by those who have suffered the amputation of some limb.

Pseū-da'phe,* or **Pseū-da'phi-a.*** [From ψευδής, "false," and ἀφή, the "sense of touch."] The same as PSEUDÆSTHESIA, which see.

Pseū-dar-thro'sis.* [From ψευδής, "false," and *arthro'sis*, "articulation."] The formation of a false joint.

Pseū-do-blep'si-a,* or **Pseū-do-blep'sis.*** [From ψευδής, "false," and βλέψις, a "beholding."] Depraved sight, in which objects are imagined, or seen different from what they are; false vision. A genus of the order *Dysæsthesiæ*, class *Locales*, of Cullen's Nosology.

Pseū-do-çy-e'sis.* [From ψευδής, "false," and κύησις, "pregnancy."] A mole, or false conception.

Pseū-do-mem'brane. [**Pseudo-membra'na;** from ψευδής, "false," and *membra'na*, a "membrane."] A false membrane. An organized layer of effused lymph, the effect of inflammation; like the membrane which is formed in croup.

Pseu'do-scope. [From ψευδής, "false," and σκοπέω, to "observe," or "see."] An instrument invented by Mr. Wheatstone for producing the conversion of the relief of any solid object to which it is directed, thus conveying to the mind a false perception of all external objects by transposition of the distances of the points which compose them. The inside of a teacup, for example, appears a solid convex body, and a small globe looks like a concave hemisphere.

Pseu'do-Vol-can'ic. Belonging to or produced by a pseudo-volcano.

Pseu'do-Vol-ca'no. A volcano which emits smoke or flame, but never lava. Applied, also, to a burning coal-mine.

Pso-ad'ĭ-cus.* [From ψόα, the "loin."] Belonging to the loins, or to the *psoæ* muscles: psoad'ic.

Pso-a-do-to'mĭ-a.* [From *pso'as*, and τέμνω, to "cut."] A cutting into the *psoas* muscles.

Pso'æ.* [Plural of *Pso'a;* Gr. ψόα.] The loins. Also applied to two pairs of muscles of the loins.

Pso'as, a*dos*.* [From ψόα, the "loin."] Of the loin or loins. Applied to two muscles of each loin, the *psoas magnus* and *parvus*.

Pso'as Ab'scess. (That is, abscess of the loins.) See LUMBAR ABSCESS.

Pso'as Mag'nus.* ("Great [Muscle] of the Loins.") A muscle arising from the last dorsal and the four superior lumbar vertebræ, and inserted into the lesser trochanter of the os femoris. It moves the thigh forward.

Pso'as Par'vus.* ("Small [Muscle] of the Loins.") A muscle arising from the last dorsal vertebra, and inserted into the brim of the pelvis: it is very often wanting. It bends the spine upon the pelvis.

Pso-i'tis, i*dis*.* [From *pso'æ*.] Inflammation of the sheath of the *psoas* muscles.

Pso'ra.* [Gr. ψώρα; Fr. *Gale*, gål, or *Rogne*, roñ.] The itch. A genus of the order *Dialyses*, class *Locales*, of Cullen's Nosology; also termed *Scabies*.

Pso-rel-co'ma, a*tis*.* [From ψώρα, the "itch," and ἕλκωμα, an "ulcer."] A scabious ulcer.

Pso-rel-co'sis.* The progress of *psorelcoma:* scabious ulceration.

Pso-ri'a-sis,* or so-re-a'sis. [From ψώρα, the "itch."] A cutaneous disease, characterized by a rough, scaly cuticle, continuous, or in separate, irregular patches; generally with fissures of the skin. Often called *scaly tetter*.

Psori'asis Dif-fu'sa.* ("Diffused Psoriasis.") A variety of *psoriasis*, attacking persons pursuing different trades, and variously denominated baker's, bricklayer's, grocer's itch, etc.

Psori'asis Gut-ta'ta.* ("Spotted Psoriasis.") Small, distinct, but irregular patches of laminated scales, with little or no inflammation round them, rarely exceeding a half an inch in diameter, having neither the raised edges nor oval or circular form of the other varieties of *lepra*.

Psori'asis Gy-ra'ta.* A species distributed in narrow patches or stripes, variously figured or gyrated.

Psori'asis In-fan-ti'lis.* ("Infantile Psoriasis.") The dry tetter affecting infants between two months and two years of age; irregular, scaly patches of various size, on the cheeks, breast, back, *nates*, and thighs.

Psori'asis In-vet-e-ra'ta.* ("Inveterate Psoriasis.") Characterized by an almost universal scaliness, with a harsh, dry, and thickened state of the skin.

Pso'ric. [Lat. **Pso'ricus;** Fr. *Galeux*, gå'luh'.) Belonging to *psora*, or itch.

Pso-ro'dēs.* [From ψώρα, the "itch."] Resembling *psora;* also, having the itch; pso'rous.

Pso-ro-i'dēs.* [From ψώρα, the "itch," and εἶδος, a "form."] Resembling *psora:* pso'roid.

Pso-roph-thăl'mĭ-a.* [From ψώρα, the "itch," and ὀφθαλμός, the "eye."] Inflammation of the eye attended with itchy ulcerations.

Pso-roph-thăl'mic. [**Psoroph-thal'micus.**] Belonging to *psorophthalmia*.

Psy-chĭ-a-tri'a.* [From ψυχή, the "soul," or "mind," and ἰατρεία, a "healing."] The medical treatment of disorders of the mind.

Psy̆'chĭ-cal. [**Psy'chicus;** from ψυχή, "soul," or "mind."] Belonging to the mind or intellect.

Psy'chical Rem'e-dies. These consist in the employment of the mental affections to promote the healthy functions of the body, or to modify the progress of disease.

Psychology, sī-kol'o-je. [**Psycholo'gia;** from ψυχή, the "soul," and λόγος, a "discourse."] The doctrine of the soul, or mind. In its larger acceptation, it is synonymous with mental philosophy.

Psy̆-cho-no-sol'o-gy̆. [**Psychonosolo'gia;** from ψυχή, the "soul," or "mind," and *nosolo'gia*, the "doctrine of diseases."] The doctrine or science of mental diseases.

Psy̆-cho-path'ic. [**Psychopath'i-**

cus.] Belonging to psychopathy, or mental disease.

Psy̆-chop'a-thy̆. [**Psychopathi'a;** from ψυχή, the "soul," or "mind," and πάθος, an "affection," a "disease."] Mental disease or affection.

Psy̆-cho'sis.* [From ψυχή, the "soul," or "mind."] Affection of the mind. Applied in the plural (*Psycho'ses*) to a class of such affections.

Psy̆-chrom'e-ter. [**Psychrom'e-trum;** from ψυχρός, "cold," "chilly," or "damp," and μέτρον, a "measure."] An instrument for measuring the amount of the aqueous vapor contained in the atmosphere.

Psy-drā'cious. [**Psydra'cius;** from *psydra'cium.*] Having *psydracia;* of the nature of a *psydracium.*

Psydracium,* si-dra'she-um. [Diminutive of ψύδραξ, a "small blister."] A minute species of pustule causing a slight elevation of the cuticle, and terminating in a laminated scab.

Ptar'mic. [**Ptar'micus;** from πταίρω, to "sneeze."] Causing to sneeze; sternutatory.

(☞ In all words beginning with *pt,* the *p* is silent.)

Pte-rig'e-nus.* [From πτερίς, the "fern," and γένω, to "be born," to "grow."] Growing upon ferns.

Pterigraphia,* tĕr-e-gra'fĭ-a, or **Pte-rig'ra-phy̆.** [From πτερίς, a "fern," and γράφω, to "write."] A description of ferns.

Ptĕr-o-car'pous. [**Pterocar'pus;** from πτερόν, a "wing," and καρπός, "fruit."] Having winged fruits.

Pterocarpus,* tĕr-o-kar'pus. [From the same.] A Linnæan genus of the class *Diadelphia,* natural order *Leguminosæ.* Also, the Pharmacopœial name (Br. Ph.) for the wood of the *Pterocarpus santalinus.*

Pterocar'pus Dra'co.* The systematic name of one of the trees which yields dragon's blood.

Pterocar'pus San-ta-li'nus.* The systematic name of the tree the wood of which is called red saunders, sanders, or sandal; termed also *Santalum rubrum.*

Ptĕr-o-cau'lis.* [From πτερόν, a "wing," and *cau'lis,* a "stem."] Having a winged stem. Applied to certain plants.

Pte-ro-i'dēs.* [From πτερόν, a "wing," and εἶδος, a "form."] Resembling a wing: pte'roid. See PTERYGOID.

Pte-roph'o-rus.* [From πτερόν, a "wing," and φέρω, to "bear."] Having wings: pteroph'orous.

Pte-rop'o-da.* [From πτερόν, a "wing," and πούς, ποδός, a "foot."] The fourth class of the *Cyclo-gangliata* or Mollusks, consisting of small, soft, floating marine animals, which swim by the contractions of two lateral musculo-cutaneous fins.

Pteropods. See PTEROPODA.

Pte-rop'o-dus.* [From the same.] Having winged feet or winged petioles. Applied to certain plants; also to an order of Mollusks. See PTEROPODA.

Ptĕr-o-sper'mus.* [From πτερόν, a "wing," and σπέρμα, a "seed."] Having winged seed or fruit, as the *Sida pterosperma.*

Ptĕr-o-sty'lus.* [From πτερόν, a "wing," and στῦλος, a "pillar," a "style."] Having the style compressed and broad in the form of a wing; pterosty'lous.

Pte-ry̆g'i-um.* [From πτέρυξ, a "wing."] A membranous excrescence on the internal canthus of the eye, expanding on the albuginea and cornea towards the pupil.

Ptĕr-y̆-go'dēs.* [From πτέρυξ, a "wing."] Having wings.

Ptĕr'y̆-goid. [**Pterygoi'des;** from πτέρυξ, a "wing," and εἶδος, a "form."] Resembling a wing.

Ptĕr-y̆-go-i'de-us.* [From the same.] Connected with the pterygoid process.

Pterygoi'deus Ex-ter'nus.* A muscle arising from the outer plate of the pterygoid process, etc., and inserted into the condyle of the lower jaw.

Pterygoi'deus In-ter'nus.* A muscle arising from the inner plate of the pterygoid process of the sphenoid bone, and inserted into the inside of the angle of the lower jaw. This and the preceding muscle move the jaw from side to side, and perform the action of grinding with the teeth.

Ptĕr'y̆-go-Phăr-y̆n-ġe'us.* A synonym of the *constrictor superior* muscle of the pharynx, because it arises from the pterygoid process of the sphenoid bone.

Pter'ygo-Staph-y̆-li'nus.* [From σταφυλή, a "grape;" also, the "uvula."] The name of a muscle arising from the pterygoid process of the sphenoid bone, and inserted into the *velum palati.*

Ptisane, tĭ-zan' or tiz'an. [**Ptis'ana;** from πτίσσω, to "bruise."] Barley pounded and made into balls; also, a drink made of farinaceous substances boiled in water and sweetened.

Pto'sis.* [From πτόω, to "fall."] A falling, or prolapsus.

Pto'sis Păl'pe-bræ.* ("Falling of

the Eyelid.") Inability to raise the upper eyelid.

Ptyalagogue, tī-al'ạ-gog. [**Ptyalago'gus;** from πτύαλον, "spittle," and ἄγω, to "carry or bring away."] Promoting or increasing the flow of saliva; termed also SIALAGOGUE.

Ptȳ'ạ-lin, or **Ptȳ'ạ-līne.** [**Ptyali'na;** from πτύαλον, "spittle."] A constituent principle peculiar to saliva, and on which its faint, sickly, or salivary odor depends.

Ptȳ'ạ-liṡm. [**Ptyalis'mus;** from πτυαλίζω, to "spit abundantly."] Increased and involuntary flow of saliva. A genus of the order *Apocenoses*, class *Locales*, of Cullen's Nosology.

Pty-ạ-loph'thī-sis.* [From πτύαλον, "spittle," and φθίσις, a "wasting."] *Tabes salivalis*, or wasting from excessive salivation.

Pty'ạ-lum.* [From πτύαλον, "spittle."] The secretion called saliva; mucus from the *bronchia:* spittle.

Pu'ber-tȳ. [**Puber'tas, a'***tis*; from *pu'beo*, to "be in the bloom of youth," to "grow to maturity."] The earliest age at which young persons are marriageable, or have the power of procreating offspring. See ÆTAS.

Pu'bēṡ,* gen. **Pu'bis.** [From the same.] The external part of the generative region, which is more or less covered with hair after puberty. Also applied to the down on leaves, stems, seeds, etc., of certain plants; pubescence.

Pu-bĕs'çence. [**Pubescen'tia;** from *pubes'co*, to "bud," or "bloom," to "have down, or incipient beard."] Fine hair, or down, closely pressed to the surface of leaves, stems, etc.

Pu-bĕs'çent. [**Pubes'cens;** from the same.] Covered with downy hair.

Pu'bic. [**Pu'bicus.**] Belonging to the pubes.

Pu-bĭ-flo'rus.* [From *pu'bes*, "down," and *flos*, a "flower."] Applied to plants having the calyx or the corolla covered with light down: pubiflo'rous.

Pu-biġ'er-ous. [**Pubiġ'erus;** from *pu'bes*, "down," or "soft hair," and *ge'ro*, to "bear."] Bearing down.

Pu'bis, Os.* ("Bone of the Pubes.") A bone constituting the anterior portion of the *Os innominatum*, but forming a separate bone in the fœtal pelvis.

Pu-den'dạ,* gen. **Pu-den-do'rum,** the plural of PUDENDUM, which see.

Puden'da Vī-ro'rum.* [From *vir*, a "man."] The male organs of generation.

Pu-den'dạ-grạ.* [From *puden'da*, the "private parts," and ἄγρα, a "seizure."] Pain in the *pudenda*.

Pu-den'dum,* gen. **Pu-den'di.** [From *pu'deo*, to "have shame, or modesty."] The genital organs, or parts of generation, of either sex, taken as a whole; also used, perhaps more correctly, in the plural (*puden'da*).

Puden'dum Mu-lĭ-e'bre* [from *mu'lier*, a "woman"]. The female parts of generation, collectively.

Pu'dic, or **Pu'dĭ-cạl.** [**Pudi'cus;** from *pu'deo*, to "have shame, or modesty."] Belonging to the *pudenda*, or genital organs.

Pu-er'pe-rạ.* [From *pu'er*, a "child," and *pa'rio*, to "bring forth."] A woman in childbed, or one who has been lately delivered.

Pu-er'pe-rạl. [**Puerpera'lis;** from *puer'pera*.] Belonging to, or consequent on, childbearing.

Puer'peral Fe'ver. [**Fe'bris Puerpera'rum.**] A severe febrile disease which sometimes occurs in the puerperal state, usually about the third day after childbirth, originating in an inflamed condition of the peritonæum. Termed also *me'tria* [from μήτρα, the "womb"].

Puer'peral Ma'nĭ-ạ. The delirious excitement occurring in puerperal fever.

Pu-er-pe'rĭ-um.* [From *puer'pera*.] The state or period of a woman in confinement.

Pu-er-pe-rop'ȳ-rạ.* [From *puerpe'rium*, "confinement in childbed," and πῦρ, a "fever."] A term for puerperal fever.

Pug. = *Pugil'lus.** A "pugil," or pinch between the finger and thumb.

Pu-ġil'lus.* [Diminutive of *pug'nus*, the "fist."] A little handful; held to be about the eighth part of an ordinary handful. See preceding article.

Pu-ġĭ-o'nĭ-form. [**Pugionifor'mis;** from *pu'gio*, a "poignard."] Dagger-shaped; having the shape of a poignard. Applied to leaves.

Pu-le'ġĭ-um.* [From *pu'lex*, a "flea."] The Pharmacopœial name (Lond. and Ed. Ph.) for the dried herb of MENTHA PULEGIUM, which see.

Pu'lex.* [Said to be derived from *pul'vis*, "dust," because they were supposed to be produced from it.] A flea; a species of insect in which a single impregnation suffices for at least six or seven generations.—(HOBLYN.) It is a curious fact, that in the warmer summer months, the young of this insect are produced viviparously; and in the cooler autumnal months, oviparously.

Pul'mo,* gen. **Pul-mo'nis** (plural **Pul-mo'nēs,** gen. **Pul-mo'num**). (Fr. *Poumon*, poo'môNG'.) A Latin word signifying a "lung," or the "lungs." See LUNGS.

Pul'mo-grades, or **Pul-mog'ra-da.*** [From *pul'mo*, a "lung," and *gra'dior*, to "go," to "advance."] The name of a tribe of Acalephans, including those gelatinous species which swim by the contraction of the vascular margin of a disk-shaped body, supposed to be their lungs.

Pul-mom'e-ter. [**Pulmom'etrum;** from *pul'mo*, the "lungs," and *μέτρον*, a "measure."] An instrument for measuring the capacity of the lungs.

Pul-mom'e-try. [**Pulmome'tria;** from *pul'mo*, the "lungs," and *μετρέω*, to "measure."] The measuring of the size or capacity of the lungs in reference to the quantity of air employed in respiration. See SPIROMETRY.

Pul'mo-na-ry. [**Pulmona'ris,** or **Pulmona'lis;** from *pul'mo*, *pulmo'nis*, the "lungs."] (Fr. *Pulmonaire*, pül'mo'nêR'.) Of the lungs, or belonging to the lungs; pulmonic.

Pul'monary Con-sump'tion. [**Phthi'sis Pulmona'lis.**] A disease which in most northern temperate climates causes more deaths than any other. Its usual symptoms are cough, emaciation, debility, and hectic fever, generally accompanied with purulent expectoration. In the later stages of this formidable malady, there is little hope of successful treatment. The aim of the physician should, therefore, be to prevent the development of its worst symptoms, by timely precautions, namely, by a careful attention to proper clothing, by a judicious employment of external irritation, by the use of a mild but nutritious and strengthening diet, and, above all, by maintaining the tone of the system by means of suitable exercise in the fresh and open air. When the strength of the patient is such as to admit of it, gentle exercise on horseback is especially to be recommended. Although a mild, dry atmosphere is always desirable, extensive observation has proved that the patient loses more by confinement to the house, than by a *regular* exposure (with proper precautions as to clothing, etc.) to all kinds of weather, except the very most inclement. See CLIMATE.

Pul'monary Plex'us. The *bronchial plexus* of nerves, or that formed at the back of the *bronchia* by the *par vagum* and great sympathetic nerves.

Pul-mo'nēs,* gen. **Pul-mo'num,** the plural of PULMO, which see.

Pul-mo'ne-us.* [From *pul'mo*, a "lung."] Applied in the plural feminine (*Pulmo'neæ*) to an order of the *Gastéropoda* which respire air through an opening in the margin of the mantle.

Pul-mon'ic. [**Pulmon'icus;** from *pul'mo*, a "lung."] Synonymous with pulmonary.

Pulmon'ic Cir-cu-lā'tion. The passage of the blood from the right side of the heart through the pulmonary arteries to the lungs, and back to the left side of the heart through the pulmonary veins. This is also called the *lesser circulation*, in order to distinguish it from the *greater circulation*, or the passage of the blood from the left side of the heart through the aorta and its ramifications, and back again through the veins to the right side of the heart.

Pul-mo-nif'er-ous. [**Pulmonif'erus;** from *pul'mo*, a "lung," and *fe'ro*, to "bear."] Bearing or having lungs or *branchia*.

Pul-mo-ni'tis, *idis*.* [From *pul'mo*, a "lung."] Inflammation of the lungs. See PNEUMONIA.

Pulp. [**Pul'pa.**] Originally, the fleshy part of meat; also, the pith of wood. Usually applied to the soft part of fruit, as distinguished from the seeds, skin, etc.

Pulp of the Teeth, or **Den'tal Pulp.** [**Pul'pa Den'tis.**] An extremely sensitive pulpy substance, of a reddish or reddish-gray color, which fills the central cavity of the teeth.

Pul'pous. [**Pulpo'sus;** from *pul'pa*, "pulp."] Having or resembling pulp.

Pul'sa-tile. [**Pulsat'ilis;** from *pul'so*, *pulsa'tum*, to "beat frequently," to "throb."] Beating; pulsating.

Pul-sa-til'la.* A common name for the *Anemo'ne pulsatil'la*, a plant which is sometimes employed as a remedy in amaurosis and in certain cutaneous affections.

Pul-sā'tion. [**Pulsa'tio,** *o'nis;* from the same.] Any throbbing sensation, resembling the beating of the pulse; the heart's action extending to the arteries, felt in any part of the body.

Pulse. [**Puls.**] Originally, "gruel," or "pottage." Applied to leguminous plants or seeds, as peas, beans, etc.

Pulse. [**Pul'sus;** from *pel'lo, pul'sum,* to "drive," to "beat," or "strike."] (Fr. *Pouls,* poo.) The beating of the arteries following the contractile action of the heart. The radial artery at the wrist is commonly made use of in order to ascertain the force, frequency, etc., of the general circulation. An examination of the pulse, taken in connection with other symptoms, is often of the greatest utility to the physician, in enabling him to determine the peculiar character of different diseases.

Not merely the *frequency* and *force,* but the *fulness, hardness,* etc., as well as the opposite characteristics, are to be carefully noted. It is, however, of the utmost importance that the practitioner should take into consideration those variations, temporary or otherwise, which are not necessarily dependent on a state of disease.

Not only may the force and frequency of the pulse be greatly increased by a mere temporary cause (such, for example, as extraordinary exertion, sudden alarm, etc.), but, owing to certain constitutional peculiarities, the pulse of some persons in a state of perfect health is uniformly much more frequent than the general average. As a general rule, the pulse in persons of an excitable temperament is considerably more frequent than in those of an opposite character; it is usually more frequent in women than in men. It is estimated that the pulse of an adult male at rest, in a state of perfect health, has from sixty-five to seventy-five beats per minute. An infant at birth has from one hundred and twenty to one hundred and forty pulsations per minute; a child a year old, from one hundred and ten to one hundred and twenty; at three years, from ninety to one hundred; at ten, from eighty or eighty-five to ninety; at puberty, about eighty. As life advances, the pulse usually becomes slower, until the infirmities of age begin, when, as a result of debility, it often increases in frequency. Of the different kinds or characters of the pulse, the following are, perhaps, the most deserving of notice:—

1. Dicrotic Pulse. [See Dicrotic.] That in which the finger is struck twice (first forcibly, then lightly) at every pulsation.

2. Filiform (or thread-like) Pulse. That in which the pulsating artery seems so narrow as to resemble a thread.

3. Gaseous Pulse. One in which the artery seems full and very soft, as if it were filled with air.

4. Hard Pulse. One which does not yield under the firm pressure of the finger.

5. Intermittent Pulse. One in which the pulsation every now and then fails, or seems altogether wanting; a common symptom in diseases of the heart, though not unfrequently resulting from the derangement of the nervous system, caused by dyspepsia.

6. Jerking Pulse. One in which the artery seems to strike the finger with a sudden start, or jerk.

7. Quick Pulse. One which has a quick or sudden beat, though the interval between the beats may be of usual length.

8. Small Pulse. One in which the pulsations are both slender and weak.

9. Tense Pulse. [From *ten'sus,* "stretched."] One in which the artery seems stretched or filled to its utmost capacity. It resembles a *hard* pulse, but is more elastic.

10. Wiry Pulse. One resembling the *filiform* pulse, with this difference, that it is very *hard,* as well as *narrow.*

Thready, or Thread-like, Pulse. See Filiform Pulse.

The significations of most of the other terms applied to the pulse (such as *bounding, feeble, frequent, full, jarring* or *vibrating, languid, soft, tremulous,* etc.) seem so simple and obvious as to require no particular explanation.

Pul-sĭ-le'gĭ-um.* [From *pul'sus,* the "pulse," and *le'go,* to "read," to "gather the sense of," hence, to "estimate."] The same as Pulsimeter, which see.

Pul-sim'e-ter. [**Pulsim'etrum;** from *pul'sus,* the "pulse," and μέτρον, a "measure."] An instrument for measuring the force or frequency of the heart or pulse.

Pul-som'e-trum.* The same as Pulsimeter.

Pul'sus Cor'dis.* ("Pulse of the Heart.") The impulse of the heart, or the shock communicated by the apex of the heart to the walls of the thorax in the neighborhood of the fifth and sixth ribs. This must not be confounded with the arterial pulse.

Pul-tā'ceous. [**Pulta'ceus;** from *puls,* "pulse," or "pap."] Of the nature of pulse or pap.

Pulv. = *Pul'vis,** a "powder," or *Pul'veres,** "powders."

Pul-ve-rā'ceous. [**Pulvera'ceus;** from *pul'vis,* a "powder," or "dust."] Covered with powder; dusty.

Pul'ver-ēs,* gen. **Pul'ver-um,** the plural of PULVIS, which see.

Pul'veres Ef-fer-vĕs-çen'tēs.* ("Effervescing Powders.") Soda Powders. Take of bicarbonate of soda, in fine powder, three hundred and sixty grains; tartaric acid, in fine powder, three hundred grains. Divide each of the powders into twelve equal parts, and keep the parts severally of the bicarbonate and of the acid in separate papers of different colors.

Pul'veres Effervescen'tes A-pe-rĭ-en'tēs.* ("Aperient Effervescing Powders.") Sedlitz Powders. Take of bicarbonate of soda, in fine powder, a troyounce; tartrate of potassa and soda, in fine powder, three troyounces; tartaric acid, in fine powder, four hundred and twenty grains. Mix intimately the bicarbonate of soda with the tartrate of potassa and soda, and divide this mixture into twelve equal parts. Then divide the tartaric acid into the same number of equal parts. Lastly, keep the parts severally of the mixture and of the acid in separate papers of different colors.

Pul-vĕr'u-lent. [**Pulverulen'tus;** from *pul'vis,* "powder," or "dust."] Covered with dust; dusty; powdery.

Pul-vi'nar.* A pillow, or cushion; hence, *pulvi'nar* (or *cervica'le*), *lu'puli,* a pillow of hops, employed for its soothing effects in mania and other diseases.

Pul'vĭ-nāt-ed. [**Pulvina'tus;** from *pulvi'nus,* a "cushion," or "pillow."] Having or resembling a cushion, or pillow; cushioned.

Pul-vin'ĭ-form. [**Pulvinifor'mis;** from the same.] Having the form of a cushion,—*i.e.* more or less hemispherical, and somewhat stuffed out.

Pul'vis,* gen. **Pul'ver-is.** (Fr. *Poudre,* poodR.) A powder formed of any medicinal substance or substances.

Pul'vis Al'o-ēs et Ca-nel'læ.* ("Powder of Aloes and Canella.") Take of Socotrine aloes, in fine powder, twelve troyounces; canella, in fine powder, three troyounces. Rub them together until they are thoroughly mixed.

Pul'vis An-tĭ-mo-nĭ-a'lis* ("Antimonial Powder"), or **Pul'vis An-tĭ-mo'nĭ-i Com-pos'ĭ-tus*** ("Compound Powder of Antimony"). A preparation composed of the peroxide of antimony and phosphate of lime. It is employed as a diaphoretic, and is intended as a substitute for James's Powder, which is similar in composition.

Pul'vis Ar-o-mat'ĭ-cus.* ("Aromatic Powder.") Take of cinnamon, in fine powder, ginger, in fine powder, each two troyounces; cardamom, deprived of the capsules and in fine powder, nutmeg, in fine powder, each a troyounce. Rub them together until they are thoroughly mixed.

Pul'vis Ip-e-cac-u-an'hæ Com-pos'ĭ-tus* ("Compound Powder of Ipecacuanha"), **Pul'vis Ipecacuan'hæ et O'pĭ-i,*** 1850 ("Powder of Ipecacuanha and Opium"), commonly known as "Dover's Powder." Take of ipecacuanha, in fine powder, opium, dried and in fine powder, each sixty grains; sulphate of potassa, a troyounce. Rub them together into a very fine powder.

Pul'vis Ja-la'pæ Com-pos'ĭ-tus.* ("Compound Powder of Jalap.") Take of jalap, in fine powder, a troyounce; bitartrate of potassa, in fine powder, two troyounces. Rub them together until they are thoroughly mixed.

Pul'vis Rhe'i Com-pos'ĭ-tus.* ("Compound Powder of Rhubarb.") Take of rhubarb, in fine powder, four troyounces; magnesia, twelve troyounces; ginger, in fine powder, two troyounces. Rub them together until they are thoroughly mixed.

Pŭm'ice, or pū'miss. [From *pu'mex, pu'micis,* a "pumice-stone."] A porous volcanic product, consisting chiefly of silica and alumina.

Pu'mĭ-cĭ-form. [**Pumicifor'mis;** from the same.] Resembling pumice-stone.

Pu-mĭ-co'sus.* [From the same.] Having or resembling pumice-stone: pu'micose.

Punc'ta,* the plural of PUNCTUM, which see.

Punc'ta Lach-rȳ-ma'lĭ-a.* ("Lachrymal Points.") Two small orifices at the edges of the eyelids near the inner angle of the eye.

Punc'tate. [**Puncta'tus;** from *punc'to, puncta'tum,* to "point," or "prick."] Dotted as if with punctures; punctured.

Punc'tum,* plural **Punc'ta.** [From *pun'go, punc'tum,* to "prick."] A point. In Geometry, that which has position but not magnitude. See STITCH.

Punc'tum Au're-um* ("Golden Point"), called also **Mac'u-la Lu'te-a*** ("Yellow Spot"). A small, orange-colored spot on the internal surface of the retina and in the direction of the axis of the eye; termed also the Spot of Soemmering.

Punc'tum Çæ'cum.* ("Blind Point or Spot.") A spot in the centre of the retina where the central artery enters the eye. A ray of light falling on this point is not perceived. Also termed PORUS OPTICUS.

Punc'tum Sa'lĭ-ens.* ("Starting or Springing Point.") A name given by some writers to the first pulsations of the heart in the embryo; but, according to others, the first moving point that appears after the fecundation of the germ.

Pu'nĭ-ca.* [From *Pu'nicus*, "belonging to Carthage, or Northern Africa."] A Linnæan genus of the class *Icosandria*, natural order *Myrtaceæ*.

Pu'nica Gra-na'tum.* The pomegranate-tree, the flowers of which, termed balaustine flowers, are used medicinally as astringents.

Pu'pa.* [From *pu'pus*, a "puppet."] The second condition of the metamorphosis of insects; the chrysalis.

Pu'pil. [**Pupil'la;** from *pu'pa*, a "girl," "baby," or "doll."] The round black opening in the centre of the iris.

Pu'pil-la-rȳ Mem'brane. [**Membra'na Pupilla'ris.**] See VELUM PUPILLÆ.

Pu-pip'a-rus.* [From *pu'pa*, a "chrysalis," and *pa'rio*, to "bring forth."] Pupip'arous; bringing forth in the *pupa* state. Applied in the plural feminine (*Pupip'aræ*) to a family of dipterous insects.

Pupivorous. See PUPIVORUS.

Pu-piv'o-rus.* [From *pu'pa*, a "chrysalis," and *vo'ro*, to "devour."] Pupiv'orous; *pupa*-devouring. Applied in the neuter plural (*Pupiv'ora*) to a family of hymenopterous insects.

Pu-poph'a-gus.* [From *pu'pa*, and φάγω, to "eat."] The same as PUPIVORUS.

Purgatif. See PURGATIVE.

Pur-gā'tion. [**Purga'tio, o'nis;** from *pur'go, purga'tum*, to "cleanse," to "purge."] A purging, or evacuating, of the bowels.

Pur'ga-tive. [**Purgati'vus;** from the same.] (Fr. *Purgatif*, pür̀gå'tēf'.) Causing purgation; increasing the alvine excretions.

Pur'ging. [**Pur'gans;** from the same.] Having the power of evacuating the bowels, etc.

Pur'ging Flax. The common name for the *Linum catharticum*.

Pu'rĭ-form. [**Purifor'mis;** from *pus, pu'ris*, "matter issuing from a sore."] Resembling pus.

Pur'pu-ra.* [From πορφύρα, "purple."] (Fr. *Pourpre*, POORPR.) A purple color. Also, a genus of univalve shellfish which secretes a purple dye. In Pathology, a disease in which there are small distinct purple specks and patches, with general debility, but not always with fever.

Pur'pura Hæm-or-rhag'ĭ-ca.* Malignant petechial fever.

Pur'pu-rāte. [**Pur'puras, a'tis.**] A combination of purpuric acid with a salifiable base.

Pur-pu'ric. [**Purpu'ricus;** from *pur'pura*, "purple."] Belonging to purple. Applied to an acid of a purple color obtained from calculi and other animal excretions.

Pur-pu'rĭ-fers. [**Purpurif'era;** from *pur'pura*, "purple," and *fe'ro*, to "bear."] The name of a family of Gasteropodous Mollusks including those species belonging to the genus *Murex*, which secrete the purple substance forming the celebrated Tyrian dye of the ancients.

Pur'pu-rin, or **Pur'pu-rīne.** [**Purpuri'na;** from *pur'pura*, "purple."] A substance prepared by boiling madder-root acted on by sulphuric acid with water and alum, and collecting the precipitate. Also found in urine.

Pur'ree. [From πυῤῥός, "yellowish red"?] A beautiful yellow pigment, brought from India. It is adapted for oil or water-color painting, and is known by the name of Indian yellow (Fr. *Jaune Indien*, zhōn ăɴᴳ'de-ăɴᴳ').

Pu'ru-lent. [**Purulen'tus.**] Consisting of pus; of the nature of pus.

Pus,* gen. **Pu'ris.** [Gr. πύον.] A bland, cream-like fluid found in abscesses, or on the surface of sores; matter.

Push. A pustule: an inflammatory swelling which differs from a boil in containing uniform and mature pus.

Pus'tu-late. [**Pustula'tus;** from *pus'tula*, a "pustule."] Having pustules; blistered.

Pus'tule. [**Pus'tula;** diminutive of *pus*.] A small globate or conoidal elevation of the cuticle, containing pus, or lymph.

Pu-ta'men,* gen. **Pu-tam'ĭ-nis.** Originally, the "shell of a nut." In Botany, the stone of a drupe, *e.g.* a peach-stone, a plum-stone. Synonymous with ENDOCARP.

Pu-ta-min'e-us.* [From *puta'men*.] Belonging to a shell, or putamen.

Pu-tre-fac'tion. [**Putrefac'tio, o**'*nis;* from *pu'tris,* "rotten," and *fi'o, fac'tus,* to "become."] The spontaneous decomposition of animal or vegetable matters; the process of putrefying; rottenness.

Pu-trĕs'çence. [**Putrescen'tia;** from *putres'co,* to "rot."] A state of rottenness or putridity.

Putrid Fever. See TYPHUS.

Py-æ'mi-a,* or **Py-o-hæ'mi-a.*** [From πῦον, "pus," and αἷμα, "blood."] Purulent blood, or a state of the blood in which pus globules are found floating among the proper blood disks.

Pȳ-æm'ic, or **Pȳ-em'ic.** [**Pyæm'icus.**] Relating to *pyæmia.*

Py-au-la-co-me'le.* [From πῦον, "pus," and *aulacome'le,* a "grooved probe."] A grooved probe for searching for matter or pus.

Pȳc-no-car'pus.* [From πυκνός, "thick," and καρπός, "fruit."] Having thick, swollen fruit.

Pȳc-no-çeph'a-lus.* [From πυκνός, "thick," and κεφαλή, the "head."] Collected together in thick heads. Applied to flowers.

Pȳc-no-sta'chȳ-us.* [From πυκνός, "thick," and σταχύς, an "ear," or "spike."] Having flowers disposed in large spikes.

Py-e-li'tis, idis.* [From πύελος, a "trough."] Inflammation of the pelvis (or *sinus*) of the kidney.

Pyemia, Pyemic. See PYÆMIA, PYÆMIC.

Pyesis. See PYOSIS.

Py'ĭ-cus.* [From πῦον, "pus."] Of or belonging to pus; py'ic.

Py'in. [**Pyi'na;** from the same.] A constituent principle of pus.

Pȳ-lŏr'ic. [**Pylor'icus.**] Belonging to the pylorus.

Pȳl-o-rid'e-us.* [From πυλωρός, the "pylorus."] Applied in the plural neuter (*Pylorid'ea*) by Blainville to a family of Mollusks having a shell gaping at the two ends.

Pȳ-lo'rus.* [From πύλη, a "gate," or "entrance," and οὖρος, a "guard," or "keeper."] Sometimes called also **Jan'ĭ-tor*** [from *jan'ua,* a "gate"]. Literal signification of both terms being "gatekeeper." The inferior aperture of the stomach, at the commencement of the duodenum.

Pȳ-o-blen'nic. [**Pyoblen'nicus;** from πῦον, "pus," and βλέννα, "mucus."] The same as MUCO-PURULENT.

Py-o-blen-nor-rhœ'a.* [From πῦον, "pus," βλέννα, "mucus," and ῥέω, to "flow."] A flow of purulent mucus.

Py-o-ġen'e-sis.* [From πῦον, "pus," and γενέσις, "production."] The secretion or formation of pus.

Pȳ-o-ġe-net'ic. [**Pyogenet'icus.**] Pertaining to *pyogenesis.* Also, the same as PYOGENIC.

Pȳ-o-ġen'ic. [**Pyogen'icus;** from πῦον, "pus," and γεννάω, to "produce."] Producing or secreting pus.

Pyohæmia. See PYÆMIA.

Py-o-i'dēs.* [From πῦον, "pus," and εἶδος, a "form."] Resembling pus: py'oid.

Py-o-me'le.* [From πῦον, "pus," and μήλη, a "probe."] The same as PYAULACOMELE, which see.

Py-o-poi-e'sis.* [From πῦον, "pus," and ποιέω, to "make."] The same as PYOGENESIS, which see.

Py-o'sis.* [Gr. πύωσις.] The progress or formation of pus. Nearly the same as PYOGENESIS and PYESIS.

Pȳr'a-mid. [Lat. **Pyr'amis, m**'*idis;* Gr. πυραμίς.] A solid contained by a triangular, square, or polygonal base, and other planes meeting in a point which is called the vertex. The planes which meet in the vertex are called the sides, which are necessarily all triangles. Pyramids are triangular, quadrangular, pentagonal, etc., according as the base is a triangle, a square, a pentagon, etc. Applied in Anatomy to a small bony projection in the cavity of the tympanum.

Pȳ-ram'ĭ-dal. [**Pyramida'lis.**] Relating to a pyramid, or formed like a pyramid.

Pyram'idal Skull. Under this name, Dr. Prichard describes that form of the skull which Blumenbach terms Mongolian, and which is most characteristically seen in the Esquimaux.

Pȳ-ram-ĭ-da'lis* ("Pyramidal"), otherwise termed **Pyramida'lis Abdom'ĭ-nis.*** A muscle arising from the pubes, and inserted into the *linea alba,* nearly half-way between the pubes and umbilicus. It assists the rectus.

Pyramidalis Femoris. See PYRIFORMIS.

Pyramida'lis Na'si.* ("Pyramidal [Muscle] of the Nose.") A slip of the *occipito-frontalis* muscle which goes down over the nasal bones and is fixed to the *compressor nasi.*

Pȳ-ram'ĭ-doid. [**Pyramidoi'des;** from *pyr'amis,* a "pyramid," and εἶδος, a "form."] Resembling a pyramid.

Pȳ-rec'tĭ-ca.* [From πυρεκτικός, "feverish," or "having fever."] The name of an order in Good's Nosology, comprising fevers of every kind.

Pȳr'e-thrum.* Pellitory. The Pharmacopœial name (U.S. Ph.) for the root of the *Anacyclus Pyrethrum.*

Pȳ-ret'ic. [**Pyret'icus;** from πυρετός, "fever."] Relating to fever; febrile.

Pȳr-e-to-ġe-ne'sĭ-ạ,* or **Pȳr-e-to-ġen'e-sis.*** [From πυρετός, "fever," and γένεσις, "generation."] The origin and formation of fever.

Pȳr-e-tog'rạ-phȳ. [**Pyretogra'phia;** from πυρετός, "fever," and γράφω, to "write."] A history or description of fever.

Pȳr-e-tol'o-ġȳ. [**Pyretolo'gia;** from πυρετός, "fever," and λόγος, a "discourse."] A treatise on fevers. Also, the doctrine or science of fevers, their nature, causes, and distinctive characters.

Pȳ-rex'ĭ-ạ,* plural **Pȳ-rex'ĭ-æ.** [From πυρέσσω, future πυρέξω, to "be feverish," to "have a fever."] The state of fever. (See FEVER.) In the plural, febrile diseases: a class of Cullen's Nosology.

Pȳ-rex'ĭ-ạl. [**Pyrexia'lis.**] Belonging to *pyrexia;* febrile.

Pȳ-rif'er-us.* [From *py'rum*, a "pear," and *fe'ro*, to "bear."] Bearing fruits in form of the pear: pyriferous. Applied as a specific name to certain plants.

Pȳr'ĭ-form, or **Pȳ'rĭ-form.** [**Pyrifor'mis;** from *py'rum*, a "pear."] Resembling a pear in shape.

Pȳr-ĭ-for'mis.* ("Pear-shaped [Muscle].") A muscle arising from the hollow of the sacrum, and inserted into the cavity at the root of the *trochanter major.* It moves the thigh. It is also called *Pyramida'lis*, or *Pyramida'lis Fem'oris.*

Pȳ-ri'tēs,* or pĭr'ĭ-tēz. [From πῦρ, "fire."] Native compounds of metals with sulphur, as iron pyrites, etc.

Pȳr-ĭ-tif'er-ous. [**Pyritif'erus;** from *pyri'tes*, and *fe'ro*, to "bear."] Containing pyrites.

Pȳr-ĭ-tol'o-ġȳ. [**Pyritolo'gia;** from πυρίτης, "pyrites," and λόγος, a "discourse."] A treatise on pyrites; that part of Mineralogy which treats of the various kinds of pyrites.

Pȳr'o-ġen. [**Pyroge'nium;** from πῦρ, "fire," and γεννάω, to "produce."] Literally, "producing fire." A term applied to the electric fluid.

Pȳr-o-ġe-ne'sĭ-ạ,* or **Pȳr-o-ġen'e-sis.*** [From πῦρ, "fire," and γένεσις, "generation."] The generation or production of fire.

Pȳr-o-ġe-net'ic. [**Pyrogenet'icus.**] Belonging to *pyrogenesia;* generating fire.

Pȳr-o-ġe'ne-us.* [From πῦρ, "fire," and γείνω, to "be born," to "be produced."] Produced by fire, or heat: pyroge'neous.

Pȳ-roġ'e-nous. [**Pyroġ'enus;** from the same.] Igneous; produced by fire. Applied to a class of rocks comprehending the volcanic and igneous strata.

Pȳr'o-lạ.* [From *py'rus*, a "pear."] A Linnæan genus of the class *Decandria*, natural order *Pyrolaceæ.* Also, the Pharmacopœial name (Ed. Ph.) of the *Chimaph'ila umbella'ta*, formerly *Pyr'ola umbella'ta.*

Pyr'ola Um-bel-la'tạ.* A former name for the *Chimaphila umbellata*, or American winter-green.

Pyrolaceæ,* pĭr-o-la'she-ē. [From *Pyr'ola*, one of the genera.] A natural order of exogenous plants, mostly herbaceous, natives of Europe, North America, and Asia. It includes the *Chimaph'ila* (Winter-green) and other tonics.

Pȳr-o-lā'ceous. [**Pyrola'ceus.**] Belonging to, or resembling, the genus *Pyrola.*

Pȳr-o-lig'ne-ous. [**Pyrolig'neus;** from πῦρ, "fire," and *lig'neus*, "of wood."] Applied to an acid obtained by the destructive distillation of wood.

Pyrolig'neous Aç'id. [**Aç'idum Pyrolig'neum.**] An acid obtained from the destructive distillation of wood. It consists of acetic acid mixed with empyreumatic oil and bitumen.

Pyrolig'neous Spir'it, called also **Pȳr-ox-ȳl'ic Spir'it.** A substance produced during the distillation of wood. It is more volatile than alcohol, but burns very well in a spirit-lamp, and is comparatively cheap.—(HOBLYN.)

Pȳ-rol'o-ġȳ. [**Pyrolo'gia;** from πῦρ, "fire," and λόγος, a "discourse."] A treatise on heat; the doctrine or theory of fire or heat; that branch of science which treats of heat.

Pȳr-o-ma'nĭ-ạ.* [From πῦρ, "fire," and μανία, "madness."] A form of insanity in which those affected have a propensity to set houses on fire.

Pȳ-rom'e-ter. [**Pyrom'etrum;** from πῦρ, "fire," and μέτρον, a "measure."] An instrument for ascertaining those higher degrees of heat to which the thermometer cannot be applied.

Pȳ-roph'o-rus.* [From πῦρ, "fire."

and φέρω, to "bear," to "produce."] An artificial substance which takes fire or burns on exposure to the air; also, an instrument for striking fire or light.

Pўr-o-sco'pĭ-um.* [From πῦρ, "fire," and σκοπέω, to "examine."] The same as PYROMETER, which see.

Pў-ro'sis.* [From πυρόω, to "burn."] Water-brash; a disease characterized by pain in the stomach, with copious eructation of a watery, insipid fluid; it is a form of *Cardialgia.* A genus of the order *Spasmi,* class *Neuroses,* of Cullen's Nosology.

Pўr-os-phy'ra.* [From πῦρ, "fire," and σφῦρα, a "hammer."] An instrument formed like a hammer, heated or plunged into hot water, and employed as a cautery to produce irritation or vesication.

Pўr'o-tech-nў. [**Pyrotech'nia;** from πῦρ, "fire," and τέχνη, "art."] The art or science of making fireworks.

Pў-rot'ic. [**Pyrot'icos,** or **Pyrot'-icus;** from πυρόω, to "burn."] Having power to burn; caustic.

Pўr-ox-ўl'ic. [**Pyroxyl'icus;** from πῦρ, "fire," and ξύλον, "wood."] Applied to acetic spirit, because obtained in the distillation of wood. See PYROLIGNEOUS SPIRIT.

Pў-rox'ў-lin, or **Pў-rox'ў-line.** [**Pyroxyli'na;** from the same.] A term applied to gun-cotton, or other substances similarly produced.

Pў-rox'ў-lous. [**Pyroxylo'sus;** from the same.] Applied to an acid of less power than the pyroxylic, obtained in the distillation of wood. See PYROLIGNEOUS.

Pўr'rhin. [**Pyrrhi'na;** from πυῤῥός, "ruddy."] Applied to a substance regarded as the chief colorant of red snow.

Py'rus.* A Linnæan genus of the class *Icosandria,* natural order *Pomaceæ.*

Pyrus Aucuparia. See SORBUS AUCUPARIA.

Py'rus Com-mu'nis.* ("Common Pear-Tree.") The systematic name of the pear-tree. The juice of its fruit, when fermented, forms perry.

Py'rus Cy-do'nĭ-a.* A former name for the *Cydonia vulgaris,* or quince-tree.

Py'rus Ma'lus.* The systematic name of the apple-tree, of all the varieties of which the common crab-tree is supposed to be the parent.

Pўx-id'ĭ-um,* or **Pўx'is.*** [Gr. πυξίς, πυξίδος, a "box."] A pod which opens by a circular horizontal line cutting off the upper part as a lid.

Q.

Q. P. = *Quan'tum pla'cet.** "As much as you please," or "as much as is thought fit."

Q. Q. H., or **Quaq. Quart. Hor.** = *Qua'que quar'tâ ho'râ.** "Every four hours."

Q. S. = *Quan'tum suf'ficit.** "As much as will suffice."

Quack'e-rў. "Mean or bad acts in physic," comprehending not only the absurd impostures of ignorant pretenders, but also unbecoming acts of professional men themselves.

Quad-ran'gu-lar. [From *qua'tuor,* "four," and *an'gulus,* an "angle."] Having four angles.

Quad'rant. [**Quad'rans;** from *qua'tuor,* "four."] Literally, the "fourth part of any thing;" usually the fourth part of a circle, or ninety degrees. Applied to an instrument of great use in practical geometry.

Quad'rant E-lec-trom'e-ter. An instrument for estimating the degree or intensity of electricity. The differences of electric intensity are denoted by an index which traverses a quadrant divided into ninety equal parts called degrees.

Quadrate. See QUADRATUS.

Quad-ra'tus.* [From *quad'ra,* a "square."] (Fr. *Carré,* kå'rå'.) Quadrate; of a square figure. Applied to certain muscles, from their shape.

Quadra'tus Fem'o-ris.* ("Square [Muscle] of the Thigh.") A muscle arising from the outer border of the tuberosity of the ischium and inserted into a ridge leading from the great trochanter. It moves the thigh backwards.

Quadra'tus Ge'næ.* ("Square [Muscle] of the Cheek.") A name given to the muscle otherwise called *depressor labii inferioris* and *platysma myodes.*

Quadra'tus Lum-bo'rum.* ("Square [Muscle] of the Loins.") A muscle arising from the crest of the ilium, and inserted into the last rib and the transverse processes of the first four lumbar vertebræ. It inclines the loins to one side.

Quad-rĭ-cap'su-lar. [**Quadricap-**

sula'ris; from *qua'tuor*, "four," and *cap'sula*, a "capsule."] Applied to a fruit formed by the union of four capsules.

Quad-rĭ-cot-ÿ-led'o-nous. [**Quadricotyledo'neus**; from *qua'tuor*, "four," and *cotyle'don*.] Applied to an embryo with four cotyledons.

Quad-rĭ-den'tate. [**Quad'ridens**, or **Quadridenta'tus**; from *qua'tuor*, "four," and *dens, den'tis*, a "tooth."] Having four teeth, or divisions. Applied to a calyx, petal, etc.

Quad-rĭ-fa'rĭ-ous. [**Quadrifa'rius**; from *qua'tuor*, "four."] Literally, "in four ways." In Botany, having leaves disposed in four vertical ranks.

Quad'rĭ-fid. [**Quadrif'idus**; from *qua'tuor*, "four," and *fin'do*, to "cleave."] Divided nearly to the middle of its length into four equal portions.

Quad-rĭ-fo'lĭ-ate. [**Quadrifolia'tus**; from *qua'tuor*, "four," and *fo'lium*, a "leaf."] Bearing four leaves.

Quad-rĭ-fo'lĭ-o-late. [**Quadrifoliola'tus**; from *qua'tuor*, "four," and *foli'olum*, a "foliole."] Composed of four folioles.

Quad-rĭ-ġem'ĭ-nus.* [From *qua'tuor*, "four," and *gem'inus*, "double."] "Four-double," or consisting of four nearly equal parts. See TUBERCULA QUADRIGEMINA.

Quad-rij'u-gate. [**Quadrij'ugus**; from *qua'tuor*, "four," and *ju'gum*, a "yoke," or "pair."] Having four pairs of folioles.

Quad-rĭ-lat'e-ral. [**Quadrilatera'lis**; from *qua'tuor*, "four," and *la'tus, lat'eris*, a "side."] A plane figure bounded by four straight lines; having four sides.

Quad-ril'o-bate. [**Quadriloba'tus**; from *qua'tuor*, "four," and *loba'tus*, "lobed."] Divided into four lobes.

Quad-rĭ-par'tīte. [**Quadripar'ti'tus**; from *qua'tuor*, "four," and *par'ti'tus*, "divided."] Divided into four parts.

Quad-rĭ-pen'nis.* [From *qua'tuor*, "four," and *pen'na*, a "wing."] Having four wings: quadripen'nate. Applied to certain insects.

Quad'rĭ-vălve. [**Quadrival'vis**; from *qua'tuor*, "four," and *val'væ*, "folding doors."] Separated into four valves, as the capsule of some plants.

Quad-ru'ma-na.* [See next article.] The name of an order of Mammalia, comprising those of which each of the four extremities is terminated by a hand, as the ape, baboon, and monkey.

Quad-ru'ma-nous. [**Quadru'manus**; from *qua'tuor*, "four," and *ma'nus*, the "hand."] Having four hands: quadru'manate.

Quad'ru-ped. [From *qua'tuor*, "four," and *pes*, a "foot."] A four-footed animal. The term is no longer used by zoologists as strictly indicative of a particular class of animals.

Quad-ru'pe-dal. [**Quad'rupes, pedis**; from the same.] Having four feet.

Quadrupl. = *Quadruplica'to.** "Four times as much."

Qual'ĭ-ta-tĭve. [From *qual'itas, qualita'tis*, "quality."] Pertaining to quality.

Qual'itative A-nal'ÿ-sis. The determination of the nature of the component parts of a chemical compound, without reference to their relative proportions.

Quarantine, kwŏr-an-teen' [**Quaranti'na**], formerly written **Quarantain.** [From the Italian *quaran'ta*, "forty;" because it usually lasted forty days.] (Fr. *Quarantaine*, kå'rōnᴳ'tĕn' or kå'rŏnᴳ'tån'.) The period during which vessels from infected or suspected ports are debarred from entering into a healthy one, and from landing their goods, crew, or passengers, unless to be confined in a lazaretto.

Quar'tan. [**Quarta'nus**; from *quar'tus*, the "fourth."] Occurring every fourth day.

Quar'tan A'gue. An intermittent fever the paroxysms of which recur every fourth day, leaving between them an interval of two days.

Quar'tīne. [**Quarti'na**; from *quar'tus*, the "fourth."] The fourth envelope of the ovule of plants.

Quartz. [Ger. *Quarz*.] Pure silex; a constituent of granite. Rock crystal is crystallized quartz.

Quart'zose. Relating to, resembling, or containing quartz; quartzous.

Quassia,* kwŏsh'e-a. The Pharmacopœial name (U.S. Ph.) for the wood of the *Simaru'ba excel'sa*, or of the *Picræ'na excel'sa* (or *Quassia excelsa*), according to the British Pharmacopœia. Quassia has, in the highest degree, all the properties of the simple or pure bitters. As a tonic, it increases the powers of the digestive organs, with little excitement to the circulatory system.

Quas'sia A-ma'ra.* A tree from which quassia wood is obtained.

Quas'sia Ex-cel'sa.* One of the trees from which quassia wood is obtained.

Quas'sin. [**Quassi'na.**] A peculiar vegetable principle obtained from quassia wood, on which the virtues of the latter are supposed to depend.

Qua-ter'na-ry̆. [**Quaterna'rius;** from *quater'ni*, "four by four."] Disposed in fours; consisting of four. In Botany, the same as TETRAMEROUS, which see.

Qua-ter'nate. [**Quaterna'tus;** from the same.] Applied to verticillate leaves arranged four by four.

Qua-ter-ni-fo'li-us.* [From *quater'ni*, "four by four," and *fo'lium*, a "leaf."] Having quaternate leaves: quaternifo'liate.

Quer-cit'ron. [From *quer'cus*, an "oak."] The bark of *Quercus tinctoria*, or *Quercus nigra*, black oak, or dyer's oak. It yields a valuable yellow coloring matter, called *quercitrin* and *quercitric* or *quercitronic* acid.

Quer'cus.* (Fr. *Chêne*, shĕn or shån.) A Linnæan genus of the class *Monœcia*, natural order *Cupuliferæ*. Also, the Pharmacopœial name (Br. Ph.) for the dried bark of the small branches and young stems of the *Quercus pedunculata* (or *Quercus robur*).

Quer'cus Al'ba.* White-oak bark. The Pharmacopœial name (U.S. Ph.) for the bark of the *Quercus alba*. It is astringent and tonic, and has sometimes proved very beneficial in the treatment of intermittents.

Quer'cus Cer'ris.* Another name for the QUERCUS INFECTORIA, which see.

Quercus Coccifera. See KERMES, ANIMAL.

Quer'cus In-fec-to'ri-a.* The systematic name of the tree which yields the gall-nuts of commerce.

Quer'cus Ni'gra.* The same as *Quercus tinctoria*.

Quer'cus Pe-dun-cu-la'ta.* A name for the *Quercus robur*.

Quer'cus Ro'bur.* The systematic name of the most valuable British oak-tree. A decoction of the acorns is reputed efficacious against dysentery and colic. Also called *Quer'cus peduncula'ta*.

Quer'cus Su'ber.* The Cork Oak. A tree growing in Southern Europe, the bark of which constitutes the spongy, semi-elastic substance known in commerce as *cork*.

Quer'cus Tinc-to'ri-a.* Black-oak bark. The Pharmacopœial name (U.S. Ph.) for the bark of the *Quercus tinctoria*. Its medical properties are similar to those of the bark of the *Quercus alba*, but it is more apt to irritate the bowels.

Quick'lime. [**Calx Vi'vum.**] Unslacked, or unquenched, lime.

Quicksilver. See HYDRARGYRUM, and MERCURY.

Quina. See QUININE.

Quina do Campo, kee'nå do kåm'po. ("Cinchona of the Plain.") The bark of *Strychnos pseudo-quina*, used in Brazil as a substitute for cinchona.

Quinaquina. See CINCHONA.

Qui'na-ry̆. [From *qui'nus*, "five by five."] Consisting of five. Applied to leaves, petals, sepals, etc. The same as PENTAMEROUS, which see.

Quinate. See KINATE.

Qui'nate. [**Quina'tus;** from *qui'ni*, "five."] Arranged by fives. Applied to leaves that are inserted five by five around the stem, and to a digitate leaf with five leaflets.

Quince. [**Cydo'nium.**] The fruit of *Py'rus Cydo'nia*.

Quin-cun'cial. [**Quincuncia'lis;** from *quin'cunx*.] Arranged in the manner of a *quincunx*.

Quin'cunx.* [From *quin'que*, "five."] A Latin term for such a disposition of five objects, that they shall occupy the four corners of a square and the point of intersection of the diagonals of the same. An arrangement of trees or other objects in rows, so that each stands opposite to the centre of the vacant space which occurs between two members of the next row.

Quin-dec'a-gon. [**Quindecago'num;** from *quin'que*, "five," δέκα, "ten," and γωνία, an "angle."] A plane figure having fifteen sides and angles.

Quin-de-cag'o-nal. [**Quindecago'nus.**] Belonging to a quindecagon.

Quin'i-a,* or **Qui-nine'** (Fr. pronunciation, kè'nèn'); also called **Qui'na,*** or **Qui-ni'na.*** One of the alkaline proximate principles (the other being *Cincho'nia*) in which the medicinal virtues of the Peruvian bark chiefly reside.

Quinia, or **Quinine, Amorphous.** See QUINOIDINE.

Quin'i-æ Sul'phas.* ("Sulphate of Quinia.") The Pharmacopœial name ‖ for a substance in the form of silky, very light crystals, which are readily soluble in alcohol, and in water acidulated with sulphuric acid. It is composed of two equivalents of *quinia* with one of sulphuric acid and eight of water. Sulphate of quinia appears to possess essentially the same medical properties as Peruvian bark, without being so apt to nauseate or oppress the stomach. In large doses it sometimes produces serious or dangerous cerebral disturbance, and has occasionally proved fatal.

Quin'iæ Va-le-ri-a'nas.* ("Valerianate of Quinine.") The Pharmacopœial name (U.S. Ph.) for a salt which crystallizes in rhomboidal tables, and has a peculiar repulsive odor and bitter taste. It seems to combine the properties of quinia with those of valerian.

Quinine. See QUINIA.

Quin'ic. [**Quin'icus.**] Applied to salts that have quinine for their base.

Quinic Acid. See KINIC ACID.

Quinicia, kwe-nish'e-ą. See QUINOIDINE.

Quin'ĭ-dīne. [**Quinid'ia.**] An alkaloid found in the *Cinchonas.*

Quinine, Sulphate of. See QUINIÆ SULPHAS.

Quin'ĭ-nism. [**Quininis'mus;** from *quinine'.*] That disturbance of the nervous system caused by large doses, or by the continued use, of the sulphate of quinine.

Quin-oi'dīne. [**Quinoi'dia,** or **Quinoidin'ia;** from *qui'na,* "quinine," and εἶδος, a "form."] A resinous substance obtained from the mother-liquor remaining after all the crystals which can be procured are separated, in the preparation of the sulphate of quinine. Also called amorphous quinine, and *quinicia.*

Quin-quan'gu-lar. [**Quinquangula'ris,** or **Quinquangula'tus;** from *quin'que,* "five," and *an'gulus,* an "angle."] Having five angles.

Quin-que-den'tate. [**Quinquedenta'tus;** from *quin'que,* "five," and *dens,* a "tooth."] Having five teeth or serratures.

Quin-que-dig'ĭ-tate. [**Quinquedigita'tus;** from *quin'que,* "five," and *dig'itus,* a "finger."] Applied to a leaf the petiole of which terminates in five folioles.

Quin'que-fid. [**Quinquef'idus;** from *quin'que,* "five," and *fin'do,* to "cleave."] Cleft into five segments.

Quin-que-flo'rus.* [From *quin'que,* "five," and *flos,* a "flower."] Having five flowers.

Quin-que-fo'lĭ-ate. [**Quinquefolia'tus;** from *quin'que,* "five," and *fo'lium,* a "leaf."] Having five leaves.

Quin-que-fo'lĭ-o-late. [**Quinquefoliola'tus;** from *quin'que,* "five," and *foli'olum,* a "foliole."] Having five leaflets.

Quin-quef'o-rus.* [From *quin'que,* "five," and *fo'ro,* to "pierce."] Having five holes: quinquef'orous.

Quin'que-ju-gus.* [From *quin'que,* "five," and *ju'gum,* a "yoke."] Applied to a pinnate leaf the petiole of which bears five pairs of folioles: quin'quejugate.

Quin'que-lo-bate. [**Quinqueloba'tus;** from *quin'que,* "five," and *lo'bus,* a "lobe."] Having five lobes.

Quin-que-loc'u-lar. [**Quinquelocula'ris;** from *quin'que,* "five," and *loc'ulus,* a "cell."] Having five cells.

Quin-que-ner'vis,* or **Quin-que-ner'vĭ-us.*** [From *quin'que,* "five," and *ner'vus,* a "nerve."] Applied to a leaf having five longitudinal nervures.

Quin-que-par'tīte. [**Quinqueparti'tus;** from *quin'que,* "five," and *parti'tus,* "divided."] Deeply parted with five segments. Applied to a calyx, etc.

Quin-que-plī'cate. [**Quinqueplica'tus;** from *quin'que,* "five," and *plica'tus,* "plaited."] Having five plaits. Applied to parts of certain plants.

Quin-que-văl'vis.* [From *quin'que,* "five," and *val'va,* a "valve."] Opening in five valves: quinquevalvate.

Quin-qui'na.* Another name for CINCHONA, which see.

Quin'sȳ, formerly **Squinan'cy.** [A corruption of *Cynan'che,* "sore-throat."] A popular term for *Cynanche tonsillaris,* or *Tonsillitis phlegmonodes.* See CYNANCHE.

Quinta Essentia (es-sen'she-ą). See QUINTESSENCE.

Quin'tan. [**Quinta'nus;** from *quin'tus,* the "fifth."] A form of intermittent, which recurs every fifth day, leaving an interval of three days between the paroxysms.

Quint-es'sence. [**Quin'ta Essen'tia.**] A term denoting in alchemical language the *fifth,* and last, or highest, essence of any natural body. It is now commonly applied to any extract which contains all the virtues of a substance in a small bulk or compass. Sometimes it is used to designate the most volatile part of a substance, as being considered the most valuable.

Quin'tīne. [**Quinti'na;** from the same.] The fifth and innermost coat of the ovule of a plant.

Quin'tu-ple. [**Quin'tuplex;** from *quin'que,* "five," and *plĭ'co,* to "fold."] Five-fold.

Quin'tu-ple-nerved, or **Quin'tu-plĭ-nerved.** [From *quin'tuplex*, "five-fold," and *ner'vus*, a "nerve."] Having two strong primary nerves on each side of the midrib, as some leaves.

Quor. = *Quo'rum.** "Of which."

Quo-tid'ĭ-an, or **Quotid'ian Fe'ver.** [**Fe'bris Quotidia'na**; from *quotid'ie*, "daily."] (Fr. *Quotidien*, ko'tè'-de-ăNG'.) Applied to a kind of intermittent fever, in which the paroxysm returns every twenty-four hours. A genus of the order *Febres*, class *Pyrexiæ*, of Cullen's Nosology.

Q. V. = *Quan'tum vis.** "As much as you will."

R.

R. = *Reç'ipe.** "Take."

Ra'bĭ-ēs.* [From *ra'bio*, to "be mad," to "rage."] A disease caused by the saliva of dogs and some other animals being absorbed into the system through a wound, bite, or scratch. In this disorder the very sight of water, or any liquid, usually causes a spasm of the pharynx, accompanied by a sense of suffocation, and an indescribable horror, whence the name *hydrophobia* (or, "dread of water"), by which it is commonly known. See HYDROPHOBIA.

Ra'bies Ca-ni'na.* ("Canine Madness.") The most common form of the disease termed hydrophobia; also called *lyssa*. See HYDROPHOBIA.

Ra'bies Fe-li'na.* ("Feline Madness.") A variety of hydrophobia produced by the bite of a rabid cat. The spastic symptoms are said to be less acute than those of canine rabies, and frequently intermitting.

Race. [From the Italian *raz'za*, which is probably from the Latin *ra'dix*, a "root."] Races of men are permanent varieties of the human species, characterized by certain prominent distinctive traits. Blumenbach distinguished the following races:—

1. The *Caucasian Race.*—Skin white, passing into flesh-color, occasionally brownish; hair wavy, of a light or dark tint; face oval, facial angle large, viz. from 80° to 85°: comprising the Europeans (excepting the Laplanders and Finns), the inhabitants of Western Asia as far as the Obi, the Ganges, and the Caspian Sea, and most of the tribes of Northern Africa.

2. *Mongolian Race.*—Skin yellow; hair black, straight, scanty; face broad, flat; glabella flat and broad: comprising the Tartars and Chinese; also the Laplanders, the Finns, the Esquimaux and Greenlanders.

3. *American Race.*—Skin brownish copper-colored; hair black, straight, and scanty. It comprises all the aborigines of America, except those included in the preceding variety.

4. *Ethiopian Race.*—Skin black, or brownish black; hair black, coarse, short, woolly or frizzly; skull narrow, long; facial angle from 70° to 75°: including all the Africans (excepting those of the Caucasian variety), also the negroes of New Holland, and those of Papua, etc.

5. *Malay Race.*—Skin black; hair black, soft, curling, and abundant; cranium moderately narrow: comprising the brown islanders of the South Sea, the inhabitants of the Sunda Isles, the Moluccas, the Philippine and Marianne Isles, and the true Malays of Malacca.

Ra-ceme'. [**Race'mus.**] Originally, a "cluster of grapes." In Botany, a form of inflorescence in which the flowers, each on its own pedicel, are arranged along a common peduncle or axis, as the currant, hyacinth, and choke-cherry.

Raç-e-mif'er-ous. [**Racemif'erus**; from *race'mus*, a "cluster of grapes," or a "raceme," and *fe'ro*, to "bear."] Bearing racemes.

Ra-cem-ĭ-flo'rus.* [From *race'mus*, a "raceme," and *flos*, a "flower."] Having clusters of flowers: racemiflo'rous.

Raç-e-mose', or **Ra-ce'mous.** [**Racemo'sus**; from *race'mus*, a "raceme."] Bearing or resembling racemes.

Rachiagra, Rachialgia, Rachialgitis. See RHACHIAGRA, RHACHIALGIA, RHACHIALGITIS, etc.

Rachis. See RHACHIS.

Ra-chi'tis, *idis.** [From ῥαχίς, the "spine."] (Fr. *Rachitisme*, rå'shè'tèzm', or *Nouure*, noo'üR'.) Properly, inflammation of the spine, but usually applied to the disease commonly known as the RICKETS, which see.

Rack. See ARRACK.

Rad. = *Ra'dix.** "Root."

Radesyge (Danish), rå'deh-sü'geh.

[From *Ra·de* (the same as the German *Räu'de*), a "scab," and *syg*, "sick," "diseased."] Also termed **Nor-we'ġi-an Lep'ro-sy̆**, and **Scan-dĭ-nā'vĭ-an Syph'ĭ-lis.** A virulent and infectious disease, particularly affecting the skin, bones, and throat.

Rā'dĭ-al. [**Radia'lis;** from *ra'dius*, a "ray."] Belonging to the radius. In Botany, belonging to the border or ray of a head of flowers.

Rā'dĭ-ant, or **Rā'dĭ-ate.** [**Ra'dians, an**'*tis;* from *ra'dio, radia'tum*, to "shine," to "emit rays," or to "radiate."] Having or emitting rays; spreading from, or arranged around, a centre. Applied to the *corona* of the *Compositæ*.

Ra-dĭ-a'ta.* [From *ra'dio, radia'tum*, to "radiate."] A grand division or sub-kingdom of animals, chiefly marine; constituting the fourth primary division of animals in the system of Cuvier. They are so called because they have their parts arranged around an axis, and on one or several radii.

Rā'dĭ-āt-ed. [**Radia'tus;** from the same.] Having rays. See RADIANT.

Rā'dĭ-ate-Veined, or **Rā'dĭ-āt-ed-Veined.** A term applied to reticulated leaves in which three or more veins of nearly equal size diverge from the base; palmately-veined.

Ra-dĭ-at-ĭ-flo'rus.* [From *ra'dius*, a "ray," and *flos*, a "flower."] Having radiated flowers.

Rā-dĭ-ā'tion. [**Radia'tio, o**'*nis;* from *ra'dius*, a "ray."] The emission of rays of light or heat from a luminous or heated body.

Rad'ĭ-cal. [**Radica'lis;** from *ra'dix, radi'cis*, a "root."] Springing from a root; relating to the root; original; total; thorough. Radical leaves are those which apparently spring from the root. As a noun, radical is used in Chemistry as synonymous with a base; thus, sulphur and phosphorus are the radicals of sulphuric and phosphoric acids.

Rad'ĭ-cant. [**Rad'icans, an**'*tis;* from *rad'icor, radica'tus*, to "take root."] Rooting. Applied to a stalk bending and taking root where it touches the earth, or striking root by fibres which do not imbibe nourishment; as the ivy.

Rad-ĭ-cā'tion. [**Radica'tio, o**'*nis;* from the same.] The act of taking root; the arrangement of the roots.

Rad'ĭ-cel. A diminutive root, or a rootlet.

Ra-di'cēs,* the plural of RADIX, which see.

Rad-ĭ-cĭ-flo'rous. [**Radiciflo'rus;** from *ra'dix*, a "root," and *flos*, a "flower."] Having flowers which grow, or appear to grow, from the root.

Ra-diç'ĭ-form. [**Radicifor'mis;** from *ra'dix*, a "root."] Resembling a root.

Rad'ĭ-cle. [**Radic'ula;** diminutive of *ra'dix*, a "root."] A little root: a rad'icule. The part of the embryo (of a plant) which becomes the root. Also applied to a fibre of the tap-root.

Rad-ĭ-cu-lĭ-for'mis.* [From *radic'ula*, a "radicle."] Having the form of radicles.

Ra-dic-u-lo'sus.* [From the same.] Having radicles.

Ra'dĭ-i,* the plural of RADIUS, which see.

Ra-di'o-lus.* [Diminutive of *ra'dius*, a "ray."] A probe; also, a sound.

Rā'dĭ-ous. [**Radio'sus;** from *ra'dio, radia'tum*, to "send out rays," to "radiate."] Emitting luminous rays; radiant.

Rad'ish, Horse. The common English name of the *Cochlearia armoracia*.

Ra'dĭ-us.* [From ῥάβδος, a "rod," "streak," or "staff."] Literally, the "spoke of a wheel:" hence, a ray of light. In Geometry, a straight line drawn from the centre to the circumference of a circle. In Anatomy, applied to one of the bones of the forearm. In Botany, the ray of a flower. See RAY.

Ra'dius Vec'tor.* In Astronomy, an imaginary straight line, drawn from the centre of attraction to the point of an orbit in which the body (planet, comet, or satellite) may be; for example, the line joining the centre of the sun with the centre of a planet.

Ra'dix,* gen. **Ra-di'cis.** [From ῥάδιξ, a "branch."] The root, or the descending axis, of a plant, or that portion which grows downwards, ordinarily fixing the plant to the soil, and absorbing nourishment from it. It is the principal organ of nutrition. It produces no other organs or parts but naked branches, which are mere repetitions of the original descending axis. Unlike the stem, the root elongates continuously from its extremity alone. See TAP-ROOT, and STEM.

Radzyge. See RADESYGE.

Rafflesiaceæ,* raf-fle-se-a'she-ē. [From *Raffle'sia*, one of the genera.] A natural order of exogenous, stemless, anomalous plants (parasites), found in the East Indies on the stems of Cissi. The flower constitutes the whole plant.

Rage, râzh. The French term for RABIES, which see.

Rain-Gauge. See PLUVIOMETER.

Rai'sin. The dried fruit of the *Vitis vinifera;* also called *Uva passa* or *passula.*

Rak. See ARRACK.

Râle, râl. (Fr. *Râler,* to "rattle in the throat.") A rattle. Applied to various kinds of sound attending the circulation of air in the bronchia and vesicles of the lungs, different from the murmur produced in health. Also termed *Rhonchus.*

Râle Crépitant, râl cRâ'pè'tŏNG'. ("Crepitating Rattle.") A pathognomonic sign, common in severe pneumonia. It has been compared to the noise of butter boiling, or to that produced by particles of salt thrown on live coals.

Râle Muqueuse, râl mü'kuz'. ("Mucous Rattle.") A sound similar to that produced by blowing through a pipe into soapy water; when very strong, it is termed *gurgling.*

Râle Sibilant, râl sè'bè'lŏNG'. ("Sibilant or Hissing Rattle.") A sound caused by the presence of only a small quantity of mucus in the ramifications of the bronchia. It has been compared to the sound produced by suddenly separating two oiled surfaces.

Râle Sonore, râl so'noR'. ("Sonorous Rattle.") A sound like that of the cooing of a dove, or sometimes the snoring of a sleeping man.

Rā'me-al. [**Ramea'lis;** from *ra'mus,* a "branch."] Relating to branches, or growing on branches.

Rament. See RAMENTUM.

Ra-men'ta,* the plural of RAMENTUM, which see.

Ram-en-tā'ceous. [**Ramenta'ceus;** from *ramen'tum,* a "shaving," or a "rament."] Covered with small, dry, membranous scales, as the *Erica ramentacea.*

Ra-men'tum,* plural **Ra-men'ta.** [From *ra'do,* to "shave," to "scrape."] Any thing which is reduced, or rubbed down, by a file; filings; raspings. Applied to a species of pubescence, consisting of thin chaffy scales.

Ra'me-us.* The same as RAMEAL, which see.

Ram-ĭ-cor'nis.* [From *ra'mus,* a "branch," and *cor'nu,* a "horn."] Having branched antennæ. Applied to certain insects.

Ra-mif'er-ous. [**Ramif'erus;** from *ra'mus,* a "branch," and *fe'ro,* to "bear."] Bearing branches.

Ram-ĭ-fĭ-cā'tion. [**Ramifica'tio, o'nis;** from *ra'mus,* a "branch," and *fa'cio,* to "make."] The division of a stem into branches; the act or mode of branching; the arrangement of branches in trees.

Ram'ĭ-fied. [**Ramifica'tus;** from the same.] Having branches; divided into branches; branched.

Ram-ĭ-flo'rous. [**Ramiflo'rus;** from *ra'mus,* a "branch," and *flos,* a "flower."] Having flowers growing upon the branches.

Ram'ĭ-form. [**Ramifor'mis;** from *ra'mus,* a "branch."] Resembling a branch.

Ramollissement, râ'mo'lèss'mŏNG'. The French term for SOFTENING, which see.

Ra-mose', or **Rā'mous.** [**Ramo'sus;** from *ra'mus,* a "branch."] Full of branches; much branched.

Ram-u-lĭ-flo'rus.* [From *ram'ulus,* a "little branch," and *flos,* a "flower."] Having flowers on the ramules, as the *Crassula ramuliflora.*

Ram'u-lose, or **Ram'u-lous.** [**Ramulo'sus;** from *ram'ulus,* a "little branch."] Bearing many branchlets.

Ram'u-lus.* [Diminutive of *ra'mus,* a "branch."] A little branch: a ra'mule.

Ra'mus,* plural **Ra'mi.** The bough, or branch of a tree or other body.

Ra-mus'cu-lus.* [Diminutive of *ra'mus,* a "branch."] A little branch or division: a ramuscule.

Ran'çid. [**Ran'cidus;** from *ran'ceo,* to "be musty, stale, and rank."] Applied to fat, oil, and any greasy body which, by absorbing oxygen from the air, has acquired a strong odor and disagreeable taste.

Ran-cid'ĭ-tў. [**Rancid'itas, a'tis;** from *ran'cidus,* "musty and stale."] The property of being RANCID, which see.

Ra-nīne', or ran'īn. [**Rani'nus;** from *ra'na,* a "frog."] Belonging to the frog. Applied to a branch of the lingual artery.

Ra-niv'o-rous. [**Raniv'orus;** from *ra'na,* a "frog," and *vo'ro,* to "devour."] Living on frogs. Applied to certain birds.

Ran'u-la.* [Diminutive of *ra'na,* a "frog:" so called from a fancied resemblance.] A fluctuating semi-transparent tumor under the tongue, resulting from accumulated saliva and mucus in the ducts of the sublingual gland.

Ranunculaceæ,* ra-nun-ku-la'she-ē, or **Ra-nun'cu-li.*** A natural order of exogenous plants, mostly herbaceous, natives of the colder parts of the world. Acridity, causticity, and poison are the general characters of this order, which comprises Aconite (*Acon'itum*), Liverwort (*Hepat'ica*), Crowfoot (*Ranun'culus*), and *Clem'atis*.

Ra-nun-cu-lā'ceous. [**Ranuncula'ceus.**] Resembling the *ranunculus*.

Ra-nun'cu-li* (Fr. *Renoncules*, rẹh-nôɴɢ'kül'), the plural of *Ranun'culus*, forming the Jussieuan name of an order of plants. See RANUNCULACEÆ.

Ra-nun'cu-lus.* Crowfoot. The Pharmacopœial name (U.S. Ph.) for the cormus and herb of the *Ranunculus bulbosus*. It was formerly, before the general introduction of the Spanish fly, much used as a vesicatory, but it is very uncertain in its operation.

Rạ-pa'çēs,* the plural of RAPAX, which see.

Ra'pax, a'cis.* [From *ra'pio*, to "seize or take by violence."] Ravenous; rapacious. Applied in the plural (*Rapa'ces*) to an order of birds; also called *Accipitres* and *Raptores*. See ACCIPITER.

Rape. [From *ra'pa*, the "turnip."] The *Brassica napus*, or wild navew.

Rape. [**Rap'tus;** from *ra'pio, rap'tum*, to "take by violence," to "ravish."] Applied in Medical Jurisprudence to the defloration of a female forcibly and against her will, or of a girl of tender age who has, as yet, in the legal sense, no will.

Rape Oil. An oil procured from rape-seed, and used in making ointments, etc.

Rạ-pha'ni-ạ.* [From *raph'anus*, the "radish."] A disease attended with spasms of the joints; supposed to have been caused by the seeds of a species of *raphanus* mixed with the grain used for food. A genus of the order *Spasmi*, class *Neuroses*, of Cullen's Nosology.

Raph'ạ-nus.* [Gr. ῥαφανίς.] The radish. A Linnæan genus of plants of the class *Tetradynamia*, natural order *Cruciferæ*.

Raphanus Rusticanus. See COCHLEARIA ARMORACIA.

Ra'phe,* or **Rha'phe.*** [From ῥάφη, a "seam," or "suture."] A cord or ridge which connects the hilum with the chalaza of some plants.

Ra'phe Cor'po-ris Cal-lo'si.* ("Suture of the Callous Body.") A linear depression along the middle of the *corpus callosum*, between two slightly elevated longitudinal bands.

Ra'phe Pĕr-ĭ-næ'i.* ("Raphe, or Suture, of the Perinæum.") An elevated line which runs along the middle of the perinæum to the anus.

Raph'ĭ-dēṡ.* [From ῥαφίς, a "needle."] The acicular crystals found in the texture of nearly all plants. They commonly consist of oxalate of lime, and often of phosphate or sulphate of lime.

Rap'tor, o'ris.* [From *ra'pio, rap'tum*, to "seize or take by violence."] Applied in the plural (*Rapto'res*) to an order of birds; also called *Accipitres* and *Rapaces*. See ACCIPITER.

Rap-to'rēṡ,* the plural of RAPTOR, which see.

Rap'tus.* [From the same.] A forcible seizure. Hence the terms *raptus-nervorum* (seizure of the nerves), or cramp, etc.

Rar-e-fac'tion. [**Rarefac'tio, o'nis;** from *ra'rus*, "thin," "rare," and *fa'cio, fac'tum*, to "make."] The act of rarefying or expanding; also, the state of being rarefied or expanded.

Rar-ĭ-cos'tus.* [From *ra'rus*, "rare," or "sparse," hence, "few," and *cos'ta*, a "rib."] Having a small number of ribs.

Rar-ĭ-flo'rus.* [From *ra'rus*, "sparse," or "few," and *flos*, a "flower."] Having few flowers.

Rar-ĭ-spi-no'sus.* [From *ra'rus*, "few," and *spi'na*, a "thorn," or "spine."] Having few spines.

Ras. = *Rasu'ræ.** "Shavings."

Rash. An eruption on the skin. See EXANTHEMA.

Ra'sor, o'ris.* [From *ra'do, ra'sum*, to "scrape," "scratch," or "shave."] Applied in the plural (*Raso'res*) to an order of birds which scratch the ground for their food, as the common hen; also called *Gallinaceæ*.

Rạ-so'rēṡ,* the plural of RASOR, which see.

Rasp'ạ-to-rỹ. [**Raspato'rium;** from *ra'do, ra'sum*?] An instrument for rasping bones. See SCALPRUM.

Ra-su'rạ.* [From *ra'do, ra'sum*, to "scrape," or "shave."] A shaving.

Ratanhy. See RHATANY.

Rate (Fr.), råt. See SPLEEN.

Ratio (ra'she-o), **o'nis.*** [From *re'or, ra'tus*, to "suppose," "judge," or "think."] Originally, "reason," "thought," "design." Proportion; rate. The proportion which one magnitude bears to another of the same kind.

Rational, rash'un-al. [**Rationa'lis;** from *ra'tio,* "reason," "method."] Conformable to reason, or to a well-reasoned plan. Often applied to a sound course of practice, as opposed to empiricism.

Rat's Bane. Arsenious acid. Also applied to the seed of the *Strychnos nux vomica.*

Rat'tle. (Fr. *Râle,* râl.) A vulgar term for the rattling sound in the throat of dying persons, arising from the accumulation of mucus, or purulent matter, in the *bronchia,* etc.

Rat'tle-snake Root. The *Polygala senega.* See SENEGA.

Rau, or **Raw, Proç'ess of.** The *processus gracilis* of the *malleus.*

Rau-ce'do, ed'inis.* [From *rau'cus,* "hoarse."] Hoarseness, caused by an inflamed state of the mucous membrane of the larynx and trachea.

Ray. [**Ra'dius.**] A term for the marginal flowers of a head (or compound flower) when they are different from the rest, as in the sunflower; also, one of the pedicels of an umbel. In Optics, a beam of light propagated in a straight line from some luminous point. Rays are distinguished into—

1. CALORIF'IC rays, which produce heat; the highest degree of caloric being found in the red ray of the prismatic spectrum.

2. LU'MINOUS rays, which impart light; the highest degree of illumination being afforded by the brightest yellow or the palest green of the prismatic spectrum.

3. CHEM'ICAL rays, which cause neither heat nor light, but produce chemical changes. The greatest chemical action is in the violet ray.

The term *ray* is also applied to the bony or cartilaginous formations, more or less numerous, which support the membranous fins of fishes. See RADIUS.

Rays, Medullary. See MEDULLARY RAYS.

Re. A Latin particle signifying "again," "back," or "against;" hence often implying resistance. Before a vowel, a *d* is added, as *redintegration* for *re-integration.*

Re-ac'tion. [**Reac'tio, o'nis;** from *re,* "again," or "back," and *a'go, ac'tum,* to "act."] Literally, "acting back or against;" also, "acting again." In Mechanics, the reciprocality of force exerted by two bodies which act mutually on or against each other. In Physiology, the "acting again" of the vital powers after they have been greatly depressed. Also applied to the effect produced on the system by irritants or stimuli, in which the vital forces seem to resist the irritating substance. The state or process of applying a reagent, or test, for detecting the presence of certain other bodies.

Re-ā'gent. [**Rea'gens, en'tis;** from the same.] A substance employed in chemical analysis to ascertain the quantity or quality of the component parts of bodies by reacting on their elements: a test.

Re-ăl'gar. The protosulphuret of arsenic; also called *Arsenicum rubrum,* or "Red Arsenic." Realgar occurs native; it may also be formed artificially, by heating arsenious acid with sulphur.

Réaumur's Scale. See THERMOMETER.

Reaumuriaceæ,* rō-mu-re-a'she-ē, or râ-o-mu-re-a'she-ē. [From *Reaumu'ria,* one of the genera.] A small natural order of exogenous shrubs, found on the coast of the Mediterranean and saline plains of Northern Asia.

Re-cēiv'er. A vessel fitted to a retort, alembic, or the like, for receiving the product of distillation.

Re-cep'ta-cle. [**Receptac'ulum;** from *recip'io, recep'tum,* to "receive."] Originally, a place to receive or keep things in. Applied to the apex of the flower-stalk, on which all the organs of a flower are situated; the axis of the flower.

Re-cep-tac'u-lum Chy'li.* ("Receptacle of the Chyle.") (Fr. *Réservoir du Chyle,* râ'zĕR'vwâR' dü shēl.) A name applied to the somewhat expanded lower portion of the thoracic duct.

Reç'i-pe.* [Imperative mood of *recip'io,* to "take."] Constantly used in the abbreviated form, ℞, as the commencement of a medical prescription.

Rec-li-nā'tion. [**Reclina'tio, o'nis;** from *recli'no, reclina'tum,* to "bend back."] One of the operations for cataract, in which the lens is thrown backwards into the middle and towards the bottom of the vitreous humor.

Re-clined', or **Rec'li-nate.** [**Reclina'tus;** from the same.] Bending downwards.

Rec're-ment [from *re,* "again," and *cer'nere, cre'tum,* to "sift," or "secrete"], or **Recrementitial** (rek-re-men-tish'al) **Hu'mor.** Literally, "a returned secretion,"—that is, a secretion, like the saliva, which, after having been separated from the blood, is again given back to it.

Rec-ru-dĕs'çence. [**Recrudes'cens;** from *recrudes'co*, to "grow raw and sore again."] A growing worse again; an increase of a disease after a temporary abatement.

Rect. = *Rectifica'tus*.* "Rectified."

Rec-tăl'ğĭ-a.* [From *rec'tum*, and ἄλγος, "pain."] Pain of the rectum. The same as PROCTALGIA.

Rec-tan'gle. [**Rectan'gulus;** from *rec'tus*, "right," and *an'gulus*, an "angle."] A right-angled parallelogram. When the adjacent sides are equal, it becomes a square.

Rec-tan'gu-lar. [**Rectangula'ris.**] Having right angles.

Rec-tem'brȳ-us.* [From *rec'tus*, "straight," and *em'bryon*, an "embryo."] Applied to a section of the *Leguminosæ*, containing those having the radicle of the embryo straight.

Rec-tĭ-fĭ-cā'tion. [**Rectifica'tio, o'nis;** from *rectif'ico*, *rectifica'tum*, to "make right."] A second or repeated distillation, in which substances are more perfectly purified.

Rec'tĭ-fied. [**Rectifica'tus;** from the same.] Made more pure, or stronger.

Rectified Spirit. See SPIRITUS RECTIFICATUS.

Rec-tĭ-lin'e-ar. [**Rectilin'eus;** from *rec'tus*, "straight," and *li'nea*, a "line."] Relating to, or bounded by, straight lines.

Rec'tĭ-nerved. [**Rectiner'vis;** from *rec'tus*, "straight," and *ner'vus*, a "nerve."] Having straight nerves or veins; parallel-veined. Applied to leaves.

Rec-tĭ-ros'tris.* [From *rec'tus*, "straight," and *ros'trum*, a "beak."] Having a straight beak. Applied to shells, birds, etc.: rectirostrate.

Rec-ti'tis, idis.* [From *rec'tum*.] Inflammation of the rectum. See PROCTITIS.

Rec-tri'cēs,* the plural of RECTRIX, which see.

Rec'trix, tri'cis,* plural **Rec-tri'cēs.** [From *re'go*, *rec'tum*, to "guide."] The plumes of the tail of birds, which, like a rudder, direct their flight.

Rec'tum.* [From *rec'tus*, "straight."] The last, nearly straight, portion of the large intestine, terminating at the anus.

Rec'tus.* [From *re'go*, *rec'tum*, to "rule."] Right; straight. Applied to muscles, etc.

Rec'tus Ab-dom'ĭ-nis.* ("Straight [Muscle] of the Abdomen.") A muscle arising from the pubes, and inserted into the three inferior true ribs and the ensiform cartilage. It pulls down the ribs in respiration.

Rec'tus Cap'ĭ-tis,* plural **Rec'ti Cap'ĭ-tis.** ("Straight [Muscles] of the Head.") The name of five muscles arising from the upper cervical vertebræ, and inserted into the occipital bone. These are the *Rec'tus cap'itis anti'cus ma'jor*, *Rec'tus cap'itis anti'cus mi'nor*, *Rec'tus cap'itis latera'lis*, *Rec'tus cap'itis posti'cus ma'jor*, and *Rec'tus cap'itis posti'cus mi'nor*.

Rec'tus Ex-ter'nus Oc'u-li.* ("External Straight [Muscle] of the Eye.") A muscle arising from the optic foramen, and inserted into the outer side of the eye. It is also named *abductor oculi*, from its turning the eye outwards.

Rec'tus Fem'o-ris.* ("Straight [Muscle] of the Thigh.") A muscle arising by two heads from the ilium and acetabulum, and inserted into the patella. It is sometimes called *rectus cruris* ("Straight [Muscle] of the Leg"). It extends the leg.

Rec'tus In-fe'rĭ-or Oc'u-li.* ("Inferior Straight [Muscle] of the Eye.") A muscle arising from the lower part of the optic foramen, and inserted opposite to the *rectus superior*. It is also named *deprimens oculi*, from its drawing the eye downwards.

Rec'tus In-ter'nus Oc'u-li.* ("Internal Straight [Muscle] of the Eye.") A muscle arising from the margin of the optic foramen, and inserted into the inner side of the eye. It is also named *adducens*, from its drawing the eye towards the nose.

Rec'tus Su-pe'rĭ-or Oc'u-li.* ("Superior Straight [Muscle] of the Eye.") A muscle arising from the upper part of the optic foramen, and inserted into the superior and fore part of the sclerotica. It is also named *attollens* or *levator oculi*, from its office of raising the eye, and the *superbus* ("proud"), from the expression which it imparts.

Re-cur'rent. [**Recur'rens, en'tis;** from *recur'ro*, to "run back."] Running back. Applied to a nerve, and to branches of arteries, nerves, etc.; also, returning at intervals.

Re-cur-vā'tion. [**Recurva'tio, o'nis;** from *recur'vo*, *recurva'tum*, to "bend back."] A bending backwards. Applied to the vertebral column.

Re-curved', or **Re-cur'vate.** [**Re-**

curva'tus, Recur'vus; from the same.] Bent or curved backwards. Applied to plants.

Re-cur-vi-fo'li-us.* [From *recur'vo*, to "bend back," and *fo'lium*, a "leaf."] Having leaves recurved or reflected at their extremity.

Red Fire. A pyrotechnical compound of nitrate of strontia, sulphur, antimony, and chlorate of potash, burning with a red flame.

Red Gum. A popular name for *Stroph'ulus intertinc'tus.*

Red Lead. Minium, or red oxide of lead.

Red Pre-cip'i-tate. The HYDRARGYRI OXYDUM RUBRUM, which see.

Red Root. One of the popular names for the *Ceano'thus America'nus*, otherwise called **New Jer'sey Tea.** A small indigenous shrub, of the Linnæan class *Pentandria*, natural order *Rhamnaceæ*, found in most parts of the United States. It has small white flowers in clusters or dense panicles, and ovate, acuminate, and serrate leaves. The root is astringent, and imparts a red color to water. During the Revolutionary War, the leaves of this plant were used as a substitute for tea, on which account it has recently attracted considerable attention. An infusion of the dried leaves and seeds has been recommended in aphthous affections of the mouth, and in the sore throat attending scarlet fever.

Red San'dal, Red Saun'ders. The wood of *Pterocar'pus santali'nus.*

Red. in pulv. = *Redac'tus in pul'verem.** "Reduced to powder."

Redig. in pulv. = *Rediga'tur in pulverem.** "Let it be reduced to powder."

Re-din'te-grate. [**Redintegra'tus;** from *re*, "again," and *in'teger*, "entire," "sound."] Restored to soundness or completeness; renovated.

Re-din-te-gra'tion. [**Redintegra'tio, o'nis;** from the same.] A restoration to soundness; a reproduction of a part of the body which has been destroyed.

Re-duc'tion. [**Reduc'tio, o'nis;** from *redu'co, reduc'tum*, to "bring back," to "reduce."] The process by which metals, changed or disguised by a union with other substances, are restored to their metallic state. It is generally applied to the restoration of metallic oxides. In Surgery, the returning of a dislocated bone into its natural situation.

Re-duc'tor, o'ris.* [From the same.] A bringer or leader back. Applied to a muscle of the vertebral column.

Re-du-pli-ca'tion. [**Reduplica'tio, o'nis;** from *re*, "again," and *du'plico, duplica'tum*, to "double."] The act of doubling. Applied to the paroxysms of ague of a double type.

Re-fi'ning. The act of purifying any thing; particularly the assaying or purifying gold and silver by separating them from other bodies which are combined with them.

Re-flect'. [From *re*, "again," or "back," and *flec'to, flec'tum* or *flex'um*, to "bend," or "turn."] To turn back. (See REFLECTION.) To double back on itself, as a membrane.

Re-flec'tion, or **Re-flex'ion.** [**Reflec'tio, o'nis;** from the same.] The act of turning back or reflecting. In Mechanics, the rebound of a body from the surface of another body against which it impinges. In Natural Philosophy, the term is applied to analogous motions of light, heat, and sound. In Obstetrics, it is applied to a bending back of the uterus. (See RETROVERSIO UTERI.) In Anatomy, to a duplicature of a membrane, etc.

Reflec'tion, An'gle of. The angle made by the line of direction of the reflected body or ray with a line which is perpendicular to the reflecting surface.

Re'flex. [**Reflex'us;** see REFLECTION.] Applied to certain actions and functions of living beings. See next article.

Re'flex Ac'tion. A term applied to those involuntary movements caused by some impression or irritation conveyed to the spinal marrow by the afferent spinal nerves, in consequence of which, an excitement or impulse is sent back by the reflex spinal nerves, producing the movements in question. Thus, an irritation of the lining membrane of the nostril causes the convulsive involuntary movement of the muscles of respiration, termed *sneezing.*

Re'flex Func'tion. Applied to certain functions of living beings, performed through the medium of the reflex nerves.

Re'flex Spi'nal Nerves. Those of the spinal system of nerves which convey motor impulses from the spinal marrow in consequence of impressions made upon the surface of the body. See REFLEX ACTION.

Re-flexed'. Bent downwards or backwards. Applied to parts of plants.

Reflexion. See Reflection.

Re'flux. [**Reflux'us;** from *re,* "back," and *flu'o, flux'um,* to "flow."] The movement of the sea when it retires after the *flux* or flow; the ebb. In Physiology, the return of the blood from the head, or from the lower half of the body, to the heart.

Re-fract'ed. In Botany, suddenly bent backwards.

Re-frac'tion. [**Refrac'tio, o'nis;** from *re,* "again," or "back," and *fran'go, frac'tum,* to "break."] The deviation of a ray of light from its original direction on entering obliquely a medium of a different density. The laws which regulate the refraction of light form the subject of that branch of Natural Philosophy called Dioptrics.

Double Refraction is a property of certain transparent minerals, etc., as Iceland spar, by which they present two images of any object seen through them. A ray of light passing through these media is separated into two distinct pencils which pursue separate courses.

Re-frac'tive. [**Refracti'vus;** from the same.] Pertaining to refraction; causing or producing refraction.

Re-frac'to-rў. [From *re,* "back," or "against," implying resistance, and *fran'go, frac'tum,* to "break," to "subdue."] Properly, "that will not or cannot be subdued." Applied to a substance which it is difficult or impossible to melt.

Re-fran-ği-bil'ĭ-tў. [**Refrangibil'itas, a'tis;** from the same.] The tendency of luminous rays to be refracted or bent in passing obliquely from one transparent medium into another, or in traversing a medium the density of which is not uniform.

Re-fran'ği-ble. [**Refrangib'ilis;** from the same.] Susceptible of refraction.

Re-frig'e-rant. [**Refrig'erans;** from *refrig'ero, refrigera'tum,* to "cool," to "chill."] Applied to medicines which cool the body or blood.

Re-frig'e-ra-to-rў. [**Refrigerato'rium;** from the same.] A vessel filled with cold water, for condensing vapors or cooling substances.

Re-ğen-e-rā'tion. [**Regenera'tio, o'nis;** from *re,* "again," or "anew," and *gen'ero, genera'tum,* to "generate."] Applied in Physiology to the reproduction of a part or substance lost by disease or injury. See Redintegration.

Re'ği-a A'qua.* ("Royal Water.") See Nitro-Muriatic Acid.

Reğ'ĭ-men, m'inis.* [From *re'go,* to "rule," or "regulate."] A Latin word signifying "government," or "regulation:" applied to the regulation of the diet. A rational and methodical course of life in respect to food, etc.

Re'ğion. [**Re'gio, o'nis.**] A particular portion of the body; especially used in reference to a particular organ or viscus, as the region of the liver, heart, kidney, etc.

Reg'u-lar. [**Regula'ris;** from *reg'ula,* a "rule."] Applied to flowers in which the members of each floral circle (*i.e.* the corolla or calyx) are alike in shape and size.

Regular Solids. See Solid.

Reg-u-lar-ĭ-flo'rus.* [From *regula'ris,* "regular," and *flos,* a "flower."] Applied to the head and the disk of the *Synantheræ,* when composed of flowers with regular corols.

Reg'u-lus.* [Diminutive of *rex, re'gis,* a "king."] A pure metal reduced from its ore.

Reg. umb. = *Re'gio umbili'ci.** "Region of the navel."

Re-gur-ği-tā'tion. [**Regurgita'tio, o'nis;** from *re,* "again," or "back," and *gur'ges,* a "flood," a "flowing."] A flowing back; a flowing the wrong way. Applied, for example, to the flowing back of the blood from the ventricles into the auricles of the heart.

Re-lā'tions, Or-gan'ic. A term applied to the relations subsisting between different parts of the animal economy. They may be ranked under three different heads:—

1. *Mechanical Relations,* or such as depend upon the position of parts, in consequence of which, if one organ be displaced (or greatly enlarged), the free and healthy operation of an adjacent organ is interfered with: thus, in cases of *prolapsus uteri,* urination is sometimes rendered difficult and painful.

2. *Functional Relations,* or those whereby the healthy condition of one organ depends upon the healthy operation of another: thus, if there be derangement in either the respiratory or digestive function, the blood fails to communicate a healthful stimulus to the heart, and the function of the latter organ becomes consequently impaired.

3. *Sympathetic Relations,* or those which depend upon the nervous sympathy subsisting between different parts. See Sympathy.

Relaxantia,* re-lax-an'she-a, **Re-**

lax'ants. (Fr. *Relâchant,* rẹh-lâ'shŏnᴳ'.) [From *relax'o, relaxa'tum,* to "loosen."] Applied to substances which relax and soften parts that are inflamed.

Rel-ax-ā'tion. [**Relaxa'tio, o'***nis;* from the same.] The act of relaxing, or state of being relaxed. In Physiology, the reverse of contraction or tension.

Re-lĭ'quĭ-æ, a'*rum.** [From *relin'quo,* to "leave."] Relics. Applied to organic remains, as fossil Zöophytes, Crustaceans, etc.

Re-me'dĭ-um Cạ-thol'ĭ-con.* A panacea. See CATHOLICON.

Rem'e-dȳ. [**Reme'dium;** from *re,* "again," and *me'deor,* to "heal."] That which is employed in the treatment of diseases, whether palliative, preventive, or curative.

Rem'ĭ-ġēṡ.* [Plural of *re'mex, rem'igis,* a "rower," or "oarsman."] Applied to strong, stiff feathers in the wings of birds, the action of which is compared to that of oars.

Re-mis'sion. [**Remis'sio, o'***nis;* from *remit'to, remis'sum,* to "remit," to "relax."] An abatement or diminution of febrile symptoms occurring between the accessions of remittent fever. Also applied to the abatement of the symptoms of continuous fever.

Re-mit'tent. [**Remit'tens;** from the same.] Applied to disorders the symptoms of which abate considerably and then return again and again until the disease is overcome or proves fatal.

Remit'tent Fe'ver. [Lat. **Fe'bris Remit'tens;** Fr. *Fièvre Rémittente,* fe-ĕvʀ' rå'mĕt'tŏNt'.) The name given to any fever which abates, but does not wholly cease, at regular intervals. See EPANETUS.

Rem'o-rạ.* [From *rem'oror,* to "hinder," or "stop."] A stoppage, or stagnation. Also applied to surgical instruments used to retain parts in their place (*in situ*).

Re-mo-tĭ-fo'lĭ-us.* [From *remo'tus,* "distant," and *fo'lium,* a "leaf."] Applied to leaves distant from each other.

Ren,* gen. **Re'nis.** The kidney; the gland by which the urine is secreted.

Re'nạl. [**Rena'lis;** from *ren,* the "kidney."] Belonging to the kidney.

Re'nal Ap'o-plex-ȳ. Another name for *Ischu'ria rena'lis.*

Renal Calculus. See NEPHROLITHOS.

Re'nal Glands or **Cap'sules.** [**Glan'dulæ** or **Cap'sulæ Rena'les.**] The renal (suprarenal) glands or atrabiliary capsules.

Ren'cu-lus.* [Diminutive of *ren,* the "kidney."] The name of each distinct lobe of the kidney in the embryo of the Mammalia.

Ren-ĭ-fo'lĭ-us.* [From *ren, re'nis,* the "kidney," and *fo'lium,* a "leaf."] Having reniform leaves: renifo'lious.

Ren'ĭ-form. [**Renifor'mis;** from *ren, re'nis,* the "kidney."] Formed like the kidney. Applied to a roundish cordate leaf, of which the lateral dimension exceeds the length from the base to the apex.

Ren'net, or **Run'net.** Applied to a fluid made by infusing the rennet-bag, or inner coat or membrane of a calf's stomach, in hot water; also to the membrane itself. It has the property of coagulating milk.

Renoncule, rẹh-nonᴳ'kül'. The French name for Ranunculus. See RANUNCULI.

Re-pand'. [**Repan'dus.**] Bowed, or waved. Applied to a leaf of which the margin is slightly waved, or sinuate.

Repanditas. See LORDOSIS.

Re-pel'lent. [**Repel'lens;** from *repel'lo,* to "beat or drive back."] Driving back. Applied to medicines which cause diseases to recede from the surface.

Re'pent. [**Re'pens;** from *re'po,* to "creep."] Creeping on the ground. Applied to plants and reptiles.

Re-per-cus'sĭve. [From *re,* "back," and *percu'tio, percus'sum,* to "strike," or "beat."] The same as REPELLENT, which see.

Repercutiens (rep-er-ku'she-ĕns), **en'***tis.** [From the same.] The same as REPELLENT, which see.

Repet. = *Repeta'tur,** or *Repetan'tur.** "Let it, or them, be repeated."

Re-plē'tion. [**Reple'tio, o'***nis;* from *rep'leo, reple'tum,* to "fill up."] The state or condition of being full, or gorged. The same as PLETHORA, which see.

Rep'lĭ-cate, or **Rep'lĭ-cā-tĭve.** [**Replicati'vus;** from *re,* "again," or "back," and *pli'co, plica'tum,* to "fold."] Folded back. Applied to æstivation when the floral organs are folded inwards upon themselves, and to vernation when the upper part of the leaves is folded back and applied to the lower.

Re'plum.* A Latin word signifying a leaf of a door. In Botany, a framelike placenta from which the valves of the pod fall away in dehiscence, as in the *Papaveraceæ,* etc.

Reprimentia,* rep-re-men'she-ạ.

[From *rep'rimo*, to "repress."] "Repressing Medicines." Remedies for fluxes; as astringents, acid stimulants, etc.

Rep'rĭ-ments. The same as REPRIMENTIA, which see.

Re-pro-duc'tion. [**Reproduc'tio, o'***nis;* from *re,* "again," and *produ'co, produc'tum,* to "bring forth," to "produce."] The production by organized bodies of others similar to themselves.

Re-pro-duc'tĭve. [**Reproducti'vus;** from the same.] Producing again; adapted for reproduction.

Reproduc'tive Or'gans of Plants. The stamens and pistils.

Rep'tant. [**Rep'tans;** from *rep'to,* to "creep."] Creeping. The same as REPENT.

Rep-tā'tion. [**Repta'tio, o'***nis;* from *rep'to, repta'tum,* to "creep."] Creeping. The mode of progression proper to serpents and certain *Invertebrata.*

Rep'tĭle. [See REPTILIS.] A cold-blooded vertebrate animal which creeps on the ground.

Rep-til'ĭ-a,* the plural of REPTILIS, which see.

Rep'tĭ-lis.* [From *re'po, rep'tum,* to "creep."] A reptile; any thing that creeps. Applied in the plural neuter (*Reptil'ia*) to a class of animals which have either no feet, as the serpents, or feet so short, as the lizards, that they creep with their bodies close to the ground.

Rep-tĭ-liv'o-rous. [**Reptiliv'orus;** from *rep'tilis,* a "reptile," and *vo'ro,* to "devour."] Eating or devouring reptiles. Applied to birds.

Re-pul'sion. [**Repul'sio, o'***nis;* from *repel'lo, repul'sum,* to "drive back," or "repel."] That power or tendency which impels the particles of matter to separate, and is in constant opposition to attraction. This repulsive force, which is inherent in all matter, is by many supposed to be produced by caloric.

Re-pul'sĭve. [**Repulsi'vus;** from the same.] Producing repulsion. Sometimes applied to double refraction when the extraordinary ray is more removed from the axis than the ordinary, and this is situated between it and the axis.

Repulsive Force. See REPULSION.

Re-sec'tion. [**Resec'tio, o'***nis;* from *res'eco, resec'tum,* to "cut off."] A variety of amputation.

Re-se'da Lu-te'o-la.* A European plant called Weld, or Dyers' Weed, which was once used as a diaphoretic and diuretic.

Resedaceæ,* res-e-da'she-ē. A small natural order of exogenous plants, mostly herbaceous, comprising the *Rese'da* (Mignonette), highly prized for its fragrance.

Réservoir du Chyle, rā-zĕr'vwår' dü shēl. The French term for RECEPTACULUM CHYLI, which see.

Re-sid'u-um.* [From *resi'deo,* to "remain."] The residue. Applied to that which is left after any process of separation or purification.

Re-sī'na,* plural **Re-si'næ.** [Gr. ῥητίνη; from ῥέω, to "flow."] A resin. The Pharmacopœial name for a vegetable solid, inflammable substance; the residuum of the turpentines of various species of *Pinus* and *Abies.*

Resi'na Al'ba.* ("White Resin.") Obtained from the *Pinus sylvestris,* etc.; also, the residuum of the distillation of turpentine in a particular state of purity.

Resi'na Fla'va.* ("Yellow Resin.") Applied to the residuum after the distillation of the volatile oil from the turpentines: sometimes called *Colopho'nia,* or *Coloph'ony,* in the United States popularly termed *rosin.*

Resi'na Ja-la'pæ* ("Resin of Jalap") is prepared in precisely the same manner as the RESINA PODOPHYLLI, which see.

Resi'na Ni'gra.* ("Black Resin.") Applied to a coarser kind of resin.

Resi'na Pod-o-phȳl'li.* ("Resin of May-Apple.") Take of May-apple, in fine powder, sixteen troyounces; alcohol, water, each a sufficient quantity. Moisten the May-apple with four fluidounces of alcohol, pack it firmly in a cylindrical percolator, and gradually pour alcohol upon it until four pints have passed, or until the filtered liquid ceases to occasion turbidness when dropped into water. Reduce the tincture to half a pint by distilling off the alcohol, mix the residue with four pints of water, separate the precipitate formed, wash it thoroughly with water, and dry it with a gentle heat. This preparation, directed by the U.S. Pharmacopœia, is essentially the same substance as PODOPHYLLIN, which see.

Re-si'næ,* the plural of RESINA, which see.

Res-i-na'tus.* [From *resi'na,* "resin."] Belonging to, or having, resin.

Reṡ-ĭ-nif'er-ous. [**Resinif'erus;** from *resi'na,* "resin," and *fe'ro,* to "bear."] Bearing or affording resin.

Reṡ'in-ĭ-form. [**Resinifor'mis;** from *resi'na,* "resin."] Having the appearance of a resin.

Res'i-noid. [**Resinoi'des;** from *resi'na*, "resin," and εἶδος, a "form."] Resembling resin.

Res-i-no'sa.* Resinous stimulants. Vegetable stimulants which owe the whole of their activity to resin.

Res'i-nous. [**Resino'sus;** from *resi'na*, "resin."] Resembling, containing, or consisting of resin.

Re-sis'tance. [**Resistan'tia;** from *resis'to*, to "stand still," to "stop," to "withstand."] Applied in Mechanics and Physiology to a force or power acting in opposition to another force or power, so as to destroy or diminish its effect.

Res Nat-u-ra'lēs.* ("Natural Things.") A term formerly applied to the elements, humors, etc. which were supposed to constitute the nature or life of man.

Res Non-nat-u-ra'lēs.* ("Non-natural Things.") Those principal things and substances which contribute to the support of life; viz., air, meat and drink, motion and rest, sleep, etc.

Res-o-lu'tion. [**Resolu'tio, o'nis;** from *resol'vo*, *resolu'tum*, to "unbind," to "resolve."] The act of resolving or solving; analysis; decomposition. One of the terminations of inflammation, in which it gradually disappears without abscess or mortification.

Re-sol'vent. [**Resol'vens;** from the same.] Applied to substances that discuss inflammatory or other tumors; discu'tient.

Res'o-nance. [From *res'ono*, to "resound."] (Fr. *Retentissement*, rẹh-tŏng'-tĕss'mŏng', or *Résonance*, rā'zo'nŏnss'.) A preternatural resounding of the voice, or its sounding in a part where it is not heard in health. A pathognomonic symptom in certain morbid conditions of the lungs.

Re-sorp'tion. [**Resorp'tio, o'nis;** from *re*, "again," and *sor'beo*, *sorp'tum*, to "drink up," to "swallow."] The absorption of a fluid or substance which has been previously deposited. Sometimes applied to the degeneration of an organ, or part, resulting in atrophy.

Re-spī-ra-bil'i-ty. [**Respirabil'itas, a'tis;** from *respi'ro*, *respira'tum*, to "breathe."] The quality of a gas proper for respiration.

Re-spī'ra-ble. [**Respirab'ilis;** from the same.] Applied to a gas fit for respiration.

Res-pi-rā'tion. [**Respira'tio, o'nis;** from the same.] The function of breathing, including both inspiration and expiration; the function by which the nutrient circulating fluid of an organized body is submitted to the influence of air for the purpose of changing its properties.

Respira'tion, Bron'chi-al. Applied to a kind of respiration in which there is a sound of air passing through the bronchial tubes without entering the minute air-cells.

Respira'tion, Cav'er-nous. That in which there is a sound of air passing from the *bronchia* into large morbid cavities, instead of the air-cells.

Respira'tion, Pu'e-rile. That in which there is a sound like the respiration of infants.

Res'pi-ra-to-ry. [**Respirato'rius;** from *respi'ro*, *respira'tum*, to "breathe."] Pertaining to respiration.

Res'piratory Mur'mur. The murmuring sound heard from the lungs of a healthy adult, produced by the penetration of the air into the pulmonary tissue and its expulsion from it.

Res'piratory Tract. The middle column of the spinal marrow, described by Sir Charles Bell as that from which the respiratory nerves originate.

Restiaceæ,* res-te-a'she-ē. [From *Res'tio*, one of the genera.] A natural order of endogenous glumaceous plants, found in South Africa and Australia.

Res-ti-for'mis.* [From *res'tis*, a "rope," or "cord."] Res'tiform; having the appearance of a cord or rope. See CORPORA RESTIFORMIA.

Re-su'pi-nate. [**Resupina'tus;** from *resupi'no*, *resupina'tum*, to "turn upside down."] Having the lower surface turned upward.

Re-sus-çi-tā'tion. [**Resuscita'tio, o'nis;** from *re*, "again," and *sus'cito*, *suscita'tum*, to "wake," to "excite," to "raise up."] The act of restoring to life those who are apparently dead.

Re-tar-dā'tion. [**Retarda'tio, o'nis;** from *retar'do*, *retarda'tum*, to "hinder," or "retard."] A stopping, or hindering. Applied to delay of childbirth.

Retch'ing. [**Vomituri'tio, o'nis.**] Continued involuntary efforts to vomit, without effect.

Re'te,* or **Re'tis.*** A net or network. Any interlacement of fibres, nerves, or vessels, like network.

Rete Malpighii. See RETE MUCOSUM.

Re'te Mi-rab'i-le.* ("Wondrous Network.") The network of blood-vessels at the base of the brain of quadrupeds.

Re'te Mu-co'sum.* ("Mucous Network.") A mucous substance between the *derma* and *epidermis*, containing the coloring matter of the skin; best exhibited in the negro.

Re'te Tes'tis.* ("Network of the Testis.") The tubular structure, or mingling of the *Tubuli recti*, on the back of the *Tunica albuginea testis*.

Re-ten'tion. [**Reten'tio, o'***nis;* from *retin'eo, reten'tum*, to "hold back," to "retain."] The keeping back, or stoppage, of any of the excretions, particularly the urine.

Retention of the Menses. See EMANSIO MENSIUM, and AMENORRHŒA.

Retentissement, rēh-tōN^o^'tēss'mōN^o^'. A French term for RESONANCE, which see.

Re-tic'u-lar. [**Reticula'ris;** from *re'te*, a "net."] Pertaining to, or resembling, a net.

Re-tic'u-lāt-ed, or **Re-tic'u-late.** [**Reticula'tus;** from the same.] Formed like a net; netted; as reticulated or netted-veined leaves, which are almost universal in exogenous plants. They present two general forms of venation, the feather-veined and the radiate-veined.

Re-tic'u-lum.* [Diminutive of *re'te*, a "net."] A little net. Applied to the second stomach of the *Ruminantia*.

Re-tif'er-ous. [**Retif'erus;** from *re'te*, a "net," and *fe'ro*, to "bear."] Marked with, or having, lines like a net.

Ret'ĭ-form. [**Retifor'mis;** from *re'te*, a "net."] Formed like a net.

Ret'ĭ-na.* [From *re'te*, a "net."] The organ of visual perception, the most internal membrane of the eye, being an expansion of the optic nerve. It consists of three layers; the external, or Jacob's membrane, the middle, or nervous, and the internal, or vascular membrane.

Ret-ĭ-nac'u-lum,* plural **Ret-ĭ-nac'u-la.** [From *retin'eo*, to "hold back."] A stay, or tie. Applied in Anatomy to the *frænum*, or fold of membrane, continued from each commissure of the ilio-cæcal and ilio-colic valves round on the inner side of the cæcum. In Botany, a viscous globular corpuscle, to which is attached the small pedicle which sustains the masses of pollen in the *Orchids*. In Surgery, it is applied to an instrument for keeping the bowels or other parts in their place in certain operations.

Ret'ĭ-nerved. [**Retiner'vis;** from *re'te*, a "net," and *ner'vus*, a "nerve."] The same as RETICULATED, which see.

Ret-ĭ-ni'tis, i*dis.** Inflammation of the retina.

Ret'ĭ-ped. [**Ret'ipes, p'e***dis;* from *re'te*, a "net," and *pes*, a "foot."] Having the skin of the legs divided into small polygonous scales. Applied to certain birds.

Re-tort'. [**Retor'ta;** from *retor'queo, retor'tum*, to "twist or turn back;" named from the bend in the neck.] A vessel made of glass, earthenware, or iron, for the purpose of distillation.

Retort, Tu'bu-lāt-ed. A retort having a small hole in the roof.

Re-trac'tĭle. [**Retrac'tilis;** from *re*, "again," or "back," and *tra'ho, trac'tum*, to "draw."] Capable of being drawn back. Applied to nails or claws when the phalanx which bears them is articulated in such a manner that, in repose, they are withdrawn to the superior part of the toe.

Re-trac-til'ĭ-tў. [**Retractil'itas, a'***tis;* from the same.] The quality of a part that is retractile.

Retrac'tion. [**Retrac'tio, o'***nis;* from the same.] The shortening of a broken limb, the contraction of the muscles forcing the broken ends of the bone to glide by each other, as in oblique fractures.

Re-trac'tor.* [From the same.] A piece of linen employed in amputation for drawing the divided muscles upward, and thus keeping every part of the wound out of the way of the saw.

Ret'ra-hens.* [From the same.] Drawing back; retracting.

Ret'rahens Au'ris.* ("Retracting [Muscle] of the Ear.") A name given to the *posterior auris* muscle, from its action in drawing back the ear.

Rétrécissement, rà'trà'sĕss'mōN^o^'. The French term for STRICTURE, which see.

Ret-ro-ce'dent. [**Retroce'dens;** from *re'tro*, "backwards," and *ce'do*, to "go," or "move."] Going back, or going from the outer part of the body to an interior organ, as gout, rheumatism, etc.

Ret'ro-curved. The same as RECURVED.

Ret'ro-flexed. [**Retroflex'us;** from *re'tro*, "backwards," and *flec'to, flex'um*, to "bend."] The same as REFLEXED.

Retroflex'io (ret-ro-flek'she-o) **U'teri.*** A bending back of the womb. Sometimes used in the same manner as RETROVERSIO UTERI.

Ret-ro-flex'ion. [**Retroflex'io, o'***nis;* from the same.] A bending backwards.

Ret'ro-grade. [**Retrog'radus;** from *re'tro,* "backwards," and *gra'dior,* to "go."] Going back or backwards; retrocedent.

Retrover'sio (ret-ro-ver'she-o) **U'teri.*** A displacement of the uterus in which the fundus is thrown downwards below the promontory of the sacrum, while the *os* and *cervix* are forced upwards and forwards against or over the *symphysis pubis.*

Ret-ro-ver'sion. [**Retrover'sio, o'***nis;* from *re'tro,* "backwards," and *ver'to, ver'sum,* to "turn."] A turning backwards. Applied to the bladder, uterus, etc.

Ret-ro-vert'ed. [From *re'tro,* "backwards," and *ver'to,* to "turn."] In Botany, turned back or over; turned upside down.

Re-tuse'. [**Retu'sus;** from *retun'do, retu'sum,* to "make blunt."] Slightly notched at a rounded apex. Applied to leaves.

Re-ver-be-rā'tion. [**Reverbera'tio, o'***nis;* from *re,* "again," or "back," and *ver'bero, verbera'tum,* to "strike," or "beat."] Reflection of light, heat, or sound.

Re-ver-ber-a-to'rĭ-um.* [From the same.] The metallic concave plate appended to lamps for the purpose of increasing the intensity of their light.

Re-ver'ber-a-to-rȳ Fur'nace. One in which, by its peculiar construction, the flame is thrown back, or reverberated, upon the substance or body exposed to its action.

Rev'e-rȳ, or **Rev'e-rie.** [Fr. *Rêver,* to "muse."] Absence of mind; a loose or extravagant train of thoughts; mental aberration. See APHELXIA.

Re-viv-ĭ-fĭ-cā'tion. [From *re,* "again," *vi'vus,* "alive," and *fa'cio,* to "make."] Making alive; recovery of life: a phenomenon occurring in some animalcules, as the *Rotifer redivivus.*

Rev'o-lute. [**Revolu'tus;** from *revol'vo, revolu'tum,* to "roll back."] Rolled back. Applied to the margins of leaves.

Rev-o-lu'tion. [**Revolu'tio, o'***nis;* from the same.] The act of revolving. In Astronomy, the movement which a heavenly body performs, between its departure from a given point in its orbit, and its return to the same point; also, the interval of time spent in such act of revolving. Also applied to the rotation of a heavenly body on its axis.

Re-vul'sant. [**Revul'sans;** from *re,* "back," and *vel'lo, vul'sum,* to "pull," or "draw;" to "draw off."] Drawing off; deriving. See DERIVATIVE.

Re-vul'sion. [**Revul'sio, o'***nis;* from the same.] Literally, a "drawing back," or "drawing off." A pulling or drawing off, as of the hair, teeth, etc. Usually applied to the action of medicines which, by producing irritation in one part, draw off diseased action from another.

Rex Met-al-lo'rum.* ("King of Metals.") An alchemical name for gold.

Rha-bar'ba-rum.* [From *Rha,* the Volga, a river in Russia, and *bar'barus,* "wild."] Tournefort's name for RHEUM, which see.

Rha-chĭ-æ'us.* [From ῥάχις, the "spine."] Belonging to the spine.

Rha-chi'a-gra.* [From ῥάχις, the "spine," and ἄγρα, a "seizure."] Gout or severe pain in the spinal region. Also spelled *Rachisagra.*

Rha-chĭ-ăl'ġĭ-a.* [From ῥάχις, the "spine," and ἄλγος, "pain."] Pain occurring in the spine, or vertebral column.

Rha-chĭ-ăl-ġĭ'tis, i*dis.** Inflammatory *rhachialgia.*

Rha-chĭ-as'mus.* [From ῥάχις, the "spine."] Applied by M. Hall to the first symptoms of epilepsy, consisting in a spasmodic action of muscles at the back of the neck.

Rha-chĭ-o-camp'sis.* [From ῥάχις, the "spine," and κάμψις, a "bending."] Curvature of the spine.

Rha-chĭ-och'ȳ-sis.* [From ῥάχις, the "spine," and χύσις, a "pouring."] Accumulation of water in the vertebral column.

Rha'chĭ-o-çy-pho'sis.* [From ῥάχις, the "spine," and κυφωσις, a "bowing."] A *gibbus,* or hump on the back.

Rha-chĭ-o-dȳn'ĭ-a.* [From ῥάχις, the "spine," and ὀδύνη, "pain."] Pain in the back, spasmodic or hæmorrhoidal, but not purely nervous.

Rha-chĭ-o-my-e-lĭ'tis, i*dis.** [From ῥάχις, the "spine," and *myeli'tis,* "inflammation of the marrow."] Inflammation of the spinal marrow.

Rha-chĭ-o-my-e-loph'thĭ-sis.* [From ῥάχις, the "spine," μυελός, "marrow," and φθίσις, "wasting."] The same as TABES DORSALIS, which see.

Rha-chĭ-o-pa-răl'ȳ-sis.* [From ῥάχις, the "spine," and *paral'ysis.*] Paralysis of the spinal marrow.

Rha-chi-ar-rheū'ma, a'tis.* [From ῥάχις, the "spine," and ῥεῦμα, a "flux," or "humor."] Applied to rheumatism of the back.

Rha'chi-o-sco-li-o'ma, atis.* [From ῥάχις, the "spine," and σκολίωμα, a "curve."] Lateral curvature of the spine.

Rha-chi-o-sco-li-o'sis.* The progress or formation of *rhachioscolioma*.

Rha-chi-ot'o-mum,* or **Rha-chi-ot'o-mus.*** [From ῥάχις, the "spine," and τέμνω, to "cut."] An instrument for opening the spinal canal: a rachiotome.

Rha-chi-ot'o-mȳ. [**Rhachiotoʹ-mia;** from the same.] Dissection of the spine.

Rha'chis,* or **Ra'chis.*** [Gr. ῥάχις.] The spine, or vertebral column. Applied in Botany to the axis of inflorescence when covered with sessile flowers, as a spike. Also, the rib, or leaf-stalk, of ferns.

Rhachisagra. See RHACHIAGRA.

Rhachitis. See RACHITIS.

Rha-co'dēs.* [From ῥάκος, a "ragged garment;" in the plural ῥάκεα, "wrinkles."] Wrinkled, or full of wrinkles.

Rha-co'ma, a'tis.* [From ῥακόω, to "tear into strips."] A rent or chapped portion of the skin. Also, a lax or pendulous condition of the scrotum.

Rha-co'sis.* The progress of *rhacoma*.

Rhag'a-dēs.* [Plural of ῥαγάς, a "rent," or "chink."] Clefts, chaps, or excoriations of the skin, especially of the anus.

Rhamnaceæ,* ram-na'she-ē, or **Rham'ni.*** A natural order of exogenous trees and shrubs, found in all parts of the world except the arctic regions. It includes the *Rham'nus fran'gula*, which yields the best charcoal for gunpowder, and *Zizyphus*, from which jujube is procured.

Rham'ni,* the plural of *Rham'nus*, forming the Jussieuan name of an order of plants. See RHAMNACEÆ.

Rham'nus.* A Linnæan genus of the class *Pentandria*, natural order *Rhamnaceæ*. Also, the Pharmacopœial name (Lond. and Dub. Ph.) of the *Rhamnus catharticus*.

Rham'nus Ca-thar'ti-cus.* The purging buckthorn.

Rhat'a-nȳ. [**Rhata'nia.**] The root of the KRAMERIA TRIANDRA, which see.

Rheg'ma, atis,* or **Rhex'is.*** [From ῥήγνυμι, to "break," or "burst."] A rent, rupture, or fracture of a part, applied to the eyeball, bones, etc.; also, the opening or bursting of an abscess.

Rheg-ma-to'dēs.* [From ῥῆγμα, a "fracture," or "rent."] Having a rent, tear, or rupture.

Rheg-ma-to-i'dēs.* [From ῥῆγμα, a "fracture," or "rent," and εἶδος, a "form."] Resembling a *rhegma*, or rent.

Rhe'ic Aç'id. [From *rhe'um*, "rhubarb."] The yellow, crystalline, granular matter of rhubarb, procured from the plant by means of ether.

Rhe'in, or **Rhe'ine.** [**Rhei'na.**] A substance obtained by treating rhubarb with ether.

Rhe-om'e-ter. [From ῥέω, to "flow," and μέτρον, a "measure."] A term employed by French writers as synonymous with galvanometer; an instrument for measuring the force of an electric current.

Rhe'um,* gen. **Rhe'i.** [Supposed to be from *Rha*, the river Volga, from the banks of which it was originally brought.] (Fr. *Rhubarbe*, rü'baRb'.) A Linnæan genus of the class *Enneandria*, natural order *Polygonaceæ*. Also, the Pharmacopœial name (U.S. Ph.) for the root of the *Rheum palmatum* and of other species of *Rheum;* but according to the British Pharmacopœia, for the root of one or more undetermined species of *Rheum*.

Rhubarb is an astringent as well as cathartic, and combines to a certain degree the virtues of a tonic with those of a purgative. It is, therefore, well adapted to cases of debility of the digestive organs in which a moderate or gentle cathartic is needed. The principal objection to it, is that it sometimes causes griping; but this may be obviated, or mitigated, by combining it with some aromatic. Rhubarb is often advantageously associated with other cathartics.

Rhe'um Pal-ma'tum.* The systematic name (U.S. Ph.) of the plant which yields rhubarb.

Rhe'um Rha-bar'ba-rum.* Linnæus's name for the *Rheum undulatum*.

Rhe'um Un-du-la'tum.* The Russian, or Siberian, rhubarb.

Rheum, rūm. [Lat. **Rheu'ma, atis;** Gr. ῥεῦμα, a "flux," or "humor," from ῥέω, to "flow."] The discharge from the nostrils or lungs, caused by cold.

Rheū-mar-thro'sis.* [From ῥεῦμα, "flux," or "humor" arising from cold, and ἄρθρον, a "joint."] Literally, "humor in the joints;" because it was formerly supposed to be caused by a morbid humor. Rheumatism of the joints.

Rheū-ma-tăl'ğĭ-a.* [From ῥεῦμα, a "flux," or "humor," and ἄλγος, "pain."] Chronic pain arising from rheumatism. See RHEUMARTHROSIS.

Rheumatic, rū-mat'ik. [**Rheumat'icus.**] Belonging to rheumatism; afflicted with rheumatism.

Rheū'ma-tĭsm. [**Rheumatis'mus;** from ῥεῦμα, a "humor" arising from cold.] (Fr. *Rhumatisme,* rü'mâ'tèzm'.) A disease (once supposed to be caused by a morbid humor) characterized by severe pains in the joints (especially when these are acted on by the muscles) and more or less heat in the part, sometimes attended with *pyrexia.* A genus of the order *Phlegmasiæ,* class *Pyrexiæ,* of Cullen's Nosology. The following varieties may be noticed:

1. ARTICULAR RHEUMATISM, occurring in the joints and muscles of the extremities. 2. LUMBAGO, occurring in the loins, and mostly shooting upwards. 3. SCIATICA, occurring in the hip-joint, with emaciation of the nates. 4. SPURIOUS PLEURISY, occurring in the muscles of the diaphragm.

Rheū-ma-tĭs'moid. [**Rheumatismoi'des;** from *rheumatis'mus,* and εἶδος, a "form."] Resembling rheumatism.

Rheū-ma-to-dy̆n'ĭ-a.* [From ῥεῦμα, "flux," or "humor," and ὀδύνη, "pain."] Synonymous with RHEUMATALGIA.

Rheū-ma-top'y̆-ra.* [From *rheumat'icus,* "rheumatic," and πῦρ, a "fever."] Rheumatic fever.

Rheū-ma-to-spaș'mus.* [From *rheumat'icus,* "rheumatic," and *spas'mus,* a "spasm."] Rheumatic spasm or cramp: rheumatospasm.

Rhi-năl'ğĭ-a.* [From ῥίν, the "nose," and ἄλγος, "pain."] Pain in the nose.

Rhi-nen-çe-phal'ĭ-cus.* [From ῥίν, the "nose," and ἐγκέφαλον, the "brain."] Connected with the nose and brain, etc.

Rhi-nen-çeph'a-lus.* [From ῥίν, the "nose," ἐν, "in," and κεφαλή, the "head."] A monster-fœtus, having the nose prolonged in form of a proboscis.

Rhi-ni'tis, *idis.** [From ῥίν, the "nose."] Inflammation of the nose.

Rhi-no-dy̆n'ĭ-a.* [From ῥίν, the "nose," and ὀδύνη, "pain."] Pain in the nose.

Rhi-no-pho'nĭ-a.* [From ῥίν, the "nose," and φωνή, the "voice."] The sound of the voice heard through the nose.

Rhī-no-plas'tic. [**Rhinoplas'ticus.**] Relating to the operation of rhinoplasty.

Rhī'no-plas-ty̆. [**Rhinoplas'tica;** from ῥίν, the "nose," and πλάσσω, to "fabricate."] Nose-making; the operation of forming a nose from the integuments of the forehead, otherwise termed the Taliacotian operation: rhinoplastics.

Rhi-no-pol'y̆-pus.* [From ῥίν, the "nose," and *pol'ypus.*] Polypus of the nose or nostrils.

Rhi-nor-rha'ğĭ-a.* [From ῥίν, the "nose," and ῥήγνυμι, to "burst forth."] Sudden and excessive bleeding from the nose. See EPISTAXIS.

Rhi'no-trix, *ichos.** [From ῥίν, the "nose," and θρίξ, a "hair."] In the plural, the *vibrissæ,* or hairs of the nose.

Rhī-zan'thous. [**Rhizan'thus;** from ῥίζα, a "root," and ἄνθος, a "flower."] Root-flowered. Applied to parasitic flowers attached by a sort of root or roots to some foster-plant. The *Raffle'sia* and *Epiphe'gus* (Beech-drops) are examples.

Rhi'zanths. The same as RHIZOGENS, which see.

Rhizobolaceæ,* ri-zo-bo-la'she-ē. A natural order of exogenous plants, consisting of a few species of very large trees, found in the hottest parts of South America. It includes the *Car'yocar Rhizob'olus.*

Rhi-zo'dēș.* [From ῥίζα, a "root."] Having roots.

Rhī'zo-ğens. [From ῥίζα, a "root," and γεννάω, to "produce."] A class of parasitical plants which have a fungus-like consistence, and are destitute of true leaves. They seem to be intermediate between endogens and thallogens.

Rhi-zoğ'e-num.* [From the same.] A peculiar organ of some *Algæ,* which increases and fixes itself by numerous roots: a rhizogen.

Rhī-zog'ra-phy̆. [**Rhizogra'phia;** from ῥίζα, a "root," and γράφω, to "write."] A description of roots.

Rhi-zo-i'dēș.* [From ῥίζα, a "root," and εἶδος, a "form."] Resembling a root: rhi'zoid.

Rhī-zol'o-ğy̆. [**Rhizolo'gia;** from ῥίζα, a "root," and λόγος, a "discourse."] A treatise on roots; that branch of Botany which treats of the roots of plants.

Rhi-zo'ma, *atis.** [From ῥιζόω, to "support by roots."] A root-stock; a perennial, horizontal, more or less subterranean and root-like stem, as that of the iris, *Acorus calamus,* etc.: a rhizome.

Rhī-zo-mor'phous. [**Rhizomor'phus;** from ῥίζα, a "root," and μορφή, "form."] Having the form of a root; root-like.

Rhizophoraceæ,* ri-zo-fo-ra'she-ē. [From *Rhizoph'ora,* one of the genera.] Mangroves. A natural order of exogenous trees and shrubs, found on the shores of tropical regions, where they root in the mud and form a dense thicket down to the verge of the sea. Some species send down roots from the branches like the Banyan.

Rhī-zoph'o-rous. [**Rhizoph'o-rus;** from ῥίζα, a "root," and φέρω, to "bear."] Bearing or having roots.

Rhi-zo-phȳl'lous. [**Rhizophyl'-lus;** from ῥίζα, a "root," and φύλλον, a "leaf."] Having leaves bearing roots.

Rhi'zu-la.* [Diminutive of ῥίζα, a "root."] The very fine roots of mushrooms: a rhizule.

Rho'dĭ-um.* [From ῥόδον, a "rose."] A metal found among the grains of crude platina; named from the rose-color of its compounds. It is of a whitish color, and very hard. Its specific gravity is about 11.

Rho-do-den'dra,* the plural of *Rhododen'dron,* forming the Jussieuan name of an order of plants, now included in ERICACEÆ, which see.

Rho-do-den'dron.* [From ῥόδον, a "rose," and δένδρον, a "tree."] A Linnæan genus of the class *Decandria,* natural order *Ericaceæ.*

Rhododen'dron Chrȳs-an'thum.* The dwarf rosebay, or yellow-flowered rhododendron: a narcotic plant, sometimes prescribed for gout, rheumatism, etc.

Rho-dog'ra-phȳ. [**Rhodogra'-phia;** from ῥόδον, a "rose," and γράφω, to "write."] A description of roses.

Rho-dol'o-ġȳ. [**Rhodolo'gia;** from ῥόδον, a "rose," and λόγος, a "discourse."] A treatise on roses; the science of roses.

Rho-do-sper'mus.* [From ῥόδον, a "rose," and σπέρμα, "seed."] Having seeds or *sporidia* of a rose color.

Rhœ'a-din. The coloring matter of the *Papaver rhœas.*

Rhœ'as, ados.* The Pharmacopœial name (Br. Ph.) for the dried petals of the *Papaver Rhœas;* the *Rhœados petala* ("petals of Rhœas") of the Edinburgh Pharmacopœia.

Rhomb, or **Rhom'bus.*** [Gr. ῥόμβος.] An oblique-angled equilateral parallelogram which has two obtuse and two acute angles.

Rhom-bĭ-fo'lĭ-us.* [From ῥόμβος, a "rhomb," and *fo'lium,* a "leaf."] Having rhombic leaves: rhombifo'liate.

Rhom'bĭ-form. [**Rhombifor'mis;** from ῥόμβος, a "rhomb."] Having the form of a rhomb.

Rhom-bip'o-rus.* [From ῥόμβος, a "rhomb," and *po'rus,* a "pore."] Having rhombiform pores.

Rhom-bo-he'dral, or **Rhom-bo-he'dri-cal.** [**Rhombohe'drus.**] Belonging to a rhombohedron.

Rhom-bo-he'dron. [**Rhombo-he'drum;** from ῥόμβος, a "rhomb," and ἕδρα, a "base."] A solid figure bounded by six equal rhomboid faces.

Rhom'boid. [**Rhomboi'des;** from ῥόμβος, a "rhomb," and εἶδος, a "form."] Resembling a rhomb. A quadrilateral figure whose opposite sides and angles are equal, but which is neither equilateral nor equiangular.

Rhom-boid'al. [**Rhomboida'lis;** from *rhomboi'des,* "resembling a rhomb."] Approaching a rhomboid in form.

Rhom-bo-i'de-us,* or rom-bo-i-de'-us. [From the same.] The name of two muscles (or of one muscle in two parts), the *major* and the *minor,* situated at the posterior inferior part of the neck and upper part of the back. They draw the scapula backwards and upwards.

Rhom'bus.* The same as RHOMB, which see.

Rhon'chus.* [Gr. ῥόγχος.] A rattling sound in the throat, or a very strong wheezing. See RÂLE.

Rhu'barb. [**Rhabar'barum,** and **Rhe'um;** supposed to be from *Rha,* the Volga, a river in Russia, and *bar'barus,* "wild;" so named because chiefly brought from Russia.] See RHEUM.

Rhu'barb, Of-fiç'ĭ-nal. The *Rheum palmatum.*

Rhu'barb, Rus'sian, Rhu'barb, Si-be'rĭ-an, Rhu'barb, Un'du-lāt-ed. The *Rheum Russicum* or *undulatum,* the *R. rhabarbarum* of Linnæus.

Rhumatisme, rü'mâ'tēzm'. The French term for RHEUMATISM, which see.

Rhus,* gen. **Rho'is.** A Linnæan genus of the class *Pentandria,* natural order *Terebinthinaceæ* or *Anacardiaceæ.* The sumach-tree. Also, a flow or discharge, as that of the *catamenia.*

Rhus Gla'brum.* Sumach. The Pharmacopœial name (U.S. Ph.) for the fruit of the *Rhus glabrum,* the properties of which are astringent and refrigerant.

Rhus Rad'ĭ-cans.* Poison Vine, or Poison Ivy. A plant which, when applied to the skin, often produces a vesicular eruption, and sometimes erysipelatous inflammation. See RHUS TOXICODENDRON.

Rhus Tox-ĭ-co-den'dron.* The systematic name of the poison sumach, otherwise called poison oak. This plant contains an acrid poisonous principle. In small doses, however, the leaves have been given as a remedy in certain cutaneous affections. Many botanists regard the *Rhus toxicodendron* and the *R. radicans* as merely varieties of one species. See RHUS RADICANS.

Rhy'as, adis.* [From ῥέω, to "flow."] A disease of the eye consisting in a decrease or defect of the *Caruncula lacrymalis*, congenital, accidental, or the result of excision, causing an incurable *epiphora*, or continual flow of tears.

Rhyncholite, rĭnk'o-līt. [**Rhyncholi'tes;** from ῥύγχος, a "beak," and λίθος, a "stone."] The petrified beak of a bird.

Rhȳn-chos'po-rus.* [From ῥύγχος, a "beak," and σπόρα, "seed."] Having seeds prolonged in the form of a beak, as the *Rondeletia*.

Rhythm, rĭTHM. [**Rhyth'mus;** from ῥυθμός, a "measured movement."] Applied to the order or proportion of time which exists between the pulsations of the heart or the movements of any organ; also to the order which prevails in the vibrations of sonorous bodies.

Rhytidosis. See RUTIDOSIS.

Rib. [**Cos'ta.**] One of the bones which enclose the chest. Also, a strong nerve or woody fibre which forms part of the framework of a leaf. See COSTA.

Riband-Shaped. See LIGULATE.

Ribbed. A term applied to leaves in which ribs or strong nerves run lengthwise.

Ri'bēs.* A Linnæan genus of the class *Pentandria*, natural order *Grossulaceæ*. The currant-bush. Sometimes also applied to the gooseberry-tribe.

Ri'bes Ni'grum.* The black-currant bush.

Ri'bes Ru'brum.* The red-currant bush, of which the white currant is only a variety.

Ribesius,* ri-be'she-ŭs. Resembling the genus *Ribes*.

Ribless. See ENERVIS.

Ricciaceæ,* rik-se-a'she-ē. [From *Ric'cia*, one of the genera.] A natural order of flowerless plants, allied to mosses and lichens.

Rice. The common name for the *Ory'za sati'va*.

Rice Pa'per. A substance which is said to be a membrane of the *Artocar'pus inci'sa*, or breadfruit-tree. It is brought from China in small pieces of various colors, and is used as a material to paint upon.

Rich-ard-so'nĭ-a̤ Sca'bra̤.* The systematic name of the white or undulated ipecacuanha.

Riç'ĭ-nāte. [**Riç'inas, a'tis.**] A combination of ricinic acid with a base.

Rĭ-cin'ic. [**Ricin'icus;** from *riç'inus.*] Applied to one of the three acids produced by the saponification of castor oil.

Riç-ĭ-no-i'dēs.* [From *riç'inus*, and εἶδος, a "form."] Resembling the *Ricinus.*

Riç'ĭ-nus.* [From *riç'inus*, a kind of tick, which its seed resembles.] A Linnæan genus of the class *Monœcia*, natural order *Euphorbiaceæ*.

Riç'inus Com-mu'nis.* ("Common Ricinus.") The castor-oil plant.

Riç'inus Vul-ga'ris.* Another name for the *Ricinus communis*.

Rick'ets, or **Ra̤-chi'tis.*** A disease of children, characterized by a large head, crooked spine and limbs, tumid abdomen, and general debility; often accompanied with precocious mental faculties. The disease appears to consist essentially in the non-deposition of phosphate of lime in the osteoid tissues. [Respecting the etymology of *Rickets*, much diversity of opinion has prevailed. Some have erroneously supposed it to be a corruption of *rachitis*. Dr. Good has, in all probability, suggested the true derivation of the word, referring it to the Anglo-Saxon *ricg* or *hric* (German *Rücken*), the "back,"—the name *rickets*, as well as *rachitis*, implying that the back, or spine, is one of the principal seats of the disease.]

Ric'tus.* [From *rin'gor, ric'tus*, to "grin."] The opening between the lips of ringent, or personate, flowers.

Riġ-ĭ-dĭ-fo'lĭ-us.* [From *riġ'idus*, "stiff," "rigid," and *fo'lium*, a "leaf."] Having rigid leaves: rigidifo'lious.

Rĭ-ġid'ĭ-tȳ. [**Rigid'itas, a'tis;** from *riġ'idus*, "stiff," "rigid."] Stiffness; inflexibility; rigidness. In Mechanics, a resistance to a change of form.

Rig'or, o'ris.* [From ῥιγέω, to "become cold."] A sudden coldness, with shivering. See ALGOR.

Ri'ma̤.* A chink, fissure, cleft, or crack.

Ri'ma Glot'tĭ-dis.* ("Cleft or Fissure of the Glottis.") The opening of the glottis, or rather of the larynx.

Ri-mose′, or **Rī′mous.** [**Rimo′sus**; from *ri′ma*, a "crack," or "chink."] Full of fissures, or cracks.

Rim′u-la.* [Diminutive of *ri′ma*, a "crack," or "chink."] A small fissure, cleft, or crack.

Ring. See ANNULUS.

Ring, Abdominal. See ABDOMINAL RING.

Ring, Fem′o-ral. [**An′nulus Femora′lis.**] An opening bounded in front by Poupart's ligament, behind by the pubes, on the outer side by the femoral vein, on the inner by Gimbernat's ligament.

Rin′gent. [**Rin′gens**; from *rin′gor*, to "grin."] Gaping; grinning. Applied to flowers.

Rin-gen-tĭ-flo′rus.* [From *rin′gens*, "grinning," or "gaping," and *flos*, a "flower."] Applied to the *calathidium* and the disk in the *Synantheræ*, when composed of ringent corollas.

Ring-like. See CRICOID.

Ring′worm. The common name of *Herpes circinatus.*

Ring′worm of the Scalp. The disease termed *Porrigo scutulata.*

Rī-pā′rĭ-ous. [**Ripa′rius**; from *ri′pa*, a "bank of a river."] Growing along rivers or water-courses. Applied to plants.

Rip′ples. A popular term in Scotland for TABES DORSALIS, which see.

Ri-so′rĭ-us.* [From *ri′deo*, *ri′sum*, to "laugh."] The "laughing" muscle of Santorini; a thin muscular plane which arises before the parotid gland, and proceeds towards the angle of the mouth, which it draws backwards and upwards, and thus contributes to give a smiling expression to the countenance.

Risus Caninus. See SARDONIC LAUGH.

Ri′sus Sar-don′ĭ-cus.* The Latin term for SARDONIC LAUGH, which see.

Ri-vin′ĭ-an Ducts. The excretory ducts of the sublingual glands, first pointed out by Rivinus.

Roast′ing. The protracted application of heat, below the fusing-point, to metallic ores, in order to expel from them the volatile ingredients, such as sulphur, carbonic acid, etc.

Rob. [From the Arabic.] A syrup made from the juice of fruits with sugar, and reduced to a greater consistency by boiling.

Ro-bin′ĭ-a Pseū′do-Aca′cia* or **Pseudacacia*** (sū-da-ka′she-a). The systematic name of the locust-tree, a native of the United States. The bark of the root is said to be emetic and cathartic.

Rob′o-rant. [**Rob′orans**; from *rob′oro*, to "make strong."] Giving strength; strengthening.

Roc-çel′la Tinc-to′rĭ-a,* or **Dy′ers' Lich′en.** The plant which yields litmus. See LICHEN ROCCELLA.

Roc-çel′lāte. [**Roccel′las, a′tis.**] A combination of roccellic acid with a base.

Roc-çel′lic. [**Roccel′licus.**] Applied to a peculiar acid discovered in the *Roccella tinctoria.*

Rocella. See ROCCELLA TINCTORIA.

Ro-chelle′ Salt. The tartrate of potash and soda.

Rock-But′ter. A common name for the substance anciently termed *Alu′men liq′uidum*, or "liquid alum."

Rock-Oil. See PETROLEUM.

Rock′-Salt. A name given to native massive salt, found in mines in various parts of the world.

Ro′dens.* [From *ro′do*, to "gnaw."] Gnawing. Applied in the plural neuter (*Roden′tia*) to an order of *Mammalia* characterized by two large incisor teeth in each jaw. It comprises the beaver, rat, squirrel, etc.

Ro′dent. [From the same.] A term applied to certain animals. See RODENS.

Rodentia,* ro-den′she-a, the neuter plural of RODENS, which see.

Rod-Shaped. See VIRGATE.

Rogne, roñ. A French name for "itch." See PSORA.

Rognetta's (rōn-yĕt′taz) **Operation.** See PHACOCYSTECTOME.

Rōll′er. A long band of linen, calico, or flannel, wound up from one or both ends.

Ronflement, rōnf′l′mōnᵍ′. The French name for "snoring." See STERTOR.

Root. See RADIX.

Root′let. A very small root or ultimate branch of a root.

Root′stock. The same as RHIZOMA, which see.

Ro-rif′er-ous. [**Ror′ifer**, or **Rorif′erus**; from *ros*, *ro′ris*, "dew," and *fe′ro*, to "bear."] Producing or bearing dew. Applied in Anatomy to vessels which pour exhaled fluids on the surface of organs.

Ro′sa.* [Gr. ῥόδον.] The Rose. A Linnæan genus of the class *Icosandria*, natural order *Rosaceæ.*

Ro′sa Ca-ni′na.* ("Dog Rose.")

Hips. The Pharmacopœial name (Br. Ph.) for the ripe fruit of the dog rose, or hip-tree; the wild-brier.

Ro'sa Cen-tĭ-fo'lĭ-a.* ("Hundred-leaved Rose.") Pale Rose, or Cabbage Rose. The Pharmacopœial name ‖ for the petals of the *Rosa centifolia*.

Ro'sa Dam-as-ce'na.* ("Damask Rose.") The *Rosa centifolia*.

Ro'sa Gal'lĭ-ca.* ("French Rose.") Red Rose. The Pharmacopœial name ‖ for the petals of the *Rosa Gallica*.

Ro'sa Pal'lĭ-da.* ("Pale Rose.") Another name for the *Rosa centifolia*.

Ro'sa Ru'bra.* ("Red Rose.") The *Rosa Gallica*.

Ro'sa Sўl-ves'tris.* ("Wood Rose.") Another name for the *Rosa canina*.

Rosaceæ,* ro-sa'she-ē. A natural order of exogenous plants (herbs or shrubs), natives chiefly of the temperate or cold climates of the northern hemisphere. This order, which is unsurpassed for beauty and perfume, comprises, among other genera, the Rose (*Ro'sa*), Raspberry (*Ru'bus*), Strawberry (*Fraga'ria*), and *Spiræ'a*.

Ro-sā'ceous. [Rosa'ceus.] Resembling a rose. Applied specially to a form of polypetalous corolla, with five short-clawed spreading petals.

Ro-saç'ic Aç'id. A name applied by Prout to a substance of a rose-color, deposited by the urine on the access of intermittent fever.

Ro-sa'lĭ-a.* [From *ro'sa*, a "rose:" named on account of its color.] An ancient name for SCARLATINA, which see.

Ros'çid. [Ros'cidus; from *ros*, "dew."] Dewy; moistened with dew.

Rose. A plant. (See ROSA.) Also, a name for erysipelas.

Rose Cam'phor. A solid oil of roses, one of the two volatile oils composing attar of roses; the other is a liquid oil. The former is a stearopten.

Rose, Christ'mas. The *Helleborus niger*.

Rose Rash. See ROSEOLA.

Ro-sel'la.* [Diminutive of *ro'sa*, a "rose."] A rosette. Applied to a mass of small leaves, of various form and color, terminating the stem of certain mosses.

Rose'ma-rў. The common name of the *Rosmarinus officinalis*.

Ro-se'o-la.* [Diminutive of *ro'sa*, a "rose."] A rose-colored rash, not contagious, and without *papulæ*, mostly symptomatic of different febrile diseases.

Rosette. See ROSELLA.

Rosin. See RESIN.

Ros-ma-ri'nus.* [From *ros*, "dew," and *mari'nus*, "belonging to the sea."] Rosemary. A Linnæan genus of the class *Diandria*, natural order *Labiatæ* or *Lamiaceæ*. Also, the Pharmacopœial name (U.S. Ph.) for the tops of the *Rosmarinus officinalis*.

Rosmari'nus Of-fiç-ĭ-na'lis.* The plant termed rosemary.

Ros'tel-late. [Rostella'tus; from *rostel'lum*, a "little beak."] Prolonged into a small rigid and sometimes crooked point.

Ros-tel'lum.* [Diminutive of *ros'trum*, a "beak."] A little beak. Applied to any similar object.

Ros'tral. [Rostra'lis.] Resembling a beak.

Ros'trate. [Rostra'tus; from *ros'trum*, a "beak."] Having a beak; beaked. Applied to plants.

Ros-trĭ-cor'nis.* [From *ros'trum*, a "beak," and *cor'nu*, a "horn."] Applied to insects having the antennæ upon a prolongation of the head.

Ros'trĭ-form. [Rostrifor'mis; from *ros'trum*, a "beak."] Formed like a beak.

Ros'trum.* A Latin word signifying the beak of a bird, or the snout of a beast. Applied to a ridge, also called the azygous process, observed on the median line of the lower aspect of the sphenoid bone. Also, the name given to certain kinds of forceps formerly used, from their resemblance to the beaks of different birds.

Ros'u-lar, or **Ros'u-late. [Rosula'rius;** from *ro'sa*, a "rose."] Shaped like a rosette; arranged as the petals of a double rose.

Rosy-Drop. See ACNE ROSACEA.

Ro-ta-çis'mus.* [Gr. ῥωτακισμός.] The harsh vibration of the letter *r*, called a "burr," common in the northern parts of England.

Ro'tate. [Rota'tus; from *ro'ta*, a "wheel."] Wheel-shaped. Applied to a form of monopetalous flowers, *e.g.* the blossom of the potato.

Ro-tā'tion. [Rota'tio, o'*nis*; from *ro'to*, *rota'tum*, to "turn round."] The act of rotating or turning round. In Astronomy, the motion of a heavenly body on its axis.

Ro-ta'tor, o'*ris*.* [From the same.] Applied to certain muscles employed in producing a circular movement.

Ro-tif'e-ra,* or **Rot'ĭ-fers.** [See

ROTIFERUS.] The second class of the *Diploneura*, or *Helminthoida*, consisting of minute soft aquatic animals, with distinct muscular and nervous systems, and having the appearance of revolving wheels produced by the rapid movement of the cilia placed round the mouth.

Rotifers. See ROTIFERA.

Ro-tif'er-us.* [From *ro'ta*, a "wheel," and *fe'ro*, to "bear."] Having, or bearing, wheels: rotiferous. See ROTIFERA.

Ro'ti-form. [**Rotifor'mis;** from *ro'ta*, a "wheel."] Having the form of a wheel.

Rott-le'ra.* Kameela. The Pharmacopœial name (U.S. Ph.) for the powder and hairs obtained from the capsules of the *Rottle'ra tincto'ria*. This medicine, the product of a plant growing in India, is said to be almost invariably successful in destroying the tape-worm. It is given in the dose of from two to four drachms, rarely, if ever, requiring to be repeated.

Rot'u-la.* [Diminutive of *ro'ta*, a "wheel."] A little wheel. Another name for the knee-pan. See PATELLA.

Rot'u-lar. [**Rotula'ris.**] Belonging to the *rotula*. Applied by Dr. Barclay as meaning towards the *rotula*, or *patella*.

Rot'u-late. [**Rotula'tus;** from *rot'ula*, a "little wheel."] Having the form of a little wheel.

Ro-tund'. [From *rotun'dus*, "round."] Having a rounded outline, as parts of some plants.

Ro-tun'date. The same as ROTUND, which see.

Ro-tun-di-fo'li-us.* [From *rotun'dus*, "round," and *fo'lium*, a "leaf."] Having round leaves: rotundifo'liate.

Rouge, roozh. A cosmetic, or dye, prepared from *Car'thamus tincto'rius*.

Rougeole, roo'zhol'. The French term for "measles." See RUBEOLA.

Rough. See SCABER.

Roughness. See SCABRITIES.

Round-Leaved. See ROTUNDIFOLIUS.

Round Lig'a-ment. [**Ligamen'tum Te'res.**] The name applied to a short ligament connecting the head of the femur with the cotyloid cavity.

Round Lig'aments. [**Ligamen'ta Rotun'da.**] Applied to two flattish cords attached to the sides of the uterus, a little below, and in front of, the origin of the Fallopian tubes.

Routinist, roo-teen'ist. [From *routine'*.] Applied to a physician who in his practice follows an unvarying routine, without taking into consideration the varieties of the disease or the peculiarities of his patient's constitution.

Roxburghiaceæ,* rox-bur-ge-a'-she-ē. A natural order of twining shrubs, found in the hotter parts of India. It consists of a single genus, the *Roxbur'ghia*. Lindley regards them as belonging to a transition class, partaking of the nature of endogens and exogens.

Roy'al Stitch. The name of an old operation for the cure of bubonocele. It consisted in putting a ligature under the neck of the hernial sac, close to the abdominal ring, and then tying that part of the sac so as to render it impervious by the adhesive inflammation thus excited.

Rubbing Sound. See BRUIT DE FROTTEMENT.

Ru-be'do, d'inis.* [From *ru'ber*, "red."] A diffused redness of the skin, as in blushing.

Ru-be-fā'cient. [**Rubefa'ciens;** from *rubefa'cio*, to "make red."] Applied to any substance which reddens and irritates without blistering the skin.

Ru-be'o-la.* [From *ru'beo*, to "blush."] (Fr. *Rougeole*, roo'zhol'.) The measles, a disease attended with inflammatory fever, dry cough, sneezing, drowsiness, and an eruption of small red points, perceptible by the touch. A genus of the order *Exanthemata*, class *Pyrexiæ*, of Cullen's Nosology.

Ru-be'o-loid. [**Rubeoloi'des;** from *rube'ola*, the "measles."] Resembling *rubeola*.

Ru'bĭ-a.* [From *ru'ber*, "red."] Madder. A Linnæan genus of the class *Tetrandria*, natural order *Rubiaceæ* or *Cinchonaceæ*. Also, the Pharmacopœial name (U.S. Ph.) for the root of the *Rubia tinctorum*.

Ru'bia Tinc-to'rum.* ("Dyers' Madder.") The systematic name of the madder-plant; the root is called *Radix rubra* ("red-root").

Rubiaceæ,* ru-be-a'she-ē. [From *Ru'bia*, one of the genera.] The Jussieuan name of an order of plants the same as CINCHONACEÆ, which see.

Ru-bĭ-ā'ceous. [**Rubia'ceus;** from *Ru'bia*.] Resembling the *Rubia*.

Ru'bĭ-an. A term sometimes applied to the coloring matter of madder. See ALIZARIN.

Ru'bĭ-cund. [**Rubicun'dus;** from

ru'beo, to "be red."] Red, reddish, or rosy.

Ru'bĭ-form. [**Rubifor'mis;** from *Ru'bus,* the "raspberry."] Having the form of a raspberry.

Ru-big'ĭ-nous, or **Ru-big'ĭ-nose.** [**Rubigino'sus;** from *rubi'go, rubig'inis,* "rust."] Having the color of rust; rusty-reddish.

Ru-bi'go,* gen. **Ru-big'ĭ-nis.** A Latin word signifying "mildew" or "rust."

Rubi'go Fer'ri.* ("Rust of Iron.") A preparation made by exposing moistened iron wire to the air until it is converted into rust. It is essentially the same as the SESQUIOXIDE OF IRON, which see.

Ru-brĭ-cau'lis.* [From *ru'ber,* "red," and *cau'lis,* a "stem."] Having a red stem: rubricau'line.

Ru-brĭ-flo'rous. [**Rubriflo'rus;** from *ru'ber,* "red," and *flos,* a "flower."] Having red flowers.

Ru'bu-la.* [Diminutive of *Ru'bus.*] The specific name for the yaws in Good's Nosology. See ANTHRACIA RUBULA.

Ru'bus.* [From *ru'ber,* "red."] A Linnæan genus of the class *Icosandria,* natural order *Rosaceæ.*

Ru'bus.* Blackberry-root. The Pharmacopœial name (U.S. Ph.) for the root of *Rubus Canadensis,* and of *Rubus villosus.*

Ru'bus Cæ'sĭ-us.* The dewberry-plant, or heath bramble, the fruit being similar to the blackberry.

Ru'bus Fru-tĭ-co'sus.* The common bramble, which yields blackberries.

Ru'bus I-dæ'us.* The systematic name of the raspberry-plant.

Ru'bȳ. [From *ru'beo,* to "be red."] A crystallized gem of various shades of red, consisting chiefly of alumina. The Oriental ruby, or red sapphire, is a rare and precious gem.

Ructatio. See RUCTUS.

Ruc-tu-o'sus.* [From *ruc'tus,* a "belch."] Having eructation or belching.

Ruc'tus.* [From ἐρεύγομαι, to "belch."] An eructation, belching, or discharge of wind from the stomach.

Rud'dle. A kind of red chalk.

Ru'de-ral. [From *ru'dus, ru'deris,* "rubbish."] Growing among rubbish. Applied to plants.

Ru'dĭ-ment. [**Rudimen'tum;** from *ru'dis,* "raw," "inexperienced."] The first instruction given to children; a first principle in science; the origin or rude state of any thing.

Ru-dĭ-men'ta-rȳ. [**Rudimenta'rius;** from the same.] Relating to rudiments. In Botany, imperfectly or incompletely developed.

Rue. The common English name for the *Ruta graveolens.*

Ru-fĭ-ner'vis.* [From *ru'fus,* "red," and *ner'vus,* a "nerve."] Having ruddy-colored nervures.

Ru'fous. [**Ru'fus.**] Brownish-red.

Ru'ga,* plural **Ru'gæ.** (Fr. *Ride,* rēd, and *Pli,* plē.) A wrinkle.

Ru-gĭ-fo'lĭ-us.* [From *ru'ga,* a "wrinkle," and *fo'lium,* a "leaf."] Having wrinkled leaves: rugifo'lious.

Rugine. See RASPATORY.

Ru-gose'. [**Rugo'sus;** from *ru'ga,* a "wrinkle."] Rugged; wrinkled.

Rum. [**Spir'itus Jamaicen'sis.**] Jamaica spirit. A well-known spirituous liquor, obtained from the sugar-cane.

Ru'mex, *icis.** Yellow Dock. A Linnæan genus of the class *Hexandria,* natural order *Polygonaceæ.* Also, the Pharmacopœial name (U.S. Ph.) for the root of the *Rumex crispus.*

Ru'mex Aç-e-to'sa.* The common sorrel, or sour-dock.

Ru'mĭ-nant, or **Ru'mĭ-nāt-ing.** [**Ru'minans;** from *ru'mino, rumina'tum,* to "chew the cud."] Chewing the cud. Applied to an order of animals. See RUMINANTIA.

Ruminantia,* ru-me-nan'she-a. [See RUMINANT.] The name of an order of Mammalia, comprising the cow, sheep, and deer. They all have four stomachs.

Ru'mĭ-nāt-ed. [Perhaps from *ru'men,* a "throat," or "opening."] Penetrated with holes or channels. Applied to the albumen of seeds.—(GRAY.)

Ru-mĭ-nā'tion. [**Rumina'tio,** *o'nis;* see RUMINANT.] Chewing the cud, or bringing up of the food, which has been swallowed, into the mouth again to be properly chewed. A physiological peculiarity of a certain order of animals.

Run'cĭ-nate. [**Runcina'tus;** from *runci'na,* a "large saw."] Notched, like a saw; with the teeth turned backwards, *i.e.* towards the base of a leaf.

Run'ner. A prostrate slender branch sent off from the base of the parent stem. It strikes root at its apex, and produces a tuft of leaves, thus giving rise to an independent plant, as in the Strawberry.

Run'ning. Popularly applied to a continual discharge or flow of pus or mucus.

Rupellensis Sal. See SAL RUPELLENSIS.

Ru-pes'trine. [From *ru'pes*, a "rock."] Growing naturally or spontaneously on rocks.

Ru'pi-a.* [From ῥύπος, "sordes."] An eruptive disease in which there are broad flat vesicles, succeeded by an ill-conditioned discharge which thickens into superficial scabs, easily detached and immediately replaced by new ones.

Rup'tile. [From *rum'po, rup'tum*, to "break," or "burst."] Bursting irregularly. Applied to parts of plants.

Rup'ture. [From the same.] A popular name for HERNIA, which see.

Ru-ric'o-lus.* [From *rus, ru'ris*, the "country," and *co'lo*, to "inhabit."] Living in the country, or fields.

Rust. [**Rubi'go, g'***inis*.] The substance which is formed on the surface of iron and some other metals when exposed to the air and moisture. The rust of iron (*rubigo ferri*) is essentially a sesquioxide (or peroxide) of iron.

Rus-tic'o-lus.* [From *rus*, the "country," and *co'lo*, to "inhabit."] Living in fields or meadows. Applied to certain birds.

Ru'ta.* Rue. A Linnæan genus of the class *Decandria*, natural order *Rutaceæ*. Also, the Pharmacopœial name (U.S. Ph.) for the leaves of the *Ru'ta grav'eolens*.

Ru'ta Grav'e-o-lens.* ("Heavy-smelling Rue.") The common rue-plant.

Rutaceæ,* ru-ta'she-ē, or **Ru'tæ.*** A natural order of exogenous plants, mostly trees or shrubs, found in many warm regions. It includes *Ru'ta* (Rue), and *Dictam'nus*, a fragrant plant which emits an inflammable vapor.

Ru-tā'ceous. [**Ruta'ceus.**] Resembling rue (*Ruta*).

Ru-the'ni-um.* A new metal discovered in native platinum in 1844. It is hard and brittle, and has a specific gravity of about 8.5.

Ru-ti-do'sis,* written also **Rhy̆t-ĭ-do'sis,*** and **Ry̆t-ĭ-do'sis.*** [From ῥυτίς, a "wrinkle."] A shrinking or puckering of the *cornea*, regarded as a certain sign of approaching death.

Ruysch (roisk), **Membrane of.** See next article.

Ruy-schi-a'na, Mem-bra'na.* ("Ruyschian Membrane," or "Membrane of Ruysch.") The internal layer of the choroid coat of the eye: first particularized by Ruysch; also called *Tunica Ruyschiana*.

Ruy'schi-i, Tu'ni-ca Cel-lu-lo'sa.* ("Cellular Coat of Ruysch.") The cellular coat of the intestines, described by Ruysch.

Rye. A kind of cereal grain, used for bread. (See SECALE.) The seeds are sometimes infected with a parasitic fungus, when they acquire medicinal and poisonous qualities. See ERGOTA.

Rye, Ergot of. See ERGOTA.

Rye, Spurred. The *Secale cornutum*, or ergot of rye.

Rytidosis. See RUTIDOSIS.

S.

S. = *Semis'sis.** "Half."

S. A., or **S. A. L.** = *Secun'dum ar'tem,** "According to art," or *Secun'dum ar'tis le'ges.** "According to the rules of art."

Sab-a-dil'la.* [From the Spanish *Cebe'da*, "barley."] Cevadilla. The Pharmacopœial name (U.S. Ph.) for the seed of *Vera'trum sabadil'la*; but according to the British Pharmacopœia, the dried fruit of the *Asagræ'a officina'lis*.

Sab-a-dil'lin. [**Sabadilli'na.**] An excessively acrid white substance obtained from the seeds of the *Veratrum sabadilla* and *Helonias officinalis*.

Sabbatia,* sab-ba'she-a. American Centaury. The Pharmacopœial name (U.S. Ph.) for the herb of the *Sabba'tia angula'ris*.

Sabi'na.* Savine. The Pharmacopœial name ‖ for the tops of *Juniperus sabina*.

Sab-u-lic'o-lus.* [From *sab'ulum*, "sand," or "gravel," and *co'lo*, to "inhabit."] Growing or living in sand.

Sab'u-line. The same as SABULOUS, which see.

Sab'u-lose. [From *sab'ulum*, "sand," or "gravel."] Growing in sand. Applied to certain plants.

Sab'u-lous. [**Sabulo'sus**; from the same.] Gritty; sandy.

Sa-bur'ra.* A Latin word for "ballast." Applied to foulness of the stomach; sordes.

Sac'cate, or **Sac'cāt-ed.** [**Sacca'tus**; from *sac'cus*, a "sac."] Contained in a membranous bag: also, formed like a sac; sac-shaped.

Sac'cha-rāt-ed. [**Sacchara'tus;** from *sac'charum,* "sugar."] Having or containing sugar.

Sac-cha-reph-ĭ-dro'sis.* [From *sac'charum,* "sugar," and *ephidro'sis,* a "sweating."] A saccharine sweating.

Sac'cha-ri Fæx.* ("Dregs of Sugar.") Treacle, or molasses.

Sac-cha-rif'er-ous. [**Saccharif'erus;** from *sac'charum,* "sugar," and *fe'ro,* to "bear."] Yielding sugar.

Sac-cha-rĭ-fĭ-cā'tion. [**Sacchariflca'tio, o'nis;** from *sac'charum,* "sugar," and *fa'cio,* to "make."] The conversion of a substance into sugar, as starch when treated by sulphuric acid.

Sac-cha-rĭ-fĭ-ca'tus.* [From the same.] Converted into sugar.

Sac'cha-rīne. [**Sacchari'nus;** from *sac'charum,* "sugar."] Belonging to sugar, or having the properties of sugar.

Sac'cha-roid. [**Saccharoi'des;** from *sac'charum,* "sugar," and εἶδος, a "form."] Resembling loaf-sugar in texture. Applied to minerals.

Sac-cha-rol'o-ġy̆. [**Saccharolo'gia;** from *sac'charum,* "sugar," and λόγος, a "discourse."] A treatise on sugar; or the science of sugar.

Sac-cha-rom'e-ter. [**Saccharom'etrum;** from *sac'charum,* "sugar," and μέτρον, a "measure."] An instrument for ascertaining the quantity of sugar in liquors, syrups, etc.

Sac'cha-rum.* [From the Arabic *Shak'ar* or *Shak'kar.*] A Linnæan genus of the class *Triandria,* natural order *Graminaceæ.* Also, the Pharmacopœial name (U.S. Ph.) for the sugar of the *Sac'charum officina'rum* refined; the *Saccharum album* of the British Pharmacopœia. See SUGAR.

Sac'charum A-cer'num.* ("Maple Sugar.") Sugar obtained from the *A'cer sacchari'num;* also called *Sac'charum Canaden'se.*

Sac'charum Al'bum.* ("White Sugar.") Refined sugar; loaf-sugar.

Sac'charum Can-a-den'se.* ("Canadian Sugar.") A name for the *Sac'charum acer'num,* or maple-sugar.

Sac'charum Com-mu'ne* ("Common Sugar"), **Sac'charum Non-pu-rĭ-fĭ-ca'tum*** ("Unpurified Sugar"). Systematic terms for moist sugar; otherwise termed Muscovado sugar.

Sac'charum Lac'tis.* ("Sugar of Milk.") The name applied to a crystalline substance obtained from whey, in hard white masses, having a sweet taste, and the specific gravity 1.5. It has been assigned a place on the primary list of the Materia Medica of the U.S. Pharmacopœia for 1860. It has also been inserted in the list of the British Pharmacopœia. Used as a bland and nutritious article of diet in certain diseases.

Sac'charum Of-fĭç-ĭ-na'le,* or **Sac'charum Of-fĭç-ĭ-na'rum.*** ("Officinal Saccharum.") Names for the sugar-cane.

Sac'charum Sa-tur'ni.* ("Sugar of Lead.") The *Acetas plumbi.*

Sac-cho-lac'tāte. [**Saccholac'tas, a'tis.**] A combination of saccholactic acid with a base.

Sac-cho-lac'tic. [**Saccholac'ticus;** from *sac'charum,* "sugar," and *lac,* "milk."] Applied to mucic acid, because first obtained from sugar of milk.

Sac-cho-lac'tic Aç'id. [**Saccholac'ticum Aç'idum.**] The same as MUCIC ACID.

Sac-çif'er-us.* [From *sac'cus,* a "sac," and *fe'ro,* to "bear."] Bearing or having a sac or sac-like appendage. Applied to plants.

Sac'çĭ-form. [**Saccifor'mis;** from *sac'cus,* a "sac."] Formed like a sac.

Sac'cu-lāt-ed. [**Saccula'tus;** from *sac'culus,* a "little sac."] Bagged, or pursed out in little expansions.

Sac'cule. [**Sac'culus;** diminutive of *sac'cus,* a "sac."] A little sac or pouch.

Sac-cu-lo'sus.* [From *sac'culus,* a "little sac."] Having little sacs.

Sac'culus Ad-ĭ-po'sus.* ("Adipose Sac.") The *bursa mucosa* of a joint.

Sac'culus Cor'dis.* ("Sac of the Heart.") A name for the pericardium.

Sac'culus (or **Sac'cus**) **Lach-ry̆-ma'lis.*** The lachrymal sac or bag, a small cavity forming the commencement of the passage which conducts the tears from the eye to the nose.

Sac'culus La-ry̆n'ġis.* ("Little Sac of the Larynx.") A pouch extending upward from the ventricle of the larynx to the upper border of the thyroid cartilage.

Sac'culus Pro'prĭ-us.* The smaller of the two sacs of the vestibulum of the ear, formed by the expansion of the auditory nerve.

Sac'cus.* A Latin word signifying a "sac."

Sa'cer Ig'nis.* ("Sacred Fire.") A term for erysipelas; also formerly applied to *Herpes exedens.*

Sa'cer Mor'bus.* ("Sacred Disease.") A name for EPILEPSY, which see.

Sa'cer Mus'cu-lus.* ("Sacred Muscle.") A designation of the *transversa'lis lumbo'rum*.

Sack. A wine formerly much used, said to be brought from the Canary Islands, and called Canary; also applied to a wine brought from Malaga in Spain.

Sā'cral. [Lat. **Sacra'lis;** Fr. *Sacré*, så'krå'.) Belonging to the sacrum. Applied by Dr. Barclay as meaning towards the sacrum.

Sa-cro-lum-ba'lis.* A muscle arising from the sacrum, etc., and inserted into the angles of the six lower ribs.

Sa'crum.* [Etymology uncertain.] The triangular bone wedged between the *Ossa innominata*, forming the posterior wall of the pelvis.

Safe'tў Lamp. A lamp invented by Sir H. Davy, consisting of a common oil-lamp, completely surrounded with a cage of fine wire gauze, for the use of miners. The gauze has the property of preventing the flame of the lamp from igniting the explosive mixture of gases which surrounds it, that portion only being burned which is within the cage.

Saf'fron. The common English name for the CROCUS SATIVUS, which see.

Saf'fron, Mea'dow. A name for the *Col'chicum autumna'le*.

Sag-a-pe'num.* [Gr. σαγάπηνον.] The Pharmacopœial name (Lond. Ph., 1851) of the gum-resin of an uncertain plant, said to be a species of *Ferula*. It is reputed to be emmenagogue and antispasmodic.

Sage. The common name of SALVIA OFFICINALIS, which see.

Sage Femme, såzh fåmm. The French for MIDWIFE, which see.

Sag'it-tal. [**Sagitta'lis;** from *sagit'ta*, an "arrow."] Relating to, or shaped like, an arrow.

Sag'ittal Su'ture. The suture which unites the parietal bones.

Sag'it-tate. [**Sagitta'tus;** from *sagit'ta*, an "arrow."] Having the shape of an arrow, as a lanceolate leaf with a lobe at the base on each side pointing backward.

Sag-it-tif'er-ous. [**Sagittif'erus;** from *sagit'ta*, an "arrow," and *fe'ro*, to "bear."] Bearing arrow-shaped objects. Applied to plants, shells, etc.

Sa-git-ti-fo'li-ous. [**Sagittifo'lius;** from *sagit'ta*, an "arrow," and *fo'lium*, a "leaf."] Having arrow-shaped leaves.

Sā'go. (Fr. *Sagou*, så'goo'.) The Pharmacopœial name (U.S. Ph.) for the prepared fecula obtained from the pith of the *Sagus Rumphii* and other species of *Sagus*. Used as a nutritious and easily digestible food in febrile affections and in convalescence from acute disorders.

Sāim. A name for the *Adeps suillus*, or hog's lard. See ADEPS.

Saint Anthony's Fire. See ERYSIPELAS.

Saint Vi'tus' Dance. A common name for CHOREA, which see.

Sal,* gen. **Sa'lis.** [From ἅλς, "salt."] Salt. Applied to a compound in definite proportions of an acid with an alkali, earth, or metallic oxide.

Sal Am-mo'ni-ac. [**Sal Ammoni'acum.**] The former name of MURIATE OF AMMONIA, which see.

Sal Ar-gen'ti.* ("Salt of Silver.") The nitrate of silver. See LUNAR CAUSTIC.

Sal Ben'zo-in.* Benzoic acid; the *Aç'idum Benzo'icum* of the British Pharmacopœia.

Sal Ca-thar'ti-cus Am-a'rus* ("Bitter Cathartic Salt"), or **Sal Ca-thar'ti-cus An-gli-ca'nus*** ("English Cathartic Salt"). Names for the sulphate of magnesia.

Sal Cathar'ticus Glau-be'ri.* ("Cathartic Salt of Glauber.") The sulphate of soda, or Glauber's salt.

Sal Chal'ў-bis.* ("Salt of Iron or Steel.") The sulphate of iron.

Sal Com-mu'nis.* ("Common Salt.") The chloride of sodium. See SODII CHLORIDUM.

Sal Cor'nu Cer'vi.* ("Salt of Hartshorn.") The SUBCARBONATE OF AMMONIA, which see.

Sal Di-u-ret'i-cus.* ("Diuretic Salt.") The acetate of potash.

Sal Ep-so-men'sis.* ("Epsom Salts.") The sulphate of magnesia.

Sal Fos'si-lis,* Sal Gem'mæ.* ("Fossil, or Rock, Salt.") The chloride of sodium, or common salt.

Sal Glauberi. See GLAUBER'S SALT.

Sal Mirabilis Glauberi. See GLAUBER'S SALT.

Sal Prunelle (proo-nĕll'). Nitre, or saltpetre, fused and poured into moulds so as to form small balls. It is sometimes prepared with a mixture of sulphate of potash. See POTASSÆ NITRAS.

Sal Ru-pel-len'sis.* [From *Rupel'la*, the Latin name of Rochelle.] The tartrate of potash and soda, or Rochelle salt.

Sal Sa-tur'ni.* ("Salt of Lead.") The acetate of lead. See PLUMBI ACETAS.

Sal Vo-lat'i-lis.* ("Volatile Salt.") The subcarbonate of ammonia.

Sa-laç'i-ty. [**Salaç'itas, a'**tis; from *sa'lax, sala'cis,* "lustful," "wanton."] Lechery; lust; orgasm.

Sā'lep. A farinaceous powder made from the root of the *Orchis morio.* It is a light and nutritious food, like tapioca.

Salicaceæ,* sa-le-ka'she-ē. [See next article.] A natural order of exogenous trees and shrubs, natives of Europe, North America, and Northern Asia. It includes the Willow *(Sa'lix)* and Poplar *(Pop'ulus).* The bark is usually astringent, tonic, and stomachic.

Sal-i-cā'ceous. [**Salica'ceus;** from *sa'lix, sal'icis,* the "willow."] Resembling the willow. Applied to an order of plants. See SALICACEÆ.

Sal-i-ca'ri-æ.* The Jussieuan name of a natural order of plants, called by some botanists LYTHRACEÆ, which see.

Sal'i-cin, or **Sal'i-cine.** [**Salici'na.**] An extremely bitter, white substance obtained from the bark of several species of *Salix.*

Sal-i-cin'e-us.* Resembling the genus *Salix:* salicineous.

Sā'li-ent. [From *sa'lio,* to "leap," to "spring," to "shoot out."] Shooting or jutting out; prominent.

Sa'lient An'gle. An angle of a polygon projecting outwards in reference to the centre of the polygon. All the angles of any regular figure, as a triangle, square, etc., are salient.

Sa-lif'er-ous. [**Salif'erus;** from *sal,* a "salt," and *fe'ro,* to "bear."] Containing or producing salt.

Sal'i-fī-a-ble. [**Salifiab'ilis;** from *sal,* a "salt," and *fi'o,* to "be made."] Having the property of forming a salt, by combination with other substances.

Sa-lig'e-nin. [**Saligeni'na;** from *salici'na,* and *ge'no,* an ancient form of *gig'no,* to "beget."] A new substance which, together with sugar, contains the elements of salicin, from which it is obtained.

Sa-līne'. [**Sali'nus;** from *sal,* "salt."] Belonging to or resembling salt; of the nature of a salt. In Botany, growing in salt places.

Sa-lī'va.* The fluid secretion of the salivary glands; spittle.

Sa-lī'val. [**Saliva'lis;** from *sali'va,* "spittle."] Relating to the saliva.

Sal'i-vant. [**Sali'vans, an'**tis; from the same.] Exciting an increased flow of the saliva: salivating.

Sal'i-va-ry. [**Saliva'rius,** and **Saliva'ris;** from the same.] Of or relating to the saliva.

Sal'ivary Glands. [**Glan'dulæ Saliva'riæ.**] The name of three glands situated on each side of the face, behind and beneath the lower jaw, for the purpose of secreting saliva. They are the *parotid,* the *sub-maxillary,* and the *sub-lingual* glands.

Sal-i-vā'tion. [**Saliva'tio, o'**nis; from *sali'va,* "spittle."] An excessive flow of the saliva, produced by the exhibition of medicines. See PTYALISMUS.

Sa'lix, icis.* [From *sa'lio,* to "spring out."] (Fr. *Saule,* sōl.) A Linnæan genus of the class *Diœcia,* natural order *Salicaceæ.* Also, the Pharmacopœial name (U.S. and Ed. Ph.) for the bark of *Salix alba, S. caprea,* and *S. fragilis.*

Sa'lix Al'ba.* The white willow.

Sa'lix Ca'pre-a.* The great round-leaved willow.

Sa'lix Frag'i-lis.* ("Brittle Willow.") The common crack willow. The bark is tonic and astringent, and has been employed in intermittents, dyspepsia, etc.

Salpetra. See SALTPETRE.

Sal-pin-gi'tis, idis.* [From *sal'pinx,* the "Eustachian tube."] Inflammation of the Eustachian tube.

Sal-pin-gys-te-ro-çy-e'sis.* [From *sal'pinx, hys'tera,* the "womb," and *cye'sis,* "pregnancy."] A term for pregnancy or fœtation partly in the Fallopian tube and partly in the uterus.

Sal'pinx, in'gis.* [Gr. σάλπιγξ, a "trumpet," or "tube."] A name for the Eustachian tube, also for the Fallopian tube.

Săl'si-fy, or **Săl'si-fi.** A name of the oyster-plant, *Tragopo'gon porrifo'lium.*

Sal'sus.* The same as SALINE, which see.

Salt. [Lat. **Sal;** Fr. *Sel,* sĕl.] The chloride of sodium. (See SODII CHLORIDUM.) Common salt. In Chemistry, a compound, in definite proportions, of an acid with an alkali, earth, or metallic oxide.

Salt, Neū'tral. A combination of an acid with an alkali, earth, or metallic oxide, so proportioned that the resulting salt has neither acid nor alkaline properties.

Salt of Lem'ons. A combination of oxalic acid with a small portion of potash, as found in wood-sorrel; also applied to crystallized citric acid.

Salt of Tar'tar. A very pure carbonate of potassa, prepared from the bitartrate of potassa, or cream of tartar.

Săl-tā'tion. [**Salta'tio, o'**nis; from

sal'to, salta'tum, to "dance," or "jump."] A dancing or leaping; synonymous with *Chorea*.

Săl'tạ-to-rў. [**Saltato'rius;** from the same.] Having the power of leaping; adapted to leaping or saltation. Applied to certain insects.

Sal-tig'rạ-dus.* [From *sal'tus*, a "leap," and *gra'dior*, to "walk."] Seizing their prey by leaping. Applied to insects.

Sâlt-pe'tre. [**Salpe'tra;** from *sal*, "salt," and *pe'tra*, a "rock."] The nitrate of potash, or nitre. See POTASSÆ NITRAS.

Salts, Sec'on-dạ-rў. Synonymous with neutral salts. See SALT, NEUTRAL.

Săl'tus.* [From *sa'lio, sal'tum*, to "leap."] A springing, or leaping. Applied in the same manner as *Subsultus tendinum*.

Sạ-lu'brĭ-ous. [**Salu'bris;** from *sa'lus*, "health."] Salutary; wholesome; conducive to health.

Sa'lus,* gen. **Sạ-lu'tis.** A Latin word signifying "health," or "safety," also "salvation."

Sal'u-ta-rў. [**Saluta'ris;** from *sa'lus*, "health."] Healthy; wholesome; favorable to health.

Salvadoraceæ,* săl-vạ-do-ra'she-ē. A natural order of exogenous trees and shrubs, found in India and Syria. It includes the *Salvado'ra Per'sica* (the mustard-tree of Scripture).

Săl-vạ-tel'lạ.* [From *sal'vo, salva'tum*, to "save."] A small vein on the back of the hand, ascending the inner side of the forearm; it contributes to form the basilic vein. Bleeding from the *salvatella* vein was once regarded as of especial efficacy in the treatment of certain diseases.

Salve. See UNGUENTUM.

Săl'ver-Shaped. Hypocrateriform. Tubular, with a border spreading flat at right angles to the tube. Applied to a form of monopetalous corolla, as that of the Phlox.

Sal'vĭ-ạ.* (Fr. *Sauge*, sōzh.) Sage. A Linnæan genus of plants of the class *Diandria*, natural order *Labiatæ;* also, the Pharmacopœial name (U.S. Ph.) for the leaves of the *Sal'via officina'lis*. It is astringent, aromatic, and tonic.

Sam'ạ-rạ.* [From *sam'ara*, or *sam'era*, the seed of the elm and other trees.] Applied in Botany to a dry, indehiscent pericarp which has an appendage like a wing, as the maple and ash. It is also called a key-fruit.

Sam'bu-cin. [**Sambuci'na.**] A peculiar substance found in the flowers of the *Sambucus nigra*.

Sam-bu'cus. [From *sambu'ca*, a musical instrument; sometimes made, it is said, of elder wood.] (Fr. *Sureau*, sü'rō'.) Elder. A Linnæan genus of the class *Pentandria*, natural order *Caprifoliaceæ.* Also, the Pharmacopœial name (U.S. Ph.) for the flowers of the *Sambu'cus Canaden'sis;* but according to the British Pharmacopœia, for those of the *Sambu'cus ni'gra*. The berries are aperient and diaphoretic; the inner bark is purgative, and in large doses emetic.

Sambu'cus Ni'grạ.* The systematic name of the medicinal (European) elder.

Samydaceæ,* sam-e-da'she-ē. [From *Samy'da*, one of the genera.] A natural order of exogenous tropical trees and shrubs, found mostly in America.

Sạ-nab'ĭ-lis.* [From *sa'no*, to "cure."] Curable; that may be cured.

Sạ-nā'tion. [**Sana'tio, o'nis;** from *sa'no, sana'tum*, to "heal."] A cure, or restoration to health; the act of healing.

San'ạ-tĭve. [**Sanati'vus.**] Healing; having a power or tendency to heal.

San-ạ-to'rĭ-um.* A synonym of SANITARIUM, which see.

San'ạ-to-rў. [**Sanato'rius;** from *sa'no, sana'tum*, to "heal."] Having power to heal.

Sanctum Semen. See SEMEN SANCTUM.

Sand. [**Are'na.**] Finely-divided silicious matter constitutes common river and sea sand. Particles of other substances are often blended with it.

Sand-Bath. See BATH.

San-dal'ĭ-form. [**Sandalifor'mis;** from *sanda'lium*, a "sandal."] Having the form of a sandal or slipper.

San'dạl-Wood. The wood of the *Pterocar'pus santali'nus* and *San'talum al'bum*, East Indian trees. It is prized for its fragrance, and is sometimes used as a medicine.

Sand'stone. A species of stratified rock, composed of agglutinated grains of sand.

Sang, sŏngᵍ. The French term for BLOOD, which see.

San-gạ-ree'. Wine and water sweetened and spiced.

Sangsue, sŏngᵍ'sü'. The French term for the leech. See HIRUDO.

San-guif'er-ous. [**Sanguif'erus;** from *san'guis*, "blood," and *fe'ro*, to "bear," or "convey."] Containing or conveying blood.

San-guĭ-fĭ-cā'tion. [**Sanguifica'tio, o**'*nis;* from *san'guis,* "blood," and *fa'cio,* to "make."] The formation of blood; the conversion of chyle into blood, or of venous into arterial blood.

San-guĭ-na'rĭ-ạ.* Blood-root. The Pharmacopœial name (U.S. Ph.) for the rhizoma of the *Sanguinaria Canadensis,* a plant of the natural order *Papaveraceæ.* The rhizoma and seeds are emetic.

Sanguine, sang'gwin. [**Sanguin'eus;** from *san'guis, san'guinis,* "blood."] Abounding with blood; warm; ardent; nearly the same as SANGUINEOUS.

San-guin'e-ous. [**Sanguin'eus;** from the same.] Relating to the blood; bloody; of the color of blood; abounding in blood. Applied to certain diseases, as sanguineous apoplexy, etc. Also applied to a particular habit or TEMPERAMENT, which see.

San-guin-ĭ-ros'tris.* [From *san'guis,* "blood," and *ros'trum,* a "beak."] Having a blood-red beak. Applied to birds.

San'guĭ-nis,* the genitive of SANGUIS, which see.

San-guin'o-lent. [**Sanguinolen'tus;** from *san'guis,* "blood."] Of a blood-red color; bloody, or tinged with blood.

San'guis,* gen. **San'guĭ-nis.** The Latin word for BLOOD, which see.

Sanguis Draconis. See DRAGON'S BLOOD.

Sanguisorbaceæ,* san-gwe-sor-ba'she-ē. A natural order of exogenous plants, found in Europe and other temperate regions. They are allied to the *Rosaceæ.* It includes the *Sanguisor'ba.*

San-guĭ-sor'be-æ.* Synonymous with SANGUISORBACEÆ, which see.

San-guĭ-su'gạ.* [From *san'guis,* "blood," and *su'go,* to "suck."] A blood-sucker; the leech, properly so called; a subdivision of the genus HIRUDO, which see.

Sanguisu'ga Med-ĭ-cĭ-na'lis,* or **Sanguisu'ga Of-fĭç-ĭ-na'lis.*** The *Hirudo medicinalis.*

Sa'nĭ-ēṡ.* [From *san'guis,* "blood"?] A thin, greenish, serous, and fetid discharge from fistulæ, ulcers, etc., sometimes tinged with blood.

Sā'nĭ-ous. [**Sanio'sus.**] Discharging sanies; of the nature of sanies.

San-ĭ-ta'rĭ-um.* [From *san'itas,* "health."] A retreat for invalids or convalescent persons, selected in reference to the salubrity of its situation. Also, an institution for the treatment of the sick.

San'ĭ-tạ-rȳ. [**Sanita'rius;** from the same.] Pertaining to, or promoting, health.

San'ĭ-tȳ. [**San'itas, a**'*tis;* from *sa'nus,* "sound," "healthy," "sane."] (Fr. *Santé,* sōNᴳ'tà'.) Health, or soundness of mind and body.

Santalaceæ,* san-tạ-la'she-ē. A natural order of exogenous plants, natives of Europe, North America, the East Indies, etc. It includes *San'talum* (Sandal-wood), which is used as a perfume and a medicine.

San'tạ-lin. The coloring principle of the wood of the *Pterocarpus santalinus,* or red saunders.

San'tạ-lum.* Red Saunders. The Pharmacopœial name (U.S. Ph.) for the wood of the *Pterocar'pus santali'nus.* See SANDAL-WOOD.

Santé. See SANITY.

San-ton'ĭ-cạ.* Levant Wormseed. The Pharmacopœial name ‖ for the unexpanded flowers and peduncles of the *Artemisia santonica, A. contra,* and of other species of *Artemisia.* It has been placed on the primary list of the Materia Medica of the U.S. Pharmacopœia for 1860. It is anthelmintic.

San'to-nin, or **San'to-nine.** [**Santoni'nạ;** from *Santon'ica.*] A vegetable principle prepared from *Artemisia santonica.*

San-to-ri'ni, Ve'næ E-mis-so'rĭ-æ.* ("Emissory [or Emunctory] Veins of Santorinus.") The different small veins which pass through the *foramina* of the cranium, communicating between the sinuses of the *dura mater* and the external veins of the head.

San-to-ri'nus, Fis'sures of. Certain small fissures in the cartilaginous portions of the *meatus auditorius externus.*

Santori'nus, Tu'ber-cles of. The small projections on the arytenoid cartilages which support the ligaments of the glottis.

Sap. [**Suc'cus.**] The juice of plants; the liquid imbibed by the roots of plants and carried up through the stem. In a crude state it consists chiefly of water and carbonic acid; but as it rises through the tissue of the stem, it dissolves the secretions it meets with in its course, and being attracted to the leaves, in which it is subjected to the influence of light, it is converted into a very different substance, called *elaborated* sap, which contains various nutritive products, as sugar, starch, proteine, etc. See SAP-WOOD.

Sa-phe'na.* [From σαφής, "manifest."] The name of two large veins of the leg, internal and external.

Sap'id. [**Sap'idus;** from *sa'pio*, to "taste."] Having or imparting taste, especially an agreeable taste; savory.

Sa-pid'i-tў. [**Sapid'itas;** from the same.] The quality of bodies which affects the organs of taste.

Sapindaceæ,* sap-in-da'she-ē. A natural order of exogenous trees and shrubs, natives of tropical regions, especially of South America. It includes the *Sapin'dus* and *Paullin'ia*. Plants of this order are generally poisonous.

Sa-pin'di,* the plural of *Sapin'dus*, forming the Jussieuan name of a natural order of plants. See SAPINDACEÆ.

Sa'po,* gen. **Sa-po'nis.** (Fr. *Savon*, sâ'vôn'.) Soap; a compound of certain principles in oils, fats, or resin, with alkalies in definite proportions. Also, the Pharmacopœial name (U.S. Ph.) for soap made with soda and olive oil.

Sa'po Du'rus.* ("Hard Soap.") The Pharmacopœial name (Ed. Ph.) for Spanish, or Castile, soap.

Sa'po Mol'lis.* ("Soft Soap.") The Pharmacopœial name (Br. Ph.) for soap made with olive oil and potash.

Sa'po Vul-ga'ris.* ("Common Soap.") A name for soap made with soda and animal oil.

Sap-o-nā'ceous. [**Sapona'ceus;** from *sa'po*, *sapo'nis*, "soap."] Of the nature or appearance of soap; soapy.

Sap-o-na'ri-a Of-fiç-i-na'lis.* Soapwort. A plant of the Linnæan class *Decandria*, natural order *Caryophyllaceæ*. The root and leaves have been used as a remedy in scrofula, cancer, secondary syphilis, jaundice, etc.

Sa-pon-i-fi-cā'tion. [**Saponifica'tio, o'**nis; from *sa'po*, *sapo'nis*, "soap," and *fa'cio*, to "make."] The conversion of oils into soap by the action of alkalies.

Sa-pon'i-form. [**Saponifor'mis;** from *sa'po*, *sapo'nis*, "soap."] Like soap in its unctuosity.

Sap'o-nin. [**Saponi'na.**] A name applied to the frothy extract of the *Sapona'ria officina'lis*.

Sap'o-nule. [**Sapon'ulus;** from *sa'po*, "soap," and ὕλη, "material."] Literally, a material out of which soap is made. A volatile or essential oil in combination with a base.

Sap-o-rif'ic. [**Saporif'icus;** from *sa'por*, "taste," and *fa'cio*, to "make."] Causing or imparting taste.

Sap'o-rous. [From *sa'por*, "taste."] The same as SAPID.

Sapotaceæ,* sap-o-ta'she-ē, or **Sa-po'tæ.*** [From *Sapo'ta*, one of the genera.] A natural order of exogenous trees and shrubs, natives of the tropics of India, Africa, and America. Some genera produce edible fruits, as the Marmalade (*Achras*).

Sa-po'tæ,* the plural of **Sa-po'ta,** forming the Jussieuan name of a natural order of plants. See SAPOTACEÆ.

Sapphire, saf'fīr. [Lat. **Sapphi'rus;** Gr. σάπφειρος.] A precious stone of a blue color. It consists essentially of crystallized alumina. The Oriental ruby is a red variety of sapphire.

Sa-pros'to-mus.* [From σαπρός, "putrid," and στόμα, a "mouth."] Having a foul or stinking breath.

Sap-Wood, or **Al-bur'num.*** The outer part of the wood of exogenous trees, which is softer and more bibulous than the heart-wood. It is through the sap-wood that the sap ascends from the root to the leaves.

Sar'çi-na.* Literally, a "pack or burden." A name sometimes given to a peculiar substance found in the contents of the stomach. Also applied to the fœtus.

Sar-çi'tis, i*dis*.* [From σάρξ, σαρκός, "flesh."] Muscular inflammation; also, acute rheumatism.

Sar'co-carp. [**Sarcocar'pium,** or **Sarcocar'pus;** from σάρξ, σαρκός, "flesh," and καρπός, "fruit."] The fleshy, or pulpy, part of a drupe, as a peach or plum.

Sar'co-çēle.* [From σάρξ, "flesh," and κήλη, a "tumor."] (Fr. *Hernie charnue*, ĕr'nè' shar'nü'.) A fleshy enlargement of the testicle; termed also *Her'nia carno'sa* ("fleshy hernia").

Sar-co'dēs.* [From σάρξ, "flesh."] Like flesh; fleshy: sarcous.

Sar'coid. [**Sarcoi'des;** from σάρξ, "flesh," and εἶδος, a "form."] Resembling flesh.

Sar-co-lem'ma, a*tis*.* [From σάρξ, "flesh," and λέμμα, a "covering."] Applied to the sheath which encloses each of the muscular fibrils.

Sar-col'o-ġў. [**Sarcolo'gia;** from σάρξ, σαρκός, "flesh," and λόγος, a "discourse."] The part of Anatomy which treats of the fleshy parts of the body.

Sar-co'ma, a*tis*,* plural **Sar-co'ma-ta.** [From σάρξ, σαρκός, "flesh."] In Pathology, a fleshy tumor; a genus of the order *Tumores*, class *Locales*, of Cullen's Nosology. Applied by Link to a fleshy part, of variable form, which surrounds the ovary of plants, or is situated upon it.

Sar-com'a-tous. [**Sarcomato'sus;** from *sarco'ma.*] Relating to, or of the nature of, sarcoma; fleshy.

Sarcomphalos. See OMPHALONCUS.

Sar-coph'a-gous. [**Sarcoph'agus;** from σάρξ, "flesh," and φάγω, to "eat."] Eating, or living on, flesh.

Sar-coph'a-gus.* [From the same.] The name given by the ancients to a kind of stone said to have the property of consuming dead bodies placed in contact with it. Also applied to a coffin made of such stone.

Sar-co-phy'ma, atis.* [From σάρξ, "flesh," and φῦμα, a "tumor."] A fleshy tumor.

Sar-cop'tēs.* [From σάρξ, "flesh," and κόπτω, to "cut," to "pierce," or "sting," as a worm or insect.] That which stings, devours, or consumes the flesh. See next article.

Sarcop'tes Hom'i-nis.* ("Consumer of the Flesh of Man.") The name given by Raspail to the *Ac'arus scabie'i*, or itch-insect. It is a parasite, belonging to the class *Arachnida*, or spiders, and is therefore not an insect in the stricter sense of the term.

Sar-co'sis.* The progress of sarcoma. Also, preternatural generation of flesh.

Sar-cot'ic. [**Sarcot'icus;** from σαρκόω, to "produce flesh."] Making, or inducing the growth of, flesh. Applied to medicines. Also, belonging to sarcoma.

Sar'cous. [From σάρξ, "flesh."] Fleshy; pertaining to flesh or muscle.

Sar-don'ic Laugh. [**Ri'sus Sardon'icus;** from σαρδονικός, "belonging to Sardinia;" so called because a certain Sardinian plant is said to have excited a similar affection.] A singular convulsive laugh. Also applied to a peculiar expression of countenance observed in tetanus, *diaphragmitis*, etc.; also termed *Spas'mus cyn'icus.*

Sar'ment. [**Sarmen'tum;** from *sar'po*, to "prune."] A runner; a long and flexible branch.

Sar-men-tā'ceous. [**Sarmenta'ceus;** from *sarmen'tum*, a "sarment."] Bearing or resembling sarments.

Sar-men-tif'er-ous. [**Sarmentif'erus;** from *sarmen'tum*, a "sarment," and *fe'ro*, to "bear."] Bearing sarments.

Sar-men'tous. [**Sarmento'sus;** from *sarmen'tum*, a "sarment."] The same as SARMENTACEOUS.

Sarraceniaceæ,* sar-ra-se-ne-a'she-ē. A natural order of exogenous herbaceous plants, found in the bogs of North America. It includes the *Sarrace'nia* (Side-Saddle Flower).

Sar'sa.* The Pharmacopœial name (Br. Ph.) for Jamaica Sarsaparilla, the dried root of *Smi'lax officina'lis.*

Sar-sa-pa-ril'la.* [Spanish, *sarça*, or *sar'za*, a "brier," and *paril'la*, a "little vine."] The Pharmacopœial name (U.S. Ph.) for the root of *Smilax officinalis*, and other species of *Smilax*. It is an alterative, much employed in the treatment of secondary syphilis and scrofulous affections.

Sar-to'ri-us.* [From *sar'tor*, a "tailor."] Belonging to a tailor. Applied to a muscle (the longest of the human body), so called because a tailor uses it in crossing his legs. It arises from the spinous process of the ilium, and is inserted into the inner tubercle of the head of the tibia.

Sarx.* [Gr. σάρξ, σαρκός.] Flesh; the muscular part of animals.

Sar'za.* [In Spanish, a "bramble," or "low shrub."] Sarsaparilla. The Pharmacopœial name (Ed. Ph.) for the root of *Smi'lax officina'lis;* the *Radix Sarsaparillæ* ("Root of Sarsaparilla") of the Dublin Pharmacopœia.

Sas'sa-fras.* The Pharmacopœial name ‖ for the root of *Sas'safras officina'le.*

Sas'safras Me-dul'la.* ("Pith of Sassafras.") The Pharmacopœial name (U.S. Ph.) for the pith of the stems of the *Sassafras officinale.* From this pith a bland mucilage is obtained, much used as an application to inflamed eyes.

Sas'safras Of-fiç-i-na'le,* or **Lau'rus Sas'safras.*** A tree of the Linnæan class *Enneandria*, natural order *Lauraceæ.* It is a native of the United States.

Sas'safras Ra-di'cis Cor'tex.* ("Bark of Sassafras Root.") The Pharmacopœial name (U.S. Ph.) for the bark of the root of the *Sassafras officinale.* It is reputed stimulant, sudorific, and diuretic.

Sat'el-līte. [**Satel'les**, gen. **Satel'litis.**] A lifeguardsman; an attendant or partisan. In Astronomy, a moon or secondary planet, which revolves around a primary planet.

Sat'ellite Veins. Veins that accompany arteries, especially those belonging to the brachial artery.

Sa-tel'li-tēs,* gen. **Sa-tel'li-tum,** the plural of *Satel'les*. See SATELLITE.

Sa-ti'e-tȳ. [**Sati'etas;** from *sa'tis*, "enough."] Surfeit; disgust for food, from having been cloyed.

Sat'in-Spar. A fibrous variety of carbonate of lime, presenting a silky appearance when polished.

Sa-ti'vus.* [From *se'ro*, *sa'tum*, to "sow," or "plant."] Growing in fields or gardens; that is, cultivated. Applied to various plants.

Sat'u-rāte. [From *sat'uro*, *satura'tum*, to "cloy," or "fill."] To fill a liquid with as much salt, or other soluble substance, as it is capable of dissolving.

Sat-u-rā'tion. [**Satura'tio, o'nis;** from the same.] The act of saturating; the state of a solvent which has dissolved as much of a soluble body as it is capable of dissolving; or the state of a compound in which its elements are combined in such proportions that a fresh quantity of either cannot be added without excess.

Sat'ur-nine. [**Saturni'nus;** from *Satur'nus*, "Saturn;" also, a term for lead.] In Chemistry, relating to lead. Also, grave or dull, as distinguished from mercurial.

Sa-tur'nus.* Saturn. An alchemical name for lead; as, *Sal Saturni* ("Salt of Lead").

Sat-ȳ-ri'a-sis.* [From σάτυρος, a "satyr."] Excessive or inordinate sexual desire in men. A genus of the order *Dysorexiæ*, class *Locales*, of Cullen's Nosology. The proper treatment for this disease consists in a mild cooling diet, accompanied by active exercise and the use of a cold bath. The term *satyriasis* has also been applied to a species of *elephantiasis*, from its hideous appearance. See ELEPHANTIASIS GRÆCORUM.

Sauge, sōzh. The French name for "sage." See SALVIA.

Saule, sōl. The French name for "willow." See SALIX.

Sau'ri-an. [**Sau'rius;** from σαῦρος, or σαύρα, a "lizard."] Relating to or resembling a lizard. Also, an animal of the lizard tribe.

Sau-rog'ra-phȳ. [**Saurogra'phia;** from σαῦρος, a "lizard," and γράφω, to "write."] A description of the saurian reptiles.

Sau'roid. [**Sauroi'des;** from σαῦρος, a "lizard," and εἶδος, a "form."] Resembling a lizard.

Sau-rol'o-ġȳ. [**Saurolo'gia;** from σαῦρος, a "lizard," and λόγος, a "discourse."] A treatise upon saurian reptiles; or the science of saurian reptiles.

Sau-roph'a-gous. [**Sauroph'agus;** from σαῦρος, a "lizard," and φάγω, to "eat."] Eating lizards and other reptiles. Applied to birds.

Saururaceæ,* sau-ru-ra'she-ē. [From *Sauru'rus*, one of the genera.] A natural order of exogenous herbaceous plants, natives of the marshes of China, India, and North America.

Sauvagesiaceæ,* sō-vazh-e-a'she-ē. [From *Sauvage'sia*, one of the genera.] A small natural order of exogenous plants (herbs or shrubs), found in South America and the West Indies.

Sa-van'na, or **Sa-van'nah.** A low, open, or grassy plain; a prairie. Applied especially to the vast plains of the valley of the Mississippi.

Sav'in. The *Juniperus sabina*.

Savon, sȧ'vòɴɢ'. The French name for "soap." See SAPO.

Saw. The Scotch popular term for any salve, or ointment. See UNGUENTUM.

Saw-Toothed. The same as SERRATE, which see.

Sax'a-tile. [**Saxat'ilis;** from *sax'um*, a "rock."] Living or growing in rocky places. Applied to plants.

Saxifragaceæ,* sax-e-fra-ga'she-ē. A natural order of exogenous herbaceous plants, natives of the mountainous regions of Europe and the northern parts of the world. It includes *Saxif'raga*. The whole order is more or less astringent.

Sax-if'ra-ġæ,* the plural of *Saxif'raga*, forming the Jussieuan name of a natural order of plants. See SAXIFRAGACEÆ.

Sax'o-nȳ Blue. An intensely deep blue, produced by a solution of indigo in concentrated sulphuric acid.

Scab. [**Crus'ta.**] A crust-like substance formed on superficial ulcerations by the concretion of the fluid matter discharged from them. Also, the same as SCABIES.

Sca'bi-ēs.* [From *sca'bo*, to "scratch."] The itch; otherwise termed *Psora*. Also, a scab.

Scā'brid. The same as SCABROUS.

Scab-ri-flo'rus.* [From *sca'ber*, "rough," and *flos*, a "flower."] Having calyces rough with hairs.

Scab-ri-fo'li-us.* [From *sca'ber*, "rough," "scabby," and *fo'lium*, a "leaf."] Having rough leaves.

Scā'brous, or **Scā'brate.** [**Sca'ber;** from *sca'bo*, to "scratch."] Rough;

rugged; rough to the touch. Applied to leaves, etc.

Sca'la,* plural **Sca'læ.** A ladder, or staircase; a scale of steps; a regular gradation.

Sca'la Tym'pa-ni.* ("Stairway of the Tympanum.") The superior of the *scalæ* of the cochlea.

Sca'la Ves-tib'u-li.* ("Stairway of the Vestibule.") The inferior of the *scalæ* of the cochlea.

Sca'læ,* gen. **Sca-la'rum,** the plural of SCALA, which see.

Sca'læ of the Coch'le-a, or **Sca'læ Coch'le-æ.*** ("Stairways of the Cochlea.") The two cavities formed by the *lamina spiralis* or spiral septum of the cochlea. They are severally designated the SCALA TYMPANI and SCALA VESTIBULI.

Sca-lăr'i-form. [**Scalarifor'mis;** from *sca'la,* a "ladder."] Having the form of a ladder.

Scalar'iform Ducts of Plants. A form of vascular tissue, differing from dotted ducts only in the form of the markings, which are like cross-bars or the rounds of a ladder.

Scâld. [From the Italian *Scalda're,* to "heat."] A lesion of some part occasioned by the application of a hot fluid.

Scâld'-Head. A common name for *Porrigo,* or ringworm of the scalp.

Scale. [Lat. **Squa'ma;** Fr. *Écaille,* ā'kal'.] One of the small laminæ which cover most fishes, serpents, the wings of certain insects, etc. In Botany, any thin, scale-like appendage. Applied in Pathology to a small, opaque, whitish lamina of morbid cuticle, running into layers or crusts, which fall off repeatedly and are soon reproduced.

Scale. [From *sca'la,* a "ladder," or "stair;" hence, something which is regularly divided.] A line or rule of definite length, divided into a given number of equal parts, which are sometimes termed degrees.

Scale-Skin. See ICHTHYOSIS.

Sca-lēne'. [**Scale'num,** neuter of **Scale'nus;** from σκαληνός, "unequal."] A figure having unequal sides. A triangle of which all the sides are unequal.

Sca-le'nus.* [From the same.] The name of two muscles, the *anticus* and the *posticus,* which bend the head and neck. They arise from the transverse processes of the vertebræ of the neck, and are inserted into the first and second ribs.

Scā'ler. An instrument used by dentists for removing the scales of tartar from the teeth.

Scalloped, skol'lopt. The same as CRENATE,—*i.e.* marked with even and rounded notches on the margin, as some leaves.

Scalp. [**Epicra'nium.**] The integuments of the skull.

Scăl'pel. [**Scalpel'lum;** from *scal'po,* to "carve," or "scrape."] A small knife, usually with a straight blade fixed firmly in the handle: used in dissecting; also in surgical operations.

Scăl'prum.* [From *scal'po,* to "scrape."] A raspatory used in trepanning. Sometimes applied to the cutting edge of the incisor teeth of a mammal. See RASPATORY.

Scal'prum Den-ta'le.* [From *dens,* a "tooth."] A file used by dentists.

Scaly. See SQUAMOSE.

Scam-mo'nĭ-a.* The scammony-plant. See CONVOLVULUS SCAMMONIA.

Scam-mo'nĭ-um.* Scammony. The Pharmacopœial name ‖ for the concrete juice of the root of the *Convol'vulus Scammo'nia.* Scammony is an active cathartic, often causing, when taken alone, griping, or other unpleasant consequences, to obviate which it is usually combined with other medicines.

Scammo'nium Sy̆-ri'a-cum.* ("Syrian Scammony.") A name for the gum resin obtained from the root of the *Convol'vulus Scammo'nia.* See SCAMMONIUM.

Scammony. See SCAMMONIUM.

Scan'dent. [**Scan'dens;** from *scan'do, scan'sum,* to "climb."] Climbing; clinging to contiguous objects for support, by tendrils, etc. Applied to plants.

Scan'sor, o'r*is.** [From the same.] A climber. Applied in the plural (*Scanso'res*) to an order of birds which have the toes arranged in pairs, two before and two behind, a conformation of the foot which is admirably adapted for climbing.

Scan-so'rēs,* the plural of SCANSOR, which see.

Scan-so'rĭ-al. A climbing bird. See SCANSOR.

Scape. [**Sca'pus;** from σκᾶπος, a "stick," or "staff;" a "stalk."] A flower-stalk which arises from the stem at or beneath the surface of the ground, as in the primrose, blood-root, etc.

Sca'pha.* [From σκάπτω, to "dig."] A skiff, or small boat. The depression or cavity of the external ear, otherwise called *Fos'sa navicula'ris.*

Scā'phoid, or skaf'oid. [**Scaphoi'-**

des; from *sca'pha*, a "skiff," and εἶδος, a "form."] Resembling a little boat; navicular.

Scap-ĭ-flo'rus.* [From *sca'pus*, a "scape," and *flos*, a "flower."] Having flowers upon a scape: scapiflo'rous.

Scap'ĭ-form. [**Scapifor'mis;** from *sca'pus*, a "scape."] Formed like a scape.

Scap'ĭ-ger,* or **Scą-pig'e-rus.*** [From *sca'pus*, a "scape," and *ge'ro*, to "bear."] Having scape-like stems: scapigerous.

Scap'u-lą.* (Fr. *Omoplate*, o'mo'-plȧt'.) The shoulder-blade; a bone which extends from the shoulder-joint towards the vertebral column. It is broad, flat, and generally triangular, in the mammalia.

Scap-u-lăl'ġĭ-ą.* [From *scap'ula*, and ἄλγος, "pain."] Pain in the scapula.

Scap'u-lạr. [**Scapula'ris.**] Of or belonging to the scapula. Applied to arteries, veins, etc.: scapulary.

Scap-u-lo-dȳn'ĭ-ą.* [From *scap'ula*, and ὀδύνη, "pain."] Applied to pain or rheumatism in the shoulder.

Scap'u-lo-Hu'me-rąl. [**Scap'ulo-Humera'lis.**] A term sometimes applied to the shoulder-joint.

Scar. (See Cicatrix.) Applied in Botany to the Hilum, which see.

Scarf'-Skin. [Perhaps from the Anglo-Saxon *Sceorp*, "clothing," or "covering."] The cuticle, or epidermis.

Scăr-ĭ-fĭ-cā'tion. [**Scarifica'tio, o'nis;** from *scarif'ico*, *scarifica'tum*, to "lance," as a sore, to "make little incisions."] The operation of making small superficial incisions, or punctures, with a lancet or scarificator, usually with a view to local depletion.

Scăr-ĭ-fĭ-cā'tor. [**Scarifica'tor, o'ris;** from the same.] An instrument used in the operation of cupping. Also, an instrument with a blunt edge, used in tooth-extraction for separating the gum from the tooth.

Scā'rĭ-ous, or **Scā'rĭ-ose.** [**Scario'sus.**] Thin, dry, and membranaceous. Applied to parts of plants.

Scar-lą-ti'ną.* [Feminine singular of *scarlati'nus*, *fe'bris* being understood.] Scarlet fever; a disease characterized by contagious fever, and a scarlet eruption on the skin in patches, ending in three or four days in desquamation of the cuticle. A genus of the order *Exanthemata*, class *Pyrexiæ*, of Cullen's Nosology. It is often accompanied with great soreness in the fauces and throat, and is then sometimes termed *Scarlati'na angino'sa* or *paristhmit'ica*. See Paristhmitis.

Scarlati'na Mą-lig'ną.* ("Malignant Scarlet Fever.") A species of scarlatina, considered to be essentially the same with *Cynan'che malig'na* (putrid sore-throat).

Scarlati'na Sim'plex.* ("Simple Scarlet Fever.") A name sometimes applied to a mild form of scarlatina, attended with little or no soreness of the throat.

Scar'lą-tīne. [Lat. **Scarlati'nus;** from the Italian *Scarlat'to*, a "deep red."] Of a deep red or scarlet color.

Scar-lą-tĭ-no-ĭ'dēs.* [From *scarlati'nus*, and εἶδος, a "form."] Resembling scarlatina (*febris*); of a scarlet color: scarlatinoid.

Scarlet Fever. See Scarlatina.

Scarred. See Cicatrizatus.

Sceleton. See Skeleton.

Sçel-o-tyr'be.* [From σκέλος, the "leg," and τύρβη, "commotion," or "agitation."] Literally, "leg-commotion." A form of shaking palsy, usually attended with a contracted state of the limbs.

Scepaceæ,* se-pa'she-ē. A small natural order of exogenous trees, natives of tropical India. It includes the *Sce'pa*.

Scheele's (sheelz) **Green.** A well-known pigment consisting of arsenite of copper.

Scherlievo, skĕr-le-ā'vo. A disease in Illyria and Dalmatia of a syphilitic character.

Sche-ro'mą.* [From σχερός, "dry land," or ξηρός, "dry."] A dry inflammation of the eye, owing to a deficiency of the lachrymal secretion.

Schin-dȳ-le'sis.* [From σχινδυλέω, to "split into small pieces."] A variety of *synarthrosis*, in which one bone is received into a slit in another, as the *vomer* into the sphenoid.

Schist, shist. [**Schis'ta;** from σχίζω, to "cleave."] A species of rock of a fissile structure, such as gneiss. Often applied to the varieties of slate.

Schis-to-car'pous. [**Schistocar'pus;** from σχίζω, to "cleave," and καρπός, "fruit."] Having fissile fruit. Applied to a family of mosses.

Schist'oid. [**Schistoi'des;** from *schis'ta*, "schist," and εἶδος, a "form."] Resembling schist.

Schis-tor'rhą-chis.* [From σχιστός, "cloven," and ῥάχις, the "spine."] In Latin, **Spi'ną Bif'ĭ-dą.** Literally, "cloven spine." Names for *Hydrorrha-*

chis, so called from the double channel which often exists through a considerable length of the vertebral column, the one channel containing the spinal marrow, the other the dropsical fluid.—(GOOD.)

Schis'tose, or **Schis'tous.** [**Schisto'sus.**] Having the structure of schist.

Schizandraceæ,* ske-zan-dra'she-ē. [From *Schizan'dra*, one of the genera.] A small natural order of exogenous shrubs, found in India, Japan, and North America.

Sçhneī-de'rĭ-ạn Mem'brane. [From *Schnei'der*, its describer.] The mucous membrane lining the interior of the nose and cavities directly connected with it. Also termed the *Pituitary membrane.*

Sçhorl. [From the Swedish *Scorl*, "brittle"?] A brittle mineral, usually occurring in black, prismatic crystals. It becomes electric by heat and friction.

Sçi-ạ-do-phȳl'lus.* [From σκιάς, a "canopy," a "parasol," and φύλλον, a "leaf."] Having leaves in the form of an umbrella or parasol.

Sçī-at'ic. [**Sciat'icus;** from *ischiat'icus*, "ischiatic."] Belonging to the *ischium*. See ISCHIATIC.

Sciat'ic Nerve, Great. [Lat. **Ner'vus Ischiat'icus Ma'jor;** Fr. *Grand Nerf Sciatique*, gRōɴᵍ nĕRf sè'ȃ'tèk'.] The termination of the sacral or sciatic plexus. It is the largest of all the nerves, and is distributed chiefly to the muscles of the thigh.

Sçi-at'ĭ-cạ.* [From *sciat'icus*, "belonging to the *ischium*."] A rheumatic affection of the hip-joint. Also, a neuralgic affection of the sacro-sciatic nerve. See ISCHIAGRA.

Scī'ence. [**Scien'tia;** from *sci'o*, to "know."] Knowledge; learning; skill. The knowledge of many persons methodically digested and arranged so as to become attainable by one. The knowledge of reasons and their conclusions constitute *abstract*, that of causes and effects and of the laws of nature, *natural*, science.

Sçil'lạ,* gen. **Sçil'læ.** [Perhaps from σκέλλω, to "dry."] Squill. A Linnæan genus of the class *Hexandria*, natural order *Liliaceæ*. Also, the Pharmacopœial name (U.S. Ph.) of the bulb of *Scilla* (or *Squilla*) *maritima*, but according to the British Pharmacopœia, of the *Urgin'ea scil'la.*

Scil'la Mạ-rit'ĭ-mạ.* The squill, or sea-onion.

Scil'læ Mạ-rit'ĭ-mæ Bul'bus.* ("Bulb of the Scilla Maritima.") See SCILLA.

Sçil'lĭ-tin. [**Scilliti'na;** from *scil'la*, "squill."] The active principle of the squill.

Scimitar-Shaped. See ACINACIFORM.

Sçin-til-lā'tion. [**Scintilla'tio, o'nis;** from *scintil'lo*, *scintilla'tum*, to "sparkle."] A sparkling, as of fire. Applied to the twinkling or tremulous motion of the fixed stars, which appear as if the rays of light coming from them were not continuous, but produced by particles succeeding each other at intervals by a vibratory movement.

Sçī'on. A young branch or shoot of a tree, especially one used for grafting.

Scĭr-rho-gas'trĭ-ạ.* [From σκίῤῥος, "scirrhus," and γαστήρ, the "stomach."] Scirrhus, or incipient cancer, of the stomach.

Scĭr'rhoid. [**Scirrhoi'des;** from σκίῤῥος, a "hard tumor," and εἶδος, "resemblance."] The same as KELOIDE, which see.

Scĭr-rho'mạ, atis.* [From σκιῤῥόω, to "harden."] The same as SCIRRHUS.

Scĭr-rho-sar'cạ.* [From *scir'rhus*, and σάρξ, "flesh."] The *Scleriasis neonatorum*, or scirrhous hardening in the flesh of new-born infants. See SCLEROMA.

Scĭr'rhous. [**Scirrho'sus;** from *scir'rhus.*] Of the nature of scirrhus, or pertaining to scirrhus.

Scĭr'rhus.* [Gr. σκίῤῥος; Fr. *Squirrhe*, or *Squirre*, skèR.] A hard, indolent tumor, mostly affecting a glandular part, but occasionally occurring in other tissues. It generally precedes cancer in the ulcerated state. A genus of the order *Tumores*, class *Locales*, of Cullen's Nosology.

Sçit-ạ-min'e-æ.* A synonym for ZINGIBERACEÆ, which see.

Sçi-u-ri'ni,* or **Sçī'u-rīneṡ.** [From *sciu'rus*, a "squirrel."] A family of Rodents, of which the genus *Sciurus* is the type. They are distinguished by their very narrow lower incisors, and by their long bushy tail.

Sçī'u-roid. [From the same.] In Botany, like a squirrel's tail.

Scleranthaceæ,* skle-ran-tha'she-ē. [From *Scleran'thus*, one of the genera.] A small natural order of exogenous plants, found in Europe, Asia, and North America. They are all weeds.

Scle-re'mạ, atis.* [From σκληρός, "hard," and *œde'ma*, a "dropsical swelling."] A hard or indurated œdema.

Scle-rem'a-tous. Belonging to *sclerema;* of the nature of *sclerema.*

Sclĕr-en-çe-pha'lĭ-a.* [From σκληρός, "hard," and ἐγκέφαλον, the "brain."] Induration of the substance of the brain.

Scle-ri'a-sis.* [From σκληρός, "hard."] An induration, or hard tumor; a scirrhus.

Sclĕr'o-gen. [From σκληρός, "hard," and γένω, to "be born," to "be produced."] The same as LIGNINE, which see.

Scle-rog'e-nus.* [From σκληρός, "hard," and γεννάω, to "produce."] Making hard; hardening or thickening.

Scle-ro'ma, atis.* [From σκληρόω, to "harden."] Properly, a hard tumor. Applied to an induration of the cellular tissue, arteries, integuments, &c.

Sclĕr-o-me'ninx.* [From σκληρός, "hard," and μῆνιγξ, a "membrane."] Literally, the "hard or tough membrane." A name for the DURA MATER, which see.

Sclĕr-oph-thăl'mĭ-a.* [From σκληρός, "hard," and ὀφθαλμός, an "eye."] Protrusion of the eyeball. Inflammation of the eye, attended with hardness.

Sclĕr-o-phyl'lus.* [From σκληρός, "hard," and φύλλον, a "leaf."] Having rigid or stiff leaves.

Sclĕr'o-pus.* [From σκληρός, "hard," and πούς, a "foot."] Having the foot or *stipes* very hard.

Sclĕr-o-sar-co'ma, atis.* [From σκληρός, "hard," and σάρκωμα, a "fleshy tumor."] A hard, fleshy excrescence.

Scle-ro'sis.* The progress of *scleroma.* Virchow defines the term to be "thickening with condensation."

Scle-ro'tal. [**Sclerota'lis;** from σκληρός, "hard."] Applied by Owen to the cartilaginous or osseous parts of the sclerotic coat of the eye.

Scle-rot'ic. [**Sclerot'icus;** from σκληρόω, to "harden."] Hard; tough.

Sclerot'ic Coat. [**Tu'nica Sclerot'ica.**] The same as SCLEROTICA, which see.

Scle-rot'ĭ-ca.* [From *sclerot'icus,* "hard."] The hard, dense, fibrous membrane of the eye, which with the cornea forms the external coat or tunic of that organ; sometimes called the *white of the eye.*

Scle-ro'tis.* A name for the SCLEROTICA, which see.

Scle-ro-ti'tis, idis.* [From *sclero'tis.*] Inflammation of the sclerotic coat of the eye.

Sco-bic'u-lar. [**Scobicula'ris;** from *scobs, sco'bis,* "sawdust."] The same as SCOBIFORM.

Scob'ĭ-form. [**Scobifor'mis;** from the same.] Applied to seeds that are fine as sawdust.

Scobs,* gen. **Sco'bis.** Any powder or dust produced by sawing, filing, &c. Also, the scoria of any metal.

Scol'e-coid. [**Scolecoi'des;** from σκώληξ, a "worm," and εἶδος, a "form."] Resembling a worm; vermiform.

Scol-e-col'o-ġy̆. [**Scolecolo'gia;** from σκώληξ, a "worm," and λόγος, a "discourse."] A treatise upon worms; the science of worms.

Sco-lĭ-o'ma, atis.* [Gr. σκολίωμα; from σκολιόω, to "crook," to "bend."] A bend or curve. Applied to a morbid curvature of the spine.

Sco-lĭ-o'sis.* [Gr. σκολίωσις; from the same.] A distortion of the spine. The progress or formation of *scolioma.*

Sco-lĭ-ot'ic. [**Scoliot'icus.**] Belonging to *scoliosis.*

Scolloped. See CRENATE, and SCALLOPED.

Sco-pa'rĭ-um.* The Pharmacopœial name (Ed. and Dub. Ph.) for the tops of *Cytisus scoparius.* See next article.

Sco-pa'rĭ-us.* [From *sco'pæ,* a "broom."] Broom. The Pharmacopœial name ‖ for the fresh tops of the *Cytisus scoparius,* otherwise termed the *Spartium scoparium,* and *Sarotham'mus scopa'rius.* Broom is diuretic and cathartic, and has often proved useful as a remedy in dropsy.

Scor'a-mis.* [From σκῶρ, "ordure."] A night-stool, or night-chair.

Scor-bu'tic. [**Scorbu'ticus.**] Relating to *scorbutus,* or scurvy, or affected with scurvy.

Scor-bu'tus.* The scurvy, a disease characterized by heaviness, dejection of spirits, bloated countenance, livid spots on the skin, offensive breath, spongy gums, with occasional hæmorrhage from the mouth and nostrils, swelling of the legs, etc. A genus of the order *Impetigines,* class *Cachexiæ,* of Cullen's Nosology; also termed *Porphyra.*

Sco'rĭ-a,* plural **Sco'rĭ-æ.** [From σκῶρ, "excrement."] Properly, the dross of melted metals. Usually applied to volcanic cinders.

Sco-rĭ-ā'ceous. [**Scoria'ceus.**] Relating to, or like, *scoria.*

Scoriæ. See SCORIA.

Sco'rĭ-form. [**Scorifor'mis;** from *sco'ria.*] Having the character or appearance of scoriæ.

Scor'pĭ-oid. [**Scorpioi'des;** from σκορπίος, a "scorpion," and εἶδος, a "form."]

Resembling a scorpion; coiled round like a scorpion, as the branches of the cyme of the Heliotrope.

Sco-tas'ma, atis.* [From σκοτάζω, to "darken."] Dimness of sight.

Scotch-Fid'dle. A vulgar term for *scabies.*

Sco-to'ma,* plural **Sco-to'ma-ta.** [From σκότος, "darkness."] Darkness before the eyes; obscurity of vision; an affection symptomatic of various diseases.

Scott's Aç'id Bath. A bath of diluted aqua regia, employed by Dr. Scott as a remedy for jaundice. The aqua regia should be compounded of three parts in measure of muriatic acid, and two of nitric acid; and in preparing them for use, a pint of the combined acid is to be mixed with a pint of water. The acid bath is to consist of three ounces of this diluted acid to every gallon of water.

Scro-bic'u-late. [**Scrobicula'tus;** from *scrobic'ulus,* a "ditch," or "cavity."] Pitted; marked with pits or cavities.

Scro-bic-u-lo'sus.* [From the same.] Synonymous with SCROBICULATE.

Scro-bic'u-lus.* [Diminutive of *scrobs,* a "ditch."] A little ditch; a pit or hollow.

Scrobic'ulus Cor'dis.* (Literally, the "Pit of the Heart.") The hollow part near the region of the heart; the pit of the stomach.

Scrof'u-la,* written also **Scroph'u-la.*** [From *scro'fa,* a "sow;" because swine are, it is said, sometimes affected with a similar disease.] (Fr. *Scrofules,* skro'fül', and *Écrouelles,* à'kroo'ēll'.) The king's evil. A disease characterized chiefly by chronic swelling of absorbent glands, particularly of the neck, behind the ears, and under the chin, tending slowly to imperfect suppuration. A genus of the order *Impetigines,* class *Cachexiæ,* of Cullen's Nosology; also termed *Struma.*

Scrof-u-lo'sis.* The morbid condition or progress of scrofula.

Scrof'u-lous. [**Scrofulo'sus.**] Having scrofula; of the nature of scrofula.

Scroph'u-la.* The same as SCROFULA, which see.

Scroph-u-la'ri-a No-do'sa.* The systematic name of the figwort, a plant of the natural order *Scrophulariaceæ.*

Scrophulariaceæ,* skrof-u-la-re-a'she-ē. [From *Scrophula'ria,* one of the genera.] A natural order of exogenous plants (herbs or shrubs), found in all parts of the world, except the coldest. They are allied to *Solanaceæ,* and are generally acrid and bitterish. Some of them are poisonous. It includes the *Digita'lis* (Foxglove) and *Calceola'ria.*

Scroph-u-la'ri-æ,* the plural of *Scrophula'ria,* forming the Jussieuan name of an order of plants. See SCROPHULARIACEÆ.

Scroph-u-lo'sis.* The same as SCROFULOSIS.

Scro'tal. [**Scrota'lis.**] Relating to the scrotum.

Scro'tal Her'ni-a. [**Her'nia Scrota'lis,** or **Her'nia Scro'ti.**] The protrusion of a part or parts of the viscera, into the scrotum; termed also *Oscheocele,* and *Scrotocele.*

Scro'ti-form. [**Scrotifor'mis;** from *scro'tum,* a "bag," or "pouch."] Pouch-shaped.

Scro'to-çēle.* [From *scro'tum,* and κήλη, a "tumor."] The same as SCROTAL HERNIA, which see.

Scro'tum,* gen. **Scro'ti.** (Literally, a "bag," or "pouch.") The common integuments which enclose the testicles as in a bag, or pouch.

Scru'ple. [**Scru'pulus;** diminutive of *scru'pus,* a "little stone."] A weight of twenty grains. See GRAMMA.

Scurf. [**Fur'fur, uris.**] Small exfoliations of the cuticle, or branlike scales which occur on the scalp or skin, after some cutaneous eruptions; dandriff. In Botany, applied to minute or branlike scales on the epidermis.

Scurvy. See SCORBUTUS.

Scu'tate. [**Scuta'tus;** from *scu'tum,* a "shield."] Shield-shaped. Applied in Zoology to a surface protected by large scales.

Scu-tel'la,* or **Scu-tel'lum.*** [Diminutive of *scu'tum,* a "shield"?] Literally, a "platter." Applied to a species of fructification, orbicular, concave, and raised at the margin, as in some lichens. Also, a small triangular piece on the back of the *mesothorax,* between the *elytra,* or the wings of insects.

Scu-tel'læ,* the plural of SCUTELLA, which see.

Scu-tel-la'ri-a.* Scullcap. The Pharmacopœial name (U.S. Ph.) for the herb of the *Scutella'ria lateriflo'ra.* It is reputed an efficacious nervine.

Scu'tel-late. [**Scutella'tus;** from *scutel'la,* "a platter."] Applied to a lichen that is covered with *scutellæ.* Having conceptacles formed like *scutellæ.*

Scu-tel′lĭ-form. [**Scutellifor′mis;** from *scutel′la*, a "platter."] Formed like a platter.

Scu-tel-lo-i′dēs.* [From *scutel′la*, a "platter," and εἶδος, a "form."] Resembling a *scutella*.

Scu-tĭ-bran-chĭ-a′tus.* [From *scu′tum*, a "shield," and *branchiæ*.] Applied in the plural neuter (*Scutobranchia′ta*) to an order of *Gasterop′oda*, in which the shell covers the animal, and particularly the *branchiæ*, like a shield.

Scu′tĭ-form. [**Scutifor′mis;** from *scu′tum*, a "shield."] Resembling a shield in form.

Scu′tĭ-ped. [**Scu′tipes, p′e**dis; from *scu′tum*, a "shield," and *pes*, a "foot."] Literally, "shield-footed." Applied to a family of birds having the forepart of the legs covered with segments of unequal horny rings, ending on each side in a groove.

Scu′toid. [**Scutoi′des;** from *scu′tum*, a "shield."] Resembling a shield; scutiform.

Sçȳb′a-lum,* plural **Sçȳb′a-la.** [From σκύβαλον, "ordure."] Dry, hard excrement that has formed into little rounded balls like sheep's dung, or somewhat larger.

Sçȳ′phĭ-form. [**Scyphifor′mis;** from σκύφος, a "cup."] Formed like a cup or goblet.

Sçy-pho-i′dēs.* [From σκύφος, a "cup," and εἶδος, a "form."] Resembling a cup: scy′phoid.

Scytoblasta. See Scytoblastema.

Sçy-to-blas-te′ma, a*tis*.* [From σκῦτος, a "skin," and βλάστημα, a "growth."] The organic growth or development of the skin; also of the *exanthemata*.

Sçy-to-blas-te′sis.* The progress of *scytoblastema*.

Se De-fen-den′do.* ("In Defending Oneself.") Applied in Medical Jurisprudence to a species of *excusable* homicide, the consequence of a lawful act done in self-preservation.

Seam. See Suture.

Sea-On′ion. The *Scil′la marit′ima*, or squill.

Search′ing. The operation of introducing a metallic instrument through the urethra into the bladder, to ascertain the presence of a calculus.

Sea-Salt. The chloride of sodium, obtained from sea-water. See Sodii Chloridum.

Sea-Sick′ness. [**Nau′sea Mari′na.**] A distressing kind of sickness, accompanied with vomiting, generally experienced at sea by those who are as yet unused to the motion of the vessel. After one has become somewhat accustomed to a sea-life, it usually abates, or ceases altogether; but there are those who, though almost constantly at sea, are always liable to a return of this affection whenever the water is unusually agitated.

Se-bā′ceous. [**Seba′ceus;** from *se′bum*, or *se′vum*, "suet."] (Fr. *Sébacé*, så′bå′så′.) Fatty; suety. Applied to glands which secrete an oily matter resembling suet.

Se-baç′ic. [**Sebaç′icus;** from *se′bum*, "suet," or "tallow."] Applied to an acid obtained from suet and other oils.

Se′bāte. [**Se′bas, a′***tis*.] A combination of sebacic acid with a base.

Se-bĭf′er-ous. [**Sebif′erus;** from *se′bum*, "suet," or "tallow," and *fe′ro*, to "bear."] Bearing or producing fat or oil. Applied to certain plants.

Se-bip′a-rous. [**Sebip′arus;** from *se′bum*, "tallow," and *pa′rio*, to "produce," or "bear."] Producing, forming, or secreting fat or oil.

Sebum. See Sevum.

Se-ca′le.* [From *se′co*, to "cut."] (Fr. *Seigle*, sĕgl or sågl.) Rye. A Linnæan genus of the class *Triandria*, natural order *Graminaceæ*.

Seca′le Ce-re-a′le.* The systematic name of common rye.

Seca′le Cor-nu′tum.* ("Horned, or Spurred, Rye.") The ergot of rye; a diseased growth, or excrescence, on the *Secale cereale*, black, and curved like the spur of a fowl. See Ergota.

Sec′a-lin. [**Secali′na.**] The gluten of the *Secale cereale*.

Sec-a-li′nus.* Belonging to the *Secale cereale*, or to the *Secale cornutum*.

Se′cant. [**Se′cans;** from *se′co*, to "cut."] "Cutting." Applied to a right line drawn from the centre of a circle to one extremity of an arc, and produced until it meets the tangent to the other extremity.

Se-cer′nent. [**Secer′nens,** or **Secreto′rius;** from *secer′no*, to "separate," or "secrete."] (Fr. *Sécrétoire*, så′krå′twar′.) Literally, "separating," and, hence, "secreting." Applied to those vessels whose function is to separate materials from the blood, either for the reproduction of the several parts of the body, or for the purpose of throwing off effete matter from the system.

Sec′ond In-ten′tion. Healing or

closing of wounds by the second intention means a cure by the processes of suppuration, granulation, and cicatrization. See FIRST INTENTION.

Second Pair (of Nerves). See OPTIC NERVE.

Sec'on-da-rў. [From *secun'dus*, "second," "inferior."] Second in order of time or place; inferior in importance, subordinate: hence, supervening, as, *secondary symptoms* of a disease; those which supervene on the primary.

Sec'ondary. Applied to a quill attached to the forearm, or second portion of the wings, of birds.

Sec'ondary Fe'ver. The fébrile condition ensuing after a crisis, or after the discharge of some morbid matter.

Sec'ondary Rocks or **Stra'ta.** A series of stratified rocks, between the primary and lowest tertiary strata.

Secondary Syphilis. See SYPHILIS.

Se-cre'ta.* [Plural of *secre'tum*, any thing secreted.] The secretions, as milk, saliva, bile, etc. See SECRETION.

Se-cre'tion. [**Secre'tio, o'***nis;* from *secer'no, secre'tum*, to "separate," or "secrete."] A natural function of the body, by which various fluids or substances are separated from the blood, differing in different organs according to their peculiar function: thus, the liver secretes the bile, the salivary glands the saliva, the kidneys the urine, etc. The term secretion is also applied to the thing secreted from the blood of an animal or the sap of a plant.

Sécrétoire. See SECERNENT.

Se-cre'to-rў, or **Se'cre-to-rў.** [**Secreto'rius.**] The same as SECERNENT, which see.

Sec'tile. [**Sec'tilis;** from *se'co, sec'tum*, to "cut."] Capable of being cut.

Sec'tio (sek'she-o) **Ca-dav'e-ris.*** ("Cutting of a Dead Body.") The dissection of a dead body: usually applied to an autopsy, or post-mortem examination.

Sectio Cæsarea. See CÆSAREAN SECTION.

Sec'tio Nўm-pha'rum.* ("Cutting of the Nymphæ.") See NYMPHOTOMY.

Sec'tion. [**Sec'tio, o'***nis;* from *se'co, sec'tum*, to "cut."] A cutting; dissection. A line made by the intersection of two planes; also, the surface formed when a solid body is cut by a plane.

Se'cund. [From *se'quor*, to "follow:" because one part seems to follow the course or example of the other.] Having all the parts turned to the same side of the axis. Applied to certain flowers, or other organs of plants.

Sec'un-dine, or **Se-cun'dine.** [**Secun'dina;** from *secun'dus*, "second."] The second or inner coat of the ovule of a plant. Applied in the plural to the afterbirth, because expelled after the fœtus.

Secundines. See SECUNDINE.

Se-cun'dum.* [From *se'quor*, to "follow."] A Latin term signifying "following," or "according to."

Se-cun'dum Ar'tem.* ("According to Art.") That is, "according to the most approved method."

Se-cu-rif'er-us.* [From *secu'ris*, an "axe," and *fe'ro*, to "bear."] Applied to certain insects provided with an instrument for cutting or preparing a place in which to deposit their eggs. Also, the same as SECURIGEROUS.

Se-cu'ri-form. [**Securifor'mis;** from *secu'ris*, an "axe."] Shaped like an axe.

Se-cu-rig'er-ous. [**Securig'erus;** from *secu'ris*, an "axe," and *ge'ro*, to "bear."] Bearing an axe, or what resembles an axe or hatchet. Applied to certain plants.

Sed. = *Se'des.** "A stool."

Sedantia. See SEDATIVES.

Se-da'tion. [**Seda'tio, o'***nis;* from *se'do, seda'tum*, to "allay."] The act of calming; the action of a sedative.

Sed'a-tive. [**Sedati'vus;** from the same.] Allaying irritability or excitement.

Sed'a-tives. [**Sedati'va,** and **Sedan'tia.**] Medicines which by their immediate influence diminish vital action. Some, being more especially directed to the circulatory system, are termed *arterial* sedatives; while others, exerting a direct influence on the nervous system, are called *nervous* sedatives.

Sed-en-ta'ri-a Os'sa.* ("Sedentary Bones.") Applied to the bones on which we sit, the *Os ischii* and *Os coccygis*.

Sed'en-ta-rў. [**Sedenta'rius;** from *se'deo*, to "sit."] Sitting habitually; requiring a sitting posture.

Sedes. See STOOL.

Sed'i-ment. [**Sedimen'tum;** from *se'deo*, to "remain," or "settle."] The particles in liquids which by their weight fall to the bottom.

Sed-i-men'ta-rў. [From the same.] Relating to, or formed by, sediment. Applied to stratified rocks formed of materials deposited from a state of suspension in water,—*i.e.* to all rocks except those of igneous origin.

Sed'litz Pow'der. A compound of

Rochelle salt, carbonate of soda, and tartaric acid, which, dissolved in water, forms an effervescing aperient liquid in imitation of Sedlitz water. See PULVERES EFFERVESCENTES APERIENTES.

Se'dum A'cre.* ("Acrid Sedum.") The systematic name of the small houseleek, a plant of the Linnæan class *Decandria*, natural order *Crassulaceæ*. It is emetic and cathartic.

Seed. [Lat. **Se'men;** Gr. σπέρμα; Fr. *Semence*, sẹh-mŏnss'.] The seed of a plant is a body produced by the agency of a flower, containing a ready-formed plantlet or germ, called the embryo. The seed, like the ovule, of which it is the fertilized and matured state, consists of a *nucleus*, or kernel, usually enclosed in two integuments, viz.: the TESTA (or Episperm), and the TEGMEN, which see. See also SEMEN.

Seed-Bud. See GERMEN, and GERM.

Seed-Coat. See ARIL.

Seed-Down. See PAPPUS.

Seed-Lobe. See COTYLEDON.

Seed-Vessel. See PERICARP.

Seeing. See VISION.

Seg'ment. [**Segmen'tum;** from *se'co*, to "cut."] A section: a part cut out of something; one of the divisions or lobes of a leaf or other organ of a plant. The segment of a circle is the part of its area comprised between a chord and the arc which it subtends.

Seg're-gāt-ed, or **Seg're-gate.** [**Segrega'tus;** from *seg'rego*, *segrega'tum*, to "separate from the flock."] Separated; insulated.

Seidlitz Powder. See SEDLITZ POWDER.

Seigle. See SECALE.

Seignette's (sàn-yetts') **Salt.** The same as Rochelle salt, which was discovered by Seignette, of Rochelle.

Sel. The French word for SALT, which see.

Selaginaceæ,* se-laj-e-na'she-ē. A natural order of exogenous plants, found in Europe and at the Cape of Good Hope. It includes the *Sela'go*.

Se-le'nĭ-āte. [**Sele'nias, a'***tis*.] A combination of selenic acid with a base.

Se-len'ic. [**Selen'icus.**] Belonging to selenium. Applied to an acid obtained from it.

Sel-e-nif'er-ous. [**Selenif'erus;** from *sele'nium*, and *fe'ro*, to "bear."] Containing selenium.

Se-le'nĭ-ous. [**Selenio'sus.**] Applied to an acid, the second degree of oxidation of selenium.

Se-le'nīte. [**Sele'nis, i'***tis*.] A combination of selenious acid with a base.

Sel'e-nīte. [**Seleni'tes;** from σελήνη, the "moon," and λίθος, a "stone:" named on account of its silvery lustre.] A species of *La'pis specula'ris*, or transparent sulphate of lime.

Sel-e-nit'ic. [**Selenit'icus.**] Applied to waters which hold in solution selenite, or sulphate of lime.

Se-le'nĭ-um.* [From σελήνη, the "moon." See TELLURIUM.] A non-metallic elementary body which resembles sulphur in chemical properties. It is brittle, opaque, tasteless, insoluble in water and unaltered by air.

Seleniuret, se-lĕn'yu-ret. [**Seleniure'tum.**] A compound of selenium with a simple body.

Sel-e-nog'ra-phȳ. [**Selenogra'phia;** from σελήνη, the "moon," and γράφω, to "write."] A description of the surface of the moon.

Sel-e-no-to-pog'ra-phȳ. [**Selenotopogra'phia;** from σελήνη, the "moon," τόπος, a "place," and γράφω, to "write."] A description of the places on the surface of the moon. See TOPOGRAPHY.

Se-li'bra,* or **Sem-ĭ-li'bra.*** [From *se'mis*, "half," and *li'bra*, a "pound."] Half a pound.

Sel'la Tur'çĭ-ca.* (Fr. *Selle Turcique*, sĕll tür'sèk'.) ("Turkish Saddle.") The small depression within the four clinoid processes of the sphenoid bone, on which the pituitary gland rests.

Sem. = *Se'men*,* "seed," or *Sem'ina*,* "seeds."

Se-meī-og'ra-phȳ. [**Semeiogra'phia;** from σημεῖον, a "sign," or "symptom," and γράφω, to "write."] A description of the signs of disease.

Se-meī-ol'o-ġȳ. [**Semeiolo'gia;** from σημεῖον, a "sign," or "symptom," and λόγος, a "discourse."] That branch of Medicine which treats of the signs or symptoms of disease; symptomatology; symbology.

Se-meī-o'sis.* [From σημειόω, to "mark."] Applied to the observation of the signs or symptoms of disease.

Se-meī-ot'ic. [**Semeiot'icus;** from *semeiot'ice*.] Belonging to the signs or symptoms of diseases.

Se-meī-ot'ics. [**Semeiot'ica,** or **Semeiot'ice;** from σημειόω, to "mark with a sign."] That branch of Medicine which treats of the signs or symptoms of diseases. See SEMEIOSIS.

Se'men,* plural **Sem'ĭ-na.** [From *se'ro*, *se'vi*, to "sow."] (Fr. *Semence*, sęh mŏnss'.) The seed of a plant. (See SEED.) Also, the seminal liquor secreted in the testicles of animals. See SPERMATOZOON.

Se'men Con'trạ.* An abbreviation of SEMEN CONTRA VERMES, which see.

Se'men con'trạ Ver'mēs.* ("Seed against Worms.") A mixture often kept in the shops on the European Continent, as a vermifuge. It consists of the unexpanded flowers of different species of *Artemisia*, mixed occasionally with the seeds.

Se'men Sanc'tum.* ("Holy Seed:" so named on account of its supposed virtues.) The seed of *Artemisia santonica*.

Semen, Slow Emission of. See BRADYSPERMATISMUS.

Semence. See SEED, and SEMEN.

Sem'i-. [From *se'mis*, "half."] A prefix denoting half.

Sem-ĭ-cir'cu-lạr Ca-nāls'. Three canals, of a form indicated by their name, in the petrous portion of the temporal bone, and opening into the *vestibulum*.

Sem-ĭ-cor'date. [From *se'mis*, "half," and *cor*, *cor'dis*, a "heart."] Half heart-shaped (divided lengthwise).

Sem-ĭ-cu'pĭ-um.* [From *se'mis*, and *cu'bo*, to "lie down."] A half-bath, or hip-bath.

Semidr. = *Semidrach'ma.** "Half a drachm."

Sem-ĭ-flos'cu-lạr. [From *se'mis*, "half," and *flos*, a "flower."] Applied to a head of flowers whose petals are ligulate.

Semih. = *Semiho'ra.** "Half an hour."

Sem-ĭ-lu'nạr. [**Semiluna'ris;** from *se'mis*, a "half," and *lu'na*, the "moon."] Resembling a half-moon, or crescent.

Semilu'nar Gan'glĭ-ạ. The ganglia formed on the sympathetic nerve as it enters the abdomen, from which nerves are distributed to the viscera; the abdominal ganglia.

Semilu'nar Valves. [**Val'vulæ Semiluna'res.**] The three valves at the commencement of the aorta; also applied to the same number at the beginning of the pulmonary artery.

Sem-ĭ-lu'nate. The same as SEMILUNAR, which see.

Sem-ĭ-mem-bra-no'sus.* [From *sem'is*, a "half," and *membra'na*, a "membrane."] ("Half-membranous [Muscle].") A muscle arising from the *tuber ischii* and inserted into the head of the tibia and into the lower part of the femur. It bends the leg.

Sem'ĭ-nạ,* gen. **Sem'ĭ-num,** the plural of SEMEN, a "seed."

Sem'ĭ-nạl. [**Semina'lis;** from *se'men*, a "seed."] Belonging to seed, or the semen; relating to seed.

Seminal Air. See AURA SEMINALIS.

Sem-ĭ-nā'tion. [**Semina'tio, o'nis;** from *se'men*, a "seed," or the "semen."] Literally, the "act of sowing seed." The natural dispersion of seeds; also, the immission of the semen *in uterum*.

Sem-ĭ-nif'er-ous. [**Seminif'erus;** from *se'men*, "seed," and *fe'ro*, to "bear."] Bearing seeds; also, conveying the seminal fluid.

Se-min'ĭ-form. [**Seminifor'mis;** from *se'men*, "seed."] Having the appearance of seed.

Se-min'u-lạ,* or **Se-min'u-lum.*** [Diminutive of *se'men*, "seed."] Often applied to the reproductive corpuscles of cryptogamous plants.

Sem-ĭ-or-bic'u-lạr. [From *sem'i*, "half," and *or'bis*, an "orb," or "circle."] Half-round; semicircular.

Sem-ĭ-o'vate. [From *sem'i*, "half," and *ova'tus*, "ovate."] Like the half of an ovate figure divided longitudinally.

Se'mis,* or **Se-mis'sis.*** The half of any thing. See SS.

Sem-ĭ-sep'tate. [From *se'mis*, a "half," and *sep'tum*, a "partition."] In Botany, having a partition reaching partly across.

Sem-ĭ-Spi-na'lēs.* [From *se'mis*, "half," and *spi'na*, a "spinous process;" because they are attached half to the spinous and half to the transverse processes.] Two muscles connected with the transverse and spinous processes of the vertebræ, and termed respectively *semispina'lis col'li*, and *semispina'lis dor'si*.

Semissis. See SEMIS.

Sem-ĭ-ten-dĭ-no'sus.* ("Semitendinous [Muscle].") The name of a muscle arising from the *tuber ischii* and inserted into the anterior tuberosity of the tibia. It bends the leg.

Sem'ĭ-te-rete. [From *sem'i*, "half," and *te'res*, "long and round."] Half cylindrical. Applied to plants.

Sem-per-vī'rent. [From *sem'per*, "always," and *vi'rens*, the present participle of *vi'reo*, to "be green."] Evergreen.

Sem-per-vi'væ.* [From *sem'per*, "always," and *vi'vus*, "alive," or "living."] The Jussieuan name of a natural order of plants. See CRASSULACEÆ.

Séné. See SENNA.

Sen'e-cạ Oil. A name given to a variety of petroleum obtained on or near Seneca Lake, in the State of New York.

It has been much used as an external application in rheumatism.

Sene'cio (se-ne'she-o) **Vul-ga'ris.*** Groundsel. A plant of the natural order *Compositæ.* It is emetic in large doses, but is seldom used. It is sometimes applied externally to painful swellings and ulcers.

Se-nec'tus, u'*tis.** [From *se'nex,* "old."] (Fr. *Vieillesse,* ve-à'yĕss'.) Old age; usually reckoned from about the sixtieth year.

Sen'e-gạ.* [From *Sen'egal.*] Seneka. The Pharmacopœial ‖ name for the root of *Polyg'ala Sen'ega.* It is a stimulating expectorant and diuretic. It was formerly regarded as a remedy for the bite of the rattlesnake, whence the popular name *snake-root.*

Sen'e-ġin. [**Senegi'na.**] An alkaline principle obtained from the root of *Polygala senega.*

Se-nĕs'çence. [**Senescen'tia;** from *senes'co,* to "grow old."] The state or progress of growing old.

Sénevé, sȧn'vȧ', or sȧ'nẹh-vȧ'. A French name for mustard. See SINAPIS.

Se'nīle. [**Seni'lis;** from *se'nex,* "old;" also, an "old man."] Of or belonging to old age; old: as, *Ætas senilis* ("old age"), *Arcus senilis* ("bow of old age"). See ARCUS SENILIS.

Sen'nạ.* (Fr. *Séné,* sȧ'nȧ'.) The Pharmacopœial name (U.S. Ph.) for the leaflets of *Cassia acutifolia, C. obovata,* and *C. elongata.* Senna is a prompt, efficient, and safe purgative, and is well adapted to those affections in which a decided but not violent impression is desired.

Sen'na Al-ex-an-dri'nạ.* ("Alexandrine Senna.") The Pharmacopœial name (Br. Ph.) for the leaves of various species of *Cassia.*

Sen'na, A-mer'ĭ-cạn. A name for the *Cassia Marilandica.*

Sen'na In'dĭ-cạ.* ("Indian Senna.") The Pharmacopœial name for the leaves of the *Cassia elongata* (Br. Ph.), or *C. officinalis* (Lond. Ph.). See SENNA.

Se-noc'u-late. [**Senocula'tus;** from *se'ni,* "six," and *oc'ulus,* an "eye."] Having six eyes.

Sen-sā'tion. [**Sensa'tio, o'***nis;* from *sen'tio, sen'sum,* to "perceive," to "think," or "feel."] The consciousness of an impression made by an external body on the organs of sense; the immediate effect produced on the mind by the contact of an external object with the nerves of sensation.

Sensations, Diseases affecting the. See ÆSTHETIC.

Sense. [**Sen'sus;** from *sen'tio, sen'sum,* to "perceive," to "think," or "feel."] A faculty by which the properties or conditions of external things are perceived. There are usually reckoned five senses: viz., sight, hearing (or audition), taste, touch, and smell, which will be noticed under their proper heads.

Sen-sĭ-bil'ĭ-tȳ. [**Sensibil'itas, a'***tis;* from the same.] That faculty by which the brain perceives an impression made upon it; the power by which living parts receive impressions from the different bodies placed in contact with them.

Sen'sĭ-ble. [**Sensib'ilis;** from the same.] Capable of sensation; perceptible by the senses; capable of exciting sensation.

Sen'sĭ-tĭve. [**Sensiti'vus;** from the same.] Endowed with feeling; easily affected; sentient.

Sen'sitive Plant. A name for the *Mimo'sa pudi'ca,* a small annual plant, remarkable for the irritability or spontaneous motion of its pinnate leaflets, which collapse and fold up when touched, or when irritated by casting on them the focus of a burning-glass. A similar change takes place on the approach of night, when the plant seems to go to sleep.

Sen-so'rĭ-ạl. [**Sensoria'lis;** from *senso'rium,* "centre of sensation," the "brain."] Belonging to the sensorium.

Sen-so'rĭ-um.* [From *sen'tio, sen'sum,* to "perceive," or "feel."] Centre of sensation; the brain; also, the collection of ganglia at the base of the brain.

Senso'rium Com-mu'ne.* ("Common Sensorium.") The common seat or centre of all the senses, where the nerves proper to the different organs of sense take their origin. Applied to the brain.

Sen'so-rȳ. [**Senso'rius;** from *sen'sus,* "sense."] A term applied to those nerves which convey impressions to the neural axis, as distinguished from the motory nerves.

Sentient, sen'she-ent. [**Sen'tiens;** from *sen'tio,* to "perceive," or "feel."] Having sensation or feeling. That which is particularly susceptible of sensation, as the extremities of the nerves.

Sentimentalism. See ALUSIA, and ELATIO.

Se'pạl. [**Sep'alum;** from *se'par,* "divided"?] A division or leaf of a calyx.

Sep'ạ-līne, or **Sep'ạ-lous.** [From *sep'alum,* a "sepal."] Relating to sepals.

Sep'ạ-loid. [**Sepaloi'des;** from

sep'alum, a "sepal," and εἶδος, a "form."] Resembling a sepal.

Sep'a-răt-ed Flow'ers. When stamens and pistils occupy separate flowers, these are called *separated*.

Sep'a-ra-to-rȳ. [**Separato'rium;** from *sep'aro, separa'tum*, to "separate."] A vessel used for separating fluids of different densities, or liquors from the materials with which they have been mixed, or the essential from the less important parts. Also, an instrument for separating the pericranium from the skull, in post-mortem examinations or dissections.

Se'pĭ-a.* A pigment prepared from a black juice secreted by the glands of the *Sepia*, or cuttle-fish, which the animal ejects to darken the water and conceal itself from its enemies. This juice was used as ink by the ancients. It forms a beautiful brown pigment with a fine grain. See next article.

Se'pĭ-a-dæ.* [From *Se'pia*, the "cuttle-fish."] A family of Mollusks of the cuttle-fish tribe. They belong to the order CEPHALOPODA, which see.

Sep'ta,* gen. **Sep-to'rum,** the plural of SEPTUM, which see.

Sep-tæ'mĭ-a.* [From σηπτός, "putrid," and αἷμα, "blood."] A morbid state of the blood, caused by septic or putrid matters received into the circulation. Essentially the same as ICHORÆMIA.

Sep'tate. [From *sep'tum*, a "partition."] Having a partition. Applied to pericarps.

Sep-tem-an-gu-la'tus.* [From *sep'tem*, "seven," and *an'gulus*, an "angle."] Having seven prominent angles.

Sep-tem-den'tate. [**Septemdenta'tus;** from *sep'tem*, "seven," and *dens*, a "tooth."] Having seven teeth. Applied to certain animals.

Sep-tem-lo'bate. [**Septemloba'tus;** from *sep'tem*, "seven," and *lo'bus*, a "lobe."] Having seven lobes.

Sep-tem-ner'vis.* [From *sep'tem*, "seven," and *ner'vus*, a "nerve."] Having seven nerves.

Sep'te-nate. [**Septena'tus;** from *septe'ni*, "seven," "by sevens."] Disposed in sevens.

Sep-ten'trĭ-o-nal. [**Septentriona'lis,** or **Septentriona'rius;** from *septen'trio*, the "north."] Northern; that which grows in or inhabits the north or northern countries.

Septfoil. See TORMENTILLA.

Septhæmia. See SEPTÆMIA.

Sep'tic. [**Sep'ticus;** from σήπω, to "putrefy."] Tending to putrefy; causing putrefaction.

Sep-tĭ-cī'dal. [**Septici'dus;** from *sep'tum*, a "fence," a "partition," and *cæ'do*, to "cut."] Dehiscent by the partitions,—*i.e.* along the lines of junction. Applied to the capsules of plants.

Sep-tif'er-ous. [**Septif'erus;** from *sep'tum*, a "partition," and *fe'ro*, to "bear."] Bearing or having septa.

Sep'tĭ-form. [**Septifor'mis;** from *sep'tum*, a "partition."] Formed like a septum.

Sep-tif'ra-gal. [**Septif'ragus;** from *sep'tum*, a "partition," and *fran'go*, to "break."] Septifragal dehiscence is a modification of either the loculicidal, or septicidal, in which the valves fall away, leaving the dissepiments attached to the axis.

Sep'tĭ-lis.* [From *sep'tum*, a "partition."] Applied to the *placentarium* when attached to the septa: sep'tile.

Sep-tu-la'tus.* [From *sep'tulum*, a "little septum."] Having *septula*.

Sep-tu-lif'er-ous. [**Septu'lifer,** or **Septulif'erus;** from *sep'tulum*, a "little septum," and *fe'ro*, to "bear."] Bearing *septula*.

Sep'tu-lum,* plural **Sep'tu-la.** [Diminutive of *sep'tum*, a "partition."] A "little septum." Applied to a lamina which divides the anther of the Orchids into two cavities.

Sep'tum,* plural **Sep'ta.** [From *se'pio, sep'tum*, to "enclose," to "fence in."] A Latin word signifying a "fence," "partition," or "enclosure." In Botany, a dissepiment. Also applied to bony, cartilaginous, or membranous partitions in the human body.

Sep'tum Au-ric-u-la'rum.* ("Partition of the Auricles.") The partition which separates the right from the left auricle of the heart.

Sep'tum Cĕr-e-bel'li.* ("Partition of the Cerebellum.") The process of the *dura mater* dividing the *cerebellum* perpendicularly into symmetrical halves.

Sep'tum Cĕr'e-bri.* ("Partition of the Brain, or Cerebrum.") The falciform process of the *dura mater*.

Sep'tum Cor'dis.* ("Partition of the Heart.") The septum or partition between the ventricles of the heart.

Sep'tum Lu'cĭ-dum.* ("Pellucid Septum.") A thin triangular partition between the lateral ventricles of the brain.

Sep'tum Na'rĭ-um.* ("Partition of the Nostrils.") The partition between the nostrils.

Sep'tum Pec-tin-ĭ-for'me.* ("Comb-like Partition.") An imperfect tendinous septum separating the *crura* of the penis.

Sep'tum Scro'ti.* ("Partition of the Scrotum.") A partition formed by the dartos, dividing the scrotum into two equal cavities and separating the testes.

Sep'tum Trans-ver'sum.* ("Transverse Partition.") The diaphragm, which separates the thorax from the abdomen. This term is also applied to the *tentorium cerebelli.*

Sep'tum Ven-tric-u-lo'rum.* ("Partition of the Ventricles.") The partition which separates the right from the left ventricle of the heart.

Seq. Luce = *Sequen'ti Lu'ce.** "The following day."

Se-que'la,* plural **Se-que'læ.** [From *se'quor,* to "follow."] A consequence or sequel. In Pathology, *sequelæ* are morbid affections which succeed to acute or severe diseases after the latter have abated.

Se-que'læ,* gen. **Seq-ue-la'rum,** the plural of SEQUELA, which see.

Se-ques'trum.* [From *seques'tro,* to "sever," to "separate."] Any dead portion of bone in a wound, abscess, or ulcer, cast off by *necrosis.*

Se'rĭ-al. [**Seria'lis;** from *se'ries,* an "order," or "row," "succession."] Following in a determinate order, or arranged in rows.

Se'rĭ-ate. [From the same.] The same as SERIAL, which see.

Sericeous, se-rish'us. [**Seriç'eus;** from *ser'icum,* "silk."] Silky; resembling silk.

Ser-ĭ-cĭ-fo'lĭ-us.* [From *ser'icum,* "silk," and *fo'lium,* a "leaf."] Having silken leaves.

Ser'ĭ-cum.* [Gr. σηρικόν.] Silk, the product of several animals, but chiefly of the *Bom'byx mo'ri,* or silkworm. In Botany, applied to a kind of soft, hairy pubescence, of a white, shining, silky appearance.

Se'rĭ-ēs.* [From *se'ro,* to "join."] A Latin word signifying an "order, or continuous succession." A geometrical series is one to which each term is a multiple of the preceding by a constant factor. *Series* is applied in Geology to a group of strata, as the "secondary series," the "transition series," the "Silurian series," etc.

Ser'o-lin. [**Serolī'na;** from *se'rum,* and *o'leum,* "oil."] An oily or fatty matter discovered in the serum of the blood.

Se-ros'ĭ-tў. [**Seros'itas, a'tis;** from *se'rum,* "whey."] The serum of the blood, or the whey of milk.

Se-rot'ĭ-nous. [**Serot'inus;** from *se'rus,* "late."] Late; late in the evening. In Botany, flowering or fruiting late. See MEMBRANA SEROTINA.

Se'rous. [**Sero'sus;** from *se'rum.*] Of the nature of serum; also, secreting serum.

Ser'pens.* [Present participle from *ser'po,* to "creep."] Creeping or winding like a serpent. Applied to a form of baldness. See AREA.

Ser-pen-ta'rĭ-a.* [From *ser'pens,* a "serpent:" so called because reputed to be an antidote for the bite of serpents.] Virginia Snakeroot, or Ser'pentary. The Pharmacopœial name ‖ for the root of *Aristolo'chia serpenta'ria,* and other species of *Aristolochia;* the *Aristolochiæ serpentariæ radix* ("root of *Aristolochia serpentaria*") of the Dublin Pharmacopœia. Serpentaria is a stimulant tonic, sometimes acting as a diaphoretic and diuretic.

Serpenta'ria Vir-ġin-ĭ-a'na.* Another name for *Aristolo'chia serpenta'ria.*

Serpentary. See SERPENTARIA.

Ser-pen'tĭ-form. [**Serpentifor'mis;** from *ser'pens, serpen'tis,* a "serpent."] Having the form of a serpent.

Ser'pen-tīne. [**Serpenti'nus;** from the same.] Pertaining to a serpent; winding about like a serpent; meandering.

Ser'pentine. [From the same.] A magnesian rock of various colors, and often speckled like a serpent's skin. It sometimes occurs crystallized, and is used for ornamental purposes. *Verd antique* is an aggregate of serpentine and marble.

Ser-pig'ĭ-nous. [**Serpigino'sus.**] Having serpigo.

Ser-pi'go, ġ'inis.* [From *ser'po,* to "creep."] Ringworm, or tetter. See HERPES.

Ser'ra.* A Latin word signifying a "saw." Applied to the serrations or tooth-like articulating processes of certain bones, as those of the cranium.

Sĕr'rate, or **Sĕr'rāt-ed.** [**Serra'tus;** from *ser'ra,* a "saw."] Beset with teeth pointing forwards, like those of a saw. Applied to leaves.

Ser-rat'ĭ-form. [**Serratifor'mis;** from the same.] Having the appearance of a saw.

Ser-rā'tion. [**Serra'tio;** from *ser'ra,*

a "saw."] A formation or structure resembling the teeth of a saw.

Sĕr'ra-ture. [From the same.] One of the teeth of a serrate leaf or body. Also, a notching or indenture in the edge of any thing.

Ser-ra'tus Mag'nus.* ("Great Serrated [Muscle].") A muscle of the lateral thoracic region, arising by fleshy serrations from the upper ribs, and inserted into the whole length of the scapula.

Serra'tus Pos-ti'cus.* ("Posterior Serrated [Muscle].") The name of two muscles of the back, *superior* and *inferior*, arising from some of the vertebræ, and inserted by serrations into several of the ribs.

Serre-Nœud (Fr.), sêr nuh. [From *serrer*, to "press," and *nœud*, a "knot."] The name of an instrument used in surgery to tighten ligatures.

Sĕr'ru-late. [**Serrula'tus**; from *ser'rula*, a "little saw."] Minutely serrated; serrate with fine teeth.

Ser'tu-lum.* [Diminutive of *ser'tum*, a "garland."] A term sometimes applied to a simple umbel.

Se'rum.* The greenish-yellow fluid constituent of blood, which separates from the crassamentum during coagulation; the *liq'uor san'guinis* deprived of its fibrin or coagulable matter; serosity. Also, the whey of milk.

Se'rum Lac'tis.* ("Serum of Milk.") Whey. See WHEY.

Serv. = *Ser'va.** "Keep, or preserve."

Ses'a-mi Fo'li-um,* or **Ses'a-mi Fo'li-a.*** Benne Leaf. The Pharmacopœial name (U.S. Ph.) for the leaves of the *Ses'amum In'dicum* and *Ses'amum orienta'le.*

Ses'a-moid. [**Sesamoi'des,** or **Sesamoi'deus;** from σήσαμον, a "seed of the sesamum," and εἶδος, a "form."] Resembling a grain of sesamum.

Ses'amoid Bones. [**Os'sa** (or **Ossic'ula**) **Sesamoi'dea.**] A designation of certain small bones found at the roots of the first joint of the thumb and of the great toe.

Ses'qui-. A prefix signifying "one and a half," as *sesqui-granum*, a "grain and a half." Used in Chemistry to indicate that an equivalent and a half of one ingredient is combined with one of another. See SESQUIOXIDE.

Sesquih. = *Sesquiho'ra.** "An hour and a half."

Ses-qui-ox'ide. Literally, a compound of one and a half proportions of oxygen with one proportion of some other body, or, which is the same, of three equivalents of oxygen and two equivalents of another body.

Sesquiox'ide of I'ron, otherwise called **Per-ox'ide of I'ron.** A preparation made by adding water of ammonia to a solution of the sulphate of iron. The precipitate deposited is the hydrated oxide of iron (the *Fer'ri ox'idum hydra'tum* of the U.S. Pharmacopœia), also termed the hydrated peroxide of iron, forming the best, if not the only, antidote for poisoning with arsenic. By exposure to heat in a covered vessel, it becomes the simple sesquioxide (or peroxide) of iron.

Ses'sile. [**Ses'silis;** from *se'deo, ses'sum*, to "sit."] Sitting close to the stem; having no petiole or peduncle. Applied to leaves and flowers.

Ses-si-li-flo'rus.* [From *ses'silis*, "sessile," and *flos*, a "flower."] Having sessile flowers: sessiliflo'rous.

Ses-si-li-fo-li-a'tus,* or **Ses-si-li-fo'li-us.*** [From *ses'silis*, "sessile," and *fo'lium*, a "leaf."] Having sessile leaves: sessilifoliate; sessilifolious.

Sesunc. = *Sesun'cia.** "An ounce and a half."

Se'ta,* plural **Se'tæ.** A bristle. In Botany, a species of pubescence covering certain plants. Also applied to the stiff hairs that issue from certain of the *Anellata* and serve in lieu of feet.

Se-tā'ceous. [**Seta'ceus;** from *se'ta*, a "bristle."] Like bristles.

Se'tæ,* the plural of SETA, which see.

Se-tif'er-ous. [**Setif'erus;** from *se'ta*, a "bristle," and *fe'ro*, to "bear."] The same as SETIGEROUS, which see.

Se'ti-form. [**Setifor'mis;** from *se'ta*, a "bristle."] Formed like a bristle.

Se-tig'er-ous. [**Set'iger,** or **Setig'erus;** from *se'ta*, a "bristle," and *ge'ro*, to "bear."] Bearing bristles.

Se'ton, or **Setaceum,*** se-ta'she-ŭm. [From *se'ta*, a "bristle," or "coarse hair," horse-hair having been originally used for setons.] A small canal, or artificial passage, made under the skin by means of an instrument called a seton-needle, carrying with it a number of threads of linen, silk, or cotton, which are daily moved forwards or backwards, in order to keep up a constant irritation and discharge.

Se-tose'. [**Seto'sus;** from *se'ta*, a "bristle."] Covered with bristles; bristly.

Set'u-la.* [Diminutive of *se'ta*, a "bristle."] A small bristle.

Sev'enth Pair [Par Sep'timum]. A pair of encephalic nerves divided into two parts: the *portio dura* ("hard portion") being distributed to the face, and hence termed *facial nerve;* and the *portio mollis* ("soft portion"), called the *auditory nerve*, sending its filaments to the ear.

Sev'enth Sense, also called **Vis'çe-ral Sense.** A term applied by some writers to the instinctive sensations arising from the ganglionic department of the nervous system.

Se'vum.* Suet. The Pharmacopœial name for the prepared fat of sheep; the *Adeps ovilli.* Tallow; fat. Also termed *Sebum.* See ADEPS.

Se'vum Çe'ti.* ("Fat of the Whale.") Spermaceti, obtained from the *Physe'ter macroceph'alus.*

Se'vum O-vil'lum.* Mutton suet.

Sex-fa'ri-ous. Six-rowed. Applied to parts of plants.

Sex'fid, or **Sex'i-fid.** [**Sex'fidus;** from *sex*, "six," and *fin'do*, to "cleave."] Divided into six portions.

Sex-flo'rus.* [From *sex*, "six," and *flos*, a "flower."] Having six flowers: sexiflo'rous.

Sex-par'tite. [From *sex*, "six," and *par'tio, parti'tum*, to "part."] Six-parted.

Sex'tant. [From *sex'tans*, the "sixth part," the limb of the instrument being a sixth part of a circle.] An instrument for measuring the angular distance of objects by reflection. It is chiefly used for nautical purposes in measuring the altitudes of celestial objects.

Sex'u-al. [**Sexua'lis;** from *sex'us*, "sex."] Belonging to sex; distinguishing the sexes.

Sex'ual Sys'tem. The system or method of classifying plants invented by Linnæus, founded on the number, position, and connection of the sexual organs.

Shad'dock. A large fruit, resembling the orange, obtained from the *Cit'rus decuma'na*, growing in the East and West Indies. It has a slightly bitterish or astringent taste, which renders it less palatable than the orange; but it is peculiarly grateful and acceptable to the stomach in the convalescence from seasickness, especially in hot climates.

Shaggy. See HIRSUTE.

Shāk'ing Pal'sy̆. The common name for the *Synclonus ballismus* of Dr. Good.

Shale. A crumbling variety of slate; indurated clay.

Sham-poo'ing. The employment of the vapor-bath, accompanied by a process of friction, kneading, and extension of the muscles, tendons, and ligaments.

Sharp. See ACUTE.

Sharp-Pointed. See CUSPIDATE, and MUCRONATE.

Sheath. [**Vagi'na.**] In Botany, a tubular body enclosing or surrounding some other.

Sheath, Med'ul-la-ry̆. A tissue of spiral vessels or ducts surrounding the pith of plants. This is no special organ, and merely represents the earliest-formed vascular tissue of the stem.

Shell. [**Crus'ta, Tes'ta.**] The calcareous skeleton which encloses the soft parts of a testaceous mollusk; an inorganic, laminated deposit of calcareous earth, more or less combined with albuminous matter. Shells are divided into univalve, bivalve, and multivalve, and are the subjects of the science of Conchology. Also, the covering of an egg.

Sher'bet. [Lat. **Sorbe'tum,** or **Sorbe'thum;** Fr. *Sorbet*, SOR'bā'.] A cooling summer drink much used in the East, made of the juice of fruits and water, variously sweetened and flavored.

Sher'ry̆. [**Vi'num Xer'icum;** from *Xeres*, a town of Spain.] The *Vinum album*, or white wine.

Shield. A name for an *apothecium.* See APOTHECIA.

Shield'-like Car'ti-lage. The *Cartilago scutiformis*, or *Cartilago thyroides.*

Shield-Shaped. See PELTATE, and SCUTIFORM.

Shin. [**Anticne'mion.**] The crest, or prominent anterior ridge, or edge, of the tibia: sometimes applied to the bone itself.

Shin'-Bone. The tibia, or large bone of the leg. See TIBIA.

Shin'gles. [From *cin'gulum*, a "girdle."] A popular name for HERPES ZOSTER, which see.

Shoot. [**Sur'culus.**] Any young or fresh branch of a plant.

Short-Sightedness. See MYOPY.

Shoulder. See ARMUS, and HUMERUS.

Shoulder-Blade. See SCAPULA.

Show, or **La'bor Show.** Popularly, the red-colored mucus discharged from the vagina shortly before childbirth.

Show'er-Bath. [**Implu'vium.**]

A mode of bathing which consists in throwing a column of water with more or less violence upon the surface of the body. When a column of water is let fall from a considerable height, it is termed by the French *Douche* (doosh). See DOUCHE.

Shrivelled. See CORRUGATED, and RUGOSE.

Shrub. [**Fru'tex.**] A woody plant with a stem branched from or near the ground, and less than five times the height of a man. A shrub which approaches a tree in size, or resembles it in aspect, is said to be *arborescent.* Also, a liquor made of acid fruits, sugar, and other substances to give a flavor, digested in rum or brandy. *Shrub* in this sense is a corruption of the Arabic *sherab* (shẹ-râb'), and is nearly the same as SHERBET.

Shrub-like. See FRUTICOSE.

Si-al'ạ-den, en*is*.* [From σίαλον, the "spittle," and ἀδήν, a "gland."] A salivary gland.

Si-ạl-ad-e-ni'tis, i*dis*.* [From *sial'aden*, a "salivary gland."] Inflammation of a salivary gland.

Si-ạl-ad-e-non'cus.* [From *sial'aden*, a "salivary gland," and ὄγκος, a "tumor."] Swelling of a salivary gland.

Sī-al'ạ-gŏgue. [**Sialago'gus;** from σίαλον, "saliva," and ἄγω, to "lead or carry off."] Having power to increase the flow of the saliva.

Si-ạ-li'nạ.* [From σίαλον, "saliva."] A term for a peculiar principle contained in the saliva: sialin.

Sī'ạ-līne. [**Siali'nus;** from σίαλον, "saliva."] Belonging to the saliva, or spittle.

Si-ạ-lo'dēs.* [From σίαλον, "saliva."] Having saliva; like saliva.

Sī'ạ-loid. [**Sialoi'des;** from σίαλον, "saliva," and εἶδος, a "form."] Resembling saliva.

Si-ạ-lo-li-thi'ạ-sis.* [From σίαλον, "saliva," and *lithi'asis*, the "formation of stone."] The formation of salival calculus.

Si-ạ-lol'ĭ-thus.* [From σίαλον, "saliva," and λίθος, a "stone."] A salival calculus.

Sī-ạ-lol'o-ġȳ. [**Sialolo'gia;** from σίαλον, "saliva," and λόγος, a "discourse."] The doctrine of the saliva; that branch of Physiology which treats of the saliva, its secretion, uses, etc.

Si-ạ-lon'cus.* [From σίαλον, "saliva," and ὄγκος, a "tumor."] A tumor under the tongue, resulting from obstruction to the flow of saliva by a salival calculus.

Si-ạ-lor-rhœ'ạ.* [From σίαλον, "saliva," and ῥέω, to "flow."] A flow of the saliva.

Sib'bens. A popular Scotch term for a disease resembling syphilis.

Sib'ĭ-lant. [**Sib'ilans;** from *sib'ilo*, to "hiss."] Making a hissing sound, or whistling.

Sic'cant. [**Sic'cans;** from *sic'co*, to "dry."] Having power to dry; drying.

Sic-çĭ-fo'lĭ-us.* [From *sic'cus*, "dry," and *fo'lium*, a "leaf."] Having a dry leaf: siccifo'lious.

Sick. [Lat. **Æ'ger;** Fr. *Malade*, mâ'lâd'.] Affected with SICKNESS, which see.

Sick'ness. [Lat. **Mor'bus,** and **Ægritu'do;** Fr. *Maladie*, mâ'lâ'dè'.] In a general sense, any kind of disease or malady involving the whole body, but applied more particularly to a nauseated state of the stomach, with or without retching and vomiting.

Sid'er-ā-tion. [**Sidera'tio, o'***nis*; from *si'dus*, a "star," or "constellation."] A sudden attack, supposed to be the result of sidereal influence. Under this term were included, by the ancients, apoplexy and paralysis; also, mortification, or *sphacelus.*

Sī-de're-ạl, or **Sid'e-rạl.** [**Side'reus,** and **Sidera'lis;** from *si'dus*, *sid'eris*, a "star."] Belonging to the stars, or signs in the heavens; starry. A sidereal day is the time in which the earth makes a complete rotation on its axis, with respect to a fixed star, or any fixed point in space.

Sid-e-ri'tēs.* [Gr. σιδηρίτης, "of or belonging to iron;" from σίδηρος, "iron," λίθος, a "stone," being understood.] A name for the magnet, or loadstone.

Sid-e-rog'rạ-phȳ. [**Siderogra'phia;** from σίδηρος, "iron," or "steel," and γράφω, to "write."] A history of iron or steel; the art or practice of engraving on steel.

Sid-e-ro-tech'nĭ-ạ.* [From σίδηρος, "iron," and τέχνη, "art."] The art of treating minerals containing iron; also, the art of working in iron.

Sienite. See SYENITE.

Sĭ-ĕr'rạ. [From *ser'ra*, a "saw."] A Spanish word signifying a "saw," but usually applied to a chain of high mountains, because at a great distance the peaks present an appearance resembling saw-teeth.

Sieve. See COLATORIUM.

Sieve-like. See COLIFORMIS, CRIBRIFORM, and ETHMOID.

Si-gault'ti-an Op-e-rā'tion. The division of the *symphysis pubis* in cases of impracticable labor from contraction or deformity, first performed by Sigault. See SYMPHYSOTOMY.

Sigh. See SUSPIRIUM.

Sight. See VISUS, and VISION.

Sight, Dimness of. See CALIGO.

Sight, Morbid. See PAROPSIS.

Sig'il-late. [**Sigilla'tus;** from *sigil'lum*, a "seal."] Marked with a seal.

Sig'moid. [**Sigmoi'des;** from Σ, and εἶδος, a "form."] Curved like the letter S; resembling the Greek letter Σ (*sigma*).

Sig'moid Flex'ure. [**Flexu'ra Sigmoi'dea.**] A name applied to that portion of the colon which is between the descending portion and the rectum.

Sig'moid Valves. [**Val'vulæ Sigmoi'deæ.**] The semilunar valves of the aorta and of the pulmonary artery.

Sign. [**Sig'num.**] Literally, a "mark." Applied to any appearance, symptom, or circumstance from which the physician is enabled to decide as to the nature or probable termination of the disease. In Pharmacy the term is applied to certain marks employed in formulæ and prescriptions, viz.: ℔ for a pound; ℥ for an ounce; ʒ for a drachm; ℈ for a scruple; ♏ for a minim. In Astronomy, it denotes a portion of the ecliptic, or zodiac, containing thirty degrees.

Sig'na.* [Imperative mood of *sig'no*, to "mark."] "Mark," or "write." A word added at the end of prescriptions to show what directions are to be copied by the druggist for the guidance of the patient or his attendant.

Si-le'ne Vir-gin'i-ca.* The systematic name of Wild Pink, a plant of the natural order *Caryophyllaceæ*. The root has been used as an anthelmintic.

Si'lex,* gen. **Sil'i-cis.** [From χάλιξ, a "stone," or "pebble"?] Flint; quartz. Sometimes synonymous with SILICA.

Sil'i-ca.* [From *si'lex*.] One of the primitive earths; a substance composed of oxygen and silicon (or silicium), and sometimes called *silicic acid*. It forms the principal ingredient of a variety of silicious minerals, among which quartz, flint, rock-crystal, and chalcedony may be considered as silica nearly pure. It predominates in granite and sandstone. Silica in its ordinary or anhydrous state is insoluble in all acids except the hydrofluoric.

Sil'i-cāte. [**Sil'icas, a'***tis*.] A combination of silicic acid with a base.

Si-liç'ic. [**Siliç'icus.**] Belonging to, or derived from, silica. Applied to an acid.

Sil-i-cif'er-ous. [**Silicif'erus;** from *sil'ica*, and *fe'ro*, to "bear."] Containing silica.

Sil'i-ci-form. [**Silicifor'mis;** from *si'lex*, *sil'icis*, "flint."] Having the form of silex, or flint.

Silicious, se-lish'e-us. [**Silicio'sus;** from *sil'ica*.] Resembling or containing silica.

Silicium,* se-lish'e-um. Another name for SILICON, which see.

Sil'i-cle, or **Sil'i-cule.** [**Silic'ula;** diminutive of *sil'iqua*, a "silique," or "pod."] A "little pod;" a short silique or short pod of *Cruciferæ*, as shepherd's-purse.

Sil'i-con. A simple, non-metallic, infusible substance which forms the base of silica. It bears a greater analogy to boron than to any other known principle. It is not acted on by any single acid, but is soluble by a mixture of nitric and hydrofluoric acids.

Sil-i-cu-li-for'mis.* Having the form of a silicle: siliculiform.

Sil-i-cu-lo'sa.* [From *silic'ula*, a "small or short silique."] The name of an order in the Linnæan class *Tetradynamia*.

Sil-i-cu-lose'. [**Siliculo'sus;** from *silic'ula*, a "silicle."] Having or resembling silicles.

Silique, se-leek'. [**Sil'iqua.**] A slender, two-valved capsule of a cruciferous plant, like those of the mustard and radish. It has two parietal placentæ from which the valves separate in dehiscence.

Sil'i-qui-form. [**Siliquifor'mis.**] Having the form of a silique.

Sil-i-quo'sa.* [From *sil'iqua*, a "silique."] Bearing siliques. Applied to an order of the Linnæan class *Tetradynamia*.

Sil-i-quose'. [**Siliquo'sus;** from *sil'iqua*, a "silique."] Having siliques, or like a silique.

Silk'worm, Aç'id of. Bombic acid.

Silk'y̆. [**Seriç'eus.**] In Botany, clothed with fine, appressed, and glossy hairs, producing a satiny surface.

Sillon, sè'yòNº'. The French term for SULCUS, which see.

Si-lu'ri-an. [**Siluria'nus;** from *Silu'res*, an ancient people of South Wales.] A name given to a series of rocks forming the upper subdivision of the sedimentary strata found below the old red sandstone, and formerly designated the *greywacke series.* These strata are well developed in that part of England and Wales formerly occupied by the Silures.

Sil'ver. [Lat. **Argen'tum;** Gr. ἄργυρος; Fr. *Argent,* an'zhŏnᵍ'.] A precious metal of a beautiful white color, malleable, ductile, and tenacious. Its specific gravity is 10.5. It is not altered by air or moisture, but is tarnished by sulphuretted hydrogen, and is soluble in nitric and in sulphuric acid. When pure, it is softer and is tarnished less readily than the silver of coin or plate. See ARGENTUM.

Silver, Fulminating. See ARGENTATE OF AMMONIA.

Silver, Nitrate of. See ARGENTI NITRAS.

Simaba Cedron. See CEDRON.

Sim-a-ru'ba.* A Linnæan genus of the class *Decandria,* natural order *Simarubaceæ.* Also, the Pharmacopœial name (U.S. Ph.) for the bark of the root of *Simaru'ba officina'lis;* (Ed. Ph.) of the *Simaru'ba ama'ra;* (Dub. Ph.) the *Simarubæ Cortex.*

Simaru'ba A-ma'ra.* The plant (Ed. Ph.) which affords simaruba-root bark.

Simaru'ba Of-fiç-i-na'lis.* The plant (U.S. and Lond. Ph.) which affords simaruba-root bark; also called *Quassia Simaruba.*

Simarubaceæ,* sim-a-ru-ba'she-ē. A natural order of exogenous trees and shrubs, natives of tropical America, India, or Africa. The species are intensely bitter. Among the products of this order are *Quassia* and *Simaru'ba,* which are valuable medicines.

Sim'i-lor. A name for PINCHBECK, which see.

Si-moon', or **Si-moom'.** A hot, arid wind, which, after passing over sandy deserts, blows in Arabia, Syria, and the adjacent countries.

Sim'ple. [**Sim'plex,** *icis;* from *si'ne pli'câ,* "without a fold:" hence, single.] The opposite of compound; uncompounded; unadulterated; pure.

Simple Affinity. See AFFINITY, SINGLE OR SIMPLE.

Simple Cerate. See CERATUM SIMPLEX.

Sim'ple Fruit. A fruit which results from a single pistil or flower. Simple fruits may be divided into *fleshy fruits,* as the grape; *stone fruits,* as the peach; and *dry fruits,* as the chesnut.

Sim'ple Leaf. A leaf which has a blade of one piece, however cleft or lobed; or, if divided, the separate portions are neither raised on stalklets of their own, nor articulated (by a joint) with the main petiole.

Sim'ples. A general name for all herbs which have any medicinal virtue.

Sim'pli-ci-cau'lis.* [From *sim'plex,* "simple," and *cau'lis,* a "stem."] Having a simple stem.

Sim'pli-ci-fo'li-us.* [From *sim'plex,* "simple," and *fo'lium,* a "leaf."] Having simple leaves.

Sim-u-lā'tion. [**Simula'tio, o'nis;** from *sim'ulo, simula'tum,* to "feign."] A counterfeiting, or pretending to be suffering under, disease; malingering.

Sinapi. See SINAPIS.

Si-na'pis.* [Gr. σίνηπι, or σίναπι; Fr. *Moutarde,* moo'tard', or *Sénevé,* sån'-vå'.] A Linnæan genus of the class *Tetradynamia,* natural order *Cruciferæ.* Also, the Pharmacopœial name (Br. Ph.) for the seeds, reduced to powder, of *Sinapis nigra* and *S. alba.* According to the Edinburgh Pharmacopœia, it is *Sinapi.*

Sina'pis Al'ba.* White Mustard. The Pharmacopœial name (U.S. Ph.) for the seed of the *Sinapis alba.* Its properties are similar to those of *Sinapis nigra.*

Sina'pis Ni'gra.* Black Mustard. The Pharmacopœial name (U.S. Ph.) for the seed of the *Sinapis nigra.* It is stimulant, emetic, and applied externally is epispastic or rubefacient.

Sina'pis Sem'i-na.* ("Seeds of Sinapis.") See SINAPIS.

Sin'a-pism. [**Sinapis'mus;** from *sina'pis,* "mustard."] A plaster or poultice made of mustard, linseed-meal, and vinegar. Used as a rubefacient.

Sin-çip'i-tal. [**Sincipita'lis;** from *sin'ciput.*] Pertaining to the sinciput.

Sin'çi-put.* The fore and upper part of the head.

Sīne. [**Si'nus.**] A right line drawn from one extremity of an arc perpendicular to the diameter of the circle passing through the other extremity.

Sin'ew. A fibrous cord which connects a muscle with a bone; a tendon. Sometimes improperly applied to a ligament which joins two bones.

Sing. = *Singulo'rum.** "Of each."

Single Affinity. See AFFINITY, SINGLE ELECTIVE.

Sin'gu-lis Di-e'bus.* [From *sin'-*

gulus, "every," and *di'es*, "day." See DIES.] "Every day." A phrase employed in directions for taking medicine.

Sin-gul'tus.* (Fr. *Hoquet*, ho'kà'.) A convulsive motion of the diaphragm and neighboring parts, popularly named hiccough or hiccup.

Sin'is-tral. [**Sinistra'lis;** from *sinis'ter*, the "left."] Belonging to, or situated on, the left.

Sin'is-trorse. [**Sinistror'sus;** from the same.] Turned to the left; twining from right to left, as the Hop and other plants.

Sin'u-ate, or **Sin'u-āt-ed.** [**Sinua'tus;** from *si'nus*, a "bay," a "recess," a "hollow."] Hollowed; strongly wavy on the margin, with alternate convexities and concavities. Applied to leaves.

Sin'u-ous. [**Sinuo'sus;** from the same.] Having sinuses; bending in and out; winding.

Si'nus.* Originally, a "bosom," "cavity," or "winding;" sometimes, a "gulf," or "bay." Applied in Surgery to the cavity of an imposthume or sore; also to a long, narrow, hollow track leading from some abscess, diseased bone, or the like. In Botany, a re-entering angle; a recess.—(GRAY.) In Geometry, a SINE, which see.

Sinus Cavernus. See CAVERNOUS SINUS.

Sinus, Inferior Longitudinal. See LONGITUDINAL SINUS, INFERIOR.

Sinus, Longitudinal. See LONGITUDINAL SINUS.

Sinus, Maxillary. See HIGHMORIANUM, ANTRUM.

Si'nus Mu-lĭ-e'bris.* A name for the vagina.

Si'nus or **Pel'vis of the Kid'ney.** A small cavity or pouch which receives the orifices of the infundibula.

Si'nus Poc-u-la'ris.* ("Cup-like Sinus.") A large lacuna in the centre of the *Caput Gallinaginis* or *Verumontanum*.

Si'nus U-ro-ġen-ĭ-ta'lis.* [See UROGENITAL.] A sinus existing in the embryo of the mammalia. It is a cavity or canal opening externally, in which the excretory ducts of the Wolffian bodies, the ureters, and the efferent parts of the generative apparatus terminate internally.

Sinuses, Lateral. See LATERAL SINUSES.

Sinuses of Morgagni. See MORGAGNI, SINUSES OF.

Si'nus-es of the Du'ra Ma'ter. Certain channels which traverse the *dura mater* in various points for the reception of the venous blood.

Si n. val. = *Si non va'leat.** "If it does not avail," or does not answer.

Si op. sit. = *Si o'pus sit.** "If there be occasion."

Sī'phon. [Lat. **Si'pho, o'**nis; Gr. σίφων, a "tube."] A bent tube, with legs or limbs of unequal length, used for drawing liquors from one vessel into another without disturbing the sediment. In Zoology, a membranous and calcareous tube which traverses the septa and the interior of a polythalamous shell.

Si-pho'nĭ-a E-las'tĭ-ca.* The systematic name of the tree which yields Indian-rubber, or caoutchouc. It belongs to the natural order *Euphorbiaceæ*.

Si-pho-nif'er-ous. [**Siphonif'erus;** from *si'pho*, a "siphon," and *fe'ro*, to "bear."] Bearing or having siphons. Applied to certain Mollusks.

Si-phon-o-bran-chĭ-a'tus.* [From σίφων, a "siphon," and βράγχια, the "*branchiæ*."] Provided with a canal, more or less elongated, which borders upon a cavity containing the *branchiæ*. Applied to certain Mollusks.

Sī-pho-nos'to-mus.* [From σίφων, a "siphon," and στόμα, a "mouth."] Having a siphon-like mouth. Applied to a family of Crustaceans.

Sĭ-ri'a-sis.* [From *Sir'ius*, the "dog-star."] A term sometimes used for sunstroke.

Sĭ-roc'co. A soft, relaxing wind, chiefly experienced in the south of Italy, in Malta and in Sicily.

Sirop, sè'ro'. (Fr.) See SYRUPUS.

Si'son Am'mi.* A plant yielding the *Am'mi ve'rum* of the shops. The seeds were formerly used as a carminative.

Sitis. See THIRST.

Sī-tol'o-ġy̆, or **Sit-ĭ-ol'o-ġy̆.** [**Sitiolo'gia;** from σῖτος, "aliment," and λόγος, a "discourse."] The doctrine or science of aliments; dietetics.

Si'um Nod-ĭ-flo'rum.* Water-Parsnip. A plant of the Linnæan class *Pentandria*, natural order *Umbelliferæ*. It is said to be diuretic, and is occasionally used in cutaneous eruptions.

Si vir. perm. = *Si vi'res permit'tant.** "If the strength will permit."

Sixth Pair. [**Par Sex'tum.**] A pair of encephalic nerves distributed to the *rectus externus oculi* muscle.

Sixth Sense. See CŒNÆSTHESIS.

Size. A name applied to the buffy coat which appears on the surface of coagulated blood drawn in inflammation.

Si'zy̆. Like glue or size. Applied to the blood when, after coagulation, it exhibits the buffy coat.

Skel'e-ton. [Lat. **Scel'eton;** Gr. *σκελετόν*, from *σκέλλω*, to "dry," to "dry up;" Fr. *Squelette*, skẹh-lĕtt'.] The bony framework of an animal designed for the support of the soft parts: usually applied to the dried bones prepared for anatomical purposes. When the bones are connected by their own ligaments, the skeleton is called natural; when joined by wires or plates of silver, etc., it is termed artificial.

Skin. [From the old German *Schin*, from the same root as *schei'nen*, to "appear;" because the skin is that part which appears or is visible.] The organ of touch, or one of the principal mediums through which we communicate with external bodies. The skin is considered to be composed of three membranes: the outermost is the scarf-skin, cuticle, or epidermis; the middle, the *rete mucosum;* and the innermost, the true skin (*cutis vera*), or *derma.*

Skin'-Bound. A peculiar condition of infants, in which the skin becomes tense, and as if too tight for the body, which is swelled and hard beneath its surface.

Skull. See Cranium.

Slag. The dross of iron or other metal.

Slashed. The same as Laciniate, which see.

Slate. A term applied to several varieties of stratified rocks which have the property of being split into thin laminæ or plates, as clay-slate, mica-slate, and roofing-slate. Clay-slate is one of the oldest stratified rocks, and is non-fossiliferous.

Slavering. See Drivelling.

Sleep. [Lat. **Som'nus;** Fr. *Sommeil*, som'mēl'.] That state of the body in which the functions of sensation and volition are suspended, while the vital functions retain their usual activity; the operations of the mind, if not at perfect rest, are disconnected with external objects.

Sleep of Plants. A term applied by Linnæus to the condition of certain plants the leaves of which are drooping and folded at night, as the Locust, *Mimosa, Oxalis*, etc.

Sleep-Disturbance. See Paroniria.

Sleep-Inducing. See Hypnotic.

Sleep-Walk'ing. The affection termed *Oneirodynia activa.*

Sleeplessness. See Agrypnia.

Sleepy. See Somnolent.

Sling. (Fr. *Écharpe*, à'sharp'.) A bandage or apparatus.

Slip. See Talea.

Slough, slŭf. A sphacelated part of the body, eventually separating from the rest.

Small-Pox. See Variola.

Smalt, or **Smaltz.** An oxide of cobalt melted with silicious earth and potash. When ground fine, it is called powder-blue. It is used in the arts and in painting earthen-ware.

Smeg'mạ, *atis.** [Gr. *σμῆγμα*, "soap."] The offensive soap-like substance produced from the sebaceous follicles around the *glans penis* and prepuce.

Smel'ling. [**Olfac'tus.**] That sense by which we perceive the odors of different bodies.

Smell, Morbid. See Parosmis.

Smilaceæ,* smi-la'she-ē. A natural order of endogenous plants (herbs or under-shrubs), found in the temperate and tropical parts of Asia and America. It includes *Smi'lax*, from several species of which the drug Sarsaparilla is procured.

Smi'lax, *acis.** [Gr. *σμίλαξ*, "bindweed."] A Linnæan genus of the class *Diœcia*, natural order *Smilaceæ.*

Smi'lax As'pe-rạ.* The plant generally supposed to produce Indian Sarsaparilla.

Smilax Officinalis. See Sarsaparilla, and Sarza.

Smi'lax Sar-sạ-pạ-ril'lạ.* The plant known as Sarsaparilla, which see.

Smooth. See Glabrous.

Snake-Root, Vir-gin'i-ạn. A common name for the *Aristolochia serpentaria.*

Sneez'ing. [**Sternuta'tio, o'***nis.*] A convulsive action of the respiratory muscles, caused by irritation of some part of the lining membrane of the nostrils; sternutation. See Reflex Action.

Snoring, Snorting. See Stertor.

Snow-Blindness. See Niphablepsia.

Soap, Castilian, Soap, Spanish. See Sapo Durus.

Soapstone. See Steatite.

Sob'o-lēs.* Originally, a young branch, an offspring. Any rudiment of a new branch.

Sob-o-lif'er-ous. [**Sobolif'erus;** from *sob'oles*, a "shoot," and *fe'ro*, to "bear."] Bearing shoots.

So'cia (so'she-ạ) **Pạ-rot'i-dis.***

("Companion of the Parotid.") The name of a second portion of the parotid gland which is frequently developed from the duct while on the masseter muscle.

So'cial. [**Socia'lis;** from *so'cius,* a "companion."] Applied to plants which grow gregariously, as grasses.

Socotrine Aloes. See ALOE SOCOTRINA.

So'da.* (Fr. *Soude,* sood.) (A word of Arabic origin.) The mineral alkali; the oxide of sodium.

So'da His-pan'i-ca.* ("Spanish Soda.") Impure soda, or the impure mineral alkali of commerce.

So'da, Mu-ri'ate of. The chloride of sodium. See SODII CHLORIDUM.

Soda, Sulphate of. See SODÆ SULPHAS.

So'da, Tar'ta-rized. A name for the tartrate of potassa and soda (*Potassæ et sodæ tartras*).

So'da Wa'ter. A beverage formed by a solution of the carbonate of soda in water, which is afterwards impregnated with more carbonic acid than is sufficient for saturation.

So'dæ A-ce'tas.* ("Acetate of Soda.") The Pharmacopœial name (U.S. Ph.) for a substance in white or colorless crystals, which effloresce in dry air, and are wholly soluble in water.

So'dæ Bo'ras* ("Borate of Soda"), or **Bo'rax.** The Pharmacopœial name (U.S. Ph.) for a substance in colorless crystals, which slightly effloresce in dry air, and are wholly soluble in water. It is a mild refrigerant and diuretic. It is much used as a flux by workers in metals.

So'dæ Car-bo'nas.* ("Carbonate of Soda.") The Pharmacopœial name (U.S. Ph.) for a substance in colorless crystals, which rapidly effloresce on exposure to the air, and fall into a white powder. It is an antacid, and much employed in cases of acidity of the stomach and bowels.

So'dæ Phos'phas.* ("Phosphate of Soda.") A substance in colorless, transparent crystals, which speedily effloresce when exposed to air. It is a mild, saline cathartic. Its taste resembles common salt, and it is therefore not likely to be rejected by delicate stomachs, like the more nauseous medicines of this class.

So'dæ Sul'phas.* ("Sulphate of Soda.") (Popularly known as **Glau'ber's Salts.**) The Pharmacopœial name (U.S. Ph.) for a substance in colorless crystals, which rapidly effloresce on exposure to the air, and ultimately fall into a white powder. Sulphate of soda is one of the most efficient saline cathartics, nearly resembling in its general properties the sulphate of magnesia, or Epsom Salts; but the latter is less disagreeable to the taste, and is therefore more generally used. See MAGNESIÆ SULPHAS.

So'dæ Sul'phis.* ("Sulphite of Soda.") A substance in white, efflorescent, prismatic crystals, soluble in four parts of cold, and in less than one part of boiling, water. It has been placed on the primary list of the Materia Medica of the U.S. Pharmacopœia for 1860.

So'dic. [**So'dicus;** from *so'dium.*] Applied to the second degree of oxidation of sodium, or sodic oxide.

So'di-i Chlo'ri-dum* ("Chloride of Sodium"), or Common Salt. The Pharmacopœial name for a white salt, permanent in the air, and almost equally soluble in cold and boiling water. It is astringent, tonic, and antiseptic.

So'di-um.* The base of soda; a metal discovered by Davy in 1808, resembling potassium in its general characters. It is soft, malleable, fusible at 190°, and burns when heated in contact with air. Its specific gravity is 0.97.

Softening. See RAMOLLISSEMENT.

Soft'en-ing of the Brain. [Lat. **Molli'ties Cer'ebri;** Fr. *Ramollissement du Cerveau,* râ'mo'lèss'mōNG' dü sěR'vō'.] Sometimes applied to a *fatty degeneration* of the substance of the brain, sometimes to a sort of *liquefaction.* The causes of this affection are often obscure; but in many instances it would seem to be produced by *embolism* of the arteries which supply the brain.

Soft Palate. See PALATUM MOLLE.

Sol.* The Sun, a name given to gold by the alchemists.

Solanaceæ,* so-la-na'she-ē. An important natural order of exogenous plants (herbaceous or shrubby), natives of all parts of the world except the arctic regions. Many of them are narcotic and poisonous. It includes the *Sola'num tubero'sum* (Potato), *Sola'num lycoper'sicum* (Tomato), *Nicotiana* (Tobacco), *Atropa belladonna,* and *Capsicum* (Cayenne Pepper).

So-la-nā'ceous. [**Solana'ceus,** or **Sola'neus.**] Resembling the *Solanum.*

Sol'a-nin, or **Sol'a-nine.** [**Solani'na;** from *Sola'num.*] An alkali obtained, when pure, in the form of a white, opaque, and sometimes pearly powder, chiefly from the *Solanum dulcamara*.

So-la'num.* A Linnæan genus of the class *Pentandria*, natural order *Solanaceæ*.

Sola'num Dul-ca-ma'ra.* The woody nightshade.

Sola'num Es-cu-len'tum.* ("Esculent Solanum.") The *Solanum tuberosum*, or potato-plant.

Sola'num Fœt'ĭ-dum.* ("Fetid Solanum.") The *Datura stramonium*, or thorn-apple.

Sola'num Le-tha'le.* ("Deadly Solanum.") Another name for the *At'ropa belladon'na*, or deadly nightshade. See BELLADONNA.

Sola'num Lig-no'sum.* ("Woody Nightshade.") Another name for the *Solanum dulcamara*. See DULCAMARA.

Sola'num Ly-co-per'sĭ-cum.* A synonym of the tomato, *Lycopersicum esculentum*.

Sola'num Tu-be-ro'sum.* The systematic name of the potato-plant, the root (or rather tuber) of which is in general use as an article of food throughout the greater part of the civilized world. It is a native of America.

So'lar. [**Sola'ris;** from *sol, so'lis*, the "sun."] Pertaining to, or derived from, the sun; measured by the sun: as, a solar day,—that is, the interval between two successive arrivals of the sun on the same meridian.

Solar Cycle. See CYCLE.

So'lar Plex'us. [**Plex'us Sola'ris.**] An assemblage of ganglia connected with the great sympathetic nerve, with interlaced and anastomosing filaments, and surrounding the two semilunar ganglia of the abdomen. It gives off numerous filaments, which accompany, under the name of plexuses, all the branches given off by the abdominal aorta.

Solar System. See SYSTEM.

Sŏl'der, or saw'der. A substance, consisting of simple or mixed metals, by which metallic bodies are firmly united with each other. Bismuth is much used in the composition of soft solders. Plumber's solder is an alloy of three parts of lead and one of tin.

Sole of the Foot. See SOLEA.

So'le-a.* [From *so'lum*, the "bottom."] A Latin word signifying a "sandal," a "slipper." In Anatomy, the sole of the foot. See PLANTA, and THENAR.

So'le-us.* [From *so'lea*, the "sole-fish."] Belonging to or resembling the sole of the foot. Applied to a muscle which arises from the head of the fibula, etc., and is inserted into the *os calcis*. It extends the foot. It has also been named *gastrocne'mius inter'nus*.

Sol'id. [**Sol'idus.**] Firm; substantial; not fluid or hollow. Applied to bodies the particles of which adhere together so firmly that they cannot be separated without some degree of force. A solid figure is that which has three dimensions, length, breadth, and thickness. Regular solids are those which are bounded by regular and equal planes. They are five in number, viz.: the tetrahedron, hexahedron (or cube), octahedron, dodecahedron, and icosihedron, which are noticed under their respective alphabetical heads.

Sol-ĭ-da'go.* Golden Rod. The Pharmacopœial name (U.S. Ph.) for the leaves of the *Solida'go odo'ra*, a plant of the natural order *Compositæ*. It is aromatic, moderately stimulant, and carminative.

Solidism. See SOLIDISTS.

Sol'ĭ-dists. A sect in medicine who refer all diseases to a morbid change in the solid parts. They maintain that the solids alone are endowed with vital properties. This theory is termed Solidism.

Sol'ids. [From *sol'idus*, "solid."] Applied to the bones, ligaments, muscles, nerves, and vessels of animals.

Sol-ĭ-dun-gu-la'ta,* or **Sol-ĭ-dun'gu-lates.** [From *sol'idus*, "solid," and *un'gula*, a "hoof."] The same as SOLIDUNGULA. See next article.

Sol-ĭ-dun'gu-lus.* [From the same.] Having solid hoofs. Applied in the plural neuter (*Solidun'gula*) to a family of *Mammifera*, having only one hoof to each foot, or having the hoof whole, as the horse, ass, etc.

Sol'ĭ-ped. [**Sol'ipes, p'edis;** from *so'lus*, "alone," or "single," and *pes*, a "foot."] Synonymous with SOLIDUNGULUS, which see.

Sol'ĭ-ta-rȳ Glands. [**Glan'dulæ Solita'riæ.**] Small, flattened, granular bodies found in the stomach and intestines.

So'lĭ-um.* A species of tape-worm. See TÆNIA SOLIUM.

Sol-Lu'nar In'flu-ence. The influence supposed to be produced on various diseases when the sun and moon are in conjunction.

Sol'stice. [**Solsti'tium;** from *sol*, the "sun," and *sto*, to "stand," to "stop."] The time at which the sun is at its greatest distance from the equator, when it seems to stop in its course southward or northward, and to stand still for a few days, which occurs twice a year, the *summer* solstice and *winter* solstice,—that is, about the 21st of June and 21st of December.

Solstitial, sol-stish'al. [**Solstitia'lis.**] Belonging to the solstice.

Sol-u-bil'i-ty. [From *sol'vo, solu'tum,* to "loosen."] Susceptibility of solution in any menstruum. Substances are soluble in proportion as their particles have a stronger attraction for the fluid which constitutes the menstruum, than for each other. They are insoluble when their particles have a stronger attraction for each other than for the menstruum.

Sol'u-ble. [**Solu'bilis;** from the same.] Susceptible of solution. In Botany, separating into parts.

So'lum.* A Latin word, signifying the "bottom," or "ground;" also the "sole of the foot."

So-lu'tion. [**Solu'tio, o'***nis;* from *sol'vo, solu'tum,* to "loosen," to "melt," to "dissolve."] The act of dissolving a solid body; the diffusion of the particles of a solid through a liquid; also, the state of a solid body which has been dissolved. Applied also to any substance dissolved in a liquid.

Solu'tion of Con-ti-nu'i-ty. The breaking down, or division, of the skin and other textures by a blow, a cutting instrument, or ulceration.

Solv. = *Sol've.** "Dissolve."

Sol'vent. [**Sol'vens;** from *sol'vo,* to "loosen," or "dissolve."] Applied to any liquor capable of dissolving bodies.

So-ma-tol'o-gy. [**Somatolo'gia;** from σῶμα, σώματος, the "body," and λόγος, a "discourse."] A treatise on the human body; anatomy.

So-ma-tot'o-my. [**Somatoto'mia;** from σῶμα, σώματος, the "body," and τέμνω, to "cut."] The same as ANATOMY, which see.

Som-nam'bu-lism. [**Somnambulis'mus;** from *som'nus,* "sleep," and *am'bulo,* to "walk."] Sleep-walking, or walking in one's sleep; a species of dreaming in which the bodily as well as the mental functions are affected.

Som-nif'e-ra.* [The neuter plural of *somnif'erus.* See next article.] Agents which cause sleep.

Som-nif'er-ous. [**Somnif'erus;** from *som'nus,* "sleep," and *fe'ro,* to "bring."] Causing or inducing sleep; hypnotic. Nearly the same as SOPORIFEROUS, which see.

Som'no-lence, or **Som'no-len-cy.** [**Somnolen'tia;** from *som'nus,* "sleep."] Sleepiness.

Som'no-lent. [**Somnolen'tus;** from the same.] Sleepy; drowsy.

Som'no-lism. [From the same.] The somnolent state induced by the manipulations termed animal magnetism.

Sonde, sônd. The French term for a SOUND, which see.

Son'i-tus.* [From *so'no, son'itum,* to "sound."] A sounding, as in the ears. See TINNITUS.

So-nom'e-ter. [**Sonom'etrum;** from *so'nus,* "sound," and μέτρον, a "measure."] An instrument for measuring the ratios of the vibrations of different sonorous bodies.

Soot. See FULIGO LIGNI.

Soot'-Drops. Hysteric Mixture. Tincture of soot, consisting of woodsoot, assafœtida, and proof-spirit; used in hysteria.

Soot-Wart. See CANCER SCROTI.

Sooty. See FULIGINOUS.

So-phis-ti-ca'tion. [**Sophistica'tio, o'***nis;* from σοφιστικός, "sophistical," "deceitful."] Adulteration of a medicine, aliment, etc.

So'pi-ens.* [From *so'pio,* to "put to sleep," to "set at rest."] Assuaging; anodyne: so'pient.

So'por, o'*ris.** Sound, deep, or profound sleep.

So-po-rif'er-ous. [**Soporif'erus;** from *so'por,* "sound sleep," and *fe'ro,* to "bring."] Inducing sound or deep sleep. See SOMNIFEROUS.

So-po-rif'ic. [**Soporif'icus;** from *so'por,* "sound sleep," and *fa'cio,* to "make."] Causing or inducing sleep.

So'po-rous, or **So-po-rose'.** [**Soporo'sus, Sopo'rus;** from *so'por,* "sound sleep."] Causing deep sleep; narcotic.

Sor'bate. [**Sor'bas, a'***tis.*] A combination of sorbic acid with a base. The same as MALATE.

Sorbet, or **Sorbetum.** See SHERBET.

Sor'bic. [**Sor'bicus;** from *Sor'bus,* the "mountain ash."] Belonging to the *Sorbus.* A name sometimes applied to malic acid, which may be procured from its berries.

Sor'bus Au-cu-pa'ri-a.* The systematic name of the Mountain Ash, which is said to contain a large quantity of hydrocyanic acid. It is called *Pyrus Aucuparia* by some writers.

Sor'des.* Literally, "filth." Applied to the foul matter discharged from ulcers; also, to filth which collects on the teeth, more particularly in certain low fevers, to foul accumulations in the stomach, etc.

Sore-Throat. See CYNANCHE.

So'ri,* the plural of **So'rus.** Heaps, or patches, as those of the spore-cases of most ferns, called in English fruit-dots.

So-ro'sis.* [From σωρός, a "collection."] A fleshy multiple fruit, like a mulberry.

Sor'rel. A popular name applied to the *Oxalis acetosella*, and also to the *Rumex acetosa*.

Sorus. See SORI.

Soude, sood. The French name for SODA, which see.

Soufre, soofR. The French name for SULPHUR, which see.

Soul. See ANIMA.

Sound. [Lat. **So'nus;** Fr. *Son*, sôNᵍ.] The effect produced on the organ of hearing by the vibrations of the air or other medium.

Sound. [From the French *sonder*, to "fathom," to "try the depth of the sea;" hence, to "try," or "examine."] An instrument for introduction through the urethra into the bladder, to ascertain whether a calculus be present.

Sourcil, sooR'sè'. The French name for "eyebrow." See SUPERCILIUM.

Sourd, sooR. The French word for DEAF, which see.

Sour-Dock. The *Rumex acetosa*.

Sous-clavière, soo klå've-êR'. The French term for SUBCLAVIAN, which see.

South'ern-wood, Tar-tā'rĭ-an. The *Artemisia santonica*.

Soymida Febrifuga. See SWIETENIA FEBRIFUGA.

Sp. = *Spir'itus.** "Spirit."

Spa, spå. A town in Belgium, near the Prussian frontier, celebrated for its mineral waters. The name is also applied to other mineral springs.

Spadiceous, spa-dish'us. [From *spa'dix.*] Bearing a spadix.

Spa'dix, i'cis.* [Gr. σπάδιξ, a "palm-branch."] A sort of fleshy spike, enveloped by a large bract or modified leaf, called a spathe, as in Indian Turnip (*Arum*).

Spain, Pellitory of. See ANTHEMIS PYRETHRUM.

Spalter. See SPELTER.

Span. The length spanned between the thumb and little finger, equal to seven or eight inches.

Spa-næ'mĭ-a.* [From σπανός, "poor," and αἷμα, "blood."] Poverty of blood; cachæmia.

Spanish Fly. See CANTHARIS.

Span'ish Liq'uo-rice. A name for coarse or common liquorice; because chiefly brought from Spain. See GLYCYRRHIZA.

Span'ish White. A name for white bismuth; nitrate of bismuth.

Spar. [From the German *Spath?*] A mineralogical term applied to certain crystallized substances which are easily broken into cubic, prismatic, or other fragments with polished surfaces.

Spar, Fluor. See FLUOR SPAR.

Spar, Heavy. A name for sulphate of baryta.

Sparse. [**Spar'sus;** from *spar'go, spar'sum*, to "strew about," to "sprinkle," to "scatter."] Applied to flowers, leaves, etc. which are scattered and generally scanty.

Spar-sĭ-flo'rous. [**Sparsiflo'rus;** from *spar'sus*, "scattered," and *flos*, a "flower."] Having scattered or few flowers.

Spar-sĭ-fo'lĭ-ate. [**Sparsifolia'tus;** from *spar'sus*, "scattered," and *fo'lium*, a "leaf."] Having scattered leaves.

Spartium,* spar'she-um. [From σπάρτη, a "rope."] A Linnæan genus of the class *Diadelphia*, natural order *Leguminosæ*.

Spar'tium Jun'ce-um.* Spanish Broom. A leguminous plant the seeds of which have been used in dropsy.

Spar'tium Sco-pa'rĭ-um.* The former systematic name of the common broom-plant; now the *Cyt'isus scopa'rius*.

Spasm. [**Spas'mus;** from σπάω, to "draw."] The sudden, involuntary contraction of muscles, or of muscular fibres; a convulsion, cramp.

1. CONSTRICTIVE SPASM is attended with contraction, rigidity, or both, as wry-neck, lock-jaw, etc. See ENTASIA.

2. CLONIC SPASM. [See CLONIC.] A violent agitation of one or more muscles in sudden and irregular snatches, as hiccough, sneezing, epilepsy, etc.

3. SYNCLONIC SPASM [*Syn'clonus*] is the simultaneous and chronic agitation of different muscles, as in St. Vitus' Dance.

4. TONIC SPASM consists in the constant contraction of a muscle, etc.

Spasma. See SPASMUS.

Spasmatic. See SPASMODIC.

Spas'mi.* [Plural of *spas'mus*, a "spasm."] Spasmodic diseases. The name of an order of the class *Neuroses* in Cullen's Nosology.

Spas-mo'dēs.* [From σπασμός, a "spasm."] Convulsive; having spasm or convulsion.

Spas-mod'ic. [**Spasmod'icus;** from *spas'mus*, a "spasm."] Relating to spasm; convulsive. See SPASMATIC.

Spas-mo-dy̆sp-nœ'a.* [From *spas'mus*, a "spasm," and *dyspnœ'a.*] Convulsive *dyspnœa* or difficulty of breathing.

Spas-mol'o-ġy̆. [**Spasmolo'gia;** from σπασμός, a "spasm," and λόγος, a "discourse."] That branch of Pathology which treats of spasms or convulsions, their character and causes.

Spas'mus Ca-ni'nus,* **Spas'mus Cy̆n'i-cus.*** ("Canine Spasm.") The *Risus Sardonicus*. See SARDONIC LAUGH.

Spas'tic. [**Spas'ticus;** from σπάω, to "draw."] Drawing to or from. Applied to the contraction of muscles, etc., from disease.

Spas'ti-ca.* [From the same.] Agents which increase the irritability of the muscles and induce spasm or convulsion.

Spa-thā'ceous. [**Spatha'ceus.**] Having a spathe; of the character or nature of a spathe.

Spathe, spāth. [Lat. **Spa'tha;** Gr. σπάθη.] Originally, a spatula; a ladle. Applied to a sheath which completely encloses the flowers before their expansion; the enveloping bract of a spadix, as in the Indian Turnip.

Spath-i-flo'rus.* [From *spa'tha*, a "spathe," and *flos*, a "flower."] Having flowers surrounded by a spathe.

Spathula. See SPATULA.

Spathulate. See SPATULATE.

Spat'u-la.* [Diminutive of *spa'tha.*] A broad instrument like a knife with blunt edges, for spreading ointments, etc.

Spat'u-late. [**Spatula'tus.**] Shaped like a spatula.

Spear-Mint. See MENTHA SATIVA.

Spear-Shaped. See LANCEOLATE.

Speç'ial Des-crip'tive Bot'a-ny̆. A scientific account of all known plants, designated by proper names and distinguished by clear and exact descriptions.

Species,* spee'shēz. [From *spe'cio*, to "see to," to "behold."] Originally, a "form," "likeness." In Natural History, an assemblage or series of similar organic beings. A species is, abstractly, the type or original of each sort of plant or animal, represented in time by a perennial succession of like individuals; or, concretely, it is the sum of such series or congeries of individuals.—(GRAY.)

Spe-cif'ic. [**Specif'icus;** from *spe'cies*, and *fa'cio*, to "make."] Literally, "that makes or constitutes a species," as in the phrase a "specific difference." Relating to species; special. Often applied to a medicine of supposed infallible efficacy in the cure of a particular species or form of disease; or to a remedy which has a *special* action on some particular organ,—for example, like that of ergot on the uterus.

Specific Gravity. See GRAVITY.

Spe-cil'lum.* [From *spe'cio*, to "behold," or "examine."] A probe.

Speç'i-men.* [From the same.] A Latin word signifying a "proof," "instance," "model," etc. Applied to plants, animals, and minerals collected for scientific purposes; and to a part of any thing exhibited as a sample.

Spec'ta-cled Snake. The *Naja vulgaris*, or *Cobra de capello*.

Spec'trum.* [From *spec'to*, to "behold."] A figure seen or imagined; a spectre. In Optics, a spectrum is an elongated image of the sun, or other luminous body, formed on a wall or screen in a darkened room, by a beam of light received through a small aperture and refracted by a glass prism. It exhibits the colors of the rainbow.

Spec'u-lar. [**Specula'ris.**] Belonging to the *speculum*.

Spec'u-lum,* plural **Spec'u-la.** [From *spe'cio*, to "behold."] Originally, a "mirror" of any kind. In Optics, a metallic mirror used in a reflecting telescope. In Surgery, an instrument for widening natural openings of passages, or keeping parts separate, so as to obtain a view of what is within. Applied also to a brilliant colored mark, forming the anterior borders of the *tectrices* of birds.

Spec'ulum Met'al. An alloy of about two parts of copper and one of tin, used for making mirrors. Its whiteness is improved by the addition of a little arsenic.

Speechlessness. See APHONIA.

Spel'trum.* ("Spelter.") A name for native impure zinc.

Sperm. See SPERMA.

Sperm'-Cell. A cell contained in the *liquor seminis*, in which spermatozoa are produced.

Sper'ma,* gen. **Sper'ma-tis.** [Gr. σπέρμα, "seed," or "semen;" Fr. *Semence*, seh-mŏnss'.] Literally, "seed." Sperm; the fecundating liquor in animals. Also applied incorrectly to spermaceti, a substance found in the head of some species of whales, and which concretes or crystallizes spontaneously on the death of the animal.

Sper-ma-çe'ti. [From *sper'ma*, and

κῆτος, the "whale."] The same as CETACEUM, which see.

Spermalogia. See SPERMATOLOGY.

Sper'ma-phore. [From σπέρμα, "seed," and φορέω, to "bear."] A name sometimes applied to the placenta and sometimes to the funiculus of the seed of a plant.

Sper'ma-ta,* the plural of SPERMA, which see.

Sper-ma-the'ca.* [From σπέρμα, "seed," or "semen," and θήκη, a "shrine."] A repository in the upper part of the oviduct in female insects, for receiving the seminal fluid of the male.

Sper-mat'ic. [**Spermat'icus;** from σπέρμα, σπέρματος, "seed," or "semen."] Relating to the semen, or seed; seminal.

Spermat'ic Ca-nal' (otherwise called the **In'gui-nal Canal'**). The oblique passage in the abdominal parietes through which is transmitted the spermatic cord. The internal and external orifices of this canal are termed respectively the internal and external *abdominal* (or *inguinal*) *rings*.

Spermat'ic Cord [**Funic'ulus Spermat'icus**], also termed **Tes-tic'u-lar Cord.** The cord by which the testicle is suspended. It consists of the vessels and nerves which pass to and from the testis, enclosed in several tunics and the few muscular fibres (or muscular fascia) known as the cremaster muscle.

Sper'ma-tin. [**Spermati'na;** from σπέρμα, "seed," or "semen."] A substance obtained from the seminal fluid of animals.

Sper'ma-tism. [**Spermatis'mus;** from σπερματίζω, to "bear or produce seed."] The emission of semen. Also, the doctrine which maintains that the germ in animals is produced by spermatic animalcules. See SPERMATOZOA.

Sper'ma-to-çēle.* [From σπέρμα, "semen," and κήλη, a "tumor."] A swelling of the testicle, or epididymis, from an accumulation of semen.

Sper'ma-to-clem'ma, atis.* [From σπέρμα, "semen," and κλέπτω, to "steal," to "pass unobserved."] *Pollutio diurna*, or involuntary escape of semen in the daytime. See SPERMATORRHŒA, and SPERMATORRHŒA DORMIENTIUM.

Sper'ma-to-derm. [**Spermatoder'ma, atis;** from σπέρμα, "seed," and δέρμα, the "skin."] The outer covering of a seed, originally the primine of the ovule.

Sper'ma-to-go'ni-a.* [From σπέρμα, "semen," and γονή, "generation."] Secretion of semen: spermatog'ony.

Sper-ma-tog'ra-phy. [**Spermatogra'phia;** from σπέρμα, "seed," and γράφω, to "write."] A description of seeds.

Sper-ma-tol'o-gy. [**Spermatolo'gia;** from σπέρμα, σπέρματος, "semen," and λόγος, a "discourse."] That branch of Physiology which treats of the secretion and nature of semen.

Sper'ma-to-po-et'ic. [**Spermatopoet'icus,** or **Spermatopœ'us;** from σπέρμα, "semen," and ποιέω, to "make," to "produce."] Producing semen; also, promoting the secretion of semen.

Sper'ma-tor-rhœ'a.* [From σπέρμα, "semen," and ῥέω, to "flow."] An involuntary emission of semen without copulation. The same as *gonorrhœa* in the strict sense.

Spermatorrhœ'a Dormien'tium* (dor-me-en'she-ŭm), called also **Gon-or-rhœ'a Dormien'tium.*** ("Seminal Emission of [those] Sleeping.") An emission of semen during sleep, most frequently the result of libidinous dreams, but sometimes caused by nervous weakness, and occasionally by simple repletion of the seminal vessels. See POLLUTION.

Sper-ma-tos'che-sis.* [From σπέρμα, "semen," and σχέσις, a "checking."] Want or suppression of semen.

Sper'ma-to-ze'mi-a.* [From σπέρμα, "semen," and ζημία, "loss."] Cessation of the seminal secretion.

Sper-ma-to-zo'a,* the plural of SPERMATOZOON, which see.

Spermatozoids. See SPERMATOZOON.

Sper'ma-to-zo'on,* plural **Sper'ma-to-zo'a;** also termed **Sper'ma-to-zo'ids.** [From σπέρμα, "semen," and ζῶον, an "animal."] Applied to numerous minute bodies discovered in the semen, formerly supposed to be animalcula. They would seem to be analogous to the pollen-tubes of plants; they are considered by physiologists to constitute the essential or fecundating principle of the semen.

Sper'mic, or **Sper'mous.** [From σπέρμα, "seed."] In Botany, relating to the seed.

Sper-mob'o-le.* [From σπέρμα, "semen," and βάλλω, to "cast."] The same as SPERMATISM, which see.

Sper'mo-derm. [**Spermoder'ma, atis,** or **Spermoder'mis, idis;** from σπέρμα, "seed," and δέρμα, the "skin."] The outer or proper seed-coat of a plant.

Spermogonia. See SPERMATOGONIA.

Sper-mol'i-thus.* [From σπέρμα, a

"seed," or "semen," and λίθος, a "stone."] A fossil seed; a spermolite. Also applied to an indurated concretion in the *vesiculæ seminales.*

Sper-mor-rhœ'a.* The same as SPERMATORRHŒA, which see.

Sphaç'e-lāt-ed. [**Sphacela'tus;** from *sphaç'elus.*] Mortified. Pertaining to, or in the state of, sphacelus.

Sphaç-e-lā'tion. [**Sphacela'tio, o'nis;** from *sphaç'elus.*] Mortification.

Sphaç-e-lis'mus.* [From σφακελίζω, to "be affected with gangrene."] Inflammation of the brain; also, mortification of some part.

Sphaç'e-loid. [**Sphaceloi'des;** from *sphaç'elus,* and εἶδος, a "form."] Resembling sphacelus.

Sphaç'e-lus.* [Gr. σφάκελος.] The complete death of a part; complete mortification. See SIDERATION.

Sphær-i-car'pus.* [From σφαῖρα, a "sphere," and καρπός, "fruit."] Having spherical fruit: sphericarpous.

Sphæ-ric-u-la'tus.* [From σφαῖρα, a "sphere."] Approaching the form of a globe or sphere.

Sphæroidalis. See SPHEROIDAL.

Sphæroides. See SPHEROID.

Sphæ-ro'ma, atis.* [From σφαῖρα, a "sphere."] A term for a globular, fleshy protuberance or tumor.

Sphæ-ro-sper'mus.* [From σφαῖρα, a "sphere," and σπέρμα, "seed."] Having round seeds: spherosper'mous.

Sphe'noid. [**Sphenoi'des;** from σφήν, a "wedge," and εἶδος, a "form."] Resembling a wedge; cuneiform.

Sphe-noi'dal. [**Sphenoida'lis;** from *sphenoi'des* os, the "sphenoid bone."] Belonging to the sphenoid bone.

Sphe'no-pal'a-tine Gan'gli-on. The largest of the cranial ganglia, situated in the pterygopalatine fossa.

Sphe-nop'te-rus.* [From σφήν, a "wedge," and πτερόν, a "wing."] Having wings like a wedge: sphenopterous. Applied to plants.

Sphe'no-Sal-pin'go-Staph-y̆-li'nus.* A designation of the *circumflexus palati* muscle, from its connection with the sphenoid bone, Eustachian tube, and uvula.

Sphe'no-Staph-y̆-li'nus.* [See STAPHYLINUS.] A designation of the *levator palati mollis,* from its arising from the sphenoid bone and being inserted into the *velum palati.*

Sphere. [Lat. **Sphæ'ra;** Gr. σφαῖρα, a "globe."] A solid body described by the revolution of a semicircle about its diameter; or it may be defined to be a body bounded by a surface of which every point is equally distant from a single point within the surface, called the centre of the sphere. In Astronomy, the sphere is the concave expanse of the heavens, which, having no definite limits, appears to the eye as the interior surface of a sphere enclosing the earth, which seems placed at the centre.

Sphĕr'i-cal. [**Sphærica'lis;** from the same.] Formed like a globe; globular; pertaining to a sphere.

Sphe'roid. [**Sphæroi'des;** from the same.] A solid generated by the revolution of an ellipse about one of its axes. If the generating ellipse revolves about its major axis, the spheroid is *prolate,* or oblong; if about its minor axis, the spheroid is *oblate,* as the planet Earth.

Sphe-roid'al, or **Sphe-roid'ic.** [**Sphæroida'lis;** from the same.] Resembling a spheroid. Applied to crystals bounded by several convex faces.

Sphe-rom'e-ter. [**Sphærom'etrum;** from σφαῖρα, a "sphere," and μέτρον, a "measure."] An instrument for measuring the curvature of a surface, chiefly that of optical glasses.

Sphĕr'ule. [**Sphær'ula;** diminutive of *sphæ'ra,* a "sphere."] A little sphere; a round, oblong, or conical conceptacle opening at the top by slits or pores.

Sphinc'ter, e'ris.* [From σφίγγω, to "bind tight," to "close."] A circular muscle which contracts the aperture to which it is attached.

Sphinc'ter A'ni.* ("Sphincter of the Anus.") A thin layer of muscular fibres surrounding the anus like an ellipse is termed *sphincter ani externus;* another layer embracing the lower extremity of the rectum is called *sphincter ani internus.*

Sphinc'ter O'ris.* ("Sphincter of the Mouth.") A name for the *orbicula'ris o'ris* muscle, situated round the mouth.

Sphy̆g'mi-cal. [**Sphyg'micus;** from σφυγμός, the "pulse."] Belonging to the pulse.

Sphy̆g-mo'dēs.* [From the same.] Having a pulse: sphygmous.

Sphy̆g-mog'ra-phy̆. [**Sphygmogra'phia;** from σφυγμός, the "pulse," and γράφω, to "write."] A description of the pulse, its nature and causes.

Sphy̆g'moid. [**Sphygmoi'des;** from σφυγμός, the "pulse," and εἶδος, a "form."] Resembling the pulse.

Sphyg-mol'o-gy. [**Sphygmolo'-gia;** from σφυγμός, the "pulse," and λόγος, a "discourse."] The doctrine or science of the pulse.

Sphyg-mom'e-ter. [**Sphygmom'-etrum;** from σφυγμός, the "pulse," and μέτρον, a "measure."] An instrument for measuring the frequency of the pulse; or, according to Hoblyn, an instrument which renders the action of the arteries apparent to the eye.

Sphyg-mos'co-pe,* or **Sphyg-mo-sco'pi-a.*** [From σφυγμός, the "pulse," and σκοπέω, to "examine."] An exploration or examination of the pulse, or of different pulses: sphygmoscopy.

Sphyg-mo-sco'pi-um.* [From the same.] A sphygmoscope, an instrument similar to the SPHYGMOMETER, which see.

Sphyg-mo-tech'ne.* [From σφυγμός, the "pulse," and τέχνη, an "art."] The art of examining the pulse.

Spi'ca.* A Latin word signifying an "ear of wheat." Applied to a mode of inflorescence. (See SPIKE.) In Surgery, a bandage somewhat like an ear of wheat or barley in shape.

Spi'cate. [**Spica'tus;** from *spi'ca*, a "spike."] Relating to, or disposed in, a spike.

Spi-ci-flo'rous. [From *spi'ca*, a "spike," and *flos*, a "flower."] Having flowers disposed in spikes.

Spi'ci-form. [**Spicifor'mis;** from *spi'ca*, a "spike."] Having the form of an ear or spike.

Spi-cig'e-rous. [**Spicig'erus;** from *spi'ca*, a "spike," and *ge'ro*, to "bear."] Bearing ears or spikes.

Spic'u-la,* plural **Spic'u-læ.** [Diminutive of *spi'ca*, a "spike."] A little spike; a spikelet. Also applied to a needle-like splinter or fragment, as of bone, etc. See ACICULA, and SPIKELET.

Spic'u-læ,* gen. **Spic-u-la'rum,** the plural of SPICULA, which see.

Spic'u-lar. [**Spicula'ris;** from *spic'ula*, a "spikelet."] Belonging to a spikelet, or like a spicula.

Spic-u-lif'er-ous. [**Spiculif'erus;** from *spic'ula*, a "spikelet," and *fe'ro*, to "bear."] Having flowers disposed in *spiculæ*.

Spi-ge'li-a.* [From *Spige'lius*, a botanist.] Pinkroot. A Linnæan genus of the class *Pentandria*, natural order *Gentianaceæ*. Also, the Pharmacopœial name (U.S. and Ed. Ph.) for the root of *Spigelia Marilandica*.

Spige'lia Mar-i-lan'di-ca.* The Indian or Carolina pink; also called *Spige'lia lonice'ra*. It is extensively used as an anthelmintic.

Spigelian Lobe. See LOBULUS SPIGELII.

Spike. [From *spi'ca*, an "ear of corn or wheat."] A prolonged indefinite inflorescence, with sessile flowers, as in the plantain and wheat. A spike is the same as a raceme, except that the flowers are sessile.

Spike'let. [**Spic'ula.**] A little spike. A secondary spike; the ultimate flower-cluster of the grasses.

Spike'nard. A perfume and stimulant medicine procured from the *Nar'dus In'dica* (or *Nardos'tachys Jataman'si*), an Indian plant.

Spike'-Stalk. [**Rha'chis.**] The receptacle of the florets in spikelets of grasses, or of the spikelets themselves.

Spi-lo'ma, a*tis*,* plural **Spi-lo'ma-ta.** [From σπῖλος, a "stain," a "blemish."] Another name for NÆVUS MATERNUS, which see.

Spi'na,* plural **Spi'næ.** Originally, a "thorn," a "prickle." The spine. Also applied to one of the spinous processes. See SPINE.

Spina Bifida. See SCHISTORRHACHIS.

Spi'na Ven-to'sa.* A disease in which matter is formed in a bone, expands its walls, and makes its way outward, sometimes insinuating itself into the cellular substance so as to render it soft and flabby, as if filled with air. See ARTHROCACE.

Spi'næ,* the plural of SPINA. See SPINE.

Spi'nal. [**Spina'lis;** from *spi'na*, the "spine."] Pertaining to the spine, or backbone. Also, belonging to or connected with the spinous processes.

Spi'nal Cen'tre. Applied by M. Hall to the spinal marrow, regarded as distinct from the nerves proceeding from it.

Spi'nal Chord. The SPINAL MARROW, which see.

Spinal Column. See VERTEBRAL COLUMN.

Spi'nal Mar'row. [**Medul'la Spina'lis.**] The medullary substance contained in the spinal or vertebral column; the spinal chord.

Spi'nal Men-in-gi'tis. A term applied to the inflammation of the *meninges*, or membranes which enclose the spinal marrow.

Spi'nal Sys'tem of Nerves. Applied to those nerves which issue from the spinal marrow considered independently of the ganglionic or cerebral systems. Those which convey impressions of irritation from the surface of the body, or from mucous surfaces, to the true spinal marrow, called Incident,—and those that convey motor phenomena from it, named Reflex spinal nerves.

Spi-na'lis Dor'si.* ("Spinal [Muscle] of the Back.") A muscle of the back which, with its fellow, forms an ellipse enclosing the spinous processes of all the dorsal vertebræ.

Spī'nate. [**Spina'tus;** from *spi'na*, a "thorn."] Having thorns; or shaped like a spine or thorn.

Spindle-Shaped. See FUSIFORM.

Spīne. [Lat. **Spi'na;** Fr. *Épine*, à'pèn'.] A thorn, or rigid prickle proceeding from the woody part of a plant. Also applied to a process or projection of bone, and hence to the backbone or vertebral column, on account of its numerous spines or projections.

Spī-nĕs'çence. [**Spinescen'tia;** from *spi'na*, a "thorn."] The state or condition of a surface covered with thorns.

Spī-nĕs'çent. [**Spines'cens;** from the same.] Becoming hard and thorny; tipped with a spine.

Spī-nif'er-ous. [**Spinif'erus;** from *spi'na*, a "thorn," and *fe'ro*, to "bear."] Bearing spines.

Spī-nĭ-fo'lĭ-ous. [**Spinifolia'tus;** from *spi'na*, a "thorn," and *fo'lium*, a "leaf."] Having spinous leaves.

Spī'nĭ-form. [**Spinifor'mis;** from *spi'na*, a "thorn."] Having the form of spines.

Spi-nig'er-us.* [From *spi'na*, a "thorn," and *ge'ro*, to "bear."] The same as SPINIFEROUS, which see.

Spin'ne-rets. The minute teats, or *mammillæ*, of the *Arachnides*. See FUSUS.

Spin'ne-rules. [From the same.] Innumerable minute tubes with which each spinneret of the *Arachnides* is studded, every one of which emits a thread of inconceivable fineness.

Spī-no-car'pous. [**Spinocar'pus;** from *spi'na*, a "thorn," and καρπός, "fruit."] Having spinous or prickly fruit.

Spī'nous, or **Spī-nose'.** [**Spino'sus;** from *spi'na*, a "thorn."] Having thorns or spines; thorny, or shaped like a thorn.

Spin-the-ris'mus.* [From σπινθηρίζω, to "emit sparks."] The sensation of an issuing of sparks from the eyes: spintherism. The same as SCINTILLATION, which see.

Spin-the-rom'e-ter. [**Spinthe-rom'etrum;** from σπινθήρ, a "spark," and μέτρον, a "measure."] An instrument for determining the size, power, and shock of electrical sparks.

Spin-the-ro'pi-a.* [From σπινθήρ, a "spark," and ὤψ, ὠπός, the "eye."] A morbid state of vision, in which there is an appearance of sparks or scintillations before the eyes.

Spin-u-lif'er-ous. [**Spinulif'erus;** from *spin'ula*, a "little spine," and *fe'ro*, to "bear."] Bearing or having small spines.

Spin-u-lose'. [**Spinulo'sus;** from *spin'ula*, a "little spine."] Having small spines: spinulous.

Spiracle. See SPIRACULUM.

Spi-rac'u-la,* the plural of SPIRACULUM, which see.

Spi-rac'u-lum,* plural **Spi-rac'u-la.** [From *spi'ro*, to "breathe."] A Latin word signifying a "breathing-hole," or a "vent." A spiracle. Applied to the respiratory pores of the skin. Proposed by Latreille as a term instead of *stigma*, to designate the exterior orifices of the tracheæ of insects.

Spi-ræ'a.* Hardhack. The Pharmacopœial name (U.S. Ph.) for the root of the *Spiræ'a tomento'sa*. It is tonic and astringent, and is sometimes used in diarrhœa, cholera infantum, etc.

Spī'ral. [**Spira'lis;** from *spi'ra*, a "coil," or "spire;" a "wreath."] Winding like the worm of a screw; winding round a cylinder and at the same time rising or advancing. Applied to a curve which winds around a point in successive convolutions. In Geometry, a name given to a class of curves distinguished by this general property, that they continually recede from a centre or pole, while they continue to revolve about it.

Spiral Arrangement of Leaves. See PHYLLOTAXIS.

Spī'ral Ban'dage. The common roller applied spirally round a limb.

Spī'ral Ves'sels, or **Spī'ral Ducts.** Membranous tubes with conical extremities, lined on the inside by a fibre twisted spirally and capable of unrolling with elasticity. They constitute a part of the vascular tissue of plants of the higher grades, and are often filled with air.

Spirit. See SPIRITUS.

Spir'it of Salt. Muriatic, or hydrochloric, acid.

Spir'it of Wine, Rec'tĭ-fied. A name for alcohol.

Spir'it of Wine, Weak'er. [**Spir'itus Ten'uior.**] A name for proof-spirit, half the strength of rectified spirit.

Spir-i-tu-o'sa et Æ-the're-a.* ("Spirituous and Ethereal [Substances].") A class of powerful and diffusible stimulants, including ardent spirits, wine, beer, and the ethers.

Spir'it-u-ous. [**Spirituo'sus;** from *spir'itus*, "spirit."] Having spirit, or full of spirit.

Spir'i-tus.* [From *spi'ro*, to "breathe."] The air received and discharged by the action of the lungs; the breath. Also, the soul, or spirit. (See ANIMA.) Also, spirit, alcohol, or a liquor containing a large proportion of it.

Spir'itus Æ'the-ris Com-pos'i-tus.* ("Compound Spirit of Ether.") Hoffmann's Anodyne. Take of ether, half a pint; alcohol, a pint; ethereal oil, six fluidrachms. Mix them. A very popular remedy both as an anodyne and antispasmodic.

Spir'itus Æ'theris Ni'tri-ci.* Nitric ether. See next article.

Spir'itus Æ'theris Ni-tro'si.* ("Spirit of Nitrous Ether.") **Spir'itus Æ'theris Ni'tri-ci,*** 1850. Commonly called **Sweet Spir'it of Ni'tre.** The Pharmacopœial name for a volatile inflammable liquid, of a pale-yellow color inclining slightly to green, having a fragrant ethereal odor free from pungency, and a sharp, burning taste. It is diaphoretic, diuretic, and antispasmodic, and is much used in febrile affections, especially such as are accompanied with nervous excitement.

Spir'itus Æ'theris Sul-phu'ri-ci.* ("Spirit of Sulphuric Ether.") (Fr. *Esprit d'Ether sulfurique*, ĕs'prè' dā'tēr' sül'fü'rēk'.) Sulphuric ether. The *Æther* of the United States and British Pharmacopœias. It is a powerful diffusible stimulant and narcotic. It is very extensively employed as an anæsthetic. See ETHER, SULPHURIC.

Spir'itus Am-mo'ni-æ.* ("Spirit of Ammonia.") The Pharmacopœial name (U.S. Ph.) for the preparation formerly known as ammoniated alcohol. It consists of a solution of caustic ammonia in diluted alcohol. It is stimulant and antispasmodic.

Spir'itus A-ni'si.* ("Spirit of Anise.") Take of oil of anise, a fluidounce; stronger alcohol, fifteen fluidounces. Dissolve the oil in the stronger alcohol.

Spir'itus Cam'pho-ræ.* ("Spirit of Camphor.") **Tinc-tu'ra Cam'phoræ,*** 1850. ("Tincture of Camphor.") Take of camphor, four troyounces; alcohol, two pints. Dissolve the camphor in the alcohol, and filter through paper.

Spir'itus Chlo-ro-for'mi.* ("Spirit of Chloroform.") Take of purified chloroform, a troyounce; stronger alcohol, six fluidounces. Dissolve the chloroform in the stronger alcohol.

Spir'itus Cin-na-mo'mi.* ("Spirit of Cinnamon.") Take of oil of cinnamon, a fluidounce; stronger alcohol, fifteen fluidounces. Dissolve the oil in the stronger alcohol.

Spir'itus Fru-men'ti.* ("Spirit of Grain.") Whiskey. The name applied to the spirit obtained from fermented grain by distillation, and containing from forty-eight to fifty-six per cent. of absolute alcohol. It has been placed on the primary list of the Materia Medica of the U.S. Pharmacopœia for 1860.

Spir'itus Gal'li-cus.* ("French Spirit.") A name for brandy.

Spir'itus Ja-mai-çen'sis.* ("Jamaica Spirit.") A name for rum.

Spir'itus Ju-nip'e-ri Com-pos'i-tus.* ("Compound Spirit of Juniper.") Take of oil of juniper, a fluidrachm and a half; oil of caraway, oil of fennel, each, ten minims; diluted alcohol, eight pints. Dissolve the oils in the diluted alcohol.

Spir'itus La-van'du-læ.* ("Spirit of Lavender.") Take of lavender, fresh, twenty-four troyounces; alcohol, eight pints; water, two pints. Mix them, and, with a regulated heat, distil eight pints.

Spir'itus Lavan'dulæ Com-pos'i-tus.* ("Compound Spirit of Lavender.") Take of oil of lavender, a fluidounce; oil of rosemary, two fluidrachms; cinnamon, in moderately fine powder, two troyounces; cloves, in moderately fine powder, half a troyounce; nutmeg, in moderately fine powder, a troyounce; red saunders, in moderately fine powder, three hundred and sixty grains; alcohol, six pints; water, two pints; diluted alcohol, a sufficient quantity. Dissolve the oils in the alcohol, and add the water. Then mix the powders, and, having moistened the mixture with a fluidounce of the alcoholic solution of the oils, pack it firmly in a conical percolator, and gradually pour upon it the remainder of the alcoholic solution, and afterwards diluted alcohol, until the filtered liquid measures eight pints.

Spir'itus Li-mo'nis.* ("Spirit of

Lemon.") Essence of Lemon. Take of oil of lemon, two fluidounces; lemon-peel, freshly grated, a troyounce; stronger alcohol, two pints. Dissolve the oil in the stronger alcohol, add the lemon-peel, macerate for twenty-four hours, and filter through paper.

Spir'itus Men'thæ Pip-er-i'tæ.* ("Spirit of Peppermint.") **Tinc-tu'ra O'le-i Men'thæ Piperi'tæ,*** 1850. ("Tincture of Oil of Peppermint.") Essence of Peppermint. Take of oil of peppermint, a fluidounce; peppermint, in coarse powder, one hundred and twenty grains; stronger alcohol, fifteen fluidounces. Dissolve the oil in the stronger alcohol, add the peppermint, macerate for twenty-four hours, and filter through paper.

Spir'itus Men'thæ Vir'i-dis.* ("Spirit of Spearmint.") **Tinc-tu'ra O'le-i Men'thæ Vir'idis,*** 1850. ("Tincture of Oil of Spearmint.") Essence of Spearmint. Take of oil of spearmint, a fluidounce; spearmint, in coarse powder, one hundred and twenty grains; stronger alcohol, fifteen fluidounces. Dissolve the oil in the stronger alcohol, add the spearmint, macerate for twenty-four hours, and filter through paper.

Spiritus Mindereri. See MINDERERI, SPIRITUS.

Spir'itus Myr'ci-æ* ("Spirit of Myrcia"), or **Bay Rum.** The name applied to the spirit obtained by distilling rum with the leaves of the *Myrcia acris*. It has been placed on the primary list of the Materia Medica of the U.S. Pharmacopœia for 1860.

Spir'itus My-ris'ti-cæ.* ("Spirit of Nutmeg.") Take of nutmeg, bruised, two troyounces; diluted alcohol, eight pints; water, a pint. Mix them, and, with a regulated heat, distil eight pints.

Spir'itus Rec-ti-fi-ca'tus.* ("Rectified Spirit.") The Pharmacopœial name (Br. Ph.) for dilute alcohol of the specific gravity 0.838, containing sixteen per cent. of water.

Spir'itus Sac'cha-ri.* ("Spirit of Sugar.") A name for RUM, which see.

Spir'itus Ten'u-i-or.* ("Thinner or Weaker Spirit.") Proof-spirit. The Pharmacopœial name (Br. Ph.) for diluted alcohol of the specific gravity 0.920, which contains forty-nine per cent. of pure alcohol.

Spir'itus Vi'ni Gal'li-ci.* ("Spirit of French Wine.") The Pharmacopœial name (U.S. Ph.) for brandy, or the spirit obtained from fermented grapes by distillation, and containing from forty-eight to fifty-six per cent. of absolute alcohol.

Spi-ro-i'dēs.* [From *spi'ra*, a "coil," or "spire."] Resembling a spire or screw: spi'roid.

Spi-rom'e-ter. [**Spirom'etrum;** from *spi'ro*, to "breathe," and μέτρον, a "measure."] An instrument for ascertaining the quantity of air inhaled or exhaled by the lungs.

Spi-rom'e-trȳ. [**Spirome'tria;** from *spi'ro*, to "breathe," and μετρέω, to "measure."] The system or means of ascertaining the quantity of air employed in respiration, etc.

Spissatus. See INSPISSATED.

Spis'si-tude. [**Spissitu'do,** *inis;* from *spis'sus*, "thick."] Thickness, or density.

Spitting of Blood. See HÆMOPTYSIS.

Spittle. See SALIVA, and SPUTUM.

Splanch'nic. [**Splanch'nicus;** from σπλάγχνον, a "viscus."] Pertaining to the viscera.

Splanch'nic Cav'i-ties. A term applied to the cavities of the cranium, chest, and abdomen.

Splanchnic Nerve. See TRI-SPLANCHNIC NERVE.

Splanch'nic Nerves. [**Ner'vi Splanch'nici.**] These are two in number on each side, distinguished into the *great*, which passes behind the stomach and terminates in the semilunar ganglion, and the *small*, which communicates with the former and terminates in the renal ganglion.

Splanch'ni-ca.* [From σπλάγχνον, a "viscus," or "bowel."] Applied by Dr. Good as the name of an order comprising diseases of the viscera directly concerned in the function of digestion.

Splanch-nog'ra-phy̆. [**Splanchnogra'phia;** from σπλάγχνον, a "viscus," and γράφω, to "write."] A description of the viscera; that part of Anatomy which treats of the viscera.

Splanch-nol'i-thus.* [From σπλάγχνον, a "viscus," and λίθος, a "stone."] Intestinal calculus: a splanch'nolith.

Splanch-nol'o-gy̆. [**Splanchnolo'gia;** from σπλάγχνον, a "viscus," and λόγος, a "discourse."] A treatise on the viscera; the science which treats of the structure and functions of the viscera.

Splanch-no-sco'pi-a.* [From σπλάγχνον, a "viscus," and σκοπέω, to "examine."] An exploration of the viscera: splanchnos'copy.

Splanch-no-sy̆m'pa-thy̆. [**Splanch-**

nosympathi'a; from σπλάγχνον, a "viscus," and συμπάθεια, "fellow-feeling."] The sympathy of the viscera among themselves, or of a viscus with other parts.

Splanch-not'o-mȳ. [**Splanchnoto'mia;** from σπλάγχνον, a "viscus," and τέμνω, to "cut."] Dissection of the viscera.

Spleen. [Lat. **Splen, e'nis, Li'en, e'nis;** Gr. σπλήν; Fr. *Rate,* rât.] A purple, or livid-colored, viscus in the left hypochondriac region. Its function has not yet been ascertained. It would seem to have a close connection with the system of lymphatics, and to be intimately concerned in the development of blood. Also, a popular term for *hypochondri'asis,* a form of melancholy, supposed to have its seat in the spleen.

Spleenwort. See ASPLENIUM.

Sple-năl'ġĭ-a.* [From σπλήν, the "spleen," and ἄλγος, "pain."] Pain in the region of the spleen.

Sple-naux'e.* [From σπλήν, the "spleen," and αὔξη, "increase."] Enlargement of the spleen.

Splen-ec-to'pĭ-a.* [From σπλήν, the "spleen," ἐκ, "out," and τόπος, a "place."] Dislocation or displacement of the spleen.

Splen-el-co'sis.* [From σπλήν, the "spleen," and ἕλκωσις, "ulceration."] Ulceration of the spleen.

Sple-nel'cus.* [From σπλήν, the "spleen," and ἕλκος, an "ulcer."] An ulcer of the spleen.

Splen-em-phrax'is.* [From σπλήν, the "spleen," and ἔμφραξις, "obstruction."] Obstruction or congestion of the spleen.

Splen'e-tic. [**Splenet'icus.**] Relating to, or affected with, the spleen; fretful; splenic. See SPLENIC.

Sple'nĭ-al. [**Splenia'lis;** from *sple'nium,* a term denoting a "compress," sometimes applied to a splint.] Applied by Owen to the *operculaire* of Cuvier, a subdivision of the mandible in cold-blooded vertebrated animals. See TYMPANOMANDIBULAR ARCH.

Splen'ic. [**Splen'icus;** from σπλήν, the "spleen."] Pertaining to the spleen.

Splen'ĭ-ca.* [From the same.] Medicines which affect the spleen.

Splen-ĭ-fĭ-cā'tion. [**Splenifica'tio, o'nis;** from σπλήν, the "spleen," and *fa'cio,* to "make."] The conversion of the lung or liver, etc., into a substance like that of the spleen.

Sple'nĭ-ous. [**Sple'nius;** from the same.] Pertaining to, or resembling, the spleen.

Sple-nī'tis, idis.* [From σπλήν, the "spleen."] Inflammation of the spleen. A genus of the order *Phlegmasiæ,* class *Pyrexiæ,* of Cullen's Nosology.

Sple'nĭ-um.* [Said to have been originally applied to a plaster of a certain description used by those sick of the spleen.] A compress; a splint. Also, ASPLENIUM, or Spleenwort.

Sple'nĭ-us.* [See preceding article.] A muscle of the back, resembling the spleen: it is single at its origin, and divides into the *splenius capitis* and the *splenius colli,* which have distinct insertions. According to some, the *splenii* muscles are so named from their lying like surgical splints (see SPLENIUM) along the side of the neck.

Splen-ĭ-zā'tion. [**Spleniza'tio, o'nis;** from the same.] Applied to the state of the lungs in one of the stages of pneumonia in which their texture resembles that of the spleen. Compare HEPATIZATION.

Sple-no'dēs.* [From σπλήν, the "spleen."] Having the spleen; of the nature of the spleen.

Splen-o-dȳn'ĭ-a.* [From σπλήν, the "spleen," and ὀδύνη, "pain."] Pain in the spleen.

Sple-nog'ra-phȳ. [**Splenogra'phia;** from σπλήν, the "spleen," and γράφω, to "write."] A description of the spleen.

Splen-o-hæ'mĭ-a.* [From σπλήν, the "spleen," and αἷμα, "blood."] Sanguineous congestion, or *hyperæmia,* of the spleen.

Sple'noid. [**Splenoi'des;** from σπλήν, the "spleen," and εἶδος, a "form."] Resembling the spleen.

Sple-nol'o-ġȳ. [**Splenolo'gia;** from σπλήν, the "spleen," and λόγος, a "discourse."] The doctrine of the spleen; that branch of Anatomy (or Physiology) which treats of the spleen.

Sple-no'ma, atis,* or **Sple-non'cus.*** [From σπλήν, the "spleen," and ὄγκος, a "tumor."] Tumor of the spleen.

Splenomalacia,* splen-o-ma-la'she-a. [From σπλήν, the "spleen," and μαλακία, "softness."] Softening of the spleen.

Sple-not'o-mȳ. [**Splenoto'mia;** from σπλήν, the "spleen," and τέμνω, to "cut."] Dissection of the spleen.

Sple-ny-per-tro'phĭ-a.* [From σπλήν, the "spleen," and *hypertro'phia.*] Hypertrophy, or morbid enlargement, of the spleen: similar to *splenoncus.*

Splint. [Lat. **Hastel'la;** Fr. *Éclisse,*

ȧ'klĕss'.] A thin piece of wood, tin, or pasteboard, used to retain fractured bones in apposition during the process of reunion.

Splint'-Bone. A name sometimes applied to the fibula, from its resemblance to a surgical splint.

Split Cloth. [**Scis'sum Lin'-teum.**] A bandage for the head, consisting of a central part and six or eight tails or heads.

Spod'u-mene. [From σποδόω, to "reduce to ashes."] A crystalline mineral found in laminated masses, consisting chiefly of alumina and silica and lithia. Before the blowpipe it exfoliates into little scales of an ash-color: hence its name.

Spon-dy̆-lăl'ġĭ-a.* [From σπόνδυλος, a "vertebra," and ἄλγος, "pain."] Pain in a vertebra.

Spon-dy̆-lar-thri'tis, idis.* [From σπόνδυλος, a "vertebra," and *arthri'tis*.] Inflammation of an articulation of the vertebræ.

Spon-dy̆-lar-throc'a-çe.* [From σπόνδυλος, a "vertebra," and *arthroc'ace*, a form of caries.] Caries of a vertebra.

Spon-dy̆-lex-ar-thro'sis.* [From σπόνδυλος, a "vertebra," and *exarthro'sis*, "luxation."] Dislocation of a vertebra.

Spon-dy̆-li'tis, idis.* [From σπόνδυλος, a "vertebra."] Inflammation of one or more of the vertebræ.

Spon-dy̆-lo-dy̆n'ĭ-a.* [From σπόνδυλος, a "vertebra," and ὀδύνη, "pain."] Pain in the body of a vertebra.

Spon-dy̆-lo-py-o'sis.* [From σπόνδυλος, a "vertebra," and *pyo'sis*.] A formation of pus in a vertebra.

Spon'dy̆-lus.* A vertebra; also, the vertex or top of the head.

Sponge, spŭnj. [See SPONGIA.] An organic, porous, marine substance, formerly supposed to be produced by minute animals termed *Polypi*. Some naturalists, however, consider sponge as a plant. According to the proposed classification of Messrs. Wilson and Cassin, the sponge is referred to a new kingdom, termed PRIMALIA, which see.

Sponge'-Tent. The SPONGIA PRÆPARATA, which see.

Spon'ġĭ-a,* plural **Spon'ġĭ-æ.** [Gr. σπόγγος, or σπογγιά; Fr. *Éponge*, ȧ'pôɴzh'.] Sponge. The Pharmacopœial name (U.S. Ph., 1850) for *Spongia officinalis*. Applied in the plural to an order or division of organized bodies. See SPONGE.

Spon'gia Of-fiç-ĭ-na'lis.* The common sponge.

Spon'gia Præp-a-ra'ta* ("Prepared Sponge"), or **Spon'gia Ce-ra'ta*** ("Waxed Sponge"). Sponge dipped into melted wax and pressed between iron plates, then, when cold, cut in pieces of any shape for dilating small openings, the wax melting by the heat of the part, and thus allowing the sponge to expand; sponge-tent.

Spon'ġĭ-æ,* the plural of SPONGIA.

Spongiform, spŭn'je-form. [**Spongifor'mis**; from *spon'gia*, a "sponge."] Having the appearance of sponge.

Spon-ġĭ-o'dēs.* The same as SPONGIOSE.

Spon'ġĭ-ole. [**Spongi'olum**; diminutive of *spon'gia*, a "sponge."] Applied to a supposed expansion of the cellular tissue at the extremity of each radicle, terminating the root. But according to Gray, "the so-called spongioles or spongelets have no existence."

Spon'ġĭ-ose. [**Spongio'sus**; from *spon'gia*, a "sponge."] Having pores like sponge; spongy.

Spongoid, spŏng'goid. [**Spongoi'-des**; from σπόγγος, a "sponge," and εἶδος, a "form."] Resembling sponge.

Spongy, spŭn'je. Resembling a sponge; of the nature of sponge.

Spon-tā'ne-ous. [**Sponta'neus**; from *spon'te*, "of one's own will."] Acting or growing of itself; voluntary. Applied to any physiological phenomenon which takes place without external agency.

Sponta'neous Com-bus'tion [**Combus'tio Sponta'nea**], or **Pre-ter-nat'u-ral Combus'tion.** A phenomenon which is said to have sometimes occurred in hard drinkers, especially those that were fat. In such Dr. Traill is stated to have found a considerable quantity of oil in the serum of the blood. Some are of opinion that the combustion may be absolutely spontaneous, while others maintain that it is necessary that the body should be brought into contact with an ignited substance.

Spo-rad'ic. [**Sporad'icus**; from σπείρω, to "sow."] Applied to diseases that are not epidemic, but attack one or at most but a few persons at a time, from causes peculiar to each case. In Botany, widely dispersed.

Spor-an-ġid'ĭ-um.* [Diminutive of *sporangi'um*, a "spore-case."] A little seed-vessel; also, the *columnella* of mosses.

Spor-an-ġĭ'o-lum.* [Diminutive of *sporangi'um*.] A small capsule on

taining a certain number of spores in a sporangium.

Spor-an-gi'um.* [From σπορά, a "seed," and ἀγγεῖον, a "vessel."] A spore-case, or membranous capsule containing the spores of cryptogamous plants.

Spore. [Lat. **Spo'ra;** Gr. σπορά, a "seed."] A body in cryptogamous plants, which is analogous to the seed of the phænogamous. A spore, in most cases, consists of a single cell.

Spor-i-dif'er-us.* [From *sporid'-ium,* and *fe'ro,* to "bear."] Bearing *sporidia.*

Spo-rid'i-um.* [From *spo'ra,* a "spore."] A body resembling a spore, occurring in algaceous plants.

Spŏr'o-carp. [From σπορά, a "seed," or "spore," and καρπός, "fruit."] A kind of sporangium, or spore-case.

Spŏr'o-gens. [From σπορά, a "spore," and γεννάω, to "produce."] A division of endogenous plants which produce spores instead of seeds.

Spo-roph'o-rous. [**Sporoph'orus;** from σπορά, a "seed," and φέρω, to "bear."] Bearing or containing seed or spores.

Spo-roph'o-rum.* [From the same.] A name for the placenta of a plant.

Spo'rule. [**Spor'ula;** diminutive of *spo'ra,* a "spore."] A small spore.

Spor-u-lif'er-ous. [**Sporulif'er-us;** from *spor'ula,* a "sporule," and *fe'ro,* to "bear."] Bearing sporules.

Sprain. [Lat. **Subluxa'tio, o'nis;** Fr. *Foulure,* foo'lür'.] (Originally, **Strain,** from the Latin *strin'go* [Fr. *étreindre*], to "bind," to "draw tight.") The sudden shifting of a joint farther than the natural conformation of bones and ligaments allows, yet not so as to produce dislocation.

Spreading. See Diffusus, and Patulous.

Spruce Fir. The *Pinus abies.*

Spt. = *Spir'itus.** "Spirit."

Spu-mĕs'çent. [From *spumes'co,* to "begin to foam" (from *spu'ma,* "froth," or "foam").] Frothy, foaming, or froth-like.

Spu'mose. The same as Spumescent.

Spur. A term applied in Botany to any tubular projection of a flower, etc.

Spurge Ol'ive. A common name for the Daphne Mezereum, which see.

Spurred. [**Calcara'tus.**] Bearing a spur. Applied to petals.

Spu'ta,* gen. **Spu-to'rum,** the plural of Sputum, which see.

Spu'tum.* [From *spu'o, spu'tum,* to "spit."] (Fr. *Crachat,* krå'shå'.) Saliva; also, the matter which is expectorated or coughed up from the chest.

Squa'lor, o'ris.* Uncleanness, filthiness, or an appearance of dejection and disorder, as from sickness or confinement.

Squa'ma,* plural **Squa'mæ.** Literally, a "scale." Applied in the plural to an order of skin-diseases.

Squā'mate. [**Squama'tus;** from *squa'ma,* a "scale."] Having scales; scaly; or resembling scales.

Squa-mif'er-ous. [**Squamif'er-us;** from *squa'ma,* a "scale," and *fe'ro,* to "bear."] Bearing, or covered with, scales.

Squa-mi-fo'li-us.* [From *squa'ma,* a "scale," and *fo'lium,* a "leaf."] Having leaves in form of imbricated scales: squamifo'lious.

Squā'mi-form. [**Squamifor'mis;** from *squa'ma,* a "scale."] Having the form or appearance of scales. See Lepidoid.

Squa-mig'er-us.* [From *squa'ma,* a "scale," and *ge'ro,* to "bear."] The same as Squamiferous, which see.

Squa-mo'sal. [**Squamo'sus;** from *squamo'sa* pars, the "squamous portion."] Applied by Owen to the homologues of the squamous portion of the temporal bone.

Squa-mose', or **Squā'mous.** [**Squamo'sus;** from *squa'ma,* a "scale."] Relating to, or resembling, a scale; having scales; scaly.

Squā'mous Su'ture. [**Sutu'ra Squamo'sa.**] The suture which unites the squamous portion of the temporal bone to the parietal.

Squam'u-la.* [Diminutive of *squa'ma,* a "scale."] A small scale; a squamule.

Squam'u-lose. [**Squamulo'sus;** from *squam'ula,* a "small scale."] Covered with small scales: squa'mulous.

Squar-rose'. [From *squar'ra,* a "small scale"?] A term applied to scales or leaves which spread widely from the axis on which they are crowded.

Squar'ru-lose. Diminutive of Squarrose.

Squill. [**Squil'la.**] The *Scilla maritima,* or sea-onion. See Scilla.

Squinting. See Strabismus.

Ss. = *Se'mis.** "A half."

St. = *Stet,** or *Stent.** "Let it (or them) stand," *i.e.* let it remain unchanged.

Stac'te.* [From στάζω, to "distil."] A name for the myrrh, because it distils or drops from the tree.

Sta'dĭ-um.* A Latin word signifying a "race-course," or a measure of length. In Medicine, a stage or period of a disease; as, *stadium calo'ris* ("stage of heat," or hot stage), *stadium frig'oris* (cold stage). See STAGE.

Staff. A carved and grooved steel instrument introduced through the urethra into the bladder, for lithotomy.

Stāge. [Lat. **Sta'dium;** Fr. *Étage*, ā'tăzh'.] The period of a disease. Applied especially to the periods of an intermittent; viz. the hot, cold, or sweating stage.

Stag'ma.* [From στάζω, to "distil."] Any distilled liquid or liquor.

Stag-nā'tion. [**Stagna'tio, o'**nis; from *stag'no, stagna'tum*, to "stand," as water in a pond.] A stoppage or retardation of the circulating fluids in any portion of the body.

Sta-lac'tic. [**Stalac'ticus;** from σταλάζω, to "flow by drops."] Flowing or oozing by drops; also, relating to a stalactite.

Sta-lac'tīte. [**Stalacti'tes;** from the same.] A conical concretion of carbonate of lime attached to the roof of calcareous caverns, and formed by the gradual dropping of water holding the lime in solution.

Stal-ac-tit'ic, or **Stal-ac-tit'ĭ-cal.** [**Stalactit'icus.**] Relating to stalactites, or of the nature of stalactites.

Sta-lag'mīte. [**Stalagmi'tes;** from *stalag'mus*, a "distillation."] A stalactitic formation of carbonate of lime found on the floors of calcareous caverns.

Sta-lag'mus.* [From σταλάζω, to "drop," to "distil."] A distillation. Formerly applied to a dropping of blood, as from the nose, etc.

Stalk. [**Cau'lis.**] The stem of a herbaceous plant, or of a flower, a leaf or leaflet.

Stalked. Furnished with a stalk or stem.

Stalk'let. A diminutive or secondary stalk.

Sta'men, *inis*,* plural **Stam'ĭ-na.** [Gr. στήμων.] Literally, "warp," or the stronger threads in weaving. Also, any thread: hence applied to the male organ of a flower, from its resemblance to a thread. It consists of the filament and anther. It is one of the *essential organs* of a flower.

Stam'ĭ-na.* [Plural of *sta'men.*] Literally, the "warp," or "strength," of the vital tissue: hence, vigor of constitution. Also, the first principles of any substance.

Stam'ĭ-nal. [**Stamina'lis.**] Pertaining to the stamen.

Stam'ĭ-nate. [From *sta'men.*] Furnished with, or relating to, stamens; also, containing stamens without any pistil. Applied to flowers.

Sta-min'e-al. [**Stamin'eus;** from *sta'men.*] Having stamens: stamineous.

Stam-ĭ-nif'er-ous. [**Staminif'erus;** from *sta'men*, and *fe'ro*, to "bear."] Bearing or having stamens.

Stam-ĭ-no'dĭ-a,* the plural of STAMINODIUM, which see.

Stam-ĭ-no'dĭ-um,* plural **Stamino'dia;** from *sta'men*, and εἶδος, a "form."] An altered and sterile stamen.

Stam'mer-ing. [**Balbu'ties, Blæs'itas, a'**tis, or **Psellis'mus.**] Interrupted articulation, caused either by emotion or reflex action.

Stan'dard. A banner, or ensign; applied to the vexillum, or upper petal, of a papilionaceous flower. Also, a criterion, test, or measure, to which something is referred: thus, the standard of comparison for gases is atmospheric air; that for solids and liquids is water.

Stan'nāte. [**Stan'nas, a'**tis.] A combination of stannic acid with a base.

Stan'ni Pul'vis.* ("Powder of Tin.") Granulated tin: used as a remedy for the tapeworm.

Stan'nic. [**Stan'nicus;** from *stan'num*, "tin."] Belonging to tin. Applied to the peroxide of tin, as if it were an acid, because soluble in alkalies.

Stan-nif'er-ous. [**Stannif'erus;** from *stan'num*, "tin," and *fe'ro*, to "bear."] Bearing or containing *stannum*, or tin.

Stan'num.* Tin. The Pharmacopœial name for powder or filings of tin. See TIN.

Stan'num Fo-lĭ-a'tum.* ("Foliated Tin.") Tin-foil. An alloy composed chiefly of tin, with a small portion of lead.

Sta-pe'dĭ-us.* Belonging to the *stapes*. Applied to a muscle arising from the interior of the pyramid and inserted into the neck of the *stapes*.

Sta'pēs, *edis*.* Literally, a "stirrup." One of the *ossicula* of the internal ear.

Staph-ĭ-sa'grĭ-a.* [From σταφίς, a "vine," and ἄγριος, "wild."] The Pharmacopœial name (Lond. and Ed. Ph.) for the seeds of *Delphin'ium staphisa'gria*,

Staph'ȳ-le.* [Gr. σταφυλή, a "grape."] The uvula.

Staphyleaceæ,* sta-fi-le-a'she-ē. [From *Staphy'lea*, one of the genera.] A small natural order of exogenous shrubs, found in Europe, Japan, and America.

Staph-ȳ-li'nus.* [From *staph'yle*, a "grape;" also, the "uvula."] Belonging to the uvula: applied to muscles: staph'yline.

Staph-ȳ-li'tis, i*dis*.* [From *staph'yle*, a "grape;" or the "uvula."] Inflammation of the uvula.

Staph-ȳ-lœ-de'ma, a*tis*.* [From *staph'yle*, a "grape," or the "uvula," and *œde'ma*.] *Œdema*, or morbid enlargement, of the uvula.

Staph-ȳ-lo'ma, a*tis*.* [From σταφυλή, a "grape;" the "uvula."] A disease of the eyeball, in which the cornea loses its transparency, rises, and even projects beyond the eyelids, like a pearl-colored tumor.

Staph-ȳ-lop-to'sis.* [From *staph'yle*, the "uvula," and *pto'sis*, a "falling."] A falling down or elongation of the uvula.

Staph-ȳ-lor'rha-phȳ. [**Staphylorrha'phia;** from σταφυλή, the "uvula," and ῥαφή, a "suture."] The operation of securing by suture the lips of a cleft uvula.

Staph-ȳ-lo'sis.* The growth or progress of *staphyloma*.

Staph-ȳ-lot'o-mȳ. [**Staphyloto'mia;** from *staph'yle*, the "uvula," and τέμνω, to "cut."] The cutting off of a portion of the UVULA, which see.

Star. See STELLA.

Star-like. See ASTEROID, and STELLATE.

Starch. [Lat. **Am'ylum,** and **Fec'ula;** Gr. ἄμυλον; Fr. *Amidon*, å'mè'dòɴᵍ'.] One of the commonest proximate principles of vegetables. It is characterized by its insipidity, and by insolubility in cold water, in alcohol, and in ether. Pure starch is a white powder without taste or smell. Starch is one of the most important and most universal of the contents of cells, and is most abundant in the internal or subterranean parts, concealed from the light, as roots, tubers, and seeds. It is the form in which nourishing matter is stored up in the plant for future use, in this respect resembling the fat of animals.

Sta'sis.* [From ἵστημι, to "stand."] A standing or settling in a place or part, as the blood at death.

Stat'ic, or **Stat'ĭ-cal.** [**Stat'icus;** from στατός, "standing," or ἵστημι, to "stand."] Having the power of keeping in a stationary condition. Applied by some writers to the *physical* phenomena exhibited in organized bodies, as contradistinguished from the *organic* or vital.

Stat'ĭ-ce.* Marsh Rosemary. The Pharmacopœial name (U.S. Ph.) for the root of the *Stat'ice Limo'nium*, variety *Carolinia'na*. It is astringent and antiseptic.

Stat'ics. [**Stat'ica;** from στατός, "standing," or ἵστημι, to "stand."] That part of Mechanics which relates to bodies considered as in a state of rest, or to the conditions under which several forces applied to a rigid body mutually destroy each other.

Stā'tion. [**Sta'tio, o'***nis*; from *sto*, *sta'tum*, to "stand," to "abide."] Primarily, the act (or position) of standing. In Botany, the locality or kind of situation in which a plant naturally grows.

Sta-tis'tics. [From *sta'tus*, a "state," "condition."] The science which exhibits the state or condition of a country or nation, principally in relation to its extent, population, productions, industry, etc.

Stat'ure. [**Statu'ra;** from *sto*, *sta'tum*, to "stand."] The height of the human figure in a standing posture.

Stau-ro-phȳl'lus.* [From σταυρός, a "cross," and φύλλον, a "leaf."] Having leaves opposed crosswise.

Staves-a'cre. The DELPHINIUM STAPHISAGRIA, which see.

Steam. [**Va'por.**] The elastic fluid into which water is converted by the continued application of heat. A cubic inch of water forms about seventeen hundred cubic inches of steam. See VAPOR.

Ste'ar,* gen. **Ste'a-tis.** [Gr. στέαρ.] Originally, "solid fat." The same as SEVUM, which see.

Ste'a-rāte. [**Ste'aras, a'***tis*.] A combination of stearic acid with a base.

Ste-ăr'ic. [**Stear'icus;** from στέαρ, "solid fat," or "tallow."] Pertaining to fat. Applied to an acid obtained from it.

Ste-ăr'ĭ-form. [**Stearifor'mis;** from the same.] Having the appearance of fat; fatty.

Ste'a-rĭne, or **Ste'a-rin.** [**Steari'na;** from the same.] That part of oils and fats which is solid at common temperatures.

Ste-a-ro-co-no'tum.* [From στέαρ,

"solid fat," and κόνις, "dust," or "powder."] A peculiar, yellow, pulverulent fat, found in the brain-mass, and said to contain phosphorus and sulphur.

Ste-a-rop'ten. [**Stearopte'num;** from στέαρ, "solid fat," and πτηνός, "volatile."] The concrete or solid portion of volatile oils.

Ste-a-ro-riç'i-nāte. [**Stearoriç'i-nas, a'**_tis._] A combination of stearoricinic acid with a base.

Ste-a-ro-ri-cin'ic. [**Stearoricin'icus.**] Applied to one of three acids produced during saponification of the _O'leum riç'ini_, or castor oil.

Ste'a-tas.* The same as STEARAS. See STEARATE.

Ste-at'i-cus.* The same as STEARICUS. See STEARIC.

Ste'a-tīne, or **Ste'a-tin.** A name for STEARIN, which see.

Ste'a-tīne. [**Steati'nus;** from στέαρ, στέατος, "solid fat."] Consisting of fat.

Ste'a-tīte. [**Steati'tes;** from the same.] A variety of talc; soapstone; a kind of unctuous stone. It is a hydrated silicate of magnesia and alumina.

Ste'a-to-çēle.* [From στέαρ, στέατος, "solid fat," and κήλη, a "tumor."] A fatty tumor in the scrotum.

Steatoconotum. See STEAROCONOTUM.

Ste-a-to'dēs.* [From στέαρ, στέατος, "solid fat."] Fatty, or full of fat.

Ste-a-to'ma, a_tis._* [From the same.] An encysted tumor containing a fatty substance: a ste'atome.

Ste-a-tom'a-tous. [**Steatomato'sus;** from _steato'ma._] Of the nature of, or belonging to, _steatoma._

Ste-a-tor-rhœ'a.* [From στέαρ, στέατος, "solid fat," and ῥέω, to "flow."] A fatty dejection from the bowels.

Ste-a-to'sis.* The progress or formation of _steatoma._

Steel. [**Cha'lybs, yb**_is._] The best, finest, and closest-grained forged iron, combined with carbon by a particular process. It is less malleable than iron, but harder, more elastic, and less liable to rust. See ACIES.

Steel Mix'ture. The same as the MISTURA FERRI COMPOSITA, which see.

Steg-no'sis.* [From στεγνόω, to "constrict," or "make costive."] Stricture or contraction of the pores and vessels; also, constipation.

Stel'la.* A Latin word signifying a "star." Applied to the rosettes of mosses.

Stel'lar. [**Stella'ris;** from _stel'la,_ a "star."] Relating to a star; starry.

Stel-la'tæ.* [Feminine plural of _stella'tus,_ "starred," or "stellate."] A natural order of plants, also known by the name of GALIACEÆ, which see.

Stel'late, or **Stel'lāt-ed.** [**Stella'tus;** from _stel'la,_ a "star."] Radiated as a star; star-shaped; arranged in rays like the points of a star. Applied to flowers, leaves, etc. Applied also to a bandage or roller wound crosswise on the back.

Stel-lif'er-ous. [**Stellif'erus;** from _stel'la,_ a "star," and _fe'ro,_ to "bear."] Having or bearing stars, or parts resembling a star. Applied to plants.

Stel'li-form. [**Stellifor'mis;** from _stel'la,_ a "star."] Having the form of a star.

Stel-lig'er-us.* [From _stel'la,_ a "star," and _ge'ro,_ to "bear."] The same as STELLIFEROUS, which see.

Stel-li-ner'vi-us.* [From _stel'la,_ a "star," and _ner'vus,_ a "nerve."] Having stellated or radiated nervures. Applied by Mirbel to leaves the nervures of which depart from the middle or centre of the lamina.

Stel'lu-la.* [Diminutive of _stel'la,_ a "star."] A little star, or foliaceous disk, which in certain mosses terminates the stems and contains the male flowers: a stel'lule.

Stel'lu-læ Ver-heȳ'nĭ-i.* ("Stars or Stellated Spots of Verheyne.") A term applied to the stellated plexuses of veins on the surface of the kidney.

Stel'lu-late. [**Stellula'tus;** from _stel'lula,_ a "little star."] The diminutive of STELLATE. Having leaves arranged in stars.

Stem. [**Cau'lis,** or **Sti'pes.**] The stalk of an herb, flower, leaf, or fruit; the stock or trunk of a tree; the ascending axis of a plant,—_i.e._ the part which grows in the opposite direction from the root. The stem is one of the fundamental or universal organs of vegetation. Its leading peculiarity is, that it is formed of a succession of similar parts (internodes) developed one upon the summit of another, each having its own independent growth. Each developing internode lengthens throughout its whole body, unlike the root, which elongates continuously from its extremity alone.

Stem'less. [**Acau'lis.**] Having no stem, or none that is obvious.

Stem'let. A little stem. Also, the first internode of the plumule.

Stenocardia. See ANGINA PECTORIS.

Sten'o-don, on'_tis_.* [From στενός, "narrow," or "close," and ὀδούς, a "tooth."] Having narrow teeth.

Ste-nog'ra-phy̆. [From στενός, "narrow," "close," and γράφω, to "write."] The art of short-hand, otherwise termed _tachygraphy_.

Ste-nol'o-bus.* [From στενός, "narrow," and λόβος, a "lobe."] Having narrow lobes.

Sten-o-pet'a-lus.* [From στενός, "narrow," and πέταλον, a "petal."] Having narrow or linear petals.

Sten-o-phy̆l'lus.* [From στενός, "narrow," and φύλλον, a "leaf."] Having narrow or linear leaves.

Ste-nop'ter-us.* [From στενός, "narrow," and πτερόν, a "wing."] Having narrow wings: stenopterous. Applied to plants.

Ste'no's (or **Ste'non's**) **Duct.** The parotid duct; a small white tube passing from the parotid gland and opening in the mouth, discovered by Steno.

Ste-no'sis.* [From στενόω, to "make narrow," or to "contract."] A contracted condition of a viscus, or vessel; as of the heart, or the larger vessels near it.

Sten-o-sto'mi-a.* [From στενός, "narrow," and στόμα, a "mouth."] Contraction of the mouth in consequence of some wound or disease.

Sten-o-tho'rax, a'_cis_.* [From στενός, "narrow," and θώραξ, the "chest."] Having a narrow chest.

Steppes, stĕps. (Russian.) The name given to the vast system of plains found in Asia, especially in Siberia, somewhat resembling the prairies of North America.

Ster-co-rā'ceous. [**Stercora'ceus;** from _ster'cus_, _ster'coris_, "ordure."] Applied to vomiting when fæces or alvine excrements are mingled with the _egesta_.

Ster-co-ra'lis,* or **Ster-co-ra'ri-us.*** [From the same.] Applied to plants that grow upon excrements or dung.

Ster-cu-li-a'ce-æ.* [From _Stercu'lia_, one of the genera.] A synonym of a natural order of plants, also called BOMBACEÆ, which see.

Stĕr-el-min'tha.* [From στερεός, "solid," and ἕλμινς, a "worm."] The name applied to two species of intestinal worms which have no true abdominal cavity, and are therefore termed solid. These are the _Tæ'nia so'lium_ and the _Bothrioceph'alus la'tus_.

Ste-re-o-dy̆-nam'ics. [**Stereodynam'ica;** from στερεός, "solid," and δύναμις, "power."] A branch of Physics which explains the laws of the movement of solid bodies.

Stĕr-e-om'e-ter. [See next article.] An instrument used for determining the specific gravity of solid bodies, porous bodies, and powders; and sometimes also of liquids.

Stĕr-e-om'e-try̆. [**Stereome'tria;** from στερεός, "solid," and μετρέω, to "measure."] The art of measuring solid bodies.

Ste-re-o-phy̆l'lus.* [From στερεός, "solid," and φύλλον, a "leaf."] Having solid or firm leaves: stereophyl'lous.

Stĕr'e-o-scope. [**Stereosco'pium;** from στερεός, "solid," and σκοπέω, to "see," to "observe."] An instrument by which two similar pictures (one being presented to each eye) are so disposed that the combined representations appear as one, and the different objects are seen in relief, as if they were solid.

Stĕr-e-o-stat'ics. [**Stereostat'ica;** from στερεός, "solid," and ἵστημι, to "stand."] That part of Physics which treats of the equilibrium of solid bodies.

Ste-rig'ma.* [From στηρίζω, to "make firm or fast."] Literally, a "base," or "foundation." Applied in Botany to the adherent base or downward prolongation of a decurrent leaf.

Stĕr'ile. [**Ster'ilis.**] Affected with sterility; barren.

Ster'ile Flow'er. A flower which has no pistil.

Ster'ile Sta'men or **Fil'a-ment.** That which is destitute of an anther.

Ste-ril'i-ty̆. [**Steril'itas, a'**_tis_; from _ster'ilis_, "barren."] Inability, whether natural or the result of disease, to procreate offspring.

Ster'nal. [**Sterna'lis.**] Belonging to the sternum. Applied by Dr. Barclay as meaning towards the sternum.

Ster-năl'gi-a.* [From _ster'num_, the "breastbone," and ἄλγος, "pain."] Pain in the sternum.

Ster'no-Clei-do-Mas-to-i'de-us.* A muscle arising by two origins from the summit of the sternum and the sternal portion of the clavicle, and inserted into the mastoid process of the temporal bone. It turns the head to one side and bends it forward.

Ster'no-Hy-o-i'de-us.* A muscle arising from the sternum and inserted into the _os hyoides_. It depresses the larynx, and furnishes a fixed point for the depressors of the jaw.

Ster'noid. [**Sternoi'des;** from

ster'num, and εἶδος, a "form."] Resembling the sternum.

Ster'no-Thy-ro-i'de-us.* A muscle arising from the sternum and inserted into the thyroid cartilage. It draws the larynx downwards.

Ster'num.* [Gr. στέρνον.] The oblong, flat bone at the fore part of the thorax: the breast-bone; also termed *Os pec'toris.* Also, the median line of the *pectus,* or inferior surface of the trunk of insects.

Ster-nu-men'tum,* or **Ster-nu-ta-men'tum.*** [From *ster'nuo, sternu'tum,* to "sneeze."] Sneezing. Also applied to a substance which causes sneezing; a snuff or a sternutatory medicine.

Ster-nu-tā'tion. [**Sternuta'tio, o'nis;** from *sternu'to, sternuta'tum,* to "sneeze often."] The act of sneezing; more particularly, frequent sneezing, which sometimes amounts to such excess as requires medical treatment.

Ster-nu'ta-to-rў. [**Sternutato'rius;** from the same.] Causing to sneeze.

Ster'tor, o'ris.* [From *ster'to,* to "snore."] (Fr. *Ronflement,* rôNᴳ'f'l-mōNᴳ'.) The loud grating sound produced in the larynx from the breathing being obstructed by accumulation of mucus in the air-passages, or otherwise. Also applied to the snoring in natural sleep caused by relaxation of the *velum palati.*

Ster'to-rous. [**Stertoro'sus.**] Belonging to, or of the nature of, *stertor.*

Ste-thæ'mĭ-a.* [From στῆθος, the "chest," or "breast," and αἷμα, "blood."] Accumulation of blood in the vessels of the lungs.

Ste-thoch'ў-sis.* [From στῆθος, the "chest," and χύσις, a "pouring," or "effusion."] The same as HYDROTHORAX, which see.

Ste-thom'e-ter. [**Stethom'etrum;** from στῆθος, the "chest," and μέτρον, a "measure."] An instrument for measuring the external movement in the walls of the chest, as a means of diagnosis in thoracic disease.

Stĕth-o-pa-ral'ў-sis.* [From στῆθος, the "chest," and *paral'ysis.*] Paralysis of the muscles of the chest.

Stĕth'o-scope. [**Stethosco'pium;** from στῆθος, the "breast," and σκοπέω, to "observe," to "examine."] A tubular instrument of various size, form, and material, for ascertaining the state of the respiration, or of the heart's action, as affected by disease.

Sthĕn'ic. [**Sthen'icus;** from σθένος, "strength."] Strong; active; robust.

Sthen'ic Dis-eaṡ'es. Those which are the result of inflammation or increased action.

Sthe-nop'ў-ra.* [From σθένος, "strength," and πῦρ, a "fever."] Sthenic or synochic fever.

Stib'ĭ-al. [**Stibia'lis;** from *stib'ium,* "antimony."] Belonging to antimony; antimonial.

Stib'ic. [**Stib'icus;** from *stib'ium,* "antimony."] Belonging to antimony. Applied to the yellow oxide of antimony, called Stibic acid.

Stib'ĭ-ous. [**Stibio'sus;** from *stib'ium,* "antimony."] Pertaining to antimony. Applied to the white oxide of antimony, called Stibious acid.

Stib'ĭ-um.* [Gr. στίβι, or στίμμι.] The ancient name for antimony.

Stic-tac'ne.* [From στικτός, "marked with points," and *ac'ne,* a "papular eruption."] The *Ac'ne puncta'ta* of Bateman; a species or variety of acne in which, according to Dr. Good, the pimples are tipped with a black dot.

Stiff-joint. See ANKYLOSIS.

Stig'ma,* plural **Stig'ma-ta.** [From στίγμα, a "mark," a "brand."] That part of the pistil which is placed at the summit of the style and receives the pollen. Also, one of the breathing-pores of insects, or the pores which admit air to their *tracheæ.* Applied in Pathology to a small red speck on the skin, without elevation of the cuticle, as if caused by a pricking instrument. Also, a natural mark or spot.

Stig'ma-ta,* the plural of STIGMA, which see.

Stig-mat'ic. [**Stigmat'icus.**] Belonging to or bearing a stigma.

Stig-mat'ĭ-form. [**Stigmatifor'mis;** from *stig'ma.*] Having the appearance of a stigma.

Stig'ma-tose. The same as STIGMATIC, which see.

Stilbaceæ,* stil-ba'she-ē. [From *Stil'be,* one of the genera.] A small natural order of exogenous shrubs, found at the Cape of Good Hope.

Stilette, ste-lĕtt'. (From the French *Stilet,* a "small dagger.") A small sharp-pointed instrument enclosed in a *cannula,* or sheath. Also, a wire kept in the flexible catheter, to give it firmness and a proper degree of curvature.

Still'born. [**Na'tus Mor'tuus,** "born dead."] Born without life.

Stil'lĭ-cĭd'ĭ-um.* [From *stil'la,* a "drop," and *ca'do,* to "fall down."] A dropping or trickling down; a flowing drop by drop. Applied especially to the urine in strangury, stricture, etc.

Stillicid'ium Lach-rȳ-ma'rum.* ("Dropping or Trickling down of Tears.") See EPIPHORA.

Stil-lin'ġĭ-a.* The Pharmacopœial name (U.S. Ph.) for the root of the *Stillin'gia sylvat'ica*. In large doses it is emetic and cathartic; in small doses, alterative.

Stimatosis. See STYMATOSIS.

Stim'u-lant. [**Stim'ulans, an'***tis;* see STIMULATE.] Stimulating. Applied to a medicine having power to excite the organic action of an animal, or increase the vital activity of an organ.

Stim'u-lāte. [From *stim'ulo, stimula'tum*, to "goad," or "urge on" (from *stim'ulus*, a "goad," or "spur").] To excite the organic action of a part of the animal economy.

Stim'u-li,* gen. **Stim-u-lo'rum,** the plural of STIMULUS, which see.

Stim'u-lus,* plural **Stim'u-li.** A Latin word signifying a "goad," "sting," or "whip." In Botany, a sting, or fine, sharp-pointed substance which easily penetrates the skin, introducing a poison into the part, as of the Nettle. In Physiology, that which rouses or excites the vital energies, whether of the whole system or of a part.

Sting. In Botany, a rigid and pointed cell borne on an expanded base or gland, which secretes an irritating fluid, as in the Nettle.

Stīpe. [**Sti'pes,** *itis;* from στύπος, a "trunk."] A stem of a fungus, fern, or palm. Also, a stalk which supports the ovary in certain plants.

Stī'pel. The stipule of a leaflet.

Stip'el-late. Furnished with stipels.

Sti-pif'er-ous. [**Stipif'erus;** from *sti'pes*, a "stipe," and *fe'ro*, to "bear."] Bearing stipes.

Stip'ĭ-tate. [**Stipita'tus;** from *sti'pes*, a "stipe."] Having a stipe, stem, or foot-stalk.

Stip'ĭ-tĭ-form, or **Stip'ĭ-form.** [**Stipifor'mis;** from *sti'pes*, a "stipe."] Shaped like a stipe.

Stip-u-lā'ceous. [From *stip'ula*, a "stipule."] Belonging to or resembling stipules.

Stip'u-lar. [**Stipula'ris;** from *stip'ula*, a "stipule."] Relating to or like a stipule.

Stip'u-late, or **Stip'uled.** [**Stipula'tus.**] Having stipules.

Stip'ule. [**Stip'ula.**] A Latin word signifying "straw," or "stubble." In Botany, a lateral and foliaceous appendage of a leaf, situated at the base of the petiole. Stipules occur in pairs.

Stip-u-lif'er-ous. [**Stipulif'erus;** from *stip'ula*, a "stipule," and *fe'ro*, to "bear."] Bearing stipules.

Stitch. [**Punc'tum.**] An acute, sudden pain, like that caused by the thrusting in of a sharp needle. See PLEURODYNIA.

Stock. [**Stirps.**] The trunk or stem of a tree or plant. Also, the original (or originals) of a lineage of animals or plants; a source of succession; a race.

Stoi-chĭ-ol'o-ġȳ, or **Stœ-chĭ-ol'o-ġȳ,** written also **Ste-chĭ-ol'o-ġȳ.** [**Stœchiolo'gia;** from στοιχεῖον, a "first principle," and λόγος, a "discourse."] Elementary knowledge; the science of first principles, or a treatise on elements.

Stoi-chĭ-om'e-trȳ. [**Stœchiome'tria;** from στοιχεῖον, an "element," and μετρέω, to "measure."] The doctrine of chemical equivalents. That part of Chemistry which treats of the relative quantities in which different substances combine with each other.

Stole. The same as STOLON, which see.

Sto'lon. [**Sto'lo, o'***nis.*] A rooting branch; a branch of a plant, which curves or falls down to the ground, where it takes root and forms an ascending stem, as in the Currant.

Stol-o-nif'er-ous. [**Stolonif'erus;** from *sto'lo*, a "stolon," and *fe'ro*, to "bear."] Bearing stolons, or suckers.

Sto'ma,* plural **Sto'ma-ta.** [From στόμα, a "mouth."] A mouth. Also, a breathing-pore; a minute orifice in the epidermis of leaves through which exhalation takes place. In the leaf of the Apple there are said to be twenty-four thousand stomata to the square inch.

Sto-mac'a-çe.* [From στόμα, a "mouth," and κακός, "bad."] See CANCRUM ORIS.

Stomacal. See STOMACHIC.

Stomach, stŭm'ak. [**Ventric'ulus,** and **Stom'achus;** from στόμα, a "mouth."] (Fr. *Estomac*, ĕs'to'mȧk'.) The membranous bag, or receptacle of the food, between the œsophagus and duodenum.

Stom'ach-Pump. (Fr. *Pompe pour l'Estomac*, pòmp poor lĕs'to'mȧk'.) An instrument used to pump out the contents of the stomach, or convey fluids into that organ when the patient is unable to swallow.

Stom'a-chal. Synonymous with STOMACHIC, which see.

Sto-mach'ic. [**Stomach'icus.**] (Fr. *Stomacal*, sto'mă'kăl'.) Belonging to the stomach; gastric. Also applied to a medicine which strengthens its healthy action.

Stomachus. See STOMACH.

Sto-map'o-dus.* [From στόμα, a "mouth," and πούς, a "foot."] Having feet near the mouth. Applied in the neuter plural (*Stomap'oda*) to an order of Crustaceans.

Sto'ma-ta,* the plural of STOMA, which see.

Sto'māte. The same as STOMA, which see.

Sto-mat'ic. [**Stomat'icus;** from στόμα, a "mouth."] A remedy for diseases of the mouth.

Stom-a-ti'tis, idis.* [From στόμα, a "mouth."] Inflammation of the mouth.

Stom-a-to-plas'tic. [**Stomato-plas'ticus.**] Belonging to stomatoplasty.

Stom'a-to-plas-tў. [**Stomato-plas'tia;** from στόμα, a "mouth," and πλάσσω, to "form."] The operation for forming an artificial mouth where the aperture has been contracted from any cause.

Stom'a-to-scope. [From στόμα, the "mouth," and σκοπέω, to "examine."] An instrument for holding open the mouth in order to facilitate examination.

Stone. See CALCULUS, and LAPIS.

Stone-Fruit. A common name for a DRUPE, which see.

Stool. [**Se'des.**] The fæces discharged from the bowels; a dejection; an evacuation. In Botany, a plant from which layers (stolons) are propagated.

Sto'rax.* A name for STYRAX, which see.

Stra-bis'mus.* [From στραβίζω, to "squint."] Squinting. An affection of the eyes in which objects are seen in an oblique manner. A genus of the order *Dyscinesiæ*, class *Locales*, of Cullen's Nosology.

Stra-bot'o-mў. [**Straboto'mia;** from στραβός, "squinting," and τομή, a "cutting."] An operation for strabismus.

Strain. See SPRAIN.

Strainer. See COLATORIUM.

Straining. See SPASMA.

Stra-min'e-ous. [From *stra'men*, "straw."] Straw-like.

Stra-mo'ni-i Fo'li-um.* ("Leaf of Stramonium.") The Pharmacopœial name (U.S. Ph.) for the leaves of *Datu'ra stramo'nium*. The *Stramo'nii Fo'lia* ("Leaves of Stramonium") of the British Pharmacopœia.

Stramo'nii Se'men.* ("Seed of Stramonium.") The Pharmacopœial name (U.S. Ph.) for the seed of the *Datu'ra stramo'nium*. It is narcotic and poisonous.

Stra-mo'ni-um.* The Pharmacopœial name (Ed. Ph.) for the herb *Datu'ra stramo'nium*.

Stran'gu-lāt-ed. [**Strangula'tus;** from *stran'gulo*, *strangula'tum*, to "choke."] Literally, "choked." Applied to irreducible hernia. In Botany, irregularly contracted.

Stran-gu-lā'tion. [**Strangula'tio, o'nis;** from the same.] (Fr. *Étranglement*, ā'tRONG'g'l-mŏNG'.) The state of choking; constriction of a part from the presence of a stricture.

Strangury, strang'gu-re. [**Stran-gu'ria;** from στράγγω, to "tie or bind tight" (or more directly from στράγξ, a "drop"), and οὖρον, the "urine."] A painful difficulty in passing water, which can be discharged only by drops.

Stra'ta,* gen. **Stra-to'rum,** the plural of STRATUM, which see.

Strat-i-fi-cā'tion. [**Stratifica'tio, o'nis;** from *stra'tum*, a "layer," and *fa'cio*, to "make."] In Chemistry, the placing of layer upon layer of different substances in a crucible, to calcine a metal, etc. In Geology, the arrangement of the rocks, earth, etc., in strata; the process of forming strata.

Strat'i-fied. [**Stratifica'tus;** from the same.] Composed of distinct strata, or layers of different materials. Applied in Geology to sedimentary rocks placed in strata which are nearly parallel, as sandstone and slate.

Strat'i-form. [**Stratifor'mis;** from *stra'tum*, a "layer."] Having the form of strata; stratified.

Stra'toid. [**Stratoi'des;** from *stra'tum*, a "layer," and εἶδος, a "form."] Resembling strata or layers.

Stra-tom'e-ter. [**Stratom'etrum;** from *stra'tum*, a "layer," and μέτρον, a "measure."] An instrument for determining in what manner geological strata press upon each other.—(MAYNE.)

Stra'tum,* plural **Stra'ta.** [From *ster'no*, *stra'tum*, to "spread," to "lay down."] A bed or layer of matter. When different rocks lie in succession upon each other, each individual forms a stratum.

Straw'bĕr-rў. The fruit of the *Fraga'ria ves'ca*. A plant of the Linnæan class *Icosandria,* natural order *Rosaceæ.*

Strem'ma.* [From στρέφω, to "twist," or "turn."] A sprain, or luxation.

Stri'a,* plural **Stri'æ.** A Latin word signifying a "groove," "furrow," or "crease." Applied in Anatomy and Zoology to longitudinal marks or lines; and sometimes, in Pathology, to the purple spots which appear under the skin in certain fevers; also called *Vibices.*

Stri'æ,* the plural of STRIA, which see.

Strī'ate. [**Stria'tus;** from *stri'o, stria'tum,* to "make furrows."] Grooved; furrowed; marked with longitudinal streaks or furrows (*striæ*).

Striated Bodies. See CORPORA STRIATA.

Strict. [From *strin'go, stric'tum,* to "bind," or "tie close."] A botanical term signifying very straight or close.

Stric'ture. [**Strictu'ra;** from the same.] (Fr. *Rétrécissement,* rà'trà'sèss'-mŏng'.) A term for a contraction in a canal, tube, or duct; as in the œsophagus, urethra, etc.

Stri'dor Den'tium* (den'she-ŭm). ("Grinding of the Teeth.") The grating noise produced by powerful attrition of the teeth of the lower jaw on those of the upper. A common symptom in gastric affections of children.

Strid'u-lous. [**Strid'ulus;** from *stri'deo,* to "crack," "creak," or "crash."] Creaking; crashing. See CYNANCHE STREPITORIA.

Strig'il,* or **Strig'ĭ-lis.*** A Latin word signifying a "curry-comb." A scraper, or flesh-brush. An instrument used in bathing.

Strig'il-lose. The same as STRIGOSE, which see.

Strī-gose'. [**Strigo'sus;** from *stri'ga,* a "small stiff hair."] Clothed with sharp and stout close-pressed hairs, or scale-like bristles (*strigæ*). Applied to plants.

Strob-ĭ-lā'ceous. [**Strobila'ceus.**] Relating to, or resembling, a strobile.

Strob'ĭle. [**Strob'ilus.**] A scaly multiple fruit resulting from the ripening of some sort of catkin. It is applied especially to the peculiar fruit of the *Coniferæ,* of which the cone of the pine-tree is an example.

Strob-ĭ-lif'er-ous. [**Strobilif'erus;** from *strob'ilus,* a "strobile," and *fe'ro,* to "bear."] Bearing strobiles

Strob'ĭ-lĭ-form. [**Strobilifor'mis;** from *strob'ilus,* a "strobile."] Resembling a strobile.

Strob-ĭ-li'tēs.* [From *strob'ilus,* a "strobile," and λίθος, a "stone"?] Fossil fruit resembling a strobile.

Stroke of the Sun. See COUP DE SOLEIL.

Stroke of the Wind. See COUP DE VENT.

Stro'ma, *atis.** [From στρῶμα, a "bed," or "couch."] The tissue which forms the bed or substance of an organ.

Strombuliferous. See STROMBULIFORM.

Strom'bu-lĭ-form. [**Strombulifor'mis;** from *strom'bulus,* diminutive of *strom'bus,* a spiral shell of a mollusk.] Contorted like a screw, or twisted spirally.

Strong'er Al'co-hol. [**Al'cohol For'tius.**] The name applied to spirit of the specific gravity 0.817. It has been placed on the primary list of the Materia Medica of the U.S. Pharmacopœia for 1860.

Stron'ġȳ-lus.* [From στρογγύλος, "globose."] A kind of worm or entozöon, found in the kidney and other viscera: a strongyle.

Stron'gylus Ġi'gas.* ("Giant Strongylus.") A very large species sometimes found in the human kidney.

Strontian, stron'she-an. [**Strontia'na;** from *Stron'tian,* in Argyleshire.] The oxide of strontium; one of the primitive earths, found in combination with carbonic acid in strontianite.

Stron'tic. [**Stron'ticus;** from *stron'tium.*] Belonging to strontium.

Strontium,* stron'she-ŭm. The metallic base of strontian.

Stro'phĭ-ole. [**Strophi'olum;** diminutive of *stro'phium,* a "garland," or "girdle."] A small curved protuberance near the hilum of some seeds.

Stroph'u-lus.* A papular eruption of various species and form, peculiar to infants.

Stroph'ulus Al'bĭ-dus.* ("White or Whitish Strophulus.") The *white gum,* a name for a variety of *Strophulus intertinctus.*

Stroph'ulus Can'dĭ-dus.* ("Shining Strophulus.") A variety in which the *papulæ* are larger, have no inflammation, but a smooth, shining surface, which gives them a lighter color than the cuticle near them.

Stroph'ulus Con-fer'tus.* ("Thick or Crowded Strophulus.") A variety in which numerous *papillæ,* varying in size, appear on different parts of the body in infants during dentition, and is therefore called *tooth-rash*.

Stroph'ulus In-ter-tinc'tus.* ("Stained or Spotted Strophulus.") A variety of *strophulus* in which the child's skin appears like printed cotton, from the various disposition of the characteristic *papulæ*, or seems covered with a red gummy exudation; therefore popularly termed *red gum*, and *red-gown*.

Stroph'ulus Vo-lat'ĭ-cus.* ("Flying Strophulus.") The wildfire rash, a species having small circular patches or clusters of *papulæ* arising successively on different parts of the body.

Struc'tu-ral Bot'a-nȳ. The branch of botanical science which treats of the structure, organization, and external conformation of plants, including Vegetable Anatomy (or PHYTOTOMY) and ORGANOGRAPHY, which see.

Struc'ture. [**Structu'ra;** from *stru'o*, *struc'tum*, to "build," to "order," to "make."] Originally, a "building." The mode of construction or putting together of any thing. In Geology and Mineralogy, the disposition of the lines of fissure or separation, from which necessarily results the form of the rock or mineral. Also, the arrangement of the organic tissues or elements of which animals and plants are composed.

Stru'ma.* A scrofulous swelling, or tumor; also, scrofula itself. Sometimes applied to *bronchocele*.

Stru-mif'er-ous. [**Strumif'erus;** from *stru'ma*, a "wen," and *fe'ro*, to "bear."] Bearing a wen or tumor. Applied to plants.

Stru-mose'. [From *stru'ma*, a "wen."] In Botany, swollen on one side; bearing a struma, or wen.

Stru'mous. [**Strumo'sus;** from *stru'ma*.] Having scrofula; scrofulous.

Struve's Lo'tion for Hoop'ing Cough. A preparation consisting chiefly of tartarized antimony and the tincture of cantharides.

Strȳch'nāte. [**Strych'nas, a'tis.**] A combination of strychnic acid with a base.

Strych'nĭ-a, Strȳch'nin, or **Strȳch'nine.** [**Strychni'na.**] The Pharmacopœial name ‖ for a peculiar alkaloid obtained from the fruit of the *Strychnos nux vomica*. It occurs in the form of a white, or grayish-white, powder, of an intensely bitter taste, nearly insoluble in water, and readily soluble in boiling alcohol. A small portion of it dissolved in officinal sulphuric acid yields, on the addition of a minute quantity of bichromate of potassa, a splendid violet color. Strychnia has, in a concentrated form, the virtues and the poisonous qualities of nux vomica.

Strȳch'nĭ-æ Sul'phas.* ("Sulphate of Strychnia.") The Pharmacopœial name (U.S. Ph.) for a white salt in colorless prismatic crystals, without odor, exceedingly bitter, readily soluble in water, sparingly soluble in alcohol, and insoluble in ether. Medical properties the same as those of STRYCHNIA.

Strȳch'nic. [**Strych'nicus.**] Applied to salts of which strychnine forms the base.

Strȳch'nos.* [Gr. στρύχνος, a species of nightshade.] (Fr. *Vomiquier*, vo'mè'-kè'à'.) A Linnæan genus of the class *Pentandria*, natural order *Loganiaceæ*.

Strych'nos Igna'tia* (ig-na'she-a). The systematic name for the tree which yields IGNATIA, which see.

Strych'nos Nux Vom'ĭ-ca.* The tree which yields the NUX VOMICA, which see.

Strychnos Tieuté. See UPAS TIEUTÉ.

Stultitia,* stul-tish'e-a. [From *stul'tus*, "foolish."] Foolishness; folly, or a certain dulness of the mind. Formerly used for FATUITY.

Stu'pa.* Literally, "tow." Applied to tow used in certain surgical dressings; also to a cloth used in fomentations: such a cloth is termed in English a *stupe*. A fomentation.

Stu-pe-fā'cient. [**Stupefa'ciens;** from *stupefa'cio*, to "render stupid."] Having power to stupefy. Formerly used in the same manner as NARCOTIC, which see.

Stu'por, o'ris.* [From *stu'peo*, to "be stupefied."] A suspension or diminished activity of the mental faculties; loss of sensibility.

Stu'por Den'tium* (den'she-um). A term sometimes applied to the affection of the teeth when they are popularly said to be "on edge."

Stut'ter-ing. Nearly the same as stammering, but in a more aggravated form.

Stȳ, or **Stȳe.** A disease of the eyelids. See HORDEOLUM.

Stȳ'late. [**Styla'tus;** from *sty'lus*, a "style."] Having a style.

Stȳle. [**Sty'lus,** a "style," an instrument which the ancients used in writing.] The columnar or slender part of a pistil above the ovary; also, a surgeon's probe.

Stylet, stè'lå'. The French name for PROBE, which see.

Stylidiaceæ,* sti-lid-e-a'she-ē. [From *Stylid'ium,* one of the genera.] A natural order of exogenous, herbaceous plants, natives of Australia.

Stȳ-lif'er-ous. [**Stylif'erus;** from *sty'lus,* a "style," and *fe'ro,* to "bear."] Bearing styles, or a style. Applied to flowers.

Stȳ'lĭ-form. [**Stylifor'mis;** from *sty'lus,* a "style," or "bodkin."] Resembling a style or bodkin; style-shaped.

Sty-lis'cus.* [From *sty'lus,* a "style," or "bodkin."] A tent in form of a bodkin.

Sty'lo-Glos'sus.* [From γλῶσσα, a "tongue."] A muscle arising from the styloid process and the stylo-maxillary ligament, and inserted into the root of the tongue. It moves the tongue laterally and backwards.

Stȳ'lo-Hȳ'al. [**Stylohya'lis;** from *styloi'des,* and *hyoi'des,* "hyoid."] Applied by Owen to the homologues of the styloid process of the temporal bone.

Stȳ'lo-Hȳ'oid. [**Sty'lo-Hyoi'deus.**] Applied to a ligament connecting the styloid process with the hyoid bone: also to a muscle. See next article.

Sty'lo-Hy-o-i'de-us.* A muscle arising from the styloid process and inserted into the *os hyoides,* which it raises.

Stȳ'loid. [**Styloi'des;** from *sty'lus,* a "style," and εἶδος, a "form."] Resembling a style, or bodkin; styliform. Applied to a process of the temporal bone, etc.

Stȳ'lo-Mast'oid. [**Sty'lo-Mastoi'deus.**] The designation of a foramen situated between the styloid and mastoid processes, through which the *portio dura* of the seventh pair of nerves passes; also, of an artery which enters that foramen.

Sty'lo-Phăr-ȳn-ġe'us.* A muscle arising from the styloid process and inserted into the pharynx and back part of the thyroid cartilage. It raises the pharynx and draws up the thyroid cartilage.

Stȳ-lo-po'dĭ-um.* [From στῦλος, a "style," and πούς, ποδός, a "foot."] An enlargement or fleshy disk at the base of a style, as in the *Umbelliferæ.*

Sty'lus.* [Gr. στῦλος, a "column," or "style."] A surgeon's probe. Also applied to the filament of the *halteres* of the *Diptera.* See STYLE.

Sty-ma-to'sis,* or **Sti-ma-to'sis.*** [From στύω, to "erect."] Violent erection of the penis, with bloody discharge.

Stȳp'sis.* [See next article.] Astriction, or constipation.

Stȳp'tic. [**Styp'ticus;** from στύφω, to "contract," to "be astringent."] Having the power of stopping hæmorrhages through an astringent quality; hæmostatic.

Styracaceæ,* stĭr-a-ka'she-ē. A natural order of exogenous trees and shrubs, found in the tropical or subtropical regions of Asia and America. It includes *Sty'rax,* from which fragrant gum resins called Storax and Benzoin are procured.

Sty'rax, a'cis.* A Linnæan genus of the class *Decandria,* natural order *Styracaceæ.* Also, the Pharmacopœial name (U.S. Ph.) for the prepared juice of *Liquidam'bar Orienta'le.* It is a stimulating expectorant.

Sty'rax Ben'zoin.* The tree which affords benzoin. See BENZOINUM.

Sty'rax Of-fiç-ĭ-na'lis.* The tree which affords the balsam *styrax,* or storax.

Sub. [Gr. ὑπό, "under."] A Latin preposition signifying "under," "beneath," or "from beneath." Before the consonants *c, f, m, p,* and *r,* the *b* is usually changed to the corresponding letter: thus, we have *succumb* for *subcumb, suffuse* for *subfuse, support* for *subport,* etc. *Sub,* as a prefix to many English words, denotes deficiency or an inferior degree; as, *sub*-acid, *sub*carbonate, etc.

Sub-a-çe'tas Cu'pri.* ("Subacetate of Copper.") See VERDIGRIS, and CUPRI SUBACETAS.

Sub-car'bo-nāte. [**Subcarbo'nas, a'tis.**] A combination of carbonic acid with a base, in which there is an excess of the latter.

Subcar'bonate of Am-mo'nĭ-a, or **Car'bo-nate of Ammo'nia.** A white, translucent salt, with a pungent odor, sometimes called *smelling salts,* or salts of hartshorn.

Sub-clā'vĭ-an. [**Subcla'vius,** or **Subclavia'nus;** from *sub,* "under," or "beneath," and *cla'vis,* the "clavicle."] (Fr. *Sous-clavière,* soo'klå've-êR'.) The designation of an artery situated under the clavicle. The *right* arises from the *arteria innominata,* the *left* separates from the aorta at the termination of its arch.

Sub-cla'vĭ-us.* [From the same.] A muscle arising from the cartilage of the first rib and inserted into the lower surface of the clavicle. It brings the clavicle and shoulder forwards and backwards.

Sub-cor'date. [From *sub,* "under," and *cor, cor'dis,* a "heart."] Slightly heart-shaped.

Sub-cu-tā'ne-ous. [**Subcuta'ne-us;** from *sub,* "under," and *cu'tis,* the "skin."] Situated just under the skin.

Su'ber-āte. [**Su'beras, a'***tis.*] A combination of suberic acid with a base.

Su-bĕr'ic. [**Suber'icus;** from *su'ber,* "cork."] Belonging to cork. Applied to an acid obtained by the action of nitric acid on cork.

Su'be-rin. [**Suberi'na.**] A name given to the cellular tissue of cork after the various soluble matters have been removed by the action of water and alcohol.

Su-be-rose', or **Sū'ber-ous.** [**Subero'sus;** from *su'ber,* "cork."] Corky; of the nature of cork.

Sub fin. coct. = *Sub fi'nem coctio'nis.** "When the boiling is nearly finished."

Sub'ject. [From *subjic'io, subjec'tum,* to "cast or place under."] Something placed under one's notice for examination or study. In Anatomy, a body for dissection.

Sub-jec'tive. [**Subjecti'vus;** from the same.] Literally, "placed under," or within [the mind]. Applied to sensations, thoughts, etc., which arise from within ourselves, and are not dependent on, or directly caused by, external impressions. (See OBJECTIVE.) Also applied to symptoms of disease noticed by the patient himself.

Sub-lĭ-ga'men, *inis.** [From *sub'ligo,* to "under-bind."] That which is applied to overcome a hernia; a kind of truss.

Sub'lĭ-mate. [**Sublima'tum.**] The product of sublimation.

Sublimate, Corrosive. See HYDRARGYRI CHLORIDUM CORROSIVUM.

Sub-lĭ-mā'tion. [**Sublima'tio, o'***nis;* from *subli'mo, sublima'tum,* to "raise up," or "sublimate."] The process by which solid substances are volatilized or raised by heat and again condensed, the product being called a sublimate when concreted in a hard mass; and flowers, when feathery, or powder-like.

Sublimed Sulphur. See SULPHUR SUBLIMATUM.

Sub-li'mis.* ("Superficial [Muscle].") A designation of the *flex'or digito'rum commu'nis* muscle, from its being more superficial than the *flexor profundus.*

Sub-lin'gual. [From *sub,* "under," and *lin'gua,* the "tongue."] Applied to a gland situated beneath the mucous membrane of the floor of the mouth on each side of the *frænum linguæ.*

Sub-lux-ā'tion. [**Subluxa'tio, o'***nis;* from *sub,* "under," "in an inferior degree," and *lux'o, luxa'tum,* to "put out of joint."] A sprain, or partial dislocation.

Sub-max'il-la-rȳ. [From *sub,* "under," and *maxil'la,* a "jaw."] Applied to a gland situated on the inner side of the ramus of the lower jaw, and to a ganglion which occurs on a level with the submaxillary gland.

Sub-men'tal. [**Submenta'lis;** from *sub,* "under," and *men'tum,* the "chin."] Applied to an artery running beneath the chin.

Sub-merged'. The same as SUBMERSED, which see.

Sub-mersed'. [**Submer'sus;** from *sub,* "under," and *mer'go, mer'sum,* to "plunge."] Growing under the water. Applied to plants.

Sub-mer'sion. [**Submer'sio, o'***nis;* from the same.] Drowning; one of the causes producing ASPHYXIA SUFFOCATIONIS, which see.

Sub-mu'rĭ-ate. [**Submu'rias, a'***tis.*] A combination of muriatic (or hydrochloric) acid with a base, having a deficiency of the acid.

Sub-o-per'cu-lar. [**Subopercula'ris;** from *suboper'culum.*] Applied by Owen to that one of the four opercular bones which is below the *interopercular* and *preopercular.*

Sub-o-per'cu-lum.* [From *sub,* "under," and *oper'culum,* a "lid."] A bony formation with which the operculum and *interoperculum* compose a sort of lid for the gills of fishes.

Sub-or'bĭ-tar. [**Suborbita'rius;** from *sub,* "under," and *or'bita,* the "orbit."] Situated under the orbitar cavity of the eye.

Sub-Or'ders. The highest divisions of natural orders, when marked by characters of such importance that it might fairly be questioned whether they ought not to be received as independent orders.

Sub-pla-cen'ta.* A name for the DECIDUA VERA, which see.

Sub'-Sâlt. Originally, a salt which contained an excess of base. This term now relates to atomic composition, a true subsalt being that in which there is less than one atom of acid to each atom of base.

Sub-scap'u-lar. [**Subscapula'ris;**

from *sub*, "under," or "beneath," and *scap'ula*, the "shoulder-blade."] Beneath the scapula, or shoulder-blade. Applied to a muscle.

Sub-scap-u-la'ris.* ("Subscapular [Muscle].") A muscle arising from all the internal surface of the scapula, and inserted into the humerus. It pulls the arm backwards and downwards.

Sub-sī'dence. [**Subsiden'tia;** from *subsi'do*, to "settle," or "sink down."] Applied to the sediment of the urine, etc. See HYPOSTASIS.

Subspecies,* sub-spē'shez. In Botany, a marked and permanent variety.

Substantia,* sub-stan'she-ạ. [From *sub'sto*, to "subsist," to "have a firm or permanent existence."] A substance or body.

Substan'tia Fer-ru-ġin'e-ạ.* ("Ferruginous Substance.") A substance found in the *rhomboid fossa* of the brain.

Substan'tia Ni'grạ.* ("Black Substance.") A dark-colored substance found near the *corpora albicantia*, in what are termed the "peduncles of the brain."

Sub'stan-tive. [**Substanti'vus;** from *substan'tia*, a "substance," "that which subsists," or stands by itself.] Applied to those coloring matters which have a strong attraction for cloth without the aid of a mordant.

Sub-stĭ-tu'tion. [**Substitu'tio, o'nis;** from *substit'uo*, *substitu'tum*, to "put in the place of another."] A term applied to those effects of chemical affinity which depend on the replacement of certain proportions of one body by the same proportions of another body.

Sub-sul'tus.* [From *subsil'io*, *subsul'tum*, to "leap or start slightly."] A start, or twitching.

Subsul'tus Ten'dĭ-num.* ("Starting, or Leaping, of the Tendons.") Convulsive twitchings of the tendons of the hands or feet, common in low nervous and typhus fevers.

Sub-tense'. [**Subten'sa;** from *sub*, "under," and *ten'do*, *ten'sum*, to "stretch," or "extend."] A right line connecting the extremities of an arc; a chord of an arc

Sub-tĕr-rā'ne-ạn. [**Subterra'neus;** from *sub*, "under," and *ter'ra*, the "earth."] In Botany, growing beneath the surface of the ground.

Sub-til-ĭ-fo'lĭ-us.* [From *subti'lis*, "fine," or "slender," and *fo'lium*, a "leaf."] Having linear leaves or folioles: subtilifo'lious.

Sub-u'ber-ēs.* [From *sub*, "under," or "at," and *u'ber*, the "pap," or "udder."] Literally, "those under or at the breast." A term applied to children not yet weaned.

Sub'u-late. [**Subula'tus;** from *sub'ula*, an "awl."] Awl-shaped; narrow and tapering to a rigid point, as the leaves of the Juniper, etc.

Sub-u-lif'er-ous. [**Subulif'erus;** from *sub'ula*, an "awl," and *fe'ro*, to "bear."] Bearing objects like awls.

Sub-u-lĭ-fo'lĭ-us.* [From *sub'ula*, an "awl," and *fo'lium*, a "leaf."] Having subulate leaves: subulifo'lious.

Sub'u-lĭ-form. [**Subulifor'mis.**] The same as SUBULATE, which see.

Suc-çe-da'ne-um.* [From *succe'do*, to "follow," or "come in place of."] A substitute. Applied to medicines, etc.

Suc'çi,* the plural of SUCCUS, which see.

Succin. See SUCCINUM.

Suc'çĭ-nāte. [**Suc'cinas, a'tis.**] A combination of succinic acid with a base.

Suc-çin'ic. [**Succin'icus;** from *suc'cinum*, "amber."] Belonging to amber. Applied to an acid obtained from it.

Suc'çĭ-nŭm.* [From *suc'cus*, "juice."] (Fr. *Succin*, sük'sᴀɴᴳ', or *Ambre*, ŏmbr.) The Pharmacopœial name for AMBER, which see.

Suc-çiv'o-rous. [**Succiv'orus;** from *suc'cus*, "juice," and *vo'ro*, to "devour."] Feeding on juice. Applied to certain insects.

Suc-cose'. The same as SUCCULENT, which see.

Suc'cu-bous. [From *sub*, "under," and *cu'bo*, to "lie."] Applied to leaves when the apex of each leaf is covered by the base of the next, as in *Jungermannia*.

Suc'cu-lent. [**Suc'culens,** or **Succulen'tus;** from *suc'cus*, "juice."] Juicy; full of juice.

Suc'cus,* plural **Suc'çi.** [From *su'go*, *suc'tum*, to "suck."] The juice of fruits, plants, roots, etc.; sap. Also applied to certain animal fluids. The term *succus* is used by the British Pharmacopœia for the juices of certain plants used in medicine: as, *Suc'cus coni'i* ("juice of conium"), *Suc'cus tarax'aci* ("juice of taraxacum"), etc.

Succus Gastricus. See GASTRIC JUICE.

Suc-cus'sion. [**Succus'sio, o'nis;** from *succu'tio*, *succus'sum*, to "shake."] Giving the trunk slight but sudden shakes, in order to produce fluctuation of a liquid suspected to exist within the chest or abdomen, and so to ascertain its presence and quantity.

Suck'er. [**Sur'culus,** a "shoot," or "scion."] In Botany, a branch of subterranean origin, which, after running horizontally and emitting roots in its course, at length rises out of the ground and forms an erect stem.

Suc'tion. [**Suc'tio, o'**nis; from *su'go, suc'tum,* to "suck."] The act of sucking. Applied to the process of raising water or other liquids in a tube by forming a partial vacuum, into which the liquid is forced by the pressure of the atmosphere.

Suc-to'rĭ-a.* [From the same.] The third class of the *Diploneura* or *Helminthoida,* comprising the *Entozoa* and other similar helminthoid animals, which have their mouth adapted for sucking.

Suc-to'rĭ-ous. [**Sucto'rius;** from the same.] Having the power of sucking.

Su-da'men, *inis,** plural **Su-dam'ĭ-na** [from *su'do, suda'tum,* to "sweat"]; also termed **Pa-pil'læ Su-do-ra'lēs.*** ("Sweat-Pimples.") Vesicles like millet-seeds, appearing in numbers, suddenly and unattended by fever, after great sweating from hard labor.

Su-dam'ĭ-na,* the plural of SUDAMEN, which see.

Su-da'rĭ-um.* [From the same.] Synonymous with SUDATORIUM.

Su-dā'tion. [**Suda'tio, o'**nis; from the same.] A sweating.

Su-da-to'rĭ-a.* [From the same.] A morbid sweating. The same as EPHIDROSIS, which see.

Su-da-to'rĭ-um.* [From the same.] A sweating-bath, or sweating-room.

Su'da-to-rȳ. [**Sudato'rius;** from the same.] Belonging to perspiration, or sweat.

Su'dor, o'ris.* [From ὕδωρ, "water," or "moisture."] (Fr. *Sueur,* sü'UR'.) Sweat, or sensible perspiration; a sweating; diaphoresis.

Sudor Anglicanus or **Anglicus.** See ANGLICUS SUDOR.

Su-do-ra'lis.* Pertaining to *sudor,* or sweat.

Su-do-rif'er-ous. [**Sudorif'erus;** from *su'dor,* "sweat," and *fe'ro,* to "bear."] Bearing sweat; serving to carry off sweat.

Su-do-rif'ic. [**Sudorif'icus;** from *su'dor,* "sweat," and *fa'cio,* to "make."] Inducing or causing sweat; diaphoretic.

Su-do-rip'a-rous. [**Sudorip'arus;** from *su'dor,* "sweat," and *pa'rio,* to "produce."] Producing, or secreting, sweat. Applied to certain glands. See next article.

Sudorip'arous Gland. [**Glan'dula Sudorip'ara,** plural **Glan'dulæ Sudorip'aræ.**] A sweat-gland, consisting of a minute tube coiled up in a globular form, situated in the subcutaneous areolar tissue.

Suet. See SEVUM.

Sueur. See SUDOR.

Suf-fĭ-men'tum,* plural **Suf-fĭ-men'ta.** [From *suf'fio,* to "perfume."] A perfume of any pleasant kind that is burned or smoked; a suf'fiment.

Suffoca'tio (suf-fo-ka'she-o) **Hȳs-tĕr'ĭ-ca,*** **Suffoca'tio U-te-ri'na.*** The *globus hystericus:* hysterical or uterine suffocation.

Suf-fo-cā'tion. [**Suffoca'tio, o'**nis; from *suffo'co, suffoca'tum,* to "choke," or "stop the breath."] (Fr. *Étouffement,* à'toof'mōNᴳ'.) The act of suffocating; death or suspended animation from privation of breath; cessation or stoppage of the breath.

Suf-fru-tēs'çent. [**Suffrutes'cens.**] Slightly shrubby; woody at the base only.

Suf'fru-tex.* [From *sub,* "under," and *fru'tex,* a "shrub."] An undershrub; a woody plant of low stature.

Suf-fru'tĭ-cose. [**Suffrutico'sus;** from *suf'frutex,* an "undershrub."] Somewhat woody; low and shrubby, as an undershrub.

Suf-fu-mĭ-gā'tion. [**Suffumiga'tio, o'**nis; from *sub,* "under," "beneath," and *fu'migo, fumiga'tum,* to "make a smoke," to "fumigate."] Literally, a "fumigation from beneath:" hence, simply, fumigation.

Suf-fu'sion. [**Suffu'sio, o'**nis; from *sub,* "under," and *fun'do, fu'sum,* to "pour," to "spread."] Literally, a pouring or spreading of blood under the surface. Applied to redness of the skin as the result of inflammation or excitement, or to extravasation of some humor, as of blood, on the eye, which is then said to be bloodshot. Applied also to cataract, formerly supposed to be the suffusion of a morbid humor within the eye.

Sugar, shŏŏg'ar. [Lat. **Sac'charum;** Fr. *Sucre,* sükR. See SACCHARUM.] A proximate principle of plants, composed of carbon, oxygen, and hydrogen. It is the most soluble form of ternary organizable matter, and exists, in plants, only in solution. It abounds in growing parts, in many stems just before flowering, as those of the sugar-cane, maple, etc., and in pulpy fruits.

Su'gar, Aç'id of, Su'gar, Es'sence of. Names for OXALIC ACID, which see.

Su'gar of Lead. The common name of PLUMBI ACETAS, which see.

Su'gar of Milk. A substance commonly used by the homœopathists as the vehicle of their medicines. It is also sometimes employed in allopathic medicine. See SACCHARUM LACTIS.

Sug'gil-lāt-ed. [**Sugilla'tus;** from *sugil'lo, sugilla'tum,* to "make black and blue."] Having, or pertaining to, suggillation.

Sug-gil-lā'tion. [**Sugilla'tio, o'nis;** from the same.] The mark left by a leech or cupping-glass; also, livid spots of various size noticed on dead bodies.

Su'ĭ-cīde. [**Suicid'ium;** from *su'i,* "of himself," and *-cid'ium,* a suffix (from *cæ'do,* to "kill," signifying "slaughter," or "slaying."] Self-murder. The voluntary taking of one's own life, often the consequence of mental disease.

Suites de Couches, swėt dẹh koosh. The French term for LOCHIA, which see.

Sŭl'cate, or **Sul'cāt-ed.** [**Sulca'tus;** from *sul'co, sulca'tum,* to "furrow."] Having deep lines lengthwise; furrowed; grooved.

Sul'çi,* gen. **Sul-co'rum,** the plural of SULCUS, which see.

Sul-cif'er-us.* [From *sul'cus,* a "furrow," and *fe'ro,* to "bear."] In Zoology, bearing or having grooves or furrows.

Sŭl'cus.* (Fr. *Sillon,* sė'yȯnᵍ'.) A groove, furrow, or trench. Applied in the plural (*sul'ci*) to grooves on the surface of bones and other organs.

Sŭl'phas Ba-ry'tæ.* ("Sulphate of Baryta.") See BARYTA.

Sul'phas Căl'cis.* ("Sulphate of Lime.") Gypsum, or plaster of Paris.

Sulphas Cupri. See CUPRI SULPHAS.

Sul'phas Fer'ri.* ("Sulphate of Iron.") A salt occurring in light-green crystals, with a strong styptic taste. Commonly called copperas, or green vitriol. In small or moderate doses, it is astringent and tonic. In an overdose it acts as an irritant poison.

Sul'phas Mag-ne'si-æ.* ("Sulphate of Magnesia.") See MAGNESIÆ SULPHAS.

Sulphas Sodæ. See SODÆ SULPHAS.

Sŭl'phāte. [**Sul'phas, a'tis.**] A combination of sulphuric acid with a base.

Sulphate of Alumina and Ammonia. See ALUMEN.

Sulphate of Alumina and Potassa. See ALUMEN.

Sulphate of Magnesia. See MAGNESIÆ SULPHAS.

Sul'phate of Nick'el. [**Nic'coli Sul'phas.**] A salt which is recommended as a tonic in cases of obstinate periodic headache. It occurs in emerald-green crystals.

Sulphate of Quinia (or **Quinine**). See QUINIÆ SULPHAS.

Sulphate of Zinc. See ZINCI SULPHAS.

Sul'phāt-ed. [**Sulpha'tus.**] Converted into salts by combination with sulphuric acid.

Sŭl'phīde. [**Sul'phis, idis.**] A combination of sulphur with a metal or other body.

Sŭl'phīte. [**Sul'phis, i'tis.**] A combination of sulphurous acid with a base.

Sŭl'pho-salt. [**Sul'phosal, alis.**] A compound, both elements of which contain sulphur, forming with one an acid, with the other a base.

Sŭl'phur,* gen. **Sul'phu-ris.** [From *sal,* or *sul,* a "salt," and πῦρ, "fire"?] (Fr. *Soufre,* soofʀ.) Brimstone. A yellow, inflammable, non-metallic, simple substance, of volcanic origin. It is a non-conductor of electricity. Its specific gravity is 1.99. Also, the Pharmacopœial name for sublimed sulphur.

Sulphur, Flowers of. See FLORES SULPHURIS.

Sul'phur Lo'tum.* ("Washed Sulphur.") The Pharmacopœial name (U.S. Ph.) for sublimed sulphur thoroughly washed with water.

Sulphur, Milk of. See SULPHUR PRÆCIPITATUM.

Sul'phur Præ-cip-ĭ-ta'tum.* ("Precipitated Sulphur.") The Pharmacopœial name for a preparation sometimes known as the Milk of Sulphur. It possesses the medical properties of sublimed sulphur. See SULPHUR SUBLIMATUM.

Sul'phur Ro-tun'dum.* ("Round Sulphur.") A name for roll brimstone.

Sul'phur Sub-lĭ-ma'tum.* ("Sublimed Sulphur.") The Pharmacopœial name (U.S. Ph.) for sublimed sulphur which is wholly volatilized by heat. Sulphur is a laxative, diaphoretic, and resolvent. It is much employed, both internally and externally, in cutaneous affections, especially in *psora,* for which it is regarded as a specific.

Sul'phu-rāt-ed. [**Sulphura'tus;** from *sul'phur.*] Applied to certain substances combined with sulphur: as, sulphurated antimony (the *Antimo'nium sulphura'tum* of the British Pharmacopœia).

Sul-phu-ra'tion. [**Sulphura'tio, o'**nis; from the same.] The state of a simple substance combined with sulphur.

Sul-phu're-ous. [**Sulphu'reus;** from the same.] Belonging to, or having the qualities of, sulphur.

Sul'phu-ret. [**Sulphure'tum;** from the same.] A combination of sulphur with an alkali, earth, or metal.

Sul'phu-ret-ted. [**Sulphure'tus.**] Made into a sulphuret, or combined with sulphur.

Sul'phuretted Hy'dro-gen. Hydro-sulphuric acid, a noxious gas, consisting of hydrogen and sulphur.

Sul-phu'ric. [**Sulphu'ricus;** from *sul'phur.*] Relating to sulphur: applied to an acid obtained from it. See next article.

Sulphu'ric Aç'id. [**Aç'idum Sulphu'ricum.**] Oil of Vitriol. A limpid, colorless, and caustic fluid, which is intensely acid in all its characters even when largely diluted. Anhydrous sulphuric acid is composed of one atom of sulphur and three of oxygen. The acid, as it usually occurs in commerce, is a compound of one atom of anhydrous acid and one of water. Specific gravity, 1.8.

Sulphuric Ether. See Ether, Sulphuric.

Sul-phu-rif'er-ous. [**Sulphurif'erus;** from *sul'phur,* and *fe'ro,* to "bear."] Bearing or containing sulphur.

Sul'phu-ris I-od'i-dum.* ("Iodide of Sulphur.") The Pharmacopœial name (U.S. Ph.) for a substance of a grayish-black color, with a crystalline radiated appearance. Made into an ointment, it has been found useful in various cutaneous affections.

Sul-phu-ro'sa.* [From *sul'phur.*] A class of resolvent spanæmics, including sulphur, the alkaline sulphurets, etc.

Sul'phu-rous. [**Sulphuro'sus;** from *sul'phur.*] Of the nature of sulphur, or containing sulphur. Applied to an acid obtained from it.

Sum. = *Su'mo,** to "take," *Sumen'dus,** to "be taken;" also *Summita'tes,** "the tops."

Su'mach. A dye-stuff obtained from the *Rhus coriaria* and *Rhus cotinus.* In calico-printing, sumach affords a yellow color. See Rhus Glabra.

Sum'bul Root. [Arabic *Sumbul,* an "ear," or "spike."] A drug recently imported from Russia and India, and employed as a remedy for cholera. Its botanical origin is unknown.

Sum'mer Com-plaint'. A popular name for *diarrhœa* (or *cholera*) *infantum.*

Sum'mi-tas,* plural **Sum-mi-ta'tēs.** [From *sum'mus,* "highest."] A term for the highest part, or top: *e.g.* of a plant.

Sun-Burning. See Æstates.

Sun-Stroke. See Coup de Soleil.

Su'per. [Gr. ὑπέρ, "above."] A Latin preposition, signifying "above," "upon," "beyond," "in addition to," or "more than."

Su-per'bus.* A Latin word signifying "proud." Sometimes applied to two muscles, the *levator menti* and *rectus superior,* from the expression of pride which their action imparts. See Rectus Superior Oculi.

Su-per-cil'i-a-ry. [**Supercilia'ris.**] Belonging to the supercilium.

Su-per-cil'i-um.* [From *su'per,* "above," and *cil'ium,* the "eyelid."] (Fr. *Sourcil,* soor'sè'.) The eyebrow.

Su-per-fe-cun-da'tion. [**Superfœcunda'tio, o'**nis; from *su'per,* "over," and *fœcun'dus,* "fruitful."] The same as Superfetation, which see.

Su-per-fe-ta'tion. [**Superfœta'tio, o'**nis; from *su'per,* "over," "in addition to," and *fœ'tus.*] A second impregnation taking place before the first has run its course; while generally denied by obstetricians, the possibility of its occurrence is maintained by many physiologists.

Su-per-im-preg-na'tion. [**Superimpregna'tio, o'**nis; from *su'per,* "over," or "in addition to," and *impregna'tio,* a "conception."] The same as Superfetation, which see.

Su-pe'ri-or.* [Comparative degree of *su'perus,* "upper," "high."] A term sometimes applied to a calyx which is adherent or adnate to the ovary; also to the ovary when it is free or not adherent.

Superior Arch, or **Superior Vertebral Arch.** See Vertebral Arch.

Supe'rior Au'ris.* ("Upper [Muscle] of the Ear.") A muscle of the external ear, arising from the aponeurosis of the *occipito-frontalis* and inserted into the back part of the anthelix. It lifts the ear upwards.

Su-per-na'tant. [**Superna'tans;** from *su'per,* "above," and *na'to,* to "swim."] Floating above or upon the surface.

Su'per-sâlt. [**Su'persal, al**is.] A salt having the acid in excess.

Su-pī-nā'tion. [**Supina'tio, o'***nis;* from *supi'no, supina'tum,* to "lay or place with the face upwards."] The act of turning the palm of the hand upwards. In Pathology, the position of a person lying on his back with the arms and legs extended.

Su-pi-na'tor, o'r*is.** [From the same.] Applied to a muscle that turns the palm of the hand upwards.

Su-pine'. [**Supi'nus,** "lying on the back," "idle."] In Botany, lying flat, with face upwards.

Sup'ple-ment. [**Supplemen'tum;** from *sup'pleo,* to "fill up," to "supply" any thing that is deficient.] Literally, the "supplying" of any thing. The supplement of an arc or angle is that which must be added to it in order to make a semicircle, or 180°.

Sup-pos'ĭ-to-rȳ. [**Supposito'rium;** from *sub,* "under," and *po'no, pos'itum,* to "place."] A substance put in the rectum to be retained there till gradually dissolved.

Suppressio Mensium,* sup-presh'e-o men'she-um. ("Suppression of the Menses.") See AMENORRHŒA, and MENOSTASIA.

Sup-pres'sion. [**Suppres'sio, o'***nis;* from *sup'primo, suppres'sum,* to "press under," to "put a stop to."] Complete stoppage, or non-secretion. In Botany, an obliteration of organs or parts.

Suppurant. See SUPPURATIVE.

Sup'pu-rāte. [**Suppu'ro, Suppura'tum;** from *sub,* "under," or "beneath," and *pus, pu'ris,* "matter."] To form matter beneath the skin or within the body; to fester.

Sup-pu-rā'tion. [**Suppura'tio, o'***nis;* from the same.] One of the terminations of inflammation by which pus is formed; a gathering of matter; a festering.

Sup'pu-ra-tives. [From the same.] Medicines which promote suppuration; a variety of epispastics, producing phlegmonous inflammation.

Su'pra. A Latin preposition, signifying "above," "superior to."

Su'pra-Ax'il-la-rȳ. [From *su'pra,* "above," and *axil'la,* an "armpit," or "axil."] Above the axil of a leaf.

Su-pra-cos-ta'lēs.* [From *su'pra,* "above," and *cos'ta,* a "rib."] A designation of the *levatores costarum* muscles, from their lying above or upon the ribs.

Su-pra-de-com-pound'. Several times compounded. Applied to leaves.

Su'pra-Ju-ras'sic. [**Supra-Juras'sicus;** from *su'pra,* "above," and *Juras'sic.*] Applied to a group of sedimentary rocks, comprehending the superior Jurassic.

Su'pra-Oc-cip'ĭ-tal. [**Supraoccipita'lis;** from *su'pra,* "above," and *occipita'lis* os, the "occipital bone."] Proposed by Owen for the large upper part of the occipital bone.

Su-pra-Or'bĭ-tal. [**Supraorbita'lis,** and **Supraorbita'rius;** from *su'pra,* "above," and *or'bita,* the "orbit."] Above the orbit: supra-orbitary.

Su-pra-re'nal. [**Suprarena'lis;** from *su'pra,* "above," and *ren,* the "kidney."] Above the kidney.

Su-pra-scap'u-lar. [**Suprascapula'ris;** from *su'pra,* "above," and *scap'ula.*] Above the scapula, or shoulder-blade.

Su-pra-spī'nal. [**Supraspina'lis,** or **Supraspina'tus;** from *su'pra,* "above," and *spi'na,* a "spine."] Above or upon the spine of the back; also, above the spine of the scapula. Applied to a muscle arising from above the spine of the scapula and inserted into the humerus. It raises the arm.

Su'ra.* The calf of the leg, consisting principally of the *sole'us* and *gastrocne'mius* muscles.

Sur'cu-lose. [From *sur'culus,* a "sucker."] Producing suckers.

Sur'cu-lus.* A Latin word signifying a "shoot," or "scion." In Botany, synonymous with SUCKER, which see.

Sur'dĭ-tȳ. [**Sur'ditas, a'***tis;* from *sur'dus,* "deaf."] Deafness; dulness of hearing.

Sur-do-mu'tĭ-tas, a'*tis.** [From *sur'dus,* "deaf," and *mu'tus,* "dumb."] The state of deafness and dumbness.

Sur'dus.* (Fr. *Sourd,* SOOR.) A Latin word signifying "deaf." Applied both to those who are entirely destitute of the sense of hearing, and to those whose hearing is imperfect.

Sureau, sü'rō'. The French name for "elder." See SAMBUCUS.

Sur'feit, sŭr'fit. [From the French *surfaire,* to "overdo."] Excess of food or drink, generally attended with a sense of nausea, oppression of the stomach, with impeded perspiration, and sometimes eruptions on the skin.

Sur'geon. [Lat. **Chirur'gus;** Gr. χειρουργός, from χείρ, the "hand," and ἔργον, a "work;" Fr. *Chirurgien,* shē'rüR'zhe ăNᴳ'.) A practitioner in surgery.

Sur'geon-A-poth'e-ca-rȳ. One who unites the practice of surgery with that of the apothecary. See GENERAL PRACTITIONER.

Sur'geon-Den'tist, or **Den'tist Prop'er** [from *dens, den'tis*, a "tooth"]. One who performs operations on the natural teeth. Used in contradistinction to a *mechanical* dentist, who prepares or adapts artificial teeth.

Sur'ge-rў. [Lat. **Chirur'gia;** Gr. χειρουργία, from χείρ, the "hand," and ἔργον, a "work."] That branch of the healing art which teaches the proper use of manual operations for the preservation or restoration of health, including such general medicinal and dietetic treatment as the proper performance of such operations may render necessary.

Sur'gĭ-cal. [**Chirur'gicus;** from the same.] Relating to surgery.

Sus,* gen. **Su'is.** [Gr. ὗς.] The hog. A genus of animals of the class *Mammalia*, order *Pachydermata*.

Sus Scro'fa.* The systematic name of the hog, the fat of which affords lard.

Sus-cep-tĭ-bil'ĭ-tў. [From *suscip'io, suscep'tum*, to "receive," or "undergo."] Sensibility; impressibility.

Suspended Animation. See ASPHYXIA.

Sus-pen'sion. [**Suspen'sio, o'***nis;* from *suspen'do, suspen'sum*, to "hang up."] The state of solid particles that are diffused in water, or other solvent, but are not dissolved, and may be separated from the solvent by filtration. Also, hanging; one of the causes producing ASPHYXIA SUFFOCATIONIS, which see.

Sus-pen-so'rĭ-um Hep'a-tis.* ("Suspensory of the Liver.") The broad ligament of the liver.

Sus-pen-so'rĭ-us Tes'tis.* ("Suspensory [Muscle] of the Testicle.") Another name for the CREMASTER muscle, which see.

Sus-pen'so-rў. [**Suspenso'rius;** from *suspen'do, suspen'sum*, to "hang up."] Suspending.

Suspen'sory. [**Suspenso'rium;** from the same.] Literally, "any thing that suspends." Usually applied to a suspensory bag, or bandage, for supporting the scrotum, that the weight of the testicles may not draw on the spermatic cord.

Sus-pĭr'ĭ-um.* [From *suspi'ro*, to "breathe deeply," to "sigh."] A Latin word signifying a "deep, short, or labored breathing;" a "sigh."

Su-sur'rus.* A whisper, or low muttering.

Su-tu'ra.* [From *su'o, su'tum*, to "sew together."] A "suture," or "seam." Applied in Anatomy to the junction of the bones of the cranium by a serrated line resembling the stitches of a seam. The following varieties of suture are especially deserving of notice:—

1. SUTU'RA DENTA'TA* ("Dentate Suture"), in which the processes are long and tooth-like, as in the interparietal suture of the skull.

2. SUTU'RA SERRA'TA* ("Serrate Suture"), in which the processes are small and fine like the teeth of a saw, as in the suture between the two portions of the frontal bone.

3. SUTU'RA LIMBO'SA* ("Bordered Suture"), in which, together with the dentated margins, there is a degree of bevelling of one, so that one bone rests on the other, as in the occipito-parietal suture.

The following are named according to their situation on the skull:—

1. SUTU'RA CORONA'LIS* ("Coronal Suture"), which passes transversely over the skull, and is named from its being situated at that part of the head upon which the *corona*, or crown, given to the conquerors in the games, was formerly placed.

2. SUTU'RA SAGITTA'LIS* ("Sagittal Suture"), which passes from the middle of the superior margin of the frontal to the angle of the occipital bone, and is named from its *arrow-like* or straight course. It is sometimes continued down the frontal bone to the nose: this part is then named the *frontal suture*.

3. SUTU'RA LAMBDOIDA'LIS* ("Lambdoidal Suture"), which begins at the termination of the sagittal suture and extends on each side to the base of the cranium: it is named from its resemblance to the Greek Λ (*lambda*).

4. SUTU'RA SQUAMO'SA* ("Squamous Suture"), which joins the squamous portion of the temporal bone to the parietal.

Sutura Coronalis. See CORONAL SUTURE.

Su'tu-ral. [**Sutura'lis;** from *sutu'ra*, a "suture."] Relating to, or having, a suture.

Su'ture. [**Sutu'ra;** from *su'o, su'tum*, to "sew together."] Literally, a "sewing," or "seam." The union of flat bones by their margins. A species of synarthrosis; a dovetailing mode of articulation, the most solid of the four forms of synarthrosis. It occurs in the union of the flat bones of the skull with each other. (See SUTURA.) In Botany, the seam (or line of opening) of a pod or capsule. In Surgery, the drawing together of the lips of a wound by sewing.

Su'ture, Dry. [**Sutu'ra Sic'ca.**] The application of a piece of adhesive plaster, having a selvage, along each side of a wound (the selvages opposing each other), and then drawing them together by sewing them with a common needle.

Su'ture, Glov'er's. The introducing of a needle and thread into one lip of the wound from within outwards; then into the other in the same way. It is now abandoned as unsuitable.

Su'ture, In-ter-rup'ted, Su'ture, Knot'ted. A number of stitches tied separately at short distances from each other, to keep together the lips of a wound.

Su'ture, Twist'ed. The winding of a ligature in the form of the figure 8 round the ends of a pin inserted through both lips of a wound.

S. V. = *Spir'itus vi'ni.** "Spirit of wine."

S. V. R. = *Spir'itus vi'ni rectifica'tus.** "Rectified spirit of wine."

Swallowing, Difficulty of. See DYSPHAGIA.

Sweat. [Lat. **Su'dor, o'***ris;* Gr. ἱδρώς; Fr. *Sueur*, sü'UR'.] Perspiration. Usually applied to excessive perspiration resulting from hard exercise, mental excitement, or medicinal applications, rather than the natural perspiration of health.

Sweating. See SUDATION.

Sweating Fever. See ANGLICUS SUDOR.

Sweating, Morbid. See EPHIDROSIS.

Sweat'ing Sick'ness. [**Su'dor Anglica'nus.**] See ANGLICUS SUDOR.

Sweet Bay. The *Lau'rus Nob'ilis*, or True Laurel. A tree of the natural order *Lauraceæ*. Its leaves and berries are fragrant, aromatic, and astringent. See BAY BERRIES.

Sweet Bread. A name for the PANCREAS, which see.

Sweet-Scent'ed Flag. A common name for the ACORUS CALAMUS, which see.

Sweet Spir'it of Ni'tre. The SPIRITUS ÆTHERIS NITROSI, which see.

Swelling. See TUMEFACTION.

Swie-te'nĭ-a Fe-brif'u-ga,* or **Soy'mĭ-da Febrif'uga.*** An East Indian tree of the Linnæan class *Decandria*, natural order *Cedrelaceæ*, or *Meliaceæ*. Its bark possesses tonic properties, and is used in India as a substitute for Peruvian bark.

Swiete'nia Ma-hag'o-ni* or **Ma-hog'a-ni.*** The systematic name of the mahogany-tree, which is a native of tropical America. It belongs to the natural order *Cedrelaceæ*.

Swine'-Pox. A species of *varicella*, in which the vesicles are pointed and the fluid clear throughout.

Swinging. See ÆORA.

Swooning. See DELIQUIUM ANIMI, LEIPOTHYMIA, and SYNCOPE.

Sword-Shaped. See ENSATE, ENSIFORM, and GLADIATE.

Syaladenitis. See SIALADENITIS.

Sy-co'ma, a*tis.** [From σῦκον, a "fig."] A term for a wart, or warty excrescence, somewhat like a fig, on the eyelid, anus, or other part of the body.

Sy-co'nĭ-um,* or **Syc'o-nus.*** [From σῦκον, a "fig."] An aggregate fruit, like the fig.

Sy-co'sis.* The growth or formation of *sycoma;* more particularly, an eruptive disease, in which there are inflamed and somewhat hard tubercles clustering together in irregular patches about the beard and on the scalp.

Sȳ'e-nīte, or **Si'e-nīte.** [From *Sye'ne*, a town in Egypt, where it is found.] A granitic aggregate of quartz, felspar, and hornblende.

Sȳl'la-bus.* [From σύν, "together," and λαμβάνω, to "take:" hence, συλλαβεῖν, to "comprehend."] An index or compendium containing the chief heads of a treatise or lecture, or of a series of lectures.

Sȳl-vat'ĭ-cus.* The same as SYLVESTRIS, which see.

Sȳl-ves'tris.* [From *syl'va*, a "wood."] Growing or living in woods or forests. Applied to various plants.

Sȳl-vic'o-lus.* [From *syl'va*, a "forest," and *co'lo*, to "inhabit."] Living in woods or forests.

Sylvii Aquæductus. See AQUEDUCT OF SYLVIUS.

Sym. A prefix having the same force as SYN, which see.

Sȳm-bleph'a-ron,* or **Sȳm-bleph'-a-rum.*** [From σύν, "together," and βλέφαρον, the "eyelid."] Adhesion of the eyelid, chiefly the upper, to the eyeball.

Sȳm'bol. [Lat. **Sym'bolum;** Gr. σύμβολον, from συμβάλλω, to "put together," to "compare."] Literally, "something compared or likened to another:" hence, a type, emblem, or sign.

Sym'bols, Chem'ĭ-cal, otherwise

termed **Chem'ical Ab-bre-vĭ-ā'tions.** An abbreviated mode of expressing the composition of bodies. The elementary substances, instead of being written at full length, are indicated by the first letter of their names, a second letter being employed when more than one substance begins with the same letter: thus, *C* stands for Carbon, *Al* for Aluminium, *As* for Arsenic, etc. See Appendix.

Sȳm-met'rĭ-cal. [Symmet'ricus; from *symme'tria,* "symmetry."] Having symmetry; formed with proper proportions. Applied to flowers which have an equal number of parts in each whorl.

Sȳm'me-trȳ. [Symme'tria; from σύν, "together," and μετρέω, to "measure."] Adaptation, or the most proper relation of the measure of parts to each other and to the whole; proportion. Also applied to the resemblance which exists in many organs that are situated on each side of the median line.

Sȳm-pa-thet'ic. [Sympathet'icus; from *sympathi'a,* "sympathy."] Having, or pertaining to, sympathy; depending on sympathy.

Sympathetic Action. See REFLEX ACTION.

Sympathet'ic Bu'bo. Inflammation of a gland arising from mere irritation, not from syphilis nor *gonorrhœa.*

Sympathetic Nerve. See TRISPLANCHNIC NERVE.

Sȳm-path'ic. [Sympath'icus.] Relating to sympathy. Synonymous with SYMPATHETIC.

Sȳm'pa-thȳ. [Sympathi'a; from συμπαθέω, to "suffer with."] The feeling or suffering in common, to which different parts of the body are subject. See RELATIONS, ORGANIC.

Sȳm-pet'a-lous. [From σύν, "together," and πέταλον, a "petal."] Applied to flowers which become somewhat monopetalous by a junction of the base of the petals with the monadelphous stamens.

Sȳm-pho-re'sis.* [From σύν, "together," and φορέω, to "carry."] Synonymous with CONGESTION, which see.

Sȳm-phor-ĭ-car'pus.* [From σύν, "together," φέρω, to "bear," and καρπός, "fruit."] Bearing fruit clustered together.

Sȳm'phȳ-sis.* [From σύν, "together," and φύω, to "produce."] The natural union of bones by means of an intervening substance; a variety of SYNARTHROSIS, which see. In Botany, a growing together of parts.

Sym'physis Pu'bis.* ("Symphysis of the Pubes.") The pubic articulation, or union of the *ossa pubis,* which are connected with each other by cartilage.

Sȳm-phȳ-sot'o-mȳ. [Symphysoto'mia; from *sym'physis* pu'bis, and τέμνω, to "cut."] The operation of cutting or dividing the *symphysis pubis;* otherwise termed the SIGAULTIAN OPERATION.

Sȳm-phȳ-ste'mo-nous. [From *sym'physis,* a "growing together," and στήμων, a "stamen."] Having the stamens united.

Sȳm'phȳ-tum Of-fiç-ĭ-na'le.* The systematic name for Comfrey, a plant of the Linnæan class *Pentandria,* natural order *Boraginaceæ.* The roots are very mucilaginous, and are used as emollients.

Sȳm-pi'e-sis.* [From σύν, "together," and πίεσις, a "pressing."] A pressing or squeezing together; compression.

Sȳm-pĭ-e-som'e-ter. [Sympiesom'etrum; from *sympi'esis,* and μέτρον, a "measure."] An instrument by which to ascertain the degree of pressure of the atmosphere; a barometer, or measurer of pressure.

Sȳmp'tom. [Sympto'ma, *atis;* from σύμπτωμα, a "chance;" hence, something accidental.] A concurring circumstance happening simultaneously with the disease, and serving to point out its nature, character, and seat.

Sȳmp-to-mat'ic. [Symptomat'icus; from the same.] Relating to symptoms. Applied to a disease which is a symptom of another.

Sȳmp'to-ma-tog'ra-phȳ. [Symptomatogra'phia; from σύμπτωμα, a "chance," or "symptom," and γράφω, to "write."] A description of the signs or symptoms of disease.

Sȳmp'to-ma-tol'o-ġȳ. [Symptomatolo'gia; from σύμπτωμα, a "chance," or "symptom," and λόγος, a "discourse."] The branch of Pathology which treats of symptoms or signs; semeiology.

Syn (σύν). A Greek preposition signifying "with," "together with;" often implying union, harmony, or symmetry. Sometimes it is *intensive.* Before β (*b*), μ (*m*), π (*p*), or φ (*ph*), the ν is usually changed to μ, and before λ (*l*) to the same letter: as, σύμβολον for σύνβολον, συμμετρία for συνμετρία, συμπάθεια for συνπάθεια, συλλογισμός for συνλογισμός, etc. When συν precedes a word beginning with σ (*s*), the ν is usually dropped: hence, we have σύστημα, and not σύνστημα.

☞ Before the Greek letters γ, κ, and

χ, the ν is changed to γ: thus, we have συγγένεσις for συνγένεσις, σύγκλονος for σύνκλονος, and σύγχυσις for σύνχυσις.

Sy̆n-an'the-ræ,* or **Sy̆n-an-the're-æ.*** [See next article.] A synonym for the COMPOSITÆ, which see.

Sy̆n-an'the-rous. [**Synanthe'reus;** from σύν, "together," and *anthe'ra*, an "anther."] Having stamens joined together by anthers, and forming a tube round the style.

Sy̆n'ap-tase. A term sometimes applied to AMYGDALIN.

Sy̆n-ar-thro'di-a.* The same as SYNARTHROSIS, which see.

Sy̆n-ar-thro'di-al. [**Synarthrodia'lis.**] Belonging to *synarthrodia.*

Sy̆n-ar-thro'sis.* [From σύν, "together," and ἄρθρον, a "joint."] An immovable joint, applied to a class of articulations, having three varieties, *Sutura, Gomphosis,* and *Symphysis.*

Sy̆n'carp. [**Syncar'pium, Syncar'pum,** or **Syncar'pus;** from σύν, "together," and καρπός, "fruit."] A compound fruit resulting from the coherence of several carpels, or fleshy ovaries.

Sy̆n-car'pous. [From the same.] Formed of two or more united carpels, as the orange.

Sy̆n-chon-dro'sis.* [From σύν, "together," and χόνδρος, a "cartilage."] A union of bones by intervening cartilage; a species of *symphysis,* as of the *pubes.*

Sy̆n-chon-drot'o-my̆. [**Synchondrotomi'a;** from *synchondro'sis,* and τέμνω, to "cut."] The operation of dividing a cartilaginous union of bones. Applied particularly to the division of the *symphysis pubis.*

Sy̆n-chron'i-cal. The same as SYNCHRONOUS.

Sy̆n'chro-nous. [**Syn'chronus;** from σύν, "together," and χρόνος, "time."] Happening at the same time. The pulsations of an artery are nearly synchronous with those of the heart.

Sy̆n'chy̆-sis.* [From συγχέω, to "confound."] A mingling, or confounding, of the humors of the eye in consequence of the rupture of the internal membrane and capsule by a blow; also, a dissolution of the vitreous humor, or destruction of its consistence.

Syn'chysis, Spark'ling. A species in which sparks flash before the eyes.

Sy̆n-cli'nal. [**Syncli'nus;** from σύν, "together," and *cli'no,* to "bend," or "incline."] Inclining or bending together, or towards each other.

Syncli'nal Ax'is. An imaginary line passing along the middle of a valley the strata of which dip in opposite directions and incline towards this line.

Sy̆n'clo-nus.* [From σύν, "together," and κλόνος, "tumultuous motion."] A genus of Good's Noslogy, comprising diseases characterized by tremulous and simultaneous clonic agitation of the muscles, more particularly when exerted under influence of the will.

Syn'clonus Bal-lis'mus.* The shaking palsy; the *Scelotyrbe festinans* of De Sauvages.

Sy̆n'co-pe.* [From σύν, intensive, and κόπτω, to "cut," or "cut short," to "strike."] (Fr. *Evanouissement,* à'vå'-nwĕss'mŏNᵍ'.) Literally, a "cutting short" of one's strength. Swooning or fainting. The state termed *Deliquium animi,* being a suspension of respiration and the heart's action, complete or partial. A genus of the order *Adynamia,* class *Neuroses,* of Cullen's Nosology.

Sy̆n-cop'tic. [**Syncop'ticus;** from *syn'cope.*] Belonging to, also causing, syncope.

Sy̆n-cot'y̆-led'o-nous. [**Syncotyled'onus;** from σύν, "together," and κοτυληδών, a "cotyledon."] Having the cotyledons soldered together.

Sy̆n-des-mi'tis, idis.* [From σύνδεσμος, a "ligament."] Inflammation of the ligaments.

Sy̆n-des-mog'ra-phy̆. [**Syndesmogra'phia;** from σύνδεσμος, a "ligament," and γράφω, to "write."] A description of the ligaments.

Sy̆n-des-mol'o-gy̆. [**Syndesmolo'gia;** from σύνδεσμος, a "ligament," and λόγος, a "discourse."] A treatise on ligaments; or the science of ligaments.

Sy̆n-des'mos.* [From σύν, "together," and δεσμός, a "band."] That which binds together: hence, a ligament.

Sy̆n-des-mo'sis.* [From σύνδεσμος, a "ligament."] Union of bones by ligament, as of the radius and ulna; a species of *symphysis.*

Sy̆n-des-mot'o-my̆. [**Syndesmoto'mia;** from σύνδεσμος, a "ligament," and τέμνω, to "cut."] Dissection of the articular ligaments.

Sy̆n-e-chi'a.* [From συνέχεια, "continuity."] Adhesion of the iris to the cornea, then termed *Synechia anterior;* or to the capsule of the lens, called *Synechia posterior.*

Sy̆n-e'ma,* more correctly **Syn-ne'ma.*** [From σύν, "together," and νῆμα, a "thread," or "filament."] A name for a column of monadelphous filaments.

Sy̆n-er'ġic. [**Syner'gicus.**] Relating to synergy.

Sy̆n'er-ġy̆. [**Synergi'a;** from *σύν*, "together," and *ἔργον*, a "work."] The combined action of several organs directed to one end, as in digestion.

Sy̆n-ġe-ne'sĭ-a.* [See next article.] A Linnæan class of plants having the anthers united in a ring or tube, as in all *Compositæ.*

Sy̆n-ġe-ne'sĭ-ous, or sin-je-nee'shŭs. [**Syngene'sius;** from *σύν*, "together," and *γένεσις*, "generation," or "production."] Literally, "produced or growing together." Having anthers united into a tube, the filaments being mostly separate and distinct.

Sy̆n-ĭ-ze'sis,* or **Sy̆n-e-zi'sis.*** [From *συνίζω*, to "sit or sink together," to "collapse," to "shrink up."] A term applied to the contraction or obliteration of the pupil of the eye. It is often congenital, but sometimes the result of disease or accident.

Sy̆n-neū-ro'sis.* [From *σύν*, "together," and *νευρόω*, to "nerve."] Union of bones by intervening membrane; a species of *symphysis.*

Sy̆n'o-cha.* [From *σύνοχος*, "unintermitted;" from *συνέχω*, to "hold together," to "continue."] A pure inflammatory fever. A genus of the order *Febres*, class *Pyrexiæ*, of Cullen's Nosology.

Sy̆n'o-chus.* [Gr. *σύνοχος*.] Applied to mixed fever. A genus of the order *Febres*, class *Pyrexiæ*, of Cullen's Nosology.

Sy̆n-od'ic, or **Sy̆n-od'ĭ-cal.** [**Synod'icus;** from *σύνοδος*, a "meeting."] Applied to a lunar month, or the time between two conjunctions of the sun and moon, consisting of twenty-nine days, twelve hours, and about forty-four minutes.

Synonym. See Synonyme.

Synonyme, or **Synonym,** sin'o-nim. [Gr. *συνώνυμος*, "of like name or meaning;" from *σύν*, "with," and *ὄνομα*, a "name."] One of two words in the same language which have the same or a similar signification. An equivalent or superseded name.

Sy̆n-on'y̆-my̆. [**Synonym'ia;** from the same.] The use of synonymes; that which relates to synonymes, or the expression of the same meaning by different words.

Sy̆n-op'sis.* [From *σύν*, "together," and *ὄψις*, a "view."] A collective view of any subject; a compendious statement; a collection of things so arranged as to present the principal parts in a general view.

Sy̆n-os-te-og'ra-phy̆. [**Synosteogra'phia;** from *σύν*, "together," *ὀστέον*, a "bone," and *γράφω*, to "write."] A description of the joints.

Sy̆n-os-te-ol'o-ġy̆. [**Synosteolo'gia;** from *σύν*, "together," *ὀστέον*, a "bone," and *λόγος*, a "discourse."] The doctrine of the joints; a treatise on the joints.

Sy̆n-os-te-oph'y̆-tum.* [From *σύν*, "together," *ὀστέον*, a "bone," and *φυτόν*, a "plant."] Congenital osseous growth: a synosteophyte.

Sy̆n-os-te-o'sis.* [From *σύν*, "together," and *ὀστέον*, a "bone."] Union of bones by ossific deposit.

Sy̆n-os-te-ot'o-my̆. [**Synosteoto'mia;** from *σύν*, "together," *ὀστέον*, a "bone," and *τέμνω*, to "cut."] Dissection of the joints.

Sy̆n-o'vĭ-a.* [Supposed to be derived from *σύν*, perhaps implying union or close resemblance, and *ᾠόν*, an "egg," on account of its resemblance to the white of an egg.] The unctuous fluid secretion of certain glands in the joints, with which the cartilaginous surfaces of the articulating heads of bones are lubricated and their motions facilitated.

Sy̆n-o'vĭ-al. [**Synovia'lis.**] Relating to the *synovia.*

Sy̆n-o-vi'tis, idis.* [From *synovia'lis*, "synovial."] Inflammation of a synovial membrane.

Sy̆n-te-no'sis.* [From *σύν*, "together," and *τένων*, a "tendon."] A kind of articulation in which the bones are connected by tendons.

Sy̆n-ther'mal. [**Synther'malus;** from *σύν*, "together with," and *θέρμη*, "heat."] Of equal heat or temperature.

Sy̆n'the-sis.* [From *σύν*, "together," and *τίθημι*, to "put," or "place."] Literally, "putting together," or composition. The formation of a compound substance by the union of several distinct elements; the opposite of *analysis.* Also, a surgical operation which consists in uniting parts which have been divided.

Sy̆n-thet'ic. [**Synthet'icus.**] Relating to synthesis, or effected by synthesis. Synthetic operations in Chemistry are those in which compounds are formed by the union of elements, or component substances.

Sy̆n'to-nin, or **Sy̆n'to-nine.** [From *συντείνω*, to "stretch," or "draw;" referring to the peculiar property of muscular fibre.] A name given by Lehmann to a peculiar substance obtained from muscular fibre by the action of dilute muriatic acid.

Sȳph-ĭ-lel′cos,* or **Sȳph-ĭ-lel′cus.*** [From *syph′ilis,* and ἕλκος, an "ulcer."] A venereal or syphilitic ulcer; a chancre.

Sȳph-ĭ-lel-co′sis.* [From *syphilel′cos.*] The growth or progress of syphilitic ulcer, or chancre.

Sȳ-phil′ĭ-dēṡ.* [From *syph′ilis.*] Skin-diseases arising from syphilis.

Sȳph-ĭ-lĭ-doch′thus.* [From *syph′ilis,* and ὄχθη, a "rising ground."] A syphilitic tubercle.

Sȳph-ĭ-lĭ-do-col-pi′tis, *idis.** [From *syph′ilis,* and *colpi′tis,* "inflammation of the vagina."] Syphilitic inflammation of the vagina.

Sȳph-ĭ-lĭ-dog′ra-phȳ. [**Syphilidogra′phia;** from *syph′ilis,* and γράφω, to "write."] A history of syphilis.

Sȳph-ĭ-lĭ-dol′o-ġȳ. [**Syphilidolo′gia;** from *syph′ilis,* and λόγος, a "discourse."] The doctrine or science of syphilis, and its treatment.

Sȳph-ĭ-lĭ-doph-thăl′mĭ-a.* [From *syph′ilis,* and *ophthal′mia.*] Syphilitic ophthalmia.

Sȳph-il-ĭ-on′thus.* [From *syph′ilis,* and ἴονθος, an "eruption on the face."] Copper-colored scaly eruption, or patches: the effect of syphilis.

Sȳph′ĭ-lis, *idis.** [Etymology uncertain.] (Fr. *Vérole,* vå′rol′.) Vulgarly called **Pox.** The true venereal disease, otherwise termed *Lues venerea,* and *Morbus Gallicus.* A genus of the order *Impetigines,* class *Cachexiæ,* of Cullen's Nosology.

Syph′ilis, Con-stĭ-tu′tion-al. The same as secondary syphilis. See next article.

Syph′ilis, Sec′on-da-rȳ. Applied to syphilis after the morbific matter has been absorbed and diffused through the system. The symptoms of this condition of the disease (termed "secondary symptoms") are ulcers in the throat, blotches on the skin, pain in the bones, etc.

Sȳph-ĭ-lit′ic. [**Syphilit′icus.**] Pertaining to syphilis.

Sȳph-il-ĭ-zā′tion. [**Syphiliza′tio,** *o′nis;* from *syph′ilis.*] Applied to the condition induced by the successive inoculation of animals with syphilitic poison.

Sȳph-ĭ-lo-çe′lis, *i′dis.** [From *syph′ilis,* and κηλίς, a "stain." or "spot."] Syphilitic patches on the skin. See Syphilionthus.

Sȳph′ĭ-loid. [**Syphiloi′des;** from *syph′ilis,* and εἶδος, a "form."] Resembling syphilis.

Sȳph-ĭ-lol′e-pis, *idis.** [From *syph′ilis,* and λεπίς, a "scale."] Syphilitic scale, or scaly eruption.

Sȳph-ĭ-loph′lȳ-sis.* [From *syph′ilis,* and φλύσις, an "eruption."] Syphilitic eruption.

Syr. = *Syru′pus.** "A syrup."

Sȳ-rin′ga Vul-ga′ris.* The systematic name of the Lilac, a plant of the natural order *Oleaceæ.* The leaves have been used as tonics and antiperiodics.

Sȳr′inġe. [Lat. **Sy′rinx;** Gr. σῦριγξ; Fr. *Seringue,* sẹh-răNg′.] An instrument for injecting liquids into any vessel or cavity.

Sȳ-rin′goid. [**Syringoi′des;** from *sy′rinx,* a "pipe," and εἶδος, a "form."] Resembling a pipe or tube.

Sȳ-rin′go-tome. [**Syringot′omum;** see Syringotomy.] An instrument for cutting fistulæ.

Sȳr-in-got′o-mȳ. [**Syringoto′mia;** from *sy′rinx,* a "pipe," or "fistula," and τέμνω, to "cut."] The operation of laying open a fistula.

Sy′rinx.* [Gr. σῦριγξ.] A pipe or fistula: a syringe.

Syr′up. [**Syru′pus;** from the Arabic *Sherab,* shẹh-råb′, a "sweet or pleasant drink;" often used for "wine."] (Fr. *Sirop,* sè′ro′.) Sugar dissolved in water; distinctively termed *Syrupus simplex,* or "simple syrup." Also, any composition of the juice of herbs, flowers, or fruits, boiled with sugar to a thick consistence.

Sy-rū′pus,* plural **Sy-ru′pi.** The Pharmacopœial name for "syrup."

☞ Only a few of the more important syrups are here given. For the rest, see U. S. Pharmacopœia, pp. 299–314.

Syru′pus Fer′ri I-od′ĭ-di* ("Syrup of Iodide of Iron"), **Liq′uor Fer′ri Iod′idi,*** 1850. Take of iodine, two troyounces, iron, in the form of wire and cut in pieces, three hundred grains, distilled water, three fluidounces, syrup, a sufficient quantity. Mix the iodide, iron, and distilled water in a flask of thin glass, shake the mixture occasionally, until the reaction ceases and the solution has acquired a green color and lost the smell of iodine. Then, having introduced a pint of syrup into a graduated bottle, heat it by means of a waterbath to 212°, and, through a small funnel inserted in the mouth of the bottle, filter into it the solution already prepared. When this has passed, close the bottle, shake it thoroughly, and, when the liquid has cooled, add sufficient syrup to make the whole measure twenty fluidounces. Lastly, again shake the bottle and transfer its contents to two-ounce vials, which must be well stopped.

Syru'pus Fus'cus.* ("Brown Syrup.") Molasses. The name applied to the impure, dark-colored syrup obtained in making sugar from the *Saccharum officinarum*. It has been placed on the primary list of the Materia Medica of the U.S. Pharmacopœia for 1860.

Syru'pus Ip-e-cac-u-an'hæ.* ("Syrup of Ipecacuanha.") Take of fluid extract of ipecacuanha, two fluidounces, syrup, thirty fluidounces. Mix them.

Syru'pus Pru'ni Vir-ġin-i-a'næ.* ("Syrup of Wild Cherry [Bark].") Take of wild cherry bark, in coarse powder, five troyounces, sugar, in coarse powder, twenty-eight troyounces, water, a sufficient quantity. Moisten the bark thoroughly with water, and allow it to stand for twenty-four hours in a close vessel; then pack it firmly in a glass percolator, and gradually pour water upon it until a pint of filtered liquid is obtained. To this, transferred to a bottle, add the sugar, and agitate occasionally until it is dissolved.

Syru'pus Rhe'i Ar-o-mat'i-cus.* ("Aromatic Syrup of Rhubarb.") Take of rhubarb, in moderately fine powder, two troyounces and a half, cloves, in moderately fine powder, cinnamon, in fine powder, each half a troyounce, nutmeg, in moderately fine powder, one hundred and twenty grains, syrup, six pints, diluted alcohol, a sufficient quantity. Mix the powders, and, having moistened the mixture with two fluidounces of diluted alcohol, introduce it into a conical percolator, and pour diluted alcohol upon it until a pint of tincture has passed. Add this to the syrup previously heated, and mix them thoroughly.

Syru'pus Sçil'læ.* ("Syrup of Squill.") Take of vinegar of squill, a pint, sugar, in coarse powder, twenty-four troyounces. Dissolve the sugar in the vinegar of squill with the aid of a gentle heat, and strain the solution while hot.

Syru'pus Scil'læ Com-pos'i-tus.* ("Compound Syrup of Squill.") Take of squill, in moderately coarse powder, seneka, in moderately fine powder, each four troyounces, tartrate of antimony and potassa, forty-eight grains, sugar, in coarse powder, forty-two troyounces, diluted alcohol, water, each a sufficient quantity. Mix the squill and seneka, and, having moistened the mixture with half a pint of diluted alcohol, allow it to stand for an hour. Then transfer it to a conical percolator and pour diluted alcohol upon it, until three pints of tincture have passed. Boil this for a few minutes, evaporate it by means of a water-bath to a pint, add six fluidounces of boiling water, and filter. Dissolve the sugar in the filtered liquid, and, having heated the solution to the boiling point, strain it while hot. Then dissolve the tartrate of antimony and potassa in the solution, while still hot, and add sufficient boiling water through the strainer to make it measure three pints. Lastly, mix the whole thoroughly together.

Sȳs-pa'si-a.* [From σύν, "together," and σπάω, to "draw."] A Greek term equivalent to the Latin *Convulsio* ("convulsion"), forming the name of a genus in Dr. Good's Nosology.

Sȳs-sar-co'sis.* [From σύν, "together," and σαρκόω, to "make strong."] Union of bones by connecting muscle.

Sȳs-tat'i-ca.* [From συνίστημι, to "place together," to "associate."] The name of an order in Good's Nosology, comprising diseases which affect the different sensorial powers simultaneously, as sleeplessness, torpor, etc.

Sȳs'tem. [Lat. **Syste'ma;** Gr. σύστημα, from συνίστημι, to "place together."] Originally, a "whole composed of a number of different parts:" hence, a regular government; the constitution of a state. A methodical collection, arrangement, or classification of many things together; a connected statement of the truths of some department of science or art. In Astronomy, a hypothesis of a certain order and arrangement of the celestial bodies, by which their apparent motions are explained. The solar system consists of the sun and all the celestial bodies whose motions are controlled by his attraction, viz., the planets, satellites, and comets.

System, Sexual. See SEXUAL SYSTEM.

Sȳs-te-mat'ic. [**Systemat'icus;** from *systema*, a "system."] According or pertaining to system or regular arrangement; methodical.

Systemat'ic Bot'a-nȳ. The second great department of botanical science, or the study of plants in their relations to one another as forming a *vegetable* *kingdom.* It treats of plants as members of a system or orderly parts of a whole, and arranges them in classes, orders, genera, and species.

Sys-tem-a-tol'o-gy. [**Systematolo'gia;** from *syste'ma*, a "system," and λόγος, a "discourse."] A treatise on the various systems; the doctrine of systems or arrangements in science.

Sys-tem'ic. [**System'icus.**] Pertaining to the whole system; belonging to the general system: as, "*systemic* circulation," used in contradistinction to "*pulmonic* circulation."

Sys'to-le.* [From συστέλλω, to "draw together," or "contract."] The contraction of the heart, by which, with its alternate dilatation (diastole), the circulation of the blood is carried on.

Sys-tol'ic. [**Systol'icus.**] Pertaining to systole.

Sys-trem'ma, atis.* [Gr. σύστρεφω, to "twist or roll together."] Applied to cramp in the muscles, or the calf of the leg.

Sys-ty'lus.* [From σύν, "together," and στῦλος, a "style."] Applied to a plant the styles of which are joined into a single column: systy'lous.

Syz'y-gy. [**Syzyg'ia;** from σύν, "together," and ζυγόν, a "yoke."] In the plural (Syzygies) the places of the moon or planets when in conjunction with, or opposition to, the sun.

T.

T Bandage. A bandage formed somewhat like the letter T, for supporting dressings in diseases of the anus, groin, perinæum, etc.

Tab'a-cum.* Tobacco. The Pharmacopœial name ‖ for the dried leaves of *Nicotiana tabacum.* See TOBACCO.

Tab'a-sheer, written also **Tabaschir.** A silicious substance found in the joints of the bamboo, sometimes fluid, but generally in a concreted state. It has been used in obstruction of the bowels.

Ta'bes.* Consumption, or wasting, of the body. A genus of the order *Marcores*, class *Cachexiæ*, of Cullen's Nosology.

Ta'bes Cox-a'ri-a.* ("Hip Consumption or Wasting.") A wasting of the thigh and leg, from abscess in the hip. Essentially the same as COXARUM MORBUS, which see.

Ta'bes Dor-sa'lis.* ("Dorsal Consumption or Wasting.") A disorder of the spinal marrow, consequent on venereal excesses.

Ta'bes Mes-en-ter'i-ca.* The *Tabes scrofulosa.*

Ta'bes Pul-mo-na'lis.* ("Pulmonary Consumption or Wasting.") See PULMONARY CONSUMPTION.

Ta'bes Scrof-u-lo'sa.* ("Scrofulous Consumption.") A disease consisting in a scrofulous affection of the mesenteric glands (hence also called *Ta'bes mesenter'ica*), connected with a morbid condition of the functions of digestion and assimilation.

Ta-bes'cent. [**Tabes'cens;** from *tabes'co*, to "waste away."] Wasting or shrivelling.

Tab'u-la Vit're-a.* ("Glassy Table.") A term applied to the internal plate of the occipital bone, on account of its brittleness.

Tab'u-lar. [From *tab'ula*, a "board," or "table."] Like a board or table. In Botany, flattened horizontally.

Taccaceæ,* tak-ka'she-ē. [From *Tac'ca*, one of the genera.] A small natural order of endogenous herbaceous plants, found in the hotter parts of India and in the tropical parts of Africa.

Ta-chyg'ra-phy. [**Tachygra'phia;** from ταχύς, "short," and γράφω, to "write."] Shorthand. See STENOGRAPHY.

Tac'tile. [**Tac'tilis;** from *tac'tus*, "touch."] Pertaining to touch.

Tac'tion. [**Tac'tio;** from *tan'go*, *tac'tum*, to "touch."] The act of touching; touch.

Tac'tus.* [From the same.] The sense of TOUCH, which see.

Tac'tus Er-u-di'tus.* ("Instructed [or Skilful] Touch.") That delicate and discriminating sense of touch resulting from the union of judgment and experience.

Tac'tus Ex-per'tus.* ("Experienced Touch.") Essentially the same as the TACTUS ERUDITUS, which see.

Tæ'ni-a.* [Gr. ταινία.] Originally, a "fillet," "band," or "riband." Applied to the tapeworm, a genus of intestinal worms having long, flat, and jointed bodies.

Tæ'nia Hip-po-cam'pi.* The CORPUS FIMBRIATUM, which see.

Tæ'nia La'ta* ("Broad Tapeworm"); also called **Both-ri-o-ceph'a-**

lus.* A worm found in the human intestines. It sometimes attains an enormous length,—fifty or sixty yards, according to some writers.

Tæ'nia Os'cu-lis Mar-gĭ-nal'ĭ-bus.* ("Tapeworm with Marginal Mouths or Foramina.") The long tapeworm, or TÆNIA SOLIUM.

Tæ'nia Sem-ĭ-cir-cu-la'ris.* ("Semicircular Band.") A narrow, fibrous, semi-transparent band, situated in the groove between the optic thalamus and corpus striatum.

Tæ'nia So'lĭ-um.* The long tapeworm; also called *Tænia osculis marginalibus*. It infests the upper part of the intestines, and is not unfrequently from twenty to thirty feet long, and is said to be sometimes much longer.

Tæ'nia Ta-ri'ni.* ("Band of Tarinus.") A yellowish horny band which lies over the *vena corpora striata* of the brain, first noticed by Tarinus. It is a thickening of the lining membrane of the ventricle.

Tæ'nĭ-oid. [**Tænioi'des;** from *tæ'nia*, a "riband."] Resembling a riband.

Taffetas Vésicant, tȧf'tȧ' vȧ'zȧ'-kŏɴᵍ'. ("Blistering Cloth.") The same as PANNUS VESICATORIUS, which see.

Ta'fĭ-a.* Rum, or the spirit obtained by distillation from the fermented juice of the sugar-cane.

Taille, tȧl. Literally, "cutting." The French term for LITHOTOMY, which see.

Tălc. [**Tal'cum.**] A foliated magnesian mineral, unctuous to the touch, used for tracing lines on cloth, etc.

Ta'le-a.* [From θαλλός, a "young shoot"?] A Latin word signifying a "graft," "cutting," "shoot," or "stock."

Taliaco'tian (tā-le-a-ko'shŭn) **Op-e-rā'tion.** An operation by which, in cases of deformity or deficiency of the nose, a new one is made by turning down a flap from the forehead, or other part of the face; first practised by Taliacotius (or Tagliacozzi). See RHINOPLASTY

Tal'ĭ-pēs, p'edis.* [From *ta'lus*, the "ankle," and *pes*, the "foot."] Applied to various kinds of the distortion commonly called club-foot.

Tal'ipes E-qui'nus* ("Equine Club-foot"), or **Horse'-Foot.** Club-foot from simple retraction of the heel, so that the ankle seems to resemble that of the horse.

Tal'ipes Val'gus.* Club-foot, with distortion outwards, or eversion.

Tal'ipes Va'rus.* Club-foot, with distortion inwards.

Tăl'low. [**Se'vum.**] Animal fat, melted and separated from the fibrous matter mixed with it.

Tăl'pa.* Literally, a "mole." Hence applied to a tumor under the skin, compared to a mole under the ground. Sometimes it signifies an encysted tumor on the head.

Ta'lus.* Literally, a "die," with which a game of dice was played. Applied to the astragalus (or ankle-bone), from its resemblance to a die.

Tamaricaceæ,* tam-a-re-ka'she-ē. A small natural order of exogenous plants (shrubs or herbs), confined to the Northern hemisphere and the Old World. It includes the *Tam'arix* (Tamarisk), *Myrica'ria*, and *Trichaurus*. Several of the species are astringent or tonic; and one, the *Tam'arix mannif'era*, yields a kind of manna, consisting of mucilaginous sugar.

Tam-a-rin'dus.* [From *tamar* (Arabic), a "date," and *In'dus*, "Indian."] A Linnæan genus of the class *Monadelphia*, natural order *Leguminosæ*. Also, the Pharmacopœial name ‖ for the preserved fruit of the *Tamarindus Indica*. It is refrigerant and laxative.

Tamarin'dus In'dĭ-ca.* ("Indian Tamarind.") The systematic name of the tamarind-tree.

Tam'a-rix Gal'lĭ-ca.* The systematic name of the common Tamarisk, a tree of the Linnæan class *Pentandria*, and natural order *Tamaricaceæ*. The bark, wood, and leaves are bitter and astringent, and have been employed in medicine.

Tam'pŏn. (French pronunciation, tŏɴ'pŏɴᵍ'.) Literally, a "plug," or "stopper." A portion of rag, sponge, etc., used in PLUGGING, which see.

Ta'mus Com-mu'nis.* The systematic name of common Black Bryony. The root is diuretic.

Tan-a-ce'tum.* Tansy. A Linnæan genus of the class *Syngenesia*, natural order *Compositæ*. Also, the Pharmacopœial name (U.S. Ph.) for the herb of the *Tanace'tum vulga're*. It is chiefly used as an anthelmintic.

Tanace'tum Vul-ga're.* The common tansy-plant; also called *Tanasia*.

Ta-na'sĭ-a.* A name for *Tanace'tum vulga're*.

Tan'ġent. [**Tan'ġens;** present participle of *tan'go*, to "touch."] Literally, "touching," or "that which touches." The tangent to a curve is a straight line which meets or touches the curve without intersecting it. In Trigonometry, a tangent is a straight line which touches a circular arc at one of its extremities, and is terminated by the production of the radius passing through the other extremity.

Tan'nāte. **[Tan'nas, a'***tis.*] A combination of tannic acid (or tannin) with a base.

Tan'nic Aç'id. The same as TANNIN, which see.

Tan'nin. **[Tanni'num;** so called from its use in tanning.] (Fr. *Acide tannique*, å'sėd' tån'nėk'.) Tannic acid (the *Aç'idum tan'nicum* of the Pharmacopœias.) The peculiar astringent principle of vegetable substances on which their power of converting skins into leather depends. It is a powerful astringent.

Tansy. See TANACETUM VULGARE.

Tan'tạ-lum.* The same as COLUMBIUM, which see.

Tapeworm. See TÆNIA.

Tapeworm, Long. See TÆNIA SOLIUM.

Tap-ĭ-o'cạ.* The Pharmacopœial name (U.S. Ph.) for the fecula of the root of the *Janipha Manihot.* As an article of food it is mild and easy of digestion, and forms an excellent diet for the sick or convalescent.

Tapping. See PARACENTESIS.

Tap'-Root. A fleshy main root tapering downwards, having a moderate thickness compared with the length, and extending in a nearly vertical direction, as in the pine, maple, parsnip, etc.

Tar. A dark-brown, viscid liquid, obtained by heating the wood of the pine or fir tree. It consists of resin, empyreumatic oil, and acetic acid.

Tar, Barbadoes. See PETROLEUM BARBADENSE.

Tăr-an-tis'mus.* [From *taran'tula,* a peculiar kind of venomous spider.] Tarantism. The morbid desire of excessive motion, or dancing, said to be excited by music in those affected by the bite of the tarantula.

Tạ-ran'tu-lạ.* A species of poisonous spider, whose bite was supposed to be cured by music.

Tạ-rax'ạ-cum.* Dandelion. The Pharmacopœial name ‖ for the root of the *Tarax'acum Dens-leo'nis.* It is slightly tonic, diuretic, and aperient, and appears to have a specific action on the liver. It has sometimes proved extremely beneficial in affections accompanied by torpidity of that organ.

Tarax'acum Cof'fee. Dandelion Coffee; a powder consisting of taraxacum-roots, cleaned, dried, and powdered, and mixed with coffee.

Tarax'acum Dens-le-o'nis.* ("Tooth of Lion.") The systematic name of the dandelion. See TARAXACUM.

Tạ-rax'is.* [From ταράσσω, to "trouble," or "confound."] A slight inflammation of the eye.

Tar-dĭ-flo'rus.* [From *tar'dus,* "slow," or "late," and *flos,* a "flower."] Flowering late.

Tardigrada. See TARDIGRADUS.

Tar-dig'rạ-dus.* [From *tar'dus,* "slow," and *gra'dus,* a "step."] Tardigrade. Moving slowly. Applied in the plural neuter (*Tardig'rada*) to certain animals, which from their peculiar construction move with excessive slowness, as the sloths.

Target-Shaped. See PELTATE, SCUTIFORM, and THYROID.

Tarini Pons. See PONS TARINI.

Tar'sạl. **[Tarsa'lis;** from *tar'sus.*] Belonging to the *tarsus;* also, to the cartilage of the eyelid.

Tar'sal Car'tĭ-la-ġes. The thin elastic plates which give shape to the eyelids.

Tar'si,* gen. **Tar-so'rum,** the plural of TARSUS, which see.

Tar-so-phy'mạ, a*tis.** [From *tar'sus,* and φῦμα, a "growth."] A morbid growth or tumor of the tarsus.

Tar-sor'rhạ-phȳ. **[Tarsorrha'phia;** from *tar'sus,* and ῥαφή, a "suture."] The uniting by suture any wound of the eyelids near the tarsus.

Tar-sot'o-mȳ. **[Tarsoto'mia;** from *tar'sus,* and τέμνω, to "cut."] A cutting of the tarsus, or cartilage of the eyelid.

Tar'sus,* plural **Tar'si.** [From ταρσός, the "instep."] That portion of the foot between the metatarsal bones and the leg, itself comprising seven bones; the instep. Also, the thin cartilage towards the edge of each eyelid, giving it firmness and shape. Applied also to a number of minute joints in insects, forming the fifth principal segment of the leg or foot.

Tar'tạr. **[Tar'tarum,** or **Tar'tarus.]** The substance which concretes on the inside of wine-casks; the impure supertartrate of potash. Also, an earthy-like substance deposited from the saliva, which becomes incrusted on the human teeth. See ODONTOLITHUS, and TOPHUS.

Tar'tar, Cream of. The bitartrate of potash. See POTASSÆ BITARTRAS.

Tar'tar E-met'ic. The tartrate of antimony and potassa (*Antimo'nii et potas'sæ tar'tras*) of the U.S. Pharmacopœia, or *Antimo'nium tartara'tum* (Br. Ph.), also termed *Antimo'nii potas'sio-tar'tras*, and *Antimo'nium tartariza'tum*. Tartar emetic is the most valuable of all the preparations of antimony. It is a powerful arterial sedative: in small doses it acts as a diaphoretic, in large quantities as an emetic, and sometimes as a cathartic.

Tar'ta-rāt-ed An'ti-mo-ny̆. [**Antimo'nium Tartara'tum.**] See TARTAR EMETIC.

Tar-tăr'ic. [**Tartar'icus.**] Applied to an acid obtained from tartar. It is refrigerant and antiseptic.

Tar'ta-rīzed An'timony. [**Antimo'nium Tartariza'tum.**] See TARTAR EMETIC.

Tar'trāte. [**Tar'tras, a'tis.**] A combination of tartaric acid with a base.

Tartrate of Antimony and Potassa. See TARTAR EMETIC.

Tartre des Dents, tartR dā dŏNᵍ. ("Tartar of the Teeth.") The French term for ODONTOLITHUS, which see.

Taste. [Lat. **Gus'tus;** Fr. *Gout*, goo.] That sense by which we perceive the savors of certain bodies upon the tongue, which is its principal organ. The lips, the inside of the cheeks, the palate, teeth, *velum pendulum palati*, pharynx, œsophagus, and even the stomach, are also susceptible of impressions by contact with the same bodies, which are termed sapid bodies.

Taste, Morbid. See PARAGEUSIS.

Taste'less A'gue-Drop. An arsenical solution, formerly in great repute, for which Fowler's solution, or the *Liquor arsenicalis*, is now substituted.

Taste'less Salt. A name for phosphate of soda.

Tau'rin. [**Tauri'na;** from ταῦρος, a "bull."] A particular animal substance in bile, first discovered in ox-gall.

Tau-ro-chol'ic. [**Taurochol'icus;** from *tau'rus*, a "bull," or "ox," and χολή, "bile."] A term applied to a peculiar acid found in the bile of the ox, associated with *glycholic* acid. The latter, or a substance nearly allied to it, is found in the human bile, in which, however, taurocholic acid appears to be wanting.

Taxaceæ,* tax-a'she-ē. A natural order of exogenous trees and shrubs, found in the milder climates of a great part of the world. It includes the *Tax'us* (Yew), and other trees which are valuable for timber.

Tax-ĭ-der'mic. [**Taxider'micus.**] Belonging to taxidermy.

Tax-ĭ-der'my̆. [**Taxider'mia;** from τάξις, "arrangement," and δέρμα, a "skin."] The art of stuffing and preserving the skins of animals so as to represent their natural appearance, habits, and attitudes in life.

Tax'is.* [From τάσσω, to "put in order."] The operation of replacing by the hand, without instruments, any parts which have quitted their natural situation, as in the reduction of hernia, etc.

Tax-ol'o-ġy̆, or **Tax-on'o-my̆.** [From τάξις, "arrangement," and λόγος, a "discourse."] The department of Botany which relates to classification.

Tax-on'o-my̆. [**Taxono'mia;** from τάξις, "arrangement," and νόμος, a "law."] The theory of classifications; the laws which preside at their construction. See TAXOLOGY.

Tax'us.* (Fr. *If*, ēf.) The Yew-tree. A tree belonging to the order or tribe *Coniferæ*. The leaves have been employed as a remedy in epilepsy.

Tea. [Lat. **The'a;** Fr. *Thé*, tā.] The dried leaves of a Chinese evergreen shrub, of which there are two varieties, the *Thea Ni'gra*, black or bohea tea, and *Thea Vir'idis*, green tea. It belongs to the Linnæan class *Polyandria*, and natural order *Ternströmiaceæ*. In the form of an infusion it is used more extensively than any other artificial beverage. It is slightly astringent, and produces a decidedly exhilarating effect on the nervous system. When taken by those who are unaccustomed to it, it causes wakefulness.

Tēar. [Lat. **Lach'ryma,** or **Lac'ryma;** Gr. δάκρυμα, or δάκρυον; Fr. *Larme*, larm.] A limpid fluid secreted by the lachrymal gland, and, in the ordinary condition of the part, diffused between the eyeball and eyelids, to facilitate their movements. A permanent and morbid excess of this secretion is termed EPIPHORA (which see). The tears are saline, with a slight alkaline reaction, turning delicate vegetable blues to green. The term tear is also applied to drops (or small pieces) of gum of a globular or semi-globular shape, having dried in the form they present on issuing from the plant.

Tech-no-cau'sis.* [From τέχνη, "art," and καῦσις, a "burning."] Artificial burning, or application of the *moxa*, hot iron, etc.

Tech-nol'o-ġȳ. [**Technolo'gia**; from τέχνη, "art," and λόγος, a "discourse."] A treatise on art or the arts, especially the useful arts: a description of the arts.

Tec-noc-to'nĭ-a.* [From τέκνον, a "child," and κτείνω, to "kill."] Child-murder, or infanticide.

Tec-tĭ-bran'chĭ-ate. [**Tectibranchia'tus**; from *tec'tus*, "covered," and *bran'chiæ*.] Having *branchiæ* more or less covered by the mantle. Applied to an order of Mollusks.

Tec-tri'cēs,* the plural of TECTRIX.

Tec'trix, *icis*.* [From *te'go*, *tec'tum*, to "cover."] Covering or hiding. Applied in the plural (*tectri'ces*) to the feathers which cover the quill-feathers and other parts of the wings of birds.

Teeth. See TOOTH.

Teeth, Grinding of. See STRIDOR DENTIUM.

Teeth, Per'ma-nent. [**Den'tes Permanen'tes.**] A term applied to the teeth of the adult, thirty-two in all. See TOOTH.

Teeth'ing. Cutting of the teeth, or dentition.

Teg'men, *inis*,* or **Teg-men'tum.*** [From *te'go*, to "cover."] A covering, whether scale or membrane, of fruits, flowers, etc.: thus, the scales covering the leaf-buds of deciduous trees of cold climates are called *tegmenta*. Applied to the inner coat of the seeds of plants. Also applied to the superior wings of insects when coriaceous or pergamentaceous, and furnished with nervures, as in the *Orthoptera*.

Teg-men'ta,* the plural of TEGMENTUM, which see.

Teg'mĭ-nate. [**Tegmina'tus.**] Enveloped in a tegmen.

Teg'u-ment. [**Tegumen'tum**; from *te'go*, to "cover."] Applied to a membrane which covers the *sori* of ferns (the *indusium*, or *involucrum*, of some authors). Also, nearly the same as INTEGUMENT.

Tégument, tā'gü'mōnᵍ'. The French term for INTEGUMENT, which see.

Teigne, tĕñ or tāñ. The French term for PORRIGO, which see.

Te'la.* A Latin word signifying a "web." Applied to a membrane or tissue.

Te'la Ad-ĭ-po'sa.* A name for ADIPOSE MEMBRANE, which see.

Te'la Cel-lu-lo'sa.* A name for CELLULAR TISSUE, which see.

Te'la Chor-o-i'de-a.* ("Choroid Web.") A membranous prolongation of the *pia mater* in the third ventricle.

Te-lan-ġĭ-ec-ta'sĭ-a,* or **Te-lan-ġĭ-ec'ta-sis.*** [From τέλος, the "end," ἀγγεῖον, a "vessel," and ἔκτασις, "extension."] Literally, an extension of the terminations of the vessels (*i.e.* of the capillaries). A term for the dilatation of the capillary vessels.

Te-lan-ġĭ-o'sis.* [From τέλος, the "end," and ἀγγεῖον, a "vessel."] Disease of the capillary vessels.

Tel-e-ol'o-ġȳ. [**Teleolo'gia**; from τέλος, "end," or "purpose," and λόγος, a "discourse."] The doctrine of final causes; *i.e.* the doctrine that the different parts of the universe have been created for a special end or purpose.

Tel'e-scope. [**Telesco'pium**; from τῆλε, "far off," and σκοπέω, to "observe," or to "see."] An optical instrument for viewing distant objects; a tube having a convex object-glass at one end, and a convex (or concave) lens at the other, placed at the distance of the sum (or difference) of their focal lengths. Telescopes are of two kinds, *refracting* and *reflecting*: the former depending on the use of properly figured lenses through which the rays of light pass; and the latter on the use of specula or polished metallic mirrors which reflect the rays.

Tellurate. See TELLURIC.

Tel'lu-rāt-ed. [**Tellura'tus.**] Applied to a gas which holds tellurium in solution.

Tel-lu'ric. [**Tellu'ricus**; from *tellu'rium*.] Belonging to tellurium. Applied to the peroxide of tellurium, which is called telluric acid, and combines with many of the metallic oxides, producing a class of compounds called Tellurates.

Tel-lu'rĭ-um.* [From *Tel'lus*, the "earth." It may be observed that many of the metals are named from the different planets. Besides the well-known examples of Mercury and Saturn (Latin *Saturnus*, a name for "lead"), we have Cerium from *Ceres*, Palladium from *Pallas*, Selenium from σελήνη, the "moon," etc.] A rare metal found in the gold-mines of Transylvania. It is white, brilliant, brittle, and easily fusible. Its specific gravity is about 6.25.

Temp. dext. = *Tem'pori dex'tro.** "To the right temple."

Tempe. See TEMPLE.

Tem'per-a-ment. [**Temperamen'tum**; from *tem'pero*, *tempera'tum*, to "mix," to "temper;" because it was supposed to depend on the mixture or apportioning of the different humors of the body.] The peculiar constitution of the body; that peculiarity of physical organization which to a certain extent influences the disposition and character of men.

Many of the old physiologists attached great importance to temperament. The different kinds have been variously distinguished by different writers: the best classification is perhaps the following:—

1. The Sanguineous (or Sanguine) Temperament, characterized by a fair and ruddy complexion, yellow, red, or light auburn hair, a full, muscular development, large, full veins, and an active pulse, all indicating an abundant supply of blood. Persons of this description, are usually, it is said, of a hopeful disposition, fond of pleasure, with strong and eager passions, but deficient in constancy of purpose, especially when the object of their pursuit can only be won by perseverance and long delay.

2. The Bilious Temperament, characterized by a preponderance of bile, indicated by a dark or sallow complexion, black hair, and a slow or moderate circulation of the blood. Persons of this temperament, it is said, are apt to be grave and thoughtful, remarkable for firmness and tenacity of purpose, capable of long endurance, constant in their attachments, implacable in their hate, etc. It has been remarked, by a modern writer, that nearly all the great tyrants mentioned in history, appear to have possessed a large share of the bilious temperament.

The term *choleric*, though often used (in accordance with its etymology) as synonymous with bilious, implies, in its popular acceptation, a certain combination of the bilious and sanguineous temperaments.

3. The Lymphatic (or Phlegmatic) Temperament, resulting, according to the old physiologists, from the predominance of lymph, or phlegm (which was regarded as the cold and watery humor of the body), in the system. It is characterized by a fair but not ruddy complexion, light hair, and a general softness or laxity of the tissues. Persons of this temperament, it is said, are apt to be of a mild and amiable disposition, but to possess little activity or force of character.

The ancients reckoned also among the temperaments the Atrabilious or Melancholic, characterized by a predominance of *black bile* (which was supposed to be secreted by the spleen), rendering the disposition melancholy and morose; and when in great excess, producing hypochondriasis. This, however, is so obviously a diseased condition of the system that it scarcely merits a place among the other temperaments, which are, properly, not forms of disease, but merely constitutional peculiarities.

To the foregoing has been added, more recently,—

4. The Nervous Temperament, characterized by the predominance of the nervous element, and by great activity or susceptibility of the great nervous centre, the brain. Persons possessing this temperament are usually distinguished by their impressibility, their capability of intense feeling or intense excitement (which is often, however, not manifested externally), and by the general activity of all those functions directly dependent upon the brain and nervous system. Literary men, especially those distinguished in poetry or imaginative literature, are usually of this temperament.

It must, however, be borne in mind, that in no instance is any one temperament to be found absolutely unmixed, but even in the most strongly-marked cases it will be qualified by elements belonging to the other temperaments,—not to speak of the modifications caused by moral or educational influences. Yet, if we take the most remarkable examples of each class,—that is, those in which the peculiar characteristics of some one temperament are most fully developed with the smallest admixture of other elements,—we shall probably find that, though much of a merely fanciful character has been written on this subject, the views of the old physiologists are not without considerable foundation in truth.

Tem'pe-rance. [**Sobri'etas,** or **Temperan'tia;** from the same.] Moderation in eating and drinking, an indispensable condition to the enjoyment of perfect health.

Temperantia,* tem-pe-ran'she-ạ. [From the same.] Agents which reduce the temperature of the body when unduly augmented, as cold, acids, certain salts, etc.

Tem'per-ate. [**Tempera'tus;** from the same.] Moderate; without excess; tempered.

Tem'per-ạ-ture. [**Temperatu'ra;**

from the same.] A definite or certain degree of sensible heat, as measured by the thermometer.

Tem'ple. [Lat. **Tem'pus,** *oris*, plural **Tem'pora;** Gr. κρόταφος; Fr. *Tempe*, tŏмp.] The lateral region of the head above a line drawn from the eye and to the ear. In Entomology, the part from each side of the posterior half of the eyes between the forehead and the vertex.

Tem'po-ra,* the plural of *tem'pus*, the temple of the head.

Tem'po-ral. [**Tempora'lis.**] Belonging to the *tempora*, or temples.

Tem-po-ra'lis.* ("Temporal [Muscle].") A muscle arising from the temporal fossa and the semicircular line bounding it, and inserted into the upper part of the coronoid process of the lower jaw. It draws the jaw upwards.

Temporary Teeth. See TOOTH.

Tem'u-lence. [**Temulen'tia;** from *teme'tum*, "strong wine."] Drunkenness; intoxication.

Te-naç'ĭ-tȳ. [**Tenaç'itas, a'***tis*; from *te'nax, tena'cis*, "tenacious."] The power of resistance which bodies oppose to efforts to break them either by shock, pressure, or traction.

Te-nac'u-lum.* [From *te'neo*, to "hold fast."] A small, hook-shaped instrument for taking up divided vessels.

Ten'dĭ-nēs,* gen. **Ten'dĭ-num,** the plural of TENDO, which see.

Ten'dĭ-nous. [**Tendino'sus;** from *ten'do, ten'dinis*, a "tendon."] Pertaining to tendons, or like tendons.

Tendo Achillis. See ACHILLIS, TENDO.

Ten'don. [**Ten'do,** *inis* or **o***nis*, plural **Ten'dines,** or **Ten'dones;** from *ten'do*, to "stretch."] A white, fibrous cord, more or less round, by which a muscle is attached to a bone; vulgarly, a "guider."

Ten'dril. [**Cir'rus.**] A tendril is commonly a thread-like, leafless branch, capable of coiling spirally, by which some climbing plants attach themselves to surrounding bodies for support. Sometimes tendrils belong to the leaves, as in the pea.

Te-nes'mus.* [From τείνω, to "stretch," or "strain."] A constant desire to go to stool, with great straining, but no discharge.

Ten-on-tog'ra-phȳ. [**Tenontogra'phia;** from τένων, τένοντος, a "tendon," and γράφω, to "write."] A description or delineation of the tendons.

Ten-on-tol'o-ġȳ. [**Tenontolo'gia;** from τένων, a "tendon," and λόγος, a "discourse."] The doctrine or science of the tendons.

Te-not'o-mȳ. [**Tenoto'mia;** from τένων, a "tendon," and τέμνω, to "cut."] The cutting of a tendon with a view to remedy certain distortions caused by muscular contractions. See LOXARTHRON.

Ten'sion. [**Ten'sio, o'***nis*; from *ten'do, ten'sum*, to "stretch."] The act of stretching or straining; the state of being stretched or drawn tight.

Ten'sĭve. [**Tensi'vus;** from the same.] Tending to stretch or make tense. Attended with a feeling of tension.

Ten'sor, o'*ris*.* [From the same.] A stretcher, or extender, or that which stretches or makes tense. Applied to certain muscles.

Ten'sor Tȳm'pa-ni.* ("Stretcher of the Tympanum.") A muscle of the tympanum which by its contraction acts upon the *membrana tympani* and modifies the sense of hearing.

Ten'sor Va-ġi'næ Fem'o-ris.* ("That which makes tense the Sheath of the Thigh.") The name of a muscle which arises from the spine of the ilium and is inserted into the *fascia lata*, whence it is also called *Fascia'lis* and *Fascia lata*. It stretches the *fascia*, etc.

Tent. [**Ten'ta, Linamen'tum, Penicil'lum;** from *ten'do, ten'sum* or *ten'tum*, to "stretch," or "spread."] A roll of lint, or piece of prepared sponge, for keeping open or dilating sores, sinuses, etc.

Tent, Sponge. See SPONGE-TENT.

Tentacle. See TENTACULUM.

Ten-tac'u-la,* the plural of TENTACULUM, which see.

Ten-tac'u-late. [**Tentacula'tus;** from *tentac'ulum*.] Having tentacula or appendages resembling tentacula.

Ten-tac'u-lum,* plural **Ten-tac'u-la.** [From *ten'to*, to "feel often."] A tentacle, or feeler. This term is used in a restricted sense to signify the long, filiform, inarticulate appendage of the mouth of *Anellata* or *Annelides*. It is also applied to all appendages, whether jointed or not, which are used as instruments of exploration and prehension.

Ten-to'rĭ-um.* [From *ten'do, ten'tum*, to "stretch."] Originally, a tent or pavilion. Applied to the horizontal process of the *dura mater* between the cerebrum and cerebellum.

Ten-u-ĭ-cos-ta'tus.* [From *ten'uis*, "slender," and *cos'ta*, a "rib."] Having slender ribs. Applied to the leaves of plants.

Ten-u-ĭ-flo'rus.* [From *ten'uis*, "slender," "thin," and *flos*, a "flower."] Having slender flowers: tenuiflo'rous.

Ten-u-ĭ-sil-ĭ-qua'tus.* [From *ten'uis*, "slender," "thin," and *sil'iqua*, a "pod."] Having slender pods.

Te'pal. [Analogous to SEPAL.] A name proposed for a leaf or part of a perianth when it is uncertain whether it belongs to the calyx or corolla.

Tep-ĭ-da'rĭ-um.* [From *tep'idus*, "lukewarm."] A warm or tepid bath.

Ter-. "Thrice." A prefix to names of salts, denoting that three atoms of acid are combined with one of base.

Tĕr-a-tol'o-gy̆. [**Teratolo'gia;** from τέρας, τέρατος, a "monster," and λόγος, a "discourse."] That branch of Physiology which treats of monsters, or the various malformations of the organic kingdoms of nature.

Ter-chlo'ride of For'my̆le. A name for CHLOROFORM, which see.

Ter'çine. [**Terci'na;** from *ter*, "thrice."] The third coat of the ovule of a plant,—*i.e.* the inner coat when the ovule has three.

Tĕr-e-bel'la.* [Diminutive of *ter'ebra*, a "gimlet."] A kind of instrument with which the posterior part of a great number of insects is provided, serving to pierce the epidermis of vegetables, or the skin of animals, in order to deposit their eggs. Also, an old name for the trepan.

Terebintaceæ,* tĕr-e-bin-ta'she-ē, or **Ter-e-bin-tha'ce-æ.*** [From *Terebin'thus*, one of the genera.] The Jussieuan name of a natural order of plants. It has been divided by Brown, and its genera have been chiefly distributed between the orders *Anacardiaceæ* and *Amyridaceæ*.

Tĕr-e-bin'thĭ-na.* ("Turpentine.") The Pharmacopœial name (U.S. Ph.) for the concrete juice of the *Pinus palustris*, and of other species of *Pinus*. It is stimulant, diuretic, anthelmintic, and, in large doses, laxative.

Terebin'thina A-mer-ĭ-ca'na.* The name for an oleo-resin from the *Pinus palustris* and *Pinus tæda*.

Terebin'thina Can-a-den'sis* ("Canada Turpentine"), or **Bal'sam of Fir.** The Pharmacopœial name ‖ for the juice of the *Abies balsamea*. It is sometimes called *Bal'samum Canaden'se*, or "Canada Balsam."

Terebin'thina Chi'a.* The Pharmacopœial name (Lond. and Ed. Ph.) for the Chian (or Cyprian) turpentine.

Terebin'thina Ven'e-ta.* The Pharmacopœial name (Ed. Ph.) for Venice turpentine, obtained from *Pinus larix*, or the larch-tree.

Terebin'thina Vul-ga'ris.* Common turpentine obtained from *Pinus sylvestris*.

Terebinthinæ Oleum. See OLEUM TEREBINTHINÆ.

Tĕr-e-bin'thĭ-nate. [**Terebinthina'tus.**] Of the nature of turpentine; containing turpentine.

Tĕr'e-bra,* and **Tĕr-e-bel'la.*** [From *ter'ebro*, to "bore."] Literally, a "borer." In Surgery, a trepan.

Terebrantia,* tĕr-e-bran'she-a. [Neuter plural of *ter'ebrans*, present participle of *ter'ebro*, to "bore."] Literally, "boring [animals]." A term applied to a section of hymenopterous insects possessing an instrument (termed *ter'ebra*, or "borer") for perforating bodies in order to deposit their eggs. Some of the *Terebrantia*, for example, the ichneumon-fly, deposit their ova in the subcutaneous fatty matter found in the larvæ and pupæ of other insects, so that their young when hatched are abundantly provided with the needful nourishment.

Te'rēs,* gen. **Tĕr'e-tis.** A Latin adjective, signifying "long and round," "terete." Applied to two muscles, the *major* and *minor*, which arise from the scapula and are inserted into the humerus. They move the arm in various directions.

Te-rete'. [From *te'res*, "long and round."] Long and round,—that is, having the cross-section circular.

Tĕr-e-tĭ-cau'lis.* [From *te'res*, "round," "terete," and *cau'lis*, a "stem."] Having a fine rounded stem.

Ter-ġem'ĭ-nate. [**Tergem'inus;** from *ter*, "thrice," and *gem'inus*, "double."] "Three times double," or thrice twin; as when a forked leaf-stalk has two leaflets at the end of each portion, and two at the division of the fork.

Ter-ġĭ-sper'mus.* [From *ter'gum*, the "back," and σπέρμα, "seed."] Bearing reproductive corpuscles on the back of the leaves; tergispermous.

Ter'mĭ-nal. [From *ter'minus*, an "end."] Relating to the end. Often applied substantively to the terminating syllable or syllables of a compound term, as *-ate* in Sulphate, *-ides* in *Conoides*. In Botany, belonging or relating to the summit.

Ter-mĭ-na'lĭ-a.* A genus of East Indian plants of the natural order *Com-*

bretaceæ. It bears a fruit called MYROBALAN, which see.

Ter-mĭ-nol'o-ġȳ. [**Terminolo'gia;** from *ter'minus*, a "term," and λόγος, a "discourse."] A treatise on the doctrine or science of technical terms belonging to the different arts and sciences; or that preliminary knowledge which teaches us to define the technical or peculiar terms employed. Often the same as Glossology.

Ter'na-rȳ. [**Terna'rius;** from *ter'nus*, "three," or "three by three."] Belonging to the number three, or consisting of three. Arranged in threes. Applied by Dalton to any chemical compound formed by the union of three atoms. See ATOMIC THEORY.

Ter'nate. [**Terna'tus;** from the same.] Arranged three by three, or united in threes; trifoliate. Applied to compound leaves, such as that of the clover.

Ter-nĭ-flo'rous. [**Terniflo'rus;** from *ter'nus*, "by threes," and *flos*, a "flower."] Having flowers disposed three by three.

Ter-nĭ-fo'lĭ-ous. [**Ternifo'lius;** from *ter'nus*, "three by three," and *fo'lium*, a "leaf."] Having verticillated leaves, three by three.

Ter-nĭ-spi'nus.* [From *ter'nus*, "three by three," and *spi'na*, a "thorn."] Bearing spines which are arranged three by three.

Ternströmiaceæ,* tern-ström-e-a'she-ē. [From *Ternströ'mia*, one of the genera.] A natural order of exogenous trees and shrubs, natives of China, Japan, India, and America. It includes the beautiful *Camel'lia Japon'ica* and the *The'a* (tea-plant), the decoction of which is a favorite beverage of the civilized world.

Tĕr'ra.* A Latin word signifying the "land;" hence, applied to the planet Earth, also to the substances termed earths. See EARTH.

Ter'ra Ja-pon'ĭ-ca.* ("Japan Earth.") See CATECHU.

Ter'ra Lem'nĭ-a.* ("Lemnian Earth.") An argillaceous substance, prepared, it is said, from the fruit of the Bao-bab tree, which has been employed as an astringent.

Ter'ra O-rel-la'na,* or **Ter'ra Or-le-a'na.*** Names for ANNOTTO, which see.

Ter'ra Pon-de-ro'sa.* ("Heavy Earth.") See BARYTA.

Ter'ræ O'le-um.* ("Oil of Earth.") A name for *petroleum.*

Tĕr-rā'que-ous. [From *ter'ra*, the "earth," and *a'qua*, "water."] Consisting of land and water.

Tĕr-rene'. [**Terre'nus;** from *ter'ra*, the "earth."] Belonging to the earth; terrestrial.

Tĕr're-ous. [**Ter'reus;** from the same.] Of the nature of earth; earthy.

Ter-ro'sus.* [From *ter'ra*, "earth."] Earthy, or full of earth.

Tertian, ter'shan. [**Tertia'nus;** from *ter'tius*, "third."] (Fr. *Tierce*, teërss'.) Applied to one of the most common forms of intermittent fever, in which the intermission lasts about forty-eight hours, and thus the paroxysm returns every third day; a genus of the order *Febris*, class *Pyrexiæ*, of Cullen's Nosology.

Tertiary, ter'she-a-re. [**Tertia'rius;** from the same.] Tertiary strata, a series of sedimentary rocks, which lie above the primary and secondary strata, and are distinguished from them by their organic remains.

Tes'sel-lāt-ed. [**Tessella'tus;** from *tessel'la*, a "small square stone."] Having square figures; chequered.

Tes'su-lar. [From *tes'sula*, diminutive of *tes'sera*, a "square," or "square tile."] Applied to a system of crystals derived from the hexahedron.

Test. [From the old French *taster* (*tâter*), to "feel," to "taste," to "try."] As a verb, it signifies to "try," or "prove." Applied in Chemistry, as a noun, to any thing by which we distinguish the chemical nature of substances from each other: thus, infusion of galls is a *test* of the presence of iron, which it renders evident by the production of a black color in water and other liquids containing that metal.

Test-Pā'per, or **Lit'mus Pa'per.** Paper dipped several times in a filtered infusion of litmus, and dried after each immersion until it is of a deep-purple color. It is used as a test of the presence of free acids or alkalies.

Tes'ta.* Originally, an "earthen pot;" also, a "shell." The outer seed-coat or integument of a seed. Also, the shell of a molluscous animal. See SHELL.

Tes'ta.* Oyster-shell. The Pharmacopœial name (U.S. Ph.) for the shell of the *Os'trea edu'lis.*

Tes'ta O'vi.* "Shell of Egg," or egg-shell.

Testacea,* tes-ta'she-a, or **Tes-ta'ceans.** [From *tes'ta*, a "shell."] An order of molluscous animals comprising those which have a calcareous shell. See SHELL.

Testaceans. See TESTACEA.

Testaceiform, tĕs-tā′she-ĭ-form. [**Testaceifor′mis;** from *tes′ta,* a "shell."] Having the form of a kind of shell.

Testaceography, tĕs-tā-she-og′ra-fe. [**Testaceogra′phia;** from *testa′ceus,* and γράφω, to "write."] A description of the *Testacea.*

Testaceology, tĕs-tā-she-ol′o-je. [**Testaceolo′gia;** from *testa′ceus,* and λόγος, a "discourse."] A treatise on the *Testacea;* the science of testaceous mollusks; Conchology.

Tes-tā′ceous. [**Testa′ceus;** from *tes′ta,* a "shell," or "earthen pot."] Belonging to, or having, a shell; of the nature of a shell. In Botany, brownish yellow, like unglazed earthen-ware.

Tĕs′tēs,* gen. **Tes′tĭ-um,** the plural of TESTIS, which see.

Tes′tes Cĕr′e-bri.* The two inferior and posterior of the *tubercula quadrigemina.*

Testicle. See TESTIS.

Testicle, Inflamed, or **Testicle, Swelled.** See ORCHITIS.

Tes-tic′u-late. [**Testicula′tus;** from *testic′ulus,* a "testicle."] Having the appearance of small testicles.

Testicular Cord. See SPERMATIC CORD.

Tes-tic′u-lus.* [Diminutive of *tes′tis.*] A testicle. See TESTIS.

Tĕs′tis,* plural **Tĕs′tēs.** [Literally, a "witness;" because they furnish evidence of one's virility.] A testicle, or gland which secretes the semen; one of two small ovoid bodies contained in the scrotum, and more immediately covered by a strong white and dense coat called *Tu′nica albugin′ea.*

Tes′tis Fœ-min′e-us,* or **Tes′tis Mu-lĭ-e′bris.*** ("Female Testicle.") A name sometimes applied to the ovary.

Tes-ti′tis, *idis.** [From *tes′tis,* a "testicle."] The same as ORCHITIS, which see.

Tes-tu′do, *inis,** plural **Tes-tu′dĭ-nēs.** [From *tes′ta,* a "shell."] A tortoise; a genus of the order *Chelonia.* Applied to a melicerous tumor of the scalp, supposed to resemble a tortoise.

Te-tan′ic. [**Tetan′icus.**] Belonging to tetanus. Also applied to a patient affected with tetanus when in the *excited* condition.

Te-tan′ĭ-ca.* [From *tet′anus.*] Agents which augment the irritability of the muscles inducing tetanus or spasm, as strychnia, etc.

Tet′a-node. [**Tetano′des;** from *tet′anus,* and εἶδος, a "form," or "resemblance."] Literally, "affected with something resembling tetanus." Applied to a patient affected with tetanus when in the unexcited state, as distinguished from his being excited or *tetanic.*—(M. HALL.)

Tet′a-noid. [**Tetanoi′des;** from the same.] Resembling tetanus.

Tet′a-nus.* [From τείνω, to "stretch."] (Fr. *Tétanos,* tā′tā′nos′.) A disease in which there is a spasmodic contraction of the muscles of voluntary motion, with tension and rigidity of the parts affected; spasm with rigidity. A genus of the order *Spasmi,* class *Neuroses,* of Cullen's Nosology.

Tet′anus Com-ple′tus.* ("Complete Tetanus.") A variety of tetanus, consisting in the spasmodic and rigid contraction of the greater number of the voluntary muscles, which thus antagonize and counteract one another.

Tetanus Emprosthotonos. See EMPROSTHOTONOS.

Tetanus Opisthotonos. See OPISTHOTONOS.

Tetanus Pleurothotonos. See PLEUROTHOTONOS.

Tet′anus Tris′mus.* A variety of tetanus, consisting in spastic rigidity of the muscles of the lower jaw; locked-jaw.

Tet′ra-. [Gr. τέτρα, for τέσσερα, "four."] A prefix denoting the number four.

Tet-ra-car′pel-la-rȳ. [From τέτρα, "four," and *car′pel.*] Consisting of four carpels.

Tet-ra-chot′o-mous. [**Tetrachot′omus;** from τέτραχα, "in four parts," and τέμνω, to "cut."] Cut or divided into four parts.

Tet-ra-dȳ-na′mĭ-a.* [From τέτρα, "four," and δύναμις, "power."] The fifteenth Linnæan class of plants, comprising those which have four long and two short stamens.

Tet-ra-dȳn′a-mous. [**Tetradyna′mius;** from the same.] Having six stamens, of which four are long and two short.

Tetraedron. See TETRAHEDRON.

Tet-ra-fo′lĭ-ate. [**Tetrafolia′tus;** from τέτρα, "four," and *fo′lium,* a "leaf."] Having bijugate leaves. Applied to a pinnate leaf with two pairs of leaflets.

Tet′ra-gon. [**Tetrago′num;** from τέτρα, "four," and γωνία, an "angle."] A figure of four angles and sides; a quadrangle.

Tet-rag'o-nal. [**Tetrago'nus.**] Belonging to a tetragon; four-angled.

Tetragoniaceæ,* tet-ra-go-ne-a'-she-ē. [From *Tetrago'nia*, one of the genera.] A natural order of exogenous succulent plants (mostly herbaceous), found in the South Sea Islands and in the tropics.

Tet-ra-gyn'i-ous. [**Tetragyn'ius;** from τέτρα, "four," and γυνή, a "woman," or "female."] Having four pistils. Applied to a Linnæan order.

Tet-rag'y-nous. The same as TETRAGYNIOUS, which see.

Tet-ra-he'dri-cal. [**Tetrahe'dricus.**] Belonging to a tetrahedron.

Tet-ra-he'dron. [**Tetrahe'drum;** from τέτρα, "four," and ἕδρα, a "base."] A solid figure bounded by four equilateral and equal triangles. It is one of the Platonic bodies, or regular solids.

Te-tram'e-rous. [From τέτρα, "four," and μέρος, a "part."] Having four parts in each whorl. Applied to flowers which have four petals, four stamens, etc. It is often printed thus: 4-merous.

Tet-ran'dri-a.* [From τέτρα, "four," and ἀνήρ, a "man," or "male."] The fourth Linnæan class of plants, comprising those which have four stamens in each flower.

Tet-ran'drous. [**Tetran'drius;** from the same.] Having four stamens.

Tet-ra-phyl'lous. [**Tetraphyl'lus;** from τέτρα, "four," and φύλλον, a "leaf."] Having four leaves.

Te-trap'o-dous. [**Tetrap'odus;** from τέτρα, "four," and πούς, a "foot."] Having four feet.

Te-trap'ter-us.* [From τέτρα, "four," and πτερόν, a "wing."] Tetrapterous; having four wings. Applied to plants.

Tet-ra-sep'a-lous. [**Tetrasep'alus;** from τέτρα, "four," and *sep'alus*, a "sepal."] Having four sepals.

Tet-ra-sper'ma-tous. [**Tetrasper'matus;** from τέτρα, "four," and σπέρμα, a "seed."] Having four seeds.

Tet-ra-ste'mo-nis.* [From τέτρα, "four," and στήμων, a "stamen."] Having four stamens.

Te-tras'ti-chous. [**Tetras'tichus;** from τέτρα, "four," and στίχος, a "row."] Disposed in four vertical ranks. Applied to leaves.

Tet-ra-sty'lous. [**Tetrasty'lus;** from τέτρα, "four," and στῦλος, a "style," or a "pillar."] Having four styles.

Tetter. See PSORIASIS.

Tet'ter, Moist (or **Hu'mid**), and **Tet'ter, Run'ning.** Popular names for IMPETIGO, which see.

Teu'cri-um Cha-mæ'drys.* Germander. A plant of the natural order *Labiatæ*. It is bitter and aromatic.

Teucrium Marum. See MARUM SYRIACUM.

Tex'ti-form. [**Textifor'mis;** from *tex'tum*, a "web," or "tissue."] Formed like a tissue or network.

Tex'tu-ral. Pertaining to a texture or tissue.

Tex'ture. [**Textu'ra;** from *tex'o*, *tex'tum*, to "weave."] See TISSUE.

Thæria. See THERIA.

Thal'a-mi,* the plural of THALAMUS.

Thal'ami Ner-vo'rum Op-ti-co'-rum.* ("Beds of the Optic Nerves.") See OPTIC THALAMUS, and CORPORA STRIATA.

Thal-a-mi-flo'rous. [**Thalamiflo'rus;** from *thal'amus*, a "bridal chamber," also "receptacle," and *flos*, a "flower."] Having the stamens and pistils inserted in the receptacle.

Thal'a-mus,* plural **Thal'a-mi.** [Gr. θάλαμος, a "chamber," or "bridal bed."] Applied to a body of white substance at the base of each lateral ventricle of the brain, which in part gives origin to the optic nerve. Also, a term for the receptacle of a flower.

Tha-las'sic. [**Thalas'sicus;** from θάλασσα, the "sea."] A geological term applied by some writers to the strata of superior sediment,—*i.e.* from the surface of the earth to the limestone.

Tha-las-si-oph'y-tus.* [From θάλασσα, the "sea," and φυτόν, a "plant."] Applied in the plural feminine (*Thalassioph'ytæ*) to the marine *Algæ*.

Thal'li,* the plural of THALLUS, which see.

Thal'lo-gen. A plant consisting of *thalli* only.

Thal-log'e-nous. [**Thallog'enus;** from *thal'lus*, and γεννάω, to "produce."] Producing *thalli*.

Thal'lo-gens. A synonyme for THALLOPHYTES, which see.

Thal'lo-phytes. [**Thalloph'ytum;** from *thal'lus*, and φυτόν, a "plant."] A natural class of cryptogamous plants, having no distinction of axis and foliage, as lichens, fungi, and algæ. Also called Thallogens.

Thal'lus,* plural **Thal'li.** [From θάλλω, to "be verdant."] A term applied to the organs of vegetation of lichens, sea-weeds, etc.

Than-a-to'dēs.* [From θάνατος, "death."] Deadly; causing death.

Than-a-to-i'dēs.* [From θάνατος, "death," and εἶδος, a "form."] Resembling death: thanatoid.

Than-a-tol'o-gy̆. [**Thanatolo'gia**; from θάνατος, "death," and λόγος, a "discourse."] Literally, a "discourse or treatise on death." That branch of Pathology which treats of the phenomena and proximate cause of death.

Thé, tȧ. The French for THEA and TEA, which see.

The'a.* The tea-shrub, of which there are several species; also, tea. See TEA.

The'a Ni'gra.* The systematic name for the plant which yields black tea, or Bohea.

The'a Vir'ĭ-dis.* The systematic name for the plant which yields green tea.

The-be'sĭ-i Fo-ram'ĭ-na.* ("Orifices of Thebesius.") Certain small orifices on the right auricle of the heart, first described by Thebesius.

The'ca.* [Gr. θήκη; from τίθημι, to "place."] Literally, "the place where any thing is kept;" hence, a case, or sheath. In Anatomy, the investing membranous covering or sheath of the spinal cord and nerves. In Botany, an anther-cell; also, the spore-case, or urn, of mosses.

The'ca Ver-te-bra'lis.* ("Vertebral Sheath.") A prolongation of the *dura mater* lined by the arachnoid membrane, which is continued down and invests the spinal cord as far as the third lumbar vertebra, and sends off a tubular process to each of the spinal nerves.

The'ca-phore. [**Thecaph'orum**; from θήκη, a "case," or "sheath," and φέρω, to "bear."] Synonymous with GYNAPHORE, which see.

The-çi'tis.*[From *the'ca*, a "sheath."] Inflammation of the sheath of a tendon.

Thec'o-dus, *on'tis.** [From θήκη, a "case," or "sheath," and ὀδούς, a "tooth."] A covered or sheathed tooth.

The'in. [**Thei'na**; from *The'a*, the "tea-plant."] A substance found in the tea-shrub, assuming the form of beautiful crystals having a large proportion of nitrogen in their composition. It is believed to be the same as *caffein*, found in coffee.

The-li'tis, *idis.** [From θηλή, a "nipple."] Inflammation of the nipples.

The'nal. [From *the'nar*.] Belonging to the palm of the hand; applied by Dr. Barclay as meaning towards the palm of the hand.

The'nar, *aris.** [Gr. θέναρ.] The palm of the hand, or the sole of the foot. Also, a muscle extending the thumb.

The-o-bro'ma Ca-ca'o.* A plant of the natural order *Sterculiaceæ*, the seeds of which, when roasted and made into paste with vanilla, constitute chocolate.

The-o-ma'nĭ-a.* [From Θεός, "God," and μανία, "madness."] Religious madness or melancholy.

The-o-ma-ni'a-cus.* Belonging to *theomania*: theomaniacal.

The'o-rem. [**Theore'ma,** *atis*; from θεωρέω, to "view," to "weigh," or "consider."] In Geometry, a truth proposed to be proved.

The-o-ret'ĭ-cal. [**Theoret'icus**; from the same.] Relating to theory; speculative; not practical.

The'o-ry̆. [Gr. θεωρία; from the same.] The abstract principles of any science or art, considered without reference to practice. In Science, a connected arrangement of facts according to their bearing on some real or hypothetical law.

Thĕr-a-pei'a,* or **Thĕr-a-pi'a.*** [From θεραπεύω, to "heal."] Synonymous with THERAPEUTICS.

Thĕr-a-peū'tic, or **Thĕr-a-peū'tĭ-cal.** [**Therapeu'ticus**; from *therapeu'tica*.] Belonging to therapeutics.

Thĕr-a-peū'tics. [**Therapeu'tice, Therapeu'tica**; from θεραπεύω, to "cure."] That branch of Medicine which treats of the application of remedies, and the curative treatment of diseases.

Thĕr-a-peū'tist. [From the same.] A person who is skilful in therapeutics, or who practises therapeutics.

Therapia. See THERAPEIA.

The'rĭ-a.* [From θήριος, "savage."] A name for RADESYGE, which see.

The-rĭ'a-ca.* [From θήρ, a "wild beast," or any wild animal.] The'riac. An antidote to poisons, or the bites of venomous animals. Also, the Pharmacopœial name (Br. Ph.) for molasses, or treacle.

The-rĭ-o-ca-tar'rhus.* [From θέρος, "summer," and *catar'rhus*, a "catarrh."] Summer catarrh, or hay-fever; hay-asthma.

The-rĭ-o'ma.* [From θήρ, a "fierce or savage animal."] A term applied to a very malignant ulcer.

The-rĭ-ot'o-my̆. [**Theriot'ome,** or **Therioto'mia**; from θηρίον, a "beast," and τέμνω, to "cut."] Dissection of the lower animals; the same as ZOOTOMY.

Ther'mæ* (occurring only in the plural). [From θέρμη, "heat."] Warm springs, or warm baths.

Ther'mal. [**Therma'lis;** from θέρμη, "heat."] Pertaining to warmth or heat, or to hot springs.

Ther-mol'o-gy̆. [**Thermolo'gia;** from θέρμη, "heat," and λόγος, a "discourse."] A treatise on heat; the science of heat.

Ther-mom'e-ter. [**Thermom'etrum;** from θέρμη, "heat," and μέτρον, a "measure."] An instrument for measuring or ascertaining the degree of temperature of different bodies, but especially of the atmosphere. Among the different kinds of thermometers, the following are the most important:

1. *Fahrenheit's* (făr'ẹn-hīts) Thermometer; the scale of which, between the freezing and boiling points of water under a medium pressure of the atmosphere, is divided into one hundred and eighty parts or degrees, the freezing point being marked 32°, and the boiling point 212°. Fahrenheit's scale is almost universally employed in England and the United States.

2. *Centigrade* Thermometer; in the scale of which there are just one hundred degrees between the freezing and boiling points of water, the former being marked 0°, or *zero*, and the latter 100°. This scale is generally used in France, and in many other countries of Continental Europe, and is perhaps the most convenient in practice.

3. *Réaumur's* (rå'ō'müʀz') Thermometer. In this scale the freezing point is marked 0°, and the boiling point 80°. In this and also in the Centigrade, the degrees are continued of the same size below and above these points, those below being reckoned negative. These different modes of graduation are easily convertible. The scale of Centigrade is reduced to that of Fahrenheit by multiplying by nine and dividing by five; that of Réaumur to that of Fahrenheit by dividing by four instead of five; or that of Fahrenheit to either of these by reversing the process. Thus,—C. $100° \times 9 = 900 \div 5 = 180° + 32° = 212°$ F.; R. $80° \times 9 = 720 \div 4 = 180° + 32° = 212°$ F.

Thermom'eter, Differen'tial (differ-en'shạl). An instrument of great use in experimental philosophy, for measuring very small differences of temperature.

Ther'mo-scope. [**Thermosco'pium;** from θέρμη, "heat," and σκοπέω, to "examine."] An instrument for measuring minute differences of temperature. The same as DIFFERENTIAL THERMOMETER. See preceding article.

The'sēs,* the plural of THESIS.

The'sis,* plural **The'sēs.** [Gr. θέσις, a "position."] A proposition, affirmative or negative, which is advanced or laid down to be supported by argument; also applied to an essay composed by a candidate for graduation in medicine or some other branch of learning or science.

Thigh. See FEMUR.

Thigh-Bone. See OS FEMORIS.

Third Pair (of Nerves). See MOTORES OCULORUM.

Thirst. [Lat. **Si'tis;** Gr. δίψα; Fr. *Soif*, swåf.] A sensation attended with a desire to drink, having its seat chiefly in the mouth and fauces, but also felt in the pharynx, œsophagus, and, in extreme cases, the stomach; all, however, modified by circumstances. When it is morbid, it is usually termed *dipsosis;* when excessive, *polydipsia*. See DIPSOSIS, and POLYDIPSIA.

Thirst, Morbid. See DIPSOSIS.

Thom-so'nĭ-ạn-ĭsm. A fanciful or empirical system of medicine introduced by Thomson, a native of New Hampshire. Thomson and his immediate followers rejected all mineral medicines: they had frequent recourse to powerful emetics (usually of lobelia), to profuse sweats from vapor-baths, and to powerfully stimulating compounds, in which capsicum was an abundant ingredient. The system has, however, been, it is said, materially modified, and more cautious treatment is now generally pursued.

Tho-rạ-çen-te'sis.* The same as THORACOCENTESIS, which see.

Tho-raç'ic. [**Thoraç'icus.**] Belonging to the thorax.

Thoraç'ic Duct. [**Duc'tus Thoraç'icus.**] The principal trunk of the absorbent vessels lying upon the dorsal vertebræ. It commences at the *receptaculum chyli*, which is formed by the junction of several large lymphatic trunks. Its contents are discharged into the left subclavian vein. At its termination there are two valves, which prevent the blood from flowing from the vein into the duct.

Tho-rac'o-çen-te'sis.* [From *tho'rax*, and κέντησις, a "pricking."] A piercing of the thorax, as in the operation for *empyema*.

Tho-rạ-cod'y̆-ne,* or **Tho-rac-o-**

ʹdŷn'ĭ-a.* [From *tho'rax*, and ὀδύνη, "pain."] Pain in the chest.

Tho-rac-o-my-o-dŷn'ĭ-a.* [From *tho'rax*, and *myodyn'ia*, "pain of a muscle."] Muscular pain in the chest.

Tho-rac-o-pa-thi'a.* [From θώραξ, θωρακός, the "chest," and πάθος, an "affection."] An affection or disease of the chest.

Tho-rac'o-ste-no'sis.* [From *tho'rax*, and στένω, to "straiten."] Coarctation or contraction of the chest.

Tho'rax, a'cis.* [Gr. θώραξ, a "breastplate."] (Fr. *Poitrine*, pwå'-trèn'.) The chest, or that part of the body between the neck and diaphragm, in the cavity of which are contained the lungs and the heart. Also, the trunk, or intermediate portion of the body of insects which bears the legs.

Tho-ri'na.* [From *Thor*, a Scandinavian idol.] An earth discovered in a rare Norwegian mineral called *thorite*. Thorina is an oxide of thorium.

Tho'ri-um.* [From the same.] A heavy gray metal which combined with oxygen forms thorina.

Thorn. [**Spi'na.**] An imperfectly developed, indurated, leafless branch of a woody plant, tapering to a point.

Thorn-Apple. See DATURA STRAMONIUM.

Thorn, E-ġŷp'tian. The ACACIA VERA, which see.

Thread. See FILAMENT.

Thread-like. See FILIFORM.

Thread-Worm. See OXYURUS.

Three-Cornered. See TRIGONAL, and TRIQUETROUS.

Three-Leaved. See TRIFOLIATE, and TRIPHYLLOUS.

Threp-sol'o-ġŷ. [**Threpsolo'gia;** from *threp'sis*, "nutrition," and λόγος, a "discourse."] A treatise on the nutrition of organized bodies; the doctrine or science of nutrition.

Thrid'a-ce. [**Thrida'cium;** from θρίδαξ, the "lettuce."] A substance obtained from lettuce, supposed to be identical with *Lactucarium*.

Throat. [Lat. **Gu'la, Gut'tur,** and **Ju'gulum;** Fr. *Gorge*, gorzh.] The common name of the pharynx; also of the anterior part of the neck, or *jugulum*. Applied in Botany to the orifice of a tubular flower or other organ.

Throm'bi,* the plural of THROMBUS, which see.

Throm-bo'dēs.* [From *throm'bus*.] Resembling or having *thrombi*: thrombous.

Throm'boid. [**Thromboi'des;** from *throm'bus*, and εἶδος, a "form."] Resembling a *throm'bus*.

Throm-bo'sis.* The formation or progress of *throm'bus*. The obstruction of vessels by a morbid product developed in the very locality of the obstruction, and thus distinguished from *embolia* (or *embolism*), which consists in the obstruction of a vessel by a piece of coagulum (or thrombus) carried into the circulation from a distant part of the system.

Throm'bus,* plural **Throm'bi.** [From θρόμβος, a "clot of blood."] A small tumor of extravasated blood after bleeding or contusion. Applied by Virchow to a coagulum, forming, from some morbific cause, usually in a small vein, and gradually prolonged into the larger veins, so that ultimately portions are broken off and carried into the circulation, thus producing what is termed *embolism*. (See EMBOLIA.) To the original thrombus (not the *prolonged* portion) he has applied the epithet *autoch'thonous* [from αὐτός, "itself," and χθών, "country," or "place"], that is, "produced in the place itself," and not derived from another part.

Thrush. A popular term for *aphthæ* on the tongue, lining membrane of the mouth, fauces, etc., of infants. See APHTHA.

Thumb. [**Pol'lex,** *icis*.] The first, or greatest, of the fingers. In Ornithology, a small bone of the *hand*, or third portion of the anterior extremity; also, the shortest toe, which has only two phalanges. Also, the first finger of the forefoot of certain reptiles.

Thun'der-bolt. A name for the BELEMNITE, which see.

Thu-rif'er-ous. [**Thurif'erus;** from *thus*, *thu'ris*, "frankincense," and *fe'ro*, to "bear."] Bearing or producing frankincense.

Thus, u'ris.* [From θύω, to "offer a sacrifice;" because it was used in making offerings to the gods.] The *Olibanum*, or true frankincense, obtained from the *Boswel'lia serra'ta*.

Thus A-mer-ĭ-ca'num.* ("American Frankincense.") The Pharmacopœial name (Br. Ph.) for common frankincense, or the concrete turpentine of the *Pinus tæda* and *Pinus palustris*.

Thu'ya (or **Thu'ja**) **Oc-çĭ-den-ta'-lis.*** *Ar'bor Vitæ* ("Tree of Life"). A tree belonging to the natural order *Coniferæ*. The leaves and twigs have been used in dropsy, intermittent fevers, etc.

Thymelaceæ,* thim-e-la'she-ē. [From *Thymelæ'a*, one of the genera.] A natural order of exogenous plants (mostly shrubs), found in Australia, South Africa, and other regions. The great feature of this order is the causticity of the bark. It includes the *Daphne Mezereum*, used as a medicine, and *Dirca* (Leatherwood).

Thy'mic. [Thym'icus.] Belonging to the *thymus* gland.

Thy-mi'tis, idis.* [From *thy'mus*.] Inflammation of the *thymus* gland.

Thy'mus.* [From θύω, to "sacrifice."] Thyme. A Linnæan genus of the class *Didynamia*, natural order *Labiatæ* or *Lamiaceæ*. In Anatomy, the *thymus* gland.

Thy'mus Gland. Situated in the neck of the fœtus, disappearing after birth as a gland.

Thy'mus Vul-ga'ris.* The systematic name of common thyme, an aromatic plant, which is reputed to be a resolvent, tonic, and stomachic. It is used in cookery more than in medicine.

Thy're-o-A-rȳt-æ-no-i-dæ'us.* A muscle arising from the thyroid and inserted into the arytenoid cartilage. It widens the glottis.

Thȳ're-o-çēle.* [From θυρεός, an "oblong shield," and κήλη, a "tumor."] Tumor or swelling of the thyroid gland. See THYREOPHYMA.

Thy're-o-Ep-ĭ-glot-tĭ-de'us.* A muscle arising from the thyroid cartilage and inserted into the side of the epiglottis. It has been divided by Albinus into the *major* and *minor*.

Thy're-o-Hy-o-i'de-us.* A muscle arising from the thyroid cartilage and inserted into the *os hyoides*. It brings the larynx and hyoid bone towards each other.

Thy-re-on'cus.* [From θυρεός, an "oblong shield," and ὄγκος, a "tumor."] A tumor of the thyroid gland. The same as THYREOCELE.

Thy're-o-phy'ma, atis.* [From θυρεός, an "oblong shield," and φῦμα, a "tumor."] An enlargement of the thyroid gland. Similar to THYREOCELE.

Thȳ'ro-Hy'al. [Thyrohya'lis; from *thy'ro-*, and *hyoi'des* os, the "hyoid bone."] Applied by Owen to the homologues of the lateral lingual bone, or larger horn of the hyoid bone.

Thȳ'roid. [Thyroi'des; from θυρεός, a "shield," and εἶδος, a "form."] Resembling a shield. See SCUTIFORM.

Thy'roid Car'tĭ-lage. The largest of the cartilages of the larynx, forming the *Pomum Adami*.

Thy'roid Gland. Situated on the cricoid cartilage, trachea, and horns of the thyroid cartilage.

Thyrse. [Lat. **Thyr'sus,** plural **Thyr'si;** Gr. θυρσός.] A compact panicle of a pyramidal, oval, or oblong outline, such as the flower-cluster of the Lilac, or a bunch of grapes.

Thyr-sif'er-ous. [Thyrsif'erus; from *thyr'sus*, a "thyrse," and *fe'ro*, to "bear."] Having or bearing thyrses.

Thyr-sĭ-flo'rus.* [From *thyr'sus*, a "thyrse," and *flos*, a "flower."] Having flowers disposed in thyrses.

Thyr'sus.* The same as THYRSE, which see.

Tib'ĭ-a.* A Latin word signifying a "pipe," or "flute." Applied to the largest bone of the leg: the shin-bone.

Tib-ĭ-æ'us.* The same as TIBIAL, which see.

Tib'ĭ-al. [Tibia'lis.] Belonging to the tibia. Applied by Dr. Barclay as meaning towards the tibia.

Tib-ĭ-a'lis.* ("Tibial.") The name of two muscles of the tibia, the *anticus* or flexor, and the *posticus*, called also *extensor tarsi tibialis*.

Tic Douloureux, tik doo'loo-roo'. (French pronunciation, tēk doo'loo'rūh'.) Severe pain affecting the nerves of the face, especially the *infra-orbitary* branches of the fifth pair.

Tick. An insect of the genus ACARUS, which see.

Tick, Domestic. The *Acarus domesticus*.

Tick, Itch. The *Acarus scabiei*.

Tide. [Originally, a "time," or "season;" because it returns at stated times.] Applied to the ebb and flow of the sea, or the periodic and alternate rise and fall of the water of the ocean, caused principally by the attraction of the moon, and modified by that of the sun.

Tierce, te-êrss'. The French name for TERTIAN, which see.

Tieuté. See UPAS TIEUTÉ.

Tĭ-ġel'la.* [Diminutive of *tig'num*, a "rafter."] That part of the embryo of a plant which unites the radicle to the cotyledon.

Tiġ'el-late. [Tigella'tus.] Supplied with a *tigella*.

Tig'lĭ-i, Gra'na.* ("Grains or Seeds of Tiglium.") The seeds of the *Croton tiglium*. See CROTON.

Tiglii, Oleum. See OLEUM TIGLII.

Tig'lĭ-um.* The specific name of the *Croton tiglium.*

Tiliaceæ,* til-e-a'she-ē. A natural order of exogenous plants, found in many tropical and temperate regions. It includes the *Til'ia* (Linden or Lime tree). The berries of some species are eatable.

Tin. [Lat. **Stan'num;** Fr. *Étain,* ā'tăNG'.] A comparatively rare, white metal, harder than lead, and very malleable. In ductility and tenacity it is inferior to most of the other malleable metals. Exposed to the air, it soon becomes superficially oxidized. Its specific gravity is 7.2. The temperature at which it melts is about 442°.

TIN'FOIL is an alloy of tin and lead in the form of a thin lamina or leaf.

Tin'ca.* The tench fish. See OS TINCÆ.

Tin'cal. Crude borax as it is imported from the East Indies in yellow, greasy crystals.

Tinct. = *Tinctu'ra.** "A tincture."

Tinc-to'rĭ-us.* [From *tin'go, tinc'tum,* to "dye."] Relating to dyeing. Applied as the specific name to the Black Oak (*Quercus tinctoria*), also called Dyer's Oak.

Tinc-tu'ra,* plural **Tinc-tu'ræ.** [From *tin'go, tinc'tum,* to "dye," to "steep."] A tincture. A solution of any medicinal substance in alcohol, or diluted alcohol, prepared by maceration, digestion, or percolation. A solution in spirit of ammonia is termed an ammoniated tincture, and a solution in ethereal spirit, an ethereal tincture.

☞ The great number of officinal tinctures, as well as the narrow limits of this work, preclude the insertion of the full Pharmacopœial directions for making this important class of preparations. It has been deemed sufficient to give, in addition to the names, the strength of the tinctures, as indicated by the relative proportions of the different medicinal substances, to a given quantity of alcohol, employed in their preparation. (For the dose of each, see TABLE OF DOSES, in the Appendix. See, also, the U.S. Pharmacopœia, pp. 314–339.)

Tinctu'ra Ac-o-ni'ti Fo'lĭ-i* ("Tincture of Leaf of Aconite"), **Tinctu'ra Aconi'ti Fo-lĭ-o'rum,*** 1850. ("Tincture of Leaves of Aconite.") Prepared with two ounces of the drug to a pint of diluted alcohol.

Tinctu'ra Aconi'ti Ra-di'cis.* ("Tincture of Aconite Root.") Prepared with six ounces of the drug to a pint of strong alcohol.

Tinctu'ra Al'o-ēs.* ("Tincture of Aloes.") Prepared with half an ounce of Socotrine aloes, and an ounce and a half of liquorice, to a pint of very dilute alcohol.

Tinctu'ra Al'oes et Mȳr'rhæ.* ("Tincture of Aloes and Myrrh.") Prepared with an ounce and a half of aloes, half an ounce of saffron, and an ounce and a half of myrrh, to a pint of strong alcohol.

Tinctu'ra Ar'nĭ-çæ.* ("Tincture of Arnica.") Prepared with three ounces of the drug to a pint of diluted alcohol.

Tinctu'ra As-sa-fœt'ĭ-dæ.* ("Tincture of Assafœtida.") Prepared with two ounces of assafœtida to a pint of strong alcohol.

Tinctu'ra Bel-la-don'næ.* ("Tincture of Belladonna.") Prepared with two ounces of the drug to a pint of diluted alcohol.

Tinctu'ra Ben-zo'ĭ-ni Com-pos'ĭ-ta.* ("Compound Tincture of Benzoin.") Prepared with an ounce and a half of benzoin, an ounce of storax, half an ounce of balsam of Tolu, two drachms of aloes, to a pint of strong alcohol.

Tinctu'ra Ca-lum'bæ* ("Tincture of Columbo"), **Tinctu'ra Co-lom'bæ,*** 1850. Prepared with two ounces of columbo to a pint of diluted alcohol.

Tinctu'ra Can'na-bis.* ("Tincture of Hemp.") Prepared with six drachms of the extract of hemp to a pint of strong alcohol.

Tinctu'ra Can-thăr'ĭ-dis.* ("Tincture of Cantharides.") Prepared with half an ounce of cantharides to a pint of diluted alcohol.

Tinctu'ra Cap'sĭ-çi.* ("Tincture of Capsicum.") Prepared with half an ounce of the drug to a pint of diluted alcohol.

Tinctu'ra Car-da-mo'mi.* ("Tincture of Cardamom.") Prepared with two ounces of the drug to a pint of diluted alcohol.

Tinctu'ra Cardamo'mi Com-pos'ĭ-ta.* ("Compound Tincture of Cardamom.") Prepared with three drachms of cardamom, two and a half drachms of cinnamon, one drachm of caraway, one ounce of honey, and half a drachm of cochineal, to one pint of diluted alcohol.

Tinctu'ra Cas-to're-i.* ("Tincture of Castor.") Prepared with one ounce of castor to a pint of strong alcohol.

Tinctu'ra Cat'e-chu.* ("Tincture of Catechu.") Prepared with an ounce and a half of catechu, and an ounce of cinnamon, to a pint of diluted alcohol.

Tinctu'ra Cin-cho'næ.* ("Tincture of Cinchona.") Prepared with three ounces of the yellow bark to a pint of diluted alcohol.

Tinctu'ra Cincho'næ Com-pos'ĭ-tạ.* ("Compound Tincture of Cinchona.") Prepared with two ounces of red bark, an ounce and a half of bitter orange-peel, three drachms of serpentaria, one drachm of saffron, and one drachm of red saunders, to twenty fluidounces of diluted alcohol.

Tinctu'ra Cin-nạ-mo'mi.* ("Tincture of Cinnamon.") Prepared with an ounce and a half of the drug to a pint of diluted alcohol.

Tinctu'ra Col'chĭ-çi* ("Tincture of Colchicum"), **Tinctu'ra Col'chici Sem'ĭ-nis,*** 1850. ("Tincture of the Seed of Colchicum.") Prepared with two ounces of the drug to a pint of diluted alcohol.

Tinctu'ra Co-ni'i.* ("Tincture of Hemlock.") Prepared with two ounces of the drug to a pint of diluted alcohol.

Tinctu'ra Cu-be'bæ.* ("Tincture of Cubebs.") Prepared with two ounces of cubebs to a pint of diluted alcohol.

Tinctu'ra Dig-ĭ-ta'lis.* ("Tincture of Digitalis.") Prepared with two ounces of the drug to a pint of diluted alcohol.

Tinctu'ra Fer'ri Chlo'ri-di.* ("Tincture of Chloride of Iron.") Estimated to contain about a drachm of the chloride of iron to an ounce of the tincture.

Tinctu'ra Gal'læ.* ("Tincture of Nutgall.") Prepared with two ounces of the drug to a pint of diluted alcohol.

Tinctu'ra Gentia'næ (jen-she-a'nē) **Com-pos'ĭ-tạ.*** ("Compound Tincture of Gentian.") Prepared with one ounce of gentian, half an ounce of bitter orange-peel, and two drachms of cardamom, to a pint of diluted alcohol.

Tinctu'ra Guai'ạ-çi.* ("Tincture of Guaiac.") Prepared with three ounces of guaiacum to a pint of strong alcohol.

Tinctu'ra Guai'aci Am-mo-nĭ-a'-tạ.* ("Ammoniated Tincture of Guaiac.") Prepared with four ounces of guaiacum to a pint and a half of aromatic spirit of ammonia.

Tinctu'ra Hel-leb'o-ri.* ("Tincture of [Black] Hellebore.") Prepared with two ounces of the drug to a pint of diluted alcohol.

Tinctu'ra Hu'mu-li.* ("Tincture of Hops.") Prepared with two ounces and a half of the drug to a pint of diluted alcohol.

Tinctu'ra Hy-os-çy'ạ-mi.* ("Tincture of Henbane.") Prepared with two ounces of the drug to a pint of diluted alcohol.

Tinctu'ra I-o-din'ĭ-i.* ("Tincture of Iodine.") Prepared with an ounce of iodine to a pint of alcohol.

Tinctu'ra Iodin'ii Com-pos'ĭ-tạ.* ("Compound Tincture of Iodine.") Prepared with half an ounce of iodine, and an ounce of iodide of potassium, to one pint of alcohol.

Tinctu'ra Ja-la'pæ.* ("Tincture of Jalap.") Prepared with three ounces of jalap to a pint of diluted alcohol.

Tinctu'ra Ki'no.* ("Tincture of Kino.") Prepared with an ounce and a half of kino to a pint of diluted alcohol.

Tinctu'ra Kra-me'rĭ-æ.* ("Tincture of Rhatany.") Prepared with three ounces of the drug to a pint of diluted alcohol.

Tinctu'ra Lo-be'lĭ-æ.* ("Tincture of Lobelia.") Prepared with two ounces of the drug to a pint of diluted alcohol.

Tinctu'ra Lu-pu-li'næ.* ("Tincture of Lupulin.") Prepared with two ounces of lupulin to a pint of strong alcohol.

Tinctu'ra Mỹr'rhæ.* ("Tincture of Myrrh.") Prepared with three ounces of myrrh to two pints of strong alcohol.

Tinctu'ra Nu'çis Vom'ĭ-çæ.* ("Tincture of Nux Vomica.") Prepared with four ounces of the drug to a pint of strong alcohol.

Tinctu'ra O'pĭ-i.* ("Tincture of Opium.") Laudanum. Prepared with ten drachms of opium to a pint of alcohol.

Tinctu'ra O'pii Aç-e-ta'tạ.* ("Acetated Tincture of Opium.") Prepared with one ounce of opium to four fluidounces of alcohol and six fluidounces of vinegar.

Tinctu'ra O'pii Cam-pho-ra'tạ.* ("Camphorated Tincture of Opium.") Paregoric. Prepared with half a drachm of opium, one scruple of camphor, half a drachm of benzoic acid, half a drachm of oil of anise-seed, one ounce of honey, to a pint of diluted alcohol.

Tinctu'ra O'pii De-o-do-ra'tạ.* ("Deodorized Tincture of Opium.") Pre pared with ten drachms of opium to a pint of alcohol.

Tinctu'ra Quas'siæ* (kwosh'e-ē). ("Tincture of Quassia.") Prepared with one ounce of quassia to a pint of diluted alcohol.

Tinctu'ra Rhe'i.* ("Tincture of Rhubarb.") Prepared with an ounce and a half of rhubarb, and two drachms of cardamom, to a pint of diluted alcohol.

Tinctu'ra Rhe'i et Sen'næ.* ("Tincture of Rhubarb and Senna.") Prepared with a half an ounce of rhubarb, one drachm of senna, half a drachm of coriander, half a drachm of fennel, one drachm of red saunders, fifteen grains of saffron, fifteen grains of liquorice, and three ounces of raisins, to a pint and a half of diluted alcohol.

Tinctu'ra San-guĭ-na'rĭ-æ.* ("Tincture of Bloodroot.") Prepared with two ounces of the drug to a pint of diluted alcohol.

Tinctu'ra Sçil'læ.* ("Tincture of Squill.") Prepared with two ounces of squill to a pint of diluted alcohol.

Tinctu'ra Ser-pen-ta'rĭ-æ.* ("Tincture of Serpentaria.") Prepared with an ounce and a half of the drug to a pint of diluted alcohol.

Tinctu'ra Stra-mo'nĭ-i.* ("Tincture of Stramonium.") Prepared with two ounces of the drug to a pint of diluted alcohol.

Tinctu'ra Tol-u-ta'na.* ("Tincture of Tolu.") Prepared with an ounce and a half of tolu to a pint of strong alcohol.

Tinctu'ra Va-le-rĭ-a'næ.* ("Tincture of Valerian.") Prepared with two ounces of valerian to a pint of diluted alcohol.

Tinctu'ra Valeria'næ Am-mo-nĭ-a'ta.* ("Ammoniated Tincture of Valerian.") Prepared with two ounces of valerian to one pint of aromatic spirit of ammonia.

Tinctu'ra Ve-ra'tri Vĭr'ĭ-dis.* ("Tincture of American Hellebore.") Prepared with eight ounces of the drug to a pint of strong alcohol.

Tinctu'ra Zin-ğĭb'e-ris.* ("Tincture of Ginger.") Prepared with four ounces of ginger to a pint of strong alcohol.

Tin'e-a.* (Fr. *Teigne*, tĕñ or tāñ.) Literally, a "moth-worm." Scaldhead. A genus of the order *Dialyses*, class *Locales*, of Cullen's Nosology; also termed *Porrigo*. It is characterized by a pustular eruption, sometimes distinct and sometimes confluent, unaccompanied with fever, the pustules drying and hardening into thick scales or scabs.

There appears to be great confusion in regard to the names applied to this disease by different writers. The genus *Tinea* of Sauvages and Cullen would seem to correspond to the species *Ecpye'sis porri'go* of Good, and the genus *Porrigo* of Willan and other writers.

Tin'ea Cap'ĭ-tis.* ("Tinea of the Head.") A term for scaldhead. See preceding article.

Tin-nĭ'tus.* [From *tin'nio, tinni'tum*, to "ring like metal."] A ringing, or tinkling.

Tinni'tus Au'rĭ-um.* ("Ringing of the Ears.") A symptom in many kinds or states of disease.

Tisane, te-zan'. See PTISANE. [From πτισάνη, "barley-water."] A decoction or infusion of slightly medicinal substances, much employed in France. Formerly applied, for the most part, to a decoction of barley.

Tisane de Feltz (fĕlts). A remedy sometimes used in cutaneous diseases; prepared from sarsaparilla, crude antimony, and isinglass.

Tis'sue. (Fr. *Tissu.*) Literally, "that which is woven;" a "web." Applied to any organized solid substance of which animals or plants are composed. In plants, the thin membranous organization of which every part is formed. See MEMBRANE.

Tissue, Adipose. See ADIPOSE MEMBRANE.

Tissue, Areolar. See AREOLAR.

Tissue, Cellular. See CELLULAR TISSUE.

Tis'sue, Com-pact'. A tissue formed by fibres placed so close together as to leave no intervals: it exists at the surface of the bones, and forms the walls of the various apertures and canals which may occur in them.

Tissue, Vascular. See VASCULAR TISSUE.

Tissue, Woody. See WOODY TISSUE.

Ti-ta'nĭ-um.* [From *Ti'tan*, a name for the "sun." See TELLURIUM.] A rare metal, found in a mineral from Cornwall called *menachanite*. It is extremely infusible, and so hard as to scratch not only glass but also crystal. In color it resembles copper. Its specific gravity is 5.8.

Tit-il-lā'tion. [**Titilla'tio, o'***nis*; from *titil'lo, titilla'tum*, to "tickle."] Tickling; the production of laughter by tickling. It has been suggested as a remedy for paralysis.

Tit-u-bā'tion. [**Tituba'tio, o'***nis;* from *tit'ubo, tituba'tum,* to "stagger," or "stumble."] A staggering or stumbling gait, dependent on disease of the spinal system.

T. O. = *Tinctu'ra O'pii.** "Tincture of Opium."

Toad-stone. See BATRACHITES.

To-bac'co. The *Nicotiana tabacum.* Tobacco unites with the powers of a sedative narcotic, those of an emetic and diuretic, and produces these effects, to a greater or less extent, to whatever surface it may be applied. Taken moderately, it calms restlessness, and produces a state of general languor, or repose, which has great charms for those accustomed to its use. In large quantities, however, it causes vertigo, stupor, fainting, nausea, vomiting, and general debility of the nervous and circulatory functions. Numerous cases are on record of its incautious use having been followed by a fatal termination. See NICOTIANA.

Tobac'co, Vir-gin'ĭ-an. The *Nicotiana tabacum.*

To-col'o-ġy̆. [**Tocolo'gia;** from τόκος, "childbirth," and λόγος, a "discourse."] That branch of Medicine which treats of parturition. See OBSTETRICS.

Tod'dy̆. Palm-wine, prepared by fermentation from palm-sugar.

Toe. See DIGITUS PEDIS.

Toise. A French measure, equal to six feet English, or two yards.

Tokology. See TOCOLOGY.

Tol'e-rance. [From *tol'ero,* to "bear," to "endure."] The power of bearing. A term employed by Rasori to denote the power of bearing large doses of powerful medicines.

Tol-u-if'e-ra.* [From *To'lu,* and *fe'ro,* to "bear."] A Linnæan genus of the class *Decandria,* natural order *Leguminosæ.*

Toluif'era Băl'sa-mum.* The tree which affords *Balsamum Tolutanum.*

To-lu-if'er-ous. [**Toluif'erus.**] Bearing Tolu balsam.

Tomato, to-mā'to. The common name of the *Lycoper'sicum esculen'tum,* or *Sola'num Lycoper'sicum,* a plant of the Linnæan class *Pentandria,* natural order *Solanaceæ.*

Tom'bac. An alloy called white copper, consisting of copper and arsenic.

To-men-tose'. [**Tomento'sus;** from *tomen'tum,* a "lock of wool."] Covered with a close and matted down, or wool.

To-men'tum.* [From τομή, a "cutting"?] Literally, a "flock of wool." Applied to certain small vessels of the brain. (See TOMENTUM CEREBRI.) In Botany, a species of pubescence, woolly or downy; a close and matted down.

Tomen'tum Cĕr'e-bri.* ("Wool of the Brain.") Applied to a great number of small vessels (supposed to resemble the fibres of wool) on the inside of the *pia mater,* and penetrating the cortical substance of the brain.

Tom-o-ma'nĭ-a.* [From τέμνω, to "cut," and μανία, "madness."] The cutting mania of certain surgeons, or eagerness to use the knife in cases which could be better cured without an operation.

Tone. [Gr. τόνος; from τείνω, to "stretch," to "draw."] Tension; tenor. In Medicine, tension or firmness.

Tongue. [Lat. **Lin'gua;** Gr. γλῶσσα; Fr. *Langue,* lŏng.] The chief organ of taste and of speech.

Tongue-Shaped. See LINGUIFORM, and LINGULATE.

Tongue-Tie. See ANKYLOGLOSSIA.

Ton'ic. [**Ton'icus;** from τείνω, to "stretch," to "draw."] Applied to rigid contraction of muscles without relaxation, termed tonic spasm. Also, increasing the tone of muscular fibre: applied to certain medicines. See TONICS.

Ton'ic Pow'er. A term for IRRITABILITY, which see.

To-niç'ĭ-ty̆. [**Toniç'itas, a'***tis;* from *ton'icus,* "belonging to or having tone."] The quality of muscular fibre in a state of action.

Ton'ics. [**Ton'ica;** from the same.] Medicines which neither immediately nor sensibly excite action like stimulants, nor depress action like sedatives, but produce a permanent, though scarcely perceptible, excitement of all the vital functions; their effects being chiefly perceived in the increased tone or vigor of the entire system.

Ton'sil. [Lat. **Tonsil'la;** Fr. *Tonsille,* tônᵍ'sēl', or *Amygdale,* å'mēg'dål'.] A small, oval, almond-shaped gland in the recess between the pillars or arches of the fauces.

Ton-sil-lī'tis, i*dis.** [From *tonsil'la,* a "tonsil."] Inflammation of the tonsils; a species of sore-throat.

Tooth, plural **Teeth.** [**Dens,** plural **Den'tes;** see DENS.] The small bones fixed in the alveolar cavities of the upper and lower jaws, designed for the purpose of seizing, cutting, tearing, or grinding the various articles which form the food of animals. True teeth are found only in the *Vertebrata*. The teeth of an adult human subject are thirty-two in number; that is, sixteen in each jaw. They consist of four kinds: 1. *Inciso'res* ("cutting" or "incisor" teeth), of which there are eight (four in each jaw); 2. *Cuspida'ti* ("pointed" or "cuspidate" teeth), four in number; 3. *Bicuspida'ti* or *Bicus'pides* ("two-pointed," "bicuspidate," or "bicuspid" teeth), eight in number; and 4. *Mola'res* ("grinding" or "molar" teeth), of which there are twelve, six in each jaw. The body and lower part of the tooth consists of a very hard and firm bone-like texture, termed *dentin* (or *dentine*); that part which projects from the alveolus, called the *corona*, or crown, being covered with *enamel*, a semi-vitreous substance, which is thickest in those parts which are most exposed to friction. The structure of the enamel is usually termed fibrous; but in fact it consists of extremely minute hexagonal columns radiating from the centre towards the surface of the tooth, an arrangement by which it is enabled to sustain a great pressure without injury. When the tooth first emerges from the gum, it is covered with a very thin layer of material termed *cemen'tum* (or "cement"), the minute structure of which corresponds almost exactly to that of bone. This layer is soon removed by attrition from the crown of the tooth, but continues through life to form the covering of the fang or root. The lower portion and roots of the teeth contain a cavity filled with what is termed *dental pulp* (*pul'pa den'tis*),—in popular language the "marrow,"—which consists of a filament of nerve, with an accompanying artery and vein, joined together by connective tissue. This pulp is extremely sensitive; and when, by the decay of the tooth, it becomes wholly or partially exposed to the air, it produces the distressing affection known as toothache, or *odontalgia*.

TEM'PORARY or DECID'UOUS TEETH. (*Den'tes Decid'ui.*) These are twenty in number: so named because they are shed between the ages of seven and fourteen, and their places supplied by the permanent or adult teeth. They are also termed Milk-Teeth, because they usually make their first appearance before the child is weaned.

The term *teeth* is applied in Botany to the segments of a serrate or dentate leaf; also to the summits of sepals which are united in the greater part of their extent.

Toothache. See ODONTALGIA, and ODONTAGRA.

Toothed. Beset with teeth which do not point towards the apex; the same as *dentate*. Applied to leaves.

Tooth'-Rash. The disease *Strophulus confertus*.

To'paz. [Gr. τοπάζιον.] A crystallized mineral, of a yellow or wine color, composed chiefly of alumina and silica. It is used in jewelry.

To-phā'ceous. [**Topha'ceus**; from *to'phus*, a "sandstone."] Of a sandy, or hard, gritty nature.

To'phus.* (Gr. τόφος.) Literally, a loose or porous stone. Applied to the calcareous matter which collects on the sides of vessels in which water is boiled. Also applied to the calcareous matter in the joints (of those affected with the gout), or in other parts of the body; likewise to the tartar on the teeth. In Surgery, a swelling particularly affecting a bone, or the periosteum.

Top'ĭ-ca.* [From τόπος, a "place."] Medicines which are applied locally: as caustics, emollients, etc.

Top'ĭ-cal. [**Top'icus**; from the same.] Pertaining to a particular part or situation of the body; local.

To-pog'ra-phy̆. [**Topogra'phia**; from τόπος, a "place," and γράφω, to "write."] A description of a place, or of the form of the surface of a limited portion of the earth.

Top'-Shaped. Inversely conical; turbinate. Applied to parts of plants.

Tor'cu-lar, a'ris.* [From *tor'queo*, to "twist," or "torture."] Literally, a "wine-press." Applied to the TOURNIQUET, which see.

Tor'cular He-roph'ĭ-li.* (Literally, "Herophilus' Wine-Press.") A term applied to an irregular cavity where the principal sinuses of the *dura mater* become confluent. The columns of blood coming in different directions were supposed to be *pressed* together in this part.

Tor'ment. [**Tor'men**, *inis*, or **Tormen'tum**; from the same.] A racking pain. Applied to iliac passion, on account of its severity.

Tor-men-til'la.* Tormentil. A Linnæan genus of the class *Icosandria*, natural order *Rosaceæ*. Also, the Pharmacopœial name for the rhizome of the *Potentil'la tormentil'la*. It is a simple and powerful astringent.

Tormentil'la E-rec'ta.* The former name for *Potentilla tormentilla.*

Tor'mĭ-na.* [Plural of *tor'men*, "torment."] Severe griping or wringing pains in the bowels; also, dysentery.

Tor'mĭ-nal. [**Tormina'lis;** from *tor'men*, "torment."] Belonging to *tormina.*

Tor-nā'do. [From the Spanish *tornear*, to "turn," or "whirl."] Literally, "whirlwind." Applied to a violent hurricane or gust of wind, which, arising suddenly from the shore, veers round to all points of the compass, and has been described as blowing from all points at once. Tornadoes are frequent in the West Indies.

To-rose'. [**Toro'sus;** from *to'rus*, a "bed;" also, a "knob," or "swelling."] In Botany, applied to a cylindrical body swollen at intervals.

Tor-pe'do.* Literally, "numbness." The name given to a genus of cartilaginous fishes, separated from the *Raiæ* of Linnæus on account of the circular form of the body, and more especially from the presence of the electrical organs, on which that form of the body mainly depends. Violent shocks are experienced on touching the living and active torpedo. There is reason to believe that the torpedo uses its electrifying or benumbing power to secure its prey, as well as to defend itself against its enemies.

Tor'pid. [**Tor'pidus;** from *tor'peo*, to "be numbed."] In a state of torpor, or numbness; incapable of action, or deprived of sensibility.

Torpidity. See TORPOR.

Tor'por, o'ris.* [See TORPID.] Deficient sensation; numbness; torpidity.

Tor-re-fac'tion. [**Torrefac'tio, o'nis;** from *tor'ridus*, "dry," "hot," and *fa'cio, fac'tum*, to "make."] The act of drying or roasting.

Tor-re-fac'tus.* Roasted. See TORREFACTION.

Tor-rĭ-cel'lĭ-an Vac'u-um. [From *Torricel'li*, inventor of the mercurial barometer.] The vacuum produced by inverting a tube of sufficient length, filled with mercury or any other fluid, in a vessel containing a portion of the same fluid, and allowing the fluid in the tube to descend until its weight is counterbalanced by that of the atmosphere. In this manner the first barometers were formed by Torricelli.

Tor'rid. [**Tor'ridus;** from *tor'reo*, to "roast," or "parch."] Parched; burned; scorched. Also, hot, parching.

Tor'rid Zone. [**Zo'na Tor'rida.**] All that space between the Tropics; so called from the scorching heat which prevails there.

Tor'sion. [**Tor'sio, o'nis;** from *tor'queo, tor'tum* and *tor'sum*, to "twist."] A twisting. Torsion of the arteries: an expedient resorted to for arresting or preventing hæmorrhage.

Tor'sion Bal'ance. A delicate electrometer, so called because its principle consists in the torsion or twisting of a single fibre of the web of a silkworm.

Tor-tĭ-col'lis.* [From *tor'queo, tor'tum*, to "twist," and *col'lum*, the "neck."] The muscular affection termed wry-neck.

Tor-tĭ'pēs, p'edis.* [From *tor'tus*, "twisted," and *pes*, a "foot."] In Botany, having the foot or pedicle much twisted: tortipede.

Tor-tu-a'lis.* [From *tor'queo, tor'tum*, to "twist," or "torment."] Tormented; suffering. Sometimes applied to the countenance of the sick.

Tor'tu-ous. [**Tortuo'sus;** from the same.] Winding; crooked; bent in different directions.

Tor-u-lose'. [**Torulo'sus;** from *tor'ulus*, a "little bed."] Swelled or bulged out in a slight degree; somewhat torose: torulous.

Tor'u-lus.* [Diminutive of *to'rus*, a "bed."] The cavity in which is implanted the base of each antenna of insects.

To'rus.* (A "bed," or "bolster.") The brawn, or thick part, of the arm or leg. Also applied to the receptacle of a flower.

Touch. [Lat. **Tac'tus;** Gr. ἁφή, and ἅψις; Fr. *Toucher*, too'shā'.] One of the five senses. That sense by which we know the physical or palpable qualities of bodies.

Touch, Morbid. See PARAPSIS.

Toucher, too'shā'. (French.) Literally, the "act of touching," or examination by touch. Applied to uterine examination with the fingers *per vaginam.*

Touch'-me-not. The same as NOLI ME TANGERE, which see.

Touch'-Wood. The popular name of the *Polyp'orus ignia'rius*, a fungus found on the willow and other trees, and also called *Agaric of the Oak.* It is used for checking hæmorrhage.

Tourmaline, toor'ma-lin. A crystallized mineral, which is so hard as to scratch glass, and becomes electric when heated. It is transparent when viewed across the thickness of a crystal, but perfectly opaque when turned in the opposite direction. It is composed chiefly of silica and alumina.

Tourniquet, tur'ne-ket. (From the French *Tourner,* to "turn.") An instrument or appliance for compressing the principal blood-vessels, to prevent hæmorrhage in amputations, wounds, etc.

Toux, too. [Lat. **Tus'sis.**] The French word for COUGH, which see.

Toux Convulsive, too kôNG'vül'sēv'. ("Convulsive Cough.") The French name for PERTUSSIS, which see.

Tox-æ'mĭ-a.* The same as TOXICOHÆMIA, which see.

Tox'ĭ-cal. [From τοξικόν, "poison."] Poisonous.

Tox-ĭ-co-den'drum.* [From τοξικόν, "poison," and δένδρον, a "tree."] Poison Oak. The Pharmacopœial name (U.S. and Dub. Ph.) for the leaves of *Rhus toxicodendron.*

Tox-ĭ-co-der-mi'tis, *idis.** [From *tox'icum,* "poison," and *der'ma,* the "skin."] A term for inflammation of the skin through contact with some acrid poison.

Tox-ĭ-co-hæ'mĭ-a,* or **Tox-æ'-mĭ-a.*** [From τοξικόν, a "poison," and αἷμα, "blood."] A contaminated state of the blood; poisoned blood.

Tox-ĭ-col'o-ġy̆. [**Toxicolo'gia;** from τοξικόν, "poison," and λόγος, a "discourse."] The doctrine or science of poisons, their nature and effects; or a treatise on poisons.

Tox-ĭ-co'sis,* plural **Tox-ĭ-co'sēs.** [From *tox'icum,* a "poison."] A term applied to diseases which are the result of poisoning.

Tox-if'er-ous. [**Toxif'erus;** from *tox'icum,* "poison," and *fe'ro,* to "bear."] Bearing or containing poison.

Tr., and **Tra.** = *Tinctu'ra.** "A tincture."

Tra-bec'u-la,* plural **Tra-bec'u-læ.** [Diminutive of *trabs,* a "beam," "pillar," or "column."] Literally, "small or minute columns." Applied to the small medullary fibres of the brain which constitute the commissures, to the fibres, like comb-teeth, constituting the *septum pectiniforme* of the *corpora cavernosa* of the penis, and to other similar structures.

Tra-bec'u-late. [From *trabec'ula,* a "small beam or bar."] Cross-barred.

Tra'che-a* (or tra-kee'a), plural **Tra'-che-æ.** [Gr. τραχεῖα, the feminine of τραχύς, "rough;" Fr. *Trachée,* tRâ'shâ'.] The windpipe. The cartilaginous and membranous canal in front of the œsophagus, extending from the larynx to the lungs, to and from which it conveys the air. Also, a spiral vessel or duct of a plant: so named from its resemblance to the windpipe, or rather to the tracheæ or air-tubes of insects. See SPIRAL VESSELS.

Tra'che-æ,* the plural of TRACHEA.

Tra'che-al. [**Trachea'lis.**] Belonging to the trachea.

Trach-e-a'lĭ-a.* A name for the croup. See TRACHEITIS.

Tra-che-a'rĭ-us.* Having tracheæ.

Tra-che-i'tis, *idis.** [From *tra'chea,* the "windpipe."] Inflammation of the trachea; another name for croup.

Tra-chel'a-gra.* [From τράχηλος, the "neck," and ἄγρα, a "seizure."] Gout, or rheumatism, in the neck.

Tra-che-lis'mus.* [From τράχηλος, the "neck."] A bending back of the neck. Proposed by M. Hall as designating the first symptoms of epilepsy, consisting in contraction of the muscles of the neck, the consequent distension of the veins causing cerebral congestion: trachelism.

Trachelitis. See TRACHEITIS.

Tra-che'lo-Mas-to-ĭ'de-us.* [From τράχηλος, the "neck," and proces'sus *mastoi'deus,* the "mastoid process."] A muscle arising from the transverse processes of the four last cervical, and sometimes of the first dorsal, vertebræ, and inserted into the mastoid process of the temporal bone. It draws the head backward or obliquely.

Tra-chen'chy̆-ma, *atis.** [From *tra'chea,* and ἔγχυμα, "tissue."] In Botany, tissue formed of spiral tubes or vessels like tracheæ. See VASCULAR TISSUE, and SPIRAL VESSELS.

Trach'e-o-tome. [**Tracheot'omus;** from *tra'chea,* the "windpipe," and τέμνω, to "cut."] An instrument for performing tracheotomy.

Tra-che-ot'o-my̆. [**Tracheoto'-mia;** from the same.] The operation of cutting into or opening the trachea. See BRONCHOTOMY.

Tra-cho'ma, *atis.** [From τραχύς, "rough."] Roughness on the internal surface of the eyelid, causing violent ophthalmia and severe pain on moving the eyelid.

Tra-chy̆-pho'nĭ-a.* [From τραχύς, "rough," and φωνή, the "voice."] Roughness of the voice.

Tra-chy̆s'ma.* The same as TRACHOMA, which see.

Trach-ȳ-sta'chȳ-us.* [From τραχύς, "rough," and στάχυς, an "ear," or "spike."] Having spikes rough with hairs.

Tra-chȳt'ic. [**Trachyt'icus;** from τραχύτης, "roughness."] Applied to a group of plutonic earths having a rough appearance.

Tractors, Metallic. See PERKINISM.

Trac'tus.* [From tra'ho, trac'tum, to "draw," or "extend."] An extension: hence, a space, or region.

Trac'tus Mo-to'rĭ-us.* ("Motor Tract.") The name given to the prolongation of the *corpora pyramidalia* through the *pons Varolii* into the *crura cerebri*. The motor nerves arise from this tract.

Trac'tus Op'tĭ-cus.* ("Optic Tract.") The circular tract, or course of the optic nerve from its origin round the *crus cerebri*.

Tractus Respiratorius. See RESPIRATORY TRACT.

Trade Winds. Winds which in the torrid zone, and often a little beyond it, blow generally from the same quarter, varying, according to circumstances, from northeast to southeast. The cause is to be ascribed to the high comparative temperature of the torrid zone, combined with the rotation of the earth. The trade winds are so named because they are often taken advantage of by those engaged in commerce to distant parts of the world.

Trag-a-can'tha.* [From τράγος, a "goat," and ἄκανθα, a "thorn," the plant being called "goat-thorn" on account of its thorny petioles.] Tragacanth. The Pharmacopœial name ‖ for the concrete juice of the *Astragalus verus*, and of other species of *Astragalus*. It is demulcent, but is little employed internally. The great viscidity which it imparts to water, renders it useful for the suspension of heavy insoluble powders.

Trag-a-can'thin. A substance found to compose the whole of gum tragacanth. Also called *Adraganthin*.

Trag'ĭ-cus.* Belonging to the *tragus*. Applied to a muscle of triangular form arising from the middle and outer part of the concha and inserted into the tip of the tragus, which it pulls forward.

Trag-o-po'gon Por-rĭ-fo'lĭ-um.* The systematic name of salsify, or oyster-plant, which belongs to the natural order *Cichoraceæ*.

Tra'gus.* [From τράγος, a "goat;" because it is in many persons covered with hair.] A part of the ear: the same as ANTILOBIUM, which see.

Trailing. See PROCUMBENT.

Trance. An ecstatic or rapt state of mind. Sometimes applied to CATALEPSY.

Trans. A Latin preposition, signifying "across," or "over," sometimes "through;" also, "from one to another."

Tran-sçen-den'tal. [**Transcendenta'lis;** from *trans*, "beyond," and *scan'do*, to "climb."] That which transcends or goes beyond the limits of actual experience.

Trans-for-mā'tion. [**Transforma'tio, o'nis;** from *trans*, "over," "from one to another," and *for'mo, forma'tum*, to "make."] Literally, the act of changing one thing or substance into another. A change of form. A morbid change in a part, consisting in the conversion of its texture into one of a different kind, as of the soft parts into bone or cartilage.

Trans-fu'sion. [**Transfu'sio, o'nis;** from *transfun'do, transfu'sum*, to "pour from one vessel into another."] The introducing of blood taken from the veins of one living animal into those of another; also, the introduction of other fluids than blood.

Tran'sit. [From *tran'seo, tran'situm*, to "pass over."] In Astronomy, the culmination, or passage of a celestial body across the meridian of any place. Also, the passage of an inferior planet across the sun's disk.

Tran-sĭ'tion Rocks. A geological term formerly applied to the older secondary series, under the idea that they were formed during the transition of the globe from the uninhabited to the inhabited state.—(BRANDE.)

Trans-lā'tion. [**Transla'tio, o'nis;** from *transfe'ro, transla'tum*, to "transfer," to "translate."] The act of transferring. See METASTASIS.

Trans-lu'cent, or **Trans-lu'çid.** [**Translu'cidus;** from *trans*, "through," and *lu'ceo*, to "shine."] Penetrable by luminous rays, but too slightly to allow of perceiving objects; semi-transparent; pellucid.

Trans-mu-tā'tion. [From *trans*, "from one to another," and *mu'to, muta'tum*, to "change."] The act of changing one thing into another. In Alchemy, the operation of changing base or imperfect metals into gold or silver.

Trans-pā'rent. [**Transpa'rens, en'tis;** from *trans*, "through," and *pa'reo*, to "appear."] Admitting the passage of the rays of light, so that objects appear or are seen through any medium; diaphanous.

Trans-pi-rā'tion. [**Transpira'tio, o'**nis; from *trans*, "through," and *spi'ro, spira'tum*, to "breathe."] The emission of vapor through the skin; insensible perspiration.

Trans-u-dā'tion. [**Transuda'tio, o'**nis; from *trans*, "through," and *su'do, suda'tum*, to "sweat."] The passing or oozing of blood, or other fluid, unaltered, through the pores of the skin, or membranes; and, so, distinguished from *perspiration*, which implies that the perspired fluid is secreted from the blood.

Trans-ver-sa'lis.* [From *trans*, "across," and *ver'to, ver'sum*, to "turn," to "direct."] The same as TRANSVERSE, which see.

Transversa'lis Ab-dom'i-nis.* ("Transverse [Muscle] of the Abdomen.") A muscle arising from the cartilages of the seven lower ribs, etc., and inserted into the *linea alba* and the crest of the ilium. It supports and compresses the bowels.

Transversa'lis Col'li.* ("Transverse [Muscle] of the Neck.") A muscle arising from the transverse processes of the second, third, fourth, fifth, and sixth, cervical vertebræ, and inserted into those of the third, fourth, fifth, sixth, and seventh upper dorsal vertebræ. It turns the neck obliquely backwards and to one side.

Transversa'lis Dor'si* ("Transverse [Muscle] of the Back"); also termed **Mul-tif'i-dus Spi'næ.*** A muscle situated in the vertebral gutters. Its use is to straighten the vertebral column, and give it a slight rotary motion.

Trans-verse'. [**Transver'sus;** see TRANSVERSALIS.] Directed or placed crosswise. Applied to muscles.

Transverse' Ax'is, in conic sections, is the diameter which passes through both foci. It is the longest diameter of an ellipse, and the shortest of an hyperbola.

Transverse' Su'ture. [**Sutu'ra Transversa'lis.**] That which passes across the face, joining the bones of the skull to those of the face.

Trans-ver'sus Au'ris* ("Transverse [Muscle] of the Ear") **of Al-bi'-nus.** A muscle arising from the prominent part of the concha and inserted opposite to the outer side of the anthelix.

Transver'sus Pe'dis.* ("Transverse [Muscle] of the Foot.") A muscle arising from the metatarsal bone of the great toe and inserted into that of the little toe.

Transver'sus Pĕr-i-næ'i.* ("Transverse [Muscle] of the Perinæum.") A muscle arising from the tuber ischii and inserted into the middle line with its fellow. It is supposed to dilate the urethra.

Tra-pe'zi-form. [**Trapezifor'mis;** from *trape'zium.*] Having the form of a trapezium. In Botany, unsymmetrically four-sided.

Tra-pe'zi-um.* [Gr. τραπέζιον; from τράπεζα, a "dinner-table."] Originally, a quadrangle. Applied in Geometry to a plane figure having four sides, of which no two are parallel. In Anatomy, the name of the first bone of the second row of the *carpus*, or wrist.

Tra-pe'zi-us.* Like a trapezium. Applied to a muscle of the neck and back. See next article.

Tra-pe'zi-us.* A muscle, so named from its form, arising from the superior transverse line of the occipital bone, from the spinous processes of the seventh cervical and of all the dorsal vertebræ, and inserted into the clavicle, the acromion, and the scapula. It draws the scapula according to the three directions of its fibres. It is also termed *Cuculla-ris* (like a hood).

Trap-e-zoid'. [**Trapezoi'des;** from τράπεζα, a "table," and εἶδος, a "form."] Resembling a trapezium. Applied to a four-sided figure of which two sides only are parallel to each other.

Trap Rock. [Swedish, *Trap'pa*, a "stair."] Applied to certain volcanic rocks, which are composed of felspar, augite, and hornblende, and are so named because they occur in large tabular masses rising one above another like the successive steps of a staircase.

Trau-mat'ic. [**Traumat'icus;** from τραῦμα, a "wound."] Relating to, or caused by, a wound; vulnerary.

Trau-mo-ty'phus.* [From τραῦμα, a "wound," and *ty'phus.*] Eisenmann's term for *hospital gangrene.*

Trea'cle. [Lat. **Sac'chari Fæx,** and **Theri'aca;** Fr. *Thériaque*, tà'rè'âk'.] A name for molasses.

Tree. [Lat. **Ar'bor;** Gr. δένδρον; Fr. *Arbre*, aRbR.] A woody plant with a single trunk, which attains at least five times the human stature.

Tree-like. See ARBORESCENT, and DENDROID.

Tre'foil. [From *tres*, "three," and *fo'lium*, a "leaf."] A name for clover. (See TRIFOLIUM PRATENSE.) It is sometimes applied to the *Hepat'ica tril'oba.*

Tre'foil, Marsh, and **Tre'foil, Wa'ter.** Common names for the *Meny-an'thes trifolia'ta,* or buck-bean.

Tremandraceæ,* tre-man-dra'she-ē. [From *Treman'dra,* one of the genera.] A small natural order of exogenous shrubs, all natives of New Holland.

Tremblement. See TREMOR.

Trem'bles. A popular term for mercurial tremor.

Tre'mens.* [From *tre'mo,* to "tremble."] Shaking; trembling. See DELIRIUM TREMENS.

Tre'mor, o'ris.* [From the same.] (Fr. *Tremblement,* tRŏM'bl-mŏNᵍ'.) An involuntary trembling.

Tre'mor Cor'dis.* ("Tremor of the Heart.") A term for palpitation of the heart.

Tre'mor Mer-cu-rĭ-a'lis* ("Mercurial Tremor"); also called **Tre'mor Me-tal'lĭ-cus.*** ("Metallic Tremor.") A form of shaking palsy; an affection of the nervous system induced by the inhalation, or other application to the body, of mercurial vapors.

Tre'mor Ten'dĭ-num.* ("Trembling of the Tendons.") A term for the shaking palsy; a morbid intermittent action of a spasmodic kind.

Tre-pan'. [**Trep'anum;** from τρυπάω, to "bore."] An instrument by which a circular portion of bone is removed from the skull.

Trep-a-nā'tion. [**Trepana'tio, o'nis;** from *trep'anum,* a "trepan."] Trepanning, or operation with the trepan.

Tre-phine'. [**Trephi'na;** perhaps from τρέπω, to "turn."] The more modern instrument for perforating, or removing a circular piece of bone from, the skull.

Tre'sis.* [From τράω, to "bore," to "pierce."] Literally, a "perforation." A wound.

Tri-. [From τρεῖς, or *tres,* "three."] A prefix denoting "three," or "thrice."

Tri-a-can'thus.* [From τρεῖς, "three," and ἄκανθα, a "spine."] Having spines disposed in threes.

Tri-a-del'phous. [**Triadel'phus;** from τρεῖς, "three," and ἀδελφος, a "brother."] Having the filaments in three brotherhoods or sets.

Tri-an'dri-a.* [From τρεῖς, "three," and ἀνήρ, ἀνδρός, a "man," or "male."] The third Linnæan class of plants, comprising those which have three stamens in each flower.

Tri-an'drous. [**Trian'drius;** from the same.] Having three stamens: triandrious.

Tri-an'gu-lar. [**Triangula'ris;** from *tri-,* "three," or "thrice," and *an'gulus,* an "angle."] Having three angles.

Tri-an-gu-la'ris La-bĭ-o'rum.* ("Triangular [Muscle] of the Lips.") A name frequently given to the *depressor anguli oris,* from its triangular shape.

Triangula'ris Ster'ni.* ("Triangular [Muscle] of the Sternum.") A muscle arising from the lower part of the sternum and ensiform cartilage and inserted into the cartilages of the third, fourth, fifth, and sixth ribs. It is also called *sterno-costalis* (*i.e.* "connected with the sternum and ribs"). It depresses the ribs.

Tri-an'thous. [**Trian'thus;** from τρεῖς, "three," and ἄνθος, a "flower."] Three-flowered. Applied to a plant the peduncles of which bear three flowers.

Tri'as. A term for the new red sandstone group of rocks. See next article.

Tri-as'sic. [**Trias'sicus;** from τρίας, a "triad."] Applied to the new red sandstone (or *trias*), because composed of three divisions.

Tri-bā'sic. [**Tribas'icus;** from *tri-,* "three," and *ba'sis,* a "base."] Having three bases. Applied to salts having three equivalents of a base to one of an acid. See BIBASIC.

Tri-cap'su-lar. [**Tricapsula'ris;** from *tri-,* "three," and *cap'sula,* a "capsule."] Applied to fruits formed by the union of three capsules.

Tri-car'pel-la-rȳ. [From τρεῖς, "three," and καρπός, "fruit."] Composed of three carpels.

Tri-car'pous. [**Tricar'pus;** from the same.] In Botany, having three ovaries.

Tri-çeph'a-lous. [**Triceph'alus;** from τρεῖς, "three," and κεφαλή, the "head."] Three-headed. Applied to plants.

Tri'ceps, *ip'itis.** [From *tri-,* "three," and *ca'put,* the "head."] Having three heads. Applied to certain muscles having three origins.

Tri'ceps Au'ris.* ("Three-headed [Muscle] of the Ear.") A name given to the *posterior auris,* because it arises by three distinct slips.

Tri'ceps Ex-ten'sor Cru'ris.* ("Three-headed Extensor of the Leg.") A large muscle which extends the leg. It has been described as consisting of—1. The *Vas'tus exter'nus,* arising from the *trochanter major* and inserted into the patella and fascia of the knee-joint. 2. The *Vas'tus inter'nus,* arising from the *trochanter minor* and inserted in like manner into the patella and fascia. 3. The *Crurœ'us*, arising from between the trochanters and inserted into the patella.

Tri'ceps Exten'sor Cu'bĭ-ti.* ("Three-headed Extensor of the Elbow.") A muscle arising by three heads from the inferior border of the scapula, and from the *os humeri*, and inserted into the olecranon. It extends the forearm.

Trĭ-chan'thus.* [From θρίξ, τριχός, the "hair," and ἄνθος, a "flower."] Having capillary or hair-like flowers.

Tri'chĭ-a,* or **Tri-chi'a-sis.*** [From θρίξ, "hair."] A disease in which the eyelashes are turned in towards the eyeball.

Tri-chĭl'ĭ-a E-met'ĭ-ca.* The Elca'ja; a tree found in Arabia and Senegal. The fruit is used as an emetic.

Tri-chi'na [from θρίξ, "hair," from its minuteness] **Spi-ra'lis.*** A species of minute entozoon found in the muscles. Death is said to be sometimes caused by it.

Tri-chis'mus.* [From θρίξ, "hair."] A hair-like and scarcely perceptible fracture of a bone.

Trich-o-căl-y̆-ci'nus.* [From θρίξ, "hair," and καλύξ, a "calyx."] Having the calyx covered with hair.

Trich-o-car'pus.* [From θρίξ, "hair," and καρπός, "fruit."] Having hairy fruit.

Trich-o-cau'lus.* [From θρίξ, "hair," and καύλος, a "stem."] Having a hairy stem.

Trich-o-ceph'a-lus [from θρίξ, "hair," and κεφαλή, the "head"] **Dis'par.*** The long thread-worm, generally found in the cæcum.

Trī'choid. [**Trichoi'des;** from θρίξ, "hair," and εἶδος, a "form."] Resembling hair.

Trī-chol'o-ġy̆. [**Tricholo'gia;** from θρίξ, "hair," and λόγος, a "discourse."] A treatise on hair, or the science of hair.

Tri-cho'ma, atis.* [From θρίξ, "hair."] *Plica*, or plaited hair; also termed *Trichia*, and *Trichiasis*. A genus of the order *Impetigines*, class *Cachexiæ*, of Cullen's Nosology.

Trich-o-phy̆l'lous. [**Trichophyl'lus;** from θρίξ, "hair," and φύλλον, a "leaf."] Having hairy leaves.

Tri-cho'sis.* [From θρίξ, τριχός, "hair."] A generic term applied by Dr. Good to diseases of the hair.

Trī-chot'o-mous. [**Trichot'omus;** from τρίχα, "threefold," and τέμνω, to "cut."] Divided into threes. In Botany, branched into threes.

Trī'chro-ĭsm. [**Trichrois'mus;** from τρεῖς, "three," and χρόα, "color."] The phenomenon of a body seeming to be of three different colors, according to the way in which the luminous rays traverse it; a phenomenon observed in certain precious stones.

Tri-chu'ris, idis.* [From θρίξ, a "hair," and οὐρά, a "tail."] The long hair-worm.

Trī-coc'cous. [**Tricoc'cus;** from τρεῖς, "three," and κόκκος, a "berry."] Having three *cocci* (separable closed cells).

Trī-cor'ne.* [From *tri-*, "three," and *cor'nu*, a "horn."] A term applied to each lateral ventricle of the brain, from its three-horned shape.

Trī-cus'pid. [**Tricus'pis, idis;** from *tri-*, "three," and *cus'pis*, a "point."] Having three points. Applied to a valve between the right auricle and ventricle of the heart.

Trī-cus'pĭ-date. [**Tricuspida'tus;** from the same.] Having three points. Applied to leaves.

Trī-den'tate. [From *tri-*, "three," and *dens*, *den'tis*, a "tooth."] Three-toothed.

Trī-en'nĭ-al. [From *tri-*, "three," and *an'nus*, a "year."] Lasting three years. Applied to plants.

Trī-fā'cial. [**Trifacia'lis;** from *tri-*, "three," and *fa'cies*, the "face."] Applied to the fifth pair of nerves, their three divisions being distributed on the face. See Trigemini.

Trī-fā'rĭ-ous. [**Trifa'rius.**] In three vertical ranks. Applied to parts of plants.

Trī'fid. [**Trif'idus;** from *tri-*, "three," or "thrice," and *fin'do*, to "cleave."] Three-cleft.

Trī-fo'lĭ-ate. [**Trifolia'tus;** from *tri-*, "three," and *fo'lium*, a "leaf."] Having three leaflets; three-leaved. Applied to a compound leaf, as that of the clover.

Trī-fo'lĭ-um Pra-ten'se.* The systematic name for red clover, a plant of the Linnæan class *Diadelphia*, natural order *Leguminosæ*.

Trī-fur'cate. [From *tres*, "three," and *fur'ca*, a "fork."] Three-forked.

Trig'a-mous. [From τρεῖς, "three," and γάμος, "marriage," or "union."] Applied to plants having on the same flower-head three sorts of flowers, staminate, pistillate, and perfect.

Tri-ġem'ĭ-ni* (*ner'vi* being understood). The "triple nerves." Also termed **Par Tri-ġem'ĭ-num,*** the "triple pair." A name for the fifth and largest pair of the encephalic nerves. It consists of three principal portions or branches, called the *ophthalmic*, the *superior maxillary*, and the *inferior maxillary*. As these three branches are principally distributed to the muscles of the face, they have been termed collectively the *trifacial* nerve.

Trī-ġem'ĭ-nus.* [From *tri-*, "three," and *gem'inus*, "twin," or "double."] Literally, "three double,"—that is, triple. Applied in the plural to a pair of nerves. See preceding article.

Trī'gon. [**Trigo'num;** from τρεῖς, "three," and γωνία, an "angle." See TRIGONE.] A figure of three angles; a triangle.

Trig'o-nal, or **Trī'go-nous.** [**Trigo'nus.**] Three-cornered, or having three angles. Applied to seeds or fruits.

Trigone (Fr.), tre-gōn' [**Trigo'nus;** from *trigo'num*]; called also the **Ves'ĭ-cal Trī'an-gle.** The small triangular space on the lining membrane of the bladder, between the orifice of the urethra and the orifices of the ureters.

Trigone Vésicale (vā'zē'kāl'), or "Vesical Triangle." See TRIGONE.

Trigonella Fœnum. See FENUGREEK.

Tri-gon-o-car'pus.* [From *trigo'nus*, "triangular," and καρπός, "fruit."] Having triangular fruit: trigonocarpous.

Trig-o-no-met'rĭ-cal. [**Trigonomet'ricus.**] Belonging to trigonometry.

Trig-o-nom'e-trȳ. [**Trigonome'tria;** from τρίγωνον, a "triangle," and μετρέω, to "measure."] Originally, the measurement of triangles, or that branch of mathematics which treats of the relations between the sides and angles of triangles. In its modern acceptation, it includes all formulæ relative to angles or circular arcs, and the lines connected with them.

Trĭ'ġȳn-ous. [**Trigyn'ius;** from τρεῖς, "three," and γυνή, a "woman," or "female."] Having three pistils; trigynious.

Trī-he'dral. [**Trihed'ricus,** or **Trihe'drus;** from τρεῖς, "three," and ἕδρα, a "base."] Having three bases or faces: trihe'drous.

Trī'labe. [From *tri-*, "three," and *la'bium*, a "lip;" or perhaps from *tri-*, and λαβεῖν, to "lay hold on;" because it takes a triple hold.] An instrument for extracting foreign bodies from the bladder through the urethra. It has at the termination three branches, or arms, which can be expanded after it is inserted into the bladder.

Trī-lat'e-ral. [From *tri-*, "three," and *la'tus, lat'eris*, a "side."] Three-sided.

Trilliaceæ,* tril-le-a'she-ē. [From *Tril'lium*, one of the genera.] A natural order of endogenous herbaceous plants, found in temperate regions.

Tril'lĭ-um.* A genus of plants of the natural order *Trilliaceæ*. The root is astringent.

Trī'lo-bate. [From *tri-*, "three," and *lo'bus*, a "lobe."] Three-lobed.

Trī-loc'u-lar. [From *tri-*, "three," and *loc'ulus*, a "cell."] Three-celled.

Trĭ'me-rous. [From τρεῖς, "three," and μερός, a "part."] Having three parts in each whorl. Applied to flowers which have three petals, three stamens, etc. It is often printed with figures: as, 3-merous.

Trī-ner'vate. [From *tri-*, "three," and *ner'vus*, a "nerve."] Three-nerved. Applied to leaves.

Triœcious, tri-ē'shŭs. [**Triœ'cius;** from τρεῖς, "three," and οἶκος, a "house," "habitation;" also, "family." See DIŒCIOUS.] Having staminate, pistillate, and perfect flowers on three different plants of the same species.

Tri-os'te-um.* Fever-root. The Pharmacopœial name (U.S. Ph.) for the root of the *Trios'teum perfolia'tum*. The root is cathartic and (in large doses) emetic.

Trī-ov'u-late. [From *tri-*, "three," and *ov'ulum*, an "ovule."] Having three ovules.

Trī-par'tĭ-ble. [From *tri-*, "three," and *par'tio, parti'tum*, to "part."] Capable of being split into three.

Trī-par'tite. [**Triparti'tus;** from the same.] Three-parted.

Trī-pet'a-lous. [From τρεῖς, "three," and πέταλον, a "petal."] Having three petals.

Trī-phȳl'lous. [**Triphyl'lus;** from τρεῖς, "three," and φύλλον, a "leaf."] Having three leaves.

Trī-pin'nate. [From *tri-*, "three," or "thrice," and *pin'na*, a "feather."] Thrice-pinnate. Applied to a leaf in which there are three series of pinnation.

Trī-pin-nat'ĭ-fid. Thrice pinnatifid.

Trip'lĭ-nerved. [**Tripliner'vis;** from *tri'plus*, "triple," and *ner'vus*, a "nerve."] Triple-nerved; triple-ribbed.

Applied to a leaf when the midrib gives off a strong primary vein or branch on each side above the base.

Trip-lo'pi-a.* [From τριπλόος, "triple," and ὄπτομαι, to "see."] Disordered vision in which objects are tripled.

Tri'pod. [From τρεῖς, "three," and πούς, ποδός, a "foot."] A stool, table, or vessel having three feet.

Tri'pod, Vi'tal. A term applied to the heart, lungs, and brain.

Tri-que'tra, Os'sa* [see next article], otherwise called **Os'sa Worm-i-a'na.*** The triangular bones sometimes found in the course of the lambdoidal suture.

Tri-que'trous. [**Trique'trus;** from *trique'tra*, a "triangle."] Triangular; having three salient angles.

Tri-sâlt'. [**Tri'sal, alis;** from *tri-*, "three," or "thrice," and *sal*, a "salt."] A salt containing three times as much acid to the same quantity of base, or three times as much base to the same quantity of acid, as the corresponding neutral salt.

Tri-sep'a-lous. [From *tri-*, "three," and *sep'alum*, a "sepal."] Composed of three sepals.

Tri-se'ri-al. [From *tres*, "three," and *se'ries*, a "row," or "order."] In three rows or ranks, one below another.

Tris'mus.* [From τρίζω, to "gnash."] Lock-jaw or locked-jaw. See TETANUS TRISMUS.

Tris'mus Nascen'tium* (nas-sen'she-um). ("Locked-Jaw of Infants.") Occurring usually within two weeks from their birth.

Tris'mus Trau-mat'i-cus.* Traumatic locked-jaw; that is, locked-jaw arising from a wound.

Tri-splanch'ni-a.* Pinel's term for an affection of the trisplanchnic or great sympathetic nerve. Applied to Oriental cholera.

Tri-splanch'nic Nerve. [**Ner'vus Trisplanch'nicus;** from τρεῖς, "three," and σπλάγχνον, a "viscus;" because it is connected with the viscera of the three great cavities of the body: viz., of the head, thorax, and abdomen.] Also called the **Great Sym-pa-thet'ic.** The name of a nerve, or, rather, a series of ganglia joined together by a multitude of nervous filaments. It extends the whole length of the trunk, and is connected by a branch with each of the thirty pairs of spinal nerves, and also with some of the encephalic nerves. Its peculiar function in the animal economy has not yet been satisfactorily explained. Bichat considered it to be the nervous system of *organic* life, as contradistinguished from the brain and spinal marrow, which, with their appropriate nerves, constitute the nervous system of *animal* life.

Tris'ti-chous. [From τρεῖς, "three," and στιχός, a "row."] In three vertical ranks. Applied to leaves.

Tri-stig-mat'ic. [From *tri-*, "three," and *stig'ma*, *stig'matis*, a "mark," or "stigma."] Having three stigmas.

Tri-sty'lous. [From *tri-*, "three," and *sty'lus*, a "style."] Having three styles.

Trit. = *Trit'ura.** "Triturate."

Tri-ter'nate. [From *tri-*, "three," or "thrice," and *ter'ni*, "three by three."] Thrice ternate. Applied to a compound leaf in which there are three series of ternation.

Trit'i-cin. [**Tritici'na.**] The gluten of wheat.

Trit'i-cum.* [From *te'ro*, *tri'tum*, to "thresh."] A Linnæan genus of the class *Triandria*, natural order *Gramineæ*.

Trit'icum Æ-sti'vum.* ("Summer Wheat.") The wheat-plant; more properly applied to the variety known as "spring wheat."

Trit'icum Hy-ber'num.* ("Winter Wheat.") The name of a species or variety commonly known as winter wheat.

Trit'icum Vul-ga're.* ("Common Wheat.") Another name for the wheat-plant. See TRITICUM ÆSTIVUM.

Tri-tox'ide. [**Tritox'ydum;** from *tri-*, and *ox'ydum*, an "oxide."] An oxide which contains one atom of base united to three atoms of oxygen.

Trit-u-ra'tion. [**Tritura'tio, o'nis;** from *te'ro*, *tri'tum*, to "rub," or "bray."] The process of reducing solid bodies to powder by continued rubbing.

Triv'i-al. [**Trivia'lis;** from *triv'ium*, a "place where three ways meet."] Originally, "much frequented:" hence, "common." The trivial name is the popular name of a plant. In Botany, used synonymously with specific, being applied to the name which is added to the generic name; for example, *Gallica* is the trivial name in the compound appellation *Rosa Gallica*.

Trocar, tro'kår. [From *trois quarts*, "three-quarters," on account of its three-sided point.] A sharp-pointed instrument used in the operation of tapping, or *paracentesis*.

Troch. = *Trochis'cus.** "A troche, or lozenge."

Tro-chan'ter, e'ris.* [From τροχάω, to "turn," or "revolve."] Applied originally to the ball on which the femur turned in its socket. Applied to two processes of the femur, major and minor. Also to the second joint of the hind leg of insects; and to the second piece of the simple limb of the *Crustaceæ*.

Trochar. See TROCAR.

Troche (trōtch), or **Troch.** See TROCHISCUS.

Tro-chid-ĭ-for'mis,* or **Tro-chĭ-for'mis.*** [From τροχός, a "wheel."] Resembling a wheel.

Troch'ĭ-nus.* [From τροχός, a "wheel."] Chaussier's term for the smaller of the two superior eminences of the *os humeri*.

Tro-chis'cus,* plural **Tro-chis'çi.** [Diminutive of τροχός, a "wheel;" because often made in the shape of a wheel.] A troche, or lozenge, usually consisting of some medicinal substance incorporated with sugar or mucilage. (See U.S. Pharmacopœia, page 339.)

Troch'ĭ-ter, e'ris.* The larger of the two eminences mentioned under TROCHINUS.

Trochlea,* trŏk'le-a. [From τροχός, a "wheel"] The fibro-cartilaginous pulley near the internal angular process of the frontal bone, through which the tendon of the *obliquus superior* muscle passes.

Troch'le-ar. [**Trochlea'ris.**] Belonging to the trochlea. In Botany, pulley-shaped.

Troch-le-a'ris.* A name for the *obli'quus supe'rior*, a muscle of the eye which passes through the trochlea.

Troch-le-a'tor, o'ris.* Applied in the plural (*Trochleato'res*) to the fourth pair of nerves, because distributed to the *trochlearis* muscle. See PATHETIC NERVES.

Troch-le-a-to'rēs,* the plural of TROCHLEATOR, which see.

Tro'choid. [**Trochoi'des;** from τροχός, a "wheel," and εἶδος, a "form."] Resembling a wheel. Applied to a movable connection of bones in which one rotates upon another.

Trompe ou Conduit d' Eustache. The French term for EUSTACHIAN TUBE, which see.

Tronc. See TRUNCUS.

Tro-pæ'o-lum Ma'jus.* The systematic name of the nasturtium, a plant of the natural order *Geraniaceæ*. It is reputed antiscorbutic.

Troph'ĭ-cal. [**Troph'icus;** from τροφή, "nourishment."] Pertaining to nutrition.

Troph-o-neu-ro'sis.* [From τροφή, "nourishment," and *neuro'sis*.] A species of fatal atrophy, in which the process of nutrition suffers from diminished nervous influence.

Troph'o-sperm. [**Trophosper'mium;** from τροφός, a "nurse," or "nourisher," and σπέρμα, a "seed."] A name for the placenta of plants.

Trop'ic. [**Trop'icus;** from τροπικός, "pertaining to a turning."] One of the two parallels of latitude on the earth, distant from the equator 23½°, and marking the utmost limit of the sun's advance northward or southward at the summer or winter solstice; so named because at this point the sun seems to stop in its northward or southward course, and *turn* backwards; the Northern is called the Tropic of Cancer, the Southern, that of Capricorn.

Trop'ĭ-cal. [Gr. τροπικός; from τροπή, a "turn," or "return."] Growing near or between the tropics; belonging to the tropics.

Trough, Pneumatic. See PNEUMATIC TROUGH.

Trousse. See TRUSS.

True Ribs. The seven superior, or the sternal, ribs, attached to the sternum by distinct cartilages.

True Spi'nal Mar'row. The spinal cord.

Truf'fle. [**Lycoper'don Tu'ber.**] A subterranean fungus used as an aliment.

Trum'pet-Shaped. Tubular, with the summit dilated. Applied to flowers.

Trun'cate, or **Trun'cāt-ed.** [**Trunca'tus;** from *trun'co, trunca'tum*, to "cut off."] In Botany, shaped as if cut off at the end. Applied to leaves. A truncated cone (or pyramid) is one whose vertex has been cut off by a plane parallel to the base.

Trunk. [Lat. **Trun'cus;** Fr. *Tronc*, trôNG.] Originally, the body, exclusive of head and extremities: now often applied to the head and body without the limbs. In Botany, the main stem or column of a tree, exclusive of its branches.

Truss. [Lat. **Brache'rium;** Fr. *Trousse*, trooss.] A support or bandage of peculiar construction, adapted to several kinds of hernia.

Tuba Eustachiana. See EUSTACHIAN TUBE.

Tuba Fallopiana. See FALLOPIAN TUBES.

Tube. [From *tu'bus*, a "pipe," or "tube."] In Botany, the portion of a calyx or corolla formed by the union of the sepals or petals.

Tube, Pollen. See POLLEN TUBE.

Tu'ber, er*is*.* [From *tu'meo*, to "swell."] A knob or excrescence. Applied in Anatomy to a hump or protuberance. In Botany, a short and thickened subterranean branch, as the edible part of the potato, popularly included under the term "root." In Surgery, a knot, enlargement, or swelling of any part.

Tuber Annulare. See PONS VAROLII.

Tu'ber Ci-ne're-um.* ("Ash-colored Tuber.") An eminence of gray substance, forming part of the floor of the third ventricle of the brain.

Tu'ber Is'chĭ-i.* ("Tuber of the Ischium.") A round knob forming that point of the ischium on which we sit: hence this bone has been named *os sedentarium* ("sedentary bone").

Tu'ber-cle. [**Tuber'culum;** diminutive of *tu'ber*, a "knob," or "swelling."] A small swelling or tumor in the substance of an organ. A morbid product occurring in various textures of the body, resulting from a peculiar morbid habit or condition of the system known as *tubercular diathesis*. In Botany, a small tuber or excrescence.

Tu'ber-cled. Bearing excrescences. Applied to plants.

Tu-ber'cu-la.* [Plural of *tuber'culum*, a "tubercle," or "little knob."] An order in Willan's Cutaneous Diseases, comprising small, hard, prominent, and circumscribed tumors, permanent or partially suppurating.

Tuber'cula Quad-ri-ġem'ĭ-na.* ("Quadruple Tubercles.") [See QUADRIGEMINUS.] Also termed **Cor'po-ra Quadrigem'ina*** ("Quadruple Bodies"), and **Em-ĭ-nen'tĭ-æ Quadrigem'inæ*** ("Quadruple Eminences, or Protuberances"). The four oval-shaped bodies situated below the posterior commissure of the brain. The two superior and larger are termed the *nates*, the other two the *testes*.

Tu-ber'cu-lar. [**Tubercula'ris;** from *tuber'culum*.] Having tubercles; tubercled.

Tuber'cular Phthis'is. Consumption caused or attended by the development of tubercles in the lungs.

Tu-ber-cu-lif'er-ous. [**Tuberculif'erus;** from *tuber'culum*, a "tubercle," and *fe'ro*, to "bear."] Bearing tubercles.

Tu-ber-cu-li'tis.* [From *tuber'culum*, a "tubercle."] Inflammation of a tubercle.

Tu-ber-cu-lo'sis.* The formation of tubercles or tuberculous disease; also applied to the morbid condition which gives rise to tubercles.

Tu-ber'cu-lum An-nu-la're.* ("Annular Protuberance:" so called because its transverse *striæ* present the appearance of numerous small rings.) A name for the PONS VAROLII, which see.

Tuberculum Loweri. See LOWERI TUBERCULUM.

Tu-be-rif'er-ous. [**Tuberif'erus;** from *tu'ber*, and *fe'ro*, to "bear."] Bearing or having tubers.

Tu-be-ros'ĭ-tȳ. [**Tuberos'itas;** from *tu'ber*, a "knob."] An eminence or process of a bone, which gives attachment to muscles or ligaments.

Tuberos'ity of the Is'chĭ-um. The same as TUBER ISCHII, which see.

Tu'ber-ous. [**Tubero'sus.**] Having tubers, or resembling tubers: tu'berose.

Tu-bif'er-ous. [**Tubif'erus;** from *tu'bus*, a "tube," and *fe'ro*, to "bear."] Bearing or having tubes.

Tu-bĭ-flo'rus.* [From *tu'bus*, a "tube," and *flos*, a "flower."] Having a tubulous corolla; that is, having the tube of the corolla very long: tubiflo'rous.

Tu'bĭ-form [**Tubifor'mis,** or **Tubæfor'mis;** from *tu'ba*, a "trumpet"]; written also **Tu'be-form.** Formed like a trumpet, or tube enlarged at one of its extremities.

Tu'biform. [**Tubifor'mis;** from *tu'bus*, a "tube."] Formed like a tube.

Tu'bu-lar. [**Tubula'ris;** from *tu'bulus*, a "little tube."] Resembling a tube; tube-shaped. Applied to a form of monopetalous corolla; as that of the *Lonice'ra* (Honeysuckle).

Tu'bu-lāt-ed, or **Tu'bu-lous.** [**Tubula'tus;** from the same.] Formed like a tube; tubular.

Tu'bule. [**Tu'bulus.**] A small tube.

Tu'bu-li.* [Plural of TUBULUS.] ("Little Tubes.") Applied to several sets of minute vessels in different situations of the body.

Tu'buli Rec'ti.* ("Straight Tubules.") From twelve to twenty small tubes which pass in parallel lines to the back and upper part of the testicle, forming there an oblong eminence termed the *Corpus Highmori* or *Corpus Highmorianum* ("Highmorian Body").

Tu'buli Sem-ĭ-nif'e-ri.* ("Seminiferous Tubules.") The small, fine, tubular threads, about the two-hundredth of an inch in diameter, which, folded on each other, compose the substance of the testicle.

Tu'buli U-rĭ-nif'e-ri.* ("Uriniferous Tubules.") The small fine vessels of a pale color and dense structure, arranged in eight or ten conical *fasciculi*, which have their bases to the circumference, and their apices, or papillæ, towards the concave edge of the kidney.

Tu'bu-lĭ-bran-chĭ-a'tus.* [From *tu'bulus*, a "tubule," and *bran'chiæ*.] Having a tubular shell for the branchiæ: tubulibran'chiate.

Tu-bu-lif'er-ous. [**Tubulif'erus;** from *tu'bulus*, a "little tube," and *fe'ro*, to "bear."] Bearing little tubes.

Tu-bu-lĭ-flo'rus.* [From *tu'bulus*, a "little tube," and *flos*, a "flower."] Having tubular flowers: tubuliflo'rous.

Tu'bu-lĭ-form. [**Tubulifor'mis.**] Formed like a small tube.

Tu-bu-lose'. [**Tubulo'sus.**] The same as TUBULAR, which see.

Tu'bu-lus,* plural **Tu'bu-li.** [Diminutive of *tu'bus*, a "tube."] A little tube: a tu'bule.

Tu'bus.* A tube, or hollow cylinder. The inferior part of a calyx or a corolla. See TUBE.

Tu'fa.* A volcanic rock, composed of an agglutination of fragmented scoriæ.

Tu-lip-if'er-ous. [**Tulipif'erus;** from *tu'lipa*, a "tulip," and *fe'ro*, to "bear."] Bearing flowers like the tulip.

Tu'lip-Tree. A common name for the *Liriođen'dron tulipif'era*. See LIRIODENDRON.

Tul'pĭ-i Văl'va.* ("Valve of Tulpius.") A name applied to the ileo-cæcal valve. See BAUHIN, VALVE OF.

Tu-me-fac'tion. [**Tumefac'tio, o'nis;** from *tumefa'cio*, *tumefac'tum*, to "make to swell."] A swelling or enlargement, from whatever cause.

Tu-mĕs'çence. [**Tumescen'tia;** from *tumes'co*, to "swell."] The same as TUMEFACTION.

Tu'mid. [**Tu'midus;** from *tu'meo*, to "swell."] Swollen, or somewhat inflated.

Tu'mor,* plural **Tu-mo'rēs.** [From *tu'meo*, to "swell."] A morbid enlargement, from whatever cause; commonly applied to a permanent swelling or enlargement. Tumors may be distinguished into the *sarcomatous*, so named from their firm fleshy feel, and the *encysted*, commonly called wens.

Tu'mor O-va'rĭ-i.* ("Tumor of the Ovary.") See OARIONCUS.

Tu-mo'rēs,* the plural of TUMOR, which see.

Tung'stāte. [**Tung'stas, a'tis.**] A combination of tungstic acid with a base.

Tung'sten. [**Tungste'nium;** from the Swedish *tung*, "heavy," and *sten*, "stone."] A white, hard, brittle metal, very difficult of fusion, and having the high specific gravity of 17.4.

Tung'stic. [**Tung'sticus;** from *tungste'nium*, "tungsten."] Belonging to tungsten. Applied to an oxide which is the first, and to an acid that is the second, degree of oxidation of tungsten.

Tu'nĭ-ca.* [Perhaps from *tu'eor*, to "defend," or "protect."] A Latin word signifying a "coat," a "tunic." Applied to a covering, membrane, etc.

Tu'nica Ad-na'ta.* ("Adnate Coat or Membrane.") A term for that part of the conjunctiva which is in contact with the eyeball.

Tu'nica Al-bu-gin'e-a Oc'u-li.* ("White Tunic of the Eye.") Applied to the tendinous expansions of the muscles that move the eye, closely connected with the sclerotic coat.

Tu'nica Albugin'ea Tes'tis.* ("White Coat of the Testicle.") A strong, white, dense membrane forming the immediate covering of the testicle. See ALBUGINEOUS.

Tu'nica A-rach-no-i'dēs.* ("Arachnoid Tunic or Membrane.") The fine, thin membrane of the brain, situated between the *dura mater* and *pia mater*.

Tunica Choroides. See CHOROID MEMBRANE.

Tu'nica Com-mu'nis.* ("Common Tunic:" so called because common to the cord and testicle.) A tunic surrounding the spermatic cord and testicle, composed of the expanded fibre of the cremaster muscle and the connecting cellular tissue.

Tunica Conjunctiva. See CONJUNCTIVUS.

Tu'nica De-cid'u-a Re-flex'a.* ("Deciduous Reflexed Membrane.") See DECIDUA REFLEXA.

Tu'nica Decid'ua U'te-ri.* ("Deciduous Membrane of the Uterus.") See DECIDUA VERA.

Tunica Jacobi. See MEMBRANA JACOBI.

Tu'nica Ret'i-na.* ("Net-form Membrane.") Another name for the RETINA, which see.

Tu'nica Vag-i-na'lis Tes'tis.* ("Vaginal Coat of the Testicle.") A pouch of serous membrane derived from the peritonæum and covering the testis.

Tu-ni-ca'ta.* [From *tu'nica*, a "tunic."] The first class of the *Cyclo-gangliata*, or Mollusks, comprising soft, aquatic acephalous animals, having their body enveloped in an elastic tunic furnished with at least two apertures.

Tu'ni-cāt-ed, or **Tu'ni-cate.** [**Tunica'tus;** from the same.] Covered; coated; having an accessory covering.

Tu'nicated Bulb. A bulb with broad scales in concentric layers, as the onion.

Turbeth (or **Turbith**) **Mineral.** See TURPETH MINERAL.

Tur'beth Plant. The *Convolvulus turpethum.*

Tur'bi-nal. [**Turbina'lis;** from *turbina'tum* os.] Proposed by Owen for the homologues of the inferior turbinated or spongy bone.

Tur'bi-nate, or **Tur'bi-nāt-ed.** [**Turbina'tus;** from *tur'bo, tur'binis*, a "top."] Formed like a top; wreathed conically from a base to a sort of apex.

Tur'binated Bones. [**Os'sa Turbina'ta.**] "Top-shaped bones." Two bones of the nostrils: so called from their being formed like a top. They are also called inferior spongy bones, and *ossa convoluta*, or "convoluted bones."

Tur'bi-ni-flo'rus.* [From *tur'bo, tur'binis*, a "top," and *flos*, a "flower."] Having turbinated flowers: turbiniflo'rous.

Tur'bi-ni-form. [**Turbinifor'mis;** from *tur'bo, tur'binis*, a "top."] The same as TURBINATED.

Turf. [**Ces'pes.**] A grassy sod; the surface of grass-lands of a smooth and uniform texture, covered with pasture-grass. The term is also sometimes applied to peat cut out of a bog.

Tur-ġĕs'çence. [From *turges'co*, to "begin to swell."] A superabundance of humors in a part; turgidity.

Turgidity. See TURGESCENCE.

Tur'gor Vi-ta'lis.* A synonym of TURGESCENCE, which see.

Tu'ri-on. [**Tu'rio, o'nis;** from *ty'ro*, a "young beginner."] The early state of a sucker or subterranean shoot, as an asparagus-shoot.

Tu-ri-o-nif'er-ous. [**Turionif'erus;** from *tu'rio*, a "turion," and *fe'ro*, to "bear."] Producing turions.

Tur'key Rhu'barb. The *Rheum palmatum.* See RHEUM.

Tur'me-ric. The root of *Curcuma longa.* See CURCUMA.

Tur'meric Pa'per. White, bibulous, and unsized paper, brushed over with tincture of turmeric, prepared by digesting one part of bruised turmeric in six parts of proof-spirit. It is often used in the chemical laboratory as a test of the presence of free alkalies and their carbonates, by which its yellow color is changed to brown.

Turn of Life. The same as CHANGE OF LIFE, which see.

Tur'ner's Ce'rate. The *Ceratum Calaminæ*, or "cerate of calamine" (Lond. and Ed. Ph.), the *Unguentum Calaminæ* of the Dublin Pharmacopœia.

Turpentine. See TEREBINTHINA.

Turpentine, Chian. See TEREBINTHINA CHIA.

Turpentine, Common. See TEREBINTHINA VULGARIS.

Turpentine, Cyprian. See TEREBINTHINA CHIA.

Turpentine, Oil of. See OIL OF TURPENTINE.

Tur'pen-tine, Spir'its of. The same as OIL OF TURPENTINE.

Turpentine, Venice. See TEREBINTHINA VENETA.

Tur'peth (or **Tur'beth**) **Min'e-ral.** [**Tur'pethum Minera'le.**] A common name for HYDRARGYRI SULPHAS FLAVA, which see.

Tur'pe-thum Ni'grum.* A name for the black oxide of mercury (*Hydrar'gyri ox'ydum cine'reum* or *ni'grum*).

Tur-quoise'. A blue precious stone found in great quantities in the Nishapoor mines in Persia, consisting chiefly of hydrated alumina.

Tu-run'da,* plural **Tu-run'dæ.** A tent or suppository.

Tushy-Stone. See TUTTY.

Tus-si-la'go Far'fa-ra.* Colt's-foot. A plant of the Linnæan class *Syngenesia*, natural order *Compositæ.* It is demulcent and expectorant.

Tus'sis.* A cough.

Tus'sis Con-vul-si'va* ("Convulsive Cough"), **Tus'sis Fe-ri'na*** ("Fierce or Savage Cough"). Names for *pertussis*, or hooping-cough.

Tus'sive. [From *tus'sis*, a "cough."] Relating to, or caused by, cough.

Tut'ty̆. [**Tu'tia.**] (Persian.) A gray oxide of zinc, vulgarly called tushy-stone.

Twin-Forked. See BIGEMINATE.

Twi'ning. [**Volu'bilis.**] Winding spirally round a support, as a twining plant.

Twink'ling. The tremulous motion of the light of the fixed stars, attributed to the unequal refraction caused by inequalities and undulations in the atmosphere. See SCINTILLATION.

Twins. [**Gem'ini.**] Two children born of one woman at the same accouchement.

Two-Ranked. See DISTICHOUS.

Ty̆ch'i-ca.* [From τύχη, an "accident."] Accidental wounds or deformities.

Ty-loph'o-ra Asth-mat'i-ca.* An East Indian plant of the natural order *Asclepiadaceæ*. The root is emetic and cathartic.

Ty-lo'sis.* [From τύλος, a "callosity."] A swollen and knotty state of the eyelids, in which their margin often loses altogether its natural form and appearance.

Ty̆-los-te-re'sis.* [From τύλος, a "callus," and στέρησις, "privation."] Extirpation or removal of a callus.

Ty̆m'pa-nal. [**Tympana'lis.**] Belonging to the tympanum.

Ty̆m'pa-nic, or tim-pan'ik. [**Tympan'icus;** from *tym'panum*, the "drum of the ear."] Relating to the tympanum.

Ty̆m-pa-ni'tēs.* [From *tym'panum*, a "drum."] Tympany; wind-dropsy. A genus of the order *Intumescentiæ*, class *Cachexiæ*, of Cullen's Nosology.

Ty̆m'pa-num.* [From τύμπανον, a "drum."] The drum, or hollow part of the *middle ear*, containing the *ossicula*.

Ty̆pe. [From *ty'pus*, a "form," or "type." See TYPUS.] In Botany, a pattern or ideal plan. The leaf is assumed as the type or pattern to which all the other organs (arising from the ascending axis) may be referred; that is, all those organs are considered as modifications or transformations of a leaf. Also, a letter, or a piece of metal moulded into the form of a letter or character.

Ty̆pe-Met'al. An alloy of lead and antimony, with a small proportion of tin, used in casting printers' types. One part of antimony to three of lead are the usual proportions.

Typhaceæ,* ti-fa'she-ē. A natural order of endogenous herbaceous plants, growing in marshes or ditches in the northern parts of the world. It includes the *Ty'pha* (Cat-tail).

Ty'phæ,* the plural of *Ty'pha*, forming the Jussieuan name of an order of plants. See TYPHACEÆ.

Ty-pho'dēs.* [From *ty'phus*.] Having, or pertaining to, typhus: ty'phous.

Ty̆'phoid. [**Typhoi'des;** from *ty'phus*, and εἶδος, a "form."] Resembling typhus.

Ty'phoid Fe'ver. [**Fe'bris Typhoi'des.**] Applied to a fever distinguished from typhus by a lesion of the intestines, but closely resembling it in other respects. By many it is thought to be typhus merely complicated with the intestinal lesion.

Ty̆'pho-Ma-lā'ri-al. A term applied to a group of fevers in which the typhoid and malarial elements are variously blended.

Ty-pho-ma'ni-a.* [From τῦφος, "stupor," and μανία, "madness."] A low, lethargic state, complicated with muttering delirium, characterizing typhus fever.

Ty̆-phoon'. [From the Chinese *ta*, "great," and *foong*, "wind."] A name given to a violent tornado or hurricane in the Chinese seas.

Ty-pho'sus.* The same as TYPHODES, which see.

Ty̆'phus.* [From τῦφος, a "heavy stupor."] A kind of continued fever, attended with great prostration of the nervous and vascular systems, with a tendency to putrefaction in the fluids, and vitiation of the secretions; putrid fever. A genus of the order *Febres*, class *Pyrexiæ*, of Cullen's Nosology.

Ty'phus Car'ce-rum.* ("Typhus of Prisons.") The jail-fever, a name for *Typhus gravior;* also called *Febris carcerum* ("fever of prisons").

Ty'phus Cas-tren'sis.* ("Camp Typhus.") A name for *Typhus gravior;* otherwise called *Febris castrensis*, or "camp fever." These names, however, must be understood to refer to European armies. Typhus, in its *unmixed character*, has seldom, if ever, made its appearance in the armies of the United States.

Ty'phus Gra'vi-or.* ("Severer Typhus.") The malignant form of typhus; also called, according to circumstances, *Febris carcerum*, and *Febris castrensis*. See the two preceding articles.

Ty'phus Mit'ior* (mish'e-or).

("Milder Typhus.") The milder form of typhus, or low fever; slow fever; also called *Febris lenta* ("slow fever"), *Febris nervosa* ("nervous fever").

Ty'phus Ner-vo'sus.* ("Nervous Typhus.") A name for *Typhus mitior; Febris nervosa.*

Ty'phus Pe-te-chĭ-a'lis* ("Petechial Typhus"), or typhus with purple spots, a name for *Typhus gravior;* called also *Febris petechialis* ("petechial fever").

Tўp'ĭ-cal, or **Tўp'ic.** [From *ty'pus*, a "type."] Representing the type, or plan; figurative; representative.

Tў-pog'ra-phў. [**Typogra'phia;** from τύπος, a "type," and γράφω, to "write."] The art of printing.

Tўp'o-lite. [**Typol'ithus;** from *ty'pus*, a "type," and λίθος, a "stone."] A stone with impressions of organic, vegetable, or animal bodies: a typolith.

Ty'pus.* [From τύπτω, to "strike," or "stamp."] Literally, a "mould," or "pattern." Applied to the form, order, and progress of fevers, etc.: a type.

Tўr-e-i'na.* [From τυρός, "cheese."] The same as CASEIN, which see.

Ty-rem'e-sis [from τυρός, "cheese," and ἔμεσις, a "vomiting"] **Infan'tium*** (in-fan'she-um). The caseous vomiting of infants.

Tўr'o-sīne. [**Tyrosi'na;** from τυρός, "cheese."] The essential ingredient of cheese. See CASEIN.

Ty-so'ni Glan'du-læ.* ("Tyson's Glandules.") The *Glandulæ odoriferæ,* small sebaceous glands around the *corona glandis* of the penis, and on the *labia pudendi* and *nymphæ.*

U.

U-læm-or-rha'ġĭ-a.* [From οὖλον, the "gum," and *hæmorrha'gia.*] Bleeding from the gums.

U-la-tro'phĭ-a.* [From οὖλον, the "gum," and *atro'phia*, "atrophy."] Wasting or shrinking away of the gums.

Ul'çer. [**Ul'cus,** *eris.*] A solution of continuity in any soft parts by ulceration on some internal or external surface.

Ul'ce-rāt-ed. [**Ulcera'tus;** from *ul'cus*, an "ulcer."] Affected with ulcers; having ulcers.

Ul-ce-rā'tion. [**Ulcera'tio, o'***nis;* from the same.] The formation of an ulcer; or that process by which ulcers are formed, consisting in the old particles of the textures affected being taken up by the absorbents more rapidly than new particles are supplied by the secerning arteries.

Ul'ce-ra-tīve. [**Ulcerati'vus;** from the same.] Pertaining to or causing ulceration.

Ul'cer-ous. [**Ulcero'sus;** from *ul'cus, ul'ceris*, an "ulcer."] Having ulcers; of the nature of an ulcer.

Ul'cus,* gen. **Ul'çe-ris.** A Latin term signifying an "ulcer."

U-liġ'ĭ-nous, or **U-liġ'ĭ-nose.** [**Uligino'sus;** from *uli'go, ulig'inis*, "moisture of the earth."] Oozy or slimy; also, growing or living in moist and marshy meadows.

U-li'tis, i*dis.** [From οὖλον, the "gum."] Inflammation of the gums.

Ulmaceæ,* ŭl-ma'she-ē. A natural order of exogenous trees and shrubs, natives of Europe, Asia, and North America. It includes the *Ul'mus* (Elm) and other timber-trees.

Ul'mic. [**Ul'micus;** from *ul'mus*, the "elm."] Belonging to the elm. Applied to an acid obtained from it.

Ul'min. [From the same.] A peculiar vegetable principle which exudes spontaneously from the trunk of a species of elm, supposed to be the *Ulmus nigra.*

Ul'mus.* (Fr. *Orme*, ORM.) A Linnæan genus of the class *Pentandria*, natural order *Ulmaceæ.* Also, the Pharmacopœial name (Br. Ph.) for the inner bark of *Ulmus campestris;* but according to the United States Pharmacopœia, the inner bark of *Ulmus fulva.*

Ul'mus Cam-pes'tris.* ("Elm of the Open Fields.") A species of European elm, the bark of which is used as a demulcent, and sometimes as a tonic, astringent, and diuretic.

Ul'na.* [From ὠλένη, the "elbow," also, the "arm."] The larger bone of the forearm; also termed *cubitus.*

Ul'nar. [**Ulna'ris;** from *ul'na.*] Belonging to the ulna or cubit; used by Dr. Barclay as meaning towards the ulna.

Ul-na'ris.* The name of two muscles of the forearm:—1. A *flexor* muscle, arising from the inner condyle of the *os humeri* and inserted into the pisiform bone. 2. An *extensor* muscle, arising from the outer condyle of the *os humeri* and inserted into the little finger.

U-lo-car-çi-no'mą, atis.* [From οὖλον, the "gum," and *carcino'ma*, "cancer."] Cancer of the gums or *alveoli*.

U-lon'cus.* [From οὖλον, the "gum," and ὄγκος, a "tumor."] A tumor or swelling of the gum.

U-lor-rha'ġi-ą.* [From οὖλον, the "gum," and ῥήγνυμι, to "burst forth."] A sudden discharge of blood from the gums.

U-lor-rhœ'ą.* [From οὖλον, the "gum," and ῥέω, to "flow."] An oozing (of blood) from the gums.

Ul'ti-mate. [From *ul'timus*, "last," or "utmost;" the superlative degree of *ul'tra*, "beyond."] The last, or farthest; extreme. See next article.

Ul'ti-mate A-nal'y̆-sis. A term applied in Chemistry to the resolution of substances into their absolute or simple elements, and opposed to *proximate analysis*, by which they are merely resolved into secondary compounds.

Ul'timate El'e-ments, or **Ul'ti-mate Prin'ci-ples.** Those which compose proximate principles; in other words, the last to which we can trace the constitution of substances. See ULTIMATE ANALYSIS, and PROXIMATE PRINCIPLES.

Ul-trą-marine (-mą-reen'). [From *ul'tra*, "beyond," and *ma're*, the "sea;" implying that its color surpasses the deep blue of the sea.] A blue powder or pigment obtained from the *lapis lazuli*, and highly prized for the beauty and permanence of its color.

-ulus, -ula, and **-ulum.** Latin terminals denoting diminutives. Compare TUBULUS, SPICULA, and ANIMALCULUM.

Umb. = *Umbili'cus.** The "navel."

Um'bel, or **Um-bel'lą.*** [Diminutive of *um'bra*, a "shade."] An umbrella-shaped inflorescence in which several flower-stalks arise from the same apparent point, so as to resemble the rays of an umbrella, as in the Milkweed, Parsley, etc.

Um'bel-late. [From *umbel'la*, an "umbel."] Bearing or having umbels.

Um'bel-let. [From the same.] A secondary or partial umbel.

Um-bel-lif'e-ræ.* [See next article.] A natural order of exogenous herbaceous plants, found mostly in temperate or cold climates, and named from the mode of inflorescence. Some are esculent, as parsnip and celery; many produce aromatic seeds, as coriander and caraway. The hemlock (*Cicuta*) and others are poisonous. Among the products of this order is *Assafœtida*.

Um-bel-lif'er-ous. [**Umbellif'erus;** from *umbel'la*, an "umbel," and *fe'ro*, to "bear."] Bearing umbels. See UMBELLIFERÆ.

Um-bel'lu-lą.* [Diminutive of *umbel'la*, an "umbel."] A little or partial umbel; an umbellule.

Um'ber. [Probably from *Om'bria*, where it was obtained.] A brown clay iron-ore, used as a pigment.

Um-bil'i-cal. [**Umbilica'lis.**] Pertaining to the umbilicus.

Umbil'ical Cord. [**Fu'nis Umbilica'lis.**] The navel-string.

Umbil'ical Re'gion. [**Mesogas'trium.**] That portion of the abdomen two or three inches above, below, and on each side of the umbilicus.

Umbilical Vesicle. See BLASTODERMIC VESICLE.

Um-bil'i-cate. [**Umbilica'tus;** from *umbili'cus*, the "navel."] Dimpled; depressed in the centre like the navel. Applied to parts of plants.

Um-bi-li'cus.* See Preface, page ix.) [From ὀμφαλικός, "pertaining to the navel"?] (Fr. *Nombril*, nôm'brè'.) The navel. In Botany, the hilum of a seed.

Um'bo-nate. [From *um'bo*, the "boss of a shield."] Bearing an *umbo*, boss, or central projection.

Um-brac'u-li-form. [From *umbrac'ulum*, a "parasol."] Umbrella-shaped. Applied to plants.

U-ną-bran'chi-us.* [From *u'nus*, "one only," and *branchiæ*.] Having *branchiæ* only on one side of the body.

Un'ci-ą.* An ounce; a weight containing eight drachms. In Troy weight, as well as in apothecaries' weight, the twelfth part of a pound.

Un'ci-form, or **Un'ci-nate.** [**Uncina'tus;** from *un'cus*, a "hook."] Hooked; shaped like a hook.

Uncinate. See UNCIFORM.

Un'date. The same as UNDULATE, which see.

Undershrub. See SUFFRUTEX.

Un'du-late, or **Un'du-lāt-ed.** [**Undula'tus;** from *un'dula*, a "little wave."] Waved or wavy; having a margin alternately concave and convex.

Un'du-lą-to-ry̆ The'o-ry̆. In Optics, the theory which maintains that the impression of light is conveyed to the eye by the vibrations or undulations of a very subtle and elastic fluid, or ether, which pervades all space and penetrates all substances, and to which the luminous body gives an impulse, which is propagated with inconceivable rapidity, as sound is conveyed through the air.

Un-e'qual-ly̆-Pin'nate. The same as IMPARI-PINNATE, which see.

Ung. = *Unguen'tum.** "Ointment."

Un'guent. [**Unguen'tum;** from *un'guo,* to "anoint."] (Fr. *Onguent,* ôɴɢ'gŏɴɢ'.) An ointment or preparation usually of the consistence of butter; a salve.

Un-guen'tum Aç'ĭ-di Tan'nĭ-ci.* ("Ointment of Tannic Acid.") Take of tannic acid, thirty grains, water, half a fluidrachm, lard, a troyounce. Rub the acid first with the water, and then with the lard, until they are thoroughly mixed, avoiding the use of an iron spatula.

Unguen'tum Ad'ĭ-pis* ("Ointment of Lard"), **Unguen'tum Sim'plex,*** 1850 ("Simple Ointment"). Take of lard, eight troyounces, white wax, two troyounces. Melt them together with a moderate heat, and stir the mixture constantly while cooling.

Unguen'tum An-tĭ-mo'nĭ-i.* ("Ointment of Antimony.") Take of tartrate of antimony and potassa, in very fine powder, one hundred and twenty grains, lard, a troyounce. Rub the powder with a little of the lard, then add the remainder and thoroughly mix them.

Unguen'tum Bel-la-don'næ.* ("Ointment of Belladonna.") Take of extract of belladonna, sixty grains, water, half a fluidrachm, lard, a troyounce. Rub the extract first with the water until rendered uniformly soft, then with the lard, and thoroughly mix them.

Unguen'tum Cre-a-so'ti.* ("Ointment of Creasote.") Take of creasote, half a fluidrachm, lard, a troyounce. Mix them.

Unguen'tum Gal'læ.* ("Ointment of Nutgall.") Take of nutgall, in fine powder, a troyounce, lard, seven ounces. Mix them.

Unguen'tum Hy-drar'gy̆-ri.* ("Ointment of Mercury.") The Pharmacopœial name ‖ for an ointment prepared by rubbing mercury with a mixture of equal parts of suet and lard until the globules can no longer be seen.

Unguen'tum Hydrar'gyri Ox'ĭ-di Ru'bri.* ("Ointment of Red Oxide of Mercury.") Take of red oxide of mercury, in very fine powder, sixty grains, ointment of lard, a troyounce. Add the oxide of mercury to the ointment previously softened with a gentle heat, and thoroughly mix them.

Unguen'tum I-o-din'ĭ-i.* ("Ointment of Iodine.") Take of iodine, twenty grains, iodide of potassium, four grains, water, six minims, lard, a troyounce. Rub the iodine and iodide of potassium first with the water, and then with the lard, until they are thoroughly mixed.

Unguen'tum Iodin'ii Com-pos'ĭ-tum.* ("Compound Ointment of Iodine.") Take of iodine, fifteen grains, iodide of potassium, thirty grains, water, thirty minims, lard, a troyounce. Rub the iodine and iodide of potassium first with the water, and then with the lard, until they are thoroughly mixed.

Unguen'tum Pi'cis Liq'uĭ-dæ* ("Ointment of Tar"), or Tar Ointment. Take of tar and suet, each twelve troyounces. Mix the tar with the suet previously melted with a moderate heat, and, having strained the mixture through muslin, stir it constantly while cooling.

Unguen'tum Plum'bi Car-bo-na'tis.* ("Ointment of Carbonate of Lead.") Take of carbonate of lead, in very fine powder, eighty grains, ointment of lard, a troyounce. Add the carbonate of lead to the ointment previously softened with a gentle heat, and thoroughly mix them.

Unguen'tum Potas'sii (po-tash'e-i) **I-od'ĭ-di.*** ("Ointment of Iodide of Potassium.") Take of iodide of potassium, in fine powder, sixty grains, water, a fluidrachm, lard, a troyounce. Dissolve the iodide of potassium in the water, and mix the solution with the lard.

Unguen'tum Sul'phu-ris.* ("Ointment of Sulphur.") Take of sublimed sulphur, a troyounce, lard, two troyounces. Mix them.

Unguen'tum Sul'phuris I-od'ĭ-di.* ("Ointment of Iodide of Sulphur.") Take of iodide of sulphur, thirty grains, lard, a troyounce. Rub the iodide of sulphur, first reduced to a fine powder, with a little of the lard, then add the remainder, and thoroughly mix them.

Unguen'tum Ve-ra'trĭ-æ.* ("Ointment of Veratria.") Take of veratria, twenty grains, lard, a troyounce. Rub the veratria with a little of the lard, then add the remainder, and thoroughly mix them.

Unguen'tum Zin'çi Ox'ĭ-di.* ("Ointment of Oxide of Zinc.") Take of oxide of zinc, eighty grains, lard, a troyounce. Mix them.

Un-guic-u-la'ta.* [From UNGUIC'-ULUS, which see.] A primary division of the class Mammalia, including those animals which have the digits armed with claws, but free for the exercise of touch upon their under-surface, as the cat, bear, and elephant.

Un-guic'u-late. [**Unguicula'tus;** from the same.] Having or resembling claws; clawed. Applied to petals.

Un-guic'u-lus.* [Diminutive of *un'guis*, a "nail," or "claw."] A little or young nail or claw.

Un'guĭ-nal. [**Unguina'lis;** from *un'guis*, a "nail," or "claw."] Belonging to the nails, or to claws or talons.

Un'guis.* [Gr. ὄνυξ; Fr. *Ongle*, ôngl.] The nail of a finger or toe; also applied to the talons or claws of birds, to the claws of certain *Crustaceæ*, etc. In Botany, the narrow part of the petal of a polypetalous corolla. In Surgery, a collection of pus in the eye.

Un'guis Os.* ("Nail-Bone.") The name of a small, very thin, and semi-transparent bone at the inner side of the orbit of the eye.

Un-gu-la'ta,* or **Un'gu-lates.** [From *un'gula*, a "hoof."] A primary division of the class Mammalia, including those species which have the digits enclosed in hoofs, the under-surface not being left free for the exercise of touch, as the horse and ox.

Un'gu-late. [**Ungula'tus;** from the same.] Having hoofs.

Ungulates. See UNGULATA.

U-nĭ-cel'lu-lar. [From *u'nus*, "one," and *cel'la*, or *cel'lula*, a "cell."] One-celled.

U-nĭ-flo-rig'er-us.* [From *u'nus*, "one," *flos*, a "flower," and *ge'ro*, to "carry."] The same as UNIFLOROUS, which see.

U-nĭ-flo'rous. [**Uniflo'rus;** from *u'nus*, "one," and *flos*, a "flower."] Bearing one flower; one-flowered.

U-nĭ-fo'lĭ-ate, or **U-nĭ-fo'lĭ-ous.** [**Unifo'lius;** from *u'nus*, "one," and *fo'lium*, a "leaf."] Having one leaf; one-leaved.

U-nĭ-lā'bĭ-ate. [From *u'nus*, "one," and *la'bium*, a "lip."] One-lipped. Applied to flowers.

U-nĭ-lat'e-ral. [From *u'nus*, "one," and *la'tus*, *lat'eris*, a "side."] One-sided.

U-nĭ-loc'u-lar. [**Unilocula'ris;** from *u'nus*, "one," and *loc'ulus*, a "cell."] Having only one cell; one-celled.

U-nĭ-ner'vate. [From *u'nus*, "one," and *ner'vus*, a "nerve."] One-nerved. Applied to leaves.

Union by First Intention. See FIRST INTENTION.

Union by Second Intention. See SECOND INTENTION.

U-nip'a-rous. [**Unip'arus;** from *u'nus*, "one," and *pa'rio*, to "bring forth."] Producing only one at a birth.

U-nĭ-pet'a-lous. [From *u'nus*, "one," and *pet'alum*, a "petal."] Having only one petal.

U-nĭ-se'rĭ-al. [From *u'nus*, "one," and *se'ries*, a "row."] In one horizontal row or whorl. Applied to parts of plants.

U-nĭ-se'rĭ-ate. The same as UNISERIAL, which see.

U-nĭ-sex'u-al. [From *u'nus*, "one," and *sex'us*, "sex."] Applied to a flower having stamens only or pistils only.

U'nĭ-vălve. [From *u'nus*, "one," and *val'va*, a "valve."] Having only one valve. Applied to pericarps, and to those Mollusks the shell of which is composed of a single piece, and is generally convoluted spirally, as the *Voluta*.

Unnamed Bones. See OSSA INNOMINATA.

U'pas. A name given in Java to several deadly poisons, the most remarkable of which are the *Bohun upas* and *Upas tieuté*. See BOHUN UPAS.

U'pas Tieu'té (te-u'tà). A poison, the product of the *Strychnos tieuté*, which owes its deadly power to *strychnia*.

U'ra-chus.* [From οὖρον, "urine," and ἔχω, to "have," or "contain;" because it was formerly supposed that in the fœtus it was a passage for the urine.] A fibrous canal or cord which extends from the bladder to the umbilicus.

U-ra-cra'sĭ-a.* [From οὖρον, "urine," and ἀκρασία, "ill temperature."] A bad quality of the urine.

U-ra-cra'tĭ-a.* [From οὖρον, "urine," and ἀκρατία, "debility."] The same as ENURESIS, which see.

U-ræ'mĭ-a.* [From *ure'a*, a constituent of urine, and αἷμα, "blood."] The presence of *urea*, or urine, in the blood.

U-ra-nis-co-plas'tĭ-ce.* [From *uranis'cus*, the "palate," and πλάσσω, to "form."] The (artificial) formation of a palate.

U-ra-nis-cor-rha'phi-a.* [From *uranis'cus*, the "palate," and ῥαφή, a "seam."] Suture of the palate.

U'ra-nite. A beautiful crystalline mineral composed chiefly of the phosphate of uranium, combined with the phosphate of lime or copper.

U-ra'ni-um.* [From the planet *U'ranus*, discovered about the same time with the metal.] A gray, brittle metal found in uranite. Its specific gravity is about 9.

U-ra-nog'ra-phy, or **Ou-ra-nog'ra-phy.** [**Uranogra'phia;** from οὐρανός, "heaven," and γράφω, to "write."] A description of the heavens and heavenly bodies.

U-ra-nol'o-gy. [**Uranolo'gia;** from οὐρανός, "heaven," and λόγος, a "discourse."] A treatise on the heavens, or the science of the heavenly bodies.

U-rar'in. [**Urari'na.**] An organic alkali found in *urari*, a poison with which the savages of America empoison the iron points of their arrows. See CURARE.

U'rate. [**U'ras, a'***tis*.] A combination of uric or lithic acid with a base.

Ur'ce-i-form. [**Urceifor'mis;** from *ur'ceus*, a "pitcher."] Formed like a pitcher.

Ur-ce-o-la'ris.* The same as URCEOLATE, which see.

Ur'ce-o-late. [**Urceola'tus;** from *urce'olus*, a "little pitcher."] Pitcher-shaped, or urn-shaped, *i.e.* hollow and contracted at the mouth. Applied to a form of monopetalous corolla, as that of the Heath.

Ur-ce-o-lif'er-ous. [**Urceolif'erus;** from *urce'olus*, a "little pitcher," and *fe'ro*, to "bear."] Having calyces like little goblets.

U-re'a.* [From *uri'na*, "urine."] A principal constituent of the urine. It is a hydrated cyanate of ammonia, composed of two equivalents each of oxygen, nitrogen, and carbon, united to four of hydrogen. It is a white, transparent, crystallizable solid.

U-re'do, d'*inis*.* [From *u'ro*, to "burn."] An itching or burning sensation of the skin which accompanies many diseases. Also applied to *urticaria*, or nettle-rash.

U-re'ni-um.* Synonymous with UREA, which see.

U-re'sis.* [From οὐρέω, to "void urine."] Micturition, or the act of passing urine.

-uret. [**-ure'tum.**] A terminal denoting combination of simple inflammable bodies with each other, or with metals.

U-re'ter, e'*ris*.* [From οὐρέω, to "pass urine."] The membranous tube through which the urine is conveyed from the kidney to the urinary bladder.

U-re-te-ral'gi-a.* [From *ure'ter*, and ἄλγος, "pain."] Pain in the ureter.

U-re-te-ri'tis, i*dis*.* [From *ure'ter*.] Inflammation of the ureter.

U-re'thra.* [From οὐρέω, to "pass urine."] The membranous canal communicating between the neck of the bladder and the external surface, and passing in the male through the entire length of the penis. The female urethra does not exceed two inches in length, and the passage is considerably larger than that of the male.

U-re'thral. [**Urethra'lis.**] Belonging to the urethra.

U-re-thral'gi-a.* [From *ure'thra*, and ἄλγος, "pain."] Pain in the urethra: urethralgy.

U-re-thri'tis, i*dis*.* [From *ure'thra*.] Inflammation in the urethra.

Urethri'tis Ve-ne're-a.* ("Venereal Inflammation of the Urethra.") A term for gonorrhœa.

U-reth-ro-plas'tic. [**Urethroplas'ticus.**] Belonging to urethroplasty.

U-reth-ro-plas'ty. [From *ure'thra*, and πλάσσω, to "form."] An operation by which a new urethra is said to have been formed by Ricord in the male: applicable to the repair of any lesion of the urethra by supplying the deficiency from the healthy parts.

U-reth-ror-rha'gi-a.* [From *ure'thra*, and ῥήγνυμι, to "burst forth."] Sudden discharge (of blood) from the urethra.

U-reth-ror-rhœ'a.* [From *ure'thra*, and ῥέω, to "flow."] A flow, as of mucus, pus, semen, etc., from the urethra.

U-re-throt'o-my. [**Urethroto'mia;** from *ure'thra*, and τέμνω, to "cut."] The division, by a cutting instrument, of urethral stricture.

U-ret'i-ca.* [From οὖρον, "urine."] Medicines which promote a discharge of urine.

U-ret'i-cus.* [From the same.] Diuretic.

Ur-gin'e-a Scil'la.* The systematic name, according to the British Pharmacopœia, of the plant which produces the squill.

U'ric. [**U'ricus;** from οὖρον, "urine."] Belonging to the urine. Applied to an acid, otherwise called Lithic acid, obtained from urine. See CALCULI, URINARY.

U-rĭ-dro'sis.* [From οὖρον, "urine," and ἱδρώς, "sweat."] Urinous sweat.

Urinæ, Ardor. See ARDOR URINÆ.

U'rĭ-nal. [From *uri'na*, "urine."] A vessel to receive urine.

U'rĭ-na-rў. [**Urina'rius;** from the same.] Relating to the urine.

U'rinary Blad'der. [Lat. **Vesi'ca Urina'ria;** Fr. *Vessie*, vå'sė'.] A membranous bag immediately behind the *symphysis pubis*, of a flattened, triangular form when contracted, of an oval figure when distended, composed of four coats,—the peritoneal, muscular, cellular, and mucous; the serous being but partial.

Urinary Calculi. See CALCULI, URINARY.

U'rĭ-nā'tion. [**Urina'tio, o'nis;** from *uri'na*, "urine."] The act of passing urine.

U'rĭne. [Lat. **Uri'na;** Gr. οὖρον.] The saline secretion of the kidneys which flows from them through the ureters into the urinary bladder.

Urine, Difficult Discharge of. See DYSURIA.

U'rine, In-con'tĭ-nence of. Inability to retain the urine. See ENURESIS.

U'rine, Re-ten'tion of. Inability to pass urine. See ISCHURIA.

Urine, Suppression of. See ISCHURIA.

U-rĭ-nif'er-ous. [**Urinif'erus;** from *uri'na*, "urine," and *fe'ro*, to "bear."] Bearing, or conveying, urine.

U-ri-nol'o-ġў. The same as UROLOGY, which see.

U'rĭ-nous, or **U-rĭ-nose'.** [**Urino'sus;** from *uri'na*, "urine."] Relating to urine, or like urine.

Ur-nig'er-ous. [**Urnig'erus;** from *ur'na*, an "urn," and *ge'ro*, to "bear."] Bearing capsules like urns.

U'ro-çēle.* [From οὖρον, "urine," and κήλη, a "tumor."] Urinous *œdema* of the scrotum.

U-roch'e-ras.* [From οὖρον, "urine," and χεράς, "sand."] The sand, or sediment, of the urine.

U-ro-çўs'tis, *idis*.* [From οὖρον, "urine," and κύστις, a "bag."] The urinary bladder.

U-ro-çўs-ti'tis, *idis*.* [From *urocys'tis*.] Inflammation of the urinary bladder.

U-ro-dĭ-al-ў-sis.* [From οὖρον, "urine," and διάλυσις, a "dissolution," or "cessation."] A cessation of the secretion of urine.

U-ro-do'chĭ-um.* [From οὖρον, "urine," and δέχομαι, to "receive."] The same as URINAL, which see.

U-ro-dўn'ĭ-a.* [From οὖρον, "urine," and ὀδύνη, "pain."] Pain during the passing of urine.

U-rœ-de'ma, *atis*.* [From οὖρον, "urine," and οἴδημα, a "swelling."] Urinous swelling.

U-ro-er-ўth'rin. [**Uroerythri'na;** from οὖρον, "urine," and ἐρυθρός, "red."] A dark-red precipitate deposited by the urine.

U-ro-ġen'ĭ-tal. [**Urogenita'lis.**] Pertaining to the urinary and genital apparatus.

U-ro-hў'al. [**Urohya'lis;** from οὐρά, a "tail," and *hyoi'des*, "hyoid."] Applied by Professor Owen to a long, slender, and pointed bone, articulated with the posterior end of the basihyal.

U-ro-lith'ic. [**Urolith'icus;** from *urol'ithus*.] Belonging to urinary calculus. Applied to an acid obtained from it.

U-rol'ĭ-thus.* [From οὖρον, "urine," and λίθος, a "stone."] A urinary calculus: a u'rolith.

U-ro-loġ'ĭ-cal. [**Urolog'icus.**] Belonging to urology.

U-rol'o-ġў. [**Urolo'gia;** from οὖρον, the "urine," and λόγος, a "discourse."] The science of the urine, or a consideration of its secretion, nature, etc.

U-ro-man-ti'a.* [From οὖρον, "urine," and μαντεία, "divination."] Prognostication from inspection of the urine. See UROSCOPIA.

U-ro-pla'nĭ-a.* [From οὖρον, "urine," and πλάνη, "wandering."] Literally, "a wandering of the urine." A secretion of urine in other parts than the proper urinary organs.

U-ro-po-e'sis.* [From οὖρον, "urine," and ποιέω, to "make."] Secretion of the urine.

U-rop-sam'mus.* [From οὖρον, "urine," and ψάμμος, "sand."] Sand, or sediment, of the urine. See UROCHERAS.

U-ror-rha'ġĭ-a.* [From οὖρον, "urine," and ῥήγνυμι, to "burst forth."] An excessive flow of urine; *diabetes*.

U-ror-rhœ'a.* [From οὖρον, "urine," and ῥέω, to "flow."] An involuntary discharge of urine; *enuresis*. Also applied to diabetes.

U-ror-rhor-rhœ'a.* [From οὖρον, "urine," and *orrhorrhœ'a*, a "flow of serum."] Excretion of serum (or albumen) with the urine, or albuminous urine, constituting the *Morbus Brightii.*

U-ros'che-o-çēle.* [From οὖρον, "urine," and *os'cheocele*, a "tumor of the scrotum."] The same as UROCELE, which see.

U-ro-sco'pĭ-a.* [From οὖρον, the "urine," and σκοπέω, to "examine."] Inspection of the urine, as a means of diagnosis.

U-ro'sēs.* [From οὖρον, "urine."] Diseases of the urinary apparatus.

U-ros'te-a-lith. [**Urosteal'ithus,** from οὖρον, "urine," στέαρ, "fat," and λίθος, a "stone."] A fatty constituent of urinary calculi.

U'rous. [**Uro'sus.**] Belonging to the urine. Applied to an oxide, or substance forming a rare ingredient in vesical calculi.

Urticaceæ,* ur-te-ka'she-ē. A natural order of exogenous plants, widely dispersed over the world, in hot and cold climates. Among them is the *Urti'ca* (Nettle). Excessive causticity in their juice is their chief characteristic. This order once included hemp, the hop-vine, the fig, mulberry, bread-fruit, etc., which are now arranged under new orders, *Cannabinaceæ, Moraceæ,* and *Artocarpaceæ.*

Ur-ti'ca Di-oi'ca* or **His'pĭ-da.*** (Fr. *Ortie*, oR'tè'.) The systematic name of the nettle, a plant of the Linnæan class *Monœcia*, natural order *Urticaceæ.*

Ur-tĭ-ca'rĭ-a.* [From *Urti'ca*, a "nettle."] The nettle-rash. An exanthematous fever characterized by an eruption like the elevations produced on the skin by the sting of a nettle. A genus of the order *Exanthemata*, class *Pyrexiæ*, of Cullen's Nosology. See UREDO.

Ur-tĭ-cā'tion. [**Urtica'tio, o'***nis;* from the same.] The whipping of a part, as a paralytic limb, with nettles, with the view of restoring sensation.

Us'ne-a.* The *Li'chen saxat'ilis*. A kind of moss or lichen, particularly that adhering to the human skull when exposed to the air in damp places. See next article.

Us'nea Cra'nĭ-i Hu-ma'ni.* ("Usnea of the Human Skull.") A plant formerly believed to possess extraordinary anti-epileptic and anti-hæmorrhagic virtues.

Usquebaugh, ŭs-kwe-baw'. The Irish name for whiskey.

Us'tion. [**Us'tio, o'***nis;* from *u'ro, us'tum*, to "burn."] A burning. Formerly used for Incineration; also, for Combustion. In Surgery, employed for Cauterization.

Us'tus.* [From the same.] Burnt. The same as calcined, or dried by fire.

U'te-ri,* the genitive of *u'terus*, signifying "of the womb:" *e.g. Cer'vix U'teri*, the "neck [or narrow part] of the womb;" *Retrover'sio U'teri*, the "retroversion of the womb," etc.

U'ter-ine. [**Uteri'nus.**] Belonging to the uterus.

Uterine Gestation. See UTERO-GESTATION.

Uterine Madness. See FUROR UTERINUS, and NYMPHOMANIA.

U-te-ri'tis, *idis.** [From *u'terus.*] Inflammation of the womb; also called *Metritis* and *Hysteritis.*

U'te-ro-Ģes-tā'tion. The period of pregnancy commencing with conception and terminating with delivery.

U-te-rot'o-mȳ. [**Uteroto'mia;** from *u'terus*, and τέμνω, to "cut."] The cutting into the uterus, as when the lips have become united by adhesive inflammation. See HYSTEROTOMY.

U'te-rus,* genitive **U'te-ri,** accusative **U'ter-um,** ablative **U'ter-o.** [From *u'ter*, a "bottle of skin or leather."] (Gr. ὑστέρα and μήτρα; Fr. *Matrice*, mȧ'tRèss' [from the Latin *Ma'trix*], or *Sein*, sȧNᵍ'.) The womb; a hollow muscular organ designed for the lodgment and nourishment of the fœtus from the moment of conception until birth. In its ordinary condition, it is a compact fleshy body, about three inches in length, two inches in its greatest breadth, shaped somewhat like a flattened pear, the narrower portion being below. The upper or broader part is termed the *fundus*, the contracted portion is called the *cervix* or neck, and the external orifice, communicating with the vagina, the *os tincæ* or *os uteri*. At the superior angles, it sends off the Fallopian tubes, which, when conception takes place, receive the ovule or ovules from the ovary and convey them to the uterus.

U'terus, In-ver'sion of the. [**Inver'sio U'teri.**] The state of the womb being turned inside out, caused by violently drawing away the placenta before it is detached by the natural process of labor.

Uterus, Retroversion of. See RETROVERSIO UTERI.

U'trĭ-cle. [**Utric'ulus,** or **Uter'-**

culus; diminutive of *u'ter*, a "bottle."] A minute cell or vesicle; also, a small, bladdery fruit.

U-tric'u-lar. [**Utricula'ris.**] Belonging to, or like, a utricle; bladder-like.

U-tric'u-late. [**Utricula'tus;** from *utric'ulus*, a "utricle."] Having utricles.

U-tric'u-li-form. [**Utriculifor'mis;** from *utric'ulus*, a "utricle."] Having the form of a utricle; shaped like a little bottle.

U-tric'u-lose, or **U-tric'u-lous.** [**Utriculo'sus;** from *utric'ulus*, a "utricle."] Having or bearing utricles. Applied to plants.

U'tri-form. [**Utrifor'mis;** from *u'ter*, a "bladder" or "bottle."] Having the form of a bottle.

U-trig'er-ous. [**Utrig'erus;** from *u'ter*, a "bladder" or "bottle," and *ge'ro*, to "bear."] Bearing objects like bottles.

U'va.* A "grape." The Pharmacopœial name (Lond. Ph.) for the dried fruit of the *Vitis vinifera;* the raisin.

U'va Pas'sa* ("Dried Grape"), or **U'væ Pas'sæ*** ("Dried Grapes"). The Pharmacopœial name (U.S. Ph. and Ed. Ph.) for the raisin. See UVA.

U'va Ur'si.* The Pharmacopœial name for the leaves of *Arctostaphylos Uva Ursi*. It is astringent and tonic, and has been extolled as an antilithic.

U've-a,* or **Tu'ni-ca U'vea.*** ("Grape-like Tunic.") [From *u'va*, a "grape."] The posterior surface of the *iris* of the eye, supposed to resemble the skin of a grape.

U-ve-i'tis, i*dis*.* [From *u'vea*.] Inflammation of the *uvea*.

U-vif'er-ous. [**Uvif'erus;** from *u'va*, a "grape," or "raisin," and *fe'ro*, to "bear."] Bearing fruits like the grape.

U'vi-form. [**Uvifor'mis;** from *u'va*, a "grape."] Shaped like a grape.

U'vu-la.* [Diminutive of *u'va*, a "grape."] The small fleshy body hanging from the *velum pendulum palati*, above the root of the tongue. It is sometimes of a preternatural length, interfering with the functions of the voice, and producing a tendency to cough. In these cases amputation may become necessary.

U'vula Ve-si'cæ.* ("Uvula of the Bladder.") The small eminence forming the apex of the *trigone*.

U'vu-lar. [**Uvula'ris.**] Belonging to the uvula.

V.

Vac-ci'na.* [From *vac'ca*, a "cow."] Cow-pox; also called *Vari'ola vacci'na*. A disease originating in the cow, with which, if the human body be inoculated, it is preserved from the contagion of small-pox.

Vac-ci-nā'tion. [**Vaccina'tio, o'nis;** from *vac'ca*, a "cow."] The minor operation of inserting matter for the production of *vaccina*, or cow-pox.

Vaccinia. See VACCINA.

Vacciniaceæ,* vak-sin-e-a'she-ē. A natural order of exogenous plants (shrubs or trees), which abound in the temperate parts of the world. It includes the *Vaccin'ium* (Whortleberry), and *Oxycoc'cus*, or *Vaccinium macrocarpon* (Cranberry).

Vac-cin'i-um Mac-ro-car'pon.* The systematic name of the common American Cranberry, a plant of the Linnæan class *Octandria*, natural order *Vacciniaceæ*.

Vaç'il-lant. [**Vacil'lans, an'tis;** from *vacil'lo*, to "move to and fro," to "waver."] Wavering. In Botany, the same as VERSATILE, which see.

Vac'u-um.* [From *vac'uus*, "void," or "empty."] That is, *vac'uum spa'tium*, an "empty space." In Physics, a portion of space void of matter. The most perfect vacuum that can be produced artificially is the TORRICELLIAN, which see.

Va-gi'na,* gen. **Va-gi'næ.** (A "sheath," or "case.") (Fr. *Vagin*, vå'-zhăng'.) The canal extending from the vulva to the uterus. The term is also applied to other parts; *e.g.* the fascia encasing or covering a limb, etc.

Vagi'na Cor'dis.* ("Case of the Heart.") The same as PERICARDIUM, which see.

Vag'i-nal. [**Vagina'lis;** from *vagi'na*.] Belonging to the vagina. In Botany, relating to a sheath.

Vaginal Coat of the Testicle. See TUNICA VAGINALIS.

Vag'i-nant. [**Vagi'nans;** from *vagi'no, vagina'tum*, to "sheathe."] Encasing; sheathing.

Vag'i-nate. [**Vagina'tus;** from the same.] Cased or sheathed.

Vag-i-ner'vi-us.* [From *va'gus,* "wandering," and *ner'vus,* a "nerve."] Having leaves the nervures of which run in all directions.

Vag-i-nif'er-ous. [**Vaginif'erus;** from *vagi'na,* a "sheath," and *fe'ro,* to "bear."] Bearing one or more sheaths.

Va-gi-ni'tis, *idis.** [From *vagi'na.*] Inflammation of the vagina.

Va-gi'tus.* [From *va'gio, vagi'tum,* to "cry as an infant."] (Fr. *Vagissement,* vå'zhĕss'mōNG'.) The crying of infants.

Vagi'tus U-ter-i'nus.* ("Uterine Crying.") The crying of the child heard, or supposed to have been heard, while yet in the passages.

Vāgue. [From *va'gus,* "wandering."] In Botany, having no definite order or direction.

Va'gus.* [From *va'go,* to "wander."] Wandering. Applied to the pneumogastric nerve, or *Nervus vagus,* otherwise called *Par vagum,* or "wandering pair." See PNEUMOGASTRIC NERVES.

Va-le-ri-a'na.* [From *Vale'rius,* who first described it.] A Linnæan genus of the class *Triandria,* natural order *Valerianaceæ.* Also, the Pharmacopœial name for the root of *Valeriana officinalis,* which is used as a nervous stimulant or antispasmodic.

Valeria'na Of-fic-i-na'lis.* ("Officinal Valerian.") The wild valerian plant.

Valeria'na Syl-ves'tris.* The same as VALERIANA OFFICINALIS.

Valerianaceæ,* va-le-re-a-na'she-ē. A natural order of exogenous herbaceous plants, abundant in Europe, Northern India, and South America. It includes the *Valeria'na,* the root of which is tonic and antispasmodic.

Va-le'ri-a-nāte. [**Valeria'nas, a'tis.**] A combination of valerianic acid with a base.

Va-le-ri-an'ic. [**Valerian'icus;** from *Valeria'na.*] Belonging to valerian. Applied to an acid obtained from it.

Val-e-tu-di-nā'ri-an, or **Val-e-tu'-di-na-ry.** [From *valetu'do,* "state or condition of body (or health)," whether good or bad.] A person who is in delicate or infirm health, or subject to frequent illness.

Văl'gus.* Having legs bent outward; crooked; awry

Val'ley. [**Val'lis.**] The name of a depression of the cerebellum, in which is lodged the commencement of the spinal marrow.

Val-săl'va, Si'nus-es of. Three prominences formed by dilatation of the walls of the aorta in the places which correspond to the sigmoid valves.

Valva. See VALVE.

Văl-vā'ceous. [**Valva'ceus.**] Applied to indehiscent fruits formed of valves with distinct sutures.

Val'væ,* the plural of *Val'va.* See VALVE.

Văl'var. [**Valva'ris;** from *val'va,* a "valve."] Belonging to a valve.

Val'vate, or **Val'vāt-ed.** [**Valva'-tus;** from the same.] Having valves; valved.

Valve. [**Val'va,** plural **Val'væ;** from *vol'vo,* to "roll," to "fold."] Originally, *valvæ* were folding doors. Applied to a fold or elongation of the lining membrane of canals, preventing the reflux of their contents. In Botany, one of the pieces into which a pod or capsule separates in dehiscence.

Valved. [**Valva'tus;** from *val'va,* a "valve."] Opening by valves.

Văl'vi-form. [**Valvifor'mis;** from *val'va,* a "valve."] Formed like a valve.

Val'vu-la,* plural **Val'vu-læ.** [Diminutive of *val'va,* a "valve."] A little valve: a val'vule.

Val'vu-læ,* gen. **Val-vu-la'rum,** the plural of VALVULA.

Val'vulæ Con-ni-ven'tēs.* The semilunar folds formed by the mucous lining of the duodenum, jejunum, and ileum.

Valvulæ Semilunares. See SEMILUNAR VALVES.

Va-na'di-um.* [From *Vanadis,* a Scandinavian deity.] A white, brittle metal, very difficult of reduction, and not oxidized by air or water. It is soluble in nitric acid and aqua regia, with which it yields solutions of a fine dark-blue color. It was first found in Sweden.

Vane-like. See VERSATILE.

Va-nil'la.* The name applied to the prepared unripe capsules of the *Vanil'la aromat'ica.* They have been placed on the primary list of the Materia Medica of the U.S. Pharmacopœia for 1860. Vanilla is a grateful aromatic, employed in confectionery, etc. It has been recommended, in the form of infusion, as a remedy in hysteria, and in certain low fevers.

Va'por,* gen. **Va-po'ris.** A Latin word signifying "steam," or "exhalation." Applied to any elastic fluid into which a liquid or solid is converted by heat. Vapors differ from gases in this respect, that they are not permanently elastic, but resume the liquid or solid form when cooled down to ordinary temperatures.

Va'por Douche (doosh). A kind of vapor-bath; properly, a column of vapor directed to a particular part.

Vap-o-ra'rĭ-um.* [From *vapo'ro*, to "send out vapor."] A vapor-bath.

Vap-o-rĭ-zā'tion. [**Vaporiza'tio, o'nis**; from the same.] The rapid conversion of a fluid into vapor by heat.

Va'pors, or **Va'pours.** A name for hypochondriasis, spleen, or depression of spirits.

Văr-ĭ-cel'la.* [Diminutive of *vari'ola*, "small-pox."] Chicken-pox, a disease characterized by an eruption of smooth, transparent, lentil-shaped, or irregular circular vesicles. A genus of the order *Exanthemata*, class *Pyrexiæ*, of Cullen's Nosology.

Văr'ĭ-çĭ-form. [**Varicifor'mis**; from *va'rix*, a "swollen vein."] Resembling a *varix*.

Văr'ĭ-co-çēle.* [From *va'rix*, and κήλη, a "tumor."] A swelling of the veins of the scrotum, or of the spermatic cord. Also, any tumor originating in a varicose vein.

Văr-ĭ-cose'. [**Varico'sus**; from *va'rix*.] Applied to veins in a state of permanent dilatation, with accumulation of dark-colored blood, the circulation of which is materially retarded in the affected vessel, which is irregular, knotted, and winding in a variety of ways.

Varicose Aneurism. See ANEURISMAL VARIX.

Va-rī'e-tȳ. [**Vari'etas, a'tis**; from *va'rius*, "changeable," "variegated."] In Natural History, this term is applied to individuals of the same species which, from the operation of different causes, as climate, food, or cultivation, present deviations from the specific type in size, color, form, etc., but have the capacity of reverting to the original typical form in successive generations on the cessation of the influences under which the variety originated.

Va-rĭ-ĭ-fo'lĭ-us.* [From *va'rius*, "diverse," and *fo'lium*, a "leaf."] Having leaves not all of the same form.

Va-rī'o-la.* [From *va'rius*, "variegated," "spotted."] (Fr. *Variole*, vå'-rē'ol', or *Petite Vérole*, peh-tēt' vå'rol'.) Small-pox. A very contagious disease characterized by *synocha* and an eruption of pustules on the third day, which suppurate about the eighth, and afterwards, drying, fall off in crusts. A genus of the order *Exanthemata*, class *Pyrexiæ*, of Cullen's Nosology.

Va-rī'o-lar. [**Variola'ris**; from *vari'ola*, "small-pox."] Pertaining to *variola*.

Va-rī'o-late. [**Variola'tus**; from the same.] Having small eminences like the pustules of small-pox.

Variole. See VARIOLA.

Vā'rĭ-o-loid. [**Varioloi'des**; from *vari'ola*, and εἶδος, a "form."] Resembling *variola*, or small-pox. Varioloid (Lat. *varioloïs*), used as a noun, is a common term for small-pox modified by previous vaccination or inoculation.

Va-ri-o-lo'is, idis.* [Diminutive of *vari'ola*.] Small-pox modified by previous vaccination. See VARIOLOID.

Va-rī'o-lous. [**Variolo'des**; from *vari'ola*, "small-pox."] Relating to small-pox; of the nature of small-pox.

Va'rix, icis.* [From *va'rus*, "crooked."] A dilated vein, generally becoming knotted and winding in its course. A genus of the order *Tumores*, class *Locales*, of Cullen's Nosology.

Varolii Pons. See PONS VAROLII.

Va'rus.* A spot or pimple on the face. See ACNE.

Va'rus.* Crooked; ill shaped. Applied to a variety of the deformity called *Tal'ipes*, or club-foot.

Va'rus Punc-ta'tus.* Applied to minute pimples common in the skin of the face, particularly of young persons, and called maggot-pimples, because a worm-like sebaceous substance may be pressed out of them.

Vas,* gen. **Va'sis,** plural **Va'sa.** A Latin word signifying any kind of vessel. Applied in Anatomy to membranous canals or tubes through which the fluids of the body are conveyed, as arteries, veins, etc.

Vas Def'e-rens.* A continuation of the *epididymis*, forming the duct which conveys the semen secreted in the testicle, into the ejaculatory duct.

Va'sa,* gen. **Va-so'rum,** the plural of VAS, which see.

Va'sa Bre'vĭ-a.* ("Short Vessels.") The small branches of the splenic artery which anastomose with others of the gastric artery, and are distributed on the large arch of the stomach.

Va'sa Cap-re-o-la'rĭ-a.* ("Tendril-like Vessels.") The spermatic vessels: so named from their tortuous course.

Va'sa Efferen'tia* (ef-fer-en'she-a). ("Efferent Vessels.") Applied generally to vessels that go out from a gland, but specially to five or six tortuous vessels which ascend obliquely backwards from the testis. See next article.

Va'sa Inferen'tia* (in-fe-ren'she-a). [From *in*, "into," and *fe'ro*, to "carry."] Applied to vessels which enter a gland, as distinguished from *vasa efferentia*, or the vessels which carry out the substance secreted by the gland.

Va'sa Se-ro'sa.* ("Serous Vessels.") A name formerly applied to (supposed) vessels so minute as not to admit the red blood-globules, and therefore containing serum only. They were considered to be a complement to the capillaries and to convey nutriment to the ultimate tissues.

Va'sa Va-so'rum.* ("Vessels of the Vessels.") The very minute arteries and veins by which the substance of larger vessels is supposed to be supplied with nourishment.

Va'sa Vor-ti-co'sa.* ("Vorticose Vessels.") Applied to the fine vascular ramifications principally connected with the veins on the external surface of the choroid coat of the eye.

Vas'cu-lar. [**Vascula'ris;** from *vas'culum*, a "little vessel."] Having, or relating to, vessels; full of vessels.

Vas'cular Plants. [**Vascula'res.**] A term applied to all plants which have vascular and woody tissues in their composition (*i.e.* all exogenous and endogenous plants). They compose one of the two grand divisions in the system of De Candolle.

Vas'cular Sys'tem. [**Syste'ma Vaso'rum.**] That part of the animal economy which relates to the vessels. Harvey took the heart as the centre, and described the two circulations as the pulmonic through the lungs, and the systemic through the system.

Vas'cular Sys'tem of Plants. That portion of the tissue of plants which is destined for the conveyance of sap or air.

Vas'cular Tis'sue. [**Trachen'chyma.**] In Botany, a modification of cellular tissue, consisting of cells transformed into vessels or tubes called dotted ducts, spiral ducts, etc. In older stems they are filled with air, except when the whole tissue is gorged with sap.

Vas-cu-lăr'ĭ-tў. [**Vascular'itas, a'tis;** from *vas'culum*, a "little vessel."] The state or property of being vascular.

Vas-cu-lo'sus.* [From *vas'culum*, a "little vessel."] Full of vessels; vascular.

Vas'cu-lum.* [Diminutive of *vas*, a "vessel."] A little vessel. See ASCIDIUM.

Vas'ĭ form Tis'sue. The same as VASCULAR TISSUE, which see.

Vas-ta'tor, o'ris.* [From *vas'to*, *vasta'tum*, to "lay waste," to "destroy."] Destroying or destructive. Applied to certain insects. See APHIS.

Vas'tus.* Literally, "large," or "vast." A term applied to two portions of the TRICEPS EXTENSOR CRURIS, which see.

Va'sum,* plural **Va'sa.** A Latin word signifying a "vessel."

Vaterian Bodies. See PACINI, CORPUSCLES OF.

Vaulted. See FORNICIFORM.

Vauqueline, vōk'lēn'. A name for STRYCHNIA, which see.

Vec'tis.* [From *ve'ho*, *vec'tum*, to "carry," or to "bear."] The lever. In Obstetrics, an instrument employed in certain cases of preternatural labor.

Vector. See RADIUS VECTOR.

Veg-e-ta-bil'ĭ-a.* ("Vegetables," or "Plants.") A name sometimes applied to the whole vegetable kingdom.

Veg'e-ta-ble. [**Vegetab'ilis;** from *ve'geo*, to "grow," to "be strong."] An organized body possessing organs of circulation and respiration, but destitute of sensation and of the power of locomotion; a plant.

Veg'etable Al-bu'men. A proximate principle found in certain parts of plants, closely resembling animal albumen. The term albumen (so called because, like the white of an egg, it encloses the embryo) is also applied to the perisperm, or substance which surrounds the embryo, in Indian corn and most other kinds of grain. It is designed to supply nourishment to the young plant.

Veg'etable A-nat'o-mў, or **Phў-tot'o-mў.** The study of the minute structure of vegetables, as revealed by the microscope.

Veg'etable E-con'o-mў. [**Œco-no'mia Vegetab'ilis.**] The orderly arrangement of the parts of living plants or vegetables.

Veg'etable Phўs-ĭ-ol'o-ġў. The department of Botany which treats of the vital actions or functions of plants. The study of the apparatus of plants, in action, endowed with life, and fulfilling the purpose for which it was intended, and also of the forces which operate in it and by it, is the province of Vegetable Physiology.—(GRAY.)

Veg-e-tal'i-ty. [**Vegetal'itas.**] A term for the aggregate of those functions or properties which are possessed by all living vegetables; also applied to such animal phenomena as are common to the vegetable kingdom.

Veg-e-tā'ri-an. One who holds the doctrine that vegetables are the only proper food for man.

Veg-e-tā'tion. [**Vegeta'tio, o'**_nis;_ from _veg'eto, vegeta'tum,_ to "quicken," or to "make strong."] The growth of plants; the process by which plants vegetate or grow. Sometimes applied to plants collectively or in general. Also, a morbid fungous excrescence which sometimes appears on the valves of the heart, or on the semilunar valves of the aorta.

Veg'e-ta-tive. [**Vegetati'vus;** from the same.] Capable of growing; relating to growth or nutrition. Applied to organic functions, _i.e._ nutrition and reproduction.

Veg'e-to-An'i-mal. [**Veg'eto-Anima'lis.**] Applied to gluten and vegetable albumen, two vegetable substances which resemble certain proximate animal principles in chemical habitudes, etc.

Veg'eto-Min'e-ral. [**Veg'eto-Minera'lis.**] Pertaining to vegetable and mineral substances.

Veg'eto-Sul-phu'ri-cus.* Applied to an acid formed by the action of sulphuric acid on sawdust of wood, or linen rags.

Ve'hi-cle. [**Vehic'ulum;** from _ve'ho,_ to "carry," in any manner.] Literally, "that which carries or conveys." A liquor, or substance, in which medicine is rendered of more easy exhibition. See EXCIPIENT.

Veil. See VELUM, and CALYPTRA.

Vein. See VENA.

Veined. [**Veno'sus.**] Having veins or nerves. In Botany, furnished with slender vascular or woody bundles, especially branching ones, or veins.

Vein'less. [**Ave'nius.**] Destitute of apparent veins.

Vein'let. [**Ven'ula.**] A little vein; one of the smaller ramifications of the veins of a leaf.

Veins, Min'e-ral. Cracks or fissures in rocks, filled with metals or other substances different from the rock itself.

Vel'lum.* [From _vel'lus,_ a "fleece of wool;" also, the "skin of an animal."] A fine kind of parchment, made of calfskin.

Ve'lum.* [From _ve'lo,_ to "hide."] A veil. Applied to several objects like a veil or screen.

Ve'lum In-ter-pos'i-tum.* ("Interposed Veil.") The choroid membrane of the brain, situated beneath the _fornix_ and above the optic _thalami._

Ve'lum Pen'du-lum Pa-la'ti.* ("Pendulous Veil or Curtain of the Palate.") Applied to the posterior part of the palate, which forms two arches, fixed laterally to the tongue and pharynx. See PALATUM MOLLE.

Ve'lum Pu-pil'læ.* ("Veil of the Pupil.") The name of a very thin membrane which covers the pupil of the eye in the fœtus; also termed _Membrana pupillaris_ ("Pupillary Membrane").

Ve'lum Ve-si'cæ U-ri-na'ri-æ.* The _trigone._

Ve-lu'ti-nous. [From the Italian _vellu'to,_ "velvet."] Velvety; covered with very fine and close soft hairs, so that the surface resembles velvet to the touch. Applied to plants.

Ve'na,* plural **Ve'næ.** A vein; a non-pulsating vessel carrying the blood, or waste portion of it, back to the heart, after it has been distributed to the system by the arteries and has given off its nutritious properties to the various organs and tissues of the body. (See CIRCULATION.) Also, one of the woody fibres which form part of the framework of leaves.

Ve'na Ar-te-ri-o'sa.* ("Arterial Vein.") Another name for the portal vein: so called because it ramifies like an artery, and conveys blood for secretion; but it is an arterial vein in another sense, being a vein to the hepatic artery, and an artery to the hepatic vein. See VENA PORTÆ.

Ve'na Ba-sil'i-ca.* ("Royal Vein.") The large vein of the arm. See BASILIC.

Ve'na Ca'va In-fe'ri-or,* or **Ve'na Ca'va As-cen'dens.*** ("Inferior or Ascending Hollow Vein.") The large vein which extends from the articulation of the fourth and fifth lumbar vertebræ to the right auricle of the heart.

Ve'na Ca'va Su-pe'ri-or* ("Superior Hollow Vein"), otherwise called **Ve'na Ca'va De-scen'dens*** ("Descending"). The grand trunk which transmits the blood of the head, the neck, the superior extremities, and part of the circulation of the thorax to the heart.

Vena Portæ. See PORTAL VEIN.

Ve'næ,* gen. **Ve-na'rum,** the plural of VENA, which see.

Venæ Alares. See ALARES VENÆ.

Ve'næ Ca'væ.* (Literally, "Hollow Veins.") The two large terminating trunks of the veins, divided into the *Vena cava superior*, and *Vena cava inferior.*

Ven-æ-sec'tio.* ("Cutting of a Vein.") See VENESECTION.

Ve-nā'tion. [**Vena'tio;** from *ve'na*, a "vein."] The mode in which veins are distributed throughout the lamina of a leaf. There are two principal modes of venation, which are characteristic of the two grand divisions of phenogamous plants, viz. RETICULATED and PARALLEL-VEINED, which see.

Ven-e-nā'tion. [From *vene'no, venena'tum*, to "poison."] The act of poisoning.

Ven-e-nif'er-ous. [**Venenif'erus;** from *vene'num*, "poison," and *fe'ro*, to "bear."] Bearing poison. Applied to plants.

Ve-ne're-al. [**Vene'reus;** from *Ve'nus*, the goddess of love.] Belonging to sexual intercourse, or venery. Also, the same as APHRODISIAC.

Vene'real Dis-ease'. [**Mor'bus Aphrodis'ius** or **Vene'reus.**] A general term for gonorrhœal as well as syphilitic affections, but more frequently applied to the latter. See SYPHILIS.

Vene'real Disease', True. Syphilis, or *Lues venerea.*

Ven'e-rȳ. [From *Ve'nus*, the goddess of love.] The pleasures of love; sexual intercourse.

Ven-e-sec'tion. [**Venæsec'tio, o'nis;** from *ve'na*, a "vein," and *se'co, sec'tum*, to "cut."] The minor operation of opening a vein with a lancet, otherwise called *phlebotomy;* a bleeding or blood-letting.

Ven'om. [Lat. **Vene'num;** Fr. *Venin*, vẹh-năNᴳ'.] Poison. Usually applied to the poison secreted by certain animals; as that of poisonous serpents, of the spider, wasp, etc.

Ven'o-mous. [From *vene'num*, "poison."] Poisonous. Usually applied to certain noxious animals.

Ve'nose. [**Veno'sus;** from *ve'na*, a "vein."] Veiny; abounding in veins.

Ve'nous. [**Veno'sus;** from the same.] Relating to the veins; contained in the veins.

Ven'ter,* gen. **Ven'tris.** A Latin term signifying the "stomach," or "belly." (Fr. *Ventre*, vŏNᴳtr.) Also applied to the "womb."

Ven'ter I'mus.* ("Lowest Belly.") Another name for the ABDOMEN, which see.

Ven-tĭ-lā'tion. [**Ventila'tio, o'nis;** from *ven'tilo, ventila'tum*, to "blow," to "fan."] The act of ventilating or renewing the air of apartments, etc.; the art of conveying currents of fresh air through apartments, or confined places, so as to maintain the atmosphere in a state of purity.

Ventouse, vŏNᴳ'tooz'. The French for "cupping-glass." See CUCURBITULA.

Ven'tral. [**Ventra'lis;** from *ven'ter*, the "belly."] Belonging to the belly; abdominal. In Botany, relating to the inner side of a simple pistil, viz. that side next the axis.

Ven'tral Su'ture (of a pistil or pericarp). The inner suture, or that next the axis of the flower.

Ventre. See VENTER, and STOMACH.

Ven'trĭ-cle. [**Ventric'ulus;** diminutive of *ven'ter*, the "belly."] Applied to certain cavities of the brain and of the heart. See HEART.

Ven'tricle of the Lăr'ȳnx. [**Ventric'ulus Laryn'gis,** plural **Ventric'uli Laryn'gis.**] A depressed fossa situated immediately above the horizontal projection of the *chorda vocalis* at each side.

Ven'trĭ-cose. [**Ventrico'sus;** from *ven'ter*, the "belly."] Having a swelled-out appearance, like a belly; big-bellied. See URCEOLATE.

Ven-tric'u-li,* gen. **Ven-tric-u-lo'rum,** the plural of VENTRICULUS.

Ventric'uli Tri-cor'nēs.* ("Three-Horned Ventricles.") A designation of the two lateral ventricles of the brain. See TRICORNE.

Ven-tric'u-lus.* [Diminutive of *ven'ter*, the "belly."] The stomach; the principal organ of digestion. See STOMACH. Also, a VENTRICLE, which see.

Ven-tril'o-quism. [From *ven'ter*, the "belly," or "stomach," and *lo'quor*, to "speak;" because it often seems as if the voice were formed in the stomach or chest, and not in the mouth.] The utterance of the voice in such manner within the mouth that, by varying its tones in imitation of the voices of others, and according to supposed distances of the speakers, but without perceptible motion of the lips, perfect illusion is produced; also called *gastrologuism.* One possessing the power of ventriloquism is termed a *ventriloquist*.

Ventriloquist. See VENTRILOQUISM.

Ven-tril'o-quous. [**Ventril'o-quus.**] Relating to, or having the power of, ventriloquism.

Ven'trose. [**Ventro'sus;** from *ven'ter*, a "belly."] Having a belly, or swellings like the belly. See GASTRODES.

Ven'u-la.* [Diminutive of *ve'na*, a "vein."] A little vein.

Ve'nus,* gen. **Ven'e-ris.** (The goddess of beauty and love.) An ancient name of copper, which was so called because this metal was originally procured in great quantities in the island of Cyprus, the favorite abode of Venus. Also, a term for sexual love. See VENEREAL.

Ve'nus, Crys'tals of. A common name for the crystallized acetate of copper.

Ver, vêr. The French for "worm." See VERMIS.

Ve-ra'tri-a,* or **Ver'a-trin, Ver-a-tri'na.*** [From *Vera'trum*.] The Pharmacopœial name ‖ for a vegetable alkali obtained from *sabadilla*. It is very poisonous.

Ve-rat'ric. [**Verat'ricus.**] Belonging to veratria.

Ve-ra'trum.* A Linnæan genus of the class *Polygamia*, natural order *Melanthaceæ*. Also, the Pharmacopœial name (Lond., Ed., and Dub. Ph.) for the root of *Veratrum album*.

Vera'trum Al'bum.* Veratrum, or white hellebore; also termed *Helleborus albus*. The Pharmacopœial name (U.S. Ph.) for the rhizoma of the *Veratrum album*. It is a violent emetic and cathartic; in small doses it is a general stimulant to the secretions.

Vera'trum Sab-a-dil'la.* The name of one of the plants which afford *sabadilla*.

Vera'trum Vir'i-de.* American hellebore. The Pharmacopœial name (U.S. Ph.) for the rhizoma of the *Veratrum viride*. It is a violent emetic.

Verbenaceæ,* ver-be-na'she-ē. A natural order of exogenous plants, common in the tropics of both hemispheres, and in the temperate parts of South America. It includes the *Verbena*, *Vitex*, and *Tectona* (Teak), a large tree of India which is perhaps the best timber for ship-building in the world.

Verd Antique, verd an-teek'. A beautiful mottled green marble, or aggregate of marble and serpentine.

Verdigris, ver'de-grēss. [Lat. **Æru'go;** Fr. *Vert-de-gris*, věr'deh-grè'.] A common name for the subacetate of copper (*Cupri subacetas*). It occurs in masses of a pale-green color, almost wholly soluble with the aid of heat in dilute sulphuric acid. It is used externally as a detergent and escharotic, and is occasionally applied to chronic eruptions, foul and indolent ulcers, and venereal warts.

Ver'di-ter. A blue pigment obtained by adding chalk or whiting to a solution of copper in nitric acid. It is a hydrated percarbonate of copper.

Ver'juice. [From the French *verd*, "green," and *jus*, "juice."] (Fr. *Verjus*, věr'zhü'.) The juice of green or unripe grapes, crab-apples, etc.

Ver'mēs,* the plural of VERMIS, which see.

Vermicelli, vĕr-me-chel'le. [From *ver'mis*, a "worm."] An Italian article of food made from a paste of wheat flour, cheese, eggs, and sugar, which paste is formed into long wormlike pieces by forcing it through holes.

Ver-mic'u-lar. [**Vermicula'ris;** from *ver'mis*, a "worm."] Wormlike in shape or appearance.

Ver-mic'u-late. [**Vermicula'tus;** from the same.] Resembling a worm.

Ver-mic-u-lā'tion. [**Vermicula'tio, o'nis;** from the same.] A peculiar motion in certain parts like the progression of a worm.

Ver-mic'u-lose, or **Ver-mic'u-lous.** [**Vermiculo'sus;** from *vermic'ulus*, a "little worm."] Having worms.

Ver'mi-form. [**Vermifor'mis;** from *ver'mis*, a "worm."] Formed like a worm; wormlike.

Ver'miform Proc'ess. [**Proces'sus Vermifor'mis.**] Applied to the process connecting the two hemispheres of the cerebellum, like an earthworm rolled up.

Ver'mi-fuge. [**Vermif'ugus;** from *ver'mis*, a "worm," and *fu'go*, to "drive away."] Having power to expel worms; anthelmintic. See ANTISCOLIC.

Ver-mil'i-on. [**Vermil'ium.**] A red pigment of remarkable beauty; the same as cinnabar, or bisulphuret of mercury.

Ver-mi-nā'tion. [**Vermina'tio, o'nis;** from *ver'mis*, a "worm."] See MALIS.

Ver'mis,* plural **Ver'mēs.** (Fr. *Ver*, vêr.) A worm. Applied in Medicine to an animal which infests the intestines of man and other animals. Among the most common and important intestinal worms may be mentioned the *As'caris lumbricoi'des*, *Oxyurus vermicularis* (or *As'caris vermicula'ris*), *Tæ'nia la'ta*, *Tæ'nia so'lium*, and *Trichoceph'alus*, which are noticed under their proper heads. Often applied in the plural (*Vermes*) somewhat loosely to a class or division of animals including leeches, earthworms, snails, etc.

Ver-miv'o-rous. [**Vermiv'orus;** from *ver'mis*, a "worm," and *vo'ro*, to "devour."] Feeding on worms and insects.

Ver-nac'u-lar. [**Vernac'ulus;** from *ver'na*, a "bondman," a "home-born servant."] Native; indigenous; pertaining to one's native country.

Ver'nal. [**Verna'lis;** from *ver*, the "spring."] Belonging to spring.

Ver-nā'tion. [**Verna'tio, o'nis;** from the same.] The disposition of nascent leaves in the bud. Also called PRÆFOLIATION.

Ver-no'nĭ-a An-thel-min'tĭ-ca.* An East Indian plant of the natural order *Compositæ*, highly commended as a bitter tonic. The seeds are used as an anthelmintic.

Vérole, vā'rol'. The French term for SYPHILIS, which see.

Ve-ron'ĭ-ca.* A Linnæan genus of the class *Diandria*, natural order *Scrophulariaceæ*, or *Pediculares*.

Veron'ica A-quat'ĭ-ca.* A name for *Veronica beccabunga*.

Veron'ica Bec-ca-bun'ga.* The systematic name of the plant brooklime, or water-pimpernel. It was formerly much employed in Medicine, but its use of latter time has been generally abandoned.

Ver-ru'ca.* A wart; a hardening of the cuticle, of various appearance. A genus of the order *Tumores*, class *Locales*, of Cullen's Nosology. Also applied to a little knob occurring on the under surface of fungi.

Ver-ru'cĭ-form. [**Verrucifor'mis;** from *verru'ca*, a "wart."] Having the form of a wart.

Vĕr'ru-cose. [**Verruco'sus;** from the same.] Warty; covered with warts: ver'rucous.

Ver-ru'cu-lose. [**Verruculo'sus;** from *verru'cula*, a "little wart."] Having small warts: verrucu'ous.

Ver'sa-tile. [**Versat'ilis;** from *ver'so*, *versa'tum*, to "turn often."] Vane-like; oscillating. Applied to an anther when the apex of the filament is attached to a point near its middle.

Ver-sic'o-lor, o'ris.* [From *ver'sus*, "changed," and *co'lor*, "color."] Changing color, or having many tints: versicolored.

Ver'te-bra,* plural **Ver'te-bræ.** [From *ver'to*, to "turn."] A peculiarly-shaped bone, twenty-four of which compose the spine, or vertebral column and canal containing the spinal marrow. Each vertebra is composed of—

1. A *body*, or the main part, forming the centre of the spine, and bearing chiefly the weight of the body. It is sometimes termed the *cen'trum*, or "centre."

2. Four *articulating processes*, by which it is joined to the next vertebra. These are sometimes called *oblique* processes, the upper ones the *ascending* oblique, the lower the *descending* oblique processes.

3. A *spinous process*, which projects directly backward, those of the different vertebræ forming with their points the ridge of the back: from their sharpness the vertebral column is called *the Spine*.

4. Two *transverse processes*, which stand out at right angles, or laterally, from the body of the vertebra.

Ver'tebra Den-ta'ta.* The *axis*, or second cervical vertebra.

Ver'te-bræ,* gen. **Ver-te-bra'rum,** the plural of VERTEBRA, which see.

Ver'tebræ, False. A term applied to the various portions of the sacrum and *os coccygis*, regarded as vertebræ joined together by ossification.

Ver'te-bral. [**Vertebra'lis.**] Belonging to a vertebra, or the vertebræ.

Ver'tebral Arch, In-fe'rĭ-or. The same as HÆMAL ARCH, which see.

Ver'tebral Arch, Su-pe'rĭ-or. Applied in Comparative Anatomy to the portion of the vertebra *above* (the animal being in its horizontal position) the *centrum*, or body, forming the bony archway or canal in which is lodged the spinal marrow.

Ver'tebral Ar'te-rȳ. [**Arte'ria Vertebra'lis.**] A large artery, so named because it passes through a bony canal formed for it by the perforations of the cervical vertebræ. This and the carotid are the arteries of the brain.

Ver'tebral Ca-nal'. [**Cana'lis Vertebra'lis.**] Applied to the canal extending through the length of the vertebral column, and containing the spinal marrow.

Ver'tebral Col'umn. [Lat. **Colum'na Vertebra'lis;** Fr. *Colonne Vertébrale*, ko'lonn' vĕr'tâ'brâl'.] Also called **Spi'nal Col'umn** [**Colum'na Spina'lis**], and **Spine** [Lat. **Spi'na**; Fr. *Echine*, â'shĕn']. The bony column which forms the posterior part of the skeleton, between the head and pelvis. It is composed of twenty-four vertebræ, divided into—

1. The *Cervical*, or those of the neck, seven in number, characterized by having their transverse processes perforated for the passage of the vertebral artery. The first of these is called the *atlas*, from its immediately supporting the head; the second, the *dentata*, *odontoïdes*, or *axis*, from its axis or toothlike process, upon which it turns; and the lowest, *vertebra prominens*, from its spinous process being so much longer than the others.

2. The *Dorsal*, or those of the back, twelve in number. These are distinguished by having articular surfaces for the heads of the ribs.

3. The *Lumbar*, or those of the loins, five in number, and distinguished by their size and the length of the transverse processes.

Vertebral Disease. See SPONDYLARTHROCACE.

Ver'tebral Gut'ter. The vertebral gutters are situated at the side of the backbone, between the spinous processes and the angles of the ribs.

Ver-te-bra'ta,* the plural neuter of VERTEBRATUS, which see.

Vertebrates. See VERTEBRATUS.

Ver-te-bra'tus.* Vertebrated; having vertebræ. Applied in the plural neuter (*Vertebra'ta*) to the first great division of the animal kingdom, having a spine formed of vertebræ movable on each other, and each perforated by an annular opening for the passage of the spinal marrow.

Ver'tex, *icis.** [From *ver'to*, to "turn."] The summit or top of any thing. In Astronomy, the same as zenith. The vertex of an angle or cone is the angular point, or that in which the sides of the angle or cone intersect. In Anatomy, the top or crown of the head.

Ver'tĭ-cal. [**Vertica'lis**; from *ver'tex*.] Pertaining to the vertex; directed up and down; perpendicular.

Ver'tĭ-cēs,* the plural of VERTEX.

Ver'tĭ-cil, or **Ver'tĭ-cel.** [**Verticil'lus**; from *ver'to*, to "turn."] A whorl; a set of organs arranged in a circle around the axis of a plant.

Ver-tiç'il-late. [**Verticilla'tus.**] Disposed in verticils; whorled. Leaves are called verticillate when three or more are ranged around each node.

Ver-tĭ-cil-lĭ-flo'rous. [**Verticilliflo'rus**; from *verticil'lus*, a "spindle," and *flos*, a "flower."] Having spikes composed of verticils.

Ver-tĭ-cil'lus,* plural **Ver-tĭ-cil'li.** A term sometimes applied to the vertebræ.

Ver-tiġ'ĭ-nous. [**Vertigino'sus.**] Relating to vertigo.

Ver'tĭ-go. [**Verti'go, ġ'inis**; from *ver'to*, to "turn."] (Fr. *Étourdissement*, â'tooR'dĕss'mōNG'.) Dizziness; swimming of the head; giddiness.

Verumontanum. See CAPUT GALLINAGINIS.

Ve-sa'nĭ-a,* plural **Ve-sa'nĭ-æ.** [From *vesa'nus*, "mad," "furious."] Madness. Applied in the plural to an order in Cullen's Nosology, including diseases in which the judgment is impaired, without coma or pyrexia.

Ve-si'ca.* [From *vas*, a "vessel."] A bladder. In ordinary acceptation, the *Vesi'ca urina'ria*, or urinary bladder. Applied also to any thing resembling a bladder.

Vesi'ca Fel'lis.* ("Bladder of the Bile.") See GALL-BLADDER.

Vesi'ca Nat-a-to'rĭ-a.* ("Swimming Bladder.") The air-bladder of fishes, etc.

Ves'ĭ-cal. [**Vesica'lis**; from *vesi'ca*, a "bladder."] Having the appearance of a bladder.

Vesicantia,* ves-e-kan'she-a. See VESICANTS.

Ves'ĭ-cants. [**Vesican'tia**; from *vesi'ca*, a "bladder;" also, a "blister."] Epispastics. Topical agents which cause the exhalation of a thin serous fluid under the cuticle.

Ves'ĭ-cāt-ing. [**Ves'icans, an'tis**; from the same.] The same as VESICATORIUS.

Ves-ĭ-cā'tion. [**Vesica'tio, o'nis**; from the same.] The action of a vesicant; the formation of a blister.

Ves-ĭ-ca-to'rĭ-um.* [From the same.] (Fr. *Vésicatoire*, vâ'zè'kâ'twâR'.) A blister, or vesicatory.

Ves-ĭ-ca-to'rĭ-us.* [From the same.] Having the property of raising a blister; blistering: ves'icatory.

Vesicatory. See VESICATORIUS, and VESICATORIUM.

Ves'ĭ-cle. [**Vesic'ula**; diminutive of *vesi'ca*, a "bladder."] Literally, a "small bladder;" usually applied to an elevation of the cuticle, containing a clear watery fluid. Applied in the plural to certain little receptacles, etc.

Ves'ĭ-cle, Ger'mĭ-nal. A nucleated vesicle, being the earliest-formed part of the ovum. Its nucleus is termed the *germinal spot.*

Ve-sic'u-la Fel'lis.* ("Bladder of the Bile.") See Gall-Bladder.

Ve-sic'u-læ,* the plural of *Vesic'ula.* See Vesicle.

Vesiculæ Graafianæ. See Graafianæ Vesiculæ.

Vesiculæ Nabothi. See Nabothi Glandulæ.

Vesic'ulæ Sem-ĭ-na'lēs.* ("Seminal Vesicles.") The two reservoirs or receptacles of the semen situated on the back and lower part of the urinary bladder.

Ve-sic'u-lar. [**Vesicula'ris;** from *vesic'ula*, a "vesicle."] Belonging to or having vesicles.

Vésicule du Fiel, vā'zē'kül' dü fe-ĕl', or **Vésicule Biliaire,** vā'zē'kül' bē'-le-ēr'. The French terms for Gall-Bladder, which see.

Ves-ĭ-cu-lif'er-ous. [**Vesiculif'erus;** from *vesic'ula*, a "vesicle," and *fe'ro*, to "bear."] Bearing vesicles.

Ve-sic'u-lous. [**Vesiculo'sus;** from *vesic'ula*, a "vesicle."] Having or resembling vesicles.

Ves'per-tine. [From *ves'per*, "evening."] Appearing or expanding in the early evening. Applied to flowers.

Ves'sel. (Fr. *Vaisseau*, vā'sō'.) A canal or conduit by which blood, chyle, etc., are conveyed through the body and organs. (See Vas.) Applied in Botany to ducts and tubes. See Spiral Vessels, and Vascular Tissue.

Vessie, vā'sē', or vĕs'sē'. The French for Urinary Bladder, which see.

Ves'tĭ-bule. [**Vestib'ulum.**] Originally, the "porch or entry to a house." Applied to the small elliptical cavity of the internal ear, behind the *cochlea*, and in front of the semicircular canals.

Veta, vā'tā, or **Puna,** poo'nā. A disease prevalent in the elevated districts of South America, supposed to be caused by breathing rarefied air; it resembles sea-sickness.

Vet'e-rĭ-na-rȳ. [**Veterina'rius;** from *ve'ho*, to "carry."] Literally, "belonging to beasts of burden." See next article.

Vet'erinary Med'ĭ-cine. [**Medici'na Veterina'ria.**] The healing art as applied to diseases in horses, cattle, etc.; anciently called *Mulo-medicina.*

Vex'il-la-rȳ. [**Vexilla'ris;** from *vexil'lum*, a "banner."] Pertaining to the vexillum. Applied to æstivation, when the vexillum embraces the other petals.

Vex'il-late. [**Vexilla'tus;** from the same.] Having a vexillum. Applied to a papilionaceous plant.

Vex-il'lum.* [From *ve'ho, vec'tum*, to "carry."] Originally, a standard or ensign. The standard or upper petal of a papilionaceous flower.

Vī-a-bil'ĭ-tȳ. [See next article.] Ability to live.

Vī'a-ble. [Lat. **Viab'ilis;** Fr. *Viable*, vē'ābl'; from *vie*, "life."] A term in Medical Jurisprudence signifying "able or likely to live." Applied to the condition of a child at birth.

Vi'æ Lach-rȳ-ma'lēs.* ("Lachrymal Passages.") A collective term for the double apparatus for the secretion and excretion of the tears. This apparatus consists of the lachrymal gland, lachrymal ducts, the *puncta lachrymalia*, lachrymal sac, and nasal canal.

Viæ Primæ. See Primæ Viæ.

Vial. See Phial.

Vī-bī'cēs.* [Plural of *vi'bex*, the "mark of a blow."] Large purple spots which appear beneath the skin in certain malignant fevers.

Vī'bra-tĭle. [**Vibrat'ilis;** from *vi'bro, vibra'tum*, to "shake," or "brandish."] Having an oscillatory motion; moving to and fro, or from side to side.

Vī-brā'tion. [**Vibra'tio, o'nis;** from the same.] A very rapid movement which an elastic and rigid rod fixed at one of its extremities, or a cord stretched at the two ends, executes in oscillating. In Mechanics, the reciprocating motion of a body, as a pendulum, musical chord, etc.

Vī'bra-to-rȳ. [**Vibrato'rius.**] Similar to Vibratile.

Vib'rĭ-o.* [From the same.] A name given to minute animalcules developed in putrefying animal fluids.

Vī-bris'sæ, a'rum and *o'rum.** [From the same.] The stiff hairs in the nostrils. Also, the stiff, long-pointed bristles which grow from the upper lip and other parts of the head of mammals.

Vī-cā'rĭ-ous. [**Vica'rius;** from *vi'cis*, "change."] Acting in the place of another, or taking the place of another: as, *vicarious secretion.*

Vicq d'Azyr (vĕk dā'zēr'), **Cen'tra**

O-va'lĭ-a of. The white substance surrounded by the gray portion of the hemispheres of the cerebrum when the upper parts are sliced off nearly on a level with the *corpus callosum*.—(MAYNE.)

Vid'ĭ-an Nerve. The third or posterior branch of the spheno-palatine.

Vie, vē. The French term for LIFE, which see.

Vieillesse, ve-ā'yĕss', or ve-ĕl'yĕss'. The French word for "old age." See SENECTUS.

Vieus'sens (ve-u'sens), **Cen'trum O-vā'le of.** The white substance surrounded by the gray or cortical portion of the cerebrum when both hemispheres are sliced off quite on a level with the *corpus callosum*.—(MAYNE.)

Vigilance. See PERVIGILIUM.

Vil-lif'er-ous. [**Villif'erus;** from *vil'lus*, "wool," or "shaggy hair," and *fe'ro*, to "bear."] Bearing long hairs. Applied to plants.

Vil-lose', or **Vil'lous.** [**Villo'sus;** from *vil'lus*, "wool," or "hair."] Shaggy with long and soft hairs. Applied to stems, etc.

Vil'lus,* plural **Vil'li.** [From *vel'lus*, a "fleece of wool"?] Originally, "hair," or the "nap of cloth." Applied in the plural to the small conical projections on the *valvulæ conniventes*, having small pores which are the mouths of the absorbent vessels. In Botany, a hairy pubescence composed of slender and soft, hair-like filaments.

Vĭ-min'e-ous. [From *vi'men*, an "osier" or "twig."] Bearing or resembling long and flexible twigs like wicker.

Vine. [**Vin'ea;** from *vi'num*, "wine."] Any trailing, climbing, or twining stem. *Vine*, originally and properly, is applied to the Grape-vine.

Vinegar. See ACETUM.

Vinegar, Mother of. See MOTHER OF VINEGAR.

Vĭ-nif'er-ous. [**Vinif'erus;** from *vi'num*, "wine," and *fe'ro*, to "bear."] Wine-bearing or wine-yielding. See VITIS VINIFERA.

Vī'nous. [**Vino'sus;** from *vi'num*, "wine."] Relating to, or resembling, wine.

Vī'num.* A Latin word for wine, the juice of the grape. See WINE.

Vinum Album. See VINUM XERICUM.

Vī'num An-tĭ-mo'nĭ-i.* ("Wine of Antimony.") See ANTIMONIAL WINE.

Vī'num Por-ten'se,* or **Vī'num Ru'brum*** ("Red Wine"), 1850. The Pharmacopœial name (U.S. Ph.) for port wine.

Vī'num Xĕr'ĭ-cum.* The Pharmacopœial name (U.S. and Br. Ph.) for sherry wine, otherwise called *Vinum album* and *Vi'num al'bum Hispa'num.*

Vī'o-la.* [From ἴον, a "violet."] A Linnæan genus of the class *Pentandria*, natural order *Violaceæ*. Also, the Pharmacopœial name (U.S. Ph.) for the herb of *Viola pedata;* (Lond. and Ed. Ph.) for the flowers of the *Vi'ola odora'ta*, or sweet violet. It is a demulcent and expectorant.

Vī'ola Ca-ni'na.* Dog Violet. A plant the root of which is emetic and cathartic.

Vī'ola Od-o-ra'ta.* The sweet violet. See VIOLA.

Violaceæ,* vi-o-la'she-ē. A natural order of exogenous plants, natives of many temperate regions. Emetic properties are generally possessed by the roots of this order, which includes the *Vi'ola* (Violet).

Vi-o-lā'ceous. [**Viola'ceus.**] Resembling the violet.

Vī'o-let, Sweet. The *Viola odorata.*

Viper, or **Vipère.** See COLUBER BERUS.

Vir,* gen. **Vi'ri.** A Latin word signifying a "man" (or "male"), as distinguished from a woman; while *Homo* signifies man (human being), when reference is made to the race without respect to sex. See HOMO.

Vī'rēs,* gen. **Vir'ĭ-ŭm.** The plural of VIS, which see.

Vĭ-rĕs'çent. [From *vires'co*, to "become green."] Somewhat green.

Vir'gate. [**Virga'tus;** from *vir'ga*, a "rod."] Having the form of a rod; wand-like.

Vir'gin Oil. The substance which flows first from the pulp of the ripe juice of the olive, on expression.

Vir-ġĭ-na'le Claus'trum.* A name sometimes applied to the HYMEN.

Vir-ġin'ĭ-an Snake'-root. The *Aristolochia serpentaria*. See SERPENTARIA.

Vir'ġin's Milk. A cosmetic prepared by mixing one drachm of simple tincture of benzoin with four ounces of water.

Vir-gul'tum.* [From *vir'ga*, a "rod."] A twig or young shoot.

Vī'ri,* gen. **Vĭ-ro'rum,** the plural of VIR, which see.

Vir'ĭ-de Æ'ris.* (The "Green of Brass.") Another term for VERDIGRIS.

Vĭr-ĭ-dĕs'çent. [From *vir'idis*, "green."] The same as VIRESCENT, which see.

Vĭr-ĭ-dĭ-flo'rus.* [From *vir'idis*, "green," and *flos*, a "flower."] Having flowers of a green color.

Vĭr'ĭ-din. [**Viridi'na;** from *vir'idis*, "green."] Proposed by De Candolle for CHROMULE, which see.

Vī'rile. [**Viri'lis;** from *vir*, a "man."] Belonging to a man; peculiar to man, as distinguished from woman.

Virile Membrum. See MEMBRUM VIRILE.

Virilis Ætas. See ÆTAS VIRILIS.

Vĭ-rĭl'ĭ-tȳ. [**Viril'itas, a'***tis;* from *vir'ilis*, "proper to man."] Manhood; full age. Usually applied to the generative power of man.

Vĭr'u-lent. [**Virulen'tus;** from *vi'rus*, a "poison."] Poisonous; malignant.

Vī'rus.* [From *vis*, plural *vi'res*, "strength."] Literally, "poison." Applied to any matter produced by disease, and capable of propagating that disease by inoculation or contagion.

Vis,* plural **Vī'rēs.** A Latin word signifying "force," or "power."

Vis a Ter'go.* Literally, "force from behind." Any impelling power.

Vis For-mạ-ti'vạ.* ("Formative Power.") The formative power or influence which is supposed to preside over the nourishment and growth of the body, and the performance of its various functions.

Vis Inertiæ* (in-er'she-ē). ("Force of Inertia.") See INERTIA.

Vis Med-ĭ-ca'trix (or **Con-ser-va'trix**) **Nạ-tu'ræ.*** The healing or preserving power of nature.

Vis Mor'tu-ạ.* ("Dead Force.") That property by which a muscle contracts after the death of the animal to which it belongs, or after it has been cut from a living body.

Vis Ner've-ạ.* ("Nervous Force or Power.") The name given by Haller to that power in the muscular fibre which enables it to receive impressions conveyed to it by the nerves.

Vis Vi'tæ,* or **Vis Vi-ta'lis.*** Vital power or force. See IRRITABILITY.

Vis'çe-rạ,* the plural of VISCUS.

Vis'çe-rạl. [**Viscera'lis;** from *vis'cus, vis'ceris*, a "bowel."] Belonging to the viscera. See SPLANCHNIC.

Vis'çid. [**Vis'cidus;** from *vis'cum*, "birdlime."] Clammy, gluey, adhesive.

Vĭs-çĭd'ĭ-tȳ, Vis-cos'ĭ-tȳ. [**Viscid'itas, a'***tis*, or **Viscos'itas, a'***tis;* from the same.] The property of adhesiveness; stickiness or clamminess.

Vis'coid. [**Viscoi'des;** from *vis'cum*, the "mistletoe," and εἶδος, a "form."] Resembling the mistletoe.

Vis'cous. [**Visco'sus;** from *vis'cum*, "birdlime."] Very glutinous; adhesive; sticky.

Vis'cus,* or **Vis'cum.*** [Gr. ἰξός, or Æol. βισκός.] The fruit of the mistletoe, or *Viscum album.* A Linnæan genus of the class *Diœcia*, natural order *Loranthaceæ.*

Vis'cus Quer'cus,* or **Vis'cum Al'bum.*** The mistletoe, a parasitical plant growing on the oak, and other trees.

Vis'cus, *eris*,* plural **Vis'çe-rạ.** Any large organ contained in the splanchnic cavities, such as the lungs, liver, spleen, etc. In the plural, it signifies entrails.

Vĭ'sion. [**Vi'sus** and **Vi'sio, o'***nis;* from *vi'deo, vi'sum*, to "see."] (Fr. *Vue*, vü.) Sight; the faculty of seeing; the act of seeing; also, something which is the object of sight; an apparition. In the act or process of vision, the lens of the eye casts an image upon the retina similar to that thrown upon the screen of a camera obscura. From the retina the impression is conveyed by the optic nerve to the brain.

Vision, Defective, or **Depraved.** See DYSOPSIA.

Vision, Distorted. See METAMORPHOPSIA.

Vision, Double. See DIPLOPIA.

Vision, Single. See MONOBLEPSIS.

Vision, Treble. See TRIPLOPIA.

Visual, vizh'u-ạl. Pertaining to, or used in, vision.

Vis'ual An'gle, in Optics, is the angle under which an object is seen, or the angle formed at the eye by the rays of light coming from the extremities of an object.

Vis'ual Rays. The lines of light coming from an object to the eye.

Visus. See VISION.

Vi'sus Trip'lex.* ("Triple Vision.") The same as TRIPLOPIA, which see.

Vi'tạ.* [From βιοτή, "life," or "means of living."] The state of existence or being; life. See LIFE.

Vi'tạ Pro'pri-ạ.* Sometimes used as synonymous with IRRITABILITY. See NISUS FORMATIVUS.

Vitaceæ,* vi-ta'she-ē, or **Vi'tēs.*** A natural order of exogenous plants (climbing shrubs), natives of the milder and hotter parts of both hemispheres.

The most important genus of this order is the *Vi'tis* (Grape-vine).

Vi'tal. [**Vita'lis;** from *vi'ta,* "life."] Belonging or essential to life.

Vi'tal Air. A name for oxygen gas.

Vital Functions. See FUNCTIONS.

Vi'tal Prin'ci-ple. [**Princip'ium Vi'tæ.**] That on which life depends; the unknown cause of life.

Vi-tal'i-ty. [From *vi'ta,* "life."] The principle of life; vital action, or vital power.

Vi'ta-lize. [From *vi'ta,* "life."] To animate; to endow with life.

Vi'tals. [**Vita'lia.**] A term applied to the heart, lungs, brain, etc.

Vi-tel-lif'er-ous. [**Vitellif'erus;** from *vitel'lus,* and *fe'ro,* to "bear."] Provided with a *vitellus.* Applied to certain plants.

Vi-tel'lo-In-tes'ti-nal Duct. [From *vitel'lus.*] A wide duct by means of which the nutritive substance of the yolk enters the alimentary canal for the nutrition of the embryo.

Vi-tel'lus.* [From *vi'ta,* "life."] The yelk or yolk of the bird's egg; also, the yelk or yolk of the *ovum,* afterwards to become the *Vesicula umbilicalis.* In Botany, the thickened embryo-sac persistent in the seed, as in *Sauru'rus.*

Vi'tes,* the plural of *Vi'tis,* forming the Jussieuan name of an order of plants. See VITACEÆ.

Vitia Conformationis,* vish'e-a kon-for-ma-she-o'nis. ("Faults or Defects of Conformation.") A term signifying malformations.

Vit-i-li'go, *inis.** A skin-disease in which there are smooth, white, glistening tubercles about the ears, neck, or face, or over the whole body, mingled with shining *papulæ.* Also, a name for leprosy.

Vi-til'i-goid. [**Vitiligoi'des;** from *vitili'go,* and εἶδος, a "form."] Resembling *vitiligo.*

Vi'tis.* A Linnæan genus of the class *Pentandria,* natural order *Vitaceæ.*

Vi'tis Vi-nif'e-ra.* ("Wine-bearing Vine.") The systematic name of the common Vine of Europe.

Vit. Ov. Sol. See V. O. S.

Vit're-ous. [**Vit'reus;** from *vi'trum,* "glass."] Of, or pertaining to, glass; glassy; hyaline.

Vit're-ous Hu'mor [**Hu'mor Vit'reus**]; called, also, **Cor'pus Vit're-um*** ("Vitreous Body"). The name applied to the transparent gelatinous substance which fills the back part of the eye behind the crystalline lens.

Vit-ri-fac'tion. The same as VITRIFICATION.

Vit-ri-fi-ca'tion. [**Vitrifica'tio, o'nis;** from *vi'trum,* "glass," and *fa'cio,* to "make."] The act or process of vitrifying, or converting into glass.

Vit'ri-ol. [**Vitri'olum;** from *vi'trum,* "glass."] A term applied to the sulphates of iron, copper, zinc, according to their respective color, as green, blue, and white vitriol; named from their glass-like appearance. Also, a popular term for sulphuric acid.

Vit'riol, Aç'id of. Sulphuric or vitriolic acid.

Vit'riol, Blue. [**Vitri'olum Cæru'leum.**] The sulphate of copper. See CUPRI SULPHAS.

Vit'riol, Green. [**Vitri'olum Vir'ide.**] The sulphate of iron; copperas.

Vit'riol, Oil of. An old name for sulphuric acid, given because it was formerly obtained by distillation from green vitriol (sulphate of iron, or copperas).

Vit'riol, White. [**Vitri'olum Al'bum.**] The common term for sulphate of zinc. See ZINCI SULPHAS.

Vit-ri-ol'ic Aç'id. Sulphuric acid.

Vitriolum. See VITRIOL.

Vit-ro'sus.* [From *vi'trum,* "glass."] The same as VITREOUS, which see.

Vi'trum.* A Latin word signifying "glass."

Vi'trum An-ti-mo'ni-i.* ("Glass of Antimony.") A reddish-brown-colored glass obtained by first calcining antimony and then melting it in a crucible. It is employed in preparing tartarized antimony.

Vivianiaceæ,* viv-e-an-e-a'she-ē. [From *Vivia'nia,* one of the genera.] A small natural order of exogenous plants, natives of Brazil and Chili.

Vi-vip'a-rous. [**Vivip'arus;** from *vi'vus,* "alive," and *pa'rio,* to "bring forth."] Bringing forth young alive. In Botany, germinating from the seed, or sprouting from a bulb, etc., while still attached to the parent plant.

Viv-i-pa'tion. [**Vivipa'tio, o'nis;** from the same.] A term applied to the mode of generation which consists in the *ovum,* when separated from the ovary, becoming attached to the maternal organs, and deriving its nourishment from them until birth. Otherwise termed viviparous generation.

Viv-i-sec'tion. [**Vivisec'tio, o'nis;** from *vi'vus,* "alive," and *se'co, sec'tum,* to "cut."] The cruel practice of cutting into or dissecting living animals.

Vo'cal. [**Voca'lis;** from *vox, vo'cis,* the "voice."] Pertaining to the voice, or uttered by the voice.

Vo'cal Chords, or **Vo'cal Lig'a-ments.** The same as CHORDÆ VOCALES, which see.

Vochyaceæ,* vo-ke-a'she-ē. [From *Vo'chya,* one of the genera.] A natural order of exogenous trees and shrubs, found in equinoctial America.

Voice. [Lat. **Vox, Vo'cis;** Gr. φωνή; Fr. *Voix,* vwå.] The sound produced in the larynx by means of the air which passes out of the trachea.

Vo-lat'ic. [**Volat'icus;** from *vo'lo, vola'tum,* to "fly."] Flying; flitting.

Vol'a-tile. [**Volat'ilis;** from the same.] Evaporating; flying off; disposed to pass off by spontaneous evaporation.

Vol'atile Al'ka-li, or **Vol'atile Salt.** The same as AMMONIA, which see.

Vol-a-til'ĭ-tў. [**Volatil'itas, a'tis;** from *volat'ilis,* "volatile."] The state of being volatile. That property by which certain bodies assume the elastic state.

Vol-a-til-ĭ-zā'tion. [**Volatiliza'tio, o'nis;** from the same.] The transformation of a solid body into gas or vapor.

Vol-can'ic. Pertaining to a volcano, or produced by a volcano.

Vol-cā'no. [From *Vulca'nus,* or *Volca'nus,* the god of fire, and of smiths: he was supposed to have his workshops in volcanic mountains.] A mountain or hill having at the top a cup-shaped cavity, called a crater, from which issue flames of fire, steam, and gases of various kinds, and sometimes streams of red-hot lava, masses of melted rock, stones, ashes, and scoriæ.

Vo-lĭ'tion. [From *vo'lo,* obsolete supine *vol'itum,* to "will," to "desire."] The act of willing, or choosing.

Vol-sel'la.* [From *vel'lo, vul'sum,* to "pull."] An instrument for removing bodies sticking in the throat; forceps. Also spelled *Vulsella.*

Vol-tā'ic. Applied to a galvanic apparatus or battery invented by Volta. See GALVANIC.

Vol'ta-ism. [**Voltais'mus.**] Galvanism, as produced by Volta's apparatus. See GALVANISM.

Vol-tam'e-ter. [**Voltam'etrum;** from *Vol'taism,* and μέτρον, a "measure."] An instrument for indicating the amount of voltaic electricity passing through it in a given time.

Vol'u-ble. [**Volu'bilis;** from *vol'vo, volu'tum,* to "roll."] Apt to roll. In Botany, turning round spirally; twining.

Vol'ume. [**Volu'men,** *inis;* from the same.] Originally, a roll of manuscript, which was the form of ancient books. A book or bundle. In Chemistry, the bulk or dimension of gases. The space which a fluid occupies is called its volume.

DEF'INITE VOL'UMES. The union of gases is always effected in simple proportions of their volumes: a volume of one gas combines with an equal volume, or twice, three, four, or five times the volume, of another gas, and in no intermediate proportion. This is called the law of *definite volumes.*

Vol'un-ta-rў. [From *volun'tas,* the "will."] Relating to the will; spontaneous; acting or moving in obedience to the will.

Vo-lute'. [From *vol'vo, volu'tum,* to "roll."] Rolled up. Applied to parts of plants.

Vol'va.* [From the same.] The membranous cover or wrapper enclosing a young fungus.

Vol'vate. [**Volva'tus.**] Provided with a *volva.*

Vol'vu-lus.* [From *vol'vo,* to "roll."] The same as ILEAC PASSION, which see.

Vo'mer, eris.* A "ploughshare." Applied to a small thin bone in the median line, forming the posterior and principal portion of the *septum narium.*

Vom'ĭ-ca,* plural **Vom'ĭ-çæ.** [From *vo'mo,* to "vomit or expectorate."] Abscess of the lungs; resolution of tubercles.

Vom'ĭ-cus.* [From the same.] Pertaining to, or causing, vomiting.

Vomiquier, vo'mė'ke-å'. The French name for STRYCHNOS, which see.

Vomissement. See VOMITING.

Vom'it. [**Vom'itus;** from *vo'mo, vom'itum,* to "vomit."] An emetic draught or powder; also, the matter rejected by vomiting. See EMETIC, and VOMITING.

Vom'it-ing. [**Vomi'tio, o'nis;** from the same.] (Fr. *Vomissement,* vo'mėss'-mōNº'.) The forcible ejection of the contents of the stomach through the œsophagus and mouth; vomition; emesis.

Vomiting of Blood. See HÆMATEMESIS.

Vomition. See VOMITING.

Vomito Nigro, vom'e-to nee'gro. ("Black Vomit.") A Spanish name for yellow fever.

Vom-i-to'ri-a.* [See next article.] Emetics; agents which produce vomiting.

Vom'i-to-ry. [**Vomito'rius;** from *vo'mo, vom'itum,* to "vomit."] Causing vomiting; emetic. See EMETIC.

Vomituritio,* vom-e-tu-rish'e-o. [From the same.] Retching; an ineffectual effort to vomit.

Vom'i-tus Cru-en'tus.* ("Bloody Vomit.") See HÆMATEMESIS.

Vo-ra'cious. [**Vo'rax, a**'*cis;* from *vo'ro,* to "devour."] Devouring; ravenous; extremely hungry.

Voracious Appetite. See VORACITY.

Vo-raç'i-ty, or **Vo-ra'cious-ness.** [From *vo'ro,* to "devour."] Greediness for food. Also, the disease termed *Bulimia.* See ADDEPHAGIA.

Vor'tex,* plural **Vor'ti-ces.** [From *ver'to,* to "turn."] A Latin word signifying a "whirlpool." In the Cartesian philosophy, vortex signifies a collection of material particles forming a fluid or ether, endowed with a rapid rotary motion about an axis.

Vor'ti-ces,* the plural of VORTEX.

V. O. S., or **Vit. Ov. Sol.** = *Vitel'lo o'vi solu'tus.** "Dissolved in the yolk of an egg."

Vox. See VOICE.

Vox Ab-sçis'sa* (literally, "voice cut off"). Loss of voice.

Vox Cholerica. See CHOLEROPHONE.

V. S. = *Venæsec'tio.** "Venesection."

Vue, vü. The French term for VISION, which see.

Vulcanization. See VULCANIZING.

Vul'ca-niz-er. A name for the steam apparatus used in vulcanizing.

Vul'ca-niz-ing. [From *Vul'can,* the god of fire.] A process by which caoutchouc and some other substances combined with sulphur, and exposed to the action of steam at a high temperature, are rendered hard and elastic like horn.

Vul-ne-ra'ri-a A'qua.* ("Vulnerary Water.") A water or lotion which promotes the healing of wounds. See ARQUEBUSADE, EAU D'.

Vul'ne-ra-ry. [**Vulnera'rius;** from *vul'nus, vul'neris,* a "wound."] Belonging to wounds. Applied to medicines which are supposed to favor the healing of wounds.

Vul'pis Mor'bus.* ("Fox Disease.") A name for ALOPECIA, which see.

Vul'tus,* anciently written **Vol'tus.** [From *vol'itum,* the old supine of *vo'lo,* to "will;" because the expression of the countenance indicates the wish or will.] A Latin word signifying the "countenance, look, or face."

Vul'va,* anciently written **Vol'va.** [From *vol'vo,* to "roll or wrap up."] Originally, "that which is wrapped round any thing;" hence, the "womb;" now applied to the fissure in the female, extending from the *mons Ven'eris* to the perinæum.

Vul'va Cĕr'e-bri.* A small aperture of the brain forming the part by which the three ventricles communicate.

Vul-vi'tis, *idis.** Inflammation of the vulva.

Vulvi'tis Blen-nor-rhag'i-ca.* A muco-purulent discharge from the mucous membrane of the vulva. See BLENNORRHAGIA.

Vul'vo-Vag'i-nal Gland. A small gland at each side of the junction of the vulva with the vagina.

W.

Wacke, wăk, or wăk'ęh. (German.) A modification of basalt.

Wadd, wŏd. A name sometimes applied to the ores of manganese; and also to plumbago.

Wakefulness. See AGRYPNIA.

Warm-Blood'ed. A term applied to mammals and birds which have a twofold circulation, *systemic* and *pulmonic.* See DIPLO-CARDIAC.

Wart. See VERRUCA.

Warty. See VERRUCOSE.

Wash. See LOTION.

Wash, Black. See BLACK WASH.

Wast'ing. [From *vas'to,* to "waste," or "destroy"?] See CONSUMPTION, EMACIATION, and TABES.

Watchfulness. See AGRYPNIA.

Watching. See PERVIGILIUM.

Water. See AQUA.

Water-Bed, Arnott's. See HYDROSTATIC BED.

Wa'ter-Brash. The common name for PYROSIS, which see.

Wa'ter-Cure. The system of medical treatment termed HYDROPATHY, which see.

Water, Distilled. See AQUA DESTILLATA.

Wa'ter-Dock. The *Ru'mex aquat'icus* or *R. Britan'nica hydrolap'athum.*

Wa'ter of Crys-tal-li-zā'tion. The water which combines with salts in the act of crystallizing.

Waters, Distilled. See AQUÆ STILLATITIÆ.

Waters, Green. See GREEN WATERS.

Waters, Mineral. See AQUÆ MINERALES.

Waters, The. The *Liquor amnii.* See PRIMITIÆ.

Wa'ter-spout. A very remarkable meteorological phenomenon observed for the most part at sea, but sometimes also on shore, though generally near the ocean. Its general appearance may be described as follows: from a dense cloud a conical pillar, which appears to consist of condensed vapor, is seen to descend with the apex downwards. When over the sea, there are usually two cones,—one projecting from the cloud, and the other from the water below it. These sometimes unite, and the junction has been observed to be accompanied by a flash of lightning.

Wa'ter-Tomes. A name for *pyrosis.*

Waved. See UNDULATE.

Wax. A name applied to various substances. (See CERA, and CERUMEN.) Vegetable wax is a ternary product of vegetation, occurring as an excretion on the surface of leaves and fruits, forming the bloom or *glaucous* surface which repels water.

Wax-Ker'nels. The popular name for irritated submaxillary glands.

Weaning. See ABLACTATION.

Wedge-Shaped. See CUNEIFORM.

Weld. A name for RESEDA LUTEOLA, which see.

Weld'ing. The act of uniting metals by the hammer at a temperature below fusion. Iron (or steel) and platinum are said to be the only metals which can be welded.

Wen. [**Lu'pia?**] An encysted tumor.

Whartonian Duct. See DUCT OF WHARTON.

Whēal. An elevation of the skin, as if produced by a stroke from a cane. See WHELK.

Whēat. The seeds of the *Trit'icum hyber'num.*

Wheel-Shaped. See ROTATE, and TROCHOID.

Wheezing. See CERCHNUS, and RHONCHUS.

Whelk. Similar to wheal; also applied to a small tubercle usually situated on the face, otherwise called IONTHUS, which see.

Whey, hwā. [**Se'rum Lac'tis.**] The fluid part of milk which remains after the separation of the curd.

Whiskey. See SPIRITUS FRUMENTI.

White Gum. The *Strophulus albidus.*

White Lead. See CERUSE, and PLUMBI CARBONAS.

White Leg. The common name for PHLEGMATIA DOLENS.

White Pre-cip'i-tate. The *Hydrar'gyrum ammonia'tum* of the United States and British Pharmacopœias, otherwise called *Hydrar'gyrum præcipita'tum al'bum* ("White Precipitated Mercury"), and *Submu'rias hydrar'gyri ammonia'ta* ("Ammoniated Submuriate of Mercury"). Used as an external application in *psora* and other cutaneous affections.

White Swell'ing. A common name for HYDRARTHRUS, which see.

White Vit'ri-ol. The sulphate of zinc. See ZINCI SULPHAS.

Whi'ten-ing. See BLANCHING. The carbonate of lime. See CHALK.

Whites. The popular name for LEUCORRHŒA, which see.

Whitlow. See ONYCHIA, and PARONYCHIA.

Whooping-Cough. See PERTUSSIS.

Whorl. See VERTICIL.

Whorled. Disposed in whorls; verticillate.

Wild. In Botany, growing spontaneously; uncultivated.

Wild Cherry. See PRUNUS VIRGINIANA.

Wild Cucumber. See MOMORDICA ELATERIUM.

Wild'fire-Rash. See STROPHULUS VOLATICUS.

Wil'lis, Chords of. [**Chor'dæ Willis'ii.**] Small, white, fibrous bands which in many places cross the superior longitudinal sinus of the brain.

Wil'lis, Cir'cle of. [**Cir'culus Willis'ii.**] See CIRCULUS.

Will-o'-the-Wisp. See IGNIS-FATUUS.

Willow. See SALIX.

Willow, Crack. See SALIX FRAGILIS.

Willow, White. See SALIX ALBA.

Wind. See FLATULENCE.

Wind-Blast. See COUP DE VENT.

Wind Drop'sȳ. A name sometimes applied to EMPHYSEMA, which see.

Wind'pipe. The trachea.

Wine. [**Vi'num.**] Properly, the fermented juice of the grape, or of fruits the juice of which resembles that of the grape. All products of spirituous fermentation are sometimes denominated wines.

Wine-Madness. See ŒNOMANIA.

Wing. In Botany, any membranous expansion. See ALA, PENNA, and PINNA.

Winged. See ALATE, and PINNATE.

Wing-like Bones. See ALARIA OSSA.

Wing-like Veins. See ALARES VENÆ.

Wing-Shaped. See ALIFORM, ALARIS, and PTERYGOIDES.

Wins'low, Fo-ra'men of. [**Fora'men Winslo'vii.**] A somewhat oval opening, through which the cavity of the omentum communicates with the general peritonæal cavity.

Wins'low, Lig'ạ-ment of. The external process of the tendon of the *semimembranosus* muscle.

Wins'low, Pos-te'rĭ-or Lig'a-ment of. Irregular bands passing obliquely over the back part of the capsular ligament of the knee-joint.

Win-te'rạ.* [Named from Captain *Winter.*] A Linnæan genus of the class *Polyandria,* natural order *Magnoliaceæ.*

Winte'ra Ar-o-mat'ĭ-cạ.* The former name of the *Dri'mys aromat'ica,* or *Dri'mys Winte'ri,* from which Winter's bark is procured. See WINTER'S BARK.

Win-te-ra'nạ Cạ-nel'lạ.* A name for *Canella alba.*

Winteranus Cortex. See WINTER'S BARK.

Win'ter-Green. The common name for the *Chimaph'ila umbella'ta;* otherwise called *Pyr'ola umbella'ta,* and *Gaulthe'ria procum'bens.*

Win'ter's Bark. [**Wintera'nus Cor'tex.**] The bark of the *Dri'mys aromat'ica,* or *Dri'mys Winte'ri;* formerly termed *Winte'ra aromat'ica.* It is a stimulant aromatic tonic.

Wirt'sung, Duct of. A name for the pancreatic duct.

Wisdom-Teeth. See DENTES SAPIENTIÆ.

Withering. See MARCESCENT.

Woad. A name for *Isatis tinctoria,* a plant formerly used to dye blue.

Wolf'fĭ-ạn Bod'ies. [**Cor'pora Wolffia'na,** or **Cor'pus Wolffia'num** in the singular.] The name given to certain bodies found in the renal region of the fœtus previous to the formation of the kidneys, the function of which they are supposed to fulfil during the early period of fœtal existence. They disappear about the ninth or tenth week of utero-gestation. They were first discovered in fowl and described by Wolff, whence their name.

Wolf's Bane. See ACONITUM NAPELLUS.

Womb. See UTERUS; also, HYSTERA, MATRIX, and METRA.

Womb, Inflammation of. See HYSTERITIS, METRITIS, and UTERITIS.

Womb, Inflammation of the Lining Membrane of. See ENDOMETRITIS, and ENDO-UTERITIS.

Womb-Passage. See VAGINA.

Womb, Retroflexion of. See RETROFLEXIO UTERI.

Womb, Retroversion of. See RETROVERSIO UTERI.

Wood. [**Lig'num.**] The hard fibrous substance of which trunks and branches of trees are chiefly composed. See SAP-WOOD, and DURAMEN.

Wood-Sor'rel. A common name of the OXALIS ACETOSELLA, which see.

Wood'ȳ Night'shade. The *Sola'num dulcama'ra.*

Wood'y Tis'sue, or **Wood'y Fi'bre.** A modification of cellular tissue, consisting of slender, transparent, membranous tubes, tapering acutely to each end, which is closed so that they have no direct communication with each other. Woody tissue constitutes a large part of trees and shrubs. It is also called *Pleuren'chyma.*

Woo-ra'rạ.* A very powerful poison obtained from Guiana. Written also CURARE, which see.

Wor'mĭ-i, Os'sạ* ("Bones of Wormius"), or **Os'sa Tri-que'trạ.*** Names applied to small triangular portions of bone which are often found in the lambdoid, and sometimes one in the squamous, suture; first pointed out by Wormius.

Worms. See VERMIS.

Worm'seed. See CHENOPODIUM ANTHELMINTICUM. Also applied to *Artemisia santonica.*

Worm'seed, Tar-tā'rĭ-ạn. A name for the seeds of *Artemisia santonica.*

Worm'wood. The common name of *Artemisia absinthium.* Its properties are tonic and anthelmintic.

Wort. An infusion of malt. It has been recommended as a remedy in scurvy.

Wound. [**Vul'nus,** *eris.*] A solution of continuity in any of the soft parts of the body, caused by external violence: it may be *contused, incised, lacerated, punctured,* or *poisoned.*

CONTUSED' WOUNDS. [*Vul'nera Contu'sa.*] Those made by a violent blow from some blunt instrument or surface.

GUN'SHOT WOUNDS. [*Vul'nera Sclopetu'ria.*] Those caused by metallic or stony bodies projected from firearms.

INCISED' WOUNDS. [*Vul'nera Inci'sa.*] Those made by a simple division of the fibres by a sharp cutting instrument, without contusion or laceration.

LAC'ERATED WOUNDS. [*Vul'nera Laçe'-era.*] Those in which the fibres, instead of being divided by a cutting instrument, have been torn asunder by violence, the edges being jagged and irregular.

PUNC'TURED WOUNDS. [*Vul'nera Puncta'ta.*] Those made by a pointed instrument, as a needle, thorn, or bayonet.

Wrapper. See VOLVA.

Wrinkled. See RUGOSE.

Wrisberg (ris'bẹrg, or vris'bĕrg), **Nerves of.** The cutaneous nerves of the arm, derived from the second and third dorsal nerves; first particularized by Wrisberg.

Wrist, rĭst. [Lat. **Car'pus;** Gr. καρπός; Fr. *Poignet*, pwån'yå', and *Carpe*, karp.] The part which connects the forearm with the hand. It includes eight bones arranged in two transverse rows, four in each row.

Wrist'-Drop. Paralysis of the extensor muscles of the hands from the poisonous local action of lead, in consequence of which the hand and wrist cannot be supported; whence the name.

Wry Neck. [**Torticol'lis.**] An involuntary fixed inclination of the head towards one of the shoulders.

X.

(☞ **X** at the beginning of a word is always to be sounded like *Z.*)

Xan-them'ạ-tin. [**Xanthæmati'na;** from ξανθός, "yellow," and *hæmati'na*, the coloring matter of logwood.] A yellow, bitter substance obtained by dissolving hæmatin in weak nitric acid.

Xan'thic. [**Xan'thicus;** from ξανθός, "yellow."] Belonging to a yellow color; yellowish.

Xan'thic Ox'ide. Another name for uric oxide, a yellowish substance sometimes found in the urine.

Xan'thin. [**Xanthi'na;** from ξανθός, "yellow."] A peculiar organic substance sometimes forming a species of urinary calculus; also called xanthic, or uric, oxide, and urinous acid. Also applied to the coloring matter of madder.

Xan-tho-car'pous. [**Xanthocar'pus;** from ξανθός, "yellow," and καρπός, "fruit."] Having yellow fruit.

Xan-tho-çeph'ạ-lus.* [From ξανθός, "yellow," and κεφαλή, a "head."] Applied to a mushroom the *capitulum* of which is yellow; also, as a specific name to animals having a yellow head.

Xan'tho-don, on'*tis.** [From ξανθός, "yellow," and ὀδούς, a "tooth."] Having yellow teeth; xanthodon'tous.

Xan'tho-ġen. [**Xanthoge'nium;** from ξανθός, "yellow," and γεννάω, to "produce."] A variety of the coloring matter of vegetables, producing a yellow color with alkalies.

Xan'tho-phy̆ll. [**Xanthophyl'lum;** from ξανθός, "yellow," and φύλλον, a "plant."] The yellow coloring matter of plants.

Xan-thor-rhi'zạ.* ("Yellow-Root.") The Pharmacopœial name (U.S. Ph.) for the root of the *Xanthorrhiza apiifolia.* It is a bitter tonic.

Xan-tho'sis.* [From ξανθός, "yellow."] A coloring matter or yellow pigment found in cancer, in irregular spots of small extent, presenting sometimes a saffron, at others an orange, tint.

Xanthoxylaceæ,* zan-thox-i-la'-she-ē. [From *Xanthox'ylum*, one of the genera.] A natural order of exogenous trees and shrubs, found in India, China, and in the temperate and tropical parts of America. The species are nearly all aromatic and pungent.

Xan-thox'y̆-lum.* Prickly Ash. The Pharmacopœial name (U.S. Ph.) for the bark of the *Xanthox'ylum fraxin'eum.* It is a stimulant, somewhat resembling guaiac and mezereon in its operation, and, like them, is frequently used as a remedy in rheumatic affections.

Xan'thu-ret. [**Xanthure'tum;**

from ξανθός, "yellow."] A combination of xanthogen with a metal.

Xĕr-o-der'ma, atis.* [From ξηρός, "dry," and δέρμα, the "skin."] A dryness and harshness of the skin, the consequence of diminished function of the sebiparous glands.

Xĕr-oph-thăl'mĭ-a.* [From ξηρός, "dry," and ὀφθαλμός, the "eye."] An inflammation of the eye without discharge.

Xi'phoid. [**Xiphoi'des;** from ξίφος, a "sword."] Resembling a sword; ensiform.

Xi'phoid Car'tĭ-lage. [**Cartila'go Xiphoi'des.**] A cartilaginous *epiphysis* forming the termination of the inferior extremity of the sternum; the ensiform cartilage.

Xī-phoi'dĭ-an. [**Xiphoidia'nus;** from *xiphoi'des* cartila'go.] Of, or belonging to, the xiphoid cartilage.

Xȳ-lo-car'pous. [**Xylocar'pus;** from ξύλον, "wood," and καρπός, "fruit."] Having woody fruit.

Xȳ-log'ra-phȳ. [From ξύλον, "wood," and γράφω, to "write," or "engrave."] The art of engraving on wood.

Xȳ'loid. [**Xyloi'des;** from ξύλον, "wood," and εἶδος, a "form."] Resembling wood. See LIGNIFORM.

Xȳ-loi'din. [**Xyloidi'na;** from the same.] A substance produced by the action of nitric acid upon starch: so named because partaking slightly of the properties of wood.

Xȳ-loph'ĭ-lous. [**Xyloph'ilus;** from ξύλον, "wood," and φιλέω, to "love."] Growing upon, or living in, decayed wood. Applied to plants and insects.

Y.

Yam. The esculent root or tuber of several species of *Dioscо'rea*, a plant which grows in the East and West Indies. The Yam forms an important article of food.

Yarrow. See ACHILLEA MILLEFOLIUM.

Yava (yå'va) **Skin.** A name given to *Elephantiasis Arabum*, from its being supposed to originate from drinking the beverage called *yava*. See ELEPHANTIASIS.

Yawning. See PANDICULATION.

Yaws. The disease termed *frambœsia*.

Yeast. See FERMENTUM CEREVISIÆ.

Yeast'-Plant. *Tor'ula Cerevis'iæ.* A microscopic fungous plant which is supposed to contribute to the process of fermentation.

Yelk. [**Vitel'lus.**] The yellow granular mass in the eggs of birds; also, the corresponding, and strictly analogous, portion of the *ovum* of mammals; also called *yolk*.

Yellow. See FLAVUS.

Yel'low Fe'ver. (Fr. *Fièvre Jaune*, fe-åvR' [or fe-ĕvR'] zhōn.) A remittent fever, with yellow skin from disorder of the hepatic system; termed also *Ty'phus ictero'des*, and *Syn'ochus ictero'des*, *Bulam* fever, *Vom'ito ni'gro*, etc.

Yel'low Wash. A lotion formed of two grains of oxymuriate of mercury to an ounce of lime-water.

Yest. See YEAST, or FERMENTUM.

Yeuk. The same as YOUK.

Yoked. See CONJUGATE.

Yolk. See YELK.

Youk. Popular (Scotch) term for *Scabies;* also called, in some districts, *Yuck.*

Youth, yooth. [A contraction of *youngth*, the "quality or state of being young," as Truth signifies the "quality of being true."] Usually employed in the same sense as *adolescence*. See ÆTAS.

Yt'trĭ-a.* [From *Ytterby*, in Sweden.] One of the primitive earths.

Yt'tric. [**Yt'tricus.**] Belonging to yttrium.

Yt'trĭ-co-Am-mon'ĭ-cus,* Yt'trĭ-co-Po-tas'sĭ-cus.* Applied to combinations of an yttric salt with a salt of ammonia and potassa.

Yt-trif'er-ous. [**Yttrif'erus;** from *yt'tria*, and *fe'ro*, to "bear."] Containing yttria.

Yt'trĭ-um.* The metallic base of yttria,—so named because it was discovered at Ytterby, in Sweden. It is of a dark-gray color.

Yu'ca. The name of a South American plant from which the natives prepare an intoxicating beverage.

Z.

Za'mĭ-ą.* A cycadaceous West Indian plant, which yields a sort of arrow-root.

Zanthic Oxide. See XANTHIC OXIDE.

Zanthin. See XANTHIN.

Ze'ą Mays.* The systematic name of the maize, or Indian corn, a plant of the Linnæan class *Monœcia*, natural order *Graminaceæ*. It is a native of America.

Zed'o-a-rў. A name given to the roots or tubers of *Kæmpfe'ria rotun'da*, or *Curcu'ma aromat'ica*. They are stimulant and carminative.

Ze'nith. (From the Arabic.) That point in the heavens directly over our heads, and opposed to the nadir.

Zē'ro. [Italian, *zero*, dzā'ro, a "cipher," or "naught."] A term generally used in reference to the thermometer, implying the point at which the graduation commences. The zero of Réaumur's and the Centigrade thermometer is the freezing point of water. The zero of Fahrenheit is 32° below the point at which water freezes.

Ze-rum'bet, Cas-su-mu'niar. An aromatic, bitter East Indian root, having tonic and stimulant properties, and similar to ginger.

Zigzag. See FLEXUOUS.

Zinc, Chloride of. See ZINCI CHLORIDUM.

Zinc, Sulphate of. See ZINCI SULPHAS.

Zin'çi Car-bo'nas* ("Carbonate of Zinc"); also called **Cal-ą-mi'ną,*** and **Cal'ą-mīne.** It is used externally in the form of a powder or cerate applied to excoriations.

Zin'çi Chlo'rĭ-dum.* ("Chloride of Zinc.") A white, deliquescent salt. It is antiseptic and powerfully escharotic.

Zin'çi Ox'ĭ-dum.* ("Oxide of Zinc.") A yellowish-white powder used as a tonic and antispasmodic.

Zin'çi Sul'phas.* ("Sulphate of Zinc.") The Pharmacopœial name ‖ for a substance in colorless crystals which effloresce on exposure to the air. It is emetic, tonic, and antispasmodic. It is sometimes called White Vitriol.

Zin'çic. [**Zin'cicus.**] Belonging to zinc.

Zin-çif'er-ous. [**Zincif'erus;** from *zin'cum*, "zinc," and *fe'ro*, to "bear."] Containing zinc.

Zin'coid. [**Zincoi'des;** from *zin'cum*, "zinc," and εἶδος, a "form."] Resembling zinc. A term applied to the platinum (or other metallic) plate which is in connection with a copper plate in the voltaic circle, and denoting the positive pole or positive electrode. The platinum plate is called *zincoid*, because it takes the place of the zinc in the voltaic circle.

Zin'cum.* Zinc. The Pharmacopœial name for a bluish-white metal having the specific gravity 6.8. It is malleable and ductile when its temperature is between 220° and 320°. After having been superficially oxidized, it long resists the further action of air and water. In commerce it is often called spelter.

Zin'ġĭ-ber,* gen. **Zin-ġib'e-ris.** [Gr. ζιγγίβερις, or ζιγγίβερ.] A Linnæan genus of the class *Monandria*, natural order *Zingiberaceæ*. Also, the Pharmacopœial name for the root of the *Zingiber officinale*. It is a grateful stimulant and carminative.

Zin'giber Of-fĭç-ĭ-na'le.* The systematic name of the ginger-plant; called, also, *Amo'mum Zin'giber*.

Zingiberaceæ,* zin-je-be-ra'she-ē. A natural order of endogenous herbaceous plants, found within the tropics. Several species of this order are valued for the aromatic stimulating properties of their roots or rhizomes. It includes *Zin'giber* (Ginger), *Alpin'ia* (Galangale), and *Curcu'ma*, from which turmeric is procured.

Zinn, Zo'nule of. A little zone on the vitreous humor of the eye, for receiving the crystalline lens; first particularized by Zinn.

Zir'con. A mineral chiefly composed of zirconia and silica, found in the sand of the rivers of Ceylon.

Zir-co'nĭ-ą.* One of the primitive earths.

Zir-co'nĭ-ąn. [**Zirconia'nus.**] Containing zircon.

Zir-con'ic. [**Zircon'icus.**] Belonging to zirconium.

Zir-co'nĭ-um.* The metallic base of zirconia. It is obtained in the form of a black powder.

Zi-za'nĭ-ą A-quat'ĭ-cą.* The systematic name of wild rice, an American plant of the natural order *Graminaceæ*. The seeds are used as food.

Ziz'ȳ-phus.* A genus of plants from which jujube paste is procured. It belongs to the natural order *Rhamnaceæ.*

Zo-an-thro'pĭ-a.* [From ζῶον, an "animal," and ἄνθρωπος, a "man."] A kind of monomania, in which a patient imagines that he is an animal.

Zo'dĭ-ac. [**Zodi'acus;** from ζώδιον, diminutive of ζῶον, an "animal:" so named because the groups of stars in it were fancied to represent the figures of various animals.] An imaginary zone or belt surrounding the heavens, extending about 8° on each side of the ecliptic, and coinciding with the region of the heavens within which the apparent motions of the sun, moon, and greater planets are confined. The zodiac is divided into twelve equal parts, called signs, designated by the names of the constellations, with the places of which the signs anciently corresponded.

Zoi-at'rĭ-ca.* [From ζῶον, an "animal," and ἰατρεία, "medical treatment."] Veterinary art, or veterinary medicine: zoiatrics.

Zo-is'mus.* [From ζῶον, an "animal."] The process of animal life: zo'ism.

Zom'ĭ-din. [**Zomidi'na;** from ζωμός, "broth or juice from meat."] A constituent of the extract of flesh.

Zo'na.* [From ζώννυμι, to "gird."] A zone or girdle. The shingles; a popular term for *Herpes zoster.*

Zo'na Pel-lu'cĭ-da.* ("Pellucid Zone.") The broad transparent ring which surrounds the yelk (or yolk) in the centre of the ovum.

Zone. [Lat. **Zo'na;** Gr. ζώνη, a "girdle," or "belt."] In Astronomy, a portion of the celestial sphere included between two parallel circles. In Geography, the terrestrial zones are the five broad spaces or belts into which the surface of the earth is divided by the two tropics and the polar circles: namely, the torrid zone, the north and south temperate zones, the north frigid zone, and the south frigid zone.

Zo'nule. [**Zon'ulus;** diminutive of *zo'na,* a "zone."] A little zone or girdle.

Zo-o-bi-o-tis'mus.* [From ζῶον, an "animal," and βίος, "life."] The condition of animals: zoobi'otism.

Zo-o-cam'bĭ-um.* [From ζῶον, an "animal," and *cam'bium,* "exchange."] The vital juices of animals, in which the blood-cells are formed; the *liquor sanguinis.*

Zo-o-chem'ĭ-cal. [**Zoochem'icus.**] Pertaining to zoochemy.

Zo-och'e-mȳ. [**Zooche'mia;** from ζῶον, an "animal," and *che'mia,* "chemistry."] Animal chemistry, or the chemical analysis of animal substances.

Zo-oġ'e-nȳ. [**Zoogen'esis,** or **Zooge'nia;** from ζῶον, an "animal," and γεννάω, to "generate."] The generating of animals, or the doctrine of the formation of animals.

Zo-o-go-nol'o-ġȳ. [**Zoogonolo'gia;** from *zoogo'nia,* "zoogony," and λόγος, a "discourse."] The doctrine of the origin or development of animal life.

Zo-og'o-nus.* [See next article.] Bearing living young, as opposed to oviparous. See VIVIPAROUS.

Zo-og'o-nȳ. [**Zoogo'nia;** from ζῶον, an "animal," and γονή, "generation."] The bearing or producing of living young.

Zo-og'ra-phȳ. [**Zoogra'phia;** from ζῶον, an "animal," and γράφω, to "write."] A description of animals.

Zo'o-līte. [**Zool'ithus;** from ζῶον, an "animal," and λίθος, a "stone."] Any specimen or part of a fossil or petrified animal.

Zo'o-lith. The same as ZOOLITE.

Zo-o-lĭ-thif'er-us.* [From *zool'ithus,* a "zoolite," and *fe'ro,* to "bear."] Containing fossil remains of animals.

Zo-o-loġ'ĭ-cal. Relating to zoology.

Zo-ol'o-ġist. One who is versed in zoology.

Zo-ol'o-ġȳ. [**Zoolo'gia;** from ζῶον, an "animal," and λόγος, a "discourse."] That branch of Natural History which treats of animals, their form, nature, and habits; the science of animals. The animal kingdom has been divided by Cuvier into four sub-kingdoms, or grand divisions, viz.:—1. *Vertebra'ta,* or Vertebrates; 2. *Mollus'ca,* or Mollusks (otherwise called *Heterogangliа'ta,* from the unsymmetrical arrangement of the ganglia, or nervous centres); 3. *Articula'ta,* or Articulated Animals, including insects, crustaceans, etc.: this division is also termed *Homogangliа'ta,* from the symmetrical arrangement of the ganglia; and, 4. *Radia'ta,* or Radiated Animals, including the star-fish, polypi, etc. For a more particular notice, see VERTEBRATA, MOLLUSCA, etc.

Zo'on.* [Gr. ζῶον; from ζάω, to "live."] A word signifying an "animal," a "living being."

Zo-on'o-mȳ. [**Zoono'mia;** from ζῶον, an "animal," and νόμος, a "law."]

The science which treats of the laws of animal organic life, or the laws which govern the organic actions of animals.

Zo-oph'a-gous. [**Zooph'agus;** from ζῶον, an "animal," and φάγω, to "eat."] Living on animal food; carnivorous.

Zo'o-phȳte. [**Zooph'ytum;** from ζῶον, an "animal," and φύτον, a "plant."] An animal plant, or body apparently intermediate between an animal and vegetable, being supposed to partake of the nature of both, but incorrectly. This term was applied by Cuvier to one of the primary divisions of animals.

Zo'o-phȳ-tog'ra-phȳ. [**Zoophytogra'phia;** from *zooph'ytum,* a "zoophyte," and γράφω, to "write."] A description of zoophytes.

Zo'o-phȳ-tol'o-ġȳ. [**Zoophytolo'gia;** from *zooph'ytum,* a "zoophyte," and λόγος, a "discourse."] A treatise on zoophytes; the science of zoöphytes.

Zo'o-psȳ-chol'o-ġȳ. [**Zoopsycholo'gia;** from ζῶον, an "animal," and *psycholo'gia,* "psychology."] The doctrine of the existence of mind in brute animals.

Zo'o-spores. [From *zo'on,* an "animal," and *spo'ra,* a "spore."] Applied to the spores or spermatozoids of certain *Algæ,* so named because they possess the power of spontaneous motion, thus resembling animals.

Zo-ot'ic. [**Zoot'icus;** from ζῶον, an "animal."] Applied to a rock or soil containing the *débris* of organized bodies.

Zo-ot'o-mist. [See next article.] One who dissects animals.

Zo-ot'o-mȳ. [**Zooto'mia;** from ζῶον, an "animal," and τέμνω, to "cut."] Dissection of the lower animals, as distinguished from the dissection of man; also, the anatomy of animals.

Zos'ter, e'ris.* [From ζώννυμι, to "gird."] A species of erysipelas which extends round the body, like a zone or girdle. See HERPES ZOSTER.

Zumology. See ZYMOLOGY.

Zȳg-a-poph'ȳ-sis.* [From ζυγός, a "yoke," or "junction," and ἀπόφυσις, an "offshoot."] The supero-lateral process of a vertebra, by which it is connected with the adjoining vertebra.

Zy-go'ma, atis.* [Gr. ζύγωμα, the "zygomatic arch."] The cheek-bone (*os jugale,* or *os malæ*).

Zȳg-o-mat'ic. [**Zygomat'icus.**] Belonging to the *zygoma.*

Zygomat'ic Arch. The bony arch which connects the malar bone with the squamosal portion of the temporal, and encloses the temporal muscle.

Zygomat'ic Proç'ess. A thin narrow projection of bone, bounding the squamous portion of the temporal bone at its base.

Zy-go-mat'ĭ-cus Ma'jor.* ("Greater Zygomatic [Muscle].") A muscle arising from the cheek-bone and inserted into the angle of the mouth.

Zygomat'icus Mi'nor.* ("Lesser Zygomatic [Muscle].") A muscle arising from the cheek-bone (a little higher up than the preceding) and inserted into the upper lip near the angle of the mouth. It is often wanting. This muscle and the preceding raise the angles of the mouth, as in laughter: hence the term *distortor oris* ("distorter of the mouth") has been applied to them.

Zygophyllaceæ,* zi-go-fil-la'she-ē. [From *Zygophyl'lum,* one of the genera.] A natural order of exogenous plants, found in the hotter parts of the world. The ligneous plants of this order are remarkable for the extreme hardness of their wood. It includes the *Guai'acum,* or *Lig'num vi'tæ.*

Zȳg-o-phȳl'lum.* [From ζυγός, a "yoke," and φύλλον, a "leaf."] Applied to a leaf composed of a pair of leaflets as if yoked together.

Zȳ-mol'o-ġȳ, or **Zu-mol'o-ġȳ.** [**Zymolo'gia;** from ζύμη, "leaven," and λόγος, a "discourse."] A treatise on fermentation, or the science of fermentation.

Zy-mo'ma, atis.* [From ζυμόω, to "ferment."] Leaven; a fermented mixture.

Zy-mo-sĭ-om'e-ter. [**Zymosiom'etrum;** from ζύμωσις, "fermentation," and μέτρον, a "measure."] An instrument for ascertaining the degrees of fermentation.

Zy-mo'sis.* [From ζυμόω, to "ferment."] Fermentation; also applied to those diseases depending on miasmata for their origin, and called endemic, epidemic, contagious, etc., as expressing also the mode in which morbid poisons act on the animal economy.

Zy-mot'ic. [**Zymot'icus;** from ζύμη, "leaven," or ζύμωσις, "fermentation."] Applied to those diseases which seem to be occasioned by a virus or poison, operating like leaven.

Z. Z. = anciently "myrrh;" now "zinziber," or ginger.

APPENDIX.

CONTENTS OF THE APPENDIX.

TABLE OF MATERIA MEDICA.

It is proper to state that for the plan of the following table the editor is indebted to Dr. George B. Wood, whose system of classification, as presented in the Syllabus of his lectures delivered at the University of Pennsylvania, has been substantially, and, indeed, with a few exceptions, rigidly, followed. One of the classes (the *Excito-Motor Stimulants*) has been introduced from Dr. Carson's "Synopsis."

The great advantages of classification in every department of science, in assisting the memory and enabling the student to take in at a single glance a multitude of associated facts, are too obvious and too generally recognized to require to be enforced by any array of argument. Nor is it necessary to dwell upon the difficulties with which every attempt to classify the infinitely varied productions of nature must necessarily be attended. The editor is fully aware that no system of classification can be devised to which some objections cannot be urged; suffice it to say, that he has, after mature deliberation, adopted that system which on the whole appeared to present the greatest advantages, and to be exposed to the fewest objections. It is proper to say, for the information of the reader, that as a number of substances occur which possess various and distinct medicinal properties, and which cannot therefore with propriety be referred to any one class exclusively, it has been deemed best to give such articles a place in two or more different classes, usually with a reference to that particular class to which they seemed to have the strongest claims. Compare **Cornus Florida,** given as a *tonic* and *astringent,* and **Plumbi Acetas,** given as an *astringent* and *arterial sedative.* When it has appeared somewhat doubtful whether an article was fairly entitled to a place in the list in which it has been inserted, a point of interrogation has been prefixed.

☞ When a reference is made from one name to another, *the name referred to is always to be sought in the same list* (section or class) *as that from which the reference is made.* For example: in the class of Astringents there is a reference from "Blackberry Root" to **Rubus,** which must be sought for in the same section (that is, among the Vegetable Astringents). It is especially important to bear this in mind when there are several sections in one class, as in the case of the Tonics, Diaphoretics, etc.

☞ It is to be observed that the following table is limited for the most part to the simple articles of the Materia Medica and such preparations as have a distinctive and peculiar character of their own: as, Calomel, Carbonic Acid Water, Turpeth Mineral, etc. The reader will not, therefore, look for those multitudinous preparations which are merely modifications as to form of the medicinal principles found in the simpler articles of the Materia Medica.

CONTENTS.

TABLE OF MATERIA MEDICA.

CLASS I.

ASTRINGENTS.

MEDICINES WHICH PRODUCE CONTRACTION OF THE LIVING TISSUES.

SECTION I.—Vegetable Astringents.

Aca'cia Cat'echu. See **Catechu.**

Aç'idum Gal'licum. (U.S. and Br. Ph.) Gallic Acid. An acid prepared from Galls, occurring in acicular prisms nearly colorless.

Aç'idum Tan'nicum. (U.S. and Br. Ph.) Tannic Acid. A pale-yellow amorphous powder, having a strongly astringent taste, obtained from nutgalls.

Alum Root. See **Heuchera.**

Ar'butus U'va Ur'si. See **Uva Ursi.**

Arctostaph'ylos Uva Ursi. See **Uva Ursi.**

Aspid'ium Fi'lix Mas. See **Filix Mas.**

Bearberry. See **Uva Ursi.**

Be'la. (Br. Ph.) Bael. The half-ripe fruit of *Æ'gle Mar'melos* dried.

Bistort. See **Polygonum Bistorta.**

Black Alder. See **Prinos.**

Blackberry Root. See **Rubus.**

Black Oak Bark. See **Quercus Tinctoria.**

Blunt-Leaved Dock. See **Rumex Obtusifolius.**

Casta'nea Pu'mila. Chinquapin. The bark is used as an astringent tonic.

Cat'echu. (U.S. Ph.) An extract prepared principally from the wood of *Acacia catechu.*

Cat'echu Ni'grum. (Br. Ph.) Black Catechu. An extract of *Acacia catechu.*

Cat'echu Pal'lidum. (Br. Ph.) Pale Catechu. An extract from the *Unca'ria gam'bir.*

Chimaph'ila. (U.S. Ph.) Pipsissewa. The leaves of the *Chimaph'ila umbella'ta.* See Class X.

Chinquapin. See **Castanea Pumila.**

Cor'nus Circina'ta. (U.S. Ph.) Round-Leaved Dogwood. See Class II., Section III.

Cor'nus Flor'ida. (U.S. Ph.) Dogwood. See Class II., Section III.

Cor'nus Seriç'ea. (U.S. Ph.) Swamp Dogwood. See Class II., Section III.

Cranesbill. See **Geranium.**

Dewberry Root. See **Rubus.**

Dios'pyros. (U.S. Ph.) Persimmon. The unripe fruit of *Dios'pyros Virginia'na.*

Dogwood. See **Cornus Florida.**

Elm Bark. See **Ulmus.**

Fern Root. See **Filix Mas,** or **Filix.**

? Fi'lix. (Br. Ph.) Fern Root. The same as **Filix Mas.**

? Fi'lix Mas. (U.S. Ph.) Male Fern. See Class XXIII.

Frostwort, or Frostweed. See **Helianthemum.**

Gal'la. (U.S. and Br. Ph.) Nutgall. Galls. A morbid excrescence upon the *Quercus infectoria.*

Gallic Acid. See **Acidum Gallicum.**

Galls, or Gall Nuts. See **Galla.**

Gera'nium. (U.S. Ph.) Cranesbill. The rhizoma of *Gera'nium macula'tum.*

Ge'um. (U.S. Ph.) Water Avens. The root of *Ge'um riva'le.*

Grana'ti Fruc'tûs Cor'tex. (U.S. Ph.) Pomegranate Rind. The rind of the fruit of *Pu'nica grana'tum.*

Hæmatox'ylon, or **Hæmatox'ylum.** (U.S. and Br. Ph.) Logwood. The wood of *Hæmatox'ylon Campechia'num.*

Hardhack. See **Spiræa.**

Helian'themum. (U.S. Ph.) Frostwort. The herb of *Helian'themum Canaden'se.*

? Hepat'ica. (U.S. Ph.) Liverwort. The leaves of *Hepat'ica America'na.*

Heuche'ra. (U.S. Ph.) Alum Root. The root of *Heuche'ra America'na.*

Ki'no. (U.S. and Br. Ph.) The inspissated juice of *Pterocar'pus marsu'pium,* and of other plants.

Krame'ria. (U.S. and Br. Ph.) Rhatany. The root of *Krame'ria trian'dra* (U.S. Ph.). The dried root of *Krameria triandra* (Br. Ph.).

Liverwort. See **Hepatica.**

Logwood. See **Hæmatoxylon.**

Lyc'opus. (U.S. Ph.) Bugleweed. The herb of *Lyc'opus Virgin'icus.*

Male Fern. See **Filix Mas.**

Marsh Rosemary. See **Statice.**

Oak Bark. See **Quercus.**

Persimmon. See **Diospyros.**

Pipsissewa. See **Chimaphila.**

Polyg'onum Bistor'ta. Bistort.

Potentil'la Tormentil'la. See **Tormentilla.**

Pri'nos. (U.S. Ph.) Black Alder. The bark of *Pri'nos verticilla'tus.*

Pterocar'pus Marsu'pium. See **Kino.**

Quer'cus. (Br. Ph.) Oak Bark. The bark of *Quer'cus peduncula'ta.*

Quer'cus Al'ba. (U.S. Ph.) White Oak Bark. The bark of *Quercus alba.*

Quer'cus Infecto'ria. See **Galla.**

Quer'cus Tincto'ria. (U.S. Ph.) Black Oak Bark. The bark of *Quercus tinctoria.*

Red Rose. See **Rosa Gallica.**

Rhatany. See **Krameria.**

Rhus Gla'brum. (U.S. Ph.) Sumach. The fruit of *Rhus glabrum.*

Rind of the Pomegranate. See **Granati Fructûs Cortex.**

Rock Rose. See **Helianthemum.**

Ro'sa Gal'lica. (U.S. and Br. Ph.) Red Rose. The petals of *Rosa Gallica.*

Round-Leaved Dogwood. See **Cornus Circinata.**

Ru'bus. (U.S. Ph.) Dewberry Root. Blackberry Root. The root of *Ru'bus Canaden'sis* and of *Ru'bus villo'sus.*

Ru'mex Obtusifo'lius. Blunt-leaved Dock.

?Sa'lix. (U.S. Ph.) Willow. The bark of *Sa'lix al'ba.* See Class II., Section III.

Spiræ'a. (U.S. Ph.) Hardhack. The root of *Spiræ'a tomento'sa.*

Stat'ice. (U.S. Ph.) Marsh Rosemary. The root of *Stat'ice Limo'nium,* variety *Carolinia'na.*

Sumach. See **Rhus Glabrum.**

Swamp Dogwood. See **Cornus Sericea.**

Tannic Acid. See **Acidum Tannicum.**

Tormentil. See **Tormentilla.**

Tormentil'la. (U.S. Ph.) Tormentil. The root of *Potentil'la tormentil'la.*

Ul'mus. (Br. Ph.) Elm Bark. See Class XIX.

U'va Ur'si. (U.S. and Br. Ph.) The leaves of *Ar'butus Uva Ursi,* or *Arctostaph'ylos Uva Ursi.*

Vi'num Porten'se. (U.S. Ph.) Port Wine. Otherwise called *Vinum rubrum* (Red Wine). See Class V.

Water Avens. See **Geum.**

White Oak Bark. See **Quercus Alba.**

SECTION II.—Mineral Astringents.

Acetate of Lead. See **Plumbi Acetas.**

Acetate of Zinc. See **Zinci Acetas.**

Aç'idum Sulphu'ricum Aromat'icum. (U.S. Ph.) Aromatic Sulphuric Acid.

Alum. See **Alumen.**

Alu'men. (U.S. and Br. Ph.) Alum. Sulphate of Alumina and Potassa. A salt in colorless crystalline masses, having an acid, sweetish, astringent taste.

A'qua Cal'cis. See **Liquor Calcis.**

Aromatic Sulphuric Acid. See **Acidum Sulphuricum Aromaticum.**

Blue Vitriol. See **Cupri Sulphas.**

Calx Chlora'ta. (Br. Ph.) Chlorinated Lime.

Calx Chlorina'ta. (U.S. Ph.) Chlorinated Lime, or Chloride of Lime.

Carbonate of Lead. See **Plumbi Carbonas.**

Cerate of Subacetate of Lead. See **Ceratum Plumbi Subacetatis.**

Cera'tum Plum'bi Subaceta'tis. (U.S. Ph.) Cerate of Subacetate of Lead. Goulard's Cerate. See Class XX.

Chlorinated Lime. See **Calx Chlorinata.**

Common Salt. See **Sodii Chloridum.**

Cu'pri Sul'phas. (U.S. and Br. Ph.) Sulphate of Copper, or Blue Vitriol. A salt occurring in blue crystals, slightly efflorescent in the air, and entirely soluble in water.

Elixir of Vitriol. See **Acidum Sulphuricum Aromaticum.**

Fer'ri Sul'phas. (U.S. and Br. Ph.) Sulphate of Iron, or Copperas. A salt in oblique rhombic prisms of a green color and styptic taste.

Lime Water. See **Liquor Calcis.**

Liq'uor Cal'cis (U.S. and Br. Ph.), otherwise called *A'qua Cal'cis.* Lime Water.

Liq'uor Fer'ri Nitra'tis. (U.S. Ph.) Solution of Nitrate of Iron.

Liq'uor Plum'bi Subaceta'tis. (U.S. Ph.) Solution of Subacetate of Lead.

Litharge. See **Plumbi Oxidum.**

Lithar'gyrum. (Br. Ph.) Litharge. Oxide of Lead.

Plum'bi Ace'tas. (U.S. and Br. Ph.) Acetate of Lead, or Sugar of Lead. A substance in colorless crystals, which effloresce on exposure to the air.

Plum'bi Carbo'nas. (U.S. and Br. Ph.) Carbonate of Lead, or White Lead. A heavy white powder, insoluble in water, but soluble in dilute nitric acid.

Plum'bi Ni'tras. (U.S. Ph.) Nitrate of Lead. See Class XXIV.

Plum'bi Ox'idum (U.S. Ph.), otherwise called *Plum'bi Ox'idum Semivit'reum.* Litharge, or Oxide of Lead.

Plum'bi Subaceta'tis Liq'uor. (Br. Ph.) See **Liquor Plumbi Subacetatis.**

So'dii Chlo'ridum. (U.S. and Br. Ph.) Chloride of Sodium, or Common Salt.

Solution of Nitrate of Iron. See **Liquor Ferri Nitratis.**

Solution of Subacetate of Lead. See **Liquor Plumbi Subacetatis.**

Sugar of Lead. See **Plumbi Acetas.**

Sulphate of Copper. See **Cupri Sulphas.**

Sulphate of Iron. See **Ferri Sulphas.**

Sulphate of Zinc. See **Zinci Sulphas.**

Zin'çi Ace'tas. (U.S. and Br. Ph.) Acetate of Zinc.

Zin'çi Sul'phas. (U.S. and Br. Ph.) Sulphate of Zinc, or White Vitriol. A salt occurring in colorless crystals, which have a strong metallic styptic taste and are soluble in water.

CLASS II.

TONICS.

MEDICINES WHICH PRODUCE A GENTLE AND PERMANENT EXCITEMENT OF ALL THE VITAL ACTIONS, THOUGH THEIR INFLUENCE IS CHIEFLY OBSERVABLE IN THE FUNCTIONS OF ORGANIC LIFE.

SECTION I.—Pure or Simple Bitters.

Agatho'tes Chiray'ta. See **Chiretta.**

Al'etris. (U.S. Ph.) Star Grass. The root of *Al'etris farino'sa.*

American Centaury. See **Sabbatia.**

American Columbo. See **Frasera.**

Bitte'ra (or *Bytte'ra*) *Febrif'uga.* Bitter Ash.

Blue Gentian. See **Gentiana Catesbæi.**

Calum'ba. (U.S. and Br. Ph.) Columbo. The root of *Coc'culus palma'tus.*

Chira'ta. (Br. Ph.) The entire plant of *Ophe'lia chira'ta.* The same as **Chiretta.**

Chiret'ta. (U.S. Ph.) Chiretta. The herb and root of *Agatho'tes chiray'ta.*

Coc'culus palma'tus. See **Calumba.**

Colomba, or Columbo. See **Calumba.**

Common European Centaury. See **Erythræa Centaurium.**

Cop'tis. (U.S. Ph.) Goldthread. The root of *Cop'tis trifo'lia.*

Erythræ'a Centau'rium. Common Centaury.

Frase'ra. (U.S. Ph.) American Columbo. The root of *Frase'ra Walte'ri.*

Gentian. See **Gentiana.**

Gentia'na. (U.S. and Br. Ph.) Gentian. The root of *Gentia'na lu'tea.*

Gentia'na Catesbæ'i. (U.S. Ph.) Blue Gentian. The root of *Gentiana Catesbæi.*

Goldthread. See **Coptis.**

Quassia. (U.S. and Br. Ph.) Quassia. The wood of *Simaru'ba excel'sa* (U.S. Ph.), or of *Picræ'na excel'sa* (Br. Ph.).

Sabba'tia. (U.S. Ph.) American Centaury. The herb of *Sabba'tia angula'ris.*

Simaru'ba. (U.S. Ph.) Simaruba. The bark of the root of *Simaru'ba officina'lis.*

Simaru'ba excel'sa. See **Quassia.**

Star Grass. See **Aletris.**

Xanthorrhi'za. (U.S. Ph.) Yellow-Root. The root of *Xanthorrhi'za apiifo'lia.*

Yellow-Root. See **Xanthorrhiza.**

SECTION II.—Bitters of Peculiar or Modified Properties.

Absin'thium. (U.S. Ph.) Wormwood. The tops and leaves of *Artemis'ia absin'thium.*

Al'etris. (U.S. Ph.) Star Grass. The root of *Al'etris farino'sa.*

Am'yris Myr'rha. See **Myrrha.**

An'themis. (U.S. and Br. Ph.) Chamomile. The dried flowers of *An'themis nob'ilis.*

An'themis Cot'ula. See **Cotula.**

Ar'butus U'va Ur'si. See Class I.

Artemis'ia Absin'thium. See **Absinthium.**

Balsamoden'dron Myr'rha. See **Myrrha.**

? Bal'samum Peruvia'num. (U.S. and Br. Ph.) Balsam of Peru. See Class XII.

Bal'samum Toluta'num. (U. S. and Br. Ph.) Balsam of Tolu. See Class XII.

Bebe'riæ Sul'phas. (Br. Ph.) Sulphate of Beberia.

Black Alder. See **Prinos.**

Black Snakeroot. See **Cimicifuga.**

Blunt-Leaved Dock. See **Rumex Obtusifolius.**

Buckbean. See **Menyanthes Trifoliata.**

Cedron. The seeds of the *Sima'ba Ce'dron.*

Chamomile. See **Anthemis.**

Cimicif'uga. (U.S. Ph.) Black Snakeroot. The root of *Cimicif'uga racemo'sa.*

Cod-Liver Oil. See **Oleum Morrhuæ.**

Cot'ula. (U.S. Ph.) Mayweed. The herb of *An'themis cot'ula, Maruta cotula.*

Elecampane. See **Inula.**

Elm Bark. See **Ulmus.**

Fern Root. See **Filix.**

Fi'lix. (Br. Ph.) Fern Root. The same as **Filix Mas.**

Fi'lix Mas. (U.S. Ph.) Male Fern. The rhizoma of *Aspid'ium Filix Mas.*

German Chamomile. See **Matricaria.**

Hardhack. See **Spiræa.**

? Helian'themum. (U.S. Ph.) Frostwort. The herb of *Helian'themum Canaden'se.*

Hemides'mus. (Br. Ph.) The root of *Hemidesmus Indicus.*

Hepat'ica. (U.S. Ph.) Liverwort. The root of *Hepatica Americana.*

Herac'leum Lana'tum. The root.

Hops. See **Humulus.**

Horehound. See **Marrubium.**

Hu'mulus. (U.S. Ph.) Hops. The strobiles of *Hu'mulus lu'pulus.*

In'ula. (U.S. Ph.) Elecampane. The root of *In'ula hele'nium.*

Lirioden'dron. (U.S. Ph.) Tuliptree Bark. The bark of *Lirioden'dron tulipif'era.*

Lu'pulus. (Br. Ph.) The same as **Humulus.**

Marru'bium. (U.S. Ph.) Horehound. The herb of *Marru'bium vulga're.*

Marsh Trefoil. See **Menyanthes Trifoliata.**

Masterwort. See **Heracleum Lanatum.**

Matrica'ria. (U.S. Ph.) German Chamomile. The flowers of *Matrica'ria chamomil'la.*

Mayweed. See **Cotula.**

Menyan'thes trifolia'ta. Buckbean, or Marsh Trefoil.

Myrrh. See **Myrrha.**

Myr'rha. (U.S. and Br. Ph.) Myrrh. The concrete juice of *Balsamoden'dron myr'rha* (U.S. Ph.); a gum-resinous exudation from the stem of *Balsamodendron myrrha* (Br. Ph.).

Nux Vom'ica. (U.S. and Br. Ph.) Nux Vomica. The seeds of *Strych'nos nux vom'ica.* See Class XXV.

O'leum Anthem'idis. (Br. Ph.) Oil of Chamomile.

? O'leum Bu'bulum. (U.S. Ph.) Neats'-foot Oil.

O'leum Mor'rhuæ. (U.S. and Br. Ph.) Cod-Liver Oil. The fixed oil obtained from the liver of *Ga'dus Mor'rhua.*

? Pa'nax. (U.S. Ph.) Ginseng. The root of *Pa'nax quinquefo'lium.*

? Parei'ra. (U.S. and Br. Ph.) See Class X.

? Polyg'ala Rubel'la. (U.S. Ph.) Bitter Polygala. The root and herb of *Polygala rubella.*

Pri'nos. (U.S. Ph.) Black Alder. See next section.

Pru'nus Virginia'na. (U.S. Ph.) Wild Cherry Bark. The bark of *Cer'asus serot'ina.*

Quer'cus. (Br. Ph.) Oak Bark. The bark of *Quer'cus peduncula'ta.*

? Quer'cus Tincto'ria. (U.S. Ph.) Black Oak Bark. See Class I.

Rhe'um. (U.S. and Br. Ph.) Rhubarb. See Class IX., Section I.

Rhubarb. See **Rheum.**

Ru'mex Cris'pus. (U.S. Ph.) Yellow Dock. The root of *Rumex crispus.*

? Ru'mex Obtusifo'lius. Blunt-Leaved Dock.

Sage. See **Salvia.**

Sal'via. (U.S. Ph.) Sage. The leaves of *Sal'via officina'lis.*

? **Scutella'ria.** (U.S. Ph.) Scull-cap. See Class IV.

? **Spiræ'a.** (U.S. Ph.) Hardhack. The root of *Spiræ'a tomento'sa.*

Strych'nos Nux Vom'ica. See **Nux Vomica.**

Tanace'tum. (U.S. Ph.) Tansy. The herb of *Tanace'tum vulga're.*

Tansy. See **Tanacetum.**

Tulip-tree Bark. See **Liriodendron.**

? **Ul'mus.** (Br. Ph.) Elm Bark. See Class XIX.

Wild Cherry Bark. See **Prunus Virginiana.**

Wormwood. See **Absinthium.**

Yellow Dock. See **Rumex Crispus.**

SECTION III.—Febrifuge Tonics.

Aç'idum Ni'tricum. (U.S. and Br. Ph.) Nitric Acid. See Section V.

Adanso'nia Digita'ta. Baobab.

Æs'culus Hippocas'tanum. Horse-chesnut.

Angustu'ra. (U.S. Ph.) The bark of *Galipe'a officina'lis.*

? **An'themis.** (U.S. and Br. Ph.) Chamomile. (See preceding section.)

Aristolo'chia. See **Serpentaria.**

Baobab. See **Adansonia Digitata.**

Bebeeru Bark. See **Nectandra.**

Boneset. See **Eupatorium.**

Cascaril'la. (U.S. and Br. Ph.) The bark of *Cro'ton eleute'ria.*

Chamomile. See **Anthemis.**

Cincho'na Fla'va. (U.S. and Br. Ph.) Yellow Cinchona. The bark of *Cincho'na calisay'a.*

Cincho'na Pal'lida. (U.S. and Br. Ph.) Pale Cinchona. The bark of *Cincho'na Condamin'ea.*

Cincho'na Ru'bra. (U.S. and Br. Ph.) Red Cinchona. The bark of an undetermined species of *Cinchona* (U.S. Ph.). The bark of *Cincho'na succiru'bra* (Br. Ph.).

Common Salt. See **Sodii Chloridum.**

Contrayerva. See **Dorstenia Contrayerva.**

Cor'nus Circina'ta. (U.S. Ph.) Round-Leaved Dogwood. The bark of *Cornus circinata.*

Cor'nus Flor'ida. (U.S. Ph.) Dogwood. The bark of *Cornus Florida.*

Cor'nus Seriç'ea. (U.S. Ph.) Swamp Dogwood. The bark of *Cornus sericea.*

Cro'ton Eleute'ria. See **Cascarilla.**

Cuspa'ria. (Br. Ph.) Cusparia Bark. The bark of *Galipe'a cuspa'ria.* The same as **Angustura.**

Dogwood. See **Cornus Florida.**

Dorste'nia Contrayer'va.

Eupato'rium. (U.S. Ph.) Thoroughwort, or Boneset. The tops and leaves of *Eupato'rium perfolia'tum,* gathered after flowering has commenced.

? **Frax'inus Excel'sior.** Common European Ash.

Galipe'a Officina'lis. See **Angustura.**

Gossyp'ium Herba'ceum. An infusion of the seeds. See Class XIII.

Magno'lia. (U.S. Ph.) The bark of *Magno'lia glau'ca,* and of other species of *Magnolia.* See Class XI., Section III.

Mahogany Tree. See **Swietenia.**

Nectan'dra. (U.S. and Br. Ph.) Bebeeru Bark, or bark of *Nectan'dra Rodie'i.*

Nitric Acid. See **Acidum Nitricum.**

Pale Cinchona. See **Cinchona Pallida.**

Phloridzin, or Phlœorizin. (A peculiar principle obtained from the bark of the apple, pear, and cherry tree.)

? **Pri'nos.** (U.S. Ph.) Black Alder. The bark of *Pri'nos verticilla'tus.*

Quer'cus Al'ba. (U.S. Ph.) White Oak Bark. See Class I.

Quin'iæ Sul'phas. (U.S. and Br. Ph.) Sulphate of Quinia.

Red Cinchona. See **Cinchona Rubra.**

Round-Leaved Dogwood. See **Cornus Circinata.**

Sa'lix. (U.S. Ph.) Willow. The bark of *Salix alba.*

Serpenta'ria. (U.S. and Br. Ph.) Serpentary, or Virginia Snakeroot. The root of *Aristolo'chia serpenta'ria,* and of other species of *Serpentaria.*

Serpentary. See **Serpentaria.**

Snakeroot, Virginia. See **Serpentaria.**

So'dii Chlo'ridum. (U.S. and Br. Ph.) Chloride of Sodium, or Common Salt. See Section V. of this class.

Spider's Web. See **Tela Araneæ.**

Sulphate of Quinia. See **Quiniæ Sulphas.**

Swamp Dogwood. See **Cornus Sericea.**

Swiete'nia Febrif'uga, and *Swiete'nia Mahog'ani* (Mahogany Tree). The bark.

? *Te'la Ara'neæ.* Spider's Web.

Thoroughwort. See **Eupatorium.**

Virginia Snakeroot. See **Serpentaria.**

White Oak Bark. See **Quercus Alba.**

Willow. See **Salix.**

Yellow Cinchona. See **Cinchona Flava.**

SECTION IV.—Aromatics.

Ac'orus Cal'amus. See **Calamus.**

Alpin'ia Cardamo'mum. See **Cardamomum.**

Ane'thum. (Br. Ph.) Dill Seed. The fruit of *Ane'thum grav'eolens.*

Angel'ica. (U.S. Ph.) Angelica. The root of *Angel'ica Archangel'ica.*

Angel'ica Atropurpu'rea. Purple Angelica.

Ani'sum. (U.S. Ph.) Anise. The fruit of *Pimpinel'la ani'sum.*

Artan'the Elonga'ta. See **Matico.**

As'arum. (U.S. Ph.) Canada Snakeroot, or Wild Ginger. The root of *As'arum Canaden'se.*

Auran'tii Ama'ri Cor'tex. (U.S. Ph.) Bitter Orange Peel. The rind of the fruit of *Ci'trus vulga'ris.*

Auran'tii Cor'tex. (Br. Ph.) Orange Peel (Bitter). The outer part of the rind (dried) of the ripe fruit of *Ci'trus bigara'dia.*

Auran'tii Dul'cis Cor'tex. (U.S. Ph.) Sweet Orange Peel. The rind of the fruit of *Ci'trus auran'tium.*

Balm. See **Melissa.**

Black Pepper. See **Piper.**

Cal'amus. (U.S. Ph.) Calamus, or Sweet Flag. The rhizoma of *Ac'orus cal'amus.*

Canada Snakeroot. See **Asarum.**

Canel'la. (U.S. Ph.) Canella. The bark of *Canel'la al'ba.*

Canel'la Al'ba. See **Canella.**

Caraway. See **Carum.**

Cardamom. See **Cardamomum.**

Cardamo'mum. (U.S. and Br. Ph.) Cardamom. The fruit (or seeds) of *Eletta'ria cardamo'mum.*

Car'ui. (Br. Ph.) Caraway. The dried fruit of *Ca'rum car'ui.*

Ca'rum. (U.S. Ph.) Caraway. The fruit of *Ca'rum car'ui.*

Caryophyl'lum. (Br. Ph.) Cloves. The unexpanded flower-buds of *Caryophyl'lus aromat'icus.* The same as **Caryophyllus.**

Caryophyl'lus. (U.S. Ph.) Cloves. The unexpanded flowers of *Caryophyl'lus aromat'icus.*

? Cata'ria. Catnep. See Class IV.

Cinnamo'mum. (U.S. and Br. Ph.) Cinnamon. The bark of *Cinnamo'mum Zeylan'icum,* and of *Cinnamo'mum aromat'icum* (U.S. Ph.). The inner bark from shoots of the *Cinnamomum Zeylanicum* (Br. Ph.).

Cinnamo'mum Zeylan'icum. See **Cinnamomum.**

Cinnamon. See **Cinnamomum.**

Ci'trus Auran'tium. See **Aurantii Dulcis Cortex.**

Cloves. See **Caryophyllus.**

Coriander. See **Coriandrum.**

Corian'drum. (U.S. and Br. Ph.) Coriander. The ripe fruit of *Corian'drum sati'vum* (U.S. Ph.). The ripe fruit, dried, of *Coriandrum sativum* (Br. Ph.).

Cube'ba. (U.S. and Br. Ph.) Cubeb, or Cubebs. The berries of *Pi'per cube'ba* (U.S. Ph.). The unripe fruit, dried, of *Cube'ba officina'lis* (Br. Ph.). See Class X.

Cubebs. See **Cubeba.**

Cumin. See **Cuminum.**

? Cumi'num, or *Cymi'num.* Cumin.

Curcu'ma. (U.S. Ph.) Turmeric. The rhizoma of *Curcu'ma lon'ga.*

Dill. See **Anethum.**

Dri'mys Winte'ri. Wintera.

Eletta'ria Cardamo'mum. See **Cardamomum.**

Euge'nia Caryophylla'ta. See **Caryophyllus.**

European Pennyroyal. See **Mentha Pulegium.**

Fennel, or Fennel Seed. See **Fœniculum.**

Fœnic'ulum. (U.S. and Br. Ph.) Fennel Seed. The fruit of *Fœnic'ulum vulga're* (U.S. Ph.). The fruit of *Fœnic'ulum dul'ce* (Br. Ph.).

Fœnic'ulum Officina'le. (Considered by some to be the same as *Fœniculum vulgare.*) See **Fœniculum.**

Gaulthe'ria. (U.S. Ph.) Partridge Berry. The leaves of *Gaulthe'ria procum'bens.*

Ginger. See **Zingiber.**

Ginseng. See **Panax.**

Golden Rod. See **Solidago.**

Hedeo'ma. (U.S. Ph.) American Pennyroyal. The herb of *Hedeo'ma pulegioi'des.*

Horsemint. See **Monarda.**

Lavan'dula. (U.S. Ph.) Lavender. The flowers of *Lavan'dula ve'ra.*

Lavan'dula Spi'ca. See **Lavandula.**

Lavan'dula Ve'ra. See **Lavandula.**

Lavender. See **Lavandula.**

Limo'nis Cor'tex. (U.S. and Br. Ph.) Lemon Peel.

Long Pepper. See **Piper Longum.**

Ma'cis. (U.S. Ph.) Mace.

Marjoram. See **Origanum Vulgare.**

Mati'ca. (Br. Ph.) Matico. The dried leaves of *Artan'the elonga'ta.* See **Matico.**

Mati'co. (U.S. Ph.) Matico. The leaves of *Artan'the elonga'ta.*

Melis'sa. (U.S. Ph.) Balm. The herb of *Melis'sa officina'lis.*

Men'tha Piperi'ta. (U.S. Ph.) Peppermint. The herb of *Mentha piperita.*

Men'tha Pule'gium. European Pennyroyal.

Men'tha Vir'idis. (U.S. Ph.) Spearmint. The herb of *Mentha viridis.*

Monar'da. (U.S. Ph.) Horsemint. The herb of *Monar'da puncta'ta.*

Myris'tica. (U.S. and Br. Ph.) Nutmeg. The kernel of the fruit of *Myris'tica fra'grans* (U.S. Ph.). The kernel of the seed of *Myris'tica officina'lis* (Br. Ph.).

Myr'tus pimen'ta. See **Pimenta.**

Nep'eta cata'ria. See **Cataria.**

Nutmeg. See **Myristica.**

Oil of Anise. See **Oleum Anisi.**

Oil of Bergamot. See **Oleum Bergamii.**

Oil of Caraway. See **Oleum Carui.**

Oil of Cinnamon. See **Oleum Cinnamomi.**

Oil of Dill. See **Oleum Anethi.**

Oil of Lavender. See **Oleum Lavandulæ.**

Oil of Lemon. See **Oleum Limonis.**

Oil of Nutmeg. See **Oleum Myristicæ.**

Oil of Peppermint. See **Oleum Menthæ Piperitæ.**

Oil of Spearmint. See **Oleum Menthæ Viridis.**

O'leum Ane'thi. (Br. Ph.) Oil of Dill.

O'leum Ani'si. (Br. Ph.) Oil of Anise.

O'leum Berga'mii. (U.S. Ph.) Oil of Bergamot. The volatile oil obtained from the rind of the fruit of *Ci'trus limet'ta.*

O'leum Car'ui. (Br. Ph.) Oil of Caraway.

O'leum Caryophyl'li. (Br. Ph.) Oil of Cloves.

O'leum Cinnamo'mi. (U.S. and Br. Ph.) Oil of Cinnamon. The volatile oil obtained from the bark of *Cinnamo'mum Zeylan'icum.*

O'leum Corian'dri. (Br. Ph.) Oil of Coriander.

O'leum Lavan'dulæ. (Br. Ph.) Oil of Lavender.

? O'leum Limo'nis. (U.S. and Br. Ph.) Oil of Lemon. The volatile oil obtained from the rind of the fruit of *Ci'trus limo'num.*

O'leum Men'thæ Piperi'tæ. (U.S. and Br. Ph.) Oil of Peppermint. The oil distilled from the fresh herb of *Mentha piperita.*

O'leum Men'thæ Vir'idis. (U.S. and Br. Ph.) Oil of Spearmint. The oil distilled from the fresh herb of *Mentha viridis.*

O'leum Monar'dæ. (U.S. Ph.) Oil of Horsemint.

O'leum Myris'ticæ. (U.S. and Br. Ph.) Oil of Nutmeg. The volatile oil obtained from the kernels of the fruit of *Myris'tica fra'grans* (U.S. Ph.). The oil distilled from Nutmeg (Br. Ph.).

O'leum Pimen'tæ. (U.S. and Br. Ph.) Oil of Pimento.

O'leum Ro'sæ. (U.S. Ph.) Oil of Rose.

? O'leum Rosmari'ni. (U.S. and Br. Ph.) Oil of Rosemary. See Class XVII.

O'leum Thy'mi. (U.S. Ph.) Oil of Thyme.

Orange Peel. See **Aurantii Cortex.**

Orig'anum Vulga're. Origanum, or Marjoram.

Pa'nax. (U.S. Ph.) Ginseng. The root of *Pa'nax quinquefo'lium.*

Partridge Berry. See **Gaultheria.**

Pennyroyal. See **Hedeoma.**

Pepper. See **Piper.**

Pepper, Long. See **Piper Longum.**

Peppermint. See **Mentha Piperita.**

Pimen'ta. (U.S. and Br. Ph.) Pimento. The unripe berries of *Euge'nia pimen'ta.*

Pimento. See **Pimenta.**

Pimpinel'la Ani'sum. See **Anisum.**

Pi'per. (U.S. and Br. Ph.) Black Pepper. The berries of *Pi'per ni'grum* (U.S. Ph.). The dried unripe berries of *Piper nigrum* (Br. Ph.).

Pi'per Cube'ba. See **Cubeba.**

Pi'per Lon'gum. Long Pepper.

Purple Angelica. See **Angelica Atropurpurea.**

Rosemary. See **Rosmarinus.**

Rosmari'nus. (U.S. Ph.) Rosemary. The tops of *Rosmari'nus officina'lis.*

Sage. See **Salvia.**

Sal'via. (U.S. Ph.) Sage. The leaves of *Sal'via officina'lis.*

Solida'go. (U.S. Ph.) Golden Rod. The leaves of *Solida'go odo'ra.*

Spearmint. See **Mentha Viridis.**

Sweet Flag. See **Calamus.**

Tanace'tum. (U.S. Ph.) Tansy. The herb of *Tanace'tum vulga're.*

Tansy. See **Tanacetum.**

Turmeric. See **Curcuma.**

Vanil'la. (U.S. Ph.) The prepared unripe capsules of *Vanil'la aromat'ica.*

Wild Ginger. See **Asarum.**

Wintera. See **Drymis Winteri.**

Wintergreen. See **Gaultheria.**

Winter's Bark. See **Drymis Winteri.**

Zin'giber. (U.S. and Br. Ph.) Ginger. The rhizoma of *Zin'giber officina'le* (U.S. Ph.). The rhizome, scraped and dried, of *Zingiber officinale* (Br. Ph.).

SECTION V.—Mineral Tonics.

Aç'idum Muriat'icum. (U.S. Ph.) Muriatic Acid. See Class VI.

Aç'idum Ni'tricum. (U.S. and Br. Ph.) Nitric Acid. *Aqua Fortis.* A strongly acid, corrosive, colorless or yellowish liquid. Specific gravity, 1.420 (U.S. Ph.). Specific gravity, 1.5 (Br. Ph.).

Aç'idum Ni'tricum Dilu'tum. (U.S. and Br. Ph.) Dilute Nitric Acid. A colorless liquid. Specific gravity, 1.068 (U.S. Ph.). Specific gravity, 1.101 (Br. Ph.).

Aç'idum Nitromuriat'icum. (U.S. Ph.) Nitromuriatic Acid. A compound of three parts, by weight, of nitric acid with five parts of muriatic acid.

Aç'idum Phosphor'icum Dilu'tum. (Br. Ph.) Dilute Phosphoric Acid.

Aç'idum Sulphu'ricum. (U.S. and Br. Ph.) Sulphuric Acid, or Oil of Vitriol. A colorless liquid of an oily appearance, intensely acid and corrosive. Specific gravity, 1.843 (U.S. Ph.), 1.846 (Br. Ph.).

Aç'idum Sulphu'ricum Aromat'icum. (U.S. and Br. Ph.) Aromatic Sulphuric Acid; otherwise called Elixir of Vitriol.

Ammoniated Copper. See **Cuprum Ammoniatum.**

Argen'ti Ni'tras. (U.S. and Br. Ph.) Nitrate of Silver. Lunar Caustic. See Class XVIII.

? Argen'ti Ox'idum. (U.S. and Br. Ph.) Oxide of Silver.

Aromatic Sulphuric Acid. See **Acidum Sulphuricum Aromaticum.**

Bismu'thi Subni'tras. (U.S. Ph.) Subnitrate of Bismuth, or White Bismuth; sometimes called White Oxide of Bismuth. See Class IV.

Bismu'thum Al'bum. (Br. Ph.) White Bismuth. The same as **Bismuthi Subnitras.**

Bisulphate of Potash. See **Potassæ Bisulphas.**

Black Oxide of Iron. See **Ferri Oxidum Magneticum.**

Blue Vitriol. See **Cupri Sulphas.**

Calamine. See **Zinci Carbonas.**

Carbonate of Zinc. See **Zinci Carbonas.**

Citrate of Iron. See **Ferri Citras.**

Citrate of Iron and Quinia. See **Ferri et Quiniæ Citras.**

Copperas. See **Ferri Sulphas.**

Cu'pri Sul'phas. (U.S. and Br. Ph.) Sulphate of Copper, or Blue Vitriol. See Class I., and XVIII.

Cu'prum Ammonia'tum. (U.S. Ph.) Ammoniated Copper.

Elixir of Vitriol. See **Acidum Sulphuricum Aromaticum.**

Fer'ri-Ammo'nio-Ci'tras. See **Ferri et Ammoniæ Citras.**

Fer'ri Carbo'nas Sacchara'ta. (Br. Ph.) Saccharated Carbonate of Iron.

Fer'ri Chlo'ridum. See Class XIII.

Fer'ri Ci'tras. (U.S. Ph.) Citrate of Iron.

Fer'ri et Ammo'niæ Ci'tras. (Br. Ph.) Citrate of Iron and Ammonia; otherwise called *Ferri-Ammonio-Citras.*

Fer'ri et Ammo'niæ Tar'tras. (U.S. Ph.) Tartrate of Iron and Ammonia.

Fer'ri et Potas'sæ Tar'tras. (U.S. Ph.) Tartrate of Iron and Potash. A substance occurring in transparent scales of a dark, ruby-red color, and wholly soluble in water.

Fer'ri et Quin'iæ Ci'tras. (Br. Ph.) Citrate of Iron and Quinia.

Fer'ri Ferrocyan'idum. (U.S. Ph.) Ferrocyanide of Iron. Pure Prussian Blue. A pigment of a rich blue color.

Fer'ri Iod'idum. (Br. Ph.) Iodide of Iron. See Classes XIII. and X.

Fer'ri Lac'tas. (U.S. Ph.) Lactate of Iron. A substance in greenish-white crystalline crusts or grains of a mild sweetish taste.

Fer'ri Ox'idum Magnet'icum. (Br. Ph.) Magnetic Oxide of Iron; otherwise called *Fer'ri Ox'idum Ni'grum*, or Black Oxide of Iron.

Fer'ri Perchlo'ridi Li'quor. (Br. Ph.) Solution of Perchloride of Iron.

Fer'ri Pernitra'tis Li'quor. (Br. Ph.) Solution of Pernitrate of Iron.

Fer'ri Perox'idum. (Br. Ph.) Peroxide (or Rust) of Iron. A powder of a dark brown color, and destitute of taste.

Fer'ri Phos'phas. (U.S. and Br. Ph.) Phosphate of Iron. A slate-colored powder, insoluble in water, but soluble in the mineral acids.

Fer'ri Pul'vis. See **Ferrum Redactum.**

Fer'ri Ramen'ta. Iron Filings.

Fer'ri Rubi'go. (Rust of Iron.) See **Ferri Peroxidum.**

Fer'ri Subcarbo'nas. (U.S. Ph.) Subcarbonate of Iron.

Fer'ri Sul'phas. (U.S. and Br. Ph.) Sulphate of Iron, or Copperas. See Class I., Section II.

Fer'ri Sul'phas Granula'ta. (Br. Ph.) Granulated Sulphate of Iron.

Ferrocyanuret of Iron. See **Ferri Ferrocyanidum.**

Fer'rum Ammonia'tum. Ammoniated Iron.

Fer'rum Redac'tum. (U.S. and Br. Ph.) Reduced Iron; otherwise called *Ferri Pulvis* (Powder of Iron).

Fer'rum Tartara'tum. (Br. Ph.) Tartarated Iron. The same as **Ferri et Potassæ Tartras.**

Iodide of Iron. See **Ferri Iodidum.**

Iodide of Zinc. See **Zinci Iodidum.**

Iron Filings. See **Ferri Ramenta.**

Lactate of Iron. See **Ferri Lactas.**

Lime Water. See **Liquor Calcis.**

Li'quor Cal'cii Chlo'ridi. (U.S. Ph.) Solution of Chloride of Lime (or Calcium). See Class X.

Li'quor Cal'cis. (U.S. and Br. Ph.) Lime Water, or Solution of Lime.

Li'quor Fer'ri Nitra'tis. (U.S. Ph.) Solution of Nitrate of Iron.

Lunar Caustic. See **Argenti Nitras.**

Magistery of Bismuth. See **Bismuthi Subnitras.**

Magnetic Oxide of Iron. See **Ferri Oxidum Magneticum.**

Mangane'sii Ox'idum. Oxide of Manganese.

Muriatic Acid. See **Acidum Muriaticum.**

Nitrate of Silver. See **Argenti Nitras.**

Nitric Acid. See **Acidum Nitricum.**

Nitromuriatic Acid. See **Acidum Nitromuriaticum.**

Oil of Vitriol. See **Acidum Sulphuricum.**

Oxide of Manganese. See **Manganesii Oxidum.**

Oxide of Zinc. See **Zinci Oxidum.**

Perchloride of Iron. See **Ferri Perchloridi Liquor.**

Peroxide of Iron. See **Ferri Peroxidum.**

Phosphate of Iron. See **Ferri Phosphas.**

Potas'sæ Bisul'phas. Bisulphate of Potash.

Precipitated Carbonate of Iron. The same as **Ferri Subcarbonas.**

Precipitated Carbonate of Zinc. See **Zinci Carbonas Præcipitata.**

Protocarbonate of Iron. The same as **Ferri Subcarbonas.**

Reduced Iron. See **Ferrum Redactum.**

Rust of Iron. (*Fer'ri Rubi'go.*) See **Ferri Peroxidum.**

Saccharated Carbonate of Iron. See **Ferri Carbonas Saccharata.**

Salt, Common. See **Sodii Chloridum.**

So'dii Chlo'ridum. (U.S. and Br. Ph.) Chloride of Sodium, or Common Salt. See Section III. of this class.

Solution of Chloride of Calcium. See **Liquor Calcii Chloridi.**

Solution of Nitrate of Iron. See **Liquor Ferri Nitratis.**

Subcarbonate of Iron. See **Ferri Subcarbonas.**

Subnitrate of Bismuth. See **Bismuthi Subnitras.**

Sulphate of Copper. See **Cupri Sulphas.**

Sulphate of Iron. See **Ferri Sulphas.**

Sulphate of Zinc. See **Zinci Sulphas.**

Sulphuric Acid. See **Acidum Sulphuricum.**

Tartarated Iron. See **Ferrum Tartaratum.**

Tartrate of Iron and Ammonia. See **Ferri et Ammoniæ Tartras.**

Tartrate of Iron and Potash. See **Ferri et Potassæ Tartras.**

White Bismuth, or White Oxide of Bismuth. See **Bismuthi Subnitras.**

White Vitriol. See **Zinci Sulphas.**

Zin'çi Carbo'nas. (Br. Ph.) Carbonate of Zinc.

Zin'çi Carbo'nas Præcipita'ta. (U.S. Ph.) Precipitated Carbonate of Zinc.

Zin'çi Iod'idum. Iodide of Zinc.

Zin'çi Ox'idum. (U.S. and Br. Ph.) Oxide of Zinc.

Zin'çi Sul'phas. (U.S. and Br. Ph.) Sulphate of Zinc. White Vitriol. See Class VIII.

CLASS III.

ARTERIAL STIMULANTS.

MEDICINES WHICH EXCITE THE CIRCULATION WITH LITTLE COMPARATIVE INFLUENCE ON THE NERVOUS SYSTEM.

Ammo'niæ Carbo'nas. (U.S. and Br. Ph.) Carbonate of Ammonia, or Sal Volatile. A substance in white translucent masses, having a pungent ammoniacal odor, and soluble in water.

? Ammo'niæ Li'quor For'tior. (Br. Ph.) Strong Solution of Ammonia. See Class XVII.

Aromatic Spirit of Ammonia. See **Spiritus Ammoniæ Aromaticus.**

? Buc'co. (Br. Ph.) Buchu. See next article.

? Bu'chu. (U.S. Ph.) Buchu, Bucco; or Bookoo. The leaves of *Baros'ma crena'ta* and other species of *Barosma.* See Class X.

Cap'sicum. (U.S. and Br. Ph.) Cayenne Pepper. The fruit of *Cap'sicum an'nuum* and of other species of *Capsicum* (U.S. Ph.). The ripe fruit, dried, of *Cap'sicum fastigia'tum* (Br. Ph.).

Carbonate of Ammonia. See **Ammoniæ Carbonas.**

Cayenne Pepper. See **Capsicum.**

? Cerevis'iæ Fermen'tum. (Br. Ph.) Yeast of Beer.

Oil of Turpentine. See **Oleum Terebinthinæ.**

O'leum Terebin'thinæ. Oil of Turpentine, or Spirits of Turpentine. The volatile oil distilled from the turpentine of *Pi'nus palus'tris* and of other species of *Pinus.* See Class X.

Phos'phorus. (U.S. Ph.) Phosphorus. A translucent, nearly colorless solid, resembling wax, without taste, but having a peculiar smell. (Poisonous except in very minute doses.)

Spirit of Ammonia. See **Spiritus Ammoniæ.**

Spir'itus Ammo'niæ. (U.S. Ph.) Spirit of Ammonia.

Spir'itus Ammo'niæ Aromat'icus. (U.S. and Br. Ph.) Aromatic Spirit of Ammonia. See Class IV.

Turpentine, Spirits of. See **Oleum Terebinthinæ.**

CLASS IV.

NERVOUS STIMULANTS (ANTISPASMODICS).

MEDICINES WHICH TO THE POWER OF STIMULATING THE HEART AND ARTERIES ADD THAT OF EXCITING THE NERVOUS SYSTEM.

Æ'ther. (U.S. and Br. Ph.) Ether; otherwise called Sulphuric Ether. Oxide of Ethyl. A very inflammable, volatile liquid obtained from alcohol and sulphuric acid.

Al'lium. (U.S. Ph.) Garlic. See Class XII.

Alum. See **Alumen.**

Alu'men. (U.S. and Br. Ph.) Alum. Sulphate of Alumina and Potassa.

Ammoniac. See **Ammoniacum.**

Ammoni'acum. (U.S. and Br. Ph.) The concrete juice of *Dore'ma ammoni'acum* (U.S. Ph.). A gum-resinous exudation from the stem of *Dorema ammoniacum* (Br. Ph.).

Ammo'niæ Carbo'nas. (U.S. and Br. Ph.) Carbonate of Ammonia. See Class III.

Ammo'niæ Hydrochlo'ras. (Br. Ph.) Hydrochlorate of Ammonia. The same as **Ammoniæ Murias.**

? Ammo'niæ Mu'rias. (U.S. Ph.) Muriate of Ammonia, or Sal Ammoniac. A white fibrous salt, with a pungent saline taste, but no smell.

Argen'ti Ni'tras. (U.S. and Br. Ph.) Nitrate of Silver, or Lunar Caustic. See Class XVIII.

Argen'ti Ox'idum. (U.S. and Br. Ph.) Oxide of Silver.

Ar'nica. (U.S. and Br. Ph.) Leopard's Bane. Arnica Root. The flowers of *Ar'nica monta'na* (U.S. Ph.). The dried root of *Arnica montana* (Br. Ph.).

Aromatic Spirit of Ammonia. See **Spiritus Ammoniæ Aromaticus.**

Assafœt'ida. (U.S. and Br. Ph.) Assafetida. The concrete juice (or gum resin) obtained from the root of the *Nar'thex assafœt'ida* (or *Fer'ula assafœt'ida*).

Bismu'thi Subni'tras. (U.S. Ph.) Subnitrate of Bismuth, or White Bismuth. A heavy white powder in minute crystalline scales.

Bismu'thum Al'bum. (Br. Ph.) White Bismuth. The same as **Bismuthi Subnitras.**

Caf'fea. (U.S. Ph.) Coffee. The seed of *Caf'fea Arab'ica.*

Cam'phora. (U.S. and Br. Ph.) Camphor. See Class V.

Carbonate of Ammonia. See **Ammoniæ Carbonas.**

Castor. See **Castoreum.**

Casto'reum. (U.S. and Br. Ph.) Castor. A peculiar concrete substance, obtained from *Cas'tor fi'ber.*

Cata'ria. (U.S. Ph.) Catnep. The leaves of *Nep'eta cata'ria.* (Carminative.)

Catnep. See **Cataria.**

Cherry Laurel. See **Laurocerasus.**

Chloride of Zinc. See **Zinci Chloridum.**

Coca. See **Erythroxylon Coca.**

Coffee. See **Caffea.**

Compound Spirit of Ether. See **Spiritus Ætheris Compositus.**

Cro'cus. (U.S. and Br. Ph.) Saffron. The stigmas of *Cro'cus sati'vus.*

? Cu'prum Ammonia'tum. (U.S. Ph.) Ammoniated Copper. See Class II.

Cypripe'dium Parviflo'rum. Ladies' Slipper.

Dore'ma Ammoni'acum. See **Ammoniacum.**

Dracon'tium. (U.S. Ph.) Skunk Cabbage. The root of *Dracon'tium fœt'idum.*

Erythrox'ylon Co'ca.

Fer'ula Assafœt'ida. See **Assafœtida.**

Gal'banum. (U.S. and Br. Ph.) See Class XII.

Garlic. See **Allium.**

Hoffmann's Anodyne. See **Spiritus Ætheris Compositus.**

Ladies' Slipper. See **Cypripedium Parviflorum.**

Laurocer'asus. (Br. Ph.) Cherry Laurel Leaves. The fresh leaves of *Pru'nus laurocer'asus.*

Leopard's Bane. See **Arnica.**

Lycopo'dium. (U.S. Ph.) The sporules of *Lycopo'dium clava'tum* and other species of *Lycopodium.* See Class X.

Mos'chus. (U.S. and Br. Ph.) Musk. A peculiar concrete substance, obtained from *Mos'chus moschif'erus* (U.S. Ph.). The inspissated secretion from the preputial follicles of the *Moschus moschiferus* (Br. Ph.).

Muriate of Ammonia. See **Ammoniæ Murias.**

Musk. See **Moschus.**

Nar'thex Assafœt'ida. See **Assafœtida.**

Nep'eta Cata'ria. See **Cataria.**

Nitrate of Silver. See **Argenti Nitras.**

Oil of Amber. See **Oleum Succini.**

Oil of Camphor. See **Oleum Camphoræ.**

Oil of Rue. See **Oleum Rutæ.**

O'leum Cam'phoræ. (U.S. Ph.) Oil of Camphor.

O'leum Ru'tæ. (Br. Ph.) Oil of Rue. The oil distilled from *Ru'ta grav'eolens.*

O'leum Suc'çini. (U.S. Ph.) Oil of Amber. The volatile oil obtained by the destructive distillation of amber.

Oxide of Zinc. See **Zinci Oxidum.**

Petro'leum. Rock Oil.

Pru'nus Laurocer'asus. See **Laurocerasus.**

Rock Oil. See **Petroleum.**

Rue. See **Ruta.**

Ru'ta. (U.S. Ph.) Rue. The leaves of *Ru'ta grav'eolens.*

Ru'tæ O'leum. See **Oleum Rutæ.**

Saffron. See **Crocus.**

Sagape'num. (Lond. Ph.) The gum resin of an unknown plant.

Scutella'ria. (U.S. Ph.) Scull-cap. The herb of *Scutella'ria lateriflo'ra.*

Skunk Cabbage. See **Dracontium.**

Spirit of Nitric Ether. See **Spiritus Ætheris Nitrosi.**

Spir'itus Æ'theris Compos'itus. (U.S. Ph.) Compound Spirit of Ether, or Hoffmann's Anodyne.

Spir'itus Æ'theris Nitro'si (U.S. and Br. Ph.); formerly *Spir'itus Æ'theris Ni'trici.* Spirit of Nitrous or Nitric Ether; otherwise called Sweet Spirit of Nitre.

Spir'itus Ammo'niæ Aromat'icus. (U.S. and Br. Ph.) Aromatic Spirit of Ammonia.

Subnitrate of Bismuth. See **Bismuthi Subnitras.**

Sweet Spirit of Nitre. See **Spiritus Ætheris Nitrosi.**

The'a Ni'gra. Black Tea.

The'a Vir'idis. Green Tea.

Valerian. See **Valeriana.**

Valeria'na. (U.S. and Br. Ph.) Valerian. The root of *Valeria'na officina'lis.*

Valerianate of Zinc. See **Zinci Valerianas.**

Vi'num. Wine.

White Bismuth. See **Bismuthi Subnitras.**

Zin'çi Chlo'ridum. (U. S. and Br. Ph.) Chloride of Zinc. See Class XVIII.

Zin'çi Ox'idum. (U.S. and Br. Ph.) Oxide of Zinc. A yellowish-white powder.

Zin'çi Valeria'nas. (U.S. and Br. Ph.) Valerianate of Zinc.

CLASS V.

CEREBRAL STIMULANTS (NARCOTICS).

MEDICINES WHICH, WITH A STIMULATING INFLUENCE OVER THE CIRCULATION AND THE GENERAL NERVOUS SYSTEM, COMBINE A PECULIAR DETERMINATION TO THE BRAIN.

Acetate of Morphia. See **Morphiæ Acetas.**

Ace'tum O'pii. (U.S. Ph.) Vinegar of Opium, or Black Drop.

Aç'idum Acet'icum Camphora'tum. Camphorated Acetic Acid.

Acrid Lettuce. See **Lactuca Virosa.**

Æ'ther. (U.S. and Br. Ph.) Ether, or Sulphuric Ether. A very inflammable volatile liquid prepared with alcohol and sulphuric acid.

Æ'ther For'tior. (U.S. Ph.) Stronger Ether.

Al'cohol. (U.S. Ph.) Alcohol. Spirit of the specific gravity 0.835 (Absolute Alcohol being 0.795).

At'ropa Belladon'na, or Deadly Nightshade. See **Belladonna,** and **Belladonnæ Folium.**

Atro'pia. (Br. Ph.) An alkaloid obtained from Belladonna Root. (A deadly poison, except in very minute doses.)

Belladon'na. (Br. Ph.) The leaves of *At'ropa belladon'na.* See next article.

Belladon'næ Fo'lium. (U.S. Ph.) Belladonna Leaf. The leaves of *At'ropa belladon'na.*

Belladon'næ Ra'dix. (U.S. and Br. Ph.) Belladonna Root.

Bittersweet. See **Dulcamara.**

Black Drop. See **Acetum Opii.**

Brandy. See **Spiritus Vini Gallici.**

Bugleweed. See **Lycopus.**

Camphor. See **Camphora.**

Cam'phora. (U.S. and Br. Ph.) Camphor. A peculiar concrete substance derived from *Cam'phora officina'rum* (U.S. Ph.). A concrete volatile oil, obtained by sublimation from the wood of *Camphora officinarum* (Br. Ph.).

Camphorated Acetic Acid. See **Acidum Aceticum Camphoratum.**

Can'nabis In'dica. (Br. Ph.) The flowering tops of Indian Hemp.

Chloroform. See **Chloroformum.**

Chlorofor'mum. (Br. Ph.) Chloroform. A colorless volatile liquid. Specific gravity, 1.496.

Chlorofor'mum Vena'le. (U.S. Ph.) Commercial Chloroform. A colorless volatile liquid varying in specific gravity from 1.45 to 1.49, obtained by distilling a mixture of chloride of lime and alcohol.

Compound Spirit of Æther. See **Spiritus Ætheris Compositus.**

Coni'i Fruc'tûs. (Br. Ph.) Hemlock Fruit.

Coni'um. (U.S. and Br. Ph.) Hemlock. The leaves of *Coni'um macula'tum* (U.S. Ph.). The fresh leaves and branches of *Conium maculatum*, gathered when the fruit begins to form (Br. Ph.). (An active poison.)

Creasote. See **Creasotum.**

Creaso'tum. (U.S. and Br. Ph.) Creasote. A peculiar substance obtained from wood tar (U.S. Ph.). A product of the distillation of wood tar (Br. Ph.).

Datu'ra Stramo'nium. See **Stramonii Folium.**

Deadly Nightshade. See **Belladonna.**

Dulcama'ra. (U.S. and Br. Ph.) Bittersweet. The stalks of *Sola'num dulcama'ra.*

Ether. See **Æther.**

Extrac'tum Can'nabis. (U.S. Ph.) Extract of Hemp. An alcoholic extract of the dried tops of *Can'nabis sati'va*, variety *In'dica.*

Extrac'tum Can'nabis In'dicæ. (Br. Ph.) Extract of Indian Hemp. See preceding article.

Hemlock Leaves and Seed. See **Conium.**

Henbane. See **Hyoscyamus.**

Henbane Leaves. See **Hyoscyami Folium.**

Henbane Seed. See **Hyoscyami Semen.**

Hops. See **Humulus.**

Hu'mulus. (U.S. Ph.) Hops. The strobiles of *Hu'mulus lu'pulus.*

Hyoscy'ami Fo'lium. (U.S. Ph.) The leaves of *Hyoscy'amus ni'ger.*

Hyoscy'ami Se'men. (U.S. Ph.) The seed of *Hyoscy'amus ni'ger.*

Hyoscy'amus. (Br. Ph.) Henbane. The same as **Hyoscyami Folium.**

Indian Hemp. See **Cannabis Indica.**

Jamaica Dogwood. See **Piscidia Erythrina.**

Lactu'ca Sati'va. See **Lactucarium.**

Lactu'ca Viro'sa. Acrid Lettuce.

Lactuca'rium. (U.S. Ph.) The concrete juice of *Lactu'ca sati'va.*

Lau'rus Cam'phora. See **Camphora.**

Lupulin. See **Lupulina.**

Lupuli'na. (U.S. Ph.) Lupulin. The yellow powder attached to the strobiles of *Hu'mulus lu'pulus.*

Lu'pulus. (Br. Ph.) Hop. The dried catkins of the female plant of *Humulus lupulus.* See **Humulus.**

Lyc'opus. (U.S. Ph.) Bugleweed. The herb of *Lyc'opus Virgin'icus.*

Mor'phia. (U.S. Ph.) A substance in the form of colorless crystals, which are inflammable and wholly dissipated by a red heat.

Mor'phiæ Ace'tas. (U.S. Ph.) Acetate of Morphia. A white powder entirely soluble in water and in alcohol.

Mor'phiæ Hydrochlo'ras. (Br. Ph.) Hydrochlorate (or Muriate) of Morphia. See next article.

Mor'phiæ Mu'rias. (U.S. Ph.) Muriate of Morphia. A substance occurring in snow-white feathery crystals.

Mor'phiæ Sul'phas. (U.S. Ph.) Sulphate of Morphia. A substance in the form of snow-white feathery crystals which are wholly soluble in water.

Muriate of Morphia. See **Morphiæ Murias.**

? Myris'tica. (U.S. and Br. Ph.) Nutmeg. See Class II., Section IV.

Nicotia'na Tab'acum. See **Tabacum.**

Nitrous Oxide (Gas). See **Oxidum Nitrosum.**

Nutmeg. See **Myristica.**

O'pium. (U.S. and Br. Ph.) Opium. The concrete (or inspissated) juice of the unripe capsules of *Papa'ver somnif'erum.*

Ox'idum Nitro'sum. Nitrous Oxide.

Papa'ver. (U.S. and Br. Ph.) Poppy Capsules.

Papa'ver Somnif'erum. See **Opium.**

Piscid'ia Erythri'na. Jamaica Dogwood.

Poison Oak, Poison Sumach. See **Rhus Toxicodendron.**

Port Wine. See **Vinum Portense.**

Pyroxylic Spirit. See **Spiritus Pyroxylicus.**

Rhœ'as. (Br. Ph.) Red Poppy Petals. The petals of *Papaver rhœas.*

Rhus Toxicoden'dron. See **Toxicodendron.**

Sola'num Dulcama'ra. See **Dulcamara.**

Spir'itus Æ'theris Compos'itus. Compound Spirit of Ether. See Class IV.

Spir'itus Frumen'ti. (U.S. Ph.) "Spirit of Grain," or Whiskey.

Spir'itus Pyroxyl'icus Rectifica'tus. (Br. Ph.) Rectified Pyroxylic Spirit.

Spir'itus Rectifica'tus. (Br. Ph.) Rectified Spirit.

Spir'itus Vi'ni Gal'lici. (U.S. Ph.) Spirit of French Wine, or Brandy.

Stramo'nii Fo'lia. (Br. Ph.) **Stramo'nii Fo'lium.** (U.S. Ph.) Leaves of Stramonium. The leaves of *Datu'ra stramo'nium.*

Stramo'nii Ra'dix. Root of Stramonium.

Stramo'nii Se'men. (U.S. Ph.) **Stramo'nii Sem'ina.** (Br. Ph.) Seed of Stramonium. The seed of *Datu'ra stramo'nium.*

Stramonium (Leaf). See **Stramonii Folium.**

Stramonium (Seed). See **Stramonii Semen.**

Stronger Ether. See **Æther Fortior.**

? Sty'rax. (U.S. Ph.) Storax.

Sulphuric Ether. See **Æther.**

Tab'acum. (U.S. and Br. Ph.) Tobacco. See Class VII.

Tobacco. See **Tabacum.**

Toxicoden'dron. (U.S. Ph.) Poison Oak. The leaves of *Rhus toxicoden'dron.*

Vinegar of Opium. See **Acetum Opii.**

Vi'num. Wine.

? Vi'num Porten'se. (U.S. Ph.) Port Wine. See Class I.

Vi'num Xer'icum. (U.S. and Br. Ph.) Sherry Wine; otherwise called *Vi'num Al'bum* (White Wine).

Wine. See **Vinum.**

Woody Nightshade. See **Dulcamara.**

CLASS VI.

ARTERIAL SEDATIVES.

MEDICINES WHICH, BY THEIR IMMEDIATE INFLUENCE, PRODUCE A REDUCTION OF THE VITAL ACTIONS. SOME OF THESE ARE DIRECTED MORE ESPECIALLY TO THE CIRCULATORY SYSTEM, WITHOUT ANY IMMEDIATE INFLUENCE UPON THE NERVOUS POWER. THOUGH SEDATIVE IN THEIR GENERAL INFLUENCE, THEY MAY BE STIMULATING TO PARTICULAR FUNCTIONS OR ORGANS.

Acetate of Lead. See **Plumbi Acetas.**

Acetic Acid. See **Acidum Aceticum.**

Aç'idum Acet'icum. (U.S. and Br. Ph.) Acetic Acid. A colorless liquid having a pungent odor and a specific gravity of 1.047 (U.S. Ph.). An acid liquid prepared from wood by destructive distillation. Specific gravity, 1.044 (Br. Ph.).

Aç'idum Cit'ricum. (U.S. and Br. Ph.) Citric Acid. A substance in colorless crystals, freely soluble in water, and soluble in alcohol (U.S. Ph.). An acid obtained from lemon-juice, in colorless right rhombic prisms (Br. Ph.).

Aç'idum Hydrochlo'ricum. (Br. Ph.) Hydrochloric Acid. The same as **Acidum Muriaticum.**

Aç'idum Muriat'icum. (U.S. Ph.) Muriatic Acid; otherwise termed Hydrochloric Acid. An aqueous solution of hydrochloric acid gas, of the specific gravity 1.160. (Refrigerant and tonic.)

Aç'idum Ni'tricum. (U.S. and Br. Ph.) Nitric Acid. See Class II.

Aç'idum Tartar'icum. (U.S. and Br. Ph.) Tartaric Acid. A substance in the form of colorless crystals.

Ammo'niæ Hydrosulphure'tum. Hydrosulphuret of Ammonia.

Antimonial Powder. See **Pulvis Antimonialis.**

Antimonial Wine. See **Vinum Antimonii.**

Antimo'nii et Potas'sæ Tar'tras. (U.S. Ph.) Tartar Emetic. See Class VIII.

Antimo'nii Ox'idum. (U.S. and Br. Ph.) Oxide of Antimony. See Class VIII.

Antimo'nii Sulphure'tum. (U.S. Ph.) Sulphuret of Antimony.

Antimo'nium Sulphura'tum. (Br. Ph.) Sulphurated Antimony. See Class XI.

Antimo'nium Tartara'tum. (Br. Ph.) Tartarated Antimony. The same as **Antimonii et Potassæ Tartras.**

Bitartrate of Potash. See **Potassæ Bitartras.**

Bo'rax. (Br. Ph.) Biborate of Soda. See **Sodæ Boras.**

Carbonate of Lead. See **Plumbi Carbonas.**

Chlorate of Potassa. See **Potassæ Chloras.**

Citric Acid. See **Acidum Citricum.**

Cream of Tartar. See **Potassæ Bitartras.**

Ferrocyanide of Potassium. See **Potassii Ferrocyanidum.**

Hydrosulphuret of Ammonia. See **Ammoniæ Hydrosulphuretum.**

Limo'nis Suc'cus. (U.S. and Br. Ph.) Lemon-Juice.

Mo'ri Suc'cus. (Br. Ph.) Mulberry-Juice. The juice of the ripe fruit of *Mo'rus ni'gra.*

Mulberry-Juice. See **Mori Succus.**

Nitrate of Potash. See **Potassæ Nitras.**

Nitre. See **Potassæ Nitras.**

Oxide of Antimony. See **Antimonii Oxidum.**

Plum'bi Ace'tas. (U.S. and Br. Ph.) Acetate of Lead, or Sugar of Lead. See Class I.

Plum'bi Carbo'nas. (U.S. and Br. Ph.) Carbonate of Lead, or White Lead. See Class I.

Potas'sæ Bitar'tras. (U.S. Ph.) Bitartrate of Potash, or Cream of Tartar. A white powder, dissolved sparingly in water.

Potas'sæ Chlo'ras. (U.S. and Br. Ph.) Chlorate of Potassa. A salt occurring in colorless tabular crystals.

Potas'sæ Ci'tras. (U.S. and Br. Ph.) Citrate of Potassa. See Class XI.

Potas'sæ Ni'tras. (U.S. and Br. Ph.) Nitrate of Potash, Nitre, or Saltpetre. A salt occurring in colorless prismatic crystals, unalterable in the air.

Potas'sæ Tar'tras Aç'ida. (Br. Ph.) Acid Tartrate of Potash. The same as **Potassæ Bitartras.**

Potas'sii Ferrocyan'idum. (U.S. Ph.) Ferrocyanide of Potassium.

Pul'vis Antimonia'lis. (Br. Ph.) Antimonial Powder. See Class XI.

Rhus Gla'brum. (U.S. Ph.) Sumach. The fruit of *Rhus glabrum.*

Saltpetre. See **Potassæ Nitras.**

So'dæ Bo'ras. (U.S. Ph.) Borate of Soda, or Borax. A salt in colorless crystals, which slightly effloresce in dry air.

Sugar of Lead. See **Plumbi Acetas.**

Sulphurated Antimony. See **Antimonium Sulphuratum.**

Sulphuret of Antimony. See **Antimonii Sulphuretum.**

Sumach. See **Rhus Glabrum.**

Tamarind. See **Tamarindus.**

Tamarin'dus. (U.S. and Br. Ph.) Tamarind. The preserved fruit of *Tamarin'dus In'dica.*

Tartar Emetic. See **Antimonii et Potassæ Tartras.**

Tartarated Antimony. See **Antimonium Tartaratum.**

Tartaric Acid. See **Acidum Tartaricum.**

Tartarized Antimony. See **Antimonii et Potassæ Tartras.**

Tartrate of Antimony and Potash. See **Antimonii et Potassæ Tartras.**

Vi'num Antimonia'le. (Br. Ph.) Antimonial Wine. The same as **Vinum Antimonii.**

Vi'num Antimo'nii. (U.S. Ph.) Antimonial Wine, or Wine of Antimony. See Class VIII.

CLASS VII.

NERVOUS SEDATIVES.

MEDICINES WHICH, IN THEIR PRIMARY OPERATION, REDUCE AT THE SAME TIME THE NERVOUS POWER AND THE FORCE OF THE CIRCULATION.

Aç'idum Hydrocyan'icum Dilu'tum. (U.S. and Br. Ph.) Diluted Hydrocyanic Acid or Prussic Acid. A colorless liquid, having a peculiar odor; specific gravity, 0.997.

Aconite. See **Aconitum.**

Aconite Root. See **Aconiti Radix.**

Aconi'tia. (U.S. and Br. Ph.) Aconitin. (A deadly poison, except in extremely minute doses.)

Aconi'ti Fo'lium. (U.S. Ph.) Aconite Leaf. The leaves of *Aconi'tum napel'lus.*

Aconi'ti Ra'dix. (U.S. and Br. Ph.) Aconite Root. The root of *Aconi'tum napel'lus* (U.S. Ph.). The dried root of *Aconitum napellus* (Br. Ph.).

Aconi'tum. (Br. Ph.) Aconite. Monkshood. The fresh leaves and flowering tops of *Aconi'tum napel'lus.*

Black Snakeroot. See **Cimicifuga.**

Cherry Laurel Leaves. See **Laurocerasus.**

? Cimicif'uga. (U.S. Ph.) Black Snakeroot. The root of *Cimicif'uga racemo'sa.* See Class II., Section II.

Cimicif'uga Racemo'sa. See **Cimicifuga.**

? Col'chicum. See Class X.

Cyanide of Potassium. See **Potassii Cyanidum.**

Cyanuret of Potassium. See **Potassii Cyanuretum.**

Digitali'num. (Br. Ph.) Digitalin. The active principle obtained from Digitalis, a white, intensely bitter substance, which is inodorous, but powerfully irritates the nostrils. (It is an active poison.)

Digita'lis. (U.S. and Br. Ph.) Digitalis. Foxglove. The leaves of *Digita'lis purpu'rea,* from plants of the second year's growth (U.S. Ph.). The dried leaf of *Digitalis purpurea,* gathered when about two-thirds of the flowers are expanded (Br. Ph.).

Foxglove. See **Digitalis.**

? Gelse'mium. (U.S. Ph.) The root of *Gelsemium sempervirens.*

Hydrocyanic Acid. See **Acidum Hydrocyanicum Dilutum.**

Laurocer'asus. (Br. Ph.) Cherry Laurel Leaves. The fresh leaves of the *Prunus laurocerasus.*

Monkshood. See **Aconitum.**

Nicotia'na Tab'acum. See **Tabacum.**

Oil of Almonds (**Oleum Amygdalæ**). See Class XIX.

Oil of Bitter Almonds. See **Oleum Amygdalæ Amaræ.**

O'leum Amyg'dalæ Ama'ræ. (U.S. Ph.) Oil of Bitter Almonds. The oil obtained by distilling with water the kernels of the fruit of *Amyg'dalus commu'nis,* variety *ama'ra.*

Potas'sii Cyan'idum. (U.S. Ph.) Cyanide of Potassium. A substance in white, opaque, amorphous pieces, having an alkaline reaction.

Potas'sii Cyanure'tum. See **Potassii Cyanidum.**

Prussic Acid. See **Acidum Hydrocyanicum.**

? *Spir'itus Pyroxyl'icus.* Pyroxylic Spirit.

Tab'acum. (U.S. and Br. Ph.) Tobacco. The dried leaves of *Nicotia'na tab'acum.*

Tobacco. See **Tabacum.**

CLASS VIII.

EMETICS.

MEDICINES CAPABLE OF PRODUCING VOMITING IN CERTAIN DOSES, AND AS AN ORDINARY RESULT.

SECTION I.—Vegetable Emetics.

Ace'tum Scil'læ. (U.S. Ph.) Vinegar of Squill. See Class XII.

Adder's Tongue. See **Erythronium.**

American Hellebore. See **Veratrum Viride.**

Apoç'ynum Androsæmifo'lium. (U.S. Ph.) Dogsbane. The root of *Apocynum androsæmifolium.*

Apoç'ynum Cannabi'num. (U.S. Ph.) Indian Hemp. The root of *Apocynum cannabinum.*

Ascle'pias Curassavi'ca. Bastard Ipecacuanha, or Blood Weed.

Ascle'pias Incarna'ta. Flesh-colored Asclepias.

Azed'arach. (U.S. Ph.) See Class IX.

Bloodroot. See **Sanguinaria.**

Blue Flag. See **Iris Versicolor.**

Buckbean. See **Menyanthes Trifoliata.**

Cephaë'lis Ipecacuan'ha. See **Ipecacuanha.**

Delphin'ium Staphisa'gria. Stavesacre.

Erythro'nium America'num. Adder's Tongue.

Eupato'rium. (U.S. Ph.) Thoroughwort, or Boneset. See Class II., Section III., and Class XI., Section I.

Euphor'bia Corolla'ta. (U.S. Ph.) Spurge, or Large-flowering Spurge. The root of *Euphorbia corollata.*

Euphor'bia Ipecacuan'ha. (U.S. Ph.) Ipecacuanha Spurge. The root of *Euphorbia ipecacuanha.*

Fever Root. See **Triosteum.**

Flesh-colored Asclepias. See **Asclepias Incarnata.**

Florentine Orris. See **Iris Florentina.**

Gille'nia. (U.S. Ph.) The root of *Gille'nia trifolia'ta,* and of *Gille'nia stipula'cea.*

Gille'nia Trifolia'ta. See **Gillenia.**

Indian Tobacco. See **Lobelia.**

Ipecacuan'ha. (U.S. and Br. Ph.) Ipecacuan. The root of *Cephaë'lis ipecacuan'ha* (U.S. Ph.). The dried root of *Cephaëlis ipecacuanha* (Br. Ph.).

Ipecacuanha Spurge. See **Euphorbia Ipecacuanha.**

I'ris Florenti'na. (U.S. Ph.) Florentine Orris. The rhizoma of *Iris Florentina.* See Class IX.

I'ris Versic'olor. (U.S. Ph.) Blue Flag. The rhizoma of *Iris versicolor.*

Lobe'lia. (U.S. and Br. Ph.) Indian Tobacco. The herb of *Lobe'lia infla'ta* (U.S. Ph.). The herb in flower, dried, of *Lobelia inflata* (Br. Ph.).

Marsh Trefoil. See **Menyanthes Trifoliata.**

Me'lia Azed'arach. See **Azedarach.**

Menyan'thes Trifolia'ta. Buckbean, or Marsh Trefoil.

Milkweed. See **Euphorbia Corollata.**

Mustard. See **Sinapis.**

Nicotia'na Tab'acum. See **Tabacum.**

Phytolac'ca. See **Phytolaccæ Baccæ.**

Phytolac'cæ Bac'cæ. (U.S. Ph.) Poke Berries. The berries of *Phytolac'ca decan'dra.*

Phytolac'cæ Ra'dix. (U.S. Ph.) Poke Root. The root of *Phytolac'ca decan'dra.*

Poke Berries. See **Phytolaccæ Baccæ.**

Poke Root. See **Phytolaccæ Radix.**

Polyg'ala Sen'ega. See **Senega.**

Pride of China, or Pride of India. See **Azedarach.**

Queen's Root. See **Stillingia.**

Sanguina'ria. (U.S. Ph.) Bloodroot. The rhizoma of *Sanguina'ria Canaden'sis.*

Scil'la. (U.S. and Br. Ph.) Squill. See Class XII.

Sen'ega. (U.S. and Br. Ph.) Seneka. See Class XII.

Seneka. See **Senega.**

Sina'pis. (Br. Ph.) Mustard. See next article.

Sina'pis Al'ba. (U.S. Ph.) White Mustard. See Class XVII.

Spurge. See **Euphorbia Corollata.**

Squill. See **Scilla.**

Stavesacre. See **Delphinium Staphisagria.**

Stillin'gia. (U.S. Ph.) The root of *Stillin'gia sylvat'ica.*

Tab'acum. (U.S. and Br. Ph.) Tobacco. See Class VII.

Tobacco. See **Tabacum.**

Trios'teum. (U.S. Ph.) Fever Root, or Wild Ipecac. See Class IX.

Vera'tria. (U.S. and Br. Ph.) An alkaloid obtained from cevadilla. A pale-gray, intensely acrid and bitter substance, without smell, but, in the most minute quantity, powerfully irritating the nostrils. (An active poison.)

Vera'trum Al'bum. (U.S. Ph.) White Hellebore. The rhizoma of *Veratrum album.*

Vera'trum Vir'ide. (U.S. Ph.) American Hellebore. The rhizoma of *Veratrum viride.*

Vinegar of Squill. See **Acetum Scillæ.**

White Hellebore. See **Veratrum Album.**

Wild Ipecac. See **Triosteum.**

SECTION II.—Mineral Emetics.

Antimonial Powder. See **Pulvis Antimonialis.**

Antimo'nii et Potas'sæ Tar'tras. (U.S. Ph.) Tartar Emetic. Tartrate of Antimony and Potassa. A salt occurring in transparent crystals, which become white and opaque on exposure to the air.

Antimo'nii Ox'idum. (U.S. and Br. Ph.) Oxide of Antimony. A white or grayish-white powder, insoluble in water.

Antimo'nii Sulphure'tum. (U.S. Ph.) Sulphuret of Antimony. Native tersulphuret of antimony, purified by fusion.

Antimo'nium Sulphura'tum. (Br. Ph.) Sulphurated Antimony. See Class XI.

Antimo'nium Tartara'tum. (Br. Ph.) Tartarated Antimony, or Tartar Emetic. The same as **Antimonii et Potassæ Tartras.**

Bichromate of Lead. See **Plumbi Bichromas.**

Bichromate of Potassa. See **Potassæ Bichromas.**

Blue Vitriol. See **Cupri Sulphas.**

Chloride of Sodium. See **Sodii Chloridum.**

Cu'pri Sul'phas. (U.S. and Br. Ph.) Sulphate of Copper, or Blue Vitriol. See Class XVIII.

Hydrar'gyri Sul'phas Fla'va. (U.S. Ph.) Yellow Sulphate of Mercury, or Turpeth Mineral. A lemon-yellow powder, sparingly soluble in water.

Oxide of Antimony. See **Antimonii Oxidum.**

Plum'bi Bichro'mas. (U.S. Ph.) Bichromate of Lead.

Potas'sæ Bichro'mas. (U.S. Ph.) Bichromate of Potassa. A substance in the form of orange-red, anhydrous, tabular crystals.

Pul'vis Antimonia'lis. (Br. Ph.) Antimonial Powder. See Class XI.

Salt. See **Sodii Chloridum.**

? So'dii Chlo'ridum. (U.S. and Br. Ph.) Chloride of Sodium, or Common Salt. See Class II., Section V.

Sulphate of Copper. See **Cupri Sulphas.**

Sulphate of Zinc. See **Zinci Sulphas.**

Sulphurated Antimony. See **Antimonium Sulphuratum.**

Sulphuret of Antimony. See **Antimonii Sulphuretum.**

Tartar Emetic. See **Antimonii et Potassæ Tartras.**

Tartarated Antimony. See **Antimonium Tartaratum.**

Tartrate of Antimony and Potassa. See **Antimonii et Potassæ Tartras.**

Turpeth Mineral. See **Hydrargyri Sulphas Flava.**

Vi'num Antimo'nii. (U.S. Ph.) Antimonial Wine, or Wine of Antimony. A solution of tartar emetic in sherry wine. See Class XI.

White Vitriol. See **Zinci Sulphas.**

Yellow Sulphate of Mercury. See **Hydrargyri Sulphas Flava.**

Zin'çi Sul'phas. (U.S. and Br. Ph.) Sulphate of Zinc, or White Vitriol. A substance occurring in colorless crystals.

CLASS IX.

CATHARTICS.

MEDICINES WHICH PRODUCE EVACUATIONS FROM THE BOWELS.

SECTION I.—Vegetable Cathartics.

? **Al'etris.** (U.S. Ph.) Star Grass. See Class II., Section II.

Al'oe Barbaden'sis. (U.S. and Br. Ph.) Barbadoes Aloes. The inspissated juice of the leaves of *Al'oe vulga'ris.*

Al'oe Capen'sis. (U.S. Ph.) Cape Aloes.

Al'oe Hepat'ica. Hepatic Aloes.

Al'oe Socotri'na. (U.S. and Br. Ph.) Socotrine Aloes. The inspissated juice of the leaves of the *Aloe Socotrina* (U.S. Ph.). The inspissated juice of the leaves of one or more undetermined species of *Aloe* (Br. Ph.).

Al'oe Vulga'ris. See **Aloe Barbadensis.**

Aloes. See **Aloe Barbadensis,** &c.

American Senna. See **Cassia Marilandica.**

A'pium Petroseli'num. See **Petroselinum.**

Apoç'ynum Cannabi'num. (U.S. Ph.) Indian Hemp. See Class VIII.

Asagræ'a Officina'lis. See **Sabadilla.**

? **Ascle'pias.** (U.S. Ph.) Butterflyweed. See Class XI.

? *Ascle'pias Incarna'ta.* Flesh-colored Asclepias.

? *Ascle'pias Syri'aca.* Common Milkweed, or Silkweed.

Ascle'pias Tubero'sa. See **Asclepias.**

Azed'arach. (U.S. Ph.) The bark of the root of *Me'lia azed'arach.*

Barbadoes Nut. See **Curcas Purgans.**

Bear's-foot. See **Helleborus Fœtidus.**

Be'la. Bael. The ripe fruit of the *Æ'gle Mar'melos.* (A bland and excellent aperient.) See Class I., Section I.

Benne Oil. See **Oleum Sesami.**

Black Hellebore. See **Helleborus.**

Bladder Senna. See **Colutea Arborescens.**

Blue Flag. See **Iris Versicolor.**

Bryony. The root of *Bryo'nia al'ba.*

Buckbean. See **Menyanthes Trifoliata.**

Buckthorn. See **Rhamnus Catharticus.**

Burdock. See **Lappa.**

Butterflyweed. See **Asclepias.**

Butternut. See **Juglans.**

Cambo'gia. (Br. Ph.) Gamboge. The gum resin of an undetermined species of *Garcin'ia.* See **Gambogia.**

Car'thamus. (U.S. Ph.) Safflower, or Dyer's Saffron. (Laxative.) See Class XI.

Cas'sia. (Br. Ph.) Purging Cassia. The pulp of the pods of *Cas'sia fis'tula.* See **Cassia Fistula.**

Cas'sia Acutifo'lia. See **Senna.**

Cas'sia Elonga'ta. See **Senna.**

Cas'sia Fis'tula. (U.S. Ph.) Purging Cassia. The fruit of *Cassia fistula.*

Cas'sia Marilan'dica. (U.S. Ph.) American Senna. The leaves of *Cassia Marilandica.*

Cas'sia Obova'ta. See **Senna.**

Castor Oil. See **Oleum Ricini.**

Celandine. See **Chelidonium Majus.**

Cevadilla. See **Sabadilla.**

Chelido'nium Ma'jus. Celandine.

Cissam'pelos Parei'ra. See **Pareira.**

Citrul'lus Colocyn'this. See **Colocynthis.**

? *Col'chicum.* See Classes XXI. and X.

Colocynth. See **Colocynthis.**

Colocyn'this. (U.S. and Br. Ph.) Colocynth. The fruit, deprived of its rind, of *Citrul'lus colocyn'this.*

Colu'tea Arbores'çens. Bladder Senna.

Common Silkweed. See **Asclepias Syriaca.**

Convol'vulus Pandura'tus. Wild Potato.

Convol'vulus Scammo'nia. See **Scammonium.**

Copai'ba. (U.S. and Br. Ph.) Copaiva. See Class X.

Copaiva. See **Copaiba.**

Croton Oil. See **Oleum Tiglii,** or **Crotonis Oleum.**

Cro'ton Tig'lium. See **Oleum Tiglii.**

Croto'nis O'leum. See **Oleum Crotonis.**

Cu'cumis Colocyn'this. See **Colocynthis.**

Cur'cas Pur'gans. Barbadoes Nut.

Delphin'ium Staphisa'gria. Stavesacre.

Dyer's Saffron. See **Carthamus.**

Elate'rium. (U.S. and Br. Ph.) A substance deposited by the juice of the fruit of *Momor'dica elate'rium* (U.S. Ph.). A sediment from the expressed juice of the fruit of *Ecba'lium officina'rum* (Br. Ph.).

Elder. See **Sambucus.**

Euon'ymus Atropurpu'reus. Wahoo.

Exogo'nium Pur'ga. See **Jalapa.**

Extract of Butternut. See **Extractum Juglandis.**

Extrac'tum Juglan'dis. (U.S. Ph.) Extract of Butternut.

Fever Root. See **Triosteum.**

Fi'cus. (U.S. and Br. Ph.) Fig. (Laxative.)

Fig. See **Ficus.**

Flesh-colored Asclepias. See **Asclepias Incarnata.**

Florentine Orris. See **Iris Florentina.**

Frax'inus Or'nus. See **Manna.**

Gamboge. See **Gambogia.**

Gambo'gia. (U.S. Ph.) Gamboge. The concrete juice of an undetermined tree.

Grat'iola Officina'lis. Hedge Hyssop.

Helleb'orus. (U.S. Ph.) Black Hellebore. The root of *Helleb'orus ni'ger.*

Helleb'orus Fœt'idus. Bear's-foot. See Class XXIII.

Honey. See **Mel.**

Horehound. See **Marrubium.**

Ipomæ'a Jala'pa, or *Ipomæ'a Pur'ga.* See **Jalapa.**

I'ris Florenti'na. (U.S. Ph.) Florentine Orris. The rhizoma of *Iris Florentina.*

I'ris Versic'olor. (U.S. Ph.) Blue Flag. The rhizoma of *Iris versicolor.*

Jala'pa. (U.S. and Br. Ph.) Jalap. The root of *Exogo'nium pur'ga,* or *Ipomæ'a jala'pa.*

Jala'pæ Resi'na. (Br. Ph.) See **Resina Jalapæ.**

Jat'ropha Pur'gans. See **Curcas Purgans.**

Ju'glans. (U.S. Ph.) Butternut. The inner bark of the root of the *Juglans cinerea.*

Lap'pa. (U.S. Ph.) Burdock. The root of *Lap'pa mi'nor.*

Leptan'dra. (U.S. Ph.) The root of *Veron'ica Virgin'ica* (otherwise called *Leptandra Virginica*).

Leptan'drin. A resinous extract from the root of *Veron'ica Virgin'ica.*

Li'num Cathar'ticum. Purging Flax.

? **Lith'iæ Ci'tras.** (Br. Ph.) Citrate of Lithia.

Man'na. (U.S. and Br. Ph.) The concrete juice, in flakes, of *Frax'inus or'nus,* and of *Frax'inus rotundifo'lia.*

? **Marru'bium.** (U.S. Ph.) Horehound. See Class II.

Marsh Trefoil. See **Menyanthes.**

May Apple. See **Podophyllum.**

Mel. (U.S. and Br. Ph.) Honey.

Me'lia Azed'arach. See **Azedarach.**

Menyan'thes Trifolia'ta. Buckbean, or Marsh Trefoil.

Molasses. See **Syrupus Fuscus.**

Momor'dica Elate'rium. See **Elaterium.**

Mustard. See **Sinapis Alba.**

O'leum Croto'nis. (Br. Ph.) Croton Oil. The same as **Oleum Tiglii.**

? **O'leum Li'ni.** (U.S. and Br. Ph.) Flaxseed or Linseed Oil. See Class XX.

O'leum Oli'væ. (U.S. and Br. Ph.) Olive Oil, or Sweet Oil. The oil expressed from the fruit of the *O'lea Europæ'a.* (Laxative.)

O'leum Riç'ini. (U.S. and Br. Ph.) Castor Oil. The oil expressed from the seeds of *Riç'inus commu'nis.*

O'leum Ses'ami. (U.S. Ph.) Benne Oil.

O'leum Terebin'thinæ. (U.S. and Br. Ph.) Oil of Turpentine. See Class X.

O'leum Tig'lii. (U.S. Ph.) Croton Oil. The oil obtained from the seeds of *Croton tiglium.*

Olive Oil. See **Oleum Olivæ.**

Parei'ra. (U.S. and Br. Ph.) Pareira Brava. The root of *Cissam'pelos parei'ra.*

Parei'ra Bra'va. See **Pareira.**

Parsley Root. See **Petroselinum.**

Petroseli'num. (U.S. Ph.) Parsley Root. (Aperient.) See Class X.

Phytolac'cæ Ra'dix. (U.S. Ph.) Poke Root. See Class VIII.

Pleurisy Root. See **Asclepias Tuberosa.**

Podophyl'li Resi'na. (Br. Ph.) See **Resina Podophylli.**

Podophyllin. See **Resina Podophylli.**

Podophyl'lum. (U.S. and Br. Ph.) May Apple. The rhizoma of *Podophyl'lum pelta'tum.*

Polyg'ala Rubel'la? (U.S. Ph.) The root and herb of *Polygala rubella.*

Pride of China, or Pride of India. See **Azedarach.**

Prune. See **Prunum.**

Pru'num. (U.S. and Br. Ph.) Prune. The dried fruit of *Pru'nus domes'tica.* (A mild laxative.)

Pru'nus Domes'tica. See **Prunum.**

Purging Cassia. See **Cassia Fistula.**

Purging Flax. See **Linum Catharticum.**

Queen's Root. See **Stillingia.**

Resi'na Jala'pæ. (U.S. Ph.) Resin of Jalap.

Resi'na Podophyl'li. (U.S. Ph.) Resin of Podophyllum.

Resi'na Scammo'nii. (U.S. Ph.) Resin of Scammony.

Rham'nus Cathar'ticus. Buckthorn.

Rhe'um. (U.S. and Br. Ph.) Rhubarb. The root of *Rhe'um palma'tum* and of other species of *Rheum* (U.S. Ph.). The root of one or more undetermined species of *Rheum* (Br. Ph.).

Rhubarb. See **Rheum.**

Ric'inus Commu'nis. See **Oleum Ricini.**

Sabadil'la. (U.S. and Br. Ph.) Cevadilla. The fruit of *Vera'trum sabadil'la* (U.S. Ph.). The dried fruit of *Asagræ'a officina'lis* (Br. Ph.).

Sambu'cus. Elder. The inner bark. See Class XI.

Sa'po. (U.S. Ph.) Soap. Soap made with soda and olive oil. (Mostly given in combination with other medicines).

Sa'po Vulga'ris. Common Soap. See **Sapo.**

Scammo'niæ Ra'dix. (Br. Ph.) Scammony Root.

Scammo'niæ Resi'na. (Br. Ph.) See **Resina Scammonii.**

Scammo'nium. (U.S. and Br. Ph.) Scammony. The concrete juice of the root of *Convol'vulus scammo'nia* (U.S. Ph.). A gum resin obtained from the living root of *Convolvulus scammonia* (Br. Ph.).

Scammony. See **Scammonium.**

? Sen'ega. (U.S. and Br. Ph.) Seneka. See Class XII.

Seneka. See **Senega.**

Sen'na. (U.S. Ph.) Senna. The leaflets of *Cas'sia acutifo'lia,* of *Cas'sia obova'ta,* and of *Cas'sia elonga'ta.*

Sen'na Alexandri'na. (Br. Ph.) Alexandrian Senna. The leaves of *Cassia lanceolata* and *Cassia obovata.*

Sen'na In'dica. (Br. Ph.) Tinnivelly Senna. The leaves of *Cassia elongata.*

Sina'pis. (Br. Ph.) Mustard. See Class XVII.

Sina'pis Al'ba. (U.S. Ph.) Mustard. (The unbroken seed is laxative.) See Class XVII.

Sina'pis Ni'gra. (U.S. Ph.) Black Mustard. See Class XVII.

Stavesacre. See **Delphinium.**

Stillin'gia. (U.S. Ph.) Queen's Root. The root of *Stillin'gia sylvat'ica.*

Sweet Oil. See **Oleum Olivæ.**

Syru'pus Fus'cus. (U.S. Ph.) "Brown Syrup," or Molasses. (Laxative.)

Tamarin'dus. (U.S. and Br. Ph.) Tamarind. (Aperient.) See Class VI.

Tarax'acum. (U.S. and Br. Ph.) Dandelion. See Class X.

? Terebin'thina. (U.S. Ph.) Turpentine. See Class X.

Theri'aca. (Br. Ph.) Treacle. The uncrystallized residue of the refining of sugar. See **Syrupus Fuscus.**

Treacle. See **Theriaca.**

Trios'teum. (U.S. Ph.) Fever Root. The root of *Trios'teum perfolia'tum.*

Turpentine. See **Terebinthina.**

Vera'tria. (U.S. and Br. Ph.) An alkaloid obtained from cevadilla. See Class VIII., Section I.

Vera'trum Al'bum. (U.S. Ph.) White Hellebore. See Class VIII., Section I.

? Vera'trum Vir'ide. (U.S. Ph.) American Hellebore. See Class VIII.

Veron'ica Virgin'ica. See **Leptandra.**

Wahoo. See **Euonymus Atropurpureus.**

White Hellebore. See **Veratrum Album.**

Wild Ipecac. See **Triosteum.**

Wild Potato. See **Convolvulus Panduratus.**

SECTION II.—Mineral Cathartics.

Acetate of Magnesia. See **Magnesiæ Acetas.**

Acetate of Potassa. See **Potassæ Acetas.**

Antimonial Powder. See **Pulvis Antimonialis.**

Bitartrate of Potassa. See **Potassæ Bitartras.**

Black Oxide of Mercury. See **Hydrargyri Oxidum Nigrum.**

Brimstone. See **Sulphur.**

Calcined Magnesia. See **Magnesia.**

Calomel. See **Calomelas.**

Calom'elas. (Br. Ph.) Calomel. Same as **Hydrargyri Chloridum Mite.**

Carbonate of Magnesia. See **Magnesiæ Carbonas.**

Chloride of Magnesium. See **Magnesii Chloridum.**

Citrate of Potassa. See **Potassæ Citras.**

Citrate of Soda. See **Sodæ Citras.**

Cream of Tartar. See **Potassæ Bitartras.**

Crystals of Tartar. See **Potassæ Bitartras.**

Epsom Salts. See **Magnesiæ Sulphas.**

Glauber's Salts. See **Sodæ Sulphas.**

Hydrar'gyri Chlo'ridum Mi'te. (U.S. Ph.) Calomel. Mild Chloride of Mercury. See Class XXI.

Hydrar'gyri Ox'idum Ni'grum. Black Oxide of Mercury. See Classes XIV. and XXI.

Li'quor Magne'siæ Citra'tis. (U.S. Ph.) Solution of Citrate of Magnesia.

Magne'sia. (U.S. and Br. Ph.) Calcined Magnesia. A white powder insoluble in water, but readily dissolved by acids without effervescence.

Magne'siæ Ace'tas. Acetate of Magnesia.

Magne'siæ Carbo'nas. (U.S. and Br. Ph.) Carbonate of Magnesia. A white substance in powder or pulverulent masses, wholly dissolved by dilute sulphuric acid.

Magne'siæ Sul'phas. (U.S. and Br. Ph.) Sulphate of Magnesia, or Epsom Salts. A salt in minute colorless crystals, which slowly effloresce on exposure to the air, and are very soluble in water.

Magne'sii Chlo'ridum. Chloride of Magnesium.

Mangane'sii Sul'phas. (U.S. Ph.) Sulphate of Manganese. (Cholagogue.)

Mild Chloride of Mercury. See **Hydrargyri Chloridum Mite.**

Muriate of Magnesia. See **Magnesii Chloridum.**

Phosphate of Soda. See **Sodæ Phosphas.**

Potas'sæ Ace'tas. (U.S. and Br. Ph.) Acetate of Potassa. See Class X.

Potas'sæ Bitar'tras. (U.S. Ph.) Bitartrate of Potassa, or Cream of Tartar. See Class VI.

Potas'sæ Ci'tras. (U.S. and Br. Ph.) Citrate of Potassa. (A cooling aperient.) See Class XI.

Potas'sæ et So'dæ Tar'tras. (U.S. Ph.) Tartrate of Potash and Soda, or Rochelle Salt. A substance in colorless transparent crystals, which are wholly and readily soluble in five parts of boiling water.

Potas'sæ Sul'phas. (U.S. and Br. Ph.) Sulphate of Potash, sometimes called Vitriolated Tartar. A salt in hard colorless crystals, unalterable in the air, sparingly soluble in water, and insoluble in alcohol.

Potas'sæ Tar'tras. (U.S. and Br. Ph.) Tartrate of Potash. A salt in white or colorless crystals, wholly and readily soluble in four parts of boiling water.

Potas'sæ Tar'tras Aç'ida. (Br. Ph.) Acid Tartrate of Potash. The same as **Potassæ Bitartras.**

?Pul'vis Antimonia'lis. (Br. Ph.) Antimonial Powder. See Class XI.

Rochelle Salt. See **Sodæ et Potassæ Tartras.**

Salt. See **Sodii Chloridum.**

So'dæ Ci'tras. Citrate of Soda.

So'dæ et Potas'sæ Tar'tras. (Br. Ph.) Tartrate of Potash and Soda, or Rochelle Salt. See **Potassæ et Sodæ Tartras.**

So'dæ Phos'phas. (U.S. and Br. Ph.) Phosphate of Soda. A salt in colorless transparent crystals, which speedily effloresce when exposed to the air. It is wholly soluble in water, but insoluble in alcohol.

So'dæ Sul'phas. (U.S. Ph.) Sulphate of Soda, or Glauber's Salts. A salt in colorless crystals, which rapidly effloresce on exposure to the air, and are wholly soluble in water.

So'dæ Tar'tras. Tartrate of Soda.

So'dii Chlo'ridum. (U.S. and Br. Ph.) Chloride of Sodium. Common Salt. See Class II., Section III.

Solution of Citrate of Magnesia. See **Liquor Magnesiæ Citratis.**

Sublimed Sulphur. See **Sulphur Sublimatum.**

Sulphate of Magnesia. See **Magnesiæ Sulphas.**

Sulphate of Manganese. See **Manganesii Sulphas.**

Sulphate of Potash. See **Potassæ Sulphas.**

Sulphate of Soda. See **Sodæ Sulphas.**

Sul'phur Lo'tum. (U. S. Ph.) Washed Sulphur. Sublimed sulphur thoroughly washed with water. See Class XI.

Sul'phur Præcipita'tum. (U.S. and Br. Ph.) Precipitated Sulphur. See Class XI.

Sul'phur Sublima'tum. (U.S. and Br. Ph.) Sublimed Sulphur. A greenish-yellow powder which is entirely volatilized by heat.

Tartrate of Potash. See **Potassæ Tartras.**

Tartrate of Potash and Soda. See **Potassæ et Sodæ Tartras.**

Tartrate of Soda. See **Sodæ Tartras.**

Vitriolated Tartar. See **Potassæ Sulphas.**

Washed Sulphur. See **Sulphur Lotum.**

CLASS X.

DIURETICS.

MEDICINES WHICH INCREASE THE SECRETION OF URINE.

A'bies Balsa'mea. See **Terebinthina.**

Acetate of Potassa. See **Potassæ Acetas.**

Acetate of Soda. See **Sodæ Acetas.**

Ace'tum Col'chici. (U.S. Ph.) Vinegar of Colchicum.

? Ace'tum Scil'læ. (U.S. Ph.) Vinegar of Squill.

? Aconite. See **Aconitum.**

? Aconi'tum. (Br. Ph.) Aconite.

American Hellebore. See **Veratrum Viride.**

Ammo'niæ Benzo'as. (U.S. and Br. Ph.) Benzoate of Ammonia.

Anacar'dium Occidenta'le. Cashew Nut. See Class XVIII.

A'pium Petroseli'num. See **Petroselinum.**

Apoç'ynum Cannabi'num. (U.S. Ph.) Indian Hemp. See Class VIII.

A'qua Aç'idi Carbon'ici. (U.S. Ph.) Carbonic Acid Water. See Class XI.

? Ar'butus U'va Ur'si. See Class I.

Armora'cia. (Br. Ph.) Horseradish Root. The fresh root of *Cochlea'ria armora'cia.* See Class XV.

Artichoke (Garden). See **Cynara Scolymus.**

Aspar'agus Officina'lis.

At'ropa Belladon'na. See **Belladonna.**

Balsam of Copaiva. See **Copaiba.**

Baros'ma Crena'ta, Baros'ma Betuli'na, etc. See **Buchu,** and **Bucco.**

Belladon'na. (Br. Ph.) The same as **Belladonnæ Folium.**

Belladonna Leaf. See **Belladonnæ Folium.**

Belladonna Root. See **Belladonnæ Radix.**

Belladon'næ Fo'lium. (U.S. Ph.) Belladonna Leaf. See Class V.

Belladon'næ Ra'dix. (U.S. and Br. Ph.) Belladonna Root. See Class V.

Biborate of Soda. See **Borax.**

Bicarbonate of Potassa. See **Potassæ Bicarbonas.**

Bitartrate of Potash. See **Potassæ Bitartras.**

Borate of Soda. See **Sodæ Boras.**

Bo'rax. (Br. Ph.) Biborate of Soda. Borax.

Broom. See **Scoparius.**

Buc'co. (Br. Ph.) Buchu. The dried leaves of *Baros'ma betuli'na, B. crenula'ta,* and *B. serratifo'lia.* See next article.

Bu'chu. (U.S. Ph.) Buchu, or Bookoo. The leaves of *Baros'ma crena'ta (Dios'ma crena'ta),* and of other species of *Barosma.*

Burdock. See **Lappa.**

Cahin'ca or *Cainca.*

Canada Turpentine. See **Terebinthina.**

Cantharides. See **Cantharis.**

Can'tharis. (U.S. and Br. Ph.) Spanish Flies, or Canthar'ides. See Class XVI.

Can'tharis Vitta'ta. Potato Flies. See Class XVI.

Cap'paris Spino'sa. Caper-Bush.

Carbonate of Potash. See **Potassæ Carbonas.**

Carbonic Acid Water. See **Aqua Acidi Carbonici.**

Caro'ta. (U.S. Ph.) Carrot Seed, and Root of Wild Carrot. *Dau'cus caro'ta.*

Cashew Nut. See **Anacardium Occidentale.**

Chimaph'ila. (U.S. Ph.) Pipsissewa. The leaves of *Chimaph'ila umbella'ta.*

Cissam'pelos Parei'ra. See **Pareira.**

Clem'atis Erec'ta (Virgin's Bower), and other species of Clematis.

Cochlea'ria Armora'cia. See **Armoracia.**

Cochlea'ria Officina'lis. Scurvy Grass.

Col'chici Cor'mus. (Br. Ph.) Colchicum Corm. The same as **Colchici Radix.**

Col'chici Ra'dix. (U.S. Ph.) Colchicum Root. See Class XXI.

Col'chici Se'men. (U.S. and Br. Ph.) Colchicum Seed. See Class XXI.

Colchicum Root. See **Colchici Radix.**

Colchicum Seed. See **Colchici Semen.**

? Convol'vulus Pandura'tus. Wild Potato. See Class IX., Section I.

Copai'ba. (U.S. and Br. Ph.) Copaiva, or Balsam of Copaiba. The juice of *Copaif'era multij'uga,* and of other species of *Copaifera* (U.S. Ph.). The oleo-resin obtained from the trunk of

Copaifera multijuga and other species of *Copaiferæ* (Br. Ph.).

Copaif'era Multij'uga. See **Copaiba.**

Copaiva. See **Copaiba.**

Coryd'alis Formo'sa. Turkey Corn.

Creasote. See **Creasotum.**

Creaso'tum. (U.S. and Br. Ph.) Creasote. See Class V.

Cube'ba. (U.S. and Br. Ph.) Cubeb, or Cubebs. The berries of *Pi'per cube'ba* (U.S. Ph.). The unripe fruit, dried, of *Cube'ba officina'lis* (Br. Ph.).

Cyn'ara Scol'ymus. Garden Artichoke.

Cyt'isus Scopa'rius. See **Scoparius.**

Dandelion. See **Taraxacum.**

Daph'ne Gnid'ium. See **Mezereum.**

Daph'ne Mezere'um. See **Mezereum.**

Dau'ci Ra'dix. Garden Carrot Root.

Dau'cus Caro'ta. See **Carota.**

Delphin'ium. (U.S. Ph.) Larkspur. The seed of *Delphin'ium consol'ida.*

? *Delphin'ium Staphisa'gria.* Stavesacre.

Digita'lis. (U.S. and Br. Ph.) Foxglove. Digitalis. See Class VII.

Dios'ma Crena'ta. See **Buchu.**

Dulcama'ra. (U.S. and Br. Ph.) Bittersweet. See Class V.

Epige'a Re'pens. Trailing Arbutus.

Erig'eron. (U.S. Ph.) Fleabane. The herb of *Erig'eron heterophyl'lum* and of *Erig'eron Philadel'phicum.*

Erig'eron Canaden'se. (U.S. Ph.) Canada Fleabane. The herb of *Erigeron Canadense.*

Erig'eron Heterophyl'lum. See **Erigeron.**

Fer'ri Iod'idum. (Br. Ph.) Iodide of Iron. See Class XIII. and Class II., Section V.

Fleabane. See **Erigeron.**

Foxglove. See **Digitalis.**

Garden Artichoke. See **Cynara Scolymus.**

Garden Carrot. See **Dauci Radix.**

Gene'va. See **Gin.**

Gin (*Gene'va*). Spirit distilled from juniper berries.

Hellebore, White. See **Veratrum Album.**

Hemides'mus. (Br. Ph.) Indian Sarsaparilla. See Class II., Section II.

Horseradish. See **Armoracia.**

Indian Hemp. See **Apocynum Cannabinum.**

Indian Sarsaparilla. See **Hemidesmus.**

? I'ris Florenti'na. (U.S. Ph.) Florentine Orris.

? I'ris Versic'olor. (U.S. Ph.) Blue Flag.

Junip'erus. (U.S. Ph.) Juniper. Juniper Berries. The fruit of *Junip'erus commu'nis.*

Junip'erus Virginia'na. (U.S. Ph.) Red Cedar. See Class XIII.

Lactu'ca Viro'sa. Acrid Lettuce.

Lap'pa. (U.S. Ph.) Burdock. See Class IX.

Larkspur. See **Delphinium.**

Leon'todon Tarax'acum. See **Taraxacum.**

Li'quor Cal'cii Chlo'ridi. (U.S. Ph.) Solution of Chloride of Calcium.

Li'quor Potas'sæ. (U.S. and Br. Ph.) Solution of Potassa. See Class XXII.

Lycopo'dium. (U.S. Ph.) The sporules of *Lycopo'dium clava'tum* and other species of *Lycopodium.*

Mastic. See **Mastiche.**

Mas'tiche. (U.S. and Br. Ph.) Mastic. Mastich. The concrete juice of *Pista'cia lentis'cus* (U.S. Ph.). A resinous exudation from the stem of *Pistacia lentiscus* (Br. Ph.).

Meadow Saffron. See **Colchici Radix,** or **Colchicum.**

Mezereon. See **Mezereum.**

Mezere'um. (U.S. and Br. Ph.) Mezereon. See Class XVI.

Nicotia'na Tab'acum. See **Tabacum.**

Nitrate of Potash. See **Potassæ Nitras.**

Oil of Copaiba. See **Oleum Copaibæ.**

Oil of Turpentine. See **Oleum Terebinthinæ.**

O'leum Copai'bæ. (U.S. and Br. Ph.) Oil of Copaiba.

O'leum Cube'bæ. (U.S. and Br. Ph.) Oil of Cubeb.

O'leum Junip'eri. (U.S. and Br. Ph.) Oil of Juniper.

O'leum Suc'çini. (U.S. Ph.) Oil of Amber. See Class IV.

O'leum Terebin'thinæ. (U.S. and Br. Ph.) Oil of Turpentine. The volatile oil distilled from the turpentine of *Pi'nus palus'tris* or *Pi'nus tæ'da.*

Parei'ra. (U.S. and Br. Ph.) Pareira Brava. The root of *Cissam'pelos parei'ra* (U.S. Ph.). The dried root of *Cissampelos pareira* (Br. Ph.).

Parieta'ria Officina'lis. Wall Pellitory.

Parsley Root. See **Petroselinum.**

Petroseli'num. (U.S. Ph.) Parsley. The root of *Petroseli'num sati'vum,* otherwise called *A'pium petroseli'num.*

Phos'phorus. (U.S. Ph.) See Class III.

Pi'nus Palus'tris. See **Terebinthina,** and **Pix Liquida.**

Pi'per Cube'ba. See **Cubeba.**

Pipsissewa. See **Chimaphila.**

Pista'cia Lentis'cus. See **Mastiche.**

Pix Li'quida. (U.S. and Br. Ph.) Tar. The impure turpentine procured by burning from the wood of *Pi'nus palus'tris* and of other species of *Pinus* (U.S. Ph.). A bituminous liquid obtained from the wood of *Pi'nus sylves'tris* and other pines by destructive distillation (Br. Ph.).

Polyg'ala Sen'ega. See **Senega.**

Potas'sæ Ace'tas. (U.S. and Br. Ph.) Acetate of Potassa. A white deliquescent salt, wholly soluble in water and alcohol.

Potas'sæ Bicarbo'nas. (U.S. and Br. Ph.) Bicarbonate of Potassa. *Sal æratus.* See Class XXII.

Potas'sæ Bitar'tras. (U.S. Ph.) Bitartrate of Potash, or Cream of Tartar. See Class VI.

Potas'sæ Carbo'nas. (U.S. and Br. Ph.) Carbonate of Potash; otherwise called Subcarbonate of Potash. See Class XXII.

Potas'sæ Ni'tras. (U.S. and Br. Ph.) Nitrate of Potash, Nitre, or Saltpetre. See Class VI.

Potato Flies. See **Cantharis Vittata.**

Red Cedar. See **Juniperus Virginiana.**

Scil'la. (U.S. and Br. Ph.) Squill. See Class XII.

Scopa'rius. (U. S. and Br. Ph.) Broom. The tops of *Cyt'isus scopa'rius* (U.S. Ph.). The tops of *Sarotham'nus scopa'rius* (Br. Ph.).

Scurvy Grass. See **Cochlearia Officinalis.**

Sen'ega. (U.S. and Br. Ph.) Seneka. See Class XII.

Seneka. See **Senega.**

? Serpenta'ria. (U.S. and Br. Ph.) Serpentary, or Virginia Snakeroot. See Class II., Section III.

So'dæ Ace'tas. (U.S. Ph.) Acetate of Soda. A substance in white or colorless crystals, which effloresce in dry air, and are wholly soluble in water.

So'dæ Bo'ras. (U.S. Ph.) Borate of Soda, or Borax. See Class VI.

? So'dæ Sul'phas. (U.S. Ph.) Sulphate of Soda, or Glauber's Salts. See Class IX.

Solution of Chloride of Calcium. See **Liquor Calcii Chloridi.**

Solution of Potassa. See **Liquor Potassæ.**

Spanish Flies. See **Cantharis.**

Spar'tium Jun'ceum. Spanish Broom.

Spirit of Nitric Ether. See **Spiritus Ætheris Nitrosi.**

Spir'itus Æ'theris Nitro'si. (U.S and Br. Ph.) Spirit of Nitrous Ether, or Sweet Spirit of Nitre. See Class IV., and Class XI., Section II.

Spir'itus Junip'eri.

Squill. See **Scilla.**

Sweet Spirit of Nitre. See **Spiritus Ætheris Nitrosi.**

? Tab'acum. (U.S. and Br. Ph.) Tobacco. See Classes VII. and V.

Tar. See **Pix Liquida.**

Tarax'acum. (U.S. and Br. Ph.) Dandelion. The root of *Tarax'acum densleo'nis.*

Terebin'thina. (U.S. Ph.) Turpentine. The concrete juice of *Pi'nus palus'tris* and of other species of *Pinus.*

Tobacco. See **Tabacum.**

Trailing Arbutus. See **Epigea Repens.**

Turkey Corn, or Turkey Pea. See **Corydalis Formosa.**

? Ul'mus Campes'tris. (Br. Ph.) Broad-leaved Elm. See Class XIX.

Vera'trum Al'bum. (U.S. Ph.) White Hellebore. See Class VIII.

Vera'trum Vir'ide. (U. S. Ph.) American Hellebore. See Class VIII.

Vi'num Col'chici. (Br. Ph.) Wine of Colchicum. The same as **Vinum Colchici Radicis.**

Vi'num Col'chici Radi'cis. (U.S. Ph.) Wine of Colchicum Root. See Class XXI.

Virginia Snakeroot. See **Serpentaria.**

Virgin's Bower. See **Clematis.**

Wall Pellitory. See **Parietaria Officinalis.**

White Hellebore. See **Veratrum Album.**

White Turpentine. See **Terebinthina.**

Wild Potato. See **Convolvulus Panduratus.**

Wine of Colchicum Root. See **Vinum Colchici Radicis.**

Wintergreen. See **Chimaphila.**

CLASS XI.

DIAPHORETICS.

MEDICINES WHICH PROMOTE PERSPIRATION. DIAPHORETICS MAY BE DIVIDED INTO NAUSEATING, REFRIGERANT, AND STIMULATING.

SECTION I.—Nauseating Diaphoretics.

Aconite. See **Aconitum.**

Aconite Root. See **Aconiti Radix.**

? **Aconi'ti Fo'lium.** (U.S. Ph.) Aconite Leaf. See Class VII.

? **Aconi'ti Ra'dix.** (U.S. and Br. Ph.) Aconite Root. See Class VII.

? **Aconi'tum.** (Br. Ph.) Aconite Leaf. See Class VII.

Aconi'tum Nape'llus. See **Aconitum.**

Antimonial Powder. See **Pulvis Antimonialis.**

Antimonial Wine. See **Vinum Antimonii.**

Antimo'nii et Potas'sæ Tar'tras. (U.S. Ph.) Tartrate of Antimony and Potassa, or Tartar Emetic. See Class VIII.

Antimo'nii Sulphure'tum. (U.S. Ph.) Sulphuret of Antimony.

Antimo'nium Sulphura'tum. (U.S. and Br. Ph.) Sulphurated Antimony, or Precipitated Sulphuret of Antimony. A tersulphuret of antimony, with a small and variable amount of the teroxide of antimony. An orange-red powder, whence it has been termed *antimo'nii sulphure'tum au'reum* (Ed. Ph.), or "golden sulphuret of antimony."

Antimo'nium Tartara'tum. (Br. Ph.) Tartarated Antimony. The same as **Antimonii et Potassæ Tartras.**

A'rum. (U.S. Ph.) Indian Turnip. See Class XII.

Button Snakeroot. See **Eryngium Aquaticum.**

Cephaë'lis Ipecacuan'ha. See **Ipecacuanha.**

? *Col'chicum.* See Classes XXI. and X.

Dragon Root. See **Arum.**

? Elecampane. See **Inula.**

Eryn'gium Aquat'icum. Button Snakeroot.

Eupato'rium. (U.S. Ph.) Thoroughwort, or Boneset. See Class II., Section III.

Indian Tobacco. See **Lobelia.**

Indian Turnip. See **Arum.**

? **In'ula.** Elecampane.

Ipecacuan'ha. (U.S. and Br. Ph.) Ipecacuan, or Ipecac. See Class VIII.

Lobe'lia. (U.S. and Br. Ph.) Indian Tobacco. See Class VIII.

Precipitated Sulphuret of Antimony. See **Antimonium Sulphuratum.**

Pul'vis Antimonia'lis. (Br. Ph.) Antimonial Powder. A powder consisting chiefly of bone-phosphate of lime and antimonious acid. Essentially the same as *James's Powder.*

Tartar Emetic. See **Antimonii et Potassæ Tartras.**

Tartrate of Antimony and Potassa. See **Antimonii et Potassæ Tartras.**

Vi'num Antimonia'le. (Br. Ph.) Antimonial Wine. See next article.

Vi'num Antimo'nii. (U.S. Ph.) Antimonial Wine, or Wine of Antimony. A solution of tartar emetic in sherry wine. See Class VIII.

Water Eryngo. See **Eryngium Aquaticum.**

SECTION II.—Refrigerant Diaphoretics.

Acetate of Ammonia (Solution of). See **Liquor Ammoniæ Acetatis.**

Ammo'niæ Aceta'tis Li'quor. (Br. Ph.) Solution of Acetate of Ammonia. See **Liquor Ammoniæ Acetatis.**

Ammo'niæ Carbo'nas. (U.S. and Br. Ph.) Carbonate of Ammonia. Sal Volatile, or Smelling Salts. See Class III.

A'qua Aç'idi Carbon'ici. (U.S. Ph.) Carbonic Acid Water. Water impregnated with five times its bulk of carbonic acid.

Carbonate of Ammonia. See **Ammoniæ Carbonas.**

Carbonic Acid Water. See **Aqua Acidi Carbonici.**

Citrate of Potassa. See **Potassæ Citras.**

Li'quor Ammo'niæ Aceta'tis. (U.S. and Br. Ph.) Solution of Acetate of Ammonia. Also called *Spir'itus Mindere'ri*, or Spirit of Mindererus.

Li'quor Ammo'niæ Citra'tis. Solution of Citrate of Ammonia.

? **Li'quor Cal'cii Chlo'ridi.** (U.S. Ph.) Solution of Chloride of Calcium. See Class X.

Li'quor Potas'sæ Citra'tis. (U.S. Ph.) Solution of Citrate of Potassa.

Nitrate of Potassa, or Nitre. See **Potassæ Nitras.**

Potas'sæ Ci'tras. (U.S. and Br. Ph.) Citrate of Potassa. See Class VI.

Potas'sæ Ni'tras. (U.S. and Br. Ph.) Nitrate of Potash, or Nitre. See Class VI.

Potas'sii Ferrocyan'idum. (U.S. Ph.) Ferrocyanide of Potassium. See Class VI.

Solution of Acetate of Ammonia. See **Liquor Ammoniæ Acetatis.**

Solution of Citrate of Ammonia. See **Liquor Ammoniæ Citratis.**

Solution of Citrate of Potassa. See **Liquor Potassæ Citratis.**

Spirit of Nitrous, or Nitric, Ether. See **Spiritus Ætheris Nitrosi.**

Spir'itus Æ'theris Nitro'si. (U.S. and Br. Ph.) Spirit of Nitrous Ether, or Sweet Spirit of Nitre (formerly Spirit of Nitric Ether). See Class IV.

Spir'itus Mindere'ri, or Spirit of Mindererus. See **Liquor Ammoniæ Acetatis.**

Sweet Spirit of Nitre. See **Spiritus Ætheris Nitrosi.**

SECTION III.—Stimulating and Alterative Diaphoretics.

Acrid Lettuce. See **Lactuca Virosa.**

Adanso'nia Digita'ta. The Baobab-tree.

American Dittany. See **Cunila Mariana.**

Ammoni'acum. (U.S. and Br. Ph.) Ammoniac. See Class XII.

? Ammo'niæ Phos'phas. (Br. Ph.) Phosphate of Ammonia.

? A'qua Ammo'niæ. (U.S. Ph.) Solution of Ammonia. See Classes XVII. and XXII.

Aristolo'chia Serpenta'ria. See **Serpentaria.**

Ascle'pias. (U.S. Ph.) Butterfly-weed. The root of *Ascle'pias tubero'sa.*

Ascle'pias Tubero'sa. See **Asclepias.**

Balm. See **Melissa.**

Baobab. See **Adansonia Digitata.**

Bark of Sassafras Root. See **Sassafras Radicis Cortex.**

Bisulphuret of Carbon, or Sulphuret of Carbon.

Boneset. See **Eupatorium.**

Burdock. See **Lappa.**

Butterflyweed. See **Asclepias.**

Calot'ropis Gigante'a. Madar, or Mudar.

Car'thamus. (U.S. Ph.) Dyer's Saffron, or Safflower. The flowers of *Car'thamus tincto'rius.*

? Col'chicum. See Classes XXI. and X.

Cro'cus. (U.S. and Br. Ph.) Saffron. See Class IV.

Cuni'la Maria'na. American Dittany.

Daph'ne Gnid'ium. See **Mezereum.**

Daph'ne Mezere'um. See **Mezereum.**

Dörste'nia Contrayer'va. (Aromatic and tonic.)

Dyer's Saffron. See **Carthamus.**

Elder. See **Sambucus.**

Eupato'rium. (U.S. Ph.) Thoroughwort, or Boneset. See Class II., Section III.

Guaiac. See **Guaiaci Resina.**

Guai'aci Lig'num. (U.S. and Br. Ph.) Guaiacum Wood. *Lignum Vitæ.* The wood of *Guai'acum officina'le.*

Guai'aci Resi'na. (U.S. and Br. Ph.) Guaiac. The concrete juice of *Guai'acum officina'le* (U.S. Ph.). The resin obtained from the stem of *Guaiacum officinale* (Br. Ph.).

Guai'acum Officina'le. See **Guaiaci Resina.**

Junip'erus Sabi'na. See **Sabina.**

Lactu'ca Viro'sa. Acrid Lettuce. See Class V.

Lap'pa. (U.S. Ph.) Burdock. See Class IX.

Lau'rus Sas'safras. See **Sassafras.**

Li'quor Ammo'niæ. (Br. Ph.) See **Aqua Ammoniæ.**

Madar. See **Calotropis Gigantea.**

Magno'lia. (U.S. Ph.) Magnolia. See Class II., Section III.

? Melis'sa. (U.S. Ph.) Balm. See Class II., Section IV.

Meze'reon. See **Mezereum.**

Mezere'um. (U.S. and Br. Ph.) Mezereon. See Class XVI.

Mudar. See **Calotropis Gigantea.**

Oil of Cajuput. See **Oleum Cajuputi.**

O'leum Cajupu'ti. (U.S. and Br. Ph.) Oil of Cajuput. The volatile oil obtained from the leaves of *Melaleu'ca cajupu'ti* (U.S. Ph.). The oil distilled from the leaves of *Melaleu'ca mi'nor* (Br. Ph.).

? Orig'anum Vulga're. Common Marjoram.

Petro'leum. Rock Oil. See Class IV.

? Polyg'ala Rubel'la. (U.S. Ph.) Bitter Polygala. See Class II., Section II.

Prickly Ash. See **Xanthoxylum.**

Rock Oil. See **Petroleum.**

Sabi'na. (U.S. and Br. Ph.) Savine. See Class XIII.

Sambu'cus. (U.S. and Br. Ph.)

Elder. The flowers of *Sambu'cus Canaden'sis* (U.S. Ph.). The fresh flowers of *Sambu'cus ni'gra* (Br. Ph.).

? **Sar'sa.** (Br. Ph.) See Class XXI.

? **Sarsaparil'la.** (U.S. Ph.) See Class XXI.

? **Sas'safras.** (Br. Ph.) Sassafras Root. The dried root of *Sas'safras officina'le.* See next article.

? **Sas'safras Radi'cis Cor'tex.** (U.S. Ph.) Sassafras Root. (Stimulant and aromatic.)

Serpenta'ria. (U.S. and Br. Ph.) Serpentary, or Virginia Snakeroot. See Class II., Section III.

Serpentary. See **Serpentaria.**

Solution of Ammonia. See **Aqua Ammoniæ.**

Sul'phur Lo'tum. (U. S. Ph.) Washed Sulphur. See Class IX., Section II.

Sul'phur Sublima'tum. (U. S. and Br. Ph.) Sublimed Sulphur. See Class IX., Section II.

Sulphuret of Carbon. The same as **Bisulphuret of Carbon.**

Thoroughwort. See **Eupatorium.**

Virginia Snakeroot. See **Serpentaria.**

Xanthox'ylum. (U.S. Ph.) Prickly Ash. The bark of *Xanthox'ylum fraxin'eum.*

CLASS XII.

EXPECTORANTS.

MEDICINES WHICH INCREASE THE SECRETION FROM THE MUCOUS MEMBRANE OF THE AIR-CELLS AND AIR-PASSAGES OF THE LUNGS OR FACILITATE ITS DISCHARGE.

Ace'tum Scil'læ. (U.S. Ph.) Vinegar of Squill.

? **Aç'idum Benzo'icum.** (Br. Ph.) A substance in feathery crystalline plates, nearly white.

Al'lium. (U.S. Ph.) Garlic. The bulb of *Al'lium sati'vum.*

Al'lium Ce'pa. Onion.

Ammoniac. See **Ammoniacum.**

Ammoni'acum. (U.S. and Br. Ph.) Ammoniac. The concrete juice of *Dore'ma Ammoni'acum* (U.S. Ph.). A gum-resinous exudation from the stem of *Dorema ammoniacum* (Br. Ph.).

Antimo'nii et Potas'sæ Tar'tras. (U.S. Ph.) Tartar Emetic. Tartrate of Antimony and Potassa. See Class VIII.

Antimo'nium Tartara'tum. (Br. Ph.) Tartarated Antimony. Tartar Emetic.

A'rum. (U.S. Ph.) Indian Turnip, or Dragon Root. The cormus of *A'rum triphyl'lum.*

Ascle'pias. (U.S. Ph.) Butterfly-weed, or Pleurisy Root. See Class XI.

Ascle'pias Syri'aca. Common Silk-weed.

Assafœt'ida. (U.S. and Br. Ph.) Assafetida. See Class IV.

Balsam of Peru. See **Balsamum Peruvianum.**

Balsam of Tolu. See **Balsamum Tolutanum.**

Bal'samum Peruvia'num. (U.S. and Br. Ph.) Balsam of Peru. The prepared juice of *Myrosper'mum Peruif'erum* (U.S. Ph.). A balsam obtained from the stem of *Myrosper'mum Perei'ræ* (Br. Ph.).

Bal'samum Toluta'num. (U.S. and Br. Ph.) Balsam of Tolu. The juice of *Myrosper'mum toluif'erum* (U.S. Ph.). A balsam obtained by incision from the stem of *Myrospermum toluiferum* (Br. Ph.).

? Benzoic Acid. See **Acidum Benzoicum.**

Benzoin. See **Benzoinum.**

Benzo'inum. (U.S. and Br. Ph.) Benzoin. The concrete juice of *Sty'rax ben'zoin* (U.S. Ph.). A resinous exudation from the stem of *Styrax benzoin* (Br. Ph.).

Black Snakeroot. See **Cimicifuga.**

Butterflyweed. See **Asclepias.**

Button Snakeroot. See **Eryngium Aquaticum.**

Cephaë'lis Ipecacuan'ha. See **Ipecacuanha.**

Cimicif'uga. (U.S. Ph.) Black Snakeroot. See Class VII.

Common Silkweed. See **Asclepias Syriaca.**

Dore'ma Ammoni'acum. See **Ammoniacum.**

Dragon Root. See **Arum.**

Elecampane. See **Inula.**

? *Eryn'gium Aquat'icum.* Button Snakeroot. See Class XI., Section I.

Fer'ula Assafœt'ida. See **Assafœtida.**

Gal'banum. (U.S. and Br. Ph.) The concrete juice of an undetermined plant (U.S. Ph.). A gum resin derived from an unascertained umbelliferous plant (Br. Ph.).

Garlic. See **Allium.**

Indian Tobacco. See **Lobelia.**

Indian Turnip. See **Arum.**

? In'ula. (U.S. Ph.) Elecampane. See Class II., Section II.

Ipecacuan. See **Ipecacuanha.**

Ipecacuan'ha. (U.S. and Br. Ph.) Ipecacuan. See Class VIII.

Lobe'lia. (U.S. and Br. Ph.) Indian Tobacco. See Class VIII.

Myrosper'mum Peruif'erum. See **Balsamum Peruvianum.**

Myrosper'mum Toluif'erum. See **Balsamum Tolutanum.**

Naph'thalin. A substance obtained from the distillation of coal tar.

Nar'thex Assafœt'ida. See **Assafœtida.**

Onion. See **Allium Cepa.**

? Pix Liq'uida. (U.S. and Br. Ph.) Tar.

Pleurisy Root. See **Asclepias.**

Polyg'ala Sen'ega. See **Senega.**

Prepared Storax. See **Styrax Præparatus.**

Scil'la. (U.S. and Br. Ph.) Squill. The bulb of *Scil'la marit'ima* (U.S. Ph.). The dried bulb of *Urgin'ea scil'la* (Br. Ph.).

Sen'ega. (U.S. and Br. Ph.) Seneka. The root of *Polyg'ala sen'ega.*

Seneka. See **Senega.**

Squill. See **Scilla.**

Storax. See **Styrax.**

Sty'rax. (U.S. Ph.) Storax. The prepared juice of *Liquidam'bar Orienta'le.*

Styrax Benzoin. See **Benzoinum.**

Sty'rax Præpara'tus. (Br. Ph.) Prepared Storax. A balsam obtained from the bark of *Liquidam'bar Orienta'le.* The same as **Styrax.**

Urgin'ea Scil'la. See **Scilla.**

Water Eryngo. See **Eryngium Aquaticum.**

CLASS XIII.

EMMENAGOGUES.

MEDICINES WHICH PROMOTE THE MENSTRUAL SECRETION.

Achille'a Millefo'lium. (U.S. Ph.) Milfoil, or Yarrow. The herb and flowers of *Achillea millefolium.*

Aga've America'na. American Aloe.

Al'oe Barbaden'sis. (U.S. and Br. Ph.) Barbadoes Aloes. See Class IX.

Al'oe Socotri'na. (U.S. and Br. Ph.) Socotrine Aloes. See Class IX.

American Aloe. See **Agave Americana.**

Balsamoden'dron Myr'rha. See **Myrrha.**

Barbadoes Aloes. See **Aloe Barbadensis.**

Biborate of Soda. See **Borax.**

Black Hellebore. See **Helleborus.**

Borate of Soda. See **Sodæ Boras.**

Bo'rax. (Br. Ph.) Borax. Biborate of Soda. See **Sodæ Boras.**

Cantharides. See **Cantharis.**

Can'tharis. (U.S. and Br. Ph.) Spanish Flies. Canthar'ides. See Class XVI.

Can'tharis Vitta'ta. Potato Flies.

Castor. See **Castoreum.**

Cas'tor Fi'ber. See **Castoreum.**

Casto'reum. (U.S. and Br. Ph.) Castor. See Class IV.

? Cata'ria. (U.S. Ph.) Catnep. See Class IV.

Cotton Root. See **Gossypii Radix.**

Fer'ri Chlo'ridum. (U. S. Ph.) Chloride of Iron; also called Perchloride of Iron.

Fer'ri Iod'idum. (Br. Ph.) Iodide of Iron. A brownish-green crystalline substance, soluble in water.

Fer'ri Subcarbo'nas. (U.S. Ph.) Subcarbonate of Iron. See Class II., Section V.

☞ Most of the preparations of Iron may sometimes be used as emmenagogues.

Gossyp'ii Ra'dix. (U.S. Ph.) Cotton Root. The root of *Gossypium herbaceum* and of other species of *Gossypium.*

Guaiac. See **Guaiaci Resina.**

Guai'aci Resi'na. (U.S. and Br. Ph.) Guaiac. See Class XI.

Guai'acum Officina'le. See **Guaiaci Resina.**

Hellebore, Black. See **Helleborus.**

Helleb'orus. (U.S. Ph.) Black Hellebore. See Class IX.

In'ula. (U.S. Ph.) Elecampane. See Class II., Section II.

Iodide of Iron. See **Ferri Iodidum.**

Iron. See **Ferri.**

Junip'erus Sabi'na. See **Sabina.**

Junip'erus Virginia'na. (U.S. Ph.) Red Cedar. The tops of *Juniperus Virginiana.*

Madder. See **Rubia.**

Milfoil. See **Achillea Millefolium.**

Myrrh. See **Myrrha.**

Myr'rha. (U.S. and Br. Ph.) Myrrh. See Class II., Section II.

Nep'eta Cata'ria. See **Cataria.**

O'leum Sabi'næ. (U.S. and Br. Ph.) Oil of Savine.

? Orig'anum Vulga're. Marjoram.

Polyg'ala Sen'ega. See **Senega.**

Potato Flies. See **Cantharis Vittata.**

Red Cedar. See **Juniperus Virginiana.**

Rosemary. See **Rosmarinus.**

Rosmari'nus. (U.S. Ph.) Rosemary. See Class II., Section IV.

? Ru'bia. (U.S. Ph.) Madder. The root of *Ru'bia tincto'rum.*

Rue. See **Ruta.**

Ru'ta. (U.S. Ph.) Rue. See Class IV.

Sabi'na. (U.S. and Br. Ph.) The tops of *Junip'erus sabi'na.*

? Sagape'num. (Lond. Ph.) The gum resin of an uncertain plant. See Class IV.

Savine. See **Sabina.**

Sen'ega. (U.S. and Br. Ph.) Seneka. See Class XII.

Seneka. See **Senega.**

So'dæ Bo'ras. (U.S. Ph.) Borate of Soda, or Borax. See Classes VI. and X.

Spanish Flies. See **Cantharis.**

Subcarbonate of Iron. See **Ferri Subcarbonas.**

Yarrow. See **Achillea Millefolium.**

CLASS XIV.

SIALAGOGUES.

MEDICINES WHICH PROMOTE THE SECRETION OF SALIVA.

Anacyc'lus Pyr'ethrum. See **Pyrethrum.**

Black Oxide of Mercury. See **Hydrargyri Oxidum Nigrum.**

Cal'amus. (U.S. Ph.) Sweet Flag. See Class II., Section IV.

Cinnabar. See **Hydrargyri Sulphuretum Rubrum.**

Hydrar'gyri Ox'idum Ni'grum. Black Oxide of Mercury.

Hydrar'gyri Sulphure'tum Ru'brum. Red Sulphuret of Mercury, or Cinnabar. (Sometimes used in *fumigation* as a rapid sialagogue.)

Hydrar'gyrum. (U.S. and Br. Ph.) (☞ Mercury, and most of its compounds, may be used as sialagogues.) See Class XXI.

Mercury. See **Hydrargyrum.**

Pellitory. See **Pyrethrum.**

Pyr'ethrum. (U.S. Ph.) Pellitory. The root of *Anacyc'lus pyr'ethrum.*

Red Sulphuret of Mercury. See **Hydrargyri Sulphuretum Rubrum.**

CLASS XV.

ERRHINES.

MEDICINES WHICH PROMOTE THE SECRETION FROM THE MUCOUS MEMBRANE OF THE NOSTRILS.

Armora'cia. (Br. Ph.) Horseradish Root. The fresh root of *Cochlea'ria armora'cia.* See Class X.

Asarabac'ca. The root and leaves of *As'arum Europæ'um.*

Bloodroot. See **Sanguinaria.**

Cochlea'ria Armora'cia. See **Armoracia.**

Convalla'ria Maja'lis. Lily of the Valley.

Euphor'bium. See Class XVI.

False Sunflower. See **Helenium Autumnale.**

Hele'nium Autumna'le. False Sunflower, or Sneezewort.

Horseradish. See **Armoracia.**

Hydrar'gyri Sul'phas Fla'va. (U.S. Ph.). Yellow Sulphate of Mercury, or Turpeth Mineral. See Class VIII.

Lily of the Valley. See **Convallaria Majalis.**

Sanguina'ria. (U.S. Ph.) Bloodroot. See Class VIII.

Sneezewort. See **Helenium Autumnale.**

Snuff—or Tobacco in powder.

Turpeth Mineral. See **Hydrargyri Sulphas Flava.**

Vera'tria. (U.S. and Br. Ph.) See Class VIII., Section I.

? Vera'trum Al'bum. (U.S. Ph.) White Hellebore.

CLASS XVI.

EPISPASTICS.

MEDICINES WHICH WHEN APPLIED TO THE SKIN PRODUCE A BLISTER.

Ace'tum Canthar'idis. Vinegar of Spanish Flies.

Aç'idum Acet'icum Glacia'le. (Br. Ph.) Glacial Acetic Acid. A colorless liquid, which is converted, when cooled to nearly 32°, into colorless, prismatic crystals. Specific gravity, 1.065.

? Anacar'dium Occidenta'le. See Class XVIII.

A'qua Ammo'niæ For'tior. (U.S. Ph.) Stronger Water (or Solution) of Ammonia. See Class XVII.

Argen'ti Ni'tras Fu'sa. (U.S. Ph.) Fused Nitrate of Silver, or Lunar Caustic.

Cantharides. See **Cantharis.**

Can'tharis. (U.S. and Br. Ph.) Spanish Flies. Cantharides. *Can'tharis vesicato'ria.*

Can'tharis Vitta'ta. Potato Flies.

Cerate of Spanish Flies. See **Ceratum Cantharidis.**

Cera'tum Canthar'idis. (U.S. Ph.) Cerate of Spanish Flies, or Blistering Cerate.

Crowfoot. See **Ranunculus.**

Daph'ne Mezere'um. See **Mezereum.**

Dir'ca Palus'tris. Leather-wood.

Emplas'trum Pi'cis cum Canthar'ide. (U.S. Ph.) Plaster of Pitch with Spanish Flies.

? Euphor'bium. (Ed. Ph.) The concrete resinous juice of undetermined species of *Euphorbia.*

Fused Nitrate of Silver. See **Argenti Nitras Fusa.**

Glacial Acetic Acid. See **Acidum Aceticum Glaciale.**

Leather-wood. See **Dirca Palustris.**

Liniment of Spanish Flies. See **Linimentum Cantharidis.**

Linimen'tum Canthar'idis. (U.S. and Br. Ph.) Liniment of Spanish Flies, or Liniment of Cantharides.

Lunar Caustic. See **Argenti Nitras Fusa.**

Mezereon. See **Mezereum.**

Mezere'um. (U.S. and Br. Ph.) Mezereon. The bark of *Daph'ne Mezere'um* and of *Daph'ne Gnid'ium* (U.S. Ph.). The dried bark of *Daphne mezereum,* or *Daph'ne laureo'la* (Br. Ph.).

Ointment of Spanish Flies. See **Unguentum Cantharidis.**

Potato Flies. See **Cantharis Vittata.**

Ranun'culus. (U.S. Ph.) Crowfoot. The cormus and herb of *Ranun'culus bulbo'sus.*

Sabadil'la. (U.S. and Br. Ph.) Cevadilla. See Class IX.

Stronger Solution of Ammonia. See **Aqua Ammoniæ Fortior.**

Unguen'tum Canthar'idis. (Br. Ph.) Ointment of Spanish Flies.

Vinegar of Spanish Flies. See **Acetum Cantharidis.**

CLASS XVII.

RUBEFACIENTS.

MEDICINES WHICH INFLAME THE SKIN WITHOUT VESICATING AS AN ORDINARY RESULT.

A'bies Canaden'sis. See **Pix Canaden'sis.**

A'bies Excel'sa. See **Pix Burgundica.**

Aç'idum Acet'icum Glacia'le. (Br. Ph.) Glacial Acetic Acid. See Class XVI.

Ammo'niæ Li'quor For'tior. (Br. Ph.) See next article.

A'qua Ammo'niæ For'tior. (U.S. Ph.) Stronger Water of Ammonia.

Armora'cia. (Br. Ph.) Horseradish Root. See Classes XV. and X.

Burgundy Pitch. See **Pix Burgundica.**

Canada Pitch. See **Pix Canadensis.**

Cap'sicum. (U.S. and Br. Ph.) Cayenne Pepper. See Class III.

Cayenne Pepper. See **Capsicum.**

Cochlea'ria Armora'cia. See **Armoracia.**

Crowfoot. See **Ranunculus.**

El'emi. (Br. Ph.) Elemi. A concrete resinous exudation: botanical source undetermined, probably from *Cana'rium commu'ne.*

Glacial Acetic Acid. See **Acidum Aceticum Glaciale.**

Horseradish. See **Armoracia.**

Liniment of Ammonia. See **Linimentum Ammoniæ.**

Linimen'tum Ammo'niæ. (U.S. and Br. Ph.) Liniment of Ammonia, or Volatile Liniment.

Li'quor Ammo'niæ. (Br. Ph.) Solution of Ammonia. The same as **Aqua Ammoniæ.**

Mustard. See **Sinapis Alba.**

Oil of Rosemary. See **Oleum Rosmarinus.**

Oil of Turpentine. See **Oleum Terebinthinæ.**

O'leum Rosmari'ni. (U.S. and Br. Ph.) Oil of Rosemary.

O'leum Sabi'næ. (U.S. and Br. Ph.) Oil of Savine. See Class XIII.

O'leum Terebin'thinæ. (U.S. and Br. Ph.) Oil of Turpentine. See Class X.

Pi'nus A'bies. See **Pix Burgundica.**

Pi'nus Canaden'sis. See **Pix Canadensis.**

Pix Burgun'dica. (U.S. and Br. Ph.) Burgundy Pitch. The prepared concrete juice of *A'bies excel'sa* (U.S. Ph.). A resinous exudation from the stem of *Abies excelsa* (Br. Ph.).

Pix Canaden'sis. (U.S. Ph.) Canada Pitch, or Hemlock Pitch. The prepared concrete juice of *A'bies Canaden'sis.*

Ranun'culus. (U.S. Ph.) Crowfoot. See Class XVI.

Sina'pis. (Br. Ph.) Mustard. *Sina'pis ni'gra* and *Sina'pis al'ba.* The seeds reduced to powder, mixed.

Sina'pis Al'ba. (U.S. Ph.) White Mustard. The seed of *Sinapis alba.*

Sina'pis Ni'gra. (U.S. Ph.) Black Mustard. The seed of *Sinapis nigra.*

Stronger Water (or Solution) of Ammonia. See **Aqua Ammoniæ Fortior.**

CLASS XVIII.

ESCHAROTICS.

SUBSTANCES WHICH DESTROY THE LIFE OF THE PART TO WHICH THEY ARE APPLIED, AND PRODUCE A SLOUGH.

Aç'idum Arsenio'sum. (U.S. and Br. Ph.) Arsenious Acid. White Arsenic, or White Oxide of Arsenic. A white powder, sparingly soluble in water, and entirely volatilized by heat. See Class XXI.

Aç'idum Chro'micum. Chromic Acid.

Aç'idum Ni'tricum. (U.S. and Br. Ph.) Nitric Acid, or Aqua Fortis. See Class II., Section V.

Aç'idum Sulphu'ricum. (U.S. and Br. Ph.) Sulphuric Acid. See Class II., Section V.

Alu'men Exsicca'tum. Dried Alum.

Anacar'dium Occidenta'le, or Cashew Nut.

Antimo'nii Terchlo'ridi Li'quor. (Br. Ph.) Solution of Terchloride of Antimony.

A'qua For'tis. See **Acidum Nitricum.**

Argen'ti Ni'tras. (U.S. and Br. Ph.) Nitrate of Silver, or Lunar Caustic. A heavy, colorless, anhydrous salt, wholly soluble in distilled water.

Arsenious Acid. See **Acidum Arseniosum.**

Bichloride of Mercury. See **Hydrargyri Chloridum Corrosivum.**

Blue Vitriol. See **Cupri Sulphas.**

Calx. (U.S. and Br. Ph.) Lime.

Cashew Nut. See **Anacardium Occidentale.**

Caustic Potash. See **Potassa Caustica.**

Caustic Soda. See **Soda Caustica.**

Chloride of Zinc. See **Zinci Chloridum.**

Chromic Acid. See **Acidum Chromicum.**

Common Caustic. See **Potassa.**

Corrosive Sublimate. See **Hydrargyri Chloridum Corrosivum.**

Creasote. See **Creasotum.**

Creaso'tum. (U. S. and Br. Ph.) Creasote. See Class V.

Cu'pri Ni'tras. Nitrate of Copper.

Cu'pri Subace'tas. (U.S. Ph.) Subacetate of Copper, or Verdigris. A substance in pale-green masses.

Cu'pri Sul'phas. (U.S. and Br. Ph.) Sulphate of Copper, or Blue Vitriol. See Class I. and II.

Dried Alum. See **Alumen Exsiccatum.**

Hydrar'gyri Chlo'ridum Corrosi'vum. (U.S. Ph.) Corrosive Chloride of Mercury, or Corrosive Sublimate. A substance in colorless crystals or crystalline masses, which are fusible by heat and entirely soluble in water, alcohol, and ether. See Class XXI.

Hydrar'gyri Nitra'tis Li'quor Aç'idus. (Br. Ph.) Acid Solution of the Nitrate of Mercury.

Hydrar'gyri Ox'idum Ru'brum. (U.S. and Br. Ph.) Red Oxide of Mercury, or Red Precipitate. An orange-red powder, entirely soluble in muriatic acid.

Hydrar'gyri Pernitra'tis Li'quor. Solution of Pernitrate of Mercury. The same as **Hydrargyri Nitratis Liquor Acidus.**

Hydrar'gyrum Corrosi'vum Sublima'tum. (Br. Ph.) The Bichloride of Mercury, or Corrosive Sublimate. See **Hydrargyri Chloridum Corrosivum.**

Iodide of Calomel.

Lime. See **Calx.**

Li'quor Potas'sæ. (U.S. and Br. Ph.) Solution of Potash.

Li'quor So'dæ. (U.S. Ph.) Solution of Soda.

Lunar Caustic. See **Argenti Nitras.**

Nitrate of Copper. See **Cupri Nitras.**

Nitrate of Silver. See **Argenti Nitras.**

Nitric Acid. See **Acidum Nitricum.**

Permanganate of Potash. See **Potassæ Permanganas.**

Plum'bi Bichro'mas. (U.S. Ph.) Bichromate of Lead. See Class VIII.

Potas'sa. (U.S. Ph.) Common Caustic. A very deliquescent alkali, soluble, with the exception of a slight residue, in alcohol and in water.

Potas'sa Caus'tica. (Br. Ph.) Caustic Potash, or Hydrate of Potash. The same as **Potassa.**

Potas'sa cum Cal'ci. Potash with Lime.

Potas'sæ Hy'dras. Hydrate of Potassa. See **Potassa Caustica.**

Potas'sæ Perman'ganas. (U.S. and Br. Ph.) Permanganate of Potash A substance in needle-shaped crystals of a deep purple color.

Red Oxide of Mercury. See **Hydrargyri Oxidum Rubrum.**

Red Precipitate. See **Hydrargyri Oxidum Rubrum.**

So'da Caus'tica. (Br. Ph.) Caustic Soda.

Solution of Pernitrate of Mercury. See **Hydrargyri Pernitratis Liquor.**

Solution of Potash. See **Liquor Potassæ.**

Solution of Soda. See **Liquor Sodæ.**

Subacetate of Copper. See **Cupri Subacetas.**

Sulphate of Copper. See **Cupri Sulphas.**

Sulphuric Acid. See **Acidum Sulphuricum.**

Verdigris. See **Cupri Subacetas.**

White Oxide of Arsenic. See **Acidum Arseniosum.**

Zin'çi Chlo'ridum. (U.S. and Br. Ph.) Chloride of Zinc. A white deliquescent salt, wholly soluble in water, alcohol, and ether.

CLASS XIX.

DEMULCENTS.

BLAND UNIRRITATING SUBSTANCES, MOST OF WHICH FORM, WITH WATER, A VISCID SOLUTION.

Aca'cia. (U.S. and Br. Ph.) Gum Arabic. The concrete juice of *Aca'cia ve'ra* and of other species of *Acacia* (U.S. Ph.). A gummy exudation from the stem of one or more undetermined species of *Acacia* (Br. Ph.).

Althæ'a. (U.S. Ph.) Marshmallow. The root of *Althæ'a officina'lis.*

Amyg'dala. (Br. Ph.) Sweet Almond, or Jordan Almond. The same as **Amygdala Dulcis.**

Amyg'dala Dul'cis. (U. S. Ph.) Sweet Almond. The kernel of the fruit of *Amyg'dalus commu'nis,* variety *dul'cis.*

Am'ylum. (U.S. and Br. Ph.) Starch, or Wheat Starch. The fecula of the seed of *Trit'icum vulga're.*

Arrow Root. See **Maranta.**

Astrag'alus Ve'rus. See **Tragacantha.**

Ave'næ Fari'na. (U.S. Ph.) Oatmeal. Meal prepared from the seeds of the *Ave'na sati'va.*

Barley. See **Hordeum.**

Be'la. (Br. Ph.) Bael. (The ripe fruit is demulcent, the unripe astringent.) See Class I.

Benne Leaves. See **Sesami Folium.**

Can'na. (U.S. Ph.) Canna Starch. The fecula prepared from the rhizoma of an undetermined species of *Canna.*

Carrageen. See **Chondrus.**

Ceta'ceum. (U.S. and Br. Ph.) Spermaceti. A crystalline, pearly-white substance (nearly pure Cetine) obtained from the oil of the *Physe'ter macroceph'alus.*

Cetra'ria. (U.S. and Br. Ph.) The *Cetra'ria Islan'dica,* or Iceland Moss. (Also slightly tonic.)

Chon'drus. (U.S. Ph.) The *Chon'drus cris'pus.* Carrageen, or Irish Moss.

Comfrey. See **Symphytum Officinale.**

Common Mallow. See **Malva Sylvestris.**

Cy'cas Circina'lis. See **Sago.**

Cydo'nia Vulga'ris. See **Cydonium.**

Cydo'nium. (U.S. Ph.) Quince Seed. The seed of *Cydo'nia vulga'ris.*

Dextrin [*Dextri'na*]. A mucilaginous substance obtained from starch.

Elm Bark. See **Ulmus.**

Extrac'tum Glycyrrhi'zæ. (U.S. Ph.) Liquorice.

? **Fi'cus.** (U.S. and Br. Ph.) Fig. See Class IX.

Fig. See **Ficus.**

Flaxseed. See **Linum.**

Glycerin, or Glycerine. See **Glycerina.**

Glyceri'na. (U.S. Ph.) Glycerin. A colorless, inodorous, syrupy liquid, of a sweet taste, soluble in water and in alcohol. Specific gravity, 1.25.

Glyceri'num. (Br. Ph.) Glycerine, or Glycerin. The same as **Glycerina.**

Glycyrrhi'za. (U.S. and Br. Ph.) Liquorice Root. The root of *Glycyrrhi'za gla'bra* (U.S. Ph.). The root or underground stem, fresh and dried, of *Glycyrrhiza glabra* (Br. Ph.).

Gum Arabic. See **Acacia.**

Hor'deum. (U.S. and Br. Ph.) Barley. The decorticated seed of *Hor'deum dis'tichon* (U.S. Ph.). *Hordeum distichum:* the seeds deprived of the husks (Br. Ph.).

Iceland Moss. See **Cetraria.**

Irish Moss. See **Chondrus.**

Jan'ipha Man'ihot, or *Jat'ropha Man'ihot.* See **Tapioca.**

Li'chen Islan'dicus. See **Cetraria.**

Li'ni Se'men. (Br. Ph.) Flaxseed. See next article.

Li'num. (U.S. Ph.) Flaxseed. The seed of *Li'num usitatis'simum.*

Liquorice. See **Extractum Glycyrrhizæ.**

Liquorice Root. See **Glycyrrhiza.**

Ly'thrum Salica'ria. Loose-strife.

Mal'va Sylves'tris. Common Mallow.

Maran'ta. (U.S. Ph.) Arrow Root. The fecula of the rhizoma of *Maran'ta arundina'cea.*

Marshmallow. See **Althæa.**

Oatmeal. See **Avenæ Farina.**

O'leum Amyg'dalæ. (Br. Ph.) Oil of Almond. The same as **Oleum Amygdalæ Dulcis.**

O'leum Amyg'dalæ Dul'cis. (U.S. Ph.) Oil of Sweet Almond.

Ory'za Sati'va. Rice.

Quince Seed. See **Cydonium.**

Rice. See **Oryza Sativa.**

Sac'charum. (U.S. Ph.) Sugar. The sugar of *Sac'charum officina'rum.*
Sa'go. (U.S. Ph.) The prepared fecula of the pith of *Sa'gus Rum'phii* and of other species of *Sagus.*
Sague'rus Rum'phii. See **Sago.**
Sa'gus Rum'phii. See **Sago.**
Sas'safras Medul'la. (U. S. Ph.) Sassafras Pith.
Ses'ami Fo'lium. (U.S. Ph.) Benne Leaf (or *Sesami Folia,* Benne Leaves). The leaves of *Ses'amum In'dicum* and of *Ses'amum Orienta'le.*
Slippery Elm Bark. See **Ulmus Fulva.**
Spermaceti. See **Cetaceum.**
Starch. See **Amylum.**
Sugar. See **Saccharum.**
Sweet Almond. See **Amygdala Dulcis.**
Sym'phytum Officina'le. Comfrey.
Tapio'ca. (U.S. Ph.) The fecula of the root of *Jan'ipha man'ihot.*
Tragacanth. See **Tragacantha.**
Tragacan'tha. (U.S. and Br. Ph.) Tragacanth. The concrete juice of *Astrag'alus ve'rus* and of other species of *Astrag'alus* (U.S. Ph.). A gummy exudation from the stem of *Astragalus verus* (Br. Ph.).
Ul'mus. (Br. Ph.) Elm Bark. The dried inner bark, deprived of its outer layers, of *Ul'mus campes'tris.*
Ul'mus Ful'va. (U.S. Ph.) Slippery Elm Bark. The inner bark of *Ulmus fulva.*
Vi'ola. (U.S. Ph.) Violet. The herb of *Vi'ola peda'ta.*
Violet. See **Viola.**

CLASS XX.

EMOLLIENTS.

SUBSTANCES WHICH HAVE THE PROPERTY OF SOFTENING AND SOOTHING AN IRRITATED SURFACE, OR ONE HARSH FROM DRYNESS.

A'deps. (U.S. Ph.) Lard. The prepared fat of *Sus scro'fa.*
A'deps Præpara'tus. (Br. Ph.) Prepared Lard. See **Adeps.**
Ave'næ Fari'na. (U.S. Ph.) Oatmeal. See Class XIX.
Cerate of Lard. See **Ceratum Adipis.**
Cera'tum Ad'ipis. (U.S. Ph.) Cerate of Lard, or Simple Cerate.
Cera'tum Ceta'cei. (U.S. Ph.) Cerate of Spermaceti.
Cera'tum Plum'bi Subaceta'tis. (U.S. Ph.) Goulard's Cerate.
Cera'tum Sapo'nis. (U.S. Ph.) Soap Cerate.
Cera'tum Sim'plex. ("Simple Cerate.") See **Ceratum Adipis.**
Ceta'ceum. (Br. Ph.) Spermaceti. See Class XIX.
Common Mallow. See **Malva Sylvestris.**
? Dau'ci Ra'dix. Garden Carrot Root.
Flaxseed. See **Linum.**
Flaxseed Oil. See **Oleum Lini.**
Garden Carrot. See **Dauci Radix.**
Goulard's Cerate. See **Ceratum Plumbi Subacetatis.**
Lime Liniment. See **Linimentum Calcis.**
Li'ni Fari'na. (U.S. and Br. Ph.) Linseed Meal.
Li'ni Se'men. (Br. Ph.) Flaxseed. See **Linum.**
Linimen'tum Cal'cis. (U.S. Ph.) Lime Liniment.
Linseed Meal. See **Lini Farina.**
Li'num. (U.S. Ph.) Flaxseed. See Class XIX.
Mal'va Sylves'tris. Common Mallow. See Class XIX.
Oatmeal. See **Avenæ Farina.**
Ointment of Rose Water. See **Unguentum Aquæ Rosæ.**
O'leum Li'ni. (U.S. and Br. Ph.) Flaxseed Oil, or Linseed Oil.
O'leum Oli'væ. (U.S. and Br. Ph.) Olive Oil, or Sweet Oil. See Class IX.
O'leum Ses'ami. (U.S. Ph.) Benne Oil. The oil of the seed of *Ses'amum In'dicum* and *Ses'amum Orienta'le.*
Olive Oil. See **Oleum Olivæ.**
(☞ Nearly all the fixed oils may be used as emollients.)
Se'vum. (U.S. Ph.) Suet. The prepared suet of *O'vis a'ries.*
Se'vum Præpara'tum. (Br. Ph.) Prepared Suet. The same as **Sevum.**
Simple Cerate. See **Ceratum Simplex.**
Simple Ointment. See **Unguentum Adipis.**
Spermaceti. See **Cetaceum.**
Sweet Oil. See **Oleum Olivæ.**

Unguen'tum Ad'ipis. (U.S. Ph.) Ointment of Lard; also called *Unguen'tum Sim'plex.*

Unguen'tum A'quæ Ro'sæ. (U.S. Ph.) Ointment of Rose Water.

Unguen'tum Sim'plex. See **Unguentum Adipis.**

Vi'ola. (U.S. Ph.) Violet. See Class XIX.

CLASS XXI.

ALTERATIVES.

MEDICINES WHICH PRODUCE GRADUALLY AND SCARCELY PERCEPTIBLY SUCH A CHANGE IN THE FUNCTIONS OF ORGANS AS TO PERMIT A HEALTHY ACTION TO TAKE THE PLACE OF DISEASE.

Aç'idum Arsenio'sum. (U.S. and Br. Ph.) Arsenious Acid, or White Arsenic. See Class XVIII.

Aç'idum Hydriod'icum. Hydriodic Acid.

Aç'idum Nitro-hydrochlo'ricum Dilu'tum. (Br. Ph.) The same as **Acidum Nitromuriaticum Dilutum.**

Aç'idum Nitromuriat'icum Dilu'tum. (U.S. Ph.) Nitromuriatic Acid. See Class II., Section V.

Aç'idum Sulphuro'sum. (U.S. and Br. Ph.) Sulphurous Acid. A colorless liquid having the odor of burning sulphur, and a sulphurous, sour, and somewhat astringent taste. (Used chiefly as an external application in cutaneous affections.)

Æ'ther Hydriod'icus. Hydriodic Ether.

Ammo'niæ Arse'nias. Arseniate of Ammonia.

? **Ammo'niæ Phos'phas.** (Br. Ph.) Phosphate of Ammonia. A substance in colorless transparent prisms which become opaque on exposure to air.

Ammoniated Mercury. See **Hydrargyrum Ammoniatum.**

Ammo'nii Iod'idum. Iodide of Ammonium.

Antimonial Powder. See **Pulvis Antimonialis.**

Antimo'nii Sulphure'tum Præcipita'tum. The same as **Antimonium Sulphuratum.**

Antimo'nii Sulphure'tum Præpara'tum.

Antimo'nium Sulphura'tum. (U.S. and Br. Ph.) Sulphurated Antimony. See Class XI.

Arseniate of Ammonia. See **Ammoniæ Arsenias.**

Arseniate of Iron. See **Ferri Arsenias.**

Arsen'ici Iod'idum. (U.S. Ph.) Iodide of Arsenic.

Arsenious Acid. See **Acidum Arseniosum.**

Black Oxide of Manganese. See **Manganesii Oxidum Nigrum.**

Black Oxide of Mercury. See **Hydrargyri Oxidum Nigrum.**

Black Sulphuret of Mercury. See **Hydrargyri Sulphuretum Nigrum.**

Bladder-wrack. See **Fucus Vesiculosus.**

Bromide of Iron. See **Ferri Bromidum.**

Bromide of Mercury. See **Hydrargyri Bromidum.**

Bromide of Potassium. See **Potassii Bromidum.**

Bromin'ii Chlo'ridum. Chloride of Bromine.

Bromin'ium. (U.S. Ph.) Bromine. A dark-red liquid having a strong odor, and entirely volatilized by heat in reddish vapor. Specific gravity, 3.0.

Cad'mii Iod'idum. Iodide of Cadmium.

Calomel. See **Hydrargyri Chloridum Mite,** and **Calomelas.**

Calom'elas. (Br. Ph.) Calomel, or the Subchloride of Mercury. A dull-white, heavy, and nearly tasteless powder, insoluble in water, alcohol, or ether.

Carburet of Iron. See **Ferri Carburetum.**

Chloride of Bromine. See **Brominii Chloridum.**

Chloride of Zinc. See **Zinci Chloridum.**

Chrysophyl'lum Glycyphlœ'um. See **Monesia.**

Cinnabar. See **Hydrargyri Sulphuretum Rubrum.**

Col'chici Cor'mus. (Br. Ph.) Colchicum Corm. The fresh corm of *Col'chicum autumna'le,* collected about the end of June. The same as **Colchici Radix.**

Col'chici Ra'dix. (U.S. Ph.) Colchicum Root. The cormus of *Col'chicum autumna'le.* See Class X.

Col'chici Semen. (U.S. Ph.) Colchicum Seed. The seed of *Col'chicum autumna'le.* See Class X.

Colchicum Root. See **Colchici Radix.**

Colchicum Seed. See **Colchici Semen.**

Corrosive Sublimate. See **Hydrargyri Chloridum Corrosivum.**

Fer'ri Arse'nias. (Br. Ph.) Arseniate of Iron.

Fer'ri Brom'idum. Bromide of Iron.

? *Fer'ri Carbure'tum.* Carburet of Iron, or Plumbago.

Fer'ri Iod'idum. (Br. Ph.) Iodide of Iron. See Class XIII.

Fu'cus Vesiculo'sus. Bladder-wrack, or Sea-wrack.

? Glycerin.

Green Iodide of Mercury. See **Hydrargyri Iodidum Viride.**

Hemides'mus. (Br. Ph.) The root of *Hemides'mus In'dicus.*

Hydrar'gyri Brom'idum. Bromide of Mercury.

Hydrar'gyri Chlo'ridum Corrosi'vum. (U.S. Ph.) Corrosive Chloride of Mercury, or Corrosive Sublimate. See Class XVIII.

Hydrar'gyri Chlo'ridum Mi'te. (U.S. Ph.) Mild Chloride of Mercury, or Calomel. A white or pale buff powder, which is tasteless and inodorous, and insoluble in water, alcohol, or ether.

Hydrar'gyri Iod'idum Ru'brum. (U.S. and Br. Ph.) Red Iodide of Mercury. A red powder which becomes yellow when heated, and red again when cold.

Hydrar'gyri Iod'idum Vir'ide. (U.S. and Br. Ph.) Green Iodide of Mercury. A greenish-yellow powder, which becomes red when heated.

Hydrar'gyri Ni'tras. Nitrate of Mercury.

Hydrar'gyri Ox'idum Ni'grum. Black Oxide of Mercury.

? Hydrar'gyri Ox'idum Ru'brum. (U.S. and Br. Ph.) Red Oxide of Mercury, or Red Precipitate. See Class XVIII.

Hydrar'gyri Sul'phas Fla'va. (U.S. Ph.) Yellow Sulphate of Mercury, or Turpeth Mineral. See Class VIII.

Hydrar'gyri Sulphure'tum Ni'grum. Black Sulphuret of Mercury, or Ethiops Mineral.

Hydrar'gyri Sulphure'tum Ru'brum. (U.S. Ph.) Red Sulphuret of Mercury, or Cinnabar.

? Hydrar'gyrum Ammonia'tum. (U.S. and Br. Ph.) Ammoniated Mercury, or White Precipitate.

Hydrar'gyrum Corrosi'vum Sublima'tum. (Br. Ph.) Corrosive Sublimate. See Class XVIII.

Hydrar'gyrum cum Cre'tâ. (U.S. and Br. Ph.) Mercury with Chalk.

Hydriodic Acid. See **Acidum Hydriodicum.**

Hydriodic Ether. See **Æther Hydriodicus.**

Hydrocot'yle Asiat'ica. Thick-leaved Penny-wort. (A remedy for leprosy.)

Iodide of Ammonium. See **Ammonii Iodidum.**

Iodide of Arsenic. See **Arsenici Iodidum.**

Iodide of Cadmium. See **Cadmii Iodidum.**

Iodide of Iron. See **Ferri Iodidum.**

Iodide of Potassium. See **Potassii Iodidum.**

Iodide of Sulphur. See **Sulphuris Iodidum.**

Iodide of Zinc. See **Zinci Iodidum.**

Iodine. See **Iodinium.**

Iodin'ium. (U.S. Ph.) Iodine. A substance in bluish-black crystalline scales having the metallic lustre. When heated, it first melts and then rises in purple vapor. Specific gravity, 4.9.

I'odum. (Br. Ph.) Iodine. The same as **Iodinium.**

Li'quor Arsen'ici Chlo'ridi. Solution of Chloride of Arsenic.

Li'quor Arsen'ici et Hydrar'gyri Iod'idi. (U.S. Ph.) Solution of Iodide of Arsenic and Mercury.

Li'quor Potas'sæ Arseni'tis. (U.S. Ph.) Solution of Arsenite of Potassa.

Mangane'sii Ox'idum Ni'grum. Black Oxide of Manganese.

Mangane'sii Sul'phas. (U.S. Ph.) Sulphate of Manganese. See Class IX.

Mercury with Chalk. See **Hydrargyrum cum Cretâ.**

Mild Chloride of Mercury. See **Hydrargyri Chloridum Mite.**

Mone'sia. An extract from the *Chrysophyl'lum glycyphlœ'um.*

Nitrate of Mercury. See **Hydrargyri Nitras.**

Ointment of Mercury. See **Unguentum Hydrargyri.**

Pills of Mercury. See **Pilulæ Hydrargyri.**

Pil'ulæ Hydrar'gyri. (U.S. Ph.) Pills of Mercury.

Plumbago. See **Ferri Carburetum.**

Potas'sæ Perman'ganas. (U.S. Ph.) Permanganate of Potash. See Class XVIII. and XXIV.

? *Potas'sæ Phos'phas.* Phosphate of Potash.

Potas'sii Brom'idum. (U.S. and Br. Ph.) Bromide of Potassium.

Potas'sii Iod'idum. (U.S. and Br. Ph.) Iodide of Potassium. It occurs in colorless crystals, readily soluble in water.

Precipitated Sulphuret of Antimony. See **Antimonium Sulphuratum.**

Pul'vis Antimonia'lis. (Br. Ph.) Antimonial Powder. See Class XI.

Red Iodide of Mercury. See **Hydrargyri Iodidum Rubrum.**

Red Oxide of Mercury. See **Hydrargyri Oxidum Rubrum.**

Red Sulphuret of Mercury. See **Hydrargyri Sulphuretum Rubrum.**

Sapona'ria Officina'lis. Soapwort.

Sar'sa. (Br. Ph.) Jamaica Sarsaparilla. The same as **Sarsaparilla.**

Sarsaparil'la. (U.S. Ph.) The root of *Smi'lax officina'lis* and of other species of *Smilax.*

Sea-wrack. See **Fucus Vesiculosus.**

Smi'lax As'pera. See **Sarsaparilla.**

Smi'lax Officina'lis. See **Sarsaparilla.**

Smi'lax Syphilit'ica. See **Sarsaparilla.**

Soapwort. See **Saponaria Officinalis.**

Solution of Arsenite of Potassa. See **Liquor Potassæ Arsenitis.**

Solution of Chloride of Arsenic. See **Liquor Arsenici Chloridi.**

Solution of Iodide of Arsenic and Mercury. See **Liquor Arsenici et Hydrargyri Iodidi.**

Stillin'gia. (U.S. Ph.) The root of *Stillin'gia sylvat'ica.*

Sulphur, in its various forms, is by some medical writers regarded as alterative. See Classes IX. and XII.

Sulphurated Antimony. See **Antimonium Sulphuratum.**

Sul'phuris Iod'idum. (U.S. Ph.) Iodide of Sulphur.

Turpeth Mineral. See **Hydrargyri Sulphas Flava.**

Unguen'tum Hydrar'gyri. (U.S. and Br. Ph.) Ointment of Mercury.

Vi'num Col'chici Radi'cis. (U.S. Ph.) Wine of Colchicum Root. See Class X.

Yellow Sulphate of Mercury. See **Hydrargyri Sulphas Flava.**

Zin'çi Chlo'ridum. (U.S. and Br. Ph.) Chloride of Zinc. See Class XVIII.

Zin'çi Iod'idum. Iodide of Zinc.

CLASS XXII.

ANTACIDS.

SUBSTANCES WHICH ARE CAPABLE OF COMBINING WITH AND NEUTRALIZING ACIDS. HENCE ALL SALIFIABLE BASES ARE ANTACIDS; BUT THE ALKALIES, ALKALINE EARTHS, AND THEIR CARBONATES, ARE ALMOST EXCLUSIVELY EMPLOYED FOR THIS PURPOSE.

Ammo'niæ A'qua. See **Aqua Ammoniæ.**

Ammo'niæ Carbo'nas. (U.S. and Br. Ph.) Carbonate of Ammonia. See Class III.

Ammo'niæ Li'quor. (Br. Ph.) Solution of Ammonia. See next article.

A'qua Ammo'niæ. (U. S. Ph.) Water (or Solution) of Ammonia.

Aromatic Spirit of Ammonia. See **Spiritus Ammoniæ Aromaticus.**

Bicarbonate of Potassa. See **Potassæ Bicarbonas.**

Bicarbonate of Soda. See **Sodæ Bicarbonas.**

Calcined Magnesia. See **Magnesia.**

Carbonate of Ammonia. See **Ammoniæ Carbonas.**

Carbonate of Lithia. See **Lithiæ Carbonas.**

Carbonate of Magnesia. See **Magnesiæ Carbonas.**

Carbonate of Potassa. See **Potassæ Carbonas.**

Carbonate of Soda. See **Sodæ Carbonas.**

Chalk. See **Creta.**

Cre'ta. (U.S. Ph.) Chalk. Native friable carbonate of lime.

Cre'ta Præpara'ta. (Br. Ph.) Prepared Chalk.

Dried Carbonate of Soda. See **Sodæ Carbonas Exsiccata.**

Fer'ri Ox'idum Hydra'tum. (U.S. Ph.) Hydrated Oxide of Iron. (An antidote to arsenious acid.)

Fer'ri Perox'idum Hydra'tum. (Br. Ph.) Hydrated Peroxide of Iron. The same as **Ferri Oxidum Hydratum.**

Hydrated Oxide of Iron. See **Ferri Oxidum Hydratum.**

Lime Water. See **Liquor Calcis.**

Li'quor Cal'cis. (U.S. and Br. Ph.) Lime Water.

Li'quor Potas'sæ. (U.S. and Br. Ph.) Solution of Potassa. See Class XVIII.

Li'quor So'dæ. (U.S. Ph.) Solution of Soda. See Class XVIII.

Lith'iæ Carbo'nas. (U.S. and Br. Ph.) Carbonate of Lithia. (A remedy for calculus.)

Magne'sia. (Br. Ph.) Calcined Magnesia. See Class IX.

Magne'siæ Carbo'nas. (U.S. and Br. Ph.) Carbonate of Magnesia. See Class IX.

? Potas'sa Sulphura'ta. (Br. Ph.) Sulphurated Potash. The same as **Potassii Sulphuretum.**

Potas'sæ Bicarbo'nas. (U.S. and Br. Ph.) Bicarbonate of Potassa, or *Sal æratus.* A substance in white, colorless crystals, permanent in the air and wholly soluble in water.

Potas'sæ Carbo'nas. (U.S. and Br. Ph.) Carbonate of Potash; otherwise called Subcarbonate of Potash. A white crystalline powder, alkaline and caustic to the taste, very deliquescent, and readily soluble in water.

? Potas'sii Sulphure'tum. (U.S. Ph.) Sulphuret of Potassium.

Prepared Chalk. See **Creta Præparata.**

Prepared Oyster Shell. See **Testa Præparata.**

Sa'po. (U.S. Ph.) Soap.

So'dæ Bicarbo'nas. (U.S. and Br. Ph.) Bicarbonate of Soda.

So'dæ Carbo'nas. (U.S. and Br. Ph.) Carbonate of Soda.

So'dæ Carbo'nas Exsicca'ta. (U.S. and Br. Ph.) Dried Carbonate of Soda.

Solution of Ammonia. See **Ammoniæ Liquor.**

Solution of Potassa. See **Liquor Potassæ.**

Spir'itus Ammo'niæ Aromat'icus. (U.S. and Br. Ph.) Aromatic Spirit of Ammonia. See Class IV.

Sulphuret of Potassium. See **Potassii Sulphuretum.**

Tes'ta O'vi. Egg Shell.

Tes'ta Præpara'ta. (U. S. Ph.) Prepared Oyster Shell.

CLASS XXIII.

ANTHELMINTICS.

SUBSTANCES WHICH HAVE THE PROPERTY OF POISONING OR DEBILITATING WORMS IN THE ALIMENTARY CANAL, AND THUS RENDERING THEM MORE EASY OF EXPULSION. IN RELATION TO THEIR MODE OF OPERATION, IT IS PROBABLE THAT SOME ACT BY A DIRECTLY POISONOUS INFLUENCE UPON THE WORM, OTHERS BY A MECHANICAL AGENCY.

? Absin'thium. (U.S. Ph.) Wormwood. See Class II.; Section II.

Asagræ'a Officina'lis. See **Sabadilla.**

Ascle'pias Curassavi'ca. Bastard Ipecacuanha, or Blood Weed. (The expressed juice.)

Aspid'ium Fi'lix Mas. See **Filix.**

Asple'nium Fi'lix Fœm'ina, otherwise called *Aspid'ium Fi'lix Fœm'ina.* Female Fern.

Azed'arach. (U.S. Ph.) See Class IX.

Bastard Ipecacuanha. See **Asclepias Curassavica.**

Bear's-foot. See **Helleborus Fœtidus.**

Blood Weed. See **Asclepias Curassavica.**

Calomel. See **Hydrargyri Chloridum Mite,** and **Calomelas.**

Calom'elas. (Br. Ph.) Calomel. See Class XXI.

Cevadilla. See **Sabadilla.**

Chamomile, German. See **Matricaria.**

Chenopo'dium. (U.S. Ph.) Wormseed. The fruit of *Chenopo'dium anthelmin'ticum.*

Chloride of Sodium. See **Sodii Chloridum.**

Cinnabar. See **Hydrargyri Sulphuretum Rubrum.**

Common Salt. See **Sodii Chloridum.**

Cowhage. See **Mucuna.**

Cus'so. (Br. Ph.) Kousso, or Koosso. The flowers of *Braye'ra anthelmin'tica.* (A remedy for the tapeworm.)

Female Fern. See **Asplenium Filix Fœmina.**

Fern Root. See **Filix.**

Fi'lix. (Br. Ph.) Fern Root. The dried rhizome of *Aspid'ium Fi'lix Mas.* See next article.

Fi'lix Mas. (U.S. Ph.) Male Fern. The rhizoma of *Aspid'ium Fi'lix Mas.*

German Chamomile. See **Matricaria.**

Grana'ti Radi'cis Cor'tex. (U.S. Ph.) Bark of Pomegranate Root. The bark of the root of *Pu'nica grana'tum.*

Grana'ti Ra'dix. (Br. Ph.) Pomegranate Root. The same as **Granati Radicis Cortex.**

Helleb'orus Fœt'idus. Bear's-foot.

Hydrar'gyri Chlo'ridum Mi'te. (U.S. Ph.) Mild Chloride of Mercury, or Calomel. See Class XXI.

? Hydrar'gyri Sulphure'tum Ru'brum. (U.S. Ph.) Cinnabar. See Class XXI.

Kame'la. (Br. Ph.) The powder of the capsules of *Rottle'ra tincto'ria.* The same as **Rottlera.**

Koosso, or Kousso. See **Cusso.**

Li'quor Ba'rii Chlo'ridi. (U.S. Ph.) Solution of Chloride of Barium.

Male Fern. See **Filix Mas.**

Matrica'ria. (U.S. Ph.) German Chamomile. The flowers of *Matrica'ria chamomil'la.*

Me'lia Azed'arach. See **Azedarach.**

Mild Chloride of Mercury. See **Hydrargyri Chloridum Mite.**

Mucu'na. (U.S. Ph.) Cowhage. The hairs of the pods of *Mucu'na pru'riens.*

Pe'po. (U.S. Ph.) Pumpkin Seed. (A remedy for the tapeworm.)

Pinkroot. See **Spigelia.**

Powder of Tin. See **Stanni Pulvis.**

Pride of China, or Pride of India. See **Azedarach.**

? Red Sulphuret of Mercury. See **Hydrargyri Sulphuretum Rubrum.**

Rottle'ra. (U.S. Ph.) Kamela, or Kameela. The powder and hairs obtained from the capsules of *Rottle'ra tincto'ria.* (A remedy for the tapeworm.)

Rottle'ra Tincto'ria. See **Rottlera,** and **Kamela.**

Sabadil'la. (U.S. and Br. Ph.) Cevadilla. See Class IX.

Salt. See **Sodii Chloridum.**

Santon'ica. (U.S. and Br. Ph.) The unexpanded flowers and peduncles of *Artemis'ia con'tra* and of other species of *Artemisia* (U.S. Ph.). The unexpanded flower-heads of an undetermined species of *Artemisia* (Br. Ph.).

Santoni'num. (U.S. and Br. Ph.) Santonin. A crystalline neutral principle obtained from *Santon'ica.*

So'dii Chlo'ridum. (U.S. and Br. Ph.) Chloride of Sodium, or Common Salt. See Class II., Section V.

Solution of Chloride of Barium. See **Liquor Barii Chloridi.**

Spige'lia. (U.S. Ph.) Pinkroot. The root of *Spige'lia Marilan'dica.*

Stan'ni Pul'vis. Powder of Tin.

Tanace'tum. (U.S. Ph.) Tansy. The herb of *Tanace'tum vulga're.*

Tansy. See **Tanacetum.**

Terebin'thina. (U.S. Ph.) Turpentine. The concrete juice of *Pi'nus palus'tris* and other species of *Pinus.* See Class X.

Turpentine. See **Terebinthina.**

Vera'trum Sabadil'la. See **Sabadilla.**

Verno'nia Anthelmin'tica. An East Indian plant. (Also extolled as a bitter tonic.)

Wormseed. See **Chenopodium.**

CLASS XXIV.

DISINFECTANTS, AND ANTISEPTICS.*

SUBSTANCES WHICH POSSESS THE POWER OF DESTROYING MORBIFIC VIRUS OR MIASM, AND OF CORRECTING A TENDENCY TO PUTRESCENCE.

Aç'idum Hydrochlo'ricum. (Br. Ph.) Hydrochloric Acid. The same as **Acidum Muriaticum.**

Aç'idum Muriat'icum. (U.S. Ph.) Muriatic Acid. (Antiseptic.) See Classes II. and VI.

---

* With a few exceptions, substances that are antiseptic may be used as disinfectants also: those not so used are noted in the list. (See **Sodii Chloridum,** etc.)

Aç'idum Ni'tricum. (U.S. and Br. Ph.) Nitric Acid. (Antiseptic.) See Class II., Section V.

Aç'idum Nitrohydrochlo'ricum. The same as **Acidum Nitromuriaticum.**

Aç'idum Nitromuriat'icum. (U.S. Ph.) Nitromuriatic Acid. See Class XXI.

Aç'idum Sulphu'ricum. (U.S. and Br. Ph.) Sulphuric Acid. (Antiseptic.) See Class II., Section V.

Aç'idum Sulphuro'sum. (Br. Ph.) Sulphurous Acid. See Class XXI.

Æ'ther. (U.S. and Br. Ph.) Ether, or Sulphuric Ether. See Class V.

Al'cohol. (U.S. Ph.) (Antiseptic.)

Alu'minæ Sul'phas. Sulphate of Alumina. (Antiseptic.)

A'qua Chlorin'ii. (U.S. Ph.) Chlorine Water, or Solution of Chlorine.

Bromin'ium. (U.S. Ph.) Bromine.

Cal'cis Sul'phis. Sulphite of Lime.

Calx. (U.S. and Br. Ph.) Lime. See Class XVIII.

Calx Chlora'ta. (Br. Ph.) Chlorinated Lime. See next article.

Calx Chlorina'ta. (U.S. Ph.) Chlorinated Lime.

Car'bo Lig'ni. (U.S. and Br. Ph.) Charcoal.

Carbolic Acid. See **Phenic Acid.**

Charcoal. See **Carbo Ligni.**

Chloride of Lime. See **Calx Chlorinata.**

Chloride of Sodium. See **Sodii Chloridum.**

Chlo'ri Li'quor. (Br. Ph.) Solution of Chlorine.

Chlorinated Lime. See **Calx Chlorinata.**

Chlorine. See **Chlorinium.**

Chlorine Water. See **Aqua Chlorinii.**

Chlorin'ii Li'quor. See **Aqua Chlorinii.**

Chlorin'ium. Chlorine.

Common Salt. See **Sodii Chloridum.**

Copperas. See **Ferri Sulphas.**

Creasote. See **Creasotum.**

Creaso'tum. (U.S. and Br. Ph.) Creasote. See Class V.

Ether. See **Æther.**

Fer'ri Sul'phas. (U.S. and Br. Ph.) Sulphate of Iron. See Class I., Section II.

Glyceri'na. (U.S. Ph.) Glycerin. (Antiseptic.) See Class XIX.

Labarraque's Disinfecting Liquid. The same as **Liquor Sodæ Chlorinatæ.**

Ledoyen's Disinfecting Fluid. A solution of Nitrate of Lead, in the proportion of a drachm of the salt to an ounce of water.

Li'quor So'dæ Chlora'tæ. See **Sodæ Chloratæ Liquor.**

Li'quor So'dæ Chlorina'tæ. (U.S. Ph.) Solution of Chlorinated Soda.

Nitrate of Lead. See **Plumbi Nitras.**

Nitre, or Nitrate of Potash. See **Potassæ Nitras.**

Nitromuriatic Acid. See **Acidum Nitromuriaticum.**

Phen'ic Acid, otherwise called Carbolic Acid. A substance obtained by distillation from the oily portion of coal tar, and resembling creasote in its chemical relations and physical properties.

Plum'bi Ni'tras. (U.S. Ph.) Nitrate of Lead.

Potas'sæ Ni'tras. (U.S. and Br. Ph.) Nitrate of Potash, or Nitre. Chiefly employed as an antiseptic.

Potas'sæ Perman'ganas. (U.S. Ph.) Permanganate of Potash. See Class XVIII.

? Sac'charum. (U.S. Ph.) Sugar. (Antiseptic.)

Salt. See **Sodii Chloridum.**

So'dæ Chlora'tæ Li'quor. (Br. Ph.) Solution of Chlorinated Soda. The same as **Liquor Sodæ Chlorinatæ.**

? So'dæ Sul'phis. (U.S. Ph.) Sulphite of Soda.

So'dii Chlo'ridum. (U.S. and Br. Ph.) Chloride of Sodium, or Common Salt. (Antiseptic.) See Class I., Section II.

Solution of Chlorinated Soda. See **Liquor Sodæ Chlorinatæ.**

Solution of Chlorine. See **Aqua Chlorinii.**

Sugar. See **Saccharum.** (Antiseptic.)

Sulphate of Iron. See **Ferri Sulphas.**

Sulphite of Lime. See **Calcis Sulphis.**

Sulphuric Ether. See **Æther.**

CLASS XXV.

EXCITO-MOTOR STIMULANTS.

SUBSTANCES WHICH POSSESS THE POWER OF EXCITING, THROUGH THE SPINAL MARROW AND MOTOR NERVES, CONTRACTION OF THE MUSCLES OF THE BODY.*

Bean of St. Ignatius. See **Ignatia.**

Borax. See **Sodæ Boras.**

Bru'cia. An alkaloid obtained from nux vomica and the bean of St. Ignatius.

Ergot. See **Ergota.**

Ergo'ta. (U.S. and Br. Ph.) Ergot. The diseased seed of *Seca'le cerea'le* (U.S. Ph.). *Secale cereale:* the grain diseased by the presence of an imperfect fungus (Br. Ph.). (Uterine.)

Extrac'tum Can'nabis. (U.S. Ph.) Extract of Hemp. (Uterine.) See Class V.

Extrac'tum Can'nabis In'dicæ. (Br. Ph.) Extract of Indian Hemp. The same as **Extractum Cannabis.**

Fa'ba Sanc'ti Igna'tii. See **Ignatia.**

Gossy'pii Ra'dix. (Uterine.) See Class XIII.

Igna'tia. (U.S. Ph.) Bean of St. Ignatius. The seed of *Strych'nos Igna'tia.*

Nitrous Oxide. See **Oxidum Nitrosum.**

Nux Vom'ica. (U.S. and Br. Ph.) The seed of *Strych'nos nux vom'ica.*

? Ox'idum Nitro'sum. Nitrous Oxide (Gas). See Class V.

Seca'le Cerea'le. See **Ergota.**

So'dæ Bo'ras. (U.S. Ph.) Borate of Soda, or Borax. (Uterine.) See Class VI. and X.

Strych'nia. (U.S. and Br. Ph.) Strychnine. An alkaloid in the form of a white or grayish-white powder, of an intensely bitter taste, obtained from *Strych'nos nux vom'ica.*

---

* Several of these substances have a special direction to the uterus, and are marked *uterine.*

INDEX TO TABLE OF MATERIA MEDICA.

☞ In the following Index, a single number placed after the name denotes the class to which the article belongs: as, "Acacia, 19," "Alcohol, 5;" when two numbers occur, separated by a comma, the first refers to the class, the second to the section: as, "Acetate of Magnesia, 9, 2;" but if the numbers are joined by an "and," different classes are referred to: thus, "Adansonia Digitata, 2, 3 and 11, 3," implies that this belongs to the *second class, third section* and also to the *eleventh class, third section*. For the sake of brevity, Arabic numerals are employed in the Index instead of the Roman which occur in the Table.

INDEX TO TABLE OF MATERIA MEDICA.

EXPLANATION OF LATIN TERMS, PHRASES, ETC.

It is not the design of the following pages to present a general view or synopsis, however brief, of the elements of Latin grammar; but simply to make such explanations as seem necessary in order that the medical student who is unacquainted with Latin may be enabled to acquire a tolerable understanding of the phrases and sentences which he is constantly meeting with in works on Anatomy, Pharmacy, etc. Thus, in the following examples, *Extensor digitorum communis, Orbicularis palpebrarum, Orbicularis oculi, Collodium cum cantharide, Emplastrum ammoniaci cum hydrargyro, Hydrargyrum cum cretâ, Pilulæ aloes et mastiches, Pilulæ aloes et myrrhæ, Pilulæ ferri compositæ, Alnus nigra, Helleborus niger*, etc. etc., the mere English scholar has presented to his mind phrases each of which must appear to him like some long, unintelligible word; and the more he examines or compares such as seem to resemble each other, the more embarrassed and perplexed he must of necessity become.

Now, it is believed that, by a few comparatively simple explanations, the student will not only be enabled to remember such phrases more easily, because he will understand their construction,—and if he has occasion to write them will know how to write them correctly,—but he will be able to apply the same principles to hundreds of other phrases or sentences which he is liable to meet with from time to time, even in the most common works relating to medicine.

The rules or principles which he will have to learn, will be found comparatively brief, as well as few in number, his chief attention being directed to *examples*, consisting for the most part of compound names or short sentences, of frequent occurrence in medical works, and which, in any case, he ought to understand, if he aims to become a well-informed physician.

Nouns.

I. Every Latin noun (with some unimportant exceptions) changes its termination (or last syllable) according to its case. There are in all six cases: those most used are the *nominative, genitive*, and *ablative*. The nominative corresponds as to signification, in all essential respects, to the English nominative; the genitive is virtually the same as the English possessive; the ablative is the same as the English objective when governed by the prepositions *with, from, in*, or *by*. Next to the nominative, the genitive is of most frequent occurrence, and therefore of the greatest importance. In many instances it may be rendered by the English possessive, but it is generally preferable to translate it by the preposition *of*. Thus, we might render *ba'sis cer'ebri*, the "brain's base;" *hu'mor oc'uli*, the "eye's humor;" *ar'ma viro'rum*, the "men's arms;" but it is more elegant and more usual to say, the "base of [the] brain,"* the "humor of [the] eye,"* the "arms of [the] men," etc. We always say, however, "hartshorn" (*i.e.* hart's horn) for *cor'nu cer'vi*, and not "horn of the hart."

II. Latin nouns have been arranged under different classes (or declensions)

* It should be observed that in Latin there is no article, though the usage of the English language requires it in many cases to be supplied. ☞ The words supplied are enclosed in brackets.

according to the formation of the genitive. The first declension comprises such as have the nominative in *-a*, the genitive in *æ*, and the ablative in *-â:* as, nom. *ammo'nia*, "ammonia;" gen. *ammo'niæ*, "of ammonia;" abl. *ammo'niâ*, "with ammonia;" nom. *calum'ba*, "columbo;" gen. *calum'bæ*, "of columbo;" abl. *calum'bâ*, "with columbo;" nom. *cre'ta*, "chalk;" gen. *cre'tæ*, "of chalk;" abl. *cre'tâ*, "with chalk;" nom. *myr'rha*, "myrrh;" gen. *myr'rhæ*, "of myrrh," etc.: hence the phrases *li'quor ammo'niæ*, "liquor (or solution) of ammonia;" *infu'sum calum'bæ*, "infusion of columbo;" *tinctu'ra myr'rhæ*, "tincture of myrrh;" *hydrar'gyrum cum cre'tâ*, "mercury with chalk," etc. See example of the first declension given below

List of the principal Latin Nouns of the First Declension, occurring in Medical Terms and Phrases.

Aca'cia.	Cam'era.	Euphor'bia.	Lam'ina.	Myr'rha.
Achille'a.	Cam'phora.	Fæc'ula.	Lap'pa.	Natu'ra.
Aconi'tia.	Canel'la.	Fari'na.	Lavan'dula.	Neb'ula.
Adyna'mia.	Can'na.	Fas'cia.	Lep'ra.	Nectan'dra.
Althæ'a.	Cap'sula.	Fib'ula.	Leptan'dra.	Neural'gia.
Alu'mina.	Caro'ta.	Fis'tula.	Li'bra.	Nym'pha.
Amen'tia.	Cascaril'la.	For'ma.	Lin'ea.	Odontal'gia.
Ammo'nia.	Cas'sia.	For'mula.	Lin'gua.	Offici'na.
Ampul'la.	Cata'ria.	Fos'sa.	Lith'ia.	Oli'va.
Amyg'dala.	Ce'ra.	Frase'ra.	Lobe'lia.	Ophthal'mia.
Anasar'ca.	Cetra'ria.	Gal'la.	Lupuli'na.	Or'bita.
Anato'mia.	Char'tula.	Gambo'gia.	Lym'pha.	Pal'ma.
Angel'ica.	Chimaph'ila.	Gaulthe'ria.	Lyt'ta.	Papil'la.
Angustu'ra.	Chiret'ta.	Gem'ma.	Mac'ula.	Parei'ra.
An'ima.	Chol'era.	Ge'na.	Magne'sia.	Patel'la.
Anten'na.	Chor'da.	Gentia'na.	Magno'lia.	Phlegma'sia.
Aor'ta.	Chore'a.	Gille'nia.	Ma'la.	Phytolac'ca.
Aph'tha.	Cicu'ta.	Glan'dula.	Mamil'la.	Pil'ula.
Apoplex'ia.	Cimicif'uga.	Glyceri'na.	Mam'ma.	Pimen'ta.
A'qua.	Cincho'na.	Glycyrrhi'za.	Ma'nia.	Placen'ta.
Ara'lia.	Col'ica.	Gut'ta.	Man'na.	Plan'ta.
Ar'nica.	Coni'tia (Conei'a).	Guttaper'cha.	Maran'ta.	Pleu'ra.
Arte'ria.	Copai'ba.	Hæmorrha'gia.	Mas'sa.	Pneumo'nia.
Assafœt'ida.	Cor'nea.	Hedeo'ma.	Mate'ria.	Pod'agra.
Atro'phia.	Coro'na.	Hepat'ica.	Mati'ca.	Polyg'ala.
Atro'pia.	Cos'ta.	Heuche'ra.	Matrica'ria.	Por'ta.
Au'ra.	Cot'ula.	Ho'ra.	Maxil'la.	Potas'sa.
Auric'ula.	Cre'ta.	Hydropho'bia.	Medeci'na.	Pso'ra.
Ave'na.	Cube'ba.	Hyste'ria.	Medul'la.	Quas'sia.
Axil'la.	Curcu'ma.	Ichthyocol'la.	Melis'sa.	Quin'ia.
Axun'gia.	Diarrhœ'a.	Igna'tia.	Membra'na.	Ra'na.
Bac'ca.	Drach'ma.	Iner'tia.	Men'tha.	Resi'na.
Baril'la.	Dulcama'ra.	Intumescen'tia.	Mi'ca.	Ro'sa.
Bary'ta.	Dysente'ria.	In'ula.	Mistu'ra.	Rottle'ra.
Belladon'na.	Dyspep'sia.	Ipecacuan'ha.	Monar'da.	Rube'ola.
Braye'ra.	Dyspnœ'a.	Jala'pa.	Mor'phia.	Ru'bia.
Bul'la.	Ecto'pia.	Krame'ria.	Mor'rhua.	Ru'ta.
Bur'sa.	Epiph'ora.	Lach'ryma.	Mucu'na.	Sabadil'la.
Caf'fea.	Ergo'ta.	Lactu'ca.	Myr'cia.	Sabba'tia.
Calum'ba.	Essen'tia.	Lacu'na.	Myris'tica.	Sabi'na.

Example of a Noun of the First Declension, declined through all the Cases.

	Singular.		Plural.
Nom.	Ve'na, *a vein.*	Nom.	Ve'næ, *veins.*
Gen.	Ve'næ, *of a vein.*	Gen.	Vena'rum, *of veins.*
Dat.	Ve'næ, *to or for a vein.**	Dat.	Ve'nis, *to or for veins.**
Acc.	Ve'nam, *a vein.*†	Acc.	Ve'nas, *veins.*†
Voc.	Ve'na, *vein* (or *O vein*).‡	Voc.	Ve'næ, *veins* (or *O veins*).‡
Abl.	Ve'nâ, *in, with, or by a vein.*	Abl.	Ve'nis, *in, with, or by veins.*

* The *dative* case invariably implies the prepositions "to" or "for" understood.

† The *accusative* corresponds nearly to the English objective when governed by a transitive verb or by certain prepositions, as *ante, post, præter*. See page 687.

‡ The vocative (from *voco, voca'tum*, to "call") corresponds to what is termed by some English grammarians the *nominative case addressed:* it is used in calling to or addressing persons, and in apostrophizing inanimate objects.

Sali'va.	Serpenta'ria.	Tab'ula.	Tra'chea.	Vanil'la.
Sal'via.	Sil'ica.	Tæ'nia.	Tragacan'tha.	Varicel'la.
Sanguina'ria.	Simaru'ba.	Tapio'ca.	Tu'nica.	Vari'ola.
Santon'ica.	So'da.	Te'la.	Ul'na.	Ve'na.
Sarsaparil'la.	Spige'lia.	Terebin'thina.	Un'cia.	Vesa'nia.
Scap'ula.	Spi'na.	Ter'ra.	Ure'thra.	Vesi'ca.
Scarlati'na.	Spiræ'a.	Tes'ta.	Uri'na.	Vi'a.
Scil'la.	Spon'gia.	Theobro'ma.	U'va.	Vi'ola.
Scrof'ula.	Stillin'gia.	Tib'ia.	U'vula.	Vi'ta.
Scutella'ria.	Stri'a.	Tinctu'ra.	Vagi'na.	Vul'va.
Sen'ega.	Sutu'ra.	Tin'ea.	Valeria'na.	Winte'ra.
Sen'na.	Syn'ocha.	Tormentil'la.	Val'va.	Xanthorrhi'za.

☞ To the foregoing list belong all Latin nouns ending in *-a* (with the exception of a small number of the third declension ending in *-ma*, as *aroma*, *exanthema*, &c.). *They are all of the feminine gender*, excepting a very few which are rarely, if ever, found in works relating to medicine.

All nouns of the preceding list that have a plural, form the plural nominative in *-æ* (like the genitive singular), the genitive plural ending in *-a'rum: e.g. auric'ula*, an "auricle;" nom. pl. *auric'ulæ*, the "auricles;" gen. pl. *auricula'rum*, "of [the] auricles;"* *pal'pebra*, an "eyelid;" nom. pl. *pal'pebræ*, the "eyelids;" gen. pl. *palpebra'rum*, "of [the] eyelids:"* hence the phrases *sep'tum auricula'rum*, "septum of [the] auricles;"* *orbicula'ris palpebra'rum*, the "circular [muscle] of [the] eyelids,"* etc.

III. Nouns ending in *-e* usually make the genitive in *-es:* as, nom. *al'oë*, "aloes;" gen. *al'oës*, "of aloes;" nom. *mas'tiche*, "mastic;" gen. *mas'tiches*, "of mastic:" *e.g. pil'ulæ al'oes et mas'tiches*, "pills of aloes and mastic." Words of this class are of Greek origin; they are usually included under the first declension in the Latin grammars, probably because they belong to the first Greek declension. Those which have a plural, form it in *-æ:* as, *ac'ne*, a kind of eruption; plural *ac'næ*.

To this class belong all Latin nouns of Greek origin having the nominative singular in *-e:* as,—

Ac'ne.	Anemo'ne.	Cat'oche.	Daph'ne.	Stat'ice.
Aga've.	Argemo'ne.	Cynan'che.	Phleg'mone.	Syn'cope;

including the compounds of *ce'le* (Gr. κήλη, a "tumor"), if not Anglicized: as, *ceratoce'le*, "hernia of the cornea;" *hepatoce'le*, "hernia of the liver," etc.

IV. Latin nouns having the genitive in *-i*, are said to belong to the second declension. They may be divided into two principal classes, those ending in *-us* and those in *-um*. Of the first class the following examples may be given: nom. *caryophyl'lus*, a name of the "clove-tree," also used for "cloves;" gen. *caryophyl'li*, "of the clove-tree," or "of cloves;" nom. *hyoscy'amus*, "henbane;" gen. *hyoscy'ami*, "of henbane;" nom. *hu'mulus*, the "hop plant," or "hops;" gen. *hu'muli*, "of hops:" hence the following terms, *o'leum caryophyl'li*, "oil of cloves;" *hyoscy'ami fo'lia*, "leaves of hyoscyamus;" *infu'sum hu'muli*, "infusion of hops." See example given below.

Example of a Masculine Noun of the Second Declension, declined through all the Cases.

	Singular.		Plural.
Nom.	Dig'itus, *a finger*.	Nom.	Dig'iti, *fingers*.
Gen.	Dig'iti, *of a finger*.	Gen.	Digito'rum, *of fingers*.
Dat.	Dig'ito, *to or for a finger*.†	Dat.	Dig'itis, *to or for fingers*.†
Acc.	Dig'itum, *a finger*.†	Acc.	Dig'itos, *fingers*.†
Voc.	Dig'ite, *finger* (or *O finger*).†	Voc.	Dig'iti, *fingers* (or *O fingers*).†
Abl.	Dig'ito, *in, with, or by a finger*.	Abl.	Dig'itis, *in, with, or by fingers*.

* See note on page 660. † See notes * † ‡ on page 661.

List of Nouns ending in -us and -os, of the Second Declension.

Acan'thus.
Ac'arus.
Aç'inus.
Acu'leus.
Agar'icus.
Al'nus (f.).
Alve'olus.
Al'veus.
Al'vus (f.).
Am'nios.
An'gulus.
An'imus.
An'nulus.
A'nus.
Artic'ulus.
Asbes'tos.
Aspar'agus.
Astrag'alus.
Bac'culus.
Bo'lus.
Bul'bus.
Cac'tus.
Cal'amus.
Cal'culus.
Capil'lus.
Car'pus.
Car'thamus.
Caryophyl'lus.
Catar'rhus.
Chirur'gus.
Chon'drus.
Chy'lus.
Chy'mus.
Cir'rus.
Ci'trus (f.).
Cla'vus.
Coc'cus.
Con'gius.
Cro'cus.
Did'ymus.
Dig'itus.
Dios'pyros (f.).
Euon'ymus.
Fascic'ulus.
Fi'cus (f., rarely m.).
Fo'cus.
Fontic'ulus.
Frax'inus (f.).
Fu'cus.
Fun'dus.
Fun'gus.
Funic'ulus.
Furun'culus.
Fu'sus.
Glo'bus.
Gy'rus.
Helleb'orus.
Hidron'osus (f.).
Hu'merus.
Hu'mulus.
Hydron'osus (f.).
Hyoscy'amus.
Ic'terus.
Junip'erus (f.).
Lapil'lus.
Lau'rus (f.).
Lec'tus.
Lob'ulus.
Lo'bus.
Loc'ulus.
Lo'cus.
Lum'bus.
Lyc'opus.
Mal'leus.
Ma'lus (f.).
Med'icus.
Metatar'sus.
Mor'bus.
Mo'rus (f.).
Mos'chus.
Mu'cus.
Mus'culus.
Mus'cus.
Myr'tus (f.).
Næ'vus.
Na'nus.
Narcis'sus.
Na'sus.
Ner'vus.
No'dus.
Nu'cleus.
Octa'rius.
Oc'ulus.
Œsoph'agus.
Ophthal'mus.
Orbic'ulus.
Pal'pus.
Papy'rus.
Pedic'ulus.
Pem'phigus.
Phos'phorus.
Pi'lus.
Pi'nus (f.).
Po'lus.
Po'rus.
Pri'nos.
Pru'nus (f.).
Psellis'mus.
Pylo'rus.
Py'rus (f.).
Ra'dius.
Ra'mus.
Ranun'culus.
Rham'nus.
Riç'inus.
Rosmari'nus.
Ru'bus.
Sac'culus.
Sac'cus.
Sa'gus.
Sambu'cus (f.).
Scir'rhus.
Scopa'rius.
Scorbu'tus.
Scru'pulus.
Som'nus.
Spas'mus.
Stim'ulus.
Stom'achus.
Suc'cus.
Sul'cus.
Syn'ochus.
Syru'pus.
Ta'lus.
Tamarin'dus.
Tar'sus.
Ter'minus.
Tet'anus.
Thal'lus.
Thy'mus.
Tris'mus.
Trun'cus.
Tu'bulus.
Ty'phus.
Ty'pus.
Ul'mus (f.).
Umbili'cus.
U'terus.
Ventric'ulus.
Ven'tus.
Vi'rus (neut.).
Vis'cus* (*the mistletoe*).
Vitel'lus.

☞ A few masculine nouns of the second declension, derived from the Greek, end in *-os:* as, *Asbes'tos*, gen. *Asbes'ti*, *Am'nios*, gen. *Am'nii*, &c.

A very small number end in *-r:* as, *can'cer*, a "crab;" gen. *can'cri*, "of a crab;" nom. plu. *can'cri*, "crabs;" gen. plu. *cancro'rum*, "of crabs:" hence the phrase *cancrorum oculi*, "crabs' eyes;" nom. *vir*, a "man;" gen. *vi'ri*, "of a man;" nom. plu. *vi'ri*, "men;" gen. plu. *viro'rum*, "of men."

These nouns are mostly masculine, but a few are feminine (marked f. in the list), consisting chiefly of the names of trees (see page 680, ☞ *note*). One (*vi'rus*) is neuter. Those which have a plural, form the nominative plural by changing *-us* of the nominative singular into *-i* (the same as the genitive singular), the genitive plural ending in *-o'rum: e.g. dig'itus*, a "finger;" nom. pl. *dig'iti*, "fingers," or the "fingers;" gen. pl. *digito'rum*, "of [the] fingers;" *oc'ulus*, "eye;" nom. pl. *oc'uli*, the "eyes;" gen. pl. *oculo'rum*, "of [the] eyes:" hence the terms *exten'sor digito'rum*, "extender of the fingers," applied to a muscle; *moto'res oculo'rum*, "movers of the eyes," the name of a pair of nerves.

Of nouns ending in *-um*, the following may serve as examples: nom. *aconi'tum*, "aconite;" gen. *aconi'ti*, "of aconite;" nom. *argen'tum*, "silver;" gen. *argen'ti*, "of silver;" nom. *dor'sum*, the "back;" gen. *dor'si*, "of [the] back;" nom. *li'num*, "flax;" gen. *li'ni*, "of flax:" hence we have *aconi'ti fo'lia*, "leaves of aconite;" *argen'ti ni'tras*, "nitrate of silver;" *longis'simus dor'si*, the "longest [muscle] of the back;" *li'ni sem'ina*, "seeds of flax" or "flaxseed." See example given below.

Example of a Neuter Noun of the Second Declension, declined in full.

	Singular.		Plural.
Nom.	Ligamen'tum, *a ligament.*	Nom.	Ligamen'ta, *ligaments.*
Gen.	Ligamen'ti, *of a ligament.*	Gen.	Ligamento'rum, *of ligaments.*
Dat.	Ligamen'to, *to or for a ligament.*	Dat.	Ligamen'tis, *to or for ligaments.*
Acc.	Ligamen'tum, *a ligament.*	Acc.	Ligamen'ta, *ligaments.*
Voc.	Ligamen'tum, *ligament.*	Voc.	Ligamen'ta, *ligaments.*
Abl.	Ligamen'to, *in, with, or by a ligament.*	Abl.	Ligamen'tis, *in, with, or by ligaments.*

* *Vis'cus*, gen. *Vis'ceris*, a "bowel" or "viscus," is of the third declension.

List of Neuter Nouns, ending in -um and -on, of the Second Declension.

Absin'thium.
Ace'tum.
Aç'idum.
Aconi'tum.
Æquilib'rium.
Albur'num.
Al'lium.
Alu'minum.
Amen'tum.
'Ammoni'acum.
Am'nion.
Amo'mum.
Am'ylum.
Ane'thum.
Animal'culum.
Ani'sum.
Antimo'nium.
An'trum.
A'pium.
Apoç'ynum.
Arca'num.
Argen'tum.
Arsen'icum.
A'rum.
As'arum.
Aspid'ium.
Asple'nium.
Auran'tium.
Au'rum.
Bal'neum.
Bal'samum.
Ba'rium.
Benzo'inum.
Biho'rium.
Bismu'thum.
Bo'rium.
Bra'chium.
Bromin'ium.
Bro'mium.
Cad'mium.
Cæ'cum.
Cal'cium.
Cam'bium.
Can'crum.
Capit'ulum.
Cap'sicum.
Cardamo'mum.
Ca'rum.
Caryophyl'lum.
Casto'reum.
Centau'rium.
Cen'trum.
Cera'tum.
Cerebel'lum.
Cer'ebrum.
Ce'rium.
Ceta'ceum.
Chenopo'dium.
Chlo'ridum.
Chlo'rium.
Chlorofor'mum.
Chro'mium.
Cil'ium.
Cinnamo'mum.
Col'chicum.
Collo'dium.
Col'lum.
Collyr'ium.
Colum'bium.
Condimen'tum.
Coni'um.
Corian'drum.
Corpus'culum.
Cra'nium.
Crassamen'tum.
Creaso'tum.
Cu'prum.
Cydo'nium.
Cypripe'dium.
Decoc'tum.
Deliq'uium.
Delir'ium.
Delphin'ium.
Didym'ium.
Dor'sum.
Dracon'tium.
Duode'num.
Efflu'vium.
Elate'rium.
Elec'trum.
Elemen'tum.
Emplas'trum.
Epigas'trium.
Epip'loon.
Eupato'rium.
Extrac'tum.
Fermen'tum.
Ferrocyan'idum.
Fer'rum.
Fi'lum.
Fluo'rium.
Fœnic'ulum.
Fo'lium.
Fræ'num.
Frumen'tum.
Ful'crum.
Gal'banum.
Gan'glion.
Gelse'mium.
Gera'nium.
Ge'um.
Gossyp'ium.
Grana'tum.
Gra'num.
Guai'acum.
Gyp'sum.
Hæmatox'ylon.
Helian'themum.
Herba'rium.
Hi'lum.
Hor'deum.
Hydrar'gyrum.
Hydroph'yton, or Hydroph'ytum.
Hypochon'drium.
Hypogas'trium.
Il'ium.
Infundib'ulum.
Infu'sum.
Insec'tum.
Intes'tinum.
Iodin'ium.
Io'dium.
Irid'ium.
Is'chium.
Jas'minum.
Ju'gulum.
Ju'gum.
Ka'lium.
La'bium.
La'brum.
Lactuca'rium.
Lanta'nium, or Lan'thanum.
Lar'dum.
Lau'danum.
Lepidoden'dron.
Ligamen'tum.
Lig'num.
Lil'ium.
Linimen'tum.
Li'num.
Lirioden'dron.
Lith'ium.
Lixiv'ium.
Lomen'tum.
Lycopo'dium.
Magne'sium.
Mandib'ulum.
Marru'bium.
Marsu'pium.
Meco'nium.
Medicamen'tum.
Me'dium.
Mem'brum.
Men'struum.
Metal'lum.
Mezere'um.
Min'ium.
Mollus'cum.
Molybdæ'num.
Momen'tum.
Mon'strum.
Na'trium.
Necta'rium.
Ni'trum.
Olecra'non.
O'leum.
Oma'sum.
Omen'tum.
Oper'culum.
O'pium.
Or'ganum.
Orig'anum.
Os'tium.
Ova'rium.
Ov'ulum.
O'vum.
Ox'ydum, or Ox'idum.
Pala'tum.
Palla'dium.
Pedilu'vium.
Perian'thium.
Pericar'dium.
Perinæ'um.
Perios'teum.
Peritonæ'um.
Pet'alum.
Petroseli'num.
Phyllo'dium.
Phytozo'on, or Phytozo'um.
Pigmen'tum.
Plat'inum.
Plum'bum.
Poc'ulum.
Podophyl'lum.
Poma'tum.
Po'mum.
Potas'sium.
Princip'ium.
Proflu'vium.
Pru'num.
Puden'dum.
Punc'tum.
Pyr'ethrum.
Quadriho'rium.
Ramen'tum.
Receptac'ulum.
Rec'tum.
Reg'num.
Reme'dium.
Retinac'ulum.
Rhe'um.
Ros'trum.
Ruthe'nium.
Sac'charum.
Sa'crum.
Sanita'rium.
San'talum.
Santoni'num.
Sarmen'tum.
Scammo'nium.
Scopa'rium.
Scro'tum.
Scutel'lum.
Sçyb'alum.
Se'bum, or Se'vum.
Secre'tum.
Sedimen'tum.
Sele'nium.
Semicu'pium.
Semiho'rium.
Senso'rium.
Sep'alum.
Sep'tum.
Seques'trum.
Ser'icum.
Se'rum.
Ses'amum.
Se'vum.
Sig'num.
Siliç'ium.
So'dium.
Spec'trum.
Spec'ulum.
Spirac'ulum.
Spu'tum.
Stan'num.
Ster'num.
Stib'ium.
Stramo'nium.
Stra'tum.
Stron'tium.
Succeda'neum.
Suc'cinum.
Sulphure'tum.
Supercil'ium.
Suspir'ium.
Sym'bolum.
Tab'acum.
Tanace'tum.
Tarax'acum.
Tar'tarum.
Tegmen'tum.
Tellu'rium.
Temperamen'tum.
Tentac'ulum.
Tento'rium.
Tig'lium.
Tita'nium.
Tomen'tum.
Toxicoden'dron.
Trape'zium.
Triho'rium.
Trios'teum.
Trit'icum.
Tuber'culum.
Tym'panum.
Unguen'tum.
Ura'nium.
Vac'uum.
Vana'dium.
Vehic'ulum.
Ve'lum.
Vene'num.
Vera'trum.
Vestib'ulum.
Vexil'lum.
Vi'num.
Vit'rum.
Xanthox'ylum.
Yt'trium.
Zin'cum.
Zirco'nium.
Zo'on.
Zooph'ytum.

☞ A number of neuter nouns of the second declension, derived from the Greek, end in *-on*: as, *Amnion* (also written *Amnios*), gen. *Amnii*, *Epip'loon*, gen. *Epip'loi*, &c. These nouns have the accusative and vocative singular like the nominative: they form the other cases, both in the singular and plural, exactly like nouns in *-um*. Some words of this class are also written with *-um*: as, *Hydroph'yton* or *Hydroph'ytum*, *Phytozo'on* or *Phytozo'um*, &c.

Nouns belonging to the preceding class are of the neuter gender, and form the nominative plural by changing *-um* of the nominative singular into *-a*, the genitive plural ending in *-o'rum: e.g. bal'neum*, a "bath;" nom. pl. *bal'nea*, "baths;" gen. pl. *balneo'rum*, "of baths;" *fo'lium*, a "leaf;" nom. pl. *fo'lia*, "leaves;" gen. pl. *folio'-rum*, "of leaves." Nouns of the second declension, whether they end in *-us* or *-um*, have the dative and ablative singular in *-o*, and the dative and ablative plural in *-is: e.g. al'vo adstric'tâ*, "with the bowels bound" (or the "bowels being bound"), or constipated; *fis'tula in a'no*, "fistula in the anus;" *in u'tero*, "in the uterus;" *cum hydrar'gyro*, "with mercury;" *mas'sa de* (or *ex*) *hydrar'gyro*, "mass [prepared] from, or out of, mercury;" *oc'ulis*, "with [or by means of] the eyes;" *cum fo'liis*, "with the leaves," etc.

☞ It may be remarked that the ablative is often governed by some preposition expressed, such as *a* or *ab*, "from" or "by;" *cum*, "with;" *de*, "from," or "of;" *e* or *ex*, "out," or "out of;" *in*, "in" or "on," etc. But the preposition is also very frequently omitted. The foregoing phrases exhibit examples of both kinds.

V. Latin nouns which form the genitive in *-is*, are said to be of the third declension*: e.g.* nom. *a'cer*, a "maple-tree;" gen. *aç'eris*, "of a maple-tree;" nom. *æ'ther*, "ether;" gen. *æ'theris*, "of ether." Sometimes, as in the examples just cited, the genitive is formed by simply adding *-is* to the nominative. Nouns having the nominative in *-ma*, form the genitive by adding *-tis:* as, *der'ma, der'-matis.* But many nouns of the third declension are more or less irregular in

---

Examples of Nouns of the Third Declension, declined in full.

	Singular.		Plural.
Nom.	A'pex (m.), *a point.*	Nom.	Ap'ices, *points.*
Gen.	Ap'icis, *of a point.*	Gen.	Ap'icum, *of points.*
Dat.	Ap'ici, *to or for a point.*	Dat.	Apiç'ibus, *to or for points.*
Acc.	Ap'icem, *a point.*	Acc.	Ap'ices, *points.*
Voc.	A'pex, *point.*	Voc.	Ap'ices, *points.*
Abl.	Ap'ice, *in, with, or by a point.*	Abl.	Apiç'ibus, *in, with, or by points.*
Nom.	Cri'nis (m.), *a lock (of hair).*	Nom.	Cri'nes, *locks.*
Gen.	Cri'nis, *of a lock.*	Gen.	Crin'ium, *of locks.*
Dat.	Cri'ni, *to or for a lock.*	Dat.	Crin'ibus, *to or for locks.*
Acc.	Cri'nem, *a lock.*	Acc.	Cri'nes, *locks.*
Voc.	Cri'nis, *lock.*	Voc.	Cri'nes, *locks.*
Abl.	Cri'ne, *in, with, or by a lock.*	Abl.	Crin'ibus, *in, with, or by locks.*
Nom.	Dens (m.), *a tooth.*	Nom.	Den'tes, *teeth.*
Gen.	Den'tis, *of a tooth.*	Gen.	Den'tium, *of teeth.*
Dat.	Den'ti, *to or for a tooth.*	Dat.	Den'tibus, *to or for teeth.*
Acc.	Den'tem, *a tooth.*	Acc.	Den'tes, *teeth.*
Voc.	Dens, *tooth.*	Voc.	Den'tes, *teeth.*
Abl.	Den'te, *in, with, or by a tooth.*	Abl.	Den'tibus, *in, with, or by teeth.*
Nom.	Hu'mor (m.), *a humor.*	Nom.	Humo'res, *humors.*
Gen.	Humo'ris, *of a humor.*	Gen.	Humo'rum, *of humors.*
Dat.	Humo'ri, *to a humor.*	Dat.	Humo'ribus, *to or for humors.*
Acc.	Humo'rem, *a humor.*	Acc.	Humo'res, *humors.*
Voc.	Hu'mor, *humor.*	Voc.	Humo'res, *humors.*
Abl.	Humo're, *in, with, or by a humor.*	Abl.	Humo'ribus, *in, with, or by humors*
Nom.	Os (neut.), *a bone.*	Nom.	Os'sa, *bones.*
Gen.	Os'sis, *of a bone.*	Gen.	Os'sium, *of bones.*
Dat.	Os'si, *to a bone.*	Dat.	Os'sibus, *to or for bones.*
Acc.	Os, *a bone.*	Acc.	Os'sa, *bones.*
Voc.	Os, *bone.*	Voc.	Os'sa, *bones.*
Abl.	Os'se, *in, with, or by a bone.*	Abl.	Os'sibus, *in, with, or by bones.*
Nom.	Re'te (neut.), *a net.*	Nom.	Re'tia (ree'she-a), *nets.*
Gen.	Re'tis, *of a net.*	Gen.	Re'tium (ree'she-um), *of nets.*
Dat.	Re'ti, *to a net.*	Dat.	Ret'ibus, *to or for nets.*
Acc.	Re'te, *a net.*	Acc.	Re'tia, *nets.*
Voc.	Re'te, *net.*	Voc.	Re'tia, *nets.*
Abl.	Re'ti, *in, with, or by a net.*	Abl.	Ret'ibus, *in, with, or by nets.*

respect to the formation of the genitive: *e.g.* nom. *æ'tas* ("age"), gen. *ætu'tis;* nom. *albu'go* ("white of the eye"), gen. *albu'ginis;* nom. *a'pex* (a "point"), gen. *ap'icis;* nom. *calx* ("lime"), gen. *cal'cis.* Therefore, in order to avoid any possibility of misunderstanding, in all cases (except those in which the genitive is formed by simply adding *-is* or *-tis*) in the following list, the genitive has been spelled out in full. The *genders*, also, have been marked, as it is impossible to lay down any rule by which they could be positively determined. A few general observations, however, respecting genders, may be useful in assisting the memory of the learner. 1. Nouns in *-or* are nearly always masculine: as, *abduc'tor, ar'dor, ca'lor, constric'tor, depres'sor, la'bor, mo'tor,* etc. The only exceptions in the list are *ar'bor* (a "tree," fem.), and *mar'mor* ("marble," neut.). 2. Nouns in *-go* are feminine: as, *æru'go, albu'go, cali'go, cartila'go, rubi'go,* etc.; all those of this last termination form the genitive in *-ĭnis.* 3. Nouns of which the nominative ends in *-is* are feminine when they signify an *action, state,* or *process:* as, *dial'ysis,* the "act of dissolving;" *diaphore'sis,* the "act or state of perspiring," etc. (from the Greek). The genitive of this class of nouns is always the same as the nominative. 4. Those ending in *-iō*, formed from a verb, are invariably feminine: as, *abduc'tio* [from the verb *abdu'co, abduc'tum*], *emis'sio* [from *emit'to, emis'sum*], etc. 5. Those ending in *-ma,* which form the genitive by adding *-tis,* are from the Greek, and are without exception neuter: as, *aro'ma, co'ma, der'ma,* etc.

☞ Nouns in *-as,* having the genitive in *-a'tis,* formed from an adjective, as *muti'tas,* "dumbness" [from *mu'tus,* "dumb"], are feminine; and, by analogy, nouns of the same termination, indicating the combination of some acid with a base, as *ace'tas* (an "acetate"), *sul'phas* (a "sulphate"), are generally regarded as feminine; but this is disputed by others, and as words of this class are exclusively modern, there is no classical authority to which we can appeal to decide the question.*

Nouns of the third declension usually change the *-is* of the genitive into *-e,* to form the ablative: as, *can'tharis,* gen. *canthar'idis,* abl. *canthar'ide; ca'ro* ("flesh"), gen. *car'nis,* abl. *car'ne,* etc. See examples of nouns of the third declension on preceding page.

If the noun is masculine or feminine, the nominative plural is formed by changing the *-is* of the genitive singular into *-es:* as, *ca'lyx,* gen. *cal'ycis,* nom. pl. *cal'yces; can'tharis,* gen. *canthar'idis,* nom. pl. *canthar'ides;* but if neuter, the genitive singular is changed to *-a* or *-ia:* as, *a'cer,* gen. *aç'eris,* nom. pl. *aç'era; an'imal,* gen. *anima'lis,* nom. pl. *anima'lia; fora'men,* gen. *foram'inis,* nom. pl. *foram'ina.* ☞ It may be stated as a universal rule that, in Latin, *neuter nouns, or adjectives, of whatever declension, form the nominative plural in -a.*

---

* In the last United States as well as in the British Pharmacopœia (just published), nouns of this class are assumed to be feminine, and the accompanying adjectives and participles have the feminine termination. Accordingly, they now say *Hydrar'gyri Sul'phas Fla'va,* and not *Hydrar'gyri Sul'phas Fla'vus,* as given in former Pharmacopœias; *Zin'ci Carbo'nas Præcipita'ta* (not *Præcipita'tus*), etc. etc.

In the Pharmacopœia recently published under the authority of the Prussian Government (*Pharmacopœia Borussica,* Berolini, 1862), instead of such terms as *Plum'bi Ace'tas, Magne'siæ Sul'phas, Zin'ci Sul'phas,* &c., *Plum'bum Acet'icum* ("Acetic [or acetated] Lead"), *Magne'sia Sulphu'rica* ("Sulphuric [or sulphurated] Magnesia"), *Zin'cum Sulphu'ricum* ("Sulphuric [or sulphurated] Zinc"), &c. are employed; but *Ace'tas Plum'bicus* ("Plumbic Acetate"). *Sul'phas Magne'sicus* ("Magnesian Sulphate"), *Sul'phas Zin'cicus* ("Zincic Sulphate"), &c., are given as synonyms, the noun, as in the examples just cited, being invariably joined with a masculine adjective.

EXPLANATION OF LATIN TERMS, PHRASES, ETC.

List of Nouns of the Third Declension.

Abdo'men, gen. Abdom'*inis* (neut.).
Abductor, gen. Abducto'*ris* (m.).
Ab'ies, Abi'*etis* (f.).
Accip'iter, Accip'it*ris* (m.).
A'cer, Aç'e*ris* (neut.).
Ace'tas, Aceta'*tis* (f.).
Acotyle'don, -*is* (f.).
Adductor, -o'*ris* (m.).
A'deps, Ad'*ipis* (m.).
A'er, A'e*ris* (m.).
Æru'go, Æru'g*inis* (f.).
Æs, Æ'*ris* (neut.).
Æstas, Æsta'*tis* (f.).
Æ'tas, Æta'*tis* (f.).
Æ'ther, Æ'the*ris* (m.).
Æ'thiops, Æ'thio*pis* (m.).
Albu'go, Albu'g*inis* (f.)
Albu'men, Albu'm*inis* (neut.).
Al'etris, Alet'ri*dis* (f.).
Alu'men, Alu'm*inis* (neut.).
Amauro'sis (*id.**) (f.).
Am'yris, Amyr'*idis* (f.).
Anal'ysis (*id.*) (f.).
Aneuris'ma, -*tis* (neut.)
An'imal, -*is* (neut.).
An'ser, -*is* (m.).
An'themis, Anthem'*idis* (f.).
An'thrax, Anthra'*cis* (m.).
A'pex, Ap'*icis* (m.).
A'phis, Aph'*idis* (f.).
A'pis (*id.*) (f.).
Aposte'ma, -*tis*.
Appen'dix, Appen'di*cis* (f.)
Ar'bor, Ar'bo*ris* (m.).
Ar'dor, -o'*ris* (m.).
Aro'ma, Aro'ma*tis* (neut.).
Arthri'tis, Arthrit'*idis* (f.).
Arun'do, Arun'd*inis* (f.).
As'caris, Ascar'*idis* (f.)
Ascle'pias, Ascle'pia*dis* (f.).
Asth'ma, -*tis* (neut.).
Athero'ma, Athero'ma*tis* (neut.).
At'las, Atla*n*'*tis* (m.).
Auri'go, Aurig'*inis* (f.)
A'vis (*id.*) (f.).
Ax'is (*id.*) (m.).
Ba'sis (*id.*) (f.).
Ber'beris (*id.*) (f.).
Bicarbo'nas, Bicarbona'*tis* (f.)
Bichro'mas, Bichroma'*tis* (f.).
Bitar'tras, Bitartra'*tis* (f.).
Bitu'men, Bitu'm*inis* (neut.).
Bom'bax, Bomba'*cis* (f.).
Bora'go, Borag'*inis* (f.)
Bo'ras, Bora'*tis* (f.).
Bo'rax, Bora'*cis* (f.).
Bu'bo, Bubo'*nis* (m.).
Buccina'tor, -o'*ris* (m.).
Cacu'men, Cacu'm*inis* (neut.).
Cada'ver, Cadav'e*ris* (neut.).
Cali'go, Calig'*inis* (f.).
Ca'lor, -o'*ris* (m.).
Calx, Cal'*cis* (m.).
Ca'lyx, Cal'y*cis* (m.).
Can'nabis (*id.*) (f.).
Can'tharis, Canthar'*idis* (f.).
Ca'put, Cap'*itis* (neut.)
Car'bo, -o'*nis* (m.).
Carbo'nas, Carbona'*tis* (f.).
Carcino'ma, -*tis* (neut.)
Cardi'tis, Cardit'*idis* (f.).
Ca'ro, Car'*nis* (f.).
Cartila'go, Cartilag'*inis* (f.).
Ceru'men, Ceru'm*inis* (neut.).
Chlo'ras, Chlora'*tis* (f.).
Chloro'sis (*id.*) (f.).
Chrys'alis, Chrysal'*idis* (f.).
Cica'trix, Cicatri'*cis* (f.).
Ci'nis, Cin'e*ris* (m.).
Ci'tras, Citra'*tis* (f.).
Clas'sis (*id.*) (f.).
Climac'ter, -e'*ris* (m.).
Coc'cyx, Coccy'*gis* (m.)
Colocyn'this, Colocyn'thi*dis* (f.).
Co'ma, -*tis* (neut.).
Constric'tor, -o'*ris* (m.)
Cop'tis, Cop'ti*dis* (f.).
Cor, Cor'*dis* (neut.).
Cor'pus, Cor'po*ris* (neut.).
Cor'tex, Cor'*ticis* (m. and f.).
Cre'mor, -o'*ris* (m.).
Cri'nis (*id.*) (m.).
Cri'sis (*id.*) (m.)
Cro'ton, -o'*nis* (m.).
Crus, Cru'*ris* (neut.).
Cu'cumis (*id.*) (m.).
Cu'tis (*id.*) (f.)
Cy'cas, Cyc'a*dis* (f.).
Cys'tis, Cys'ti*dis* (f.).
Dens, Den'*tis* (m.).
Depres'sor, -o'*ris* (m.).
Der'ma, -*tis* (neut.).
Diabe'tes, Diabe'*tis*.
Diær'esis (*id.*) (f.).
Diagno'sis (*id.*) (f.).
Dial'ysis (*id.*) (f.).
Diaphore'sis (*id.*) (f.).
Diaphrag'ma, -*tis* (neut.).
Diath'esis (*id.*) (f.)
Dicotyle'don, -*is* (f.).
Digita'lis (*id.*) (f.).
Dila'tor, -o'*ris* (m.).
Diplo'ma, -*tis* (neut.).
Distor'tor, -o'*ris* (m.).
Dorema (neut.).
Do'sis (*id.*) (f.).
E'bur, Eb'o*ris* (neut.).
Ecchymo'ma, -*tis* (neut.).
Ecchymo'sis (*id.*) (f.).
Elephanti'asis (*id.*) (f.)
Empye'sis (*id.*) (f.).
Empyreu'ma, -*tis* (neut.)
Endosmo'sis (*id.*) (f.).
En'ema, Enem'a*tis* (neut.).
Enteri'tis (*id.*) (f.).
Epis'chesis (*id.*) (f.).
Epistax'is (*id.*) (f.).
Erec'tor, -o'*ris* (m.).
Erig'eron, -*tis* (neut.).
Erysip'elas, Erysipel'a*tis* (neut.).
Exanthe'ma, Exanthem'a*tis* (neut.).
Exosto'sis (*id.*) (f.).
Exten'sor, -o'*ris* (m.).
Falx, Fal'*cis* (f.).
Fe'bris (*id.*) (f.).
Fel, Fel'*lis* (neut.).
Fe'mur, Fem'o*ris* (neut.).
Filix, Fil'*icis* (f.).
Flex'or, -o'*ris* (m.).
Flos, Flo'*ris* (m.).
Flu'or, Fluo'*ris* (m.).
Fo'mes, Fom'*itis* (m.).
Fons, Fon'*tis* (m.).
Fora'men, Foram'*inis* (neut.).
For'ceps, For'ci*pis* (f.).
For'nix, For'ni*cis* (m.).
Fri'gus, Frig'o*ris* (neut.).
Frons, Fron'*dis* (f.).
Frons, Fron'*tis* (f.).
Fru'tex, Fru'*ticis* (m.).
Fuli'go, Fulig'*inis* (f.).
Fu'nis (*id.*) (m.).
Fur'fur, -*is* (m.).
Gastri'tis, Gastrit'*idis* (f.).
Gen'esis (*id.*) (f.).
Ge'nus, Gen'e*ris* (neut.).
Ger'men, Ger'm*inis* (neut.).
Glans, Glan'*dis* (f.).
Glu'ten, Glu'*tinis* (neut.).
Gra'men, Gram'*inis* (neut.).
Gram'ma, -*tis* (neut.).
Gran'do, Gran'd*inis* (f.).
Hæmop'tysis (*id.*) (f.).
Ha'lo, Halo'*nis* (m.).
He'lix, Hel'i*cis*.
He'par, Hep'a*tis* (neut.).
Her'pes, Herpe'*tis* (m.)
Hiru'do, Hiru'd*inis* (f.)
Hu'mor, -o'*ris* (m.).
Hydras'tis, Hydras'ti*dis* (f.).
Hy'drops, Hydro'*pis* (m.).
Hydrotho'rax, -a'*cis* (m.).
Hypochondri'asis (*id.*) (f.).
Ig'nis (*id.*) (m.).
Ima'go, Imag'*inis* (f.).
Impeti'go, Impetig'*inis* (f.).
In'dex, In'di*cis* (m. and f.).
In'guen, In'gu*inis* (neut.).
I'ris, Ir'*idis* (f.).
I'ter, It*in*'e*ris* (neut.).
Je'cur, Jec'o*ris* (neut.)
Ju'glans, Juglan'*dis* (f.).
Jus, Ju'*ris* (neut.).
Juven'tus, Juventu'*tis* (f.).
La'bor, Labo'*ris* (m.).
Lac, Lac'*tis* (neut.).
Lanu'go, Lanu'g*inis* (f.).
Lapis, Lap'*idis* (m.).
Lar'ynx, Laryn'*gis* (f.).
La'tex, Lat'*icis* (m.).
Legu'men, Legu'm*inis* (neut.).
Lens, Len'*tis* (f.).
Leon'todon, -*tis* (neut.)
Leva'tor, -o'*ris* (m.).
Lichen, Liche'*nis* (m.).
Li'en, Lie'*nis* (m.).
Li'mon, Limo'*nis* (m.).
Li'quor, -o'*ris* (m.).
Li'vor, -o'*ris* (m.).
Lix, Li'*cis* (f.).
Lu'es, Lu'*is* (f.).
Lumba'go, Lumbag'*inis* (f.).
Ma'cis, Maç'*idis* (f.).
Mag'nes, Magne'*tis* (m.).
Mar'cor, -o'*ris* (m.).
Mar'mor, Mar'mo*ris* (neut.).
Mas, Ma'*ris* (m.).
Ma'trix, Matri'*cis* (f.).
Medica'men, Medicam'*inis* (neut.).
Mel, Mel'*lis* (neut.).
Mens, Men'*tis* (f.).
Men'sis (*id.*) (m.).
Menyan'thes, Menyan'th*is*.
Mias'ma, -*tis* (neut.).
Moli'men, Molim'*inis* (neut.).
Mors, Mor'*tis* (f.).

* *Id.* placed after the noun denotes that the genitive is the same (*idem*) as the nominative.

Mos, Mo'*ris* (m.), *manner* or *custom*.
Mo'tor, -o'*ris* (m.).
Mucila'go, Mucilag'*inis* (f.).
Mu'rias, Muria'*tis* (f.).
Mur'mur, -*is* (neut.).
Mu'titas, Mutita'*tis* (f.)
Narco'ma, -*tis* (neut.).
Na'ris (*id.*) (f.).
Nata'tor, -o'*ris* (m.).
Neuro'sis (*id.*) (f.).
Ni'tras, Nitra'*tis* (f.).
Nox, Noc'*tis* (night) (f.).
Nu'trix, Nutri'*cis* (f.).
Nux, Nu'*cis* (f.).
Ob'stetrix, Obstetri'*cis* (f.).
Oc'ciput, Occip'*itis* (neut.).
On'yx, On'y*chis* (m. and f.).
Or'do, Or'*dinis* (m.).
Ori'go, Orig'*inis* (f.).
Os, O'*ris* (neut.).
Os, Os'*sis* (neut.).
O'vis (*id.*) (f.).
Ox'alas, Oxala'*tis* (f.).
Pa'nax, Pan'a*cis* (f.).
Pan'creas, Pancre'a*tis* (neut.).
Pa'nis (*id.*) (m.).
Papa'ver, Papav'er*is* (neut.).
Paral'ysis (*id.*) (f.).
Pa'ries, Pari'e*tis* (m.).
Pathe'ma, -*tis* (neut.).
Pec'ten, Pec'*tinis* (m. and neut.).
Pec'tus, Pec'to*ris* (neut.).
Pel'vis (*id.*) (f.).
Pe'po, Pepo'*nis* (m.).
Perman'ganas, -a'*tis* (f.).
Pertus'sis (*id.*) (f.).
Pes, Pe'*dis* (m.).
Pes'tis (*id.*) (f.).
Pha'lanx, Phalan'*gis* (f.).
Phar'ynx, Pharyn'*gis* (f.).
Phos'phas, Phospha'*tis* (f.).
Phthi'sis (*id.*) (f.).
Pi'per, Pip'er*is* (neut.).
Pis'cis (*id.*) (m.).
Pix, Pi'*cis* (f.).
Planta'go, Plantag'*inis* (f.).
Plas'ma, -*tis* (neut.).
Pneuma, -*tis* (neut.).
Pol'lex, Pol'*licis* (m.).
Pon'dus, Pon'de*ris* (neut.).
Pons, Pon'*tis* (m.).
Pop'les, Pop'*litis* (m.).
Porri'go, Porrig'*inis* (f.).
Pris'ma, Pris'ma*tis* (neut.).
Probos'cis, Probos'ci*dis* (f.).
Prona'tor, -o'*ris* (m.).
Propa'go, Propag'*inis* (f.).
Pruri'go, Prurig'*inis* (f.).
Pu'bes, Pu'b*is* (f.).
Pul'mo, Pulmo'*nis* (m.).
Pul'vis, Pul'ver*is* (m.).
Pus, Pu'*ris* (neut.).
Puta'men, Putam'*inis* (neut.).
Pyr'amis, Pyram'i*dis* (f.).
Pyro'sis (*id.*) (f.).
Qua'drans, Quadran'*tis* (m.).
Ra'chis, Ra'cheos (f.).
Ra'dix, Radi'*cis* (f.).
Reg'imen, Regim'*inis* (neut.).
Ren, Re'*nis* (m.).
Re'te, Re'*tis* (neut.).
Retrac'tor, -o'*ris* (m.).
Rha'chis, Rha'*cheos*. See Rachis.
Rheu'ma, -*tis* (neut.).
Rhizo'ma, -*tis* (neut.).
Rhus, Rho'*is* (f. and m.)
Ri'gor, -o'*ris* (m.).
Rota'tor, -o'*ris* (m.).
Rubi'go, Rubig'*inis* (f.)
Ru'mex, Ru'm*icis* (m.)
Sal, Sa'l*is* (m.).
Sa'lix, Sal'i*cis* (f.).
San'guis, San'gui*nis* (m.).
San'itas, Sanita'*tis* (f.).
Sa'po, Sapo'*nis* (m.).
Sarco'ma, Sarco'ma*tis* (neut.).
Sarx, Sar'*cos* (f.).
Scan'sor, -o'*ris* (m.).
Se'des, Se'*dis* (f.).
Se'men, Sem'*inis* (neut.).
Senec'tus, Senectu'*tis* (f.).
Serpi'go, Serpig'*inis* (f.).
Si'lex, Sil'*icis* (m. or f.)
Sil'icas, Silica'*tis* (f.).
Sina'pis (*id.*) (f.).
Si'phon or Si'pho, o'*nis* (m.).
Si'tis (*id.*) (f.).
Sol, So'*lis* (m.).
Solida'go, Solidag'*inis* (f.).
So'por, -o'*ris* (m.).
Spa'dix, Spadi'*cis* (m.).
Spas'ma, Spas'ma*tis* (neut.).
Sper'ma, -*tis* (neut.).
Sphinc'ter, -e'*ris* (m.)
Sta'men, Stam'*inis* (neut.).
Ste'ar, Ste'a*tis* (neut.).
Ster'tor, -o'*ris* (m.).
Stig'ma, Stig'ma*tis* (neut.).
Sto'ma, -*tis* (neut.).
Sto'rax, Stora'*cis* (m.).
Stu'por, -o'*ris* (m.).
Sty'rax, Styra'*cis* (m. and f.).
Su'dor, Sudo'*ris* (m.).
Sul'phas, Sulpha'*tis* (f.).
Sul'phis, Sulphi'*tis* (f.).
Sul'phur, Sul'phur*is* (neut.).
Sympto'ma, -*tis* (neut.)
Synop'sis (*id.*) (f.).
Syn'thesis (*id.*) (f.).
Syph'ilis, Syphil'*idis* (f.).
Syste'ma, -*tis* (neut.).
Ta'bes, Ta'b*is* (f.).
Tax'is (*id.*) (f.).
Tec'trix, Tectri'*cis* (f.).
Teg'men, Teg'm*inis* (neut.).
Tem'pus, Tem'po*ris* (neut.).
Ten'do, Ten'*dinis* (m.).
Ten'sor, -o'*ris* (m.).
Tes'tis (*id.*) (m. or f.).
Testu'do, Testu'd*inis* (f.).
The'nar, Then'ar*is* (neut.).
The'sis (*id.*) (f.).
Tho'rax, Thora'*cis* (m.)
Thus, Thu'*ris* (neut.).
Tor'men, Tor'm*inis* (neut.).
Tre'mor, -o'*ris* (m.).
Tricho'ma, -*tis*.
Trochan'ter, -e'*ris* (m.)
Tu'ber, Tu'ber*is* (neut.).
Tu'mor, -o'*ris* (m.).
Ul'cus, Ul'çe*ris* (neut.).
Un'guis (*id.*) (m.).
Ure'do, Ured'*inis* (f.).
Ure'ter, Urete'*ris* (m.).
Va'por, -o'*ris* (m.).
Va'rix, Var'i*cis* (m.).
Vas, Va'*sis* (neut.), pl. of second declension.
Ven'ter, Ven'*tris* (m.).
Ve'nus, Ven'*eris* (f.).
Ver'mis (*id.*) (m.).
Ver'tex, Ver'*ticis* (m.).
Vis (*id.*) (f.), pl. Vi'res.
Vis'cus, Vis'çe*ris* (neut.).
Vi'tis (*id.*) (f.).
Vo'mer, -*is* (m.).
Vor'tex, Vor'*ticis* (m.).
Vox, Vo'*cis* (f.).
Vul'nus, Vul'n*eris* (neut.).
Zin'giber, Zingib'er*is* (neut.).

To these may be added the very numerous class of nouns in -*io*, derived from the supines of verbs by simply dropping the -*um* of the supine and substituting -*io*: for example, from *abdu'co*, *abduct-um*, to "abduct," we have *abduc'tio*, "abduction;" from *adhæ'reo*, *adhæ'sum*, to "adhere," we have *adhæ'sio*, "adhesion," &c. All such nouns are of the feminine gender; they invariably form the genitive by adding -*nis* to the nominative: *e.g.* *abduc'tio*, *abductio'nis*, *adhæsio*, *adhæsio'nis*, and so on. It may be observed that English nouns in -*ion*—such as *caution*, *depression*, *lotion*, *motion*, *occasion*, *retention*, *repulsion*, *tension*, &c. &c.—are, with scarcely an exception, derived from Latin nouns of the class alluded to, by simply dropping the -*is* of the genitive; as, *motio*, gen. *motion-is*, "motion;" *tensio*, gen. *tension-is*, "tension," &c.

VI. Latin nouns having the nominative in -*us* or -*u*, and the genitive like the nominative, are said to be of the fourth declension: *e.g.* nom. *a'cus*, a "needle;" gen. *a'cus*, "of a needle." Some grammarians suppose that the original form of the genitive was -*uis*, and that this was afterwards contracted into -*us*. Be this as it may, it is usual, in order to mark the difference between the nominative and genitive, to write the latter with a circumflex accent, which is a common sign of contraction: *e.g.* nom. *duc'tus*, a "duct;" gen. *duc'tûs*, "of a duct." So we have—nom. *cor'nus flo'rida*, gen. *cor'nûs flo'ridæ;* nom. *quer'cus al'ba*, gen. *quer'cûs al'bæ*, etc.: hence the terms *decoc'tum cor'nûs flo'ridæ* ("decoction of dogwood"), *decoc'tum quer'cûs al'bæ* ("decoction of white oak [bark]"). Nouns of this class form the ablative in *-u*, the nominative plural in *-us*, and the genitive plural in *-uum:* thus, *a'cus*, a "needle," has in the ablative *a'cu*, "in, with, from, or by a needle;" nom pl. *a'cus*, "needles;" gen. pl. *ac'uum*, "of needles;" *duc'tus*, a "duct;" abl. *duc'tu*, "with a duct;" nom. pl. *duc'tus*, "ducts;" gen. pl. *duc'tuum*, "of ducts," etc Nouns having the nominative singular in *-u*, are of the neuter gender, and have the same termination in all the cases of the singular. Like all neuter nouns of whatever declension, they form their plural in *-a: e.g. ge'nu*, a "knee;" gen. *ge'nu* or *ge'nûs*, "of a knee;" abl. *ge'nu*, "with a knee;" nom. pl. *gen'ua*, "knees," gen. pl *gen'uum*, 'of knees." *Cor'nu* (a "horn") is declined in precisely the same manner: hence we have the terms *cor'nu cer'vi*, "hart's horn;" *cor'nua u'teri*, "horns of the uterus;" *gen'ua val'ga*, "crooked or distorted knees," etc.

List of the most important Nouns of the Fourth Declension.

Abor'tus.	Cor'nu (neut.).	Gus'tus.	Pas'sus.	Si'tus.
Absces'sus.	Cor'nus (f.).	Hab'itus.	Plex'us.	Spir'itus.
A'cus.	Cu'bitus.	Hal'itus.	Po'tus.	Subsul'tus.
Afflux'us.	Decu'bitus.	Haus'tus.	Proces'sus.	Tac'tus.
Appara'tus.	Descen'sus.	Ic'tus.	Prolap'sus.	Tinni'tus.
Aquæduc'tus.	Duc'tus.	Lu'sus.	Pul'sus.	Trac'tus.
Ar'cus.	Fla'tus.	Ma'nus.	Quer'cus (f.).	Tran'situs.
Ascen'sus.	Flux'us.	Mo'tus.	Ri'sus.	Vic'tus.
Audi'tus.	Fœ'tus.	Ni'sus.	Sen'sus.	Vi'sus.
Co'itus.	Fruc'tus.	Olfac'tus.	Sex'us.	Vom'itus.
Congres'sus.	Ge'nu (neut.).	Par'tus.	Si'nus.	Vul'tus.

It may be observed that all Latin nouns ending in *-us*, and derived from the supine of a verb by simply changing *-m* to *-s*, are of the fourth declension and masculine gender: *e.g. audi'tus*, "hearing" [from *au'dio, audi'tum*, to "hear"]; *duc'tus*, a "duct," or "canal" [from *du'co, duc'tum*, to "lead," to "convey"]; *ic'tus*, a "stroke" [from *i'co, ic'tum*, to "strike"]; *par'tus*, "parturition" [from *pa'rio, par'tum*, to "bring forth"]; *pas'sus*, a "step" (*i.e.* an "opening" or "extension of the legs") [from *pan'do, pan'sum* or *pas'sum*, to "open," "expand," or "ex-

Examples of Nouns of the Fourth Declension, declined in full.

Fructus, *fruit* (masc.).

	Singular.		Plural.
Nom.	Fruc'tus, *fruit.*	Nom.	Fruc'tus, *fruits.*
Gen.	Fruc'tûs, *of fruit.*	Gen.	Fruc'tuum, *of fruits.*
Dat.	Fruc'tui, *to or for fruit.*	Dat.	Fruc'tibus, *to or for fruits.*
Acc.	Fruc'tum, *fruit.*	Acc.	Fruc'tus, *fruits.*
Voc.	Fruc'tus, *fruit.*	Voc.	Fruc'tus, *fruits.*
Abl.	Fruc'tu, *in, with, or by fruit.*	Abl.	Fruc'tibus, *in, with, or by fruits.*

Cornu, *a horn* (neut.).

Nom.	Cor'nu, *a horn.*	Nom.	Cor'nua, *horns.*
Gen.	Cor'nûs *or* Cor'nu,* *of a horn.*	Gen.	Cor'nuum, *of horns.*
Dat.	Cor'nu, *to or for a horn.*	Dat.	Cor'nibus, *to or for horns.*
Acc.	Cor'nu, *a horn.*	Acc.	Cor'nua, *horns.*
Voc.	Cor'nu, *horn.*	Voc.	Cor'nua, *horns.*
Abl.	Cor'nu, *in, with, or by a horn.*	Abl.	Cor'nibus, *in, with, or by horns.*

* Always *cor'nu* in medical phrases: *e.g. rasu'ræ cor'nu cer'vi* (not *cor'nûs cer'vi*), "shavings of hartshorn."

tend"]; *plex'us*, a "knitting together," a "network" [from *plec'to, plex'um*, to "knit," to "intertwine"]; *po'tus*, a "drink," or "drinking" [from *po'to, pota'tum* or *po'tum*, to "drink"], etc. etc.*

VII. Latin nouns having the nominative in *-es* and the genitive in *-e'i* are of the fifth declension. They form the ablative in *-e*, the nominative plural like the nominative singular, the genitive plural in *-e'rum*, and the ablative plural in *-e'bus*: *e.g.* nom. *di'es*, a "day;" gen. *die'i*, "of a day;" abl. *di'e*, "in a day;" nom. pl. *di'es*, "days;" gen. *die'rum*, "of days;" abl. pl. *die'bus*, "in, on, or with days:" so, nom. *res*, a "thing;" gen. *re'i*, abl. *re*, nom. pl. *res*, gen. pl. *re'rum*, abl. pl. *re'bus*, etc. etc.: hence the phrases, *alter'nis die'bus*, "on alternate days;" *re'rum natu'ra*, the "nature of things;" *res con'tra natu'ram*, "things against nature," etc. Nouns of the fifth declension are feminine, excepting *dies*, a "day," which is usually masculine,† but sometimes feminine. See examples given below.

List of Nouns of the Fifth Declension.

A'cies.	Ca'ries.	Gla'cies.	Proflu'vies.	Sca'bies.
Balbu'ties.	Di'es.	Inglu'vies.	Ra'bies.	Spe'cies.
Calvi'ties.	Fa'cies.	Ma'cies.	Res.	Spes.
Cani'ties.	Fi'des.	Molli'ties.	Sa'nies.	Superfic'ies.

Indeclinable Nouns.

Some Pharmacopœial (Latinized) names are indeclinable: that is to say, the termination remains the same through all the cases: *e.g.* nom. *Mati'co*, gen. *Mati'co*, etc.: hence the phrase, *Infu'sum Mati'co*, "infusion of matico:"‡ so *Al'cohol, Azed'arach, Bu'chu* (or *Buc'co*), *Cat'echu, Cus'so* (or *Koos'so*), *El'emi, Ki'no, Sa'go, Sas'safras*, etc. Accordingly, we have *Tinctu'ra Bu'chu, Tinctu'ra Cat'echu, Unguen'tum El'emi, Tinctu'ra Kino*, etc. The gender of the greater number of these nouns would seem to be undetermined; it is important, however, to observe that *Alcohol* is always neuter; therefore we must say, *Al'cohol Dilu'tum, Al'cohol For'tius*, etc., not *Al'cohol Dilu'tus* or *For'tior*.

Nouns of the Fifth Declension, declined in full.

Singular.		Plural.	
Nom.	Di'es, *a day.*	Nom.	Di'es, *days.*
Gen.	Die'i, *of a day.*	Gen.	Die'rum, *of days.*
Dat.	Die'i, *to a day.*	Dat.	Die'bus, *to days.*
Acc.	Di'em, *a day.*	Acc.	Di'es, *days.*
Voc.	Di'es, *day.*	Voc.	Di'es, *days.*
Abl.	Di'e, *in, with, or by a day.*	Abl.	Die'bus, *in, with, or by days.*
Nom.	Res, *a thing.*	Nom.	Res, *things.*
Gen.	Re'i, *of a thing.*	Gen.	Re'rum, *of things.*
Dat.	Re'i, *to a thing.*	Dat.	Re'bus, *to things.*
Acc.	Rem, *a thing.*	Acc.	Res, *things.*
Voc.	Res, *thing.*	Voc.	Res, *things.*
Abl.	Re, *in, with, or by a thing.*	Abl.	Re'bus, *in, with, or by things.*

* Hence the phrases *ma'nia a po'tu*, "madness from drinking;" *in par'tu*, "in parturition;" *in si'tu*, "in situation;" *in tran'situ*, "in passage;" *pa'ri pas'su*, "with an equal step or pace,"—that is, "proceeding side by side."

† In stating that *dies* is usually masculine, it is simply meant that the Roman authors commonly join it with a masculine adjective. It is scarcely necessary to observe that this, like all other questions relating to language, is to be decided by the *usage of the best writers or speakers*. As an illustration of the power of usage, it may be remarked that in English the *sun*, in poetical language, is always masculine, the *moon* always feminine; and any one would be laughed at who should speak of the sun as "she" or the moon as "he." Yet in German the moon is always masculine and the sun always feminine. The only explanation to be given is that the usage of the language has made it so.

‡ *Mati'ca*, however, the Pharmacopœial name of the same substance (according to the British Pharmacopœia), is declinable, and belongs to the first declension, making the genitive in *-æ*: as, *Infusum Maticæ, Tinctura Maticæ*, etc.

Adjectives.

Latin adjectives may be divided into two great classes, namely, those of the first and second declensions, and those of the third declension.

VIII. Adjectives of the first class have the masculine in *-us*, the feminine in *-a*, and the neuter in *-um*, the feminine corresponding exactly to nouns of the first declension; the masculine and neuter corresponding to nouns of the second declension in *-us* and *-um* respectively. Accordingly, if an adjective of this class—take *la'tus*, "broad," for example—is to be joined to a masculine noun, it retains its first termination in *-us* (the usual form in which such words are given in the dictionaries); if to a feminine noun, *-us* must be changed into *-a;* if to a neuter noun, into *-um:* hence we have *mus'culus la'tus*, a "broad muscle;" *fas'cia la'ta*, a "broad fascia;" *ligamen'tum la'tum*, a "broad ligament;" because *mus'culus* is masculine, *fas'cia*, feminine, and *ligamen'tum*, neuter. The cases of the adjectives, both singular and plural, are in these examples formed precisely in the same manner as the nouns to which they are joined. Accordingly we have in the

Genitive:
Mus'culi la'ti, "of the broad muscle."
Fas'ciæ la'tæ, "of the broad fascia."
Ligamen'ti la'ti, "of the broad ligament."

Ablative:
Mus'culo la'to, "with or in the broad muscle."
Fas'ciâ la'tâ, "with or in the broad fascia."
Ligamen'to la'to, "with or in the broad ligament."

Nominative plural:
Mus'culi la'ti, "broad muscles."
Fas'ciæ la'tæ, "broad fasciæ."
Ligamen'ta la'ta, "broad ligaments."

Genitive plural:
Musculo'rum lato'rum, "of the broad muscles."
Fascia'rum lata'rum, "of the broad fasciæ."
Ligamento'rum lato'rum, "of the broad ligaments."

In like manner, if the noun should be of the third declension, the adjective changes so as to correspond in gender and case as well as number (though it does *not* change according to the declension).

Nominative singular:
Ten'do la'tus, a "broad tendon."
Cartila'go la'ta, a "broad cartilage."
Os la'tum, a "broad bone."

Genitive:
Ten'dinis la'ti, "of a broad tendon."
Cartilag'inis la'tæ, "of a broad cartilage."
Os'sis la'ti, "of a broad bone."

Ablative:
Ten'dine la'to, "with or in a broad tendon."
Cartilag'ine la'tâ, "with or in a broad cartilage."
Os'se la'to, "with or in a broad bone."

Nominative plural:
Ten'dines la'ti, "broad tendons."
Cartilag'ines la'tæ, "broad cartilages."
Os'sa la'ta, "broad bones."

Genitive plural:
Ten'dinum lato'rum, "of broad tendons."
Cartilag'inum lata'rum, "of broad cartilages."
Os'sium lato'rum, "of broad bones."

Ablative plural:
Tendin'ibus la'tis, "with broad tendons."
Cartilagin'ibus la'tis, "with broad cartilages."
Os'sibus la'tis, "with broad bones."

List of the most important Adjectives of the First and Second Declensions.

Acera'ceus, *resembling the maple.*
Acer'bus, *harsh.*
Acet'icus, *acetic.*
Aç'idus, *acid.*
Acti'vus, *active.*
Æ'quus, *equal.*
Aera'tus (part.*), *aerated.*
Æthe'reus, *ethereal.*
Africa'nus, *African.*
Ai'dicus (or Æ'dicus), *pertaining to the pudenda.*
Al'bus, *white.*
Al'gidus, *cold, or chilled with cold.*
Ama'rus, *bitter.*
America'nus, *American.*
Amœ'nus, *pleasant.*
Anella'tus, *having small rings.*
An'glicus, *English.*
Annula'tus, *annulated, having rings.*
Anseri'nus, *of or pertaining to a goose.*
Anti'cus, *anterior.*
Anti'quus, *ancient.*
Antisep'ticus, *antiseptic.*
Aquo'sus, *aqueous.*
Ar'duus, *difficult, arduous.*
Ar'idus, *arid, dry.*
Articula'tus, *articulated.*
Asiat'icus, *Asiatic.*
Aton'icus, *atonic.*

* Part., an abbreviation for "participle."

Bo'nus, *good.*
Bovi'nus, *of or pertaining to an ox.*
Brevis'simus, *shortest.*
Calcina'tus (part.), *calcined.*
Cal'idus, *warm.*
Cal'vus, *bald.*
Can'didus, *white.*
Cani'nus, *canine.*
Ca'nus, *hoary or white.*
Carbon'icus, *carbonic.*
Caus'ticus, *caustic.*
Ca'vus, *hollow.*
Cenot'icus, *pertaining to evacuations.*
Chem'icus, *chemical.*
Cinchona'ceus, *resembling the* Cinchona.
Cine'reus, *ash-colored.*
Cinet'icus, *pertaining to motion, or to the muscles.*
Cla'rus, *clear.*
Clin'icus, *clinic.*
Clusia'ceus, *resembling the* Clusia.
Cœli'acus, *cœliac.*
Complex'us (part.), *complicated, complex.*
Compos'itus (part.), *compound.*
Con'cavus, *concave.*
Conci'sus (part.), *sliced, or cut into small pieces.*
Contu'sus (part.), *bruised.*
Convex'us, *convex.*
Corda'tus, *cordate.*
Corrosi'vus, *corrosive.*
Crit'icus, *critical.*
Crucif'erus, *cross-bearing, or bearing flowers having the form of a cross.*
Crystalli'nus, *crystalline.*
Cur'vus, *crooked.*
Cuta'neus, *cutaneous.*
Dec'imus, *tenth.*
Denuda'tus (part.), *denuded.*
Depura'tus (part.), *purified.*
Diffu'sus (part.), *diffuse, diffused.*
Dilu'tus (part.), *dilute, diluted.*
Diptera'ceus, *resembling the* Dipterocarpus.
Dissec'tus (part.), *dissected.*
Diur'nus, *diurnal.*
Domes'ticus, *domestic.*
Dras'ticus, *drastic.*
Du'rus, *hard.*
Dynam'icus, *dynamic.*
Eclec'ticus, *eclectic.*
Elas'ticus, *elastic.*
Elec'tricus, *electric.*
Epidem'icus, *epidemic.*
Equi'nus, *equine.*
Erudi'tus (part.), *instructed, learned.*
Europæ'us, *European.*
Fal'sus, *false.*
Farino'sus, *mealy.*
Febrif'ugus, *febrifuge.*
Feli'nus, *feline.*
Finit'imus, *neighboring.*
Fix'us (part.), *fixed.*
Fla'vus, *yellow.*
Flor'idus, *flowery.*
Flu'idus, *fluid.*
Fœt'idus, *stinking.*
Ful'vus, *tawny.*
Fu'sus, *fused.*
Gal'licus, *French.*
Galvan'icus, *galvanic.*
Gas'tricus, *gastric.*
Gem'inus, *double.*
Gener'icus, *generic.*
Glau'cus, *gray or glaucous.*
Gramina'ceus, *resembling grass.*
Gra'tus, *pleasing, palatable.*
Grav'idus, *pregnant.*
Hæmat'icus, *hæmatic.*
Hec'ticus, *hectic.*
Hepat'icus, *hepatic.*
Huma'nus, *human.*
Hyber'nus, *wintry.*
Idiopath'icus, *idiopathic.*
Ili'acus, *iliac.*
Imagina'rius, *imaginary.*
Impu'rus, *impure.*
In'dicus, *Indian, or belonging to India.*
Inflamma'tus, *inflamed.*
Innomina'tus, *unnamed.*
Insa'nus, *insane.*
Inten'sus, *intense.*
Inval'idus, *invalid.*
Involunta'rius, *involuntary.*
Iod'icus, *iodic.*
Irida'ceus, *resembling the* Iris.
Isomor'phus, *isomorphous.*
Lac'ticus, *lactic.*
Lar'gus, *broad or large.*
Latis'simus, *broadest.*
La'tus, *broad.*
Laura'ceus, *resembling the* Laurus.
Lax'us, *loose.*
Lilia'ceus, *resembling the lily.*
Liq'uidus, *liquid.*
Liv'idus, *livid.*
Loba'tus, *lobed.*
Longis'simus, *longest.*
Lon'gus, *long.*
Lo'tus (part.), *washed.*
Lu'cidus, *lucid.*
Lymphat'icus, *lymphatic.*
Magnet'icus, *magnetic.*
Mag'nus, *great.*
Mal'icus, *malic.*
Ma'lus, *evil, bad.*
Malva'ceus, *resembling the* Malva.
Marit'imus, *maritime.*
Mas'culus, *masculine.*
Matu'rus, *mature.*
Max'imus, *greatest.*
Media'nus, *median.*
Med'icus, *medical.*
Min'imus, *least.*
Mor'bidus, *morbid.*
Mul'tus, *many.*
Muriat'icus, *muriatic.*
Myrta'ceus, *resembling the myrtle.*
Narcot'icus, *narcotic.*
Nervo'sus, *nervous.*
Neurot'icus, *neurotic.*
Ni'tricus, *nitric.*
Noctur'nus, *nocturnal.*
No'nus, *ninth.*
No'vus, *new.*
Obli'quus, *oblique.*
Obscu'rus, *obscure.*
Occul'tus, *occult.*
Octa'vus, *eighth.*
Odo'rus, *odorous, fragrant.*
Olea'ceus, *resembling the* Olea (*olive*).
Opa'cus, *opaque.*
Op'ticus, *optic, optical.*
Op'timus, *best.*
Orchida'ceus, *resembling the* Orchis.
Organ'icus, *organic.*
Oxal'icus, *oxalic.*
Pal'lidus, *pallid, pale.*
Papavera'ceus, *resembling the poppy.*
Parotide'us, *parotid.*
Parti'tus (part.), *divided.*
Par'vus, *small.*
Pathet'icus, *pathetic.*
Pau'cus, plu. Pau'ci, *few*
Pellu'cidus, *pellucid.*
Perac'tus (part.), *finished or completed.*
Perfora'tus (part.), *perforated.*
Peristal'ticus, *peristaltic.*
Peronæ'us, *peroneal.*
Phosphor'icus, *phosphoric.*
Phys'icus, *physical.*
Pi'ceus, *of pitch.*
Pinna'tus, *pinnate.*
Pla'nus, *plane, flat.*
Pneumat'icus, *pneumatic.*
Pneumon'icus, *pneumonic.*
Poma'ceus, *resembling the apple.*
Posti'cus, *posterior.*
Præcipita'tus (part.), *precipitated.*
Præpara'tus (part.), *prepared.*
Præscrip'tus (part.), *prescribed or directed.*
Pri'mus, *first.*
Profun'dus, *deep, profound.*
Pulmon'icus, *pulmonic.*
Purifica'tus (part.), *purified.*
Purpu'reus, *purple.*
Pu'rus, *pure.*
Pyrec'ticus, *relating to pyrexia.*
Quadra'tus, *square.*
Quan'tus, *as much as.*
Quarta'nus, *quartan.*
Quar'tus, *fourth.*

Example of an Adjective of the First and Second Declensions ending in -us, declined in full.

	Singular.				Plural.		
	Masc.	Fem.	Neut.		Masc.	Fem.	Neut.
Nom.	La'tus,	la'ta,	la'tum (*broad*).	Nom.	La'ti,	la'tæ,	la'ta.
Gen.	La'ti,	la'tæ,	la'ti.	Gen.	Lato'rum,	lata'rum,	lato'rum.
Dat.	La'to,	la'tæ,	la'to.	Dat.	La'tis,	la'tis,	la'tis.
Acc.	La'tum,	la'tam,	la'tum.	Acc.	La'tos,	la'tas,	la'ta.
Voc.	La'te,	la'ta,	la'tum.	Voc.	La'ti,	la'tæ,	la'ta.
Abl.	La'to,	la'tâ,	la'to.	Abl.	La'tis,	la'tis,	la'tis

☞ In like manner are declined all adjectives and participles ending in *-us*, excepting *u'nus, a'lius* ("other"), *nul'lus, so'lus, to'tus*, and *ul'lus*. See page 676.

Quin'tus, *fifth.*
Quotidia'nus, *daily.*
Rab'idus, *rabid.*
Ranuncula'ceus, *resembling the* Ranunculus.
Rectifica'tus (part.), *rectified.*
Rec'tus, *straight.*
Redac'tus (part.), *reduced.*
Reflex'us (part.), *reflected, reflexed, or reflex.*
Rheumat'icus, *rheumatic.*
Rig'idus, *rigid.*
Rotun'dus, *round.*
Sali'nus, *saline.*
Saliva'rius, *salivary.*
Sanguin'eus, *sanguineous.*
Sa'nus, *sound, sane.*
Sati'vus, *cultivated.*
Scale'nus, *scalene.*
Sciat'icus, *sciatic.*
Sclerot'icus, *sclerotic.*
Secre'tus, *secreted.*
Secun'dus, *second.*
Sedati'vus, *sedative.*
Sep'ticus, *septic.*
Sep'timus, *seventh.*
Serra'tus, *serrate.*
Sex'tus, *sixth.*
Sic'cus, *dry.*
Sol'idus, *solid.*
Sol'itus, *usual.*
Somnif'erus, *sleep-producing.*
Spasmod'icus, *spasmodic.*
Spermat'icus, *spermatic.*
Spino'sus, *thorny.*
Sponta'neus, *spontaneous.*
Spu'rius, *spurious.*
Sublima'tus (part.), *sublimed or sublimated.*
Sulphu'ricus, *sulphuric.*
Sur'dus, *deaf.*
Sympathet'icus, *sympathetic.*
Tan'tus, *so much.*
Tep'idus, *tepid.*
Tertia'nus, *tertian.*
Ter'tius, *third.*
Thorac'icus, *thoracic.*
Tincto'rius, *pertaining to dyers, or dyeing.*
Transver'sus, *transverse.*
Trigem'inus, *triple.*
Ul'timus, *last, final.*
Us'tus (part.), *burnt or calcined.*
Val'idus, *valid, strong.*
Va'nus, *vain.*
Va'rius, *various.*
Va'rus, *bow-legged.*
Venena'tus, *envenomed.*
Vertebra'tus, *vertebrated.*
Ve'rus, *true.*
Vesicato'rius, *causing blisters.*
Virginia'nus, *Virginian.*

Adjectives in -er.

Æ'ger, *sick.*
As'per, *rough.*
Cre'ber, *frequent.*
Gla'ber, *smooth.*
In'teger, *whole, entire.*
La'cer, *torn, lacerated.*
Ma'cer, *lean.*
Ni'ger, *black.*
Pul'cher, *beautiful.*
Ru'ber, *red.*
Sa'cer, *sacred.*
Sca'ber, *rough.*
Te'uer, *tender.*

IX. Adjectives of the third declension are generally declined in all respects like nouns of the third declension having the same termination and gender: thus, adjectives in *-is* (as *mi'tis*, "mild") are declined like *cri'nis*, except that they have the ablative singular in *-i*; those in *-e*, like *re'te*; those in *-ns* (*e.g. ar'dens*, "burning"), like *dens*; those in *-ex* (as *sim'plex*, "simple"), like *a'pex*, etc. (See page 665.)

This class of adjectives may be conveniently subdivided into two sections: 1. Those ending in *-is* having the neuter in *-e*: as, *abdomina'lis*, "abdominal;" *labia'lis*, "labial;" *orbicula'ris*, "circular," etc. 2. Those terminating in two consonants: as, *astrin'gens* ("astringent"), *ser'pens* ("creeping"), *medica'trix** ("healing"), etc.

X. Those of the first section have the masculine and feminine alike, with the

Example of an Adjective of the First and Second Declensions in -er, declined in full.†

	Singular. Masc.	Fem.	Neut.		Plural. Masc.	Fem.	Neut.
Nom.	Ru'ber,	ru'bra,	ru'brum (*red*).	Nom.	Ru'bri,	ru'bræ,	ru'bra.
Gen.	Ru'bri,	ru'bræ,	ru'bri.	Gen.	Rubro'rum,	rubra'rum,	rubro'rum.
Dat.	Ru'bro,	ru'bræ,	ru'bro.	Dat.	Ru'bris,	ru'bris,	ru'bris.
Acc.	Ru'brum,	ru'bram,	ru'brum.	Acc.	Ru'bros,	ru'bras,	ru'bra.
Voc.	Ru'ber,	ru'bra,	ru'brum.	Voc.	Ru'bri,	ru'bræ,	ru'bra.
Abl.	Ru'bro,	ru'brâ,	ru'bro.	Abl.	Ru'bris,	ru'bris,	ru'bris.

Example of an Adjective of the Third Declension, declined in full.

	Singular. Masc.	Fem.	Neut.		Plural. Masc.	Fem.	Neut.
Nom.	Mi'tis,	mi'tis,	mi'te (*mild*).	Nom.	Mi'tes,	mi'tes,	mitia (mish'e-a).
Gen.	Mi'tis,	mi'tis,	mi'tis.	Gen.	Mit'ium,	mit'ium,	mit'ium (mish'e-um).
Dat.	Mi'ti,	mi'ti,	mi'ti.	Dat.	Mit'ibus,	mit'ibus,	mit'ibus.
Acc.	Mi'tem,	mi'tem,	mi'te.	Acc.	Mi'tes,	mi'tes,	mit'ia.
Voc.	Mi'tis,	mi'tis,	mi'te.	Voc.	Mi'tes,	mi'tes,	mit'ia.
Abl.	Mi'ti,	mi'ti,	mi'ti.	Abl.	Mit'ibus,	mit'ibus,	mit'ibus.

* *X* is properly a *double* consonant, being composed of *cs* (or *ks*). Compare the English word small-pox, formerly written *small pocks.*

† In like manner are declined nearly all adjectives in *-er*; but *as'per*, *la'cer*, and *te'ner* take an additional syllable in the feminine and neuter gender, and in the cases after the nominative: as, *lac'era, lac'erum, lac'eri*, etc. (not *lac'ra, lac'rum*). For *Al'ter*, see page 676.

genitive like the nominative masculine (or feminine), the neuter nominative ending always in *-e*. These adjectives are very numerous, and are constantly met with in anatomical and botanical names: as, *carun'cula* (f.) *lachryma'lis*, the "lachrymal caruncle;" *mus'culus* (m.) *orbicula'ris*, or simply *orbicula'ris*, the "circular muscle;" *os* (n.) *orbicula're*, "orbicular bone;" *os lachryma'le*, "lachrymal bone;" *Sanguina'ria* (f.) *Canaden'sis* ("bloodroot"), *As'arum* (n.) *Canaden'se* ("Canada snakeroot, or wild ginger"). It will be seen by the foregoing examples that adjectives in *-is* are applied indifferently to masculine and feminine nouns, but if applied to neuter nouns the termination changes to *-e*.

List of the most important Adjectives of the Third Declension.

Abdomina'lis, *abdominal.*
Abnor'mis, *abnormal.*
Aborig'enis, *aboriginal.*
Acau'lis, *stemless.*
Accidenta'lis, *accidental.*
Accli'vis, *sloping upwards.*
A'cris, *sharp.*
Agres'tis, *belonging to a field, growing in the fields.*
Ala'ris, *wing-like.*
Albuminen'sis, *pertaining to albumen, containing albumen.*
Alluvia'lis, *alluvial.*
Angula'ris, *angular.*
Anima'lis, *animal.*
Annula'ris, *annular.*
Antifebri'lis, *antifebrile.*
Arcifor'mis, *arciform.*
Areola'ris, *areolar.*
Armilla'ris, *armillary.*
Arsenica'lis, *arsenical.*
Arteria'lis, *arterial.*
Articula'ris, *articular.*
Arven'sis, *growing in fields.*
Auricula'ris, *auricular.*
Austra'lis, *southern.*
Axilla'ris, *axillary.*
Bilia'ris, *biliary.*
Borea'lis, *northern.*
Brachia'lis, *brachial.*
Bre'vis, *short.*
Bronchia'lis, *bronchial.*
Bul'liens, *boiling.*
Campes'tris, *growing in a plain.*
Canaden'sis, *Canadian.*
Capilla'ris, *capillary.*
Capita'lis, *belonging to the head, capital.*
Castren'sis, *of camps.*
Cauda'lis, *caudal.*
Cellula'ris, *cellular.*
Centra'lis, *central.*
Cerea'lis, *cereal.*
Cerebra'lis, *cerebral.*
Cervica'lis, *cervical.*
Chinen'sis, *Chinese.*
Cilia'ris, *ciliary.*
Columna'ris, *columnar.*
Commu'nis, *common.*
Con'color (gen. Concolo'ris), *of one (or the same) color.*
Contrac'tilis, *contractile.*
Cordia'lis, *cordial.*
Corona'lis, *coronal.*
Corpuscula'ris, *corpuscular.*
Cortica'lis, *cortical.*
Costa'lis, *costal.*
Crania'lis, *cranial.*
Crura'lis, *crural.*
Decli'vis, *descending.*
Denta'lis, *dental.*
Digita'lis, *digital.*
Dorsa'lis, *dorsal.*
Duc'tilis, *ductile.*
Dul'cis, *sweet.*
Ebul'liens, *boiling.*
Erec'tilis, *erectile.*
Exuvia'lis, *exuvial.*
Facia'lis, *facial.*
Fascia'lis, *fascial.*
Febri'lis, *febrile.*
Femora'lis, *femoral.*
Fer'tilis, *fertile.*
Fer'vens, *hot, or boiling.*
Filifor'mis, *filiform.*
Fis'silis, *fissile.*
Flex'ilis, *flexile.*
Flora'lis, *floral.*
Fluvia'lis, *fluvial.*
Fluviat'ilis, *fluviatile.*
Fœta'lis, *fetal.*
Fos'silis, *fossil.*
Frag'ilis, *fragile.*
Fronta'lis, *frontal.*
Genita'lis, *genital.*
Graç'ilis, *slender, soft.*
Gran'dis, *great.*
Granula'ris, *granular.*
Gra'vis, *heavy, severe.*
Hæma'lis, *hæmal.*
Horizonta'lis, *horizontal.*
Humera'lis, *humeral.*
Humora'lis, *humoral.*
Hyema'lis, *wintry.*
Imbeç'ilis, *imbecile.*
Immob'ilis, *immovable.*
Iner'mis, *unarmed.*
Infanti'lis, *infantile.*
Inflammab'ilis, *inflammable.*
Inframaxilla'ris, *inframaxillary.*
Infrascapula'ris, *infrascapular.*
Inguina'lis, *inguinal.*
Intercal'aris, *intercalary.*
Intercosta'lis, *intercostal.*
Interspina'lis, *interspinal.*
Interstitia'lis, *interstitial*
Intervertebra'lis, *intervertebral.*
Intestina'lis, *intestinal.*
Jugula'ris, *jugular.*
Labia'lis, *labial.*
Lachryma'lis, *lachrymal.*
Lactea'lis, *lacteal.*
Larva'lis, *larval.*
Latera'lis, *lateral.*
Letha'lis, *lethal.*
Linea'ris, *linear.*
Littora'lis, *littoral.*
Lobula'ris, *lobular.*
Loca'lis, *local.*
Locula'ris, *locular.*
Lumba'ris, *lumbar.*
Luna'ris, *lunar.*
Magistra'lis, *magistral.*
Mala'ris, *malar.*
Mammilla'ris, *mammillary.*
Mandibula'ris, *mandibular.*
Margina'lis, *marginal.*
Maxilla'ris, *maxillary.*
Medicina'lis, *medicinal.*
Medulla'ris, *medullary.*
Menstrua'lis, *menstrual.*
Menta'lis, *mental.*
Mercuria'lis, *mercurial.*
Meridiona'lis, *meridional.*
Minera'lis, *mineral.*
Mi'tis, *mild.*
Mola'ris, *molar.*
Mulie'bris, *pertaining to women, female.*
Multicau'lis, *having many stems.*
Muscula'ris, *muscular.*
Nasa'lis, *nasal.*
Natura'lis, *natural.*
Neura'lis, *neural.*
Neutra'lis, *neutral.*
Nob'ilis, *noble.*
Nodula'ris, *nodular.*
Occidenta'lis, *occidental.*
Occipita'lis, *occipital.*
Officina'lis, *officinal.*
Ora'lis, *oral.*
Orbicula'ris, *circular.*
Orbita'lis, *orbital.*
Orienta'lis, *oriental.*
Ova'lis, *oval.*
Palma'ris, *palmar.*
Palus'tris, *belonging to swamps; growing in swamps.*
Papilla'ris, *papillary.*
Parieta'lis, *parietal.*
Pectina'lis, *like a comb.*
Pectora'lis, *pectoral.*
Peren'nis, *perennial.*
Perinæa'lis, *perinæal.*
Permeab'ilis, *permeable.*
Placenta'lis, *placental.*
Planta'ris, *plantar.*
Pluvia'lis, *pluvial.*
Pocula'ris, *pocular.*
Pola'ris, *polar.*
Porten'sis, *belonging to Oporto, in Portugal.*
Potentia'lis, *potential.*
Praten'sis, *growing in meadows.*
Prehen'silis, *prehensile.*
Primordia'lis, *primordial.*
Puerpera'lis, *puerperal.*
Pulmona'ris, *pulmonary.*
Pyramida'lis, *pyramidal.*
Quadrangula'ris, *quadrangular.*

Quadrilatera'lis, *quadrilateral.*
Radia'lis, *radial.*
Radica'lis, *radical.*
Rationa'lis, *rational.*
Rectangula'ris, *rectangular.*
Rena'lis, *renal.*
Renifor'mis, *reniform.*
Retrac'tilis, *retractile.*
Rhomboida'lis, *rhomboidal.*
Riva'lis, *growing in or near a stream.*
Rupes'tris, *growing on rocks.*
Saliva'ris, *salivary.*
Saluta'ris, *salutary.*
Saxat'ilis, *growing in rocky places.*
Scapula'ris, *scapular.*
Semiluna'ris, *semilunar.*
Semina'lis, *seminal.*
Seni'lis, *senile.*
Ses'silis, *sessile.*
Solu'bilis, *soluble.*
Spectab'ilis, *admirable, worth seeing.*
Spherica'lis, *spherical.*
Spina'lis, *spinal.*
Spira'lis, *spiral.*
Stamina'lis, *staminal.*
Ster'ilis, *sterile.*
Sua'vis, *sweet, agreeable.*
Subli'mis, *superficial, high.*
Sylves'tris, *growing in forests, sylvan.*
Synovia'lis, *synovial.*
Tempora'lis, *temporal.*
Termina'lis, *terminal.*
Tex'tilis, *textile.*
Therma'lis, *thermal.*
Tibia'lis, *tibial.*
Trachea'lis, *tracheal.*
Transversa'lis, *transverse.*
Triangula'ris, *triangular.*
Trifacia'lis, *trifacial.*
Trivia'lis, *trivial.*
Tubercula'ris, *tubercular.*
Umbilica'lis, *umbilical.*
Unguina'lis, *unguinal.*
Vascula'ris, *vascular.*
Ventra'lis, *ventral.*
Versat'ilis, *versatile.*
Versic'olor (gen. Versicolo'ris), *having various colors.*
Vertebra'lis, *vertebral.*
Viab'ilis, *viable.*
Vir'idis, *green.*
Viri'lis, *of or pertaining to a man.*
Viscera'lis, *visceral.*
Vita'lis, *vital.*
Volat'ilis, *volatile.*

Adjectives belonging to the second section (*i.e.* ending in two consonants) have the masculine, feminine, and neuter alike both in the nominative and genitive: as, *mor'bus ser'pens*, a "creeping disease;" *a'rea ser'pens*,* a "creeping baldness;" *an'imal ser'pens*, a "creeping animal." In the genitive, we should have *mor'bi serpen'tis*, "of a creeping disease;" *a'reæ serpen'tis*, "of a creeping baldness;" *anima'lis serpen'tis*, "of a creeping animal."†

Adjectives of the third declension form the masculine and feminine plural by changing *-is* of the genitive singular into *-es*, and the neuter by changing it into *-ia*: *e.g. mus'culus ala'ris*, a "winged or wing-shaped muscle;" *ve'na ala'ris*, a "winged vein;" *os ala're*, a "winged bone;" nom. pl. *mus'culi ala'res*, "winged muscles;" *ve'næ ala'res*, "winged veins;" *os'sa ala'ria*, "winged bones." The genitive plural ends in *-ium* in all three genders: *e.g. musculo'rum ala'rium*, "of winged muscles;" *vena'rum ala'rium*, "of winged veins;" *os'sium ala'rium*, "of winged bones" (see Alaris and Alares, in the dictionary). In like manner, we should have, in the plural, *mor'bi serpen'tes*, "creeping diseases;" *ve'næ serpen'tes*, "creeping or winding veins;" *anima'lia serpen'tia*, "creeping animals."

Comparison of Adjectives.

Adjectives of the comparative degree are of the third declension; they have the masculine and feminine termination in *-or* (declined like *humor*: see example on page 665): *e.g. mi'tis*, "mild," has *mi'tior* in the comparative; hence, *ty'phus mi'tior*,

Example of an Adjective (participle) of the Third Declension in -ns, declined in full.

	Singular.				Plural		
	Masc.	Fem.	Neut.		Masc.	Fem.	Neut.
Nom.	Ser'pens,	ser'pens,	ser'pens, *winding.*	Nom.	Serpen'tes,	serpen'tes,	serpen'tia.
Gen.	Serpen'tis,	serpen'tis,	serpen'tis.	Gen.	Serpen'tium,	serpen'tium,	serpen'tium (contracted serpen'tum or serpen'tûm).
Dat.	Serpen'ti,	serpen'ti,	serpen'ti.	Dat.	Serpen'tibus,	serpen'tibus,	serpen'tibus.
Acc.	Serpen'tem,	serpen'tem,	ser'pens.	Acc.	Serpen'tes,	serpen'tes,	serpen'tia.
Voc.	Ser'pens,	ser'pens,	ser'pens.	Voc.	Serpen'tes,	serpen'tes,	serpen'tia.
Abl.	Serpen'te,	serpen'te,	serpen'te.	Abl.	Serpen'tibus,	serpen'tibus,	serpen'tibus.

* A term used by Celsus for a form of baldness the progress of which was supposed to resemble the creeping or winding of a serpent. See Ophiasis, in the dictionary.

† Nearly all adjectives of this termination (*-ns*) are in fact participles: thus, *astrin'gens*, "astringent," is the present participle of *astrin'go*, to "bind," to "contract;" *emol'liens*, "emollient," is derived in like manner from *emol'lio*, to "soften;" *demul'cens*, "demulcent," from *demul'ceo*, to "soothe," etc.: likewise the examples previously given: viz., *ar'dens*, "burning," *fer'vens*, "boiling," and *ser'pens*, "creeping," are from *ar'deo*, to "burn," *fer'veo*, to "boil," to "be hot," and *ser'po*, to "creep," respectively.

"milder typhus." In like manner *for'tis*, "strong," has in the comparative *for'tior*, "stronger;" *gra'vis*, "heavy," "severe," makes *gra'vior*, "severer;" *ten'uis*, "thin," or "weak," makes *ten'uior*, "weaker," and so on. Several adjectives form the comparative irregularly, but it always terminates in *-or*, and is declined as above stated: *e.g. mag'nus*, "great," has for its comparative, *ma'jor*, "greater;" *par'vus*, "little," has *mi'nor*, "less;" *bo'nus*, "good," *me'lior*, "better;" *ma'lus*, "bad," *pe'jor*, "worse." The neuter is always formed by changing the masculine and feminine termination (*-or*) into *-us:* as, *mi'tius, gra'vius, for'tius, ma'jus, mi'nus, me'lius, infe'rius, supe'rius:* hence, *la'bium infe'rius*, "lower lip;" *la'bium supe'rius*, "upper lip;" *al'cohol for'tius*, "stronger alcohol." The genitive, dative, and ablative neuter are the same as the masculine: as, *la'bii inferio'ris*, "of the lower lip;" *cum al'cohol forio're*, "with stronger alcohol."

The superlative degree of Latin adjectives usually terminates in *-issimus:* as, *mitis'simus*, "mildest;" *gravis'simus*, "severest;" *fortis'simus*, "strongest;" *latis'simus*, "broadest" (from *la'tus*, "broad"); but most of those adjectives (viz. *mag'nus, par'vus*, etc.) which have an irregular comparative, form the superlative also irregularly: as, *max'imus*, "greatest;" *min'imus*, "least;" *op'timus*, "best;" *pes'simus*, "worst." *Su'perus*, "high," makes *supre'mus* (or *sum'mus*), "highest;" *in'ferus*, "low," *in'fimus* (or *i'mus*), "lowest."

Numeral Adjectives.

U'nus, *one.*	Duod'ecim, *twelve.*	Vigin'ti du'o, or Du'o et vigin'ti, } *twenty-two.*
Du'o, *two.*	Tred'ecim, *thirteen.*	Trigin'ta, *thirty.*
Tres, *three.*	Quatuor'decim, *fourteen.*	Quadragin'ta, *forty.*
Qua'tuor, *four.*	Quin'decim, *fifteen.*	Quinquagin'ta, *fifty.*
Quin'que, *five.*	Sex'decim, *sixteen.*	Sexagin'ta, *sixty.*
Sex, *six.*	Septen'decim, *seventeen.*	Septuagin'ta, *seventy.*
Sep'tem, *seven.*	Octod'ecim, *eighteen.*	Octogin'ta, *eighty.*
Oc'to, *eight.*	Novem'decim, *nineteen.*	Nonagin'ta, *ninety.*
No'vem, *nine.*	Vigin'ti, *twenty.*	Cen'tum, *a hundred.*
De'cem, *ten.*	Vigin'ti u'nus, or U'nus et vigin'ti, } *twenty-one.*	Mil'le, *a thousand.*
Un'decim, *eleven.*		

Unus, "one."*

Singular.

	Masc.	Fem.	Neut.
Nom.	U'nus,	u'na,	u'num.
Gen.	Uni'us,	uni'us,	uni'us.
Dat.	U'ni,	u'ni,	u'ni.
Acc.	U'num,	u'nam,	u'num.
Voc.	U'ne,	u'na,	u'num.
Abl.	U'no,	u'nâ,	u'no.

Duo, "two."

Plural.

	Masc.	Fem.	Neut.
Nom.	Du'o,	du'æ,	du'o.
Gen.	Duo'rum,	dua'rum,	duo'rum.
Dat.	Duo'bus,	dua'bus,	duo'bus.
Acc.	Du'os, or du'o,	du'as,	du'o.
Voc.	Du'o,	du'æ,	du'o.
Abl.	Duo'bus,	dua'bus,	dua'bus.

Tres, "three."

Plural.

	Masc.	Fem.	Neut.
Nom.	Tres,	tres,	tri'a.
Gen.	Tri'um,	tri'um,	tri'um.
Dat.	Tri'bus,	tri'bus,	tri'bus.
Acc.	Tres,	tres,	tri'a.
Voc.	Tres,	tres,	tri'a.
Abl.	Tri'bus,	tri'bus,	tri'bus.

Alter, "another."

Singular.

	Masc.	Fem.	Neut.
Nom.	Al'ter,	al'tera,	al'terum.
Gen.	Alteri'us,	alteri'us,	alteri'us.
Dat.	Al'teri,	al'teri,	al'teri.
Acc.	Al'terum,	al'teram,	al'terum.
Voc.	Al'ter,	al'tera,	al'terum.
Abl.	Al'tero,	al'terâ,	al'tero.

Plural.

	Masc.	Fem.	Neut.
Nom.	Al'teri,	al'teræ,	al'tera.
Gen.	Altero'rum,	altera'rum,	altero'rum
Dat.	Al'teris,	al'teris,	al'teris.
Acc.	Al'teros,	al'teras,	al'tera.
Voc.	Al'teri,	al'teræ,	al'tera.
Abl.	Al'teris,	al'teris,	al'teris.

* *To'tus*, the "whole," *nul'lus*, "no," *so'lus*, "alone," and *ul'lus*, "any," are declined in the same manner.

Pronouns.

Is, ea, id, "he," "she," or "it."

	Singular.				Plural.		
	Masc.	Fem.	Neut.		Masc.	Fem.	Neut.
Nom.	Is,	e'a,	id,	Nom.	I'i,	e'æ,	e'a.
Gen.	E'jus,	e'jus,	e'jus,	Gen.	Eo'rum,	ea'rum,	eo'rum.
Dat.	E'i,	e'i,	e'i,	Dat.	E'is, or i'is,	e'is, or i'is,	e'is, or i'is.
Acc.	E'um,	e'am,	id,	Acc.	E'os,	e'as,	e'a.
Voc.	——	——	——	Voc.	——	——	——
Abl.	E'o,	e'â,	e'o,	Abl.	E'is, or i'is,	e'is, or i'is,	e'is, or i'is.

Nom.	Hic,	hæc,	hoc, *this.*	Nom.	Hi,	hæ,	hæc, *these.*
Gen.	Hu'jus,	hu'jus,	hu'jus, *of this.*	Gen.	Ho'rum,	ha'rum,	ha'rum, *of these.*
Dat.	Huic, *to or for this.*	huic,	huic (pron. hïk),	Dat.	His,	his,	his, *to or for these.*
Acc.	Hunc,	hanc,	hoc, *this.*	Acc.	Hos,	has,	hæc, *these.*
Voc.	Hic,	hæc,	hoc, *this.*	Voc.	Hi,	hæ,	hæc, *these.*
Abl.	Hoc,	hâc,	hoc, *in, by, or with this.*	Abl.	His,	his,	his, *in, by, or with these.*

Nom.	Qui, *who or which.*	quæ,	quod,	Nom.	Qui, *who or which.*	quæ,	quæ,
Gen.	Cu'jus, *whose or of which.*	cu'jus,	cu'jus,	Gen.	Quo'rum, *whose or of which.*	qua'rum,	qua'rum,
Dat.	Cui, *to whom or to which.*	cui,	cui (pron. ki),	Dat.	Qui'bus, *to whom or to which.*	qui'bus,	qui'bus,
Acc.	Quem, *whom or which.*	quam,	quod,	Acc.	Qui, *whom or which.*	quæ,	quæ,
Voc.	——	——	——	Voc.	——	——	——
Abl.	Quo, *in, by, or with whom or which.*	qua,	quo,	Abl.	Qui'bus, *in, by, or with whom or which.*	qui'bus,	qui'bus,

☞ The lists of Latin nouns, adjectives, etc. on the foregoing pages contain, it is believed, all the most important words of this kind which the student will be likely to meet with in works relating to Anatomy, Pharmacy, etc. Especial care has been taken to make the lists complete with respect to Pharmacopœial names and the terms commonly used in writing prescriptions.*

Remarks on the Use and Application of Latin Adjectives.

It has already been shown (on page 671) that Latin adjectives change their terminations so as to agree with the nouns to which they are joined, in GENDER, NUMBER, and CASE. It is important to observe that this agreement is equally necessary whether the noun be understood or expressed: for example, the adjective *æ'ger* ("sick," or "suffering") if joined with *vir* (a "man") will, of course, retain its masculine form; if with *fœm'ina* (a "woman"), it is changed to *æ'gra*, according to the rule already explained; also, if the adjective be used without a noun, as is frequently the case, to denote a "patient,"† we must always write *æ'ger*, if we mean a male, and *æ'gra*, if we mean a female patient. Hence we have the following important rule:—

☞ Whenever an adjective, participle, or adjective pronoun is used without any noun expressed, it must invariably be put in the gender, number, and case of the noun (whatever this may be) which is understood. Accordingly, all the names of

* It may be observed that the signification of the nouns is not given in the lists, because, with few if any exceptions, they will be found defined in the Dictionary. But, as only a part of the adjectives are given in the Dictionary under their own heads, and since the lists, if they contained the signification of only a portion, would have an irregular and unsightly appearance, it has been deemed best to give the meaning of the adjectives in all cases.

† "Patient" is merely an Anglicized form of the Latin *pa'tiens* [from *pa'tior, pas'sus,* to "suffer"], and signifies a "suffering" or "sick" person.

the muscles formed from adjectives (of which there are a great number), as, *cru-ræ'us, glutæ'us, hyoglos'sus, sarto'rius, semimembrano'sus, latis'simus dor'si, quadra'-tus lumbo'rum, rec'tus oc'uli,* etc., must have the masculine termination, because *mus'culus* (a "muscle"), the understood noun, is of the masculine gender. So the adjectives forming the names of nerves must be masculine, because *ner'vus* (a "nerve") is masculine: *e.g. accesso'rius Willis'ii* (in the plural, *accesso'rii Wil-lis'ii*), *hypoglos'sus, pathet'ici, trigem'ini,* etc.

One of the most important applications of the rule above stated, is to the names of the divisions, classes, or orders in the different departments of science. In Botany the natural orders are generally formed from adjectives in *-a'ceus:* as, *Acera'ceus, Clusia'ceus, Lilia'ceus, Papavera'ceus,* etc., the terminations of which are changed to agree with the noun *plan'tæ* ("plants") understood, in the nominative plural feminine. Accordingly, *Acera'ceæ* signifies "[plants] allied to, or resem-bling, the maple;" *Clusia'ceæ* "[plants] allied to, or resembling, the *Clusia;*" *Lilia'ceæ,* those "resembling the lily;" *Papavera'ceæ,* those "resembling the poppy," etc. etc.

It may be observed, however, that the orders of Jussieu are, with a few excep-tions, named from the plural of certain nouns: as, *Ac'era* (plural of *A'cer*), the "maples;" *Lil'ia* (plural of *Lil'ium*), the "lilies;" *Al'gæ* (plural of *Al'ga*), "sea-weeds;" *Mus'ci* (plural of *Mus'cus,*) "mosses," etc. etc.

The Linnæan classes (which are of Greek derivation) consist of adjectives (such as *monan'drius,* "having one stamen;" *pentan'drius,* "having five stamens;" *dec-an'drius,* "having ten stamens," etc.) in the neuter plural agreeing with *phy'ta,* or φυτά (the plural of *phy'ton,* or φυτόν, the Greek term for a "plant"), understood. By some, however, they are considered to be nouns (or adjectives used as nouns, *clas'sis,* a "class," being understood) in the feminine singular. On this supposi-tion, *Monan'dria* is equivalent to *clas'sis Monan'dria,* the "Monandrian class," or that comprising flowers having a single stamen; *Pentan'dria* is the "Pentandrian class," or that comprising flowers with five stamens, and so on. But it is preferable to consider these classes as formed of adjectives in the plural; for so they will har-monize with the names of the divisions and classes in Zoology, Nosology, etc., where they are always in the plural.

The divisions, classes, and orders of the animal kingdom are formed of adjec-tives with the neuter plural termination in *-a;* because *An'imal* (plural *Anima'lia*), the understood noun, is of the neuter gender: *e.g. Vertebra'ta,* "vertebrated [ani-mals];" *Mollus'ca,* "molluscous [animals];" *Articula'ta,* "articulated [animals];" *Radia'ta,* "radiated [animals];" *Mamma'lia,* "[animals] furnished with mammæ;" *Cephalop'oda,* "[animals] having the head furnished with feet," the designation of an order of mollusks, the most highly organized of all invertebrate animals (see CEPHALOPODA, in the Dictionary).

With respect to the classification of diseases, great diversity prevails. Cullen, like Jussieu, generally took the names of his classes and orders from the plurals of nouns: as, *Pyrex'iæ* (plural of *Pyrex'ia,* a "febrile affection"), *Neuro'ses* (plural of *Neuro'sis,* a "nervous disease"), *Spas'mi* (plural of *Spas'mus,* a "spasm"), *Tumo'res* (plural of *Tu'mor,* a "tumor"), etc.; though one of his classes, *Loca'les,* is formed from the adjective *loca'lis* ("local"), *mor'bi* ("diseases") being under-stood. Dr. Good gives a neuter termination to all his classes and orders: as, *Hæmat'ica* (from *hæmat'icus,* "pertaining to the blood"), *Cœnot'ica* (from *cœnot'i-*

cus, "pertaining to evacuations"), etc. etc., the neuter noun *pathem'ata* (plural of *pathe'ma*, an "affection," or "disease") being understood. But it is now, perhaps, more usual to put the adjective in the masculine plural, agreeing with *mor'bi* (plural of *mor'bus*, a "disease"): *e.g. Zymot'ici*, "zymotic [diseases];" *Chrot'ici*, "skin [diseases]," etc.*

It must be borne in mind that the rule respecting the agreement of adjectives with nouns (see pp. 671, 677) applies not merely to the construction of sentences, but even to the shortest Latin phrase which may form the name of a bone, a plant, or a chemical substance: as, *Os* (n.) *innomina'tum*, *Cor'nus* (f.) *Flor'ida*, *Fer'rum redac'tum*, *Syru'pus fus'cus*, etc.

If, in writing any Latin name or phrase, the student should feel the slightest doubt, he should first ascertain the declension, gender, etc. of the word, which he can readily do by a reference to the lists on the foregoing pages. If the nominative of the noun ends in *-a*, it is in all probability of the first declension, feminine gender; let him then consult the list on page 661; if in *-um*, it is of the second declension, neuter gender (see list on page 664); if in *-us*, it is probably of the masculine gender, second declension, in which case let him refer to the list on page 663 (if not found there, to that on 669); for nouns of any other termination, let him examine the list of nouns of the third declension on pages 667 and 668, or to those of the fifth declension on page 670. Suppose, for example, he is in doubt whether to write for "washed sulphur," *sulphur lotum* or *sulphur lotus:* by turning to the list of the third declension, he will find that *sulphur* is neuter, and he will therefore know that the participle *lotus*, "washed," must have the neuter termination in *-um* for the nominative case. If he wishes to use the genitive case, he will change *sulphur* to *sulphuris*, and *lotum* to *loti*. The application of the rule to botanical names is usually very easy; but it would be better in all cases of uncertainty for him to examine every point and make assurance doubly sure, not only for the satisfaction of being correct, but also that he may acquire a HABIT OF ACCURACY, an element in the character of an accomplished physician or pharmacist, the importance of which can scarcely be over-estimated.†

---

* See Dr. Farr's classification of diseases as exhibited in LYON's "Hospital Practice," and other works.

† In a large majority of cases, botanical (and zoological) names consist of a noun constituting the genus, joined with an adjective (usually denoting some characteristic of the plant) forming the specific name: for example, in *Cap'sicum an'nuum* (the "annual Capsicum"), the specific term *annuum* is used to distinguish it from other species which are biennial or perennial; so *A'rum triphyl'lum*, the "three-leaved Arum," *Cincho'na pal'lida*, "pale Cinchona," etc. etc. In a number of instances, however, *the specific name is formed of a noun* (not unfrequently the name of some obsolete genus), in which case it does not necessarily agree in gender with the generic name. The following list embraces the most important names of this class:—

Aca'cia Cat'echu.
Achille'a Millefo'lium.
Aconi'tum Napel'lus.
Ac'orus Cal'amus.
Æs'culus Hippocas'tanum.
Agatho'tes Chiray'ta.
Alis'ma Planta'go.
Amo'mum Zin'giber.
Anacyc'lus Pyr'ethrum.
An'themis Cot'ula.
Antirrhi'num Lina'ria.
A'pium Petroseli'num.
Ar'butus U'va Ur'si (or Arctostaph'ylos U'va Ur'si).
Aristolo'chia Serpenta'ria.
Artemis'ia Absin'thium.
Aspid'ium Fi'lix Mas.
Asple'nium (or Aspid'ium) Fi'lix Fœm'ina.
At'ropa Belladon'na.
Balsamoden'dron Myr'rha.
Cas'sia Fis'tula.
Cephaë'lis Ipecacuan'ha.
Cincho'na Calisay'a.
Cissam'pelos Parei'ra.
Citrul'lus Colocyn'this.
Ci'trus Auran'tium.
Ci'trus Limet'ta.
Convol'vulus Jala'pa.
Convol'vulus Scammo'nia.
Cro'ton Eleuthe'ria (or Cro'ton Cascaril'la).
Cro'ton Tig'lium.
Cucur'bita Pe'po.
Cyn'ara Scol'ymus.
Cyt'isus Scopa'rius.
Daph'ne Gnid'ium.
Daph'ne Mezere'um.
Datu'ra Stramo'nium.
Dau'cus Caro'ta.
Delphin'ium Consol'ida.
Delphin'ium Staphisa'gria.
Eletta'ria Cardamo'mum.
Euge'nia (or Myr'tus) Pimen'ta.
Euphor'bia Ipecacuan'ha.

ON WRITING PRESCRIPTIONS.

In most countries of Europe, as well as in the United States, it is customary to write medical prescriptions in Latin. It is generally conceded that the interests of science are promoted by the usage which prevails among different nations, of writing the scientific names of plants, animals, etc. in a language which is understood, to a greater or less extent, throughout the civilized world, and which is not subject to the variations, and consequent uncertainty of meaning, to which all living languages are in some degree liable. There appears to be no good reason why the names or terms used in Pharmacy should constitute any exception to a principle so generally recognized. It has been urged as a more practical argument in favor of the custom of writing prescriptions in Latin, that a person travelling in foreign

---

Exogo′nium Pur′ga.
Fer′ula Assafœt′ida.
Hed′era He′lix.
Hu′mulus Lu′pulus.
I′lex Aquifo′lium.
In′ula Hele′nium.
Ipomæ′a Jala′pa.
Junip′erus Sabi′na.
Lau′rus Sas′safras.
Leon′todon Tarax′acum.
Lirioden′dron Tulipif′era.

Momor′dica Elate′rium.
Nar′thex Assafœt′ida.
Nicotia′na Tab′acum.
Œnan′the Phellan′drium.
Pa′nax Quinquefo′lium.
Pimpinel′la Ani′sum.
Pimpinel′la Saxif′raga.
Pista′cia Lentis′cus.
Polyg′ala Sen′ega.
Polyg′onum Bistor′ta.
Potentil′la Tormentil′la.

Pterocar′pus Marsu′pium.
Pu′nica Grana′tum.
Py′rus Ma′lus.
Rhus Toxicoden′dron.
Sola′num Dulcama′ra.
Stat′ice Limo′nium.
Tarax′acum Dens-leo′nis.
Theobro′ma Caca′o.
Vera′trum Sabadil′la.
Verbas′cum Thap′sus.
Ze′a Mays.

It may be remarked that the general usage of scientific writers requires that the generic name should begin with a capital, but the specific name, if an adjective (and not derived from a proper name), should, when it occurs in a regular sentence, invariably begin with a small letter: as, *Al′etris farino′sa*, *A′rum triphyl′lum*, etc. But if the adjective is derived from some proper name, as *Canaden′sis* (from Canada), *Europæ′us* (from Europa), and *Philadel′phicus* (from Philadelphia), then, of course, both the specific and generic name should commence with a capital: as, *As′arum Canaden′se*, *As′arum Europæ′um*, *Erig′eron Philadelph′icum*. Also, when the specific name, as those in the foregoing list, is a noun, it should always begin with a capital.*

☞ The specific names of the various species of *Meloe* (sometimes used synonymously with *Cantharis*), all having a masculine termination (as, *Meloe niger*, *M. vesicatorius*, etc.), might seem at first sight to deviate from the rule that the specific term if an adjective must agree in gender with the generic name; for *Meloe*, according to all recognized rules, ought to be feminine. But the mistake of supposing *Meloe* (a term of modern origin) to be masculine, having been made by those who first used the word, has since been almost universally followed by scientific writers. So that rather than unsettle the established usage respecting this group of names, we ought perhaps to recognize *Meloe* as the sole instance of a noun ending in *-e* and forming the genitive in *-es*, and yet of the masculine gender.

In a few instances the specific name of plants is formed of a noun in the genitive case: as, *Cam′phora officina′rum* (the "Camphor of the shops"), *Ca′rum Car′ui* (which can scarcely be translated, the second word being the genitive of *Car′uon*, which signifies essentially the same as *Carum*), *Dri′mys Winte′ri* (the "Drimys of [Captain] Winter," who first brought this species into notice), *Gentia′na Catesbæ′i* (the "Gentian of Catesby"), *Ru′bia tincto′rum* ("Dyers' Madder"), etc. In the foregoing examples the second noun in the genitive has the force of an adjective: *Cam′phora officina′rum* may be translated "officinal Camphor," *Gentia′na Catesbæ′i*, "Catesbæan Gentian;" so we say in English, "Arabian spices," or "spices of Arabia," etc.

---

* The specific name of the common tulip-tree (*Lirioden′dron Tulipif′era*) is sometimes written with a small letter for its initial; but this is manifestly incorrect, for though *tulipif′era* may sometimes be an adjective, it cannot be so in this connection, otherwise it must agree with the generic name in the neuter gender, and we should then have *Lirioden′dron tulipif′erum*. The fact is, that *Tulipifera* itself was formerly a generic name, formed of the adjective *tulipiferus* ("tulip-bearing"), agreeing with *Ar′bor* ("tree") understood. ☞ It may here be observed that *all the Latin names of trees are feminine*. *Lirioden′dron* and *Rhododen′dron*, the only important apparent exceptions, are not properly Latin words, since they have the pure Greek termination in *-on*. *Liriodendron* is of modern origin; *Rhododendron* is to be found in Roman writers, but they were so averse to have the name of a tree with a neuter termination, that Pliny writes it *Rhododen′dros*, thus converting it into a feminine noun. Some of the names of trees are of different declensions: *e.g.* *Cor′nus*, usually of the fourth, is sometimes of the second; *Pi′nus* appears to be used about equally in the second and fourth; but the gender remains the same, being always feminine in the works of the best writers

countries, if taken sick, might die before a prescription written in his native tongue could be interpreted. But, whatever weight may be attached to the arguments by which the practice is sought to be defended, the fact that it is sanctioned by so large a portion of the civilized world, and that it is in a manner recognized both by the United States and British Pharmacopœias, in which the officinal names of medicines are always given in Latin, makes it absolutely necessary for the student of Medicine or Pharmacy, who aspires to a respectable rank in his profession, to bestow some attention upon this subject.

The word prescription is from the Latin *præ*, "before," or "beforehand," and *scri'bo*, to "write," and signifies, strictly speaking, something written out beforehand to serve as a guide or direction to others; but it is also applied to any formal directions, whether written or spoken, which a physician may give for promoting or restoring the health of his patient. He may prescribe blood-letting or exercise, and his directions to this effect constitute his prescription; but the application of the term is usually restricted to written directions (also called *formulæ*) for compounding and administering medicines. Formulæ are of two kinds, viz.: *officinal*, including the directions for the preparation of medicines published in Pharmacopœias; and *extemporaneous* (or *magistral*), denoting those which the physician writes out for some particular occasion.

A simple formula is one which contains but a single officinal preparation: as,

℞ Extracti Hyoscyami ....ʒj.
Fiant pilulæ xii.

("Take of Extract of Hyoscyamus a drachm. Let twelve pills be made [of it].")

A compound formula is one containing two or more officinal preparations: as,

℞ Magnesiæ Sulphatis..ʒij.
Infusi Sennæ..℥j.
Misce.

("Take of the Sulphate of Magnesia two drachms, of the Infusion of Senna an ounce. Mix [them].")

The principal medicine in a formula is termed the *basis;* that which assists or promotes the action of the basis is called an *auxiliary* or *adjuvant* (*ad'juvans*); that which corrects some objectionable quality is termed a *corrective* (*cor'rigens*); and that which is used to give a form convenient for administering the whole, is the *excipient*, or *vehicle*, or *constituent* (*excip'iens*, *vehic'ulum*, or *constit'uens*), as illustrated in the following formula:—

℞ Aloes............. ....ʒss (*basis*).
Hydrargyri Chloridi Mitis ....gr. vj. (*auxiliary*).
Olei Anisi..guttas v. (*corrective*).
Syrupi quantum sufficit (*excipient*) ut fiant pilulæ xii.

("Take of Aloes a half drachm, of the Mild Chloride of Mercury six grains, of Oil of Anise five drops, of Syrup a sufficient quantity so that twelve pills may be made.")

Any one who has a tolerable understanding of English grammar will have little difficulty in writing prescriptions correctly, if he will carefully attend to the following rules and directions.

RULE FIRST.—Whenever the *quantity* of any medicine or material is mentioned, the name of the material must always be put in the genitive case: thus, in the following example:—

℞ Eupatorii...℥j.
Aquæ Ferventis (*or* Bullientis)...Oj.
Macera per horas duas et cola.

("Take of Eupatorium an ounce, of boiling water a pint. Macerate for two hours and strain.")

Nota bene: it is necessary to write *Eupatorii* (not *Eupatorium*), and *Aquæ ferventis* (not *Aqua fervens*), since we cannot say, in English, "an ounce Eupatorium," any more than we can say, "a pint boiling water." The genitive termination in the Latin is even more indispensable than the preposition "of" is in the English; because in certain cases the "of" may be understood if it has previously been expressed: thus, we might say, "Take of Eupatorium an ounce, boiling water a pint." But the genitive termination in Latin can never thus be understood, but must *always be expressed:* indeed, it exactly corresponds in this respect to the regular form of the English possessive. It would be very ridiculous to say, in English, "John's and William books," or "Cowper's and Milton poems," on the ground that the *s* and *apostrophe* (which are, in fact, the English genitive or possessive termination) are to be *understood* after the second name: it is equally absurd to suppose that the Latin genitive termination can ever be understood when not expressed. We have dwelt longer upon this point, because physicians not wholly ignorant of the Latin tongue frequently commit the ridiculous blunder here alluded to. They may judge how their Latin would strike a good classical scholar, from the impression made on their own minds by such specimens of English as those cited above.

If the writer of a prescription cannot afford to take the trouble to be correct, it would perhaps be better for him to use abbreviated names or terms, thus:—

℞ Magnes. Sulph......................ʒij.
Infus. Senn...........................℥j.

℞ Eupator......................................℥j.
Aq. Fervent...................................Oj.

by which expedient he would, at least, shelter himself from criticism. But we would strongly recommend to those students whose ambition it is to excel in their profession, bravely to master the difficulty at the outset, and, if they afterwards think proper to employ such abbreviated terms, let them do so rather to economize time than to conceal their ignorance. The liability to mistakes, however, on the part of the druggist who puts up the prescription, is not a little increased by a resort to such abbreviations, and, if they are used at all, particular care should be taken that every letter be written distinctly. ☞ The same, or greater, caution is needed with respect to writing the signs for *ounce, drachm,* etc.; for cases might readily occur, in which the substitution of an ounce for a drachm of some particular medicine might be attended with fatal consequences.

Many of the names used in Pharmacy are compound: as, *Extractum Hyoscyami* ("Extract of Hyoscyamus"), *Infusum Sennæ* ("Infusion of Senna"), *Magnesiæ Sulphas* ("Sulphate of Magnesia"). In each of these examples there is a noun in the nominative joined with one in the genitive case, the latter qualifying the former somewhat in the manner of an adjective; for "Infusion of Senna" has precisely the same meaning as "Senna Infusion," if we use "Senna" as an adjective: so *Aqua Creasoti,* "Creasote Water" (literally, "Water of Creasote"), *Aqua Rosæ,* "Rose Water" (literally, "Water of Rose"). It is to be observed that in prescriptions this qualifying noun (which is always in the genitive case, though it is sometimes put first, and sometimes second) must remain unchanged. For example: if we wish to introduce the term "Sulphate of Magnesia" (*Magnesiæ Sulphas*) into a formula, *Magnesiæ*, which is the qualifying word, must remain always in the genitive, whatever may be the form of the sentence in which it occurs; but the other term, *Sulphas*, is to be changed according to circumstances, or as the meaning of the writer may require. If, as before observed, the quantity of any substance be mentioned, the substance itself must be put in the genitive: as, "of the Sulphate of Magnesia one ounce" (*Magnesiæ Sulphatis* ℥j). But suppose, the quantity having been previously determined, he should have occasion to speak of combining the "Infusion of Senna with Sulphate of Magnesia:" he should then write *Infusum* (or *Infusi*, according to the nature of the sentence) *Sennæ cum Magnesiæ Sulphate*. Here it will be seen that while the qualifying term (*Magnesiæ*) remains the same, the other term (*Sulphas*) is put in the ablative case, being governed by the preposition *cum*, "with." If the learner should ask why the preposition does not govern *Magnesiæ*, seeing it comes next to it, the answer is that the SENSE, or MEANING, forbids it: the meaning is "with the sulphate," not "with magnesia," the latter term being governed in the genitive by "of." Should we put "magnesia" in the ablative and "sulphate" in the genitive, we should have "with magnesia of sulphate," which is simply nonsense.*

It may here be remarked that in Latin it matters comparatively little in what order the words stand, provided each is in its proper case: thus, we may say *Sulphas Magnesiæ*, or *Magnesiæ Sulphas*, though the latter is more usual. We might also say either *Cum Sulphate Magnesiæ*, or *Cum Magnesiæ Sulphate*, since, whichever arrangement of words we use, the cases of each remain the same. So, frequently, in English, we may change the *order* of the words, provided we preserve the sense. We may say either the "brain's base," or the "base of the brain," "hartshorn" (hart's horn), or the "horn of the hart;" but the Latin language admits of transposition to a much greater extent, even when precisely the same words are made use of. Thus, for the "Compound Powder of Rhubarb," we might say, in Latin, either *Compositus Pulvis Rhei*, *Rhei Compositus Pulvis*, *Pulvis Compositus Rhei*, *Rhei Pulvis Compositus*, or *Pulvis Rhei Compositus*, and the meaning would be precisely the same whichever arrangement of the words we might adopt. But, though each form is grammatically correct, euphony requires the last; for by either of the other arrangements the two words *pulvis* and *compositus*, both ending in *s*, would come

---

* To make this subject perfectly clear, it may be well to restate the same principle in different words. When it is directed to put any compound name into the genitive, accusative, etc., the direction *always has reference to that part which is in the* NOMINATIVE, as the name stands in the Pharmacopœia. Thus, in the following examples, *Potas'sæ Carbo'nas*, *Decoc'tum Chimaph'ilæ*, *Extrac'tum Can'nabis Purifica'tum*, etc., "Carbonas," "Decoctum," and "Extractum purificatum" would alone be changed; if to the genitive, we should have "Carbonatis," "Decocti," and "Extracti purificati" (for, as "purificatum" agrees with "Extractum," it must change with it): if to the ablative, "Carbonate," "Decocto," and "Extracto purificato."

☞ Some compound Pharmacopœial names consist of a noun joined with one or more adjectives: as, *Syru'pus Toluta'nus* (U.S. Ph.), "Syrup of Tolu;" *Vi'num Antimonia'le* (Br. Ph.), "Antimonial Wine;" *Pilu'læ Cathar'ticæ Compos'itæ* (U.S. Ph.), "Compound Cathartic Pills." In writing such names, it is only necessary to take care that the adjective always agrees with the noun in number, gender, and case. If the noun is put in the genitive, the adjective must be so likewise: as, ℞ *Syrupi Tolutani fluidunciam* ("Take of Syrup of Tolu a fluidounce"); ℞ *Vini Antimonia'lis fluidrachmam* ("Take of Antimonial Wine a fluidrachm"). It is to be observed that *Toluta'nus* ("of, or pertaining to, Tolu") is declined like *la'tus* (page 672), and *Antimonia'le* like *mi'te* (neuter of *mi'tis*, page 673). But, should we have occasion to say, "To this mixture add the Syrup of Tolu," then both noun and adjective must be put in the accusative, as follows: *Huic misturæ adde Syrupum Tolutanum*.

together, producing a disagreeable alliteration. True, this might also be avoided by the form *Compositus Rhei Pulvis*; but it is usually considered preferable in Latin to place the noun before the adjective or participle.*

Variations with respect to the arrangement of the different words in a phrase are, in fact, not uncommon. Thus, for the "Bark of Pomegranate Root," our Pharmacopœia has *Granati Radicis Cortex,* while the Prussian Pharmacopœia (referred to in a note on page 666) has *Cortex Radicis Granati;* other similar examples might be cited.

RULE SECOND.—The terms which indicate the *quantity* of any material in the prescription—such, for example, as "pound," "ounce," "drachm," "scruple," "grain," "pint," "drop," or "minim," etc.—must invariably be put in the accusative case, being directly governed by the active verb *recipe,* "take."† Although these measures of quantity are usually represented by signs (as ℥, ʒ, ℈, O, etc.), which can have no distinction of case, yet the student ought to be able to write them out should occasion require; for if he is acquainted only with the signs, he will scarcely be able to read a prescription written out in full, and cases might occur in which this would be highly important: thus, he might be applied to to interpret a prescription written by another physician. He who would aspire to an honorable rank in his profession, whether as a physician or pharmacist, must not be content with knowing merely what is absolutely necessary, but should use every means within his power to become thoroughly accomplished in the different branches of his vocation.

In order clearly to explain the application of the rules above given, it may be useful to cite a number of examples. Suppose one should wish to write out in full the Latin of the following:—

Take of Sulphate of Magnesia two drachms.
of Infusion of Senna a fluidounce.
Mix.

Now, according to Rule First, the *material* itself must be put in the genitive: we should then have *Magnesiæ Sulphatis* (the genitive of *Magnesiæ Sulphas*), and *Infusi Sennæ* (the genitive of *Infusum Sennæ*). According to Rule Second, the word denoting the *quantity* must be put in the accusative: therefore we must write *drachmas* (the accusative plural of *drachma,* a "drachm:" see the declension of *Vena* on page 661), and *fluidunciam* (the accusative singular of *fluiduncia,* a "fluidounce.") The whole, written out in full, without signs or abbreviations, would then stand as follows:—

Recipe Magnesiæ Sulphatis drachmas duas
Infusi Sennæ fluidunciam.
Misce.

The principle is, of course, the same however the quantities may vary: thus, we might substitute *six* drachms for *two,* and *three* ounces for *one,* in which case the

* Compare the following names occurring in the United States Pharmacopœia,—*Pilulæ Saponis Compositæ* ("Compound Pills of Soap"); *Tinctura Opii Acetata* ("Acetated Tincture of Opium"), *Mistura Ferri Composita* ("Compound Mixture of Iron"), *Infusum Gentianæ Compositum* ("Compound Infusion of Gentian"), *Hydrargyrum Ammoniatum* ("Ammoniated Mercury"), *Hydrargyri Oxidum Rubrum* ("Red Oxide of Mercury"), in all of which the participle or adjective is placed after the noun.

† It will be seen that the principle is precisely the same as in English grammar: thus, when we say, in English, "Take of Infusion of Senna an ounce," it is not the noun "Infusion," but "ounce," which is governed in the objective by the verb "take;" "Infusion" being governed by the preposition "of."

noun "fluidounce" (*fluiduncia*) would still be in the accusative, the only change being from the singular to the plural, while the terms representing the materials would remain unchanged. The prescription would then stand—

Recipe Magnesiæ Sulphatis drachmas sex.*
Infusi Sennæ fluiduncias tres.
Misce.

Again: suppose we wish to put into Latin the following:—

Take of the Carbonate of Magnesia a drachm.
of the Powder of Rhubarb fifteen grains.
of Peppermint Water two fluidounces.
Let a mixture be made, of which a tablespoonful may be given every two hours.

We must first put the materials in the genitive. *Magnesiæ Carbonas* will then be changed to *Magnesiæ Carbonatis; Pulvis Rhei*, to *Pulveris Rhei; Aqua Menthæ Piperitæ*, to *Aquæ Menthæ Piperitæ*. The quantities being put in the accusative, *drachma* is changed to *drachmam, granum* to *grana* (the accusative plural), *fluiduncia* to *fluiduncias* (also accusative plural). The prescription would then stand—

℞ Magnesiæ Carbonatis drachmam.
Pulveris Rhei grana quindecim.
Aquæ Menthæ Piperitæ fluiduncias duas.
Fiat mistura, cujus detur cochleare magnum omni bihorio.

Again, write the following in Latin:—

Take of the Mixture of Ammoniac three fluidounces.
of the Tincture of Castor half a fluidrachm.
of Syrup of Tolu half a fluidounce.
of Tincture of Opium five drops.
of Cinnamon Water a fluidounce.
Let a mixture be made. Of this a dessert-spoonful may be taken every three hours.

Putting the materials in the genitive, we shall have to change *Mistura Ammoniaci* to *Misturæ Ammoniaci, Tinctura Castorei* to *Tincturæ Castorei, Syrupus Tolutanus* to *Syrupi Tolutani, Tinctura Opii* to *Tincturæ Opii*, and *Aqua Cinnamomi* to *Aquæ Cinnamomi*. Putting the quantities in the accusative, we must write, for "three fluidounces," *fluiduncias tres;* "half a fluidrachm," *fluidrachmam dimidiam;*† "half a fluidounce," *fluidunciam dimidiam;*† "five drops," *guttas quinque;* "a fluidounce," *fluidunciam.*

The whole prescription would then be as follows:—

Recipe Misturæ Ammoniaci fluiduncias tres.
Tincturæ Castorei fluidrachmam dimidiam.
Syrupi Tolutani fluidunciam dimidiam.
Tincturæ Opii guttas quinque.
Aquæ Cinnamomi fluidunciam.
Fiat mistura. Hujus sumatur cochleare medium omni trihorio.

---

* The learner will bear in mind that the Latin numerals after *tres* ("three") are indeclinable; that is, the termination remains the same through all the cases.

† It is to be observed that in Latin they rarely say the "half *of* a thing," but commonly use 'half," as well as "whole," simply as an adjective: thus, they say *totus orbis*, the "whole world," *urbs tota*, the "whole city:" in like manner, they would say *dimidius orbis* (or *orbis dimidius*), "half the world," *urbs dimidia*, "half the city," &c. In writing, however, the phrase an "ounce and a half," they do not say *unciam et dimidiam*, but usually *unciam* (or *uncia*) *cum semisse*, an "ounce together with [its] half." They likewise say *sesquiuncia* and *sescuncia* (see page 691).

It will be observed that in the last two examples, *directions* have been added respecting the dose, and the time when it should be taken. It is, however, generally preferable—and it is the almost universal custom in this country—to write the directions in English. The latter part of these prescriptions might then be changed as follows:—

Fiat mistura. Signa.* Let a tablespoonful be given every two hours.
Fiat mistura. Signa.* Let a dessert-spoonful of this be taken every three hours.

As, however, the United States have become a place of resort for persons from every part of the world, and it is, therefore, important that our physicians and pharmacists should not be wholly ignorant of the customs of other countries, the two following rules relating to the proper mode of writing Latin directions, have been added.

RULE THIRD.—In the directions appended to a prescription, the terms used for the purpose of indicating the time WHEN (or AT WHICH) the medicine should be taken, must be put in the ablative case.† For example: —

℞ Massæ de hydrargyro grana sex.
Opii grana tria.
Permisce (vel misce accuratè) et divide in pilulas duodecim. Harum una sumatur omni nocte.

("Take of Blue Mass (literally, "of the mass [prepared] from Mercury") six grains,
of Opium three grains.
Mix thoroughly (or mix carefully) and divide into twelve pills. Of these let one be taken every night.")

Recipe Decocti Cetrariæ octarium.
Hujus sumatur poculum omni trihorio.

("Take of Decoction of Iceland Moss a pint. Of this let a cupful be taken every three hours.")

Recipe Magnesiæ drachmam.
Aquæ Menthæ Piperitæ fluiduncias sex.
Misce.
Capiat cochleare minimum omni horâ.

("Take of Magnesia a drachm.
of Peppermint Water six fluidounces.
Mix [them].
Let him [the patient] take a teaspoonful every hour.")

So, if we have occasion to use for the same purpose such terms as the following, "half an hour" (*semiho'ra*), an "hour and a half" (*sesquiho'ra*), "two hours" (*biho'rium*) [*i.e.* the "space of two hours"], "three hours" (*triho'rium*), these Latin nouns (with their adjectives) must be put in the ablative: *e.g. om'ni semiho'râ*, "every half-hour," *omni bihorio*, "every two hours," *quartâ quâque horâ*, "every fourth hour," *quâque semihorâ*, "every half-hour," *quâque sesquihorâ*, "every hour and a half," etc. etc. So, if we should wish to say, "at night," we must write *noc'te* (the ablative of *nox*, "night"), "at evening," *ves'pere* (the ablative of *vesper*), etc. In like manner, we say *horâ somni*, "at the hour of sleep," or *horâ decubitûs*, "at

* The imperative mood of *signo*, to "mark," or "write."
† *Mane*, "in the morning," commonly regarded as an adverb, is perhaps the ablative case of some obsolete noun. *Vespere*, "in the evening," though usually called an adverb, appears to be nothing more than the ablative singular of *vesper*, "evening," a noun of the third declension.

the hour (or time) of going to bed," that is, "at bedtime;" *horâ sextâ,* "at the sixth hour," or at six o'clock; *mediâ nocte,* "at midnight." If we use the noun in the plural, the rule is the same: *e.g. alternis diebis,* "every other day:" literally, "on alternate days;" *singulis noctibus,* "in each of the nights," that is, "every night;" in all of which examples, as it will be seen, the noun and adjective (whenever it has an adjective) are put in the ablative.

RULE FOURTH.—Nouns or adjectives showing HOW LONG any process or course is to be continued, must be put in the accusative, usually governed by *per,* "through," "during," or "for:" as, *macera per horam,* "macerate for an hour," *continuetur per sex dies,* "let it be continued for six days," *coque per quadrantem horæ,* "boil for a quarter of an hour," etc.

Prepositions governing the Accusative.

Ad, *to,* or *at;* also, *according to:* as, *ad defectio'nem an'imi,* "to fainting."

An'te, *before:* as, *an'te decu'bitum,* "before lying down:" *i.e.* before going to bed.

Con'tra, *against:* as, *con'tra ver'mes,* "against worms:" *i.e.* anthelmintic.

In, when it signifies *to,* or *into,** governs the accusative: as, *te're in pul'verem,* "rub or grind to a powder;" *contun'de in mas'sam,* "beat into a mass."

In'fra, *below:* as, *in'fra or'bitam,* "below or beneath the orbit."

In'ter, *between:* as, *in'ter scap'ulas,* "between the shoulders."

In'tra, *in,* or *within:* as, *in lin'teum consu'tum,* "sewed up in linen" (applied to certain powders, poultices, etc.).

Per, *through, by, during, for:* as, *per ho'ram,* "for an hour," etc.

Post, *after:* as, *post par'tum,* "after parturition."

Præ'ter, *beyond, exceeding:* as, *præ'ter natu'ram,* "beyond or contrary to [the usual course of] nature."

Secun'dum, *according to:* as, *secun'dum ar'tem,* "according to [the rules] of art."

Sub, *near, towards:* as, *sub fi'nem,* "near the end."

Su'per, *on,* or *upon:* as, *su'per pan'num* (or *alu'tam*) *exten'de,* "spread upon cloth (or leather)."

Prepositions governing the Ablative.

A, ab, or abs, *from, by:* as, *vis a ter'go,* "force from behind;" *ab eâ par'te,* "from that part."

Cum, *with:* as, *hydrar'gyrum cum cre'tâ,* "mercury with chalk."

De, *from, of:* as, *de di'e in di'em,* "from day to day."

E, or ex, *out, from, out of:* as, *detraha'tur e brach'io san'guis,* "let blood be drawn from the arm;" *mas'sa ex hydrar'gyro,* "mass [prepared] out of mercury."

In, when it signifies simply *in* or *on** (and cannot be rendered by *into*): as, *in ventric'ulo,* "in the stomach;" *in u'tero,* "in the uterus."

Pro, *for, according to:* as, *suma'tur pro po'tu,* "let it be taken for [or as] a drink;" *pro re na'tâ,* "according to circumstances."

Sub, when it signifies simply *under* or *beneath,* without any idea of motion *to* or *towards* a place or thing (see *note* to *In*).

The table following comprises the most important of those Latin verbs which are likely to be used in writing prescriptions, directions, etc. By observing the power or signification of the different moods and tenses, as explained at the beginning of the table (see *Do, da're, Co'lo, cola're,* etc.), the learner will be able to apply the same to such other verbs as he may meet with. Thus, if he knows that *det'raho* signifies to "draw" (compare *ex'traho,* of the third conjugation), he would know that *det'rahat* must mean "he may draw," or "let him draw," and *detraha'tur* (in

* To make the proper distinction between *in* governing the accusative, and *in* governing the ablative, at first seems difficult; but it is only necessary to consider the sense in which it is used. Whenever there is an idea of passing or changing from one *place* or *state into another, in* is followed by the accusative: *e.g. red'ige in pul'verem,* "reduce to powder:" here, the idea implies a change from one *state* to another; so *injicia'tur in ventric'ulum,* "let it be thrown into the stomach," in which case the change is from one *place* to another. But if we speak of a thing being already in a certain place or state, the preposition is invariably followed by the ablative: as, *in ventric'ulo,* "in the stomach;" *in u'tero,* "in the uterus;" *in pul'vere,* "in powder or dust." In English, speaking familiarly, we sometimes use "in" for "into," but in writing Latin we must always consider the idea as above explained; for, whether we say, pour the liquor *in* the bottle, or *into* the bottle, the meaning is the same; therefore we must say in Latin, *fun'de liquo'rem in lage'nam,* never *in lage'nâ.*

	Active Voice.			Passive Voice.			
	Indicative present. Infinitive present.	*Imperative.*	*Subjunctive pres.*	*Infinitive.*	*Subjunctive present.*	*Future participle.*	*Past participle.*
First Conjugation.	Do, da're, to "give."	da, "give."	det,* he "may give," or "let [him] give."	da'ri, to "be given."	de'tur,* it "may be given," "let [it] be given," or "let [there] be given."	dan'dus, to "be given."	da'tus, "given."
	Co'lo, cola're, to "strain."	co'la, "strain."	co'let,* he "may strain," or "let [him] strain."	cola'ri, to "be strained."	cole'tur,* it "may be strained," "let [it] be strained," or "let [there] be strained."	colan'dus, to "be strained."	cola'tus, "strained."
	Adminis'tro, administra're, to "administer."	adminis'tra.	adminis'tret.	administra'ri.	administre'tur.	administran'dus.	administra'tus.
	Ag'ito, agita're, to "shake."	ag'ita.	ag'itet.	agita'ri.	agite'tur.	agitan'dus.	agita'tus.
	Ap'plico, applica're, to "apply."	ap'plica.	ap'plicet.	applica'ri.	applice'tur.	applican'dus.	applica'tus.
	Contin'uo, continua're, to "continue."	contin'ua.	contin'uet.	continua'ri.	continue'tur.	continuan'dus.	continua'tus.
	Evapo'ro, evapora're, to "evaporate."	evapo'ra.	evapo'ret.	evapora'ri.	evapore'tur.	evaporan'dus.	evapora'tus.
	Explo'ro, explora're, to "examine."	explo'ra.	explo'ret.	explora'ri.	explore'tur.	exploran'dus.	explora'tus.
	Inha'lo, inhala're, to "inhale."	inha'la.	inha'let.	inhala'ri.	inhale'tur.	inhalan'dus.	inhala'tus.
	Maç'ero, macera're, to "macerate."	maç'era.	maç'eret.	macera'ri.	macere'tur.	maceran'dus.	macera'tus.
	Mandu'co, manduca're, to "chew."	mandu'ca.	mandu'cet.	manduca'ri.	manduce'tur.	manducan'dus.	manduca'tus.
	Pa'ro, para're, to "prepare."	pa'ra.	pa'ret.	para'ri.	pare'tur.	paran'dus.	para'tus.
	Per'sto, -a're, to "persevere," or "continue."	per'sta.	per'stet.				
	Po'to, pota're, to "drink."	po'ta.	po'tet.	pota'ri.	pote'tur.	potan'dus.	pota'tus and po'tus.
	Præp'aro, præpara're, to "prepare."	præp'ara.	præp'aret.	præp'ari.	præpare'tur.	præparan'dus.	præpara'tus.
	Pul'vero, pulvera're, to "pulverize."	pul'vera.	pul'veret.	pulvera'ri.	pulvere'tur.	pulveran'dus.	pulvera'tus.
	Pur'go, purga're, to "purge."	pur'ga.	pur'get.	purga'ri.	purge'tur.	purgan'dus.	purga'tus.
	Ren'ovo, renova're, to "renew."	ren'ova.	ren'ovet.	renova'ri.	renove'tur.	renovan'dus.	renova'tus.
	Ser'vo, serva're, to "keep."	ser'va.	ser'vet.	serva'ri.	serve'tur.	servan'dus.	serva'tus.
	Sig'no, signa're, to "mark," or "write."	sig'na.	sig'net.	signa'ri.	signe'tur.	signan'dus.	signa'tus.
	Sto, sta're, to "stand."	sta.	stet.				
	Usur'po, usurpa're, to "use," or "take."	usur'pa.	usur'pet.	usurpa'ri.	usurpe'tur.	usurpan'dus.	usurpa'tus
Second Conjugation.	Admo'veo, admove're, to "apply" (literally, to "move to").	ad'move, "apply."	admo'veat,* he "may apply," or "let [him] apply."	admove'ri, "to be applied."	admovea'tur, "it may be applied," "let [it] be applied," or "let [there] be applied."	admoven'dus, "to be applied."	admo'tus, "applied."
	Adhib'eo, adhibe're, to "apply," to "give."	ad'hibe.	adhib'eat.	adhibe'ri.	adhibea'tur.	adhiben'dus.	adhib'itus.
	Admis'ceo, admisce're, to "mix with."	admis'ce.	admis'ceat.	admis'ceri.	admiscea'tur.	admiscen'dus.	admix'tus, or admis'tus.
	Au'geo, auge're, to "increase" or "augment."	au'ge.	au'geat.	auge'ri.	augea'tur.	augen'dus.	auc'tus.
	Ca'veo, cave're, to "take care" or "beware," to "shun."	ca've.	cave'at.	cave'ri.	cavea'tur.	caven'dus.	cau'tus.
	Cie'o, cie're, to "excite."	ci'e.	ci'eat.	cie'ri.	ciea'tur.	cien'dus.	ci'tus.
	Commis'ceo, commisce're, to "mix with," or to "mix together."	commis'ce.	commis'ceat.	commisce'ri.	commiscea'tur.	commiscen'dus.	commix'tus, or commis'tus.
	Exhib'eo, -e're, to "administer."	ex'hibe.	exhib'eat.	exhibe'ri.	exhibea'tur.	exhiben'dus.	exhib'itus.
	Fo'veo, fove're, to "foment," or "apply fomentations to."	fo've.	fo'veat.	fove'ri.	fovea'tur.	foven'dus.	fo'tus.
	Mis'ceo, misce're, to "mix."	mis'ce.	mis'ceat.	misce'ri.	miscea'tur.	miscen'dus.	mix'tus, or mis'tus.
	Mo'veo, move're, to "move," to "stir."	mo've.	mo'veat.	move'ri.	movea'tur.	moven'dus.	mo'tus.
	Permis'ceo, permisce're, to "mix through" or "mix thoroughly."	permis'ce.	permis'ceat.	permisce'ri.	permiscea'tur.	permiscen'dus.	permix'tus, or permis'tus.
	Promo'veo, -e're, to "excite," or "promote."	promo've.	promo'veat.	promove'ri.	promovea'tur.	promoven'dus.	promo'tus.
	Respon'deo, responde're, to "answer," as when a medicine produces the effect desired.	respon'de.	respon'deat.				

* The literal signification is, "he may give." "it may be given," "he may apply," "it may be applied," &c.; but in medical language it is usually employed as third person of the imperative: *e.g.* "let him give," "let it be given," "let him apply."

	Active Voice.			Passive Voice.			
	Indicative present. Infinitive present.	*Imperative.*	*Subjunctive pres.*	*Infinitive.*	*Subjunctive present.*	*Future participle.*	*Past participle.*
	Adjiç'io, adjiç'ere, to "add," or "add to."	ad'jice.	adjiç'iat, he "may add," or "let [him] add."	ad'jici, to be "added."	adjiçia'tur, it "may be added," "let [it] be added," or "let [there] be added."	adjiçien'dus, to "be added."	adjec'tus, "added."
Third Conjugation.	Ad'do, ad'dere, to "add."	ad'de.	ad'dat.	ad'di.	adda'tur.	adden'dus.	ad'ditus.
	Appo'no, appo'nere, to "put to," or "apply."	appo'ne.	ap'ponat.	appo'ni.	appona'tur.	apponen'dus.	appos'itus.
	Bi'bo, bib'ere, to "drink."	bi'be.	bi'bat.	bi'bi.	biba'tur.	biben'dus.	bib'itus.
	Ca'pio, cap'ere, to "take."	ca'pe.	ca'piat.	ca'pi.	capia'tur.	capien'dus.	cap'tus.
	Col'luo, -ere, to "wash," or "wash thoroughly."	col'lue.	col'luat.	col'lui.	collua'tur.	colluen'dus.	collu'tus.
	Conci'do, conci'dere, to "slice," or "cut into small pieces."	conci'de.	conci'dat.	conci'di.	concida'tur.	conciden'dus.	conci'sus.
	Concu'tio, concu'tere, to "shake," or "agitate."	con'cute.	concu'tiat.	con'cuti.	concutia'tur.	concutien'dus.	concus'sus.
	Confiç'io, confiç'ere, to "make up," or "make" (literally to "make together").	con'fice.	confiç'iat.	con'fici.	conficia'tur.	conficien'dus.	confec'tus.
	Con'tero, conter'ere, to "rub together."	con'tere.	con'terat.	con'teri.	contera'tur.	conteren'dus.	contri'tus.
	Contun'do, contun'dere, to "beat together," to "bruise."	contun'de.	contun'dat.	contun'di.	contunda'tur.	contunden'dus.	contu'sus.
	Co'quo, coq'uere, to "boil," or "cook."	co'que.	co'quat.	co'qui.	coqua'tur.	coquen'dus.	coc'tus.
	De'coquo, decoq'uere, to "boil down."	de'coque.	de'coquat.	de'coqui.	decoqua'tur.	decoquen'dus.	decoc'tus.
	Dig'ero, diger'ere, to "digest."	dig'ere.	dig'erat.	dig'eri.	digera'tur.	digeren'dus.	diges'tus.
	Div'ido, divid'ere, to "divide."	div'ide.	div'idat.	div'idi.	divida'tur.	dividen'dus.	divi'sus.
	Ex'primo, -ere, to "press out," or "express."	ex'prime.	ex'primat.	ex'primi.	exprima'tur.	exprimen'dus.	expres'sus.
	Ex'traho, extrah'ere, to "extract."	ex'trahe.	ex'trahat.	ex'trahi.	extraha'tur.	extrahen'dus.	extrac'tus.
	Faç'io, faç'ere, to "make."	fac.	faç'iat.	fie'ri.*	fi'at.*	facien'dus.	fac'tus.
	Fun'do, fun'dere, to "pour."	fun'de.	fun'dat.	fun'di.	funda'tur.	funden'dus.	fu'sus.
	Man'do, man'dere, to "chew."	man'de.	man'dat.	man'di.	manda'tur.	manden'dus.	man'sus.
	Mit'to, mit'tere, to "send," to "cause to pass."	mit'te.	mit'tat.	mit'ti.	mitta'tur.	mitten'dus.	mis'sus.
	Po'no, po'nere, to "put," or "place."	po'ne.	po'nat.	po'ni.	pona'tur.	ponen'dus.	pos'itus.
	Præscri'bo, præscri'bere, to "prescribe."	præscri'be.	præscri'bat.	præscri'bi.	præscriba'tur.	præscriben'dus.	præscrip'tus.
	Ra'do, rad'ere, to "scrape," or "rasp."	ra'de.	ra'dat.	ra'di.	rada'tur.	raden'dus.	ra'sus.
	Recip'io, recip'ere, to "take."	reç'ipe.	recip'iat.	reç'ipi.	recip'iatur.	recipien'dus.	recep'tus.
	Red'igo, redig'ere, to "reduce."	red'ige.	red'igat.	red'igi.	rediga'tur.	redigen'dus.	redac'tus.
	Rep'eto, repet'ere, to "repeat."	rep'ete.	rep'etat.	rep'eti.	repeta'tur.	repiten'dus.	repeti'tus.
	Sol'vo, sol'vere, to "dissolve."	sol've.	sol'vat.	sol'vi.	solva'tur.	solven'dus.	solu'tus.
	Su'mo, su'mere, to "take."	su'me.	su'mat.	su'mi.	suma'tur.	sumen'dus.	sump'tus.
	Te'ro, ter'ere.	te're.	te'rat.	te'ri.	tera'tur.	teren'dus.	tri'tus.
	U'ro, u'rere, to "burn."	u're.	u'rat.	u'ri.	ura'tur.	uren'dus.	us'tus.
	Vo'mo, vom'ere, to "vomit."	vo'me.	vo'mat.	vo'mi.	voma'tur.	vomen'dus.	vom'itus.
4th.	Deglu'tio, degluti're, to "swallow."	deglu'ti.	deglu'tiat.	degluti'ri.	deglutia'tur.	deglutien'dus.	degluti'tus.
	Dor'mio, dormi're, to "sleep."	dor'mi.	dor'miat.				
	Hau'rio, hauri're, to "drink," or "swallow."	hau'ri.	hau'riat.	hauri'ri.	hauria'tur.	haurien'dus.	haus'tus.
	Par'tio, parti're, to "divide."	par'ti.	par'tiat.	parti'ri.	partia'tur.	partien'dus.	parti'tus.

* Properly speaking, *facio* has no passive form, this being supplied by the irregular neuter verb *fio*, which will be noticed more particularly on next page.

☞ The infinitive and future participle passive—*e.g. dari* and *dandus*, *colari* and *colandus*, etc.—are translated into English by the same words, "to be given," "to be strained," but there is an essential difference between the two: the first is the simple infinitive, as occurs in such phrases as the following:—*jussit dari*, "he ordered it to be given;" *potest facile colari*, "it can easily be strained:" but the other always implies that something *must* or *ought* to be done: as, *Hujus misturæ danda sunt cochlearia duo*, "of this mixture two spoonfuls are to be given," or "must be given."

the passive), "it may be drawn," or "let it be drawn." So *rejiç'io*, to "reject" (compare *adjiç'io*), if put in the subjunctive present (*rejiç'iat*), would signify "he [or it] may reject;" in the passive (*rejicia'tur*), "it may be rejected," etc. So *ejiç'io*, to "eject;" *injiç'io*, to "inject [or throw into]," etc. etc. It is important, however, always to note the conjugation to which a verb belongs; for while those of the first conjugation form the present subjunctive third person in *-et* (or *-ent*), the others form it in *-at* (or *-ant*). We need scarcely remark, that if the student wishes fully to master this branch of the subject, he will have to commence the study of Latin in earnest, which, indeed, he ought by all means to do, if his circumstances and time permit. The comparatively brief instructions here given, are intended for those who have not time to study the subject very fully; or else to teach such as may already possess some knowledge of Latin, how to apply that knowledge most advantageously in their medical and pharmaceutical studies.

It should be observed that the third person plural of the subjunctive present (as well as of several other tenses) is formed by inserting *n* before the *t* of the singular: thus, *det*, "he may give;" *dent*, "they may give;" so *ca'piat* or *su'mat*, "he may take;" *ca'piant* or *su'mant*, "they may take." In like manner, in the passive, *n* is added to form the plural: accordingly, *de'tur, capia'tur, suma'tur*, are changed to *den'tur, capian'tur, suman'tur*, etc.

Fi'o, fi'eri, an irregular verb, signifying to "be made," to "become," to "be," is much used in prescriptions, but nearly always in the subjunctive present: as, singular, *fi'at*, "it may be made," "let it be made," or "let there be made;" plural, *fi'ant*, "they may be made," "let them be made," or "let there be made:" *e.g. fi'at mistu'ra*, "let a mixture be made;" *fi'ant pilu'læ duod'ecim*, "let twelve pills be made," etc.

The following are some of the most important Latin terms and phrases (not hitherto explained) used in prescriptions, directions, etc.:—

Absen'te fe'bre, "fever being absent" (or "in the absence of fever").

Ad lib'itum, "at or according to the pleasure [of the patient]."

Adstan'te fe'bre, "fever being present."

Al'iquot (indeclinable), "some," "several."

A'na (abbreviated *aa*), "of each." See Ana, in the Dictionary.

Bid'uum, "the space of two days."

Bis in di'e, "twice a day."

Cochlea're am'plum lar'gum or *mag'num*,* a "tablespoonful" (literally, a "large or big spoon").

Cochlea're me'dium or *mod'icum*, a "dessertspoonful" (literally, a "middle or moderate [sized] spoon").

Cochlea're min'imum, a "teaspoonful" (literally, the "smallest spoon:" *i.e.* a spoon of the smallest size); also termed *Cochlea're par'vum* or *par'vulum*, a "small spoon."

Cochlea'tim, "by spoonfuls."

Cras, "to-morrow."

Cucurbit'ula cruen'ta, } a "cupping-glass." See these terms in
Cucurbit'ula sic'ca, } the Dictionary.

Cy'athus (second declension, masculine), a "wineglass" or "wineglassful."

De di'e in di'em, "from day to day."

Do'nec, "until."

Dum fe'bris ab'sit, "while the fever is absent."

Dum fe'bris ad'stet, "while the fever is on or present."

Ejus'dem, "of the same" (gen. of *i'dem*).

Fe'bre duran'te, or *duran'te fe'bre*, the "fever continuing" (*i.e.* "if the fever continues").

Fo'tus, a "fomentation" (fourth declension).

Frustilla'tim, "in small pieces."

Gutta'tim, "drop by drop."

Haus'tus, a "draught" (fourth declension).

He'ri, "yesterday."

Ho'ris alter'nis, or *alter'nis ho'ris*, "every other hour."

In'dies, "daily," or "from day to day."

In promp'tu, "in readiness."

Jule'pus, jule'pum, or *jula'pium*, a "julep."

Lage'na, a "bottle."

Le'ni fo'co, "by a gentle fire."

Len'to ig'ne, "by a slow fire."

Manip'ulus, a "handful."

---

* When *cochlea're* is used by itself,—that is, without any qualifying word, such as *me'dium*, or *min'imum*,—it is to be understood as signifying a "tablespoonful." It would, however, be better always to mention the kind of spoonful; for even when the medicine is of that character that a little more or less might not be attended with any serious consequences, it is always satisfactory to the patient or attendants to have explicit directions.

Mi'ca pa'nis, "crumb of bread."
Mo're sol'ito, "in the usual manner."
Pan'nus lin'teus, a "linen cloth."
Per sal'tum, "by a leap or spring:" applied to blood when it flows from the vein in a jet.
Phi'ala, a "vial or phial."
Ple'no ri'vo, "in a full stream."
Post ci'bum, "after eating" (literally, "after food").
Pro ratio'ne, "in proportion to:" as, *pro im'petûs ratio'ne*, "in proportion to the violence of the attack."
Prout, "according as."
Quan'tum suf'ficit, or *quan'tum suffi'ciat*, a "sufficient quantity" (literally, "as much as suffices," or "as much as may suffice").
Quan'tum vis, "as much as you choose" (literally, "as much as you will").
Qua'ter in di'e, "four times a day."
Quotid'ie, "daily."
Semiho'ra,* "half an hour."
Se'mis, gen. *semis'sis*, a "half."
Semiun'cia,* "half an ounce."
Septima'na (first declension), a "week."
Sescun'cia,* or *Sesquiun'cia** (better *Un'cia cum semis'se*), an "ounce and a half."
Sesquiho'ra,* an "hour and a half."
Sta'tim, "immediately."
Subin'de, "now and then."
Ter in di'e, or *ter di'e*, "three times a day."
Trid'uum, the "space of three days."
U'tor, u'ti, "to use." This verb (which is called a "*depo'nent* verb," that is, one having a passive form with an active signification), instead of governing the accusative, like most other active verbs, always governs the ablative: *e.g. uta'tur linimen'to cal'cis*, "let him use, or make use of, lime liniment;" *utan'tur lotio'nibus cre'bris*, "let them use frequent lotions." N.B.—*Lo'tio* may be used either in the sense of a "wash," or the "act of washing."

* It may be observed as a universal rule, that when a simple noun forms the termination of a compound, the latter is declined in the same manner as the simple word: thus, *fluidun'cia, semiun'cia, sesquiun'cia*, etc. are declined precisely like *un'cia;* and *semiho'ra, sesquiho'ra*, etc. like *ho'ra:* so *merid'ies*, "mid-day," is declined like *di'es*, "day;" and *pertus'sis*, "hooping-cough," like *tussis*, a "cough." If, however, the termination is changed, it is obvious that the declension must be different; *biho'rium, triho'rium*, etc., being neuter nouns of the second declension, are declined like *ligamentum*, on page 663.

TABLE OF DOSES,

FOR ADULTS.

[See Dose, in the Dictionary.]

Absinthium ℈j. to ℈ij.
Acetum colchici f ʒj. to f ʒij.
Acetum scillæ f ʒss. to f ʒj.
Achillea millefolium ℈j. to ℈ij.
Acid. acetic. dilutum f ʒj. to f ℥ss.
Acid. arseniosum $\frac{1}{16}$ to $\frac{1}{8}$ of a gr.
Acid. benzoicum gr. x. to ʒss.
Acid. carbolicum gr. ij. to gr. v.
Acid. citricum gr. x. to ʒss.
Acid. hydrocyanic. dilut ♏j. to ♏iv.
Acid. lacticum f ʒss. to f ʒij.
Acid. muriaticum dilut ♏x. to ♏xxx.
Acid. nitric. dilut ♏x. to ♏xxx.
Acid. phosphoricum dilut ♏x. to f ʒj.
Acid. sulphuric. dilut ♏x. to ♏xxx.
Acid. tannicum gr. j. to gr. v.
Acid. tartaricum gr. v. to ʒss.
Aconitia gr. $\frac{1}{100}$ to gr. $\frac{1}{50}$.
Aconiti folium gr. j. to gr. ij.
Aconiti radix gr. ss. to gr. j.
Æther ♏xx. to ♏lx.
Æther fortior ♏xx. to f ʒj.
Æther sulphuricus ♏xx. to f ʒj.
Aletris gr. v. to gr. x.
Allium ʒss. to ʒij.
Aloe gr. iij. to gr. xv.
Althæa ʒj. to ℥ss.
Alumen gr. v. to ℈j.
Aluminæ et ammon. sul gr. v. to ℈j.
Ammoniacum gr. x. to ℈j.
Ammoniæ carbonas gr. v. to ℈j.
Ammoniæ murias gr. v. to ℈j.
Ammoniæ valerianas gr. ij. to gr. viii.
Anethum gr. xv. to ʒj.
Angelica ʒss. to ʒj.
Angustura gr. x. to gr. xxx.
Anisum gr. xv. to ʒj.
Anthemis ℈j. to ʒij.
Ant. et pot. tart. *diaph* gr. $\frac{1}{12}$ to gr. $\frac{1}{4}$.
Ant. et pot. tart. *emetic* gr. j. to gr. iij.
Antimonii oxidum gr. j. to gr. iij.
Antimon. sulph. præcip gr. j. to gr. iij.
Apocynum cannab. (pulv.) gr. xv. to gr. xxx.
Aqua acidi carbon *ad libitum.*
Aq. ammo. (dilut. in water) ♏x. to ♏xxx.
Aqua cinnamomi f ℥ss. to f ℥ij.
Aqua creasoti f ʒj. to f ʒij.
Aqua fœniculi f ℥j. to f ℥iv.
Aqua laurocerasi ♏xxx. to f ʒj.
Aqua menthæ piperitæ f ℥j. to f ℥iv.
Aqua menthæ viridis f ℥j. to f ℥iv.
Aqua rosæ *ad libitum.*
Aralia nudicaulis ℈j. to ʒj.
Aralia spinosa ℈j. to ʒj.
Argenti nitras $\frac{1}{8}$ gr. to gr. ij.
Argenti oxidum $\frac{1}{2}$ gr. to gr. ij.
Armoraciæ radix ℈j. to ʒj.
Arnica gr. v. to gr. x.
Arsenici iodidum $\frac{1}{16}$ to $\frac{1}{8}$ of a gr.
Arum gr. x. to ʒss.
Asarum gr. xx. to gr. xxx.
Asclepias gr. xx. to ʒj.
Assafœtida gr. v. to ℈j.
Atropia gr. $\frac{1}{100}$ to gr. $\frac{1}{50}$.
Atropiæ sulphas gr. $\frac{1}{100}$ to gr. $\frac{1}{50}$.
Aurantii amari cortex ʒss. to ʒj.
Azedarach (decoc.) (for a child) a tablespoonful.
Balsamum Peruvianum gr. x. to ʒss.
Balsamum Tolutanum gr. x. to ʒss.
Barii chloridum. See Liquor Barii Chloridi
Belladonnæ folia gr. j. to gr. v.
Belladonnæ radix gr. ss. to gr. iij.
Benzoinum gr. x. to ʒss.
Berberin gr. j. to gr. x.
Bismuthi subcarbonas gr. v. to gr. xlv.
Bismuthi subnitras gr. v. to ʒj.
Bistortæ radix gr. x. to ʒss.
Brominium gr. $\frac{1}{2}$ to gr. ij.
Brucia gr. $\frac{1}{8}$ to gr. $\frac{1}{4}$.
Buchu gr. xx. to ʒj.
Cadmii sulphas gr. ss. to gr. ij.
Calamus gr. x. to ʒj.
Calcis carbonas præcip gr. x. to ʒss.
Calumba gr. x. to ℈j.
Camphora gr. j. to gr. x.
Canella gr. x. to ʒss.
Cantharis gr. ss. to gr. j.
Capsicum gr. ij. to gr. x.
Cardamomum gr. v. to ℈j.
Carthamus (infus.) f ℥ij. to f ℥iv.
Carum ℈j. to ʒj.
Caryophyllus gr. v. to ℈j.
Cascarilla gr. x. to ʒss.
Cassia fistula ʒij. to ℥j.
Cassia Marilandica ʒj. to ʒiij.
Castoreum gr. v. to ℈j.
Cataria ʒj. to ʒij.
Catechu gr. v. to ℥ss.
Cetaceum gr. xv. to ʒiss.
Chenopodium ℈j. to ℈ij.
Chimaphila ʒss. to ʒj.
Chiretta gr. x. to gr. xx.
Chloroformum purific ♏v. to ♏xl.
Cimicifuga gr. x. to ʒss.
Cinchona pulv ʒss. to ℥ss.
Cinchoniæ sulphas gr. j. to gr. v.
Cinnamomi oleum ♏j. to ♏iv.
Cinnamomum gr. v. to ℈j.
Colchici radix gr. j. to gr. v.
Colchici semen gr. j. to gr. iij.
Confectio aromatica gr. x. to ʒj.
Confectio aurantii corticis ʒj. to ℥j.
Confectio opii gr. x. to ℈ij.
Confectio rosæ ʒj. to ℥j.
Confectio sennæ ʒj. to ℥ss.
Conium gr. ij. to gr. v.
Contrayervæ radix gr. x. to ʒj.
Copaiba ♏xv. to f ʒj.
Coptis (pulv.) gr. x. to gr. xxx. (Tinct.) f ʒs to f ʒj.
Coriandrum ℈j. to ʒj.
Cornus (pulv.) ℈j. to ʒj.
Cornus circinata (pulv.) ℈j. to ʒj.

Cornus sericea (pulv.).........℈j. to ʒj.
Cotula, infusion.................f℥j. to f℥ij.
Creta præparata...............gr. x. to ʒss.
Crocus ....gr. x. to gr. xxx.
Cubeba............................ʒj. to ʒiij.
Cumini semina..................℈j. to ʒj.
Cupri subacetas.................used externally.
Cupri sulphas, *emetic*.........gr. v. to gr. x.
Cupri sulphas, *tonic*..........gr. ¼ to gr. j.
Cuprum ammoniatum........gr. ¼ to gr. iv.
Curcuma..........................gr. v. to ʒss.
Cuspariæ cortex................gr. v. to ℈j.
Cusso (or Koosso)...............ʒss.
Cydonium.........................*ad libitum.*
Cypripedium......................gr. x. to gr. xv.
Decoct. cetrariæ.................f℥ij. to f℥iij.
Decoct. chimaphilæ............f℥ij. to f℥iij.
Decoct. cinchonæ...............f℥j. to f℥ij.
Decoct. cornûs floridæ.........f℥j. to f℥ij.
Decoct. dulcamaræ.............f℥ss. to f℥ij.
Decoct. hæmatoxyli............f℥j. to f℥ij.
Decoct. quercûs alb...........f℥j. to f℥ij.
Decoct. sarsaparillæ...........f℥iij. to f℥vi.
Decoct. sarsaparillæ comp...f℥iij. to f℥vi.
Decoct. senegæ..................f℥j. to f℥ij.
Decoct. uvæ ursi................f℥j. to f℥ij.
Delphinium (tinct. of seed)..♏x. to ♏xxx.
Digitalin ....gr. 1/60 to gr. 1/30.
Digitalis (folia).................gr. ⅛ to gr. iij.
Diospyros (dried)...............ʒj. to ʒij.
Dracontium ....gr. x. to gr. xx.
Dulcamara........................gr. xx. to ʒj.
Elaterium.........................gr. ⅛ or ¼ to gr. j.
Ergota ....gr. v. to gr. xxx.
Erigeron (infus.)................f℥ij. to f℥iij.
Erigeron Canadense (pulv.)..gr. xx. to ʒj.
Euonymus (pulv.)...............℈j. to ʒj.
Eupatorium (pulv.)............gr. x. to gr. xxx.
Euphorbia corollata, *emetic*..gr. x. to gr. xx.
Extract. absinth................gr. x. to ℈j.
Extract. aconiti..................gr. ss. to gr. j.
Extract. aconiti alcohol......gr. ¼ to gr. j. or ij.
Extract. aloes. ....gr. v. to gr. xv.
Extract. anthemidis fluid...♏xx. to fʒj.
Extract. arnicæ alcohol.....gr. ½ to gr. j.
Extract. belladonnæ ....gr. ¼ to gr. ij.
Ext. belladonnæ alcohol.....gr. ¼ to gr. ij.
Extract. buchu fluidum......fʒj.
Extract. cannabis...............gr. ¼ to gr. v.
Extract. cimicifugæ fluid...fʒss.
Extract. cinchonæ.............gr. x. to ʒss.
Extract. cinchonæ fluid......fʒss. to fʒj.
Extract. colchici acet.........gr. ½ to gr. ij.
Ext. colchici rad. fluid........♏v. to ♏xv.
Ext. colchici seminis fluid..♏v. to ♏xv.
Extract. colocynth. alcoh...gr. iij. to gr. vi.
Ext. colocynth. comp.........gr. v. to ℈j.
Extract. conii....................gr. ij. to gr. x.
Extract. conii alcohol.........gr. j. to gr. iv.
Extract. conii fluidum........♏v. to ♏x.
Extract. digitalis alcohol....gr. ss. to gr. ij.
Extract. dulcamaræ............gr. v. to gr. x.
Ext. dulcamaræ fluidum.....♏xx. to fʒj.
Extract. ergotæ fluidum.....♏x. to fʒss.
Extract. gentianæ.............gr. v. to ℈j.
Ext. gentianæ fluidum........fʒss. to fʒj
Extract. glycyrrhizæ.........*ad libitum.*
Extract. graminis..............gr. v. to gr. xx.
Extract. hæmatoxyli..........gr. x. to ʒss.
Extract. hellebori alcohol...gr. v. to gr. xv.
Extract. humuli.................gr. v. to ℈j.
Extract. hyoscyami...........gr. ij. to gr. x.
Extract. hyoscyami alcoh...gr. j. to gr. iv.
Ext. hyoscyami fluidum.....♏v. to ♏x.
Extract. ignatiæ alcohol.....gr. ¼ to gr. ½.
Extract. ipecacuan. fluid.....♏j. to ♏xx.
Extract. jalapæ..................gr. v. to gr. xx.
Extract. juglandis.............gr. xv. to gr. xxx.
Extract. krameriæ.............gr. x. to gr. xx.
Extract. lactucæ.................gr. ij. to gr. xv.
Extract. lupulinæ fluidum..♏v. to ♏x.
Ext. nucis vomicæ alcoh.....gr. ½ to gr. ij.
Extract. opii......................gr. ½ to gr. j.
Extract. papaveris.............gr. ij. to gr. x.
Extract. podophylli............gr. v. to gr. xv.
Ext. pruni Virgin. fluidum..fʒj.
Extract. quassiæ...............gr. iij. to gr. v.
Extract. rhei......................gr. v. to gr. xx.
Extract. rhei alcohol..........gr. v. to gr. xx.
Extract. rhei fluidum.........fʒss. to fʒj.
Extract. sarsaparillæ.........gr. x. to ʒj.
Extract. sarsap. fluidum.....fʒj.
Extract. senegæ alcohol.....gr. v. to gr. xv.
Extract. sennæ fluidum......f℥ss.
Extract. serpentariæ fluid...fʒss. to fʒj.
Ext. spigeliæ et sen. fluid...fʒij.
Extract. spigeliæ fluid........fʒj.
Extract. stramonii.............gr. j. to gr. ij.
Extract. stramonii alcoh.....gr. ½ to gr. j.
Extract. taraxaci...............gr. x. to ʒj.
Extract. taraxaci fluidum...fʒj. to fʒij.
Extract. uva ursi fluidum...fʒj to fʒij.
Extract. valerianæ alcoh....gr. v. to gr. x.
Extract. valerianæ fluid.....fʒj.
Ext. veratri virid. fluid......♏v. to ♏x.
Ext. zingiberis fluidum......♏x. to ♏xx.
Ferri chloridum.................gr. iij. to gr. v.
Ferri citras.......................gr. iij. to gr. vj.
Ferri et ammoniæ citras.....gr. iij. to gr. vj.
Ferri et ammon. sulphas.....gr. x. to gr. xv.
Ferri et ammon. tartras......gr. x. to ʒss.
Ferri et potassæ tartras......gr. x. to ʒss.
Ferri et quiniæ citras.........gr. v.
Ferri ferrocyanidum..........gr. ij. to gr. v.
Ferri lactas.......................gr. ij. to gr. x.
Ferri oxidum hydrat. (as an
antidote to arsenic).........f℥ss. to f℥iv.
Ferri phosphas..................gr. iij. to gr. x.
Ferri pulvis.......................gr. j. to gr. iij.
Ferri pyrophosphas............gr. iij. to gr. x.
Ferri subcarbonas.............gr. v. to ℈j.
Ferri sulphas.....................gr. ij. to gr. vj.
Ferri sulphas exsiccata......gr. j. to gr. v.
Ferrum ammoniatum.........gr. iij. to gr. x.
Ferrum redactum..............gr. j. to gr. iij.
Ficus...............................*ad libitum.*
Filicis radix......................ʒj. to ʒij.
Fœniculi semina...............℈j. to ʒj.
Frasera (pulv.)..................gr. xx. to ʒj.
Galbanum ....gr. v. to gr. xv.
Galla (pulv.).....................gr. x. to gr. xx.
Gambogia..........................gr. j. to gr. iij.
Gaultheria (infus.).............f℥ij.
Gelsemium ....gr. v. to gr. xx.
Gentiana ....gr. v. to ℈j.
Gentiana Catesbæi (pulv.)...gr. x. to gr. xxx.
Geranium (pulv.)...............gr. x. to gr. xxx.
Geum, decoction................f℥j. to f℥ij.
Gillenia (pulv.).................gr. xx. to gr. xxx
Glycerina ....fʒj. to fʒij.
Gossypii radix....................gr. v. to gr. xxx.
Granati cortex...................℈j. to ʒj.
Guaiaci lignum..................ʒj. to ʒij.
Guaiaci resina...................gr. x. to ℈j.
Hedeoma...........................ʒj. to ʒij.
Helianthemum extractum..gr. j. to gr. ij.
Helleborus ....gr. v. to ℈j.
Hepatica (infus.)................℥ij. to ℥iv.

Drug	Dose
Heuchera	ʒj. to ʒij.
Humulus	gr. v. to ℈j.
Hydrarg. chlorid. corrosiv.	gr. $\frac{1}{16}$ to gr. $\frac{1}{4}$.
Hydr. chlor. mite, *alterat.*	gr. $\frac{1}{12}$ to gr. $\frac{1}{2}$.
Hydr. chlor. mite, *cathar.*	gr. v. to ℈j.
Hydrarg. cyanidum	gr. $\frac{1}{16}$ to gr. $\frac{1}{8}$.
Hydrarg. iodidum rubrum	gr. $\frac{1}{16}$ to gr. $\frac{1}{4}$.
Hydrarg. iodidum viride	gr. $\frac{1}{2}$ to gr. iij. or iv.
Hydrarg. oxidum nigrum	gr. j. to gr. iij.
Hydrarg. oxidum rubrum	used externally.
Hydr. sulphas flava, *emet.*	gr. ij. to gr. v.
Hydrarg. sulphuret. nigr.	gr. v. to ℈j.
Hydrargyrum ammoniat.	used externally.
Hydrargyrum cum cretâ	gr. iij. to gr. x.
Hydrastis	gr. xv. to gr. xxx.
Hyoscyami folium	gr. iij. to gr. x.
Hyoscyami semen	gr. j. to gr. v.
Ignatia (pulv.)	gr. iij. to gr. v.
Infusum angusturæ	f℥j. to f℥ij.
Infusum anthemidis	f℥j. to f℥ij.
Infusum buchu	f℥j. to f℥ij.
Infusum calumbæ	f℥j. to f℥ij.
Infusum capsici	f℥ss. to f℥j.
Infusum caryophylli	f℥j. to f℥ij.
Infusum cascarillæ	f℥j. to f℥ij.
Infusum catechu comp.	f℥j. to f℥ij.
Infusum cinchonæ flavæ	f℥j. to f℥ij.
Infusum cinchonæ rubræ	f℥j. to f℥ij.
Infusum digitalis	fʒij. to f℥ss.
Infusum eupatorii	f℥j. to f℥ij.
Infusum gentianæ comp.	f℥ss. to f℥ij.
Infusum humuli	f℥j. to f℥ij.
Infusum juniperi	f℥ij. to f℥iv.
Infusum krameriæ	f℥j. to f℥ij.
Infusum lini comp.	*ad libitum.*
Infusum pareiræ	f℥j. to f℥ij.
Infusum picis liquidæ	f℥j. to f℥ij.
Infusum pruni Virginianæ	f℥ij. to f℥iij.
Infusum quassiæ	f℥ss. to f℥ij.
Infusum rhei	f℥ss. to f℥ij.
Infusum rosæ comp.	f℥ss. to f℥ij.
Infusum salviæ	f℥ij.
Infusum sennæ	f℥ij. to f℥iv.
Infusum serpentariæ	f℥j. to f℥ij.
Infusum simarubæ	f℥ss. to f℥ij.
Infusum spigeliæ	f℥ij. to f℥viij.
Infusum taraxaci	f℥ij.
Infusum valerianæ	f℥ij.
Infusum zingiberis	f℥ij.
Inula	℈j. to ʒj.
Iodinium	gr. $\frac{1}{4}$ to gr. ij.
Ipecacuanha, *diaphoretic*	gr. ss. to gr. ij.
Ipecacuanha, *emetic*	gr. x. to gr. xxx.
Iris versicolor	gr. x. to gr. xx.
Jalapa	gr. x. to ℈j.
Juniperus	℈j. to ʒj.
Juniperus Virginiana	no dose.
Kino	gr. x. to ʒss.
Koosso, or Kousso. See Cusso.	
Krameria (extract)	gr. x. to gr. xx.
Lactucarium	gr. v. to gr. x.
Lappa	ʒj. to ʒij.
Lauri baccæ	gr. x. to ℈j.
Leptandra (pulv.)	gr. xv. to ʒj.
Leptandrin	gr. $\frac{1}{4}$ to gr. j.
Limonis cortex	*adjuvant.*
Linum catharticum	℈j. to ʒj.
Liquor ammoniæ. See Aqua Ammoniæ.	
Liquor ammoniæ acetatis	fʒij. to f℥ss.
Liquor barii chloridi	♏iij. to ♏x.
Liquor calcis	f℥j. to f℥iv.
Liquor calcis chloridi	♏xx. to fʒj.
Liquor ferri citratis	♏v. to ♏x.
Liquor ferri iodidi. See Syrupus Ferri Iodidi.	
Liquor ferri nitratis	♏v. to ♏xv. or xx.
Liquor iodinii comp.	♏v. to ♏xxx.
Liquor magnesiæ citratis	f℥xij.
Liquor morphiæ sulphatis	fʒss. to fʒij.
Liquor potassæ	♏v. to ♏xx.
Liquor potassæ arsenitis	♏v. to ♏xx.
Liquor potassæ carbonatis	♏x. to fʒj.
Liquor potassæ citratis	f℥ss.
Liquor sodæ	♏v. to ♏xx.
Liriodendron (pulv.)	ʒj. to ʒij.
Lithiæ carbonas	gr. v. to gr. x.
Lobelia, *emetic*	gr. v. to ℈j.
Lupulina	gr. v. to gr. x.
Lycopus	$\frac{1}{2}$ pt. to 1 pt.
Macis	℈j. to ʒss.
Magnesia	℈j. to ʒj.
Magnesiæ carbonas	ʒj. to ʒij.
Magnesiæ sulphas	℥ss. to ℥j.
Magnolia (pulv.)	ʒss. to ʒj.
Manganesii carbonas	gr. v.
Manganesii sulphas, *cath.*	ʒj. to ʒij.
Manna	℥ss. to ℥j.
Marrubium	℈j. to ʒj.
Mastiche	gr. x. to ʒss.
Matico (pulv.)	ʒss. to ʒij.
Matricaria	ʒj. to ℥ss.
Melissa	ʒj. to ʒij.
Mentha piperita	ʒj. to ʒij.
Mezereum	gr. x. to ʒss.
Mistura ammoniaci	f℥ss.
Mistura amygdalæ	f℥ij. to f℥viii.
Mistura assafœtidæ	f℥ss. to f℥ij.
Mistura chloroformi	fʒss. to fʒj.
Mistura cretæ	f℥ss.
Mistura ferri comp.	f℥ss.
Mistura glycyrrhizæ comp.	a tablespoonful.
Mistura potassæ citratis	f℥ss.
Monarda	ʒj. to ʒij. See Oleum Monardæ.
Morphia	gr. $\frac{1}{8}$ to gr. $\frac{1}{2}$.
Morphiæ acetas	gr. $\frac{1}{8}$ to gr. $\frac{1}{2}$.
Morphiæ murias	gr. $\frac{1}{8}$ to gr. $\frac{1}{2}$.
Morphiæ sulphas	gr. $\frac{1}{8}$ to gr. $\frac{1}{2}$.
Moschus	gr. j. to gr. x.
Mucilago acaciæ	fʒij. to f℥j.
Mucilago sassafras	fʒij. to f℥j.
Mucuna (syrup)	fʒij. to fʒiv.
Myristica	gr. x. to ʒss.
Myrrha	gr. x. to ℈j.
Nectandra	gr. ij. to gr. v.
Nux vomica	gr. v.
Oleoresina capsici	gr. $\frac{1}{8}$ to gr. $\frac{1}{2}$.
Oleoresina cubebæ	♏ij. to ♏x.
Oleoresina lupulinæ	♏j. to ♏iij.
Oleoresina piperis	♏ $\frac{1}{4}$ to ♏j.
Oleoresina zingiberis	♏ $\frac{1}{4}$ to ♏j.
Oleum amygdalæ amaræ	♏ $\frac{1}{4}$ to ♏j.
Oleum amygdalæ dulcis	fʒj. to f℥ss.
Oleum anisi	♏v. to ♏xv.
Oleum anthemidis	♏v. to ♏x.
Oleum cajuputi	♏j. to ♏ij.
Oleum camphoræ	♏j. to ♏v.
Oleum cari	♏j. to ♏viii
Oleum caryophylli	♏j. to ♏v.
Ol. chenopodii (for child)	♏v. to ♏x.
Oleum cinnamomi	♏j. to ♏v.
Oleum copaibæ	♏x. to ♏xv.
Oleum cubebæ	♏vi. to ♏xii.
Oleum erigerontis Canad.	♏j. to ♏v.
Oleum fœniculi	♏v. to ♏x.
Oleum gaultheriæ	♏j. to ♏iij.
Oleum hedeomæ	♏j. to ♏v.
Oleum juniperi	♏v. to ♏xv.
Oleum lavandulæ	♏j. to ♏v.
Oleum limonis	♏i. to ♏v.

Drug	Dose
Oleum lini	f ʒij. to f ℥j.
Oleum menthæ piperitæ	♏v. to ♏x.
Oleum menthæ viridis	♏v. to ♏x.
Oleum monardæ	♏ij. to ♏iij.
Oleum morrhuæ	f ʒij. to f ℥j.
Oleum myristicæ	♏j. to ♏v.
Oleum olivæ	f ʒij. to f ℥ij.
Oleum origani	♏j. to ♏v.
Oleum pimentæ	♏ij. to ♏vi.
Oleum pulegii	♏i. to ♏v.
Oleum ricini	f ℥ss. to f ℥j.
Oleum rosmarini	♏ij. to ♏v.
Oleum sabinæ	♏j. to ♏v.
Oleum sassafras	♏j. to ♏v.
Oleum sesami	f ʒj. to f ℥ss.
Oleum succini rectificatum	♏v. to ♏xv.
Oleum tabaci	♏ ¼ to ♏ ½.
Oleum terebinthinæ, *anth*	f ʒj. to f ℥ss.
Oleum terebinthinæ, *diur.*	♏x. to f ʒss.
Oleum theobromæ	ʒj. to ℥ss.
Oleum thymi	♏v. to ♏x.
Oleum tiglii	♏ss. to ♏j.
Oleum valerianæ	♏ij. to ♏v.
Opium	gr. ½ to gr. iij.
Oxymel	f ʒj. to f ℥ss.
Oxymel scillæ	f ʒss. to f ʒij.
Panax	ʒss. to ʒj.
Papaver	ʒj. to ʒij.
Pareira	gr. xx. to ʒj.
Pepo	℥j.
Petroselinum	applied externally.
Phytolaccæ baccæ (tinct.)	f ʒj.
Pil. aloes	gr. iv. to gr. x.
Pil. aloes et assafœtidæ	gr. viii. to ℈j.
Pil. aloes et mastiches	gr. v. to gr. x.
Pil. aloes et myrrhæ	gr. v. to gr. xv.
Pil. antimonii compos	gr. iij. to gr. vi.
Pil. assafœtidæ	gr. v. to gr. x.
Pil. cathart. compos	gr. iij. to gr. x.
Pil. copaibæ	gr. x. to gr. xx.
Pil. ferri carbonatis	gr. x. to ʒss.
Pil. ferri compositæ	pil. i. to pil. ij.
Pil. ferri iodidi	pil. j. to pil. iij.
Pil. galbani comp	gr. x. to gr. xx.
Pil. hydrarg. *alterative*	gr. j. to gr. v.
Pil. hydrarg. *cathartic*	gr. v. to gr. xv.
Pil. opii	pil. ½ to pil. j.
Pil. quiniæ sulphatis	pil. j. to pil. v.
Pil. rhei	gr. x. to gr. xxx.
Pil. rhei compositæ	gr. x. to ℈j.
Pil. saponis compositæ	gr. iij. to gr. xviii.
Pil. scillæ comp	gr. v. to ℈ss.
Pimenta	gr. v. to ℈ij.
Piper	gr. v. to ℈j.
Piperina	gr. ½ to gr. ij.
Pix liquida	gr. xx. to ʒj.
Plumbi acetas	gr. ½ to gr. v.
Plumbi iodidum	gr. ½ to gr. iij. or iv.
Plumbi nitras	gr. ¼ to gr. ½.
Podophyllum	about gr. xx.
Polygala rubella	gr. x. to gr. xxx.
Potassa. See Liquor Potassæ.	
Potassa cum calce	externally.
Potassæ acetas	℈j. to ʒj.
Potassæ bicarbonas	gr. xv. to ʒj.
Potassæ bichromas, *emetic*	gr. ½ to gr. ¾.
Potassæ bisulphas	℈j. to ʒij.
Potassæ bitartras, *aper*	ʒj. to ʒij.
Potassæ bitartras, *cath*	℥ss.
Potassæ carbonas	℈ss. to ʒss.
Potassæ carbonas pur	gr. x. to gr. xxx.
Potassæ chloras	gr. x. to gr. xxx.
Potassæ citras	gr. xv. to gr. xxx.
Potassæ et sodæ tartras	ʒij. to ℥j.
Potassæ nitras	gr. v. to ℈j.
Potassæ permanganas	gr. ½ to gr. ij.
Potassæ sulphas	℈j. to ʒij.
Potassæ tartras	ʒj. to ℥ss.
Potassii bromidum	gr. iij. to gr. x.
Potassii cyanidum	gr. $\frac{1}{16}$ to gr. ⅛.
Potassii ferrocyanidum	gr. v. to gr. xv.
Potassii iodidum	gr. ij. to gr. x.
Potassii sulphuretum	gr. ij. to gr. x.
Prinos (pulv.)	gr. xx. to ʒj.
Prunus Virginiana (pulv.)	gr. xx. to ʒj.
Pulv. aloes et canellæ	gr. x. to ℈j.
Pulv. aromaticus	gr. x. to ℈j.
Pulv. ipecacuan. compos	gr. v. to gr. xv.
Pulv. jalapæ compositæ	gr. xxx. to ʒj.
Pulv. rhei compos	ʒss. to ʒj.
Pyrethrum	gr. iij. to gr. x.
Quassia	gr. x. to ʒss.
Quercus alba	℈j. to ʒj.
Quercus tinctoria	gr. x. to ʒss.
Quiniæ sulphas	gr. j. to gr. xv.
Quiniæ valerianas	gr. j. to gr. ij.
Resina jalapæ	gr. ij. to gr. x.
Resina podophylli, *alter*	gr. ¼ to gr. j.
Resina podophylli, *cathar*	gr. j. to gr. v.
Resina scammonii	gr. ij. to gr. x.
Rheum	gr. x. to ʒss.
Rhus glabrum	gr. ij. to gr. x.
Rosa centifolia	*ad libitum.*
Rosa Gallica	℈j. to ʒj.
Rosmarinus	gr. x. to ʒss.
Rottlera (pulv.)	ʒij. to ʒiv.
Rubia	gr. x. to ʒss.
Rubus (pulv.)	gr. xv. to gr. xxx.
Ruta	℈j. to ℈ij.
Sabadilla	gr. v. to gr. xxx.
Sabbatia (pulv.)	gr. xx. to ʒj.
Sabina	gr. v. to gr. x.
Saccharum lactis	*adjuvant.*
Salicina	gr. iij. to gr. vi.
Salix	gr. x. to ʒss.
Salvia (pulv.)	gr. xv. to gr. xxx.
Sambucus	ʒj. to ʒij.
Sanguinaria, *emetic*	gr. x. to gr. xx.
Santonica	gr. x. to gr. xxx.
Santoninum	gr. j. to gr. iv.
Sapo	gr. v. to ℈j.
Sarsaparilla	℈j. to ʒj.
Sassafras medulla	℈j. to ʒj.
Sassafras radicis cortex	ʒj. to ʒij.
Scammonium	gr. ij. to gr. x.
Scilla	gr. j. to gr. v.
Scoparius (pulv.)	gr. v. to gr. xv.
Scutellaria	ʒij.
Senega	gr. x. to ʒss.
Senna	ʒss. to ʒij.
Serpentaria	gr. x. to ℈j.
Sesami folium	*ad libitum.*
Simaruba	℈j. to ʒj.
Sinapis alba	℈j. to ʒij.
Sinapis nigra	℈j. to ʒij.
Sodæ acetas	℈j. to ʒij.
Sodæ bicarbonas	℈ss. to ʒss.
Sodæ boras	gr. v. to ʒss.
Sodæ et potassæ tartras. See Potassæ et Sodæ Tartras.	
Sodæ nitras	gr. v. to gr. xx.
Sodæ phosphas	℥ss. to ℥ij.
Sodæ sulphas	ʒij. to ℥j.
Sodæ sulphis	ʒss. to ʒj.
Solidago, infusion	f ℥ij. to f ℥iv.
Spigelia	gr. x. to ℈ij.
Spiræa, *extract*	gr. v. to gr. xv.
Spiritus ætheris comp	f ʒss. to f ʒij.

Drug	Dose
Spiritus ætheris nitrosi	f ʒss. to f ʒj.
Spiritus ætheris sulphurici	f ʒss. to f ʒj.
Spiritus ammoniæ	f ʒss. to f ʒj.
Spiritus ammoniæ aromat.	f ʒss. to f ʒj.
Spiritus anisi	f ʒss. to f ʒj.
Spiritus camphoræ	♏v. to f ʒj.
Spiritus chloroformi	f ʒss. to f ʒj.
Spiritus cinnamomi	f ʒj. to f ʒij.
Spiritus frumenti	f ℥ss. to f ℥j.
Spiritus juniperi comp	f ʒj. to f ℥ss.
Spiritus lavandulæ	♏xxx. to f ʒj.
Spiritus lavandulæ comp	f ʒss. to f ʒij.
Spiritus limonis	f ʒj. to f ʒij.
Spiritus menthæ piperitæ	f ʒss. to f ʒij.
Spiritus menthæ viridis	f ʒss. to f ʒij.
Spiritus myrciæ	used externally.
Spiritus myristicæ	f ʒss. to f ʒij.
Spiritus rosmarini	♏xxx. to f ʒj.
Spiritus vini Gallici	f ʒij. to f ℥ss.
Spongia usta	ʒss. to ʒj.
Stannum	ʒj. to ʒij.
Staphisagriæ semina	gr. iij. to gr. x.
Statice	gr. xv. to ʒss.
Stillingia (pulv.)	gr. x. to gr. xxx.
Stramonii folium	gr. ij. to gr. v.
Strychnia	gr. $\frac{1}{24}$ to gr. $\frac{1}{8}$.
Strychniæ sulphas	gr. $\frac{1}{24}$ to gr. $\frac{1}{8}$.
Styrax	gr. x. to ʒss.
Sulphur lotum	ʒss. to ʒij.
Sulphur præcipitatum	ʒss. to ʒij.
Sulphur sublimatum	ʒj. to ʒiij.
Sulphuris iodidum	used externally.
Syrupus aurantii cortex	f ʒj. to f ʒiv.
Syrupus ferri iodidi	♏xx. to ♏l.
Syrupus ipecacuanhæ	ʒj. to ℥j.
Syrupus krameriæ	ʒij. to ℥ss.
Syrupus lactucarii	f ʒj. to f ʒij.
Syrupus papaveris	f ʒss. to f ʒij.
Syrupus pruni Virginianæ	f ℥ss.
Syrupus rhamni	f ʒj. to f ℥j.
Syrupus rhei	f ℥j. to f ℥ij.
Syrupus rhei aromaticus	f ℥ss. to f ℥j.
Syr. sarsaparillæ comp	f ℥ss.
Syrupus scillæ	f ʒss. to f ʒj.
Syr. scillæ comp. *expect*	♏xx. to f ʒj.
Syrupus senegæ	f ʒj. to f ʒij.
Syrupus sennæ	f ʒij. to f ℥j.
Tabacum (infus.)	♏xl. to ♏lx.
Tamarindus	ʒiv. to ℥ij.
Taraxacum	ʒij. to ʒiv.
Terebinthina	℈ss. to ʒj.
Terebinthina Canadensis	♏v. to ♏x.
Testa præparata	gr. x. to ʒss.
Tinct. aconiti folii	♏xv. to ♏xxx.
Tinct. aconiti radicis	♏iij. to ♏x.
Tinct. aloes	f ℥ss. to f ℥iss.
Tinct. aloes et myrrhæ	f ʒj. to f ʒij.
Tinct. arnicæ	♏xx. to f ʒj.
Tinct. assafœtidæ	f ʒj. to f ʒij.
Tinct. aurantii	f ʒj. to f ʒij.
Tinct. belladonnæ	♏x. to ♏xxx.
Tinct. benzoini comp	f ʒj. to f ʒij.
Tinct. calumbæ	f ʒj. to f ʒij.
Tinct. camphoræ. See Spiritus Camphoræ.	
Tinct. cannabis	♏v. to ♏xx.
Tinct. cantharidis	♏xx. to f ʒj.
Tinct. capsici	♏x. to f ʒj.
Tinct. cardamomi	f ʒj. to f ʒij.
Tinct. cardamomi comp	f ʒj. to f ʒij.
Tinct. castorei	f ʒss. to f ʒj.
Tinct. catechu	f ʒj. to f ʒij.
Tinct. cinchonæ	f ʒj. to f ʒij.
Tinct. cinchonæ comp	f ʒj. to f ℥ss.
Tinct. cinnamomi	f ʒj. to f ʒiij.
Tinct. colchici	f ʒss. to f ʒij.
Tinct. conii	♏xx. to ♏xl.
Tinct. cubebæ	f ʒj. to f ʒij.
Tinct. digitalis	♏v. to ♏xx.
Tinct. ferri chloridi	♏x. to ♏xx.
Tinct. gallæ	f ʒj. to f ʒiij.
Tinct. gentianæ comp	f ʒj. to f ℥ss.
Tinct. guaiaci	f ʒj. to f ʒij.
Tinct. guaiaci ammon	f ʒj. to f ʒij.
Tinct. hellebori	♏x. to f ʒj.
Tinct. humuli	f ʒij. to f ℥ss.
Tinct. hyoscyami	♏xx. to f ʒj.
Tinct. iodinii	♏x. to ♏xl.
Tinct. iodinii comp	♏x. to ♏xxx.
Tinct. jalapæ	f ʒj. to f ʒij.
Tinct. kino	f ʒj. to f ʒij.
Tinct. krameriæ	f ʒj. to f ʒij.
Tinct. lobeliæ, *emetic*	f ℥ss.
Tinct. lobeliæ, *expectorant*	f ʒss. to f ʒj.
Tinct. lupulinæ	f ʒj. to f ʒij.
Tinct. myrrhæ	f ʒss. to f ʒj.
Tinct. nucis vomicæ	♏v. to ♏xx.
Tinct. opii	♏x. to ♏xl.
Tinct. opii acetata	♏x. to ♏xxx.
Tinct. opii camphorata	f ʒj. to f ℥ss.
Tinct. opii deodorata	gr. x. to gr. xl.
Tinct. quassiæ	f ʒj. to f ʒij.
Tinct. rhei	f ʒj. to f ℥ss.
Tinct. rhei et gentianæ	f ℥ss. to f ℥j.
Tinct. rhei et sennæ	f ℥ss. to f ℥j.
Tinct. sang. *exp.* and *alt.*	♏xxx. to ♏lx.
Tinct. scillæ	♏x. to f ʒss.
Tinct. sennæ et jalapæ	f ℥ss. to f ℥j.
Tinct. serpentariæ	f ʒj. to f ʒij.
Tinct. stramonii	♏x. to ♏xx.
Tinct. tolutana	f ʒss. to f ʒj.
Tinct. valerianæ	f ʒj. to f ʒiij.
Tinct. valerianæ ammon	f ʒj. to f ʒij.
Tinct. veratri viridis	♏v. to ♏xx.
Tinct. zingiberis	f ʒss. to f ʒj.
Tormentilla	℈ss. to ʒss.
Toxicodendron	gr. j. to gr. x.
Tragacantha	gr. x. to ʒj.
Triosteum	gr. xv. to gr. xxx.
Ulmus fulva	*ad libitum.*
Uva ursi	ʒss. to ʒj.
Valeriana	℈j. to ʒj.
Veratria	gr. $\frac{1}{16}$ to gr. $\frac{1}{8}$.
Veratrum album	gr. j. to gr. ij.
Veratrum viride	gr. ij. to gr. v.
Vinum aloes	f ʒj. to f ℥ss.
Vinum antimonii, *expect*	♏x. to f ʒss.
Vinum colchici radicis	♏x. to f ʒss.
Vinum colchici seminis	ʒj. to ʒij.
Vinum ergotæ	ʒj. to ʒij.
Vin. ipecacuanhæ, *diaph*	♏x. to f ʒss.
Vin. ipecacuanhæ, *emetic*	f ʒij. to f ℥j.
Vinum opii	♏v. to ♏xxx.
Vinum rhei	f ʒij. to f ℥ss.
Xanthorrhiza	℈j. to ʒj.
Xanthoxylum (pulv.)	gr. x. to gr. xxx.
Zinci carbonas præcip	gr. j. to gr. v.
Zinci chloridum	used externally.
Zinci oxydum	gr. j. to gr. vi.
Zinci sulphas, *emetic*	gr. x. to gr. xv.
Zinci sulphas, *tonic*	gr. $\frac{1}{2}$ to gr. ij.
Zinci valerianas	gr. j. to gr. ij.
Zingiber	gr. v. to ʒss.

TABLE OF CHEMICAL SYMBOLS.

Element	Symbol	Element	Symbol
Aluminum	Al.	Mercury (Hydrargyrum)	Hg.
Antimony (Stibium)	Sb.	Molybdenum	Mo.
Arsenic	As.	Nickel	Ni.
Barium	Ba.	Nitrogen	N.
Bismuth	Bi.	Osmium	Os.
Boron	B.	Oxygen	O.
Bromine	Br.	Palladium	Pd.
Cadmium	Cd.	Phosphorus	P.
Cæsium	Cs.	Platinum	Pt.
Calcium	Ca.	Potassium (Kalium)	K.
Carbon	C.	Rhodium	R.
Cerium	Ce.	Rubidium	Rb.
Chlorine	Cl.	Ruthenium	Ru.
Chromium	Cr.	Selenium	Se.
Cobalt	Co.	Silicon	Si.
Columbium (Tantalum)	Ta.	Silver (Argentum)	Ag.
Copper (Cuprum)	Cu.	Sodium (Natrium)	Na.
Didymium	Di.	Strontium	Sr.
Fluorine	F.	Sulphur	S.
Gold (Aurum)	Au.	Tellurium	Te.
Hydrogen	H.	Thallium	Tl.(?)
Indium	In.(?)	Thorium	Th.
Iodine	I.	Tin (Stannum)	Sn.
Iridium	Ir.	Tungsten (Wolframium)	W.
Iron (Ferrum)	Fe.	Uranium	U.
Lantanium	La.	Vanadium	V.
Lead (Plumbum)	Pb.	Yttrium	Y.
Lithium	L.	Zinc	Zn.
Magnesium	Mg.	Zirconium	Zr.
Manganese	Mn.		

Thus, HO is the representative or *formula* of water: that is, one equivalent of hydrogen (H) combined with one equivalent of oxygen (O). AsO_3 is the formula of arsenious acid, a compound consisting of one equivalent of arsenic and three equivalents of oxygen. NO_5 is the representative of anhydrous nitric acid, indicating that it is composed of one equivalent of nitrogen (N) combined with five equivalents of oxygen (O). The number of equivalents of an elementary substance is usually indicated by a small depressed figure following the symbol, as seen in the previous examples; but the number of equivalents of any compound is denoted by a large figure placed before the formula: thus, $3\ HO + 2\ NO_5$ is the *formula* of the officinal (hydrated) nitric acid, indicating that it is composed of three equivalents of water (HO) combined with two equivalents of nitric acid (NO_5).

TABLE OF DISPUTED PRONUNCIATIONS; WITH THE PRINCIPAL AUTHORITIES IN FAVOR OF EACH.

The design of the following Table is not merely or principally to gratify the curiosity of the reader, but rather, by showing *how* VERY FEW *points there are of any importance, about which the best scientific and classical authorities differ*, to convince the student that in his efforts to attain a correct pronunciation of scientific terms, he is not pursuing a chimera, but acquiring an accomplishment which will be highly appreciated by the truly learned in every part of the world. (See Preface.)

Ancone'us; Dunglison, Hooper. **Anco'neus;** Mayne. **Anconæ'us;** Kraus.*

Aristolo'chia; Gray, White and Riddle,† Wittstein. **Aristolochi'a;**‡ Dunglison, Hooper, Mayne.

Cad'mia; Ainsworth, Webster, Worcester. **Cadmi'a;** Dunglison, Hooper, Mayne. **Cadmi'a** or **Cad'mia;**‡ White and Riddle.

Cad'mium; Brande, Webster, Worcester. **Cadmi'um;** Dunglison, Hooper, Mayne.

Dioscore'a; Gray, Wittstein. **Diosco'rea;** Hooper, Mayne. **Dioscore'a** or **Diosco'rea;** Dunglison.

Hydrange'a;§ Wittstein. **Hydran'gea;** Gray. **Hydrange'a** or **Hydran'gea;** Dunglison.

Larynge'al; Dunglison, Hooper, Mayne. **Laryn'geal;** Worcester. **Larynge'al** or **Laryn'geal;** Webster.

Larynge'us; Dunglison, Hooper, Mayne. **Laryn'geus;** Kraus.

Lochi'a; Mayne. **Lo'chia;** Hooper. **Lochi'a** or **Lo'chia;** Dunglison.

Madar. See **Mudar.**

Menin'geal; Mayne, Worcester. **Meninge'al** or **Menin'geal;** Dunglison.

Mezere'um; Mayne, Wittstein. **Meze'reum;** U.S. Pharmacopœia. **Meze'reum** or **Mezere'um;** Dunglison.

Mŭ-dar' (*Calot'ropis gigante'a*); Thompson.‖ **Mūdar;** Ainslie.¶

Olec'ranon; Hooper. **Olecra'non;**** Kraus, Mayne. **Olec'ranon** or **Olecra'non;** Dunglison.

---

* Author of the "Kritisch-Etymologisches Medicinisches Lexikon," Göttingen, 1826.

† Editors of an excellent "Latin-English Dictionary" recently published by Longman, London.

‡ It may be remarked that, with respect to the most important root in *Aristolochia* (*lochia*), usage was divided among the Greeks themselves. Some writers have λοχεία (*locheia*), others, λοχία (*lochĭa*); so *Cadmia* has two forms in Greek, καδμεία and καδμία.

§ It is to be observed that the penultimate accent is given to this name considered simply as a Latin (or classical) word.

‖ Author of an excellent Oordoo (Hindostanee) Dictionary, published at Serampore in 1838. This pronunciation (mŭ-dar') is not only supported by the original Hindostanee spelling, but it is confirmed by the prevailing English spelling, *Madar*, which can scarcely be reconciled with the supposition that the *u* in the first syllable is long. See *Calotropis Gigantea* in Wood & Bache's Dispensatory.

¶ Author of a valuable work entitled "Materia Indica," London, 1826.

** Liddell and Scott give the penultima as undoubtedly long—ὠλεκρᾶνον. General usage, however, seems to be in favor of *Olec'ranon;* and if we may attach any weight to the Greek accent, this pronunciation can at least be defended. (See Preface, p. viii.)

Parotide'a; Dunglison, Hooper. **Parotid'ea** (*Parotid'eus*); Mayne. **Parotidæ'a**; Cullen.

Pem'phigus; Hooper, Kraus. **Pemphi'gus;** Mayne. **Pem'phigus** or **Pemphi'gus;** Dunglison.

Pharynge'al; Dunglison, Hooper. **Pharyn'geal;** Mayne, Worcester. **Pharyn'geal** or **Pharynge'al;** Webster.

Pharynge'us: Dunglison, Hooper. **Pharyn'geus;*** Kraus, Mayne.

Plat'inum; Brande, Dunglison, Worcester. **Plati'num;** Mayne. **Plat'inum** or **Plati'num;** Webster.

Syru'pus; Mayne, U. S. Pharmacopœia. **Syr'upus;** Kraus. **Syr'upus** or **Syru'pus;** Dunglison.

☞ There is one class of names, about the pronunciation of which considerable diversity prevails, that have not been introduced into the preceding table, because there seems reason to believe that the diversity in question has rather been the result of inadvertency than of any deliberate difference of judgment among scientific writers. We allude to those terminating in *-era* derived from a proper name in *-er:* as, *Brayera* (from Brayer), *Frasera* (from Fraser), *Heuchera* (from Heucher), etc. Some of our best authorities are not always consistent with themselves with respect to this class of names, but, if we mistake not, the general tendency is decidedly in favor of the penultimate accent. The United States Pharmacopœia gives *Braye'ra* and *Frase'ra* with the penultimate accent, but *Heu'chera* with the antepenultimate. The last is, not improbably, an oversight; for though something might be said in favor of making a difference between *Brayera* and the other two names, inasmuch as the last syllable of *Brayer* is long in French, there can be no good reason for making a distinction between *Frasera* and *Heuchera*, as the last syllable in both *Fraser* and *Heucher* is short. But the reason would not be a good one in any case; the name of LUTHER, the celebrated Reformer, has the last syllable short in German (*Lu'thĕr*), yet when Latinized becomes *Luthe'rus*, and in the Italian and Spanish, cognate languages, it is always *Lute'ro*.† In consideration of all these reasons and facts, we have deemed it best to adopt a uniform rule, and always to place the accent on the penultima of names of the class above referred to: *e.g. Braye'ra, Frase'ra, Heuche'ra, Rottle'ra*, etc. etc.

---

* In this instance, Dr. Mayne, who is generally so accurate in regard to his Latin and Greek quantities, would seem to be guilty of a palpable inconsistency, since he gives the parallel term *Laryngeus* with the penultima long. It is, however, proper to observe that this whole class of words (including *Anconeus, Parotideus*, etc.) are doubtful as to the length of the penultima, which there seems to be no means of determining positively. Even the light of analogy, dubious at best, utterly fails us here: while *gigante'us* has the penultima unquestionably long, *ce'reus, cine'reus, ido'neus*, etc. have it short.

† It is a great mistake to suppose that a Latinized modern name must follow either the quantity or accent of the original. This indeed is the exception, the contrary being the general rule; at least with respect to names of Teutonic origin: *Fred'eric* makes *Frederi'cus, Hen'ry* (German, Hein'rich), *Henri'cus, Lud'wig, Ludovi'cus, Mil'ton, Milto'nus*, etc.

CLASSIFICATION OF DISEASES ACCORDING TO CULLEN'S NOSOLOGY.

CLASS I.—PYREX'IÆ.

ORDER I.—**Fe'bres.**
II.—**Phlegma'siæ.**
III.—**Exanthem'ata.**
IV.—**Hæmorrha'giæ.**
V.—**Proflu'via.**

CLASS II.—NEURO'SES.

ORDER I.—**Co'mata.**
II.—**Adyna'miæ.**
III.—**Spas'mi.**
IV.—**Vesa'niæ.**

CLASS III.—CACHEX'IÆ.

ORDER I.—**Marco'res.**
II.—**Intumescen'tiæ.**
III.—**Impetig'ines.**

CLASS IV.—LOCA'LES.

ORDER I.—**Dysæsthe'siæ.**
II.—**Dysorex'iæ.**
III.—**Dyscine'siæ.**
IV.—**Apoceno'ses.**
V.—**Epis'cheses.**
VI.—**Tumo'res.**
VII.—**Ecto'piæ.**
VIII.—**Dial'yses.**

CLASS I.

PYREXIÆ.

ORDER I.—FE'BRES. *Fevers.*

Section I.—Intermitten'tes. *Intermittents.*

Genus 1.—Tertia'na. *Tertian.*
Genus 2.—Quarta'na. *Quartan.*
Genus 3.—Quotidia'na. *Quotidian.*

Section II.—Contin'uæ. *Continued Fevers.*

Genus 4.—Syn'ocha. *Pure inflammatory fever.*
Genus 5.—Ty'phus. *Typhus.*
Genus 6.—Syn'ochus.

ORDER II.—PHLEGMA'SIÆ. *Inflammations.*

Genus 1.—Phlogo'sis. *Inflammation (of a particular form).*
Genus 2.—Ophthal'mia. *Ophthalmy.*
Genus 3.—Phreni'tis. *Phrenzy, or brain fever.*
Genus 4.—Cynan'che. *Sore throat.*
Genus 5.—Pneumo'nia. *Inflammation of the lungs.*

Genus 6.—Cardi'tis. *Inflammation of the heart.*
Genus 7.—Peritoni'tis. *Inflammation of the peritonæum.*
Genus 8.—Gastri'tis. *Inflammation of the stomach.*
Genus 9.—Enteri'tis. *Inflammation of the bowels.*
Genus 10.—Hepati'tis. *Inflammation of the liver.*
Genus 11.—Spleni'tis. *Inflammation of the spleen.*
Genus 12.—Nephri'tis. *Inflammation of the kidney.*
Genus 13.—Cysti'tis. *Inflammation of the bladder.*
Genus 14.—Hysteri'tis. *Inflammation of the womb.*
Genus 15.—Rheumatis'mus. *Rheumatism.*
Genus 16.—Odontal'gia. *Toothache.*
Genus 17.—Pod'agra. *Gout.*
Genus 18.—Arthropuo'sis (or Arthropyo'sis). *Pus in a joint.*

ORDER III.—EXANTHEM'ATA. *Exanthematous Eruptions.*

Genus 1.—Erysip'elas. *Erysipelas.*
Genus 2.—Pes'tis. *The Plague.*

Genus 3.—Vari'ola. *Small-Pox.*
Genus 4.—Varicel'la. *Chicken-Pox.*
Genus 5.—Rube'ola. *Measles.*
Genus 6.—Milia'ria. *Miliary fever.*
Genus 7.—Scarlati'na. *Scarlet fever.*
Genus 8.—Urtica'ria. *Nettle-rash.*
Genus 9.—Pem'phigus. *Vesicular fever.*
Genus 10.—Aph'tha. *Superficial ulcer of the mouth.*

ORDER IV.—HÆMORRHA'GIÆ. *Hæmorrhages.*

Genus 1.—Epistax'is. *Bleeding at the nose.*
Genus 2.—Hæmop'tysis. *Spitting of blood.*
Genus 3.—Hæmor'rhois. *The Piles.*
Genus 4.—Menorrha'gia. *Menorrhagy.*

ORDER V.—PROFLU'VIA. *Morbid Discharges, or Fluxes.*

Genus 1.—Catar'rhus. *Catarrh.*
Genus 2.—Dysente'ria. *Dysentery.*

CLASS II.

NEUROSES. *Nervous Diseases.*

ORDER I.—CO'MATA. *Soporose Diseases.*

Genus 1.—Apoplex'ia. *Apoplexy.*
Genus 2.—Paral'ysis. *Palsy.*

ORDER II.—ADYNA'MIÆ. *Diseases consisting of a loss or deficiency of the Vital Power.*

Genus 1.—Syn'cope. *Fainting.*
Genus 2.—Dyspep'sia. *Indigestion.*
Genus 3.—Hypochondri'asis. *Vapors, or low spirits.*
Genus 4.—Chloro'sis. *Green-sickness.*

ORDER III.—SPAS'MI. *Spasms.*

Genus 1.—Tet'anus. *Tetanus.*
Genus 2.—Tris'mus. *Locked-jaw.*
Genus 3.—Convul'sio. *Convulsion.*
Genus 4.—Chore'a. *St. Vitus' Dance.*
Genus 5.—Rapha'nia.
Genus 6.—Epilep'sia. *Epilepsy.*
Genus 7.—Palpita'tio. *Palpitation.*
Genus 8.—Asth'ma. *Asthma.*
Genus 9.—Dyspnœ'a. *Difficulty of breathing (not asthmatic).*
Genus 10.—Pertus'sis. *Hooping-cough.*
Genus 11.—Pyro'sis. *Water-brash.*
Genus 12.—Col'ica. *Colic.*
Genus 13.—Chol'era. *Cholera.*
Genus 14.—Diarrhœ'a. *Diarrhœa.*
Genus 15.—Diabe'tes. *Diabetes.*
Genus 16.—Hyste'ria. *Hysterics.*
Genus 17.—Hydropho'bia.

ORDER IV.—VESA'NIÆ. *Mental Derangements.*

Genus 1.—Amen'tia. *Idiocy, or Imbecility.*
Genus 2.—Melancho'lia. *Melancholy.*
Genus 3.—Ma'nia. *Madness, Delirium without fever.*
Genus 4.—Oneirodyn'ia. *Nightmare, or Somnambulism.*

CLASS III.

CACHEXIÆ. *Cachectic Diseases.*

ORDER I.—MARCO'RES. *Emaciations.*

Genus 1.—Ta'bes. *Wasting, or Decline.*
Genus 2.—Atro'phia. *Atrophy.*

ORDER II.—INTUMESCEN'TIÆ. *Intumescence.* (Swelling of a part or the whole of the body without inflammation.)

Genus 1.—Polysar'cia. *Excessive corpulence.*
Genus 2.—Pneumato'sis. *Windy swelling?*
Genus 3.—Tympani'tes. *Wind dropsy, or emphysema.*
Genus 4.—Physome'tra. *Windy swelling of the womb.*
Genus 5.—Anasar'ca. *General dropsy.*
Genus 6.—Hydroceph'alus. *Dropsy of the brain.*
Genus 7.—Hydrorachi'tis (or Hydrorrhachi'tis). *Dropsy of the spine.*
Genus 8.—Hydrotho'rax. *Dropsy of the chest.*
Genus 9.—Asci'tes. *Dropsy of the belly.*
Genus 10.—Hydrome'tra. *Dropsy of the womb.*
Genus 11.—Hydroce'le. *Dropsy of the testicle.*
Genus 12.—Physco'nia. *Enlargement of the abdomen.*
Genus 13.—Rachi'tis. *Rickets.*

ORDER III.—IMPETIG'INES. *Cachectic Condition of the Skin or External Portion of the Body.*

Genus 1.—Scroph'ula [Scrof'ula]. *Scrofula.*
Genus 2.—Syph'ilis. *Venereal disease.*
Genus 3.—Scorbu'tus. *Scurvy.*
Genus 4.—Elephanti'asis.
Genus 5.—Lep'ra. *Leprosy.*
Genus 6.—Frambœ'sia. *The Yaws.*
Genus 7.—Tricho'ma. *Hair-disease.*
Genus 8.—Ic'terus. *Jaundice.*

CULLEN'S NOSOLOGY.

CLASS IV.

LOCALES. *Local Diseases.*

ORDER I.—DYSÆSTHE'SIÆ. *Depraved or Defective Perceptions.*

Genus 1.—Cali'go. *Dimness of sight,* or *blindness.*

Genus 2.—Amauro'sis. *Amaurosis.*

Genus 3.—Dyso'pia, or Dysop'sia. *Painful or defective vision.*

Genus 4.—Pseudoblep'sis. *False or depraved vision.*

Genus 5.—Dyseco'ia, or Dysecœ'a. *Deafness.*

Genus 6.—Paracu'sis. *Morbid or depraved hearing.*

Genus 7.—Anos'mia. *Loss of the sense of smell.*

Genus 8.—Ageus'tia. *Loss of taste.*

Genus 9.—Anæsthe'sia. *Loss of feeling or touch.*

ORDER II.—DYSOREX'IÆ. *Depraved Appetites.*

Genus 1.—Bulim'ia. *Insatiable hunger.*

Genus 2.—Polydip'sia. *Excessive (morbid) thirst.*

Genus 3.—Pi'ca. *Depraved or perverted appetite.*

Genus 4.—Satyri'asis. *Excessive (morbid) sexual desire in males.*

Genus 5.—Nymphoma'nia. *Excessive (morbid) sexual desire in females.*

Genus 6.—Nostal'gia. *Homesickness.*

Genus 7.—Anorex'ia. *Want of appetite.*

Genus 8.—Adip'sia. *A morbid absence of thirst.*

Genus 9.—Anaphrodis'ia. *Absence of sexual desire or of genital power.*

ORDER III.—DYSCINE'SIÆ. *Defective or Imperfect Power of Motion.*

Genus 1.—Apho'nia. *Loss of voice.*

Genus 2.—Mu'titas. *Dumbness.*

Genus 3.—Parapho'nia. *Depraved or diseased voice, referring to the sounds as uttered in the larynx.*

Genus 4.—Psellis'mus. *Defective or depraved articulation.*

Genus 5.—Strabis'mus. *Squinting, or Cross-Eye.*

Genus 6.—Contractu'ra. *Contracture.*

ORDER IV.—APOCENO'SES. *Morbid Evacuations.*

Genus 1.—Profu'sio. *Hæmorrhage.*

Genus 2.—Ephidro'sis. *Excessive morbid perspiration.*

Genus 3.—Epiph'ora. *A superabundant secretion of tears.*

Genus 4.—Ptyalis'mus. *Salivation.*

Genus 5.—Enure'sis. *Incontinency of urine.*

Genus 6.—Gonorrhœ'a. *Discharge from the urethra.*

ORDER V.—EPIS'CHESES. *Suppression of Excretions.*

Genus 1.—Obstipa'tio. *Constipation, or Costiveness.*

Genus 2.—Ischu'ria. *Retention or stoppage of the urine.*

Genus 3.—Dysu'ria. *Difficult or painful discharge of urine.*

Genus 4.—Dyspermatis'mus. *Imperfect or deficient discharge of semen.*

Genus 5.—Amenorrhœ'a. *Absence or stoppage of the menstrual discharge.*

ORDER VI.—TUMO'RES. *Tumors.*

Genus 1.—Aneuris'ma. *Aneurism.*

Genus 2.—Va'rix. *Enlarged or swollen veins.*

Genus 3.—Ecchymo'ma. *Suggilation or suffusion of blood into the areolar tissue.*

Genus 4.—Scir'rhus (Schir'rus). *Schirrus.*

Genus 5.—Can'cer. *Cancer.*

Genus 6.—Bu'bo. *Bubo.*

Genus 7.—Sarco'ma. *Sarcoma.*

Genus 8.—Verru'ca. *Wart.*

Genus 9.—Cla'vus. *Corn.*

Genus 10.—Lu'pia. *Wen.*

Genus 11.—Gan'glion. *A hard, movable tumor on a tendon.*

Genus 12.—Hyd'atis. *Hydatid.*

Genus 13.—Hydrar'thrus. *White swelling.*

Genus 14.—Exosto'sis. *Tumor of a bone.*

ORDER VII.—ECTO'PIÆ. *Displacements, or Protrusions.*

Genus 1.—Her'nia. *Rupture.*

Genus 2.—Prolap'sus. *Prolapse.*

Genus 3.—Luxa'tio. *Luxation.*

ORDER VIII.—DIAL'YSES. *Solutions of Continuity.*

Genus 1.—Vul'nus. *Wound.*

Genus 2.—Ul'cus. *Ulcer.*

Genus 3.—Her'pes. *Tetter, or Serpigo.*

Genus 4.—Tin'ea. *Scalled-head.*

Genus 5.—Pso'ra. *Itch.*

Genus 6.—Fractu'ra. *Fracture.*

Genus 7.—Ca'ries. *Decay or ulceration of a bone.*

CLASSIFICATION OF DISEASES ACCORDING TO GOOD'S NOSOLOGY.

CLASS I.

CŒLI'ACA. *Diseases of the Digestive Function.*

ORDER I.—ENTER'ICA. *Diseases affecting the Alimentary Canal.*

Genus 1.—Odon'tia. *Misdentition, or diseases affecting the teeth.*
Genus 2.—Ptyalis'mus. *Ptyalism, or diseases affecting the salivary secretion.*
Genus 3.—Dyspha'gia. *Difficulty of swallowing.*
Genus 4.—Dipso'sis. *Morbid thirst.*
Genus 5.—Limo'sis. *Morbid appetite.*
Genus 6.—Col'ica. *Colic.*
Genus 7.—Copros'tasis. *Costiveness.*
Genus 8.—Diarrhœ'a. *Looseness.*
Genus 9.—Chol'era. *Cholera.*
Genus 10.—Enterol'ithus. *Intestinal concretions.*
Genus 11.—Helmin'thia. *Worms.*
Genus 12.—Proc'tica. *Diseases affecting the anus or rectum.*

ORDER II.—SPLANCH'NICA. *Diseases affecting the Collatitious Viscera,*—i.e. *the Liver, Spleen, Pancreas, &c.*

Genus 1.—Ic'terus. *Yellow jaundice.*
Genus 2.—Melæ'na. *Melena.*
Genus 3.—Cholol'ithus. *Gall-stone.*
Genus 4.—Parabys'ma. *Visceral turgescence.*

CLASS II.

PNEUMATICA. *Diseases of the Respiratory Function.*

ORDER I.—PHON'ICA. *Diseases affecting the Vocal Avenues.*

Genus 1.—Cory'za. *Nasal catarrh.*
Genus 2.—Pol'ypus. *Polypus.*
Genus 3.—Rhon'chus. *Rattling in the throat.*
Genus 4.—Apho'nia. *Dumbness.*
Genus 5.—Dyspho'nia. *Dissonance of the voice.*
Genus 6.—Psellis'mus. *Dissonant speech.*

ORDER II.—PNEUMON'ICA. *Diseases affecting the Lungs.*

Genus 1.—Bex. *Cough.*
Genus 2.—Laryngis'mus. *Laryngic suffocation.*
Genus 3.—Dyspnœ'a. *? Difficulty of breathing, anhelation.*
Genus 4.—Asth'ma. *Asthma.*
Genus 5.—Ephial'tes. *Incubus.*
Genus 6.—Sternal'gia. *Suffocative breast-pang.*
Genus 7.—Pleural'gia. *Pain in the side.*

CLASS III.

HÆMATICA. *Diseases of the Sanguineous Function.*

ORDER I.—PYREC'TICA. *Fevers.*

Genus 1.—Ephem'era. *Diary fever.*
Genus 2.—An'etus. *Intermittent fever. Ague.*
Genus 3.—Epan'etus. *Remittent fever.*
Genus 4.—Ene'cia. *Continued fever.*

ORDER II.—PHLOGOT'ICA. *Inflammations.*

Genus 1.—Aposte'ma. *Aposteme, or Abscess.*
Genus 2.—Phleg'mone. *Phlegmon.*
Genus 3.—Phy'ma. *Tuber.*
Genus 4.—Ion'thus. *Whelk.*
Genus 5.—Phly'sis.
Genus 6.—Erythe'ma. *Inflammatory blush.*
Genus 7.—Empres'ma. *Visceral inflammation.*
Genus 8.—Ophthal'mia. *Ophthalmy.*
Genus 9.—Catar'rhus. *Catarrh.*
Genus 10.—Dysente'ria. *Dysentery.*
Genus 11.—Bucne'mia. *Tumid leg.*
Genus 12.—Arthro'sia. *Articular inflammation.*

ORDER III.—EXANTHEMAT'ICA. *Eruptive Fevers.*

Genus 1.—Enanthe'sis. *Rash exanthem.*
Genus 2.—Emphly'sis. *Ichorous exanthem.*
Genus 3.—Empye'sis. *Pustulous exanthem.*
Genus 4.—Anthra'cia. *Carbuncular exanthem.*

ORDER IV.—DYSTHET'ICA. *Cachectic Diseases.*

Genus 1.—Pletho'ra. *Plethora.*
Genus 2.—Hæmorrha'gia. *Hæmorrhage.*
Genus 3.—Maras'mus. *Emaciation.*
Genus 4.—Melano'sis.
Genus 5.—Stru'ma. *Scrofula.*
Genus 6.—Car'cinus. *Cancer.*
Genus 7.—Lu'es. *Venereal disease.*

Genus 8.—Elephanti'asis. *Elephant-skin.*
Genus 9.—Catacau'sis. *Catacausis.*
Genus 10.—Por'phyra. *Scurvy.*
Genus 11.—Exan'gia.
Genus 12.—Gangræ'na. *Gangrene.*
Genus 13.—Ul'cus. *Ulcer.*

CLASS IV.

NEUROTICA. *Diseases of the Nervous Function.*

ORDER I.—PHREN'ICA. *Diseases affecting the Intellect.*

Genus 1.—Ecphro'nia. *Insanity.*
Genus 2.—Empathe'ma. *Ungovernable passion.*
Genus 3.—Alu'sia. *Illusion,* or *Hallucination.*
Genus 4.—Aphel'xia. *Revery.*
Genus 5.—Paronir'ia. *Sleep-disturbance.*
Genus 6.—Mo'ria. *Fatuity.*

ORDER II.—ÆSTHET'ICA. *Diseases affecting the Sensations or Perceptions.*

Genus 1.—Parop'sis. *Morbid sight.*
Genus 2.—Paracu'sis. *Morbid hearing.*
Genus 3.—Paros'mis. *Morbid smell.*
Genus 4.—Parageu'sis. *Morbid taste.*
Genus 5.—Parap'sis. *Morbid touch.*
Genus 6.—Neural'gia. *Nerve-ache, or pain in the nerves.*

ORDER III.—CINET'ICA. *Diseases affecting the Muscles.*

Genus 1.—Enta'sia. *Constrictive spasm.*
Genus 2.—Clo'nus. *Clonic spasm.*
Genus 3.—Syn'clonus. *Synclonic spasm.*

ORDER IV.—SYSTAT'ICA. *Diseases affecting several or all the Sensorial Powers simultaneously.*

Genus 1.—Agryp'nia. *Sleeplessness.*
Genus 2.—Dyspho'ria. *Restlessness.*
Genus 3.—Antipathi'a. *Antipathy.*
Genus 4.—Cephalæ'a. *Headache.*
Genus 5.—Di'nus. *Dizziness.*
Genus 6.—Syn'cope. *Syncope.*
Genus 7.—Syspa'sia. *Comatose spasm.*
Genus 8.—Ca'rus. *Torpor.*

CLASS V.

GENETICA. *Diseases of the Sexual Function.*

ORDER I.—CENOT'ICA. *Diseases affecting the Fluids.*

Genus 1.—Parame'nia. *Mismenstruation.*
Genus 2.—Leucorrhœ'a. *Whites.*
Genus 3.—Blenorrhœ'a. *Gonorrhœa.*
Genus 4.—Spermorrhœ'a. *Seminal flux.*
Genus 5.—Galac'tia. *Mislactation.*

ORDER II.—ORGAS'TICA. *Diseases affecting the Orgasm.*

Genus 1.—Chloro'sis. *Green-sickness.*
Genus 2.—Prœo'tia. *Genital precocity.*
Genus 3.—Lagne'sis. *Lust.*
Genus 4.—Agene'sia. *Male sterility.*
Genus 5.—Apho'ria. *Female sterility.*
Genus 6.—Ædopto'sis. *Genital prolapse.*

ORDER III.—CARPOT'ICA. *Diseases affecting the Impregnation.*

Genus 1.—Paracye'sis. *Morbid pregnancy.*
Genus 2.—Parodyn'ia. *Morbid labor.*
Genus 3.—Eccye'sis. *Extra-uterine fœtation.*
Genus 4.—Pseudocye'sis. *Spurious pregnancy.*

CLASS VI.

ECCRITICA. *Diseases of the Excernent Function.*

ORDER I.—MESOT'ICA. *Diseases affecting the Parenchyma.*

Genus 1.—Polysar'cia. *Corpulency.*
Genus 2.—Emphy'ma. *Tumor.*
Genus 3.—Paros'tia. *Misossification.*
Genus 4.—Cyrto'sis. *Contortion of the bones.*
Genus 5.—Osthex'ia. *Osthexy.*

ORDER II.—CATOT'ICA. *Diseases affecting Internal Surfaces.*

Genus 1.—Hy'drops. *Dropsy.*
Genus 2.—Emphyse'ma. *Inflation, wind dropsy.*
Genus 3.—Paru'ria. *Mismicturition.*
Genus 4.—Lith'ia. *Urinary calculus.*

ORDER III.—ACROT'ICA. *Diseases affecting the External Surface.*

Genus 1.—Ephidro'sis. *Morbid sweat.*
Genus 2.—Exanthe'sis. *Cutaneous blush.*
Genus 3.—Exor'mia. *Papulous skin.*
Genus 4.—Lepido'sis. *Scale-skin.*
Genus 5.—Ecphly'sis. *Blains.*
Genus 6.—Ecpye'sis. *Humid scall.*
Genus 7.—Ma'lis. *Cutaneous vermination.*
Genus 8.—Ecphy'ma. *Cutaneous excrescence.*
Genus 9.—Tricho'sis. *Morbid hair.*
Genus 10.—Epichro'sis. *Macular skin.*

www.ingramcontent.com/pod-product-compliance
Lightning Source LLC
LaVergne TN
LVHW052205200926
848481LV00001B/34
9781425568832